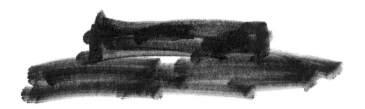

D1604535

COLD SPRING HARBOR SYMPOSIA ON QUANTITATIVE BIOLOGY

VOLUME LXX

L2QOXO

COLD SPRING HARBOR SYMPOSIA
ON QUANTITATIVE BIOLOGY

VOLUME LXX

Molecular Approaches to
Controlling Cancer

www.cshl-symposium.org

Meeting Organized by Bruce Stillman and David Stewart
COLD SPRING HARBOR LABORATORY PRESS
2005

COLD SPRING HARBOR SYMPOSIA ON QUANTITATIVE BIOLOGY VOLUME LXX

©2005 by Cold Spring Harbor Laboratory Press
International Standard Book Number 0-87969-773-3 (cloth)
International Standard Book Number 0-87969-774-1 (paper)
International Standard Serial Number 0091-7451
Library of Congress Catalog Card Number 34-8174

COLD SPRING HARBOR SYMPOSIA ON QUANTITATIVE BIOLOGY
Founded in 1933 by
REGINALD G. HARRIS
Director of the Biological Laboratory 1924 to 1936
Previous Symposia Volumes

I (1933) Surface Phenomena
II (1934) Aspects of Growth
III (1935) Photochemical Reactions
IV (1936) Excitation Phenomena
V (1937) Internal Secretions
VI (1938) Protein Chemistry
VII (1939) Biological Oxidations
VIII (1940) Permeability and the Nature of Cell Membranes
IX (1941) Genes and Chromosomes: Structure and Organization
X (1942) The Relation of Hormones to Development
XI (1946) Heredity and Variation in Microorganisms
XII (1947) Nucleic Acids and Nucleoproteins
XIII (1948) Biological Applications of Tracer Elements
XIV (1949) Amino Acids and Proteins
XV (1950) Origin and Evolution of Man
XVI (1951) Genes and Mutations
XVII (1952) The Neuron
XVIII (1953) Viruses
XIX (1954) The Mammalian Fetus: Physiological Aspects of Development
XX (1955) Population Genetics: The Nature and Causes of Genetic Variability in Population
XXI (1956) Genetic Mechanisms: Structure and Function
XXII (1957) Population Studies: Animal Ecology and Demography
XXIII (1958) Exchange of Genetic Material: Mechanism and Consequences
XXIV (1959) Genetics and Twentieth Century Darwinism
XXV (1960) Biological Clocks
XXVI (1961) Cellular Regulatory Mechanisms
XXVII (1962) Basic Mechanisms in Animal Virus Biology
XXVIII (1963) Synthesis and Structure of Macromolecules
XXIX (1964) Human Genetics
XXX (1965) Sensory Receptors
XXXI (1966) The Genetic Code
XXXII (1967) Antibodies
XXXIII (1968) Replication of DNA in Microorganisms
XXXIV (1969) The Mechanism of Protein Synthesis

XXXV (1970) Transcription of Genetic Material
XXXVI (1971) Structure and Function of Proteins at the Three-dimensional Level
XXXVII (1972) The Mechanism of Muscle Contraction
XXXVIII (1973) Chromosome Structure and Function
XXXIX (1974) Tumor Viruses
XL (1975) The Synapse
XLI (1976) Origins of Lymphocyte Diversity
XLII (1977) Chromatin
XLIII (1978) DNA: Replication and Recombination
XLIV (1979) Viral Oncogenes
XLV (1980) Movable Genetic Elements
XLVI (1981) Organization of the Cytoplasm
XLVII (1982) Structures of DNA
XLVIII (1983) Molecular Neurobiology
XLIX (1984) Recombination at the DNA Level
L (1985) Molecular Biology of Development
LI (1986) Molecular Biology of *Homo sapiens*
LII (1987) Evolution of Catalytic Function
LIII (1988) Molecular Biology of Signal Transduction
LIV (1989) Immunological Recognition
LV (1990) The Brain
LVI (1991) The Cell Cycle
LVII (1992) The Cell Surface
LVIII (1993) DNA and Chromosomes
LIX (1994) The Molecular Genetics of Cancer
LX (1995) Protein Kinesis: The Dynamics of Protein Trafficking and Stability
LXI (1996) Function & Dysfunction in the Nervous System
LXII (1997) Pattern Formation during Development
LXIII (1998) Mechanisms of Transcription
LXIV (1999) Signaling and Gene Expression in the Immune System
LXV (2000) Biological Responses to DNA Damage
LXVI (2001) The Ribosome
LXVII (2002) The Cardiovascular System
LXVIII (2003) The Genome of *Homo sapiens*
LXVIX (2004) Epigenetics

Front Cover (*Paperback*): Detail of a French anticancer poster, "Vaincre le Cancer," by Bernard Vellemot (courtesy of the National Library of Medicine).

Authorization to photocopy items for internal or personal use, or the internal or personal use of specific clients, is granted by Cold Spring Harbor Laboratory Press, provided that the appropriate fee is paid directly to the Copyright Clearance Center (CCC). Write or call CCC at 222 Rosewood Drive, Danvers, MA 01923 (978-750-8400) for information about fees and regulations. Prior to photocopying items for educational classroom use, contact CCC at the above address. Additional information on CCC can be obtained at CCC Online at http://www.copyright.com/

All Cold Spring Harbor Laboratory Press publications may be ordered directly from Cold Spring Harbor Laboratory Press, 500 Sunnyside Boulevard, Woodbury, NY 11797-2924. Phone: 1-800-843-4388 in Continental U.S. and Canada. All other locations: (516) 422-4100. FAX: (516) 422-4097. E-mail: cshpress@cshl.edu. For a complete catalog of all Cold Spring Harbor Laboratory Press publications, visit our World Wide Web Site http://www.cshlpress.com/

Web Site Access: Institutions that have purchased the hardcover edition of this book are entitled to online access to the companion Web site at www.cshl-symposium.org. For assistance with activation, please contact Kathy Cirone, CSHL Press Subscription Manager, at cironek@cshl.edu.

Symposium Participants

ABATE-SHEN, CORY, Dept. of Medicine, UMDNJ-Robert Wood Johnson Medical School, Piscataway, New Jersey

ABURATANI, HIROYUKI, Lab. for Systems Biology and Medicine, University of Tokyo, Tokyo, Japan

ACKERMAN, ANN

ADAMS, DAVID, Dept. of Informatics, The Wellcome Trust Sanger Institute, Hinxton, Cambridge, United Kingdom

ADAMS, JERRY, Molecular Genetics of Cancer, Walter and Eliza Hall Institute of Medical Research, Melbourne, Victoria, Australia

AIKHIONBARE, FELIX, Dept. of Medicine, Morehouse School of Medicine, Atlanta, Georgia

AL-HAJJ, MUHAMMAD, Oncology Disease Area, Novartis Institutes for BioMedical Research, Cambridge, Massachusetts

ALBERTS, BRUCE, Dept. of Biochemistry and Biophysics, University of California, San Francisco

ALLIO, THERESA, Dept. of Mouse Genome Informatics, The Jackson Laboratory, Bar Harbor, Maine

ALLISON, JAMES, Immunology Program, Howard Hughes Medical Institute, Memorial Sloan-Kettering Cancer Center, New York, New York

AMARIGLIO, NINETTE, Dept. of Pediatric Hematology and Oncology, Chaim Sheba Medical Center, Tel Hashomer, Israel

AMSON, ROBERT, Dept. of Cancer Research, Molecular Engines Laboratories, Paris, France

ANDL, CLAUDIA, Dept. of Medicine and Genetics, University of Pennsylvania, Philadelphia

ANN, DAVID, Dept. of Molecular Pharmacology and Toxicology, University of Southern California, Los Angeles, California

ANTONOVA, LILIA, Dept. of Pathology and Molecular Medicine, Queen's University, Kingston, Ontario, Canada

ARAI, YOSHIO, Dept. of Radiation Oncology, Veteran's Administration Medical Center, University of Pittsburgh, Pittsburgh, Pennsylvania

ARMANIOS, MARY, Dept. of Oncology, Johns Hopkins University School of Medicine, Baltimore, Maryland

ARNONE, MARC, Dept. of Oncology Biology, GlaxoSmithKline, Collegeville, Pennsylvania

ARVA, NICOLETA, Dept. of Biology, Hunter College, City University of New York, New York

ASHKENAZI, AVI, Dept. of Molecular Oncology, Genentech, Inc., South San Francisco, California

ASHWORTH, ALAN, The Breakthrough Breast Cancer Research Centre, Chester Beatty Laboratories, Institute of Cancer Research, London, United Kingdom

ATTAR, RICHARDO, Dept. of Oncology Drug Discovery, Bristol-Myers Squibb, Princeton, New Jersey

ATTARDI, LAURA, Dept. of Radiation Oncology, Stanford University, Stanford, California

AUBIN, REMY, Div. of Cell and Molecular Biology, Health Products and Food Biologicals Branch, Centre for Biologics Research, Health Canada, Ottawa, Ontario, Canada

AUSTIN, RICK, Dept. of Biology, Amgen, Inc., South San Francisco, California

BADER, ANDREAS, Dept. of Molecular and Experimental Medicine, The Scripps Research Institute, La Jolla, California

BAGCHI, ANINDYA, Cold Spring Harbor Laboratory, Cold Spring Harbor, New York

BAKIN, ANDREI, Dept. of Cancer Genetics, Roswell Park Cancer Institute, Buffalo, New York

BALLESTEROS, ANITA, *Cancer Cell*, Cell Press, Cambridge, Massachusetts

BANSAL, SANJAY, Dept. of Pharmacology and Therapeutics, Roswell Park Cancer Institute, Buffalo, New York

BARBACID, MARIANO, Centro Nacional de investigaciones Ontologica, Madrid, Spain

BARGONETTI, JILL, Dept. of Biological Sciences, Hunter College, City University of New York, New York

BARNHART, BRYAN, Dept. of Cancer Biology, University of Pennsylvania, Philadelphia

BAYLIN, STEPHEN, Oncology Center, Johns Hopkins University School of Medicine, Baltimore, Maryland

BEACHY, PHILIP, Dept. of Molecular Biology and Genetics, Johns Hopkins University School of Medicine, Baltimore, Maryland

BENEZRA, ROBERT, Dept. of Cell Biology, Memorial Sloan-Kettering Cancer Center, New York, New York

BENTIVEGNA, STEVEN, Dept. of Pharmacogenomics, Pfizer, Inc., Groton, Connecticut

BENTON, GEOFFREY, Dept. of Pathology, University of California, San Francisco

BENVENUTI, SILVIA, The Oncogenomics Center, Institute for Cancer Research and Treatment, Candiolo, Torino, Italy

BENZINGER, ANNE, Dept. of Molecular Oncology, Max-Planck-Institute for Biochemistry, Martinsried, Germany

BERBERICH, MATTHEW, Dept. of Molecular Biophysics and Biochemistry, Yale University, New Haven, Connecticut

BERNARDS, RENÉ, Dept. of Molecular Carcinogenesis, The Netherlands Cancer Institute, Amsterdam, The Netherlands

BERNS, ANTON, Dept. of Molecular Genetics, The Netherlands Cancer Institute, Amsterdam, The Netherlands

BEVERLY, LEVI, Dept. of Molecular and Cellular Oncogenesis, The Wistar Institute, Philadelphia, Pennsylvania

BIHANI, TEERU, Dept. of Molecular Pharmacology and Cancer Therapeutics, Roswell Park Cancer Institute, Buffalo, New York

BILLOTTET, CLOTILDE, Dept. of Cell Signalling, Ludwig Institute for Cancer Research, London, United Kingdom

BISHOP, J. MICHAEL, Dept. of Microbiology, University of California, San Francisco

BISSELL, MINA, Div. of Life Sciences, Lawrence Berkeley National Laboratory, Berkeley, California

BITTINGER, MARK, Dept. of Target Support and Validation, Merck Research Laboratories, Boston, Massachusetts

BLANK, JUTTA, Dept. of Discovery Technologies, Novartis Institutes for BioMedical Research, Basel, Switzerland

BLUME-JENSEN, PETER, Dept. of Molecular Oncology, Merck Research Laboratories, Boston, Massachusetts

BOMMI-REDDY, ARCHANA, Dept. of Medical Oncology, Dana-Farber Cancer Institute, Boston, Massachusetts

BORZILLO, GARY, Dept. of Cancer Biology, Pfizer, Inc., Groton, Connecticut

BRACHMANN, SASKIA, Dept. of Medical Oncology, Dana-Farber Cancer Institute, Boston, Massachusetts

BRADY, MARK, Dept. of Surgery and Oncology, University of Liverpool, Liverpool, United Kingdom

BRAHMBHATT, HIMANSHU, Dept. of Cancer Research, EnGeneIC Pty, Ltd., Sydney, New South Wales, Australia

BRENNER, SYDNEY, The Salk Institute for Biological Studies, La Jolla, California

BRIESEWITZ, ROGER, Dept. of Pharmacology, Ohio State University, Columbus, Ohio

BRUGGE, JOAN, Dept. of Cell Biology, Harvard Medical School, Boston, Massachusetts

BRUMMER, TILMAN, Cancer Research Program, Garvan Institute of Medical Research, Darlinghurst, Sydney, New South Wales, Australia

BURGESS, DARREN, Cold Spring Harbor Laboratory, Cold Spring Harbor, New York

BURNS, ALEXANDER, Metabolic Diseases Branch, National Institute of Diabetes and Digestive and Kidney Diseases, National Institutes of Health, Bethesda, Maryland

BUTT, ALISON, Cancer Research Program, Garvan Institute of Medical Research, Darlinghurst, Sydney, New South Wales, Australia

CAI, WEI-WEN, Dept. of Molecular and Human Genetics, Baylor College of Medicine, Houston, Texas

CAMPBELL, ROBERT, Dept. of Scientific Computing, Serono Research Institute, Rockland, Massachusetts

CAMPISI, JUDITH, Div. of Life Sciences, Lawrence Berkeley National Laboratory, Berkeley, California

CAO, LIU, Genetics of Development and Diseases Branch, National Institute of Diabetes and Digestive and Kidney Diseases, National Institutes of Health, Bethesda, Maryland

CAPOBIANCO, ANTHONY, Dept. of Molecular and Cellular Oncogenesis, The Wistar Institute, Philadelphia, Pennsylvania

CAPUTTO, BEATRIZ, Dept. of Biological Chemistry, CIQUIBIC, National University of Córdoba, Córdoba, Argentina

CARMANY, GEORGE

CARRIERE, CATHERINE, Dept. of Medicine, Dartmouth Medical School, Lebanon, New Hampshire

CHAN, KELVIN, Dept. of Obstetrics and Gynecology, University of Hong Kong, Hong Kong

CHEN, EMILY, Dept. of Cell Biology, The Scripps Research Institute, La Jolla, California

CHEUNG, ANN, Center for Cancer Research, Massachusetts Institute of Technology, Cambridge, Massachusetts

CHODANKAR, RAJAS, Prostate Cancer Center, Cedars-Sinai Medical Center, Los Angeles, California

CHONG, SHAORONG, Dept. of Research, New England BioLabs, Inc., Beverly, Massachusetts

CHOU, CHEN-KUNG, Dept. of Life Science, Chang Gung University, Tao-Yuan, Taiwan, Republic of China

COCHRAN, ANDREA, Dept. of Protein Engineering, Genentech, Inc., South San Francisco, California

COCHRAN, BRENT, Dept. of Physiology, Tufts University School of Medicine, Boston, Massachusetts

COLLIER, LARA, Dept. of Genetics, Cell Biology and Development, Cancer Center, University of Minnesota, Minneapolis

COMB, MICHAEL, President, Cell Signaling Technology, Beverly, Massachusetts

CONNELL, LAUREEN, *Genes & Development*, Cold Spring Harbor Laboratory Press, Cold Spring Harbor, New York

COOMBER, DAVID, Institute of Molecular and Cellular Biology, Proteos, Singapore

COOPMAN, PETER, Unité Mixte de Recherche, Centre National de la Recherche Scientifique, University of Montpellier, Montpellier, France

COQUERET, OLIVER, Cancer Center Paul Papin, INSERM, Angers, France

CORMIER, CATHERINE, Cold Spring Harbor Laboratory, Cold Spring Harbor, New York

COURTNEIDGE, SARA, Cell Adhesion and Extracellular Matrix Program, The Burnham Institute, La Jolla, California

COVELLO, KELLY, Dept. of Cell and Developmental Biology, University of Pennsylvania, Philadelphia

CRAWFORD, SARAH, Dept. of Biology, Southern Connecticut State University, New Haven, Connecticut

CRAWFORD, YONGPING, Dept. of Angiogenesis Research, Genentech, Inc., South San Francisco, California

CULLINAN, EMILY, Dept. of Oncology, Lexicon Genetics, Inc., The Woodlands, Texas

CURTIS, DANIEL, Dept. of Developmental and Molecular Pathways, Novartis Institutes for BioMedical Research, Cambridge, Massachusetts

DACKOUR, RADUWAN, Dept. of Otolaryngology, Long Island Jewish Medical Center, New Hyde Park, New York

DAI, CHENGKAI, Whitehead Institute for Biomedical Research, Cambridge, Massachusetts

DAKIC, ALEKSANDAR, Dept. of Immunology, Walter and Eliza Hall Institute of Medical Research, Parkville, Victoria, Australia

DANKORT, DAVID, Cancer Research Institute, Comprehensive Cancer Center, University of California, San Francisco

DAS, BIKUL, Dept. of Hematology and Oncology, Hospital for Sick Children, Toronto, Ontario, Canada

DE LANGE, TITIA, Dept. of Cell Biology and Genetics, Rockefeller University, New York, New York

DEPINHO, RONALD, Dept. of Medical Oncology, Dana-

Farber Cancer Institute, Boston, Massachusetts

DE SAUVAGE, FREDERIC, Dept. of Molecular Oncology, Genentech, Inc., South San Francisco, California

DEY, ANWESHA, Institute of Molecular and Cell Biology, Proteos, Singapore

DICKINS, ROSS, Cold Spring Harbor Laboratory, Cold Spring Harbor, New York

DILLIN, ANDREW, Lab. of Molecular and Cell Biology, The Salk Institute for Biological Studies, La Jolla, California

DI MARCOTULLIO, LUCIA, Dept. of Experimental Medicine and Pathology, University La Sapienza, Rome, Italy

DRAETTA, GIULIO, Dept. of Cancer Research, Merck Research Laboratories, Boston, Massachusetts

DRAGESET, VILDE, Dept. of Genetics, The Norwegian Radium Hospital, Oslo, Norway

DU, YI-CHIEH NANCY, Dept. of Cancer Biology and Genetics, Memorial Sloan-Kettering Cancer Center, New York, New York

DUAN, ZHENFENG, Dept. of Hematology and Oncology, Massachusetts General Hospital, Boston, Massachusetts

EBERT, JOAN, Cold Spring Harbor Laboratory Press, Woodbury, New York

EILERS, MARTIN, Institute of Molecular Biology and Tumor Research, University of Marburg, Marburg, Germany

EINBOND, LINDA, Dept. of Rehabilitation Medicine, Columbia University, New York, New York

EISENMAN, ROBERT, Div. of Basic Sciences, Fred Hutchinson Cancer Research Center, Seattle, Washington

ELLEDGE, STEPHEN, Dept. of Genetics, Harvard Medical School, Boston, Massachusetts

EMERY, CAROLINE, Dept. of Medical Oncology, Dana-Farber Cancer Institute, Boston, Massachusetts

ENOMOTO, TAKEHARU, Lineberger Comprehensive Cancer Center, University of North Carolina, Chapel Hill

EPPING, MIRJAM, Dept. of Molecular Carcinogenesis, The Netherlands Cancer Institute, Amsterdam, The Netherlands

EPSTEIN, CHARLES, Cambridge Genomics Center, Sanofi-Aventis, Cambridge, Massachusetts

ERDMANN, DIRK, Dept. of Oncology, Novartis Pharma AG, Basel, Switzerland

ERNKVIST, MIRA, Dept of Oncology and Pathology, Karolinska Institute, Stockholm, Sweden

EVAN, GERARD, Dept. of Cellular and Molecular Pharmacology, Cancer Research Institute, Comprehensive Cancer Center, University of California, San Francisco

FAGA, GIOVANNI, Dept. of Experimental Oncology, European Institute of Oncology, Milan, Italy

FAN, HUNG, Dept. of Molecular Biology and Biochemistry, Cancer Research Institute, University of California, Irvine

FEINBERG, ANDREW, Epigenetics Unit, Johns Hopkins University School of Medicine, Baltimore, Maryland

FERBEYRE, GERARDO, Dept. of Biochemistry, Université de Montréal, Montréal, Québec, Canada

FERO, MATTHEW, Div. of Clinical Research, Fred Hutchinson Cancer Research Center, Seattle, Washington

FLANNERY, ANGELA, Dept. of Genetic Research and Development, AstraZeneca, Macclesfield, United Kingdom

FLAVELL, MADLYN, Guilford, Connecticut

FLAVELL, RICHARD, Dept. of Immunobiology, Yale University School of Medicine, New Haven, Connecticut

FOLKMAN, JUDAH, Dept. of Surgery, Children's Hospital, Harvard Medical School, Boston, Massachusetts

FOREMAN, KENNETH, Dept. of Cancer Chemistry, OSI Pharmaceuticals, Inc., Farmingdale, New York

FOURNIER, ALAINA, Dept. of Pharmacology, University of Pennsylvania, Philadelphia

FRIDMAN, JORDAN, Dept. of Preclinical Biology, Incyte Corporation, Wilmington, Delaware

FRIEDMAN, LORI, Dept. of Research, Genentech, Inc., South San Francisco, California

FRIEND, STEPHEN, Dept. of Molecular Profiling and Cancer Research, Merck Research Laboratories, West Point, Pennsylvania

FUTREAL, ANDREW, Cancer Genome Project, The Wellcome Trust Sanger Institute, Hinxton, Cambridge, United Kingdom

GALAKTIONOV, KONSTANTIN, Dept. of Molecular and Human Genetics, Baylor College of Medicine, Houston, Texas

GALLOWAY, DENISE, Dept. of Cancer Biology, Fred Hutchinson Cancer Research Center, Seattle, Washington

GANN, ALEXANDER, Cold Spring Harbor Laboratory Press, Woodbury, New York

GANN, LILIAN, Cold Spring Harbor Laboratory, Cold Spring Harbor, New York

GAO, ZHIJIAN, Dept. of Hematology and Oncology, Massachusetts General Hospital, Boston, Massachusetts

GAO, HUI, Biosciences NOVUM, Karolinska Institute, Huddinge, Sweden

GARY, SYDNEY, Cold Spring Harbor Laboratory, Cold Spring Harbor, New York

GEIGER, THOMAS, Dept. of Molecular Genetics, The Netherlands Cancer Institute, Amsterdam, The Netherlands

GERHARD, DANIELA, National Cancer Institute, National Institutes of Health, Bethesda, Maryland

GIBSON, NEIL, Dept. of Research, OSI Pharmaceuticals, Inc., Farmingdale, New York

GIL, GERMAN, Dept. of Pediatrics, Robert Wood Johnson Medical School, Cancer Institute of New Jersey, New Brunswick, New Jersey

GIL, JESUS, Cold Spring Harbor Laboratory, Cold Spring Harbor, New York

GIRNUN, GEOFFREY, Dept. of Cancer Biology, Dana-Farber Cancer Institute, Harvard Medical School, Boston, Massachusetts

GODBOLE, MADAN, Dept. of Endocrinology, Sanjay Gandhi Postgraduate Institute of Medical Sciences, Lucknow, India

GOELET, PHILLIP, Road to the Cure, San Diego, California

GOLDBERG, ITZHAK, Dept. of Radiation Oncology, Long Island Jewish Medical Center, New Hyde Park, New York

GONZALEZ, MICHAEL, Medical Research Council Cancer Cell Unit, Hutchison/MRC Research Centre, Cambridge, United Kingdom

GORDAN, JOHN, Abramson Family Cancer Research Institute, University of Pennsylvania, Philadelphia, Pennsylvania

GOROVITS, NAIRA, Cold Spring Harbor Laboratory, Cold Spring Harbor, New York

GORRINI, CHIARA, Dept. of Experimental Oncology,

European Institute of Oncology, Milan, Italy

GRADI, ALESSANDRA, Dept. of Molecular Oncogenesis, Regina Elena Cancer Institute, Rome, Italy

GRAEBER, THOMAS, Dept. of Molecular and Medical Pharmacology, University of California, Los Angeles

GRAHAM, ROBERT, Victor Chang Cardiac Research Institute, Darlinghurst, Sydney, Australia

GRAUSENBURGER, REINHARD, Dept. of Medical Biochemistry, Medical University of Vienna, Vienna, Austria

GRAY, JOE, Lawrence Berkeley National Laboratory, Berkeley, California and University of California, San Francisco

GREIDER, CAROL, Dept. of Molecular Biology and Genetics, Johns Hopkins University School of Medicine, Baltimore, Maryland

GROSSEL, MARTHA, Dept. of Zoology, Connecticut College, New London, Connecticut

GRUBER, MICHAELA, Abramson Family Cancer Research Institute, University of Pennsylvania, Philadelphia

GRUBOR, VLADIMIR, Cold Spring Harbor Laboratory, Cold Spring Harbor, New York

GRUENEBERG, DORRE, RNAi Consortium, Broad Institute, Massachusetts Institute of Technology, Cambridge, Massachusetts

GUARDIOLA-SERRANO, FRANCISCA, Dept. of Molecular Hematology, University of Frankfurt Medical School, Frankfurt am Main, Germany

GUO, BING, Dept. of Oncology Research, Wyeth, Pearl River, New York

GUO, AILAN, Dept. of Research, Cell Signaling Technology, Beverly, Massachusetts

GUPTA, PIYUSH, Dept. of Biology, Whitehead Institute for Biomedical Research, Massachusetts Institute of Technology, Cambridge, Massachusetts

HA, TAEKJIP, Dept. of Physics, University of Illinois, Urbana

HABER, DANIEL, Cancer Center, Massachusetts General Hospital, Charlestown, Massachusetts

HABIB, TANIA, Dept. of Comparative Medicine, University of Washington, Seattle

HAGEMEIER, CHRISTIAN, Children's Hospital, Charité, Humboldt-University, Berlin, Germany

HAHN, MEINHARD, Dept. of Molecular Genetics, German Cancer Research Center, Heidelberg, Germany

HALEY, JOHN, Dept. of Translational Research, OSI Pharmaceuticals, Inc., Farmingdale, New York

HALL, MARK, Dept. of Biochemistry, St. Jude Children's Research Hospital, Memphis, Tennessee

HALL, IRA, Cold Spring Harbor Laboratory, Cold Spring Harbor, New York

HAMLIN, JOYCE, Dept. of Biochemistry and Molecular Genetics, School of Medicine, University of Virginia, Charlottesville

HAN, TAE-HEE, Dept. of Molecular Cell Biology, Sungkyunkwan University School of Medicine, Suwon, South Korea

HANAHAN, DOUGLAS, Dept. of Biochemistry and Biophysics, University of California, San Francisco

HANNON, GREGORY, Cold Spring Harbor Laboratory, Cold Spring Harbor, New York

HARLOW, ED, Dept. of Biological Chemistry and Molecular Pharmacology, Harvard University School of Medicine, Boston, Massachusetts

HARRIS, CRAFFORD, Dept. of Drug Discovery, R.W. Johnson Pharmaceutical Research Institute, Raritan, New Jersey

HE, LIN, Cold Spring Harbor Laboratory, Cold Spring Harbor, New York

HEMANN, MICHAEL, Cold Spring Harbor Laboratory, Cold Spring Harbor, New York

HERBERT, TASINO, Dept. of Biology, Southern Connecticut State University, New Haven, Connecticut

HERGOVICH LISZTWAN, JOANNA, Novartis Pharma AG, Basel, Switzerland

HERMAN, JAMES, Bunting Blaustern Cancer Research Center, Sidney Kimmel Comprehensive Cancer Center, Johns Hopkins University School of Medicine, Baltimore, Maryland

HERMEKING, HEIKO, Dept. of Molecular Oncology, Max-Planck-Institute for Biochemistry, Martinsried, Germany

HERSCHKOWITZ, JASON, Dept. of Genetics and Molecular Biology, University of North Carolina, Chapel Hill

HEUER, TIMOTHY, Dept. of Cellular Pharmacology, Exelixis, Inc., South San Francisco, California

HICKEY, MICHELE, Dept. of Cell and Molecular Biology, University of Pennsylvania, Philadelphia

HICKS, JAMES, Cold Spring Harbor Laboratory, Cold Spring Harbor, New York

HILL, REGINALD, Dept. of Genetics, Lineberger Comprehensive Cancer Center, University of North Carolina, Chapel Hill

HILLAN, KENNETH, Dept. of Research, Genentech, Inc., South San Francisco, California

HIPPO, YOSHITAKA, Cold Spring Harbor Laboratory, Cold Spring Harbor, New York

HOFFMANN, INGRID, Dept. of Cell Cycle Control and Carcinogenesis, German Cancer Research Center, Heidelberg, Germany

HOHENADL, CHRISTINE, Research Institute of Virology and Biomedicine, University of Veterinary Medicine, Vienna, Austria

HOLST, CHARLES, Dept. of Molecular Oncology, Genentech, Inc., South San Francisco, California

HU, ZHIYUAN, Dept. of Genetics, Lineberger Comprehensive Cancer Center, University of North Carolina, Chapel Hill

HUANG, CHI-YING, Dept. of Molecular and Genomic Medicine, National Health Research Institutes, Zhunan, Taiwan, Republic of China

HUANG, FEI, Dept. of Oncology Biomarkers and Clinical Discovery Technology, Bristol-Myers Squibb, Princeton, New Jersey

HUGHES, CHRISTINA, Dept. of Medical Oncology, Dana-Farber Cancer Institute, Boston, Massachusetts

IACOVIDES, DEMETRIS, Comprehensive Cancer Center, University of California, San Francisco

IANARI, ALESSANDRA, Dept. of Experimental Medicine and Pathology, University La Sapienza, Rome, Italy

IGGO, RICHARD, Dept. of Molecular Oncology, Swiss Institute for Experimental Cancer Research, Epalinges, Switzerland

INGLIS, JOHN, Cold Spring Harbor Laboratory Press, Woodbury, New York

ISHIDA, SEIKO, Dept. of Biochemistry, Comprehensive Cancer Center, University of California, San Francisco

ISHOV, ALEXANDER, Dept. of Anatomy and Cell Biology, University of Florida, Gainesville

ITO, YOSHIAKI, RUNX Study Group, Institute of Molecular and Cell Biology, Proteos, Singapore

ITOH, REINA, Dept. of Tumor Virology, Research Institute for Microbial Disease, Osaka University, Osaka, Japan

IWAKUMA, TOMOO, Dept. of Molecular Genetics, M.D. Anderson Cancer Center, University of Texas, Houston

IWATA, KENNETH, Dept. of Cancer Research, OSI Pharmaceuticals, Inc., Uniondale, New York

JACKS, TYLER, Center For Cancer Research, Howard Hughes Medical Institute, Massachusetts Institute of Technology, Cambridge, Massachusetts

JAKUBCZAK, JOHN, Pfizer Global Research and Development, Pfizer, Inc., Groton, Connecticut

JANE-VALBUENA, JUDIT, Dept. of Medical Oncology, Dana-Farber Cancer Institute, Boston, Massachusetts

JAT, PAMJIT, Dept. of Neurodegenerative Disease, Institute of Neurology, University College, London, United Kingdom

JECHLINGER, MARTIN, Dept. of Cancer Biology and Genetics, Memorial Sloan-Kettering Cancer Center, New York, New York

JI, PENG, Dept. of Developmental and Molecular Biology, Albert Einstein College of Medicine, Bronx, New York

JOHNSON, LEISA, Dept. of Molecular Biology, Genentech, Inc., South San Francisco, California

JOHNSON, MARK

JOHNSON, TOM, Dept. of Radiation Oncology, Stanford University, Stanford, California

JOUKOV, VLADIMIR, Dept. of Cancer Biology, Dana-Farber Cancer Institute, Boston, Massachusetts

JOYCE, JOHANNA, Dept. of Cancer Biology and Genetics, Memorial Sloan-Kettering Cancer Center, New York, New York

JUNTTILA, MELISSA, Dept. of Medical Biochemistry, University of Turku, Turku, Finland

KACZMAREK, LEONARD, Dept. of Pharmacology, Yale University School of Medicine, New Haven, Connecticut

KAELIN, WILLIAM, Dept. of Adult Oncology, Dana-Farber Cancer Institute, Boston, Massachusetts

KAKUMOTO, KYOKO, Dept. of Molecular Oncology, Osaka Bioscience Institute, Osaka, Japan

KALLURI, RAGHU, Dept. of Medicine, Beth Israel Deaconess Medical Center, Boston, Massachusetts

KALPANA, GANJAM, Dept. of Molecular Genetics, Albert Einstein College of Medicine, Bronx, New York

KALRA, DEEPAK, Dept. of Cardiology, Children's Hospital, Harvard Medical School, Boston, Massachusetts

KAMATA, TOHRU, Dept. of Molecular Biology and Biochemistry, Shinshu University School of Medicine, Matsumoto, Japan

KAN, JULIE, Dept. of Cancer Biology, OSI Pharmaceuticals, Inc., Farmingdale, New York

KANG, HYUNG-GYOO, Dept. of Pathology, Children's Hospital, University of Southern California, Los Angeles, California

KANNIUS-JANSON, MARIE, Dept. of Cell and Molecular Biology, Gothenburg University, Gothenburg, Sweden

KARLSEDER, JAN, Dept. of Regulatory Biology, The Salk Institute for Biological Studies, La Jolla, California

KARRETH, FLORIAN, Abramson Family Cancer Research Institute, University of Pennsylvania, Philadelphia

KASTAN, MICHAEL, Dept. of Hematology and Oncology, St. Jude Children's Research Hospital, Memphis, Tennessee

KENNY, PARAIC, Div. of Life Sciences, Lawrence Berkeley National Laboratory, Berkeley, California

KIBERTSIS, PAULA, *Science*, American Association for the Advancement of Science, Washington, D.C.

KIM, JIYOUNG, Dept. of Biochemistry, Tufts University School of Medicine, Boston, Massachusetts

KIM, MARIANNE, Dept. of Medicine, Mount Sinai School of Medicine, New York, New York

KING, MARY-CLAIRE, Div. of Medical Genetics, University of Washington, Seattle

KIVIHARJU, TAIJA, Molecular Cancer Biology Program, University of Helsinki, Helsinki, Finland

KIYOKAWA, ETSUKO, Dept. of Tumor Virology, Research Institute for Bacterial Diseases, University of Osaka, Osaka, Japan

KOGISO, TOMOMI, International Medical Center of Japan, Tokyo, Japan

KONDURI, SANTHI, Dept. of Pharmacology and Therapeutics, Roswell Park Cancer Instititute, Buffalo, New York

KOTANIDES, HELEN, Dept. of Molecular and Cell Biology, ImClone Systems, Inc., New York, New York

KRUCHER, NANCY, Dept. of Biology, Pace University, Pleasantville, New York

KUILMAN, THOMAS, Dept. of Molecular Genetics, The Netherlands Cancer Institute, Amsterdam, The Netherlands

KUMAR, CHANDRA, Dept. of Tumor Biology, Schering-Plough Research Institute, Kenilworth, New Jersey

KURKI, SARI, Molecular Cancer Biology Program, University of Helsinki, Helsinki, Finland

LADANYI, MARC, Dept. of Pathology, Memorial Sloan-Kettering Cancer Center, New York, New York

LAMONTAGNE, KENNETH, Drug Discovery, Johnson and Johnson Pharmaceutical Research and Development, Raritan, New Jersey

LANDER, ERIC, The Broad Institute, Massachusetts Institute of Technology, Cambridge, Massachusetts

LANE, KEARA, Center for Cancer Research, Massachusetts Institute of Technology, Cambridge, Massachusetts

LANE, DAVID, Executive Director, Institute of Molecular and Cell Biology, Proteos, Singapore

LEE, CHANG WOO, Research Institute, National Cancer Center, Goyang, South Korea

LEE, SOYOUNG, Dept. of Hematology and Oncology, Charité, Universitätsmedizin Berlin, Berlin, Germany

LEES, JACQUELINE, Dept. of Biology, Center for Cancer Research, Massachusetts Institute of Technology, Cambridge, Massachusetts

LEHMKUHL, KRISTINA, Dept. of Biological Sciences, Ohio University, Athens, Ohio

LENG, MEI, Dept. of Biochemistry, Baylor College of Medicine, Houston, Texas

LEPRINCE, DOMINIQUE, Lille Institute of Biology, Centre National de la Recherche Scientifique, Lille, France

LETAI, ANTHONY, Dept. of Medical Oncology, Dana-

Farber Cancer Institute, Boston, Massachusetts

LEVINE, ARNOLD, School of Natural Sciences, Institute for Advanced Studies, Princeton, New Jersey

LI, XINGNAN, Dept. of Cell Biology, University of Alabama, Birmingham

LI, RONG, Dept. of Biochemistry and Molecular Genetics, University of Virginia, Charlottesville

LIN, ATHENA, Dept. of Pharmacology and Therapeutics, Roswell Park Cancer Institute, Buffalo, New York

LIN, LING, Metabolic Diseases Branch, National Institute of Diabetes and Digestive and Kidney Diseases, National Institutes of Health, Bethesda, Maryland

LINDEMANN, RALPH, Lab. of Gene Regulation, Cancer Immunology Program, Peter MacCallum Cancer Centre, East Melbourne, Victoria, Australia

LIU, HUIPING, Ben May Institute for Cancer Research, University of Chicago, Chicago, Illinois

LIU, JIANHONG, Dept. of Biology, MethylGene, Inc., Montréal, Québec, Canada

LIU, KUN-HSIANG, Dept. of Genomics, Biomedical Engineering Center, Industrial Technology Research Institute, Hsinchu, Taiwan, Republic of China

LIU, XIANGDONG, Dept. of Drug Discovery and Development, Incyte Corporation, Wilmington, Delaware

LIU, XUESONG, Dept. of Cancer Research, Abbott Laboratories, Abbott Park, Illinois

LIU, XUESONG, Dept. of Oncology, Lexicon Genetics, Inc., The Woodlands, Texas

LIU, YING, Dept. of Cancer and Immunogenetics, Weatherall Institute of Molecular Medicine, J.R. Hospital, Oxford, United Kingdom

LIU, ZHAOLI, Dept. of Cell Biology, University of Alabama, Birmingham

LIVINGSTON, DAVID, Dept. of Cancer Biology, Dana-Farber Cancer Institute, Harvard School of Medicine, Boston, Massachusetts

LOWE, SCOTT, Howard Hughes Medical Institute, Cold Spring Harbor Laboratory, Cold Spring Harbor, New York

LU, XIN, Dept. of Molecular Biology, Princeton University, Princeton, New Jersey

LU, XIN, Lab. of Tumour Suppression, Ludwig Institute for Cancer Research, London, United Kingdom

LUCIANI, GLORIA, Dept. of Internal Medicine, Medical University of Vienna, Vienna, Austria

LUK, JOHN, Dept. of Surgery, University of Hong Kong, Hong Kong

LYONS, JESSE, Comprehensive Cancer Center, University of California, San Francisco

LÜSCHER, BERNHARD, Dept. of Biochemistry and Molecular Biology, RWTH University, Aachen, Germany

MACDIARMID, JENNIFER, Dept. of Cancer Research, EnGeneIC Pty, Ltd., Sydney, New South Wales, Australia

MACDONALD, GWEN, Dept. of Biochemistry, Cancer Research Institute, Queen's University, Kingston, Ontario, Canada

MACLEOD, KAY, Ben May Institute for Cancer Research, University of Chicago, Chicago, Illinois

MAJID, ANEELA, Toxicology Unit, Medical Research Council, Leicester, United Kingdom

MAJUMDER, SADHAN, Dept. of Molecular Genetics, M.D. Anderson Cancer Center, University of Texas, Houston

MARCUS, EMILIE, *Cell*, Cell Press, Cambridge, Massachusetts

MARGALIT, OFER, Dept. of Pediatric Hematology and Oncology, Chaim Sheba Medical Center, Tel-Hashomer, Israel

MARINE, JEAN-CHRISTOPHE, Lab. for Molecular Cancer Biology, Flanders Interuniversity Institute for Biotechnology, Ghent, Belgium

MARKOVINA, STEPHANIE, Dept. of Medicine and Hematology, University of Wisconsin, Madison

MARSHALL, DEBORAH, Dept. of Oncology Research, Centocor, Inc., Radnor, Pennsylvania

MARTE, BARBARA, *Nature*, Nature Publishing Group, London, United Kingdom

MARTIN, STEVEN, Dept. of Molecular and Cell Biology, University of California, Berkeley

MARTINS, CARLA, Comprehensive Cancer Center, University of California, San Francisco

MASSAGUÉ, JOAN, Dept. of Cell Biology, Genetics Program, Memorial Sloan-Kettering Cancer Center, New York, New York

MASUDA, KAZUHIRO, BioFrontier Laboratories, Kyowa Hakko Kogyo Co., Ltd., Tokyo, Japan

MATAPURKAR, ANAGHA, Cold Spring Harbor Laboratory, Cold Spring Harbor, New York

MAZUREK, ANTHONY, Cold Spring Harbor Laboratory, Cold Spring Harbor, New York

MCCORMICK, FRANK, Cancer Research Institute, Comprehensive Cancer Center, University of California, San Francisco

MCLEAN, ADELE, Dept. of Molecular Genetics, Institute of Biomedical and Life Sciences, University of Glasgow, Glasgow, Scotland, United Kingdom

MCMAHON, MARTIN, Cancer Research Institute, Comprehensive Cancer Center, University of California, San Francisco

MEANI, NATALIA, FIRC Institute of Molecular Oncology Foundation, European Institute of Oncology, Milan, Italy

MEDICO, ENZO, Institute for Cancer Research and Treatment, University of Torino School of Medicine, Candiolo, Torino, Italy

MELLMAN, IRA, Dept. of Cell Biology, Yale University School of Medicine, New Haven, Connecticut

MENDOZA, MICHAEL, Div. of Digestive Diseases, University of California, Los Angeles

MENON, RADHA, Dept. of Immunology and Molecular Diagnostics, Federal Drug Administration, Rockville, Maryland

MEYERSON, MATTHEW, Dept. of Molecular Oncology, Dana-Farber Cancer Institute, Boston, Massachusetts

MILLER, ABIGAIL, Cancer Research Institute, Comprehensive Cancer Center, University of California, San Francisco

MILLS, ALEA, Cold Spring Harbor Laboratory, Cold Spring Harbor, New York

MIRANTI, CINDY, Dept. of Microbiology, Van Andel Research Institute, Grand Rapids, Michigan

MISCHEK, DANIELA, Research Institute of Virology and Biomedicine, University of Veterinary Medicine, Vienna, Austria

MITRA, KOYEL, Dept. of Molecular Genetics, Albert Einstein College of Medicine, Bronx, New York

MITTAL, VIVEK, Cold Spring Harbor Laboratory, Cold Spring Harbor, New York

MOHI, M. GOLAM, Dept. of Medicine, Div. of Hematology and Oncology, Beth Israel Deaconess Medical Center, Boston, Massachusetts

MONKKONEN, MIA, Molecular Cancer Biology Program, University of Helsinki, Helsinki, Finland

MOORES, SHERI, Dept. of Oncology and Supportive Care, GlaxoSmithKline, Collegeville, Pennsylvania

MORFORD, LORRI, Dept. of Microbiology, Immunology and Molecular Genetics, University of Kentucky, Lexington

MORI, SEIICHI, Institute for Genome Sciences and Policy, Duke University, Durham, North Carolina

MORONI, MARIA CRISTINA, Dept. of Experimental Oncology, European Institute of Oncology, Milan, Italy

MORRISON, DEBRA, Dept. of Medicine, Mount Sinai School of Medicine, New York, New York

MORRISON, SEAN, Howard Hughes Medical Institute, University of Michigan, Ann Arbor

MROCZKOWSKI, BARBARA, Dept. of Structural Biology, Pfizer Global Research and Development, Pfizer, Inc., San Diego, California

MU, DAVID, Cold Spring Harbor Laboratory, Cold Spring Harbor, New York

MUJTABA, SYED, Dept. of Physiology and Biophysics, Mount Sinai School of Medicine, New York, New York

MURPHY, DANIEL, Cancer Research Institute, Comprehensive Cancer Center, University of California, San Francisco

MUTHUSWAMY, SENTHIL, Cold Spring Harbor Laboratory, Cold Spring Harbor, New York

MYSINGER, CYNTHIA, Cancer Research Institute, University of California, San Francisco

NAGAHARA, HIKARU, Sanno Hospital, International University of Health and Welfare, Tokyo, Japan

NAHLE, ZAHER, Dept. of Internal Medicine, Washington University, St. Louis, Missouri

NAKADA, DAISUKE, Div. of Biological Science, Nagoya University Graduate School of Science, Nagoya, Japan

NAKADE, KOJI, BioResource Center, RIKEN, Ibaraki, Japan

NAKAGAMA, HITOSHI, Div. of Biochemistry, National Cancer Center Research Institute, Tokyo, Japan

NARAMURA, MAYUMI, Dept. of Medicine, ENH Research Institute, Evanston, Illinois

NARITA, MASAKO, Cold Spring Harbor Laboratory, Cold Spring Harbor, New York

NARITA, MASASHI, Cold Spring Harbor Laboratory, Cold Spring Harbor, New York

NAVIN, NICHOLAS, Cold Spring Harbor Laboratory, Cold Spring Harbor, New York

NEILL, USHMA, *Journal of Clinical Investigation*, Columbia University, New York, New York

NICASSIO, FRANCESCO, FIRC Institute Molecular Oncology Foundation, European Institute of Oncology, Milan, Italy

NILSSON, JEANETTE, Dept. of Cell and Molecular Biology, Gothenburg University, Gothenburg, Sweden

NOLAN, DANIEL, Cold Spring Harbor Laboratory, Cold Spring Harbor, New York

NUNEZ, SABRINA, Cold Spring Harbor Laboratory, Cold Spring Harbor, New York

OH, HYUN JUNG, Dept. of Biological Sciences, Korea Advanced Institute of Science and Technology, Daejeon, South Korea

OH, SANG-PHIL, Dept. of Biological Sciences, Korea Advanced Institute of Science and Technology, Daejeon, South Korea

OHTA, NORIO, BioFrontier Laboratories, Kyowa Hakko Kogyo Co., Ltd., Tokyo, Japan

OLIVE, KENNETH, Abramson Family Cancer Research Institute, University of Pennsylvania, Philadelphia

OLOFSSON, BEATRIX, Dept. of Biochemistry, Drexel University College of Medicine, Philadelphia, Pennsylvania

ONEYAMA, CHITOSE, Lab. of Molecular Oncology, Osaka Bioscience Institute, Osaka, Japan

OPAVSKY, RENE, Dept. of Human Cancer Genetics, Ohio State University, Columbus, Ohio

O'SHEA, CLODAGH, Comprehensive Cancer Center, University of California, San Francisco

OZER, HARVEY, University Hospital Cancer Center, UMDNJ-New Jersey Medical School, Newark, New Jersey

PALAKURTHI, SANGEETHA, Dept. of Cancer Bioscience, AstraZeneca, Waltham, Massachusetts

PANDOLFI, PIER-PAOLO, Memorial Sloan-Kettering Cancer Center, New York, New York

PAPAGEORGIS, PANAGIOTIS, Dept. of Genetics and Genomics, Boston University School of Medicine, Boston, Massachusetts

PARADA, LUIS, Center for Developmental Biology, Southwestern Medical Center, University of Texas, Dallas

PARK, JAEHONG, Dept. of Biological Chemistry and Molecular Pharmacology, Institute of Proteomics, Harvard Medical School, Cambridge, Massachusetts

PAVLETICH, NIKOLA, Structural Biology Program, Memorial Sloan-Kettering Cancer Center, New York, New York

PENDE, MARIO, Necker Institute, INSERM, Paris, France

PERSSON, JENNY, Dept. of Laboratory Medicine, Div. of Pathology, Lund University, Malmö, Sweden

PERVIN, SHEHLA, Dept. of Obstetrics and Gynecology, University of California, Los Angeles

PETERS, GORDON, Dept. of Molecular Oncology, London Research Institute, London, United Kingdom

PETERSON, JANE, Div. of Extramural Research, National Human Genome Research Institute, National Institutes of Health, Bethesda, Maryland

PHAN, VERNON, Cancer Research Institute, Comprehensive Cancer Center, University of California, San Francisco

PHILBRICK, WILLIAM, Technical Advisory Committee, Yale University School of Medicine, New Haven, Connecticut

PICCINI, ANTONELLA, Cold Spring Harbor Laboratory, Cold Spring Harbor, New York

PICKERING, CURTIS, Dept. of Pathology, University of California, San Francisco

PIERCE, AISLING, Dept. of Molecular Biology, National Institute for Cellular Biotechnology, Dublin City University, Dublin, Ireland

PODSYPANINA, KATRINA, Dept. of Cell Biology, Memorial Sloan-Kettering Cancer Center, New York, New York

POLAKIEWICZ, ROBERTO, Dept. of Research, Cell Signaling Technology, Beverly, Massachusetts

POLITI, KATERINA, Dept. of Cancer Biology and Genetics, Memorial Sloan-Kettering Center, New York, New York

POLLOCK, MILA, Cold Spring Harbor Laboratory Library, Cold Spring Harbor, New York

PONDER, BRUCE, Dept. of Oncology, Hutchison/MRC Research Centre, Cambridge, United Kingdom

POORTINGA, GRETCHEN, Div. of Research, Peter MacCallum Cancer Centre, East Melbourne, Victoria, Australia

PORTER, JESS, School of Medicine, University of Pennsylvania, Philadelphia

POWERS, SCOTT, Cold Spring Harbor Laboratory, Cold Spring Harbor, New York

PRIVES, CAROL, Dept. of Biological Sciences, Columbia University, New York, New York

QIAN, YUEWEI, Lilly Research Laboratories, Eli Lilly and Company, Indianapolis, Indiana

QUON, KIM, Dept. of Biology, Amgen, Inc., South San Francisco, California

RABBITTS, PAMELA, Dept. of Medicine, Medical School, University College, London, United Kingdom

RABBITTS, TERENCE, Lab. of Molecular Biology, Medical Research Council, Cambridge, United Kingdom

RABINOVSKY, ROSALIA, Dept. of Medical Oncology, Dana-Farber Cancer Institute, Boston, Massachusetts

RAFFANIELLO, ROBERT, Dept. of Medical Laboratory Sciences, School of Health Professions, Hunter College, City University of New York, New York

RAMSEY, MATTHEW, Dept. of Genetics, University of North Carolina, Chapel Hill

RAUCH, JENS, Molecular Oncology Clinical Cooperation Group, Ludwig-Maximilians University of Munich, Munich, Germany

RAUHALA, HANNA, Institute of Medical Technology, University of Tampere, Tampere, Finland

RECHAVI, GIDEON, Dept. of Pediatric Hematology and Oncology, Chaim Sheba Medical Center, Tel-Hashomer, Israel

REPELLIN, CLAIRE, Dept. of Molecular Genetics, University of Glasgow, Glasgow, Scotland, United Kingdom

RICHARDSON, CELESTE, Dept. of Oncology, Novartis Institutes for BioMedical Research, Cambridge, Massachusetts

RICHMOND, JODI, Dept. of Pharmacogenomics, Pfizer, Inc., Groton, Connecticut

RIKOVA, KLARISA, Dept. of Research, Cell Signaling Technology, Beverly, Massachusetts

ROBERTS, CHARLES, Dept. of Pediatric Oncology, Dana-Farber Cancer Institute, Boston, Massachusetts

ROCHE, SERGE, Centre de Recherches de Biochimie Macromoléculaire, Centre National de la Recherche Scientifique, Montpellier, France

RODRIGUEZ, ELENA, Dept. of Molecular and Cell Biology, University of California, Berkeley

RODRIGUEZ, ROBERTO, Dept. of Vascular Biology, Children's Hospital, Boston, Massachusetts

ROOF, DAVID, Dept. of Molecular and Cell Biology, Cytokinetics, Inc., South San Francisco, California

ROTTMANN, SABINE, Dept. of Cell and Cancer Biology, Genomics Institute of the Novartis Research Foundation, San Diego, California

ROZENBLATT-ROSEN, ORIT, Dept. of Molecular Oncology, Dana-Farber Cancer Institute, Boston, Massachusetts

RUEFLI-BRASSE, ASTRID, Dept. of Biology, Amgen, Inc., South San Francisco, California

RUGGIERI, ROSAMARIA, Dept. of Oncology and Cell Biology, North Shore-Long Island Jewish Institute for Medical Research, Manhasset, New York

RUSSO, GIAN-LUIGI, Dept. of Biochemistry, Istituto Scienze dell'Alimentazione, Avellino, Italy

RYEOM, SANDRA, Dept. of Cell Biology, Harvard University School of Medicine, Boston, Massachusetts

SABAPATHY, KANAGA, Div. of Cellular and Molecular Research, National Cancer Centre, Singapore

SACCHI, NICOLETTA, Dept. of Cancer Genetics, Roswell Park Cancer Institute, Buffalo, New York

SAFRAN, MICHAL, Dept. of Adult Oncology, Dana-Farber Cancer Institute, Boston, Massachusetts

SAITO, TSUYOSHI, Dept. of Pathology, Memorial Sloan-Kettering Cancer Center, New York, New York

SANSAL, ISABELLE, Dept. of Medical Oncology, Dana-Farber Cancer Institute, Boston, Massachusetts

SANTARIUS, THOMAS, Cancer Genome Project, The Wellcome Trust Sanger Institute, Hinxton, Cambridge, United Kingdom

SAPLIS, RACHEL, Dept. of Genetics, Cellular Biology, and Development, Cancer Center, University of Minnesota, Minneapolis

SARAMAKI, OUTI, Dept. of Cancer Genetics, Institute of Medical Technology, University of Tampere, Tampere, Finland

SAUNDERS, DARREN, Cancer Research Program, Garvan Institute of Medical Research, Darlinghurst, Sydney, New South Wales, Australia

SAUNUS, JODI, School of Molecular and Microbial Sciences, University of Queensland, St. Lucia, Australia

SAWYERS, CHARLES, Dept. of Medicine, University of California, Los Angeles

SAYEED, SHEIKH, Dept. of Pharmacology and Therapeutics, Roswell Park Cancer Institute, Buffalo, New York

SCHAFFER, JAMES, Dept. of Healthcare Information Technology, Philips Research, Briarcliff Manor, New York

SCHLEGEL, ROBERT, Dept. of Oncology, Novartis Institutes for BioMedical Research, Cambridge, Massachusetts

SCHLIEKELMAN, MARK, Dept. of Genetics, University of North Carolina, Chapel Hill

SCHMITT, CLEMENS, Dept. of Hematology and Oncology, Max-Delbrück-Center for Molecular Medicine, Berlin, Germany

SCHNEIDER, GÜNTER, Dept. of Internal Medicine, Technical University of Munich, Munich, Germany

SCHUBERT, CHARLOTTE, *Nature Medicine*, Nature Publishing Group, New York, New York

SCHWEIZER, LIANG, Dept. of Oncology Drug Discovery, Bristol-Myers Squibb, Princeton, New Jersey

SCOTT, CLARE, Cold Spring Harbor Laboratory, Cold Spring Harbor, New York

SEBASTIAN, THOMAS, Lab. of Protein Dynamics and Signaling, National Cancer Institute, Frederick, Maryland

SELIVANOVA, GALINA, Microbiology and Tumor Biology Center, Karolinska Institute, Stockholm, Sweden

SELLERS, WILLIAM, Div. of Neoplastic Disease Mechanisms, Dana-Farber Cancer Institute, Harvard Medical School, Boston, Massachusetts

SERRANO, MANUEL, Centro Nacional de investigaciones Ontologica, Madrid, Spain

SHACHAF, CATHERINE, Dept. of Medical Oncology, Stanford University, Stanford, California

SHERR, CHARLES, Dept. of Tumor Cell Biology, Howard Hughes Medical Institute, St. Jude Children's Research Hospital, Memphis, Tennessee

SHI, HUA, Dept. of Molecular Biology and Genetics, Cornell University, Ithaca, New York

SHIEH, SHEAU-YANN, Institute of Biomedical Sciences, Academia Sinica, Taipei, Taiwan, Republic of China

SHIH, HSIU-MING, Institute of Biomedical Sciences, Academia Sinica, Taipei, Taiwan, Republic of China

SHIMIZU, TAKESHI, Dept. of Biochemistry and Molecular Biology, Pennsylvania State University, University Park, Pennsylvania

SHUKLA, NEERAV, Dept. of Pediatrics, Memorial Sloan-Kettering Cancer Center, New York, New York

SHUREIQI, IMAD, Dept. of Clinical Cancer Prevention, M.D. Anderson Cancer Center, University of Texas, Houston

SIBSON, DAVID, J.K. Douglas Laboratories, Clatterbridge Cancer Research Trust, Clatterbridge Hospital, Bebington, Wirral, United Kingdom

SIDENIUS, NICOLAI, Dept. of Transcriptional Mechanisms, FIRC Institute of Molecular Oncology Foundation, Milan, Italy

SILVA, RICARDO, Dept. of Hematology and Oncology, St. Jude Children's Research Hospital, Memphis, Tennessee

SILVESTRE, DAVID, Dept. of Biological Chemistry, CIQUIBIC, National University of Córdoba, Córdoba, Argentina

SIMIN, KARL, Dept. of Genetics, Lineberger Comprehensive Cancer Center, University of North Carolina, Chapel Hill

SLACK, FRANK, Dept. of Molecular, Cellular, and Developmental Biology, Yale University, New Haven, Connecticut

SLAMON, DENNIS, Dept. of Medicine, Hematology and Oncology, University of California, Los Angeles

SLATE, DORIS, Dept. of Scientific Licensing, Johnson and Johnson Pharmaceutical Research and Development, San Diego, California

SLIWKOWSKI, MARK, Dept. of Translational Oncology, Genentech, Inc., South San Francisco, California

SMALL, MICHAEL, Div. of Extramural Research, National Cancer Institute, National Institutes of Health, Bethesda, Maryland

SMIRNOV, DENIS, Dept. of Research and Development, Immunicon Corp., Huntingdon Valley, Pennsylvania

SOENGAS, MARIA, Dept. of Dermatology, University of Michigan, Ann Arbor

SONG, YURONG, Dept. of Genetics, Lineberger Comprehensive Cancer Center, University of North Carolina, Chapel Hill

SPARMANN, ANKE, Dept. of Molecular Genetics, The Netherlands Cancer Institute, Amsterdam, The Netherlands

SPECTOR, DAVID, Cold Spring Harbor Laboratory, Cold Spring Harbor, New York

SPECTOR, MONA, Cold Spring Harbor Laboratory, Cold Spring Harbor, New York

STEWART, DAVID, Meetings and Courses Programs, Cold Spring Harbor Laboratory, Cold Spring Harbor, New York

STILLMAN, BRUCE, President and CEO, Cold Spring Harbor Laboratory, Cold Spring Harbor, New York

SUH, KWANG, Lab. of Cellular Carcinogenesis and Tumor Promotion, National Cancer Institute, National Institutes of Health, Bethesda, Maryland

SUKEZANE, TAIKO, Lab. of Molecular Oncology, Osaka Bioscience Institute, Osaka, Japan

SWAIN, AMANDA, Sect. of Gene Function and Regulation, Institute of Cancer Research, London, United Kingdom

SYMONS, MARC, Dept. of Oncology and Cell Biology, North Shore-Long Island Jewish Institute for Medical Research, Manhasset, New York

SÜLTMANN, HOLGER, Dept. of Molecular Genome Analysis, German Cancer Research Center, Heidelberg, Germany

TANAKA, HISASHI, Div. of Basic Sciences, Fred Hutchinson Cancer Research Center, Seattle, Washington

TARABAN, VADIM, Tenovus Research Laboratory, University of Southampton, Southampton, United Kingdom

TELERMAN, ADAM, Dept. of Cancer Research, Molecular Engines Laboratories, Paris, France

TERAI, KENTA, Dept. of Tumor Virology, Research Institute for Microbial Diseases, Osaka University, Osaka, Japan

TERZIAN, TAMARA, Dept. of Molecular Genetics, Sect. of Cancer Genetics, M.D. Anderson Cancer Center, University of Texas, Houston

TESSIER-LAVIGNE, MARC, Dept. of Research, Genentech, Inc., South San Francisco, California

TEWS, BJOERN, Dept. of Molecular Genetics, German Cancer Research Center, Heidelberg, Germany

THEILLET, CHARLES, Genotypes et Phenotypes Tumoraux, INSERM, Montpellier, France

THIAGALINGAM, SAM, Dept. of Medicine and Genetics, Boston University School of Medicine, Boston, Massachusetts

THOMPSON, CRAIG, Abramson Family Cancer Research Institute, University of Pennsylvania, Philadelphia

THUERIGEN, DIRK, Div. of Molecular Genetics, German Cancer Research Center, Heidelberg, Germany

TLSTY, THEA, Dept. of Pathology, School of Medicine, University of California, San Francisco

TRABONI, CINZIA, Dept. of Biochemistry, Institute for Research in Molecular Biology, Pomezia, Italy

TREANOR, LOUISE, Dept. of Pathology, Unversity of Edinburgh, Edinburgh, Scotland, United Kingdom

TSAI, HSIN-YUE, Dept. of Biochemistry, Ohio State University, Columbus, Ohio

TSE, ARCHIE, Dept. of Medicine, Memorial Sloan-Kettering Cancer Cancer, New York, New York

TSUCHIHASHI, ZENTA, Dept. of Pharmacogenomics, Bristol-Myers Squibb, Princeton, New Jersey

TSUCHIYA, NAOTO, Dept. of Biochemistry, National Cancer Center Research Institute, Tokyo, Japan

TUVESON, DAVID, Dept. of Hematology and Oncology, Abramson Family Cancer Research Institute, University of Pennsylvania, Philadelphia

UREN, ANTHONY, Dept. of Molecular Genetics, The Netherlands Cancer Institute, Amsterdam, The Netherlands

UZIEL, TAMAR, Dept. of Tumor Cell Biology, St. Jude Children's Research Hospital, Memphis, Tennessee

VAFAI, SCOTT, Dept. of Cancer Biology, Dana-Farber Cancer Institute, Boston, Massachusetts

VAN DYCK, FREDERIK, Dept. of Human Genetics, Lab. for Molecular Oncology, University of Leuven, Leuven, Belgium

VAN DYKE, TERRY, Dept. of Biochemistry, University of North Carolina, Chapel Hill

VAN LOHUIZEN, MAARTEN, Dept. of Moleular Genetics, The Netherlands Cancer Institute, Amsterdam, The Netherlands

VARMUS, HAROLD, President and CEO, Memorial Sloan-Kettering Cancer Center, New York, New York

VENKATARAMAN, CHANDRASEKAR, Dept. of Cancer Research, Eli Lilly and Company, Indianapolis, Indiana

VIGNERON, ARNAUD, Cancer Center Paul Papin, INSERM, Angers, France

VILENCHIK, MARIA, Dept. of Oncology, Hoffmann-La Roche, Inc., Nutley, New Jersey

VILLANUEVA, JESSIE, Dept. of Pharmacology, University of Pennsylvania, Philadelphia

VINCENT, SYLVIE, Dept. of Molecular Technology, AVEO Pharmaceuticals, Cambridge, Massachusetts

VINSON, CHARLES, Lab. of Metabolism, National Institutes of Health, Bethesda, Maryland

VREDEVELD, LIESBETH, Dept. of Molecular Genetics, The Netherlands Cancer Institute, Amsterdam, The Netherlands

WALLACE, DOUGLAS, Center for Molecular and Mitochondrial Medicine and Genetics, University of California, Irvine

WANG, GREG, Biomedical Sciences Program, School of Medicine, University of California at San Diego, La Jolla

WANG, LIANG, Cold Spring Harbor Laboratory, Cold Spring Harbor, New York

WATNICK, RANDOLPH, Dept. of Surgery, Children's Hospital, Harvard Medical School, Boston, Massachusetts

WEI, GANG, Dept. of Tumorigenesis, Lankenau Institute for Medical Research, Wynnewood, Pennsylvania

WEINMANN, ROBERTO, Dept. of Oncology Drug Discovery, Bristol-Myers Squibb, Princeton, New Jersey

WEINREICH, MICHAEL, Van Andel Research Institute, Grand Rapids, Michigan

WEISSMAN, SHERMAN, Dept. of Genetics, Yale University School of Medicine, New Haven, Connecticut

WENDEL, HANS-GUIDO, Cold Spring Harbor Laboratory, Cold Spring Harbor, New York

WERB, ZENA, Dept. of Anatomy, University of California, San Francisco

WESTBROOK, TREY, Dept. of Genetics, Harvard University School of Medicine, Boston, Massachusetts

WILKINSON, JOHN, Unit for Laboratory Animal Medicine, University of Michigan, Ann Arbor

WINTER, CHRISTOPHER, Dept. of Target Support and Validation, Merck Research Laboratories, Boston, Massachusetts

WITTE, OWEN, Howard Hughes Medical Institute, Institute for Stem Cell Biology and Medicine, University of California, Los Angeles

WONG, SUNNY, Dept. of Biology, Massachusetts Institute of Technology, Cambridge, Massachusetts

WORKMAN, PAUL, Dept. of Cancer Therapeutics, Institute of Cancer Research, Sutton, Surrey, United Kingdom

XIA, MINGXUAN, Dept. of Biomedical Genetics, University of Rochester Medical Center, Rochester, New York

XIONG, YUE, Dept. of Biochemistry and Biophysics, University of North Carolina, Chapel Hill

XU, JUN, Dept. of Oncology Research, Wyeth, Pearl River, New York

XU, LEI, Center for Cancer Research, Massachusetts Institute of Technology, Cambridge, Massachusetts

XU, QING, Dept. of Medical Oncology, Dana-Farber Cancer Institute, Boston, Massachusetts

XU, RUI-MING, Cold Spring Harbor Laboratory, Cold Spring Harbor, New York

XU, XINGZHI, Dept. of Biology, Beckman Research Institute, City of Hope Medical Center, Duarte, California

YAMACI, REZAN, Dept. of Molecular Biology and Genetics, Bogazici University, Istanbul, Turkey

YAMADA, N. ALICE, Dept. of Biosciences, Lawrence Livermore National Laboratory, Livermore, California

YAMASAKI, LILI, Dept. of Biological Sciences, Columbia University, New York, New York

YANCOPOULOS, GEORGE, Regeneron Pharmaceuticals, Inc., Tarrytown, New York

YANG, QUAN, Dept. of Therapeutics, IBEX Pharmaceuticals, Inc., Montréal, Québec, Canada

YARDEN, RONIT, Dept. of Surgical Oncology, Chaim Sheba Medical Center, Tel-Hashomer, Israel

YIM, SUN HEE, Lab. of Metabolism, National Cancer Institute, National Institutes of Health, Bethesda, Maryland

YOON, SUNG OK, Dept. of Cellular Immunology, Ochsner Clinic Foundation, Jefferson, Louisiana

ZENDER, LARS, Cold Spring Harbor Laboratory, Cold Spring Harbor, New York

ZHANG, HONGBING, Dept. of Hematology, Brigham and Women's Hospital, Harvard Medical School, Boston, Massachusetts

ZHANG, QIAN, Dept. of Genetics, Biochemistry, and Biophysics, Lineberger Comprehensive Cancer Center, University of North Carolina, Chapel Hill

ZHANG, XIAOSHAN, Dept. of Molecular Genetics, M.D. Anderson Cancer Center, University of Texas, Houston

ZHANG, YANPING, Dept. of Radiation Oncology, University of North Carolina, Chapel Hill

ZHOU, ZONGXIANG, Dept. of Biomedical Sciences, Cornell University, Ithaca, New York

VAN DER MEIJDEN, CAROLINE, Cold Spring Harbor Laboratory, Cold Spring Harbor, New York

VAN DE WETERING, CHRISTOPHER, Dept. of Pathology, University of Iowa Hospitals and Clinics, Iowa City

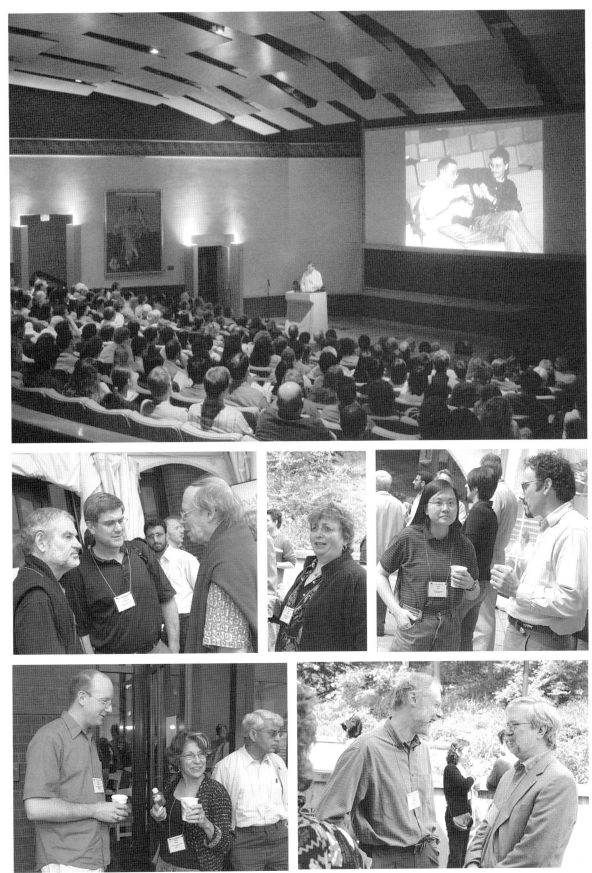

First row: Craig Thompson delivering eulogy for Stanley Korsmeyer (on screen, S. Korsmeyer [*l*] and M. Hengartner [*r*])
Second row: R. Eisenman, C. Thompson, and J. Adams; Z. Werb; J. Kan, G. Borzillo
Third row: P. Kenny, M. Bissell, M. Godbole; J. Inglis, J. Allison

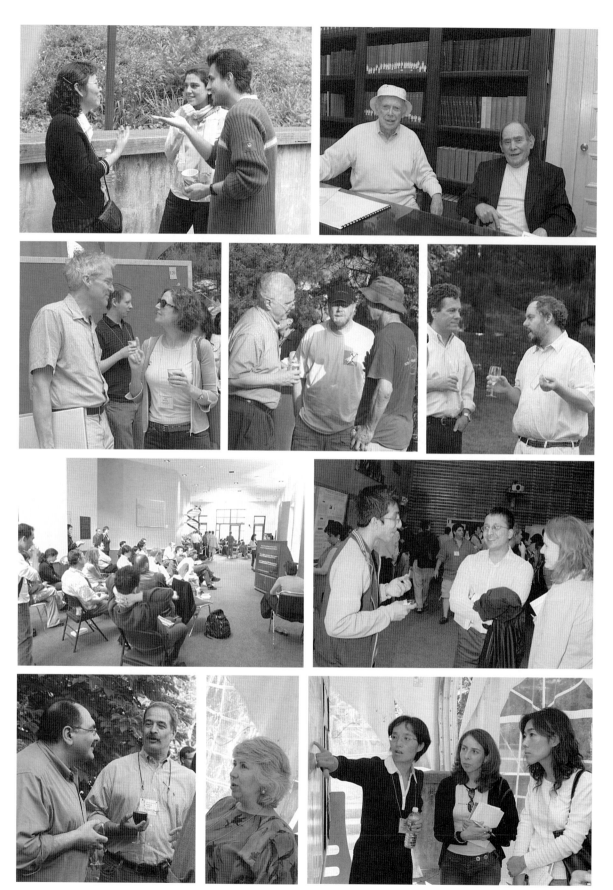

First row: L. Schweizer, R. Scotillo, M. Jechlinger; J.D. Watson, S. Brenner
Second row: R. Bernards, T. de Lange; B. Alberts, E. Harlow, H. Varmus; S. Lowe, S. Elledge
Third row: Watching Symposium in Grace lobby; G. Gupta, P. Gupta, R. Saplis
Fourth row: G. Enikolopov, R. Attar; T. Tlsty; Y. Song, S.O. Yoon, J. Villanueva

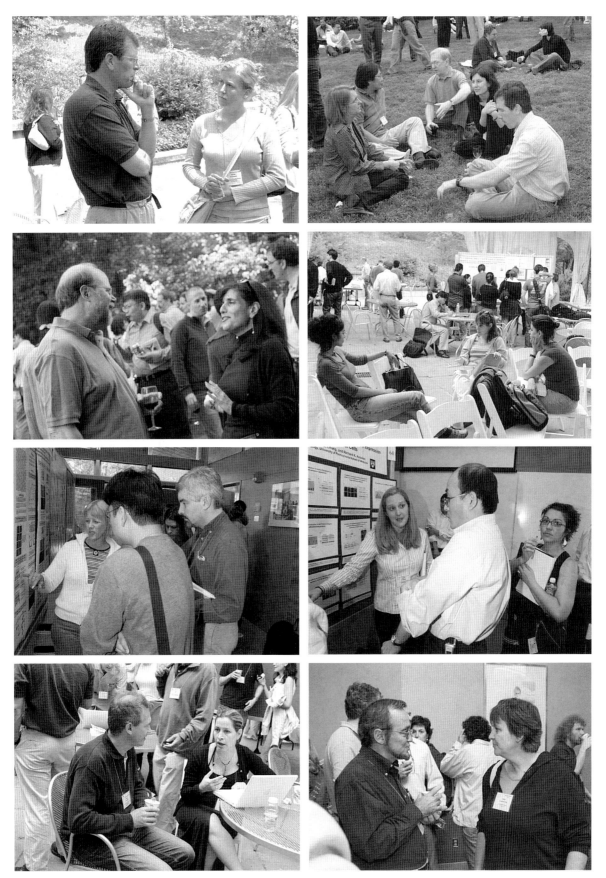

First row: B. Luscher, S. Rottmann; C. Schubert, K. Quon, G. Peters, C. Martins, M. Fero
Second row: E. Harlow, D. Esposito; Under the tent
Third row: C. Miranti, S. Wong, E. Medico; A. Fournier, H.-G. Kang, I. Sansal
Fourth row: P. Coopman, R. Yarden; M. Barbacid, S. Courtneidge

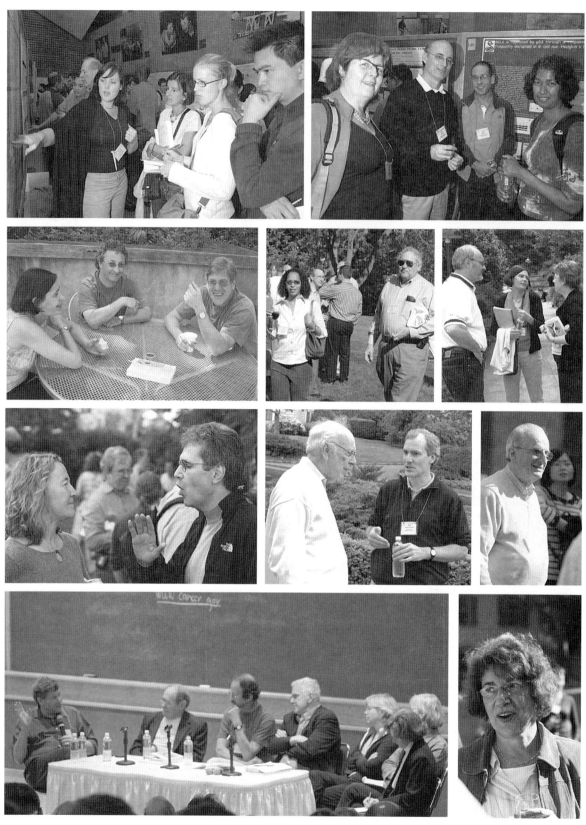

First row: G. MacDonald, S. Benvenuti, J. Saunus, K. Chan; C. Shachaf, O. Margalit, G. Rechavi, N. Amariglio
Second row: J. Lees, G. Evan, C. Sherr; J. Bargonetti, H. Ozer; M. Kastan, J. Lees, T. Van Dyke
Third row: C. Greider, R. DePinho; J.D. Watson, M. Tessier-Lavigne; J. Folkman
Fourth row: Cancer Genome Project Discussion Panel (*l–r*) E. Lander, S. Brenner, H. Varmus, B. Alberts, J. Brugge, J. Peterson, A. Barker; C. Prives

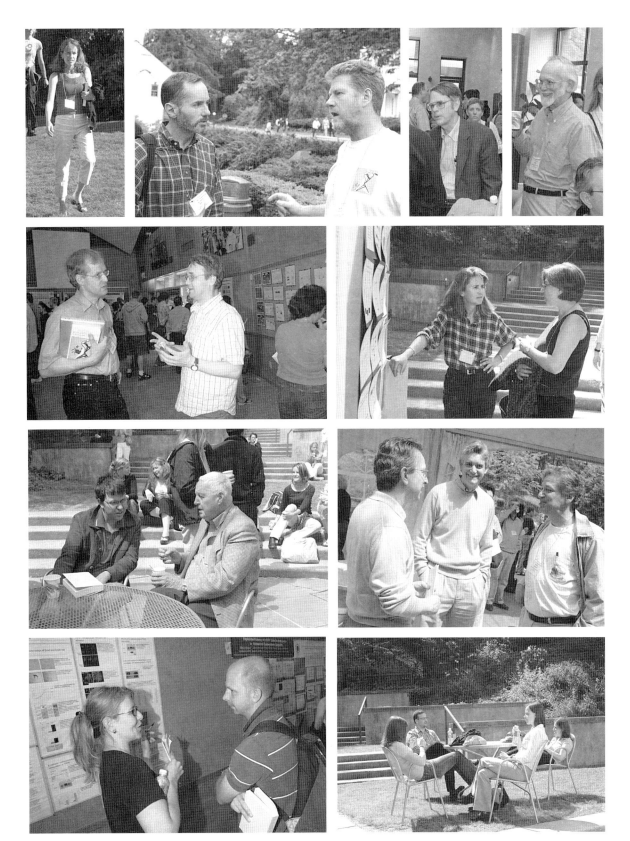

First row: L. Attardi; K. Hillan, D. Stewart, sporting the Symposium T-shirt; D. Wallace; M. Bishop
Second row: M. Eilers, M. Van Lohuizen; A. Gradi, N. Sacchi
Third row: H.-G. Wendell, B. Clarkson; J. Massagué, B. Stillman, R. Benezra
Fourth row: C. Andl, D. Thuerigen; M. Hickey, K. Olive, K. Covello, M. Gruber

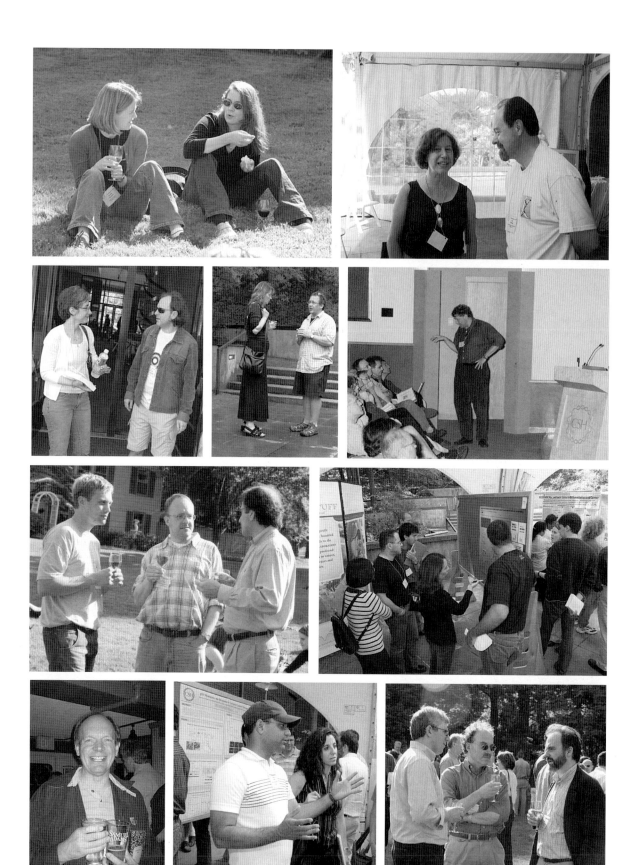

First row: H. Rauhala, O. Saramaki; N. Sacchi, L. Parada
Second row: A. Ballesteros, A. Ashworth; B. Marte, G. Hannon; E. Lander
Third row: B. Tews, M. Hahn, D. Spector; Posters under the tent
Fourth row: D. Lane; R. Kalluri; M. Meyerson, D. Haber, M. Ladanyi

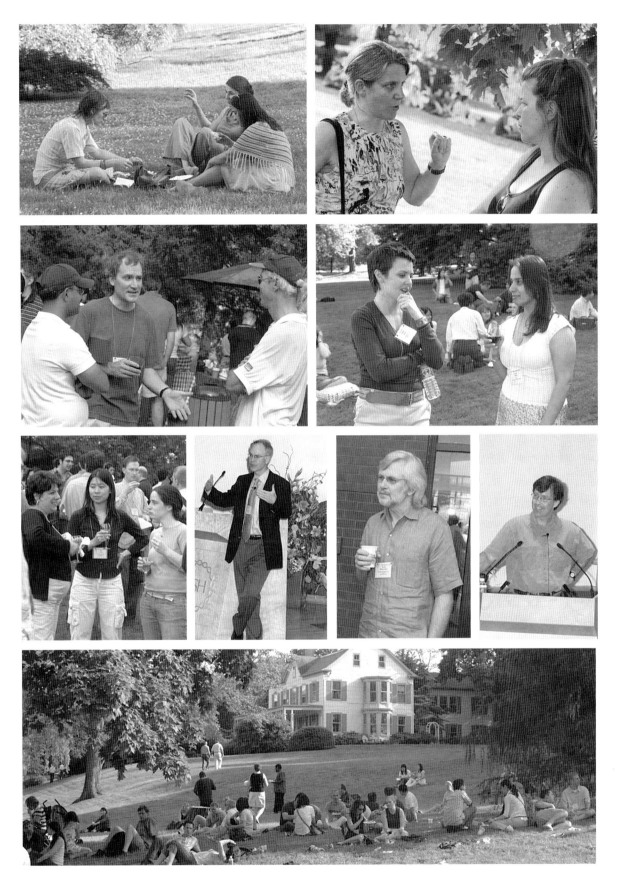

First row: G. Poortinga, C. Billottet, A. Majid; C. Scott, S. Smith
Second row: R. Kalluri, M. Tessier-Lavigne, D. Hanahan; A. Majid, M. Junttila
Third row: C. Abate-Shen, A. Cheung, K. Lane; C. Sawyers, Dorcas Cummings Lecture; F. McCormick; T. Jacks giving Summary
Fourth row: Symposium picnic

Dedication

Stan Korsmeyer passed away on March 31, 2005, at the age of 54. Ironically, he died of lung cancer. He had been looking forward to attending this meeting focused on molecular approaches to controlling cancer, a subject he dedicated his life to. Despite being gravely ill, he registered for the meeting. In the meeting book, he is listed as one of the participants and, in spirit, he was.

Stan grew up on a hog farm in southern Illinois. He did not start out to be a research scientist. In college, he became interested in science and decided to go to medical school. He went through internship and residency at the University of California, San Francisco, followed by a fellowship at the NIH. He arrived in Bethesda at the time when physicians were first learning molecular biology and applying it to cancer research. In those days, the cancer research meeting was the Cold Spring Harbor Symposium on Viral Oncogenes. It was through the scientific exchange at that meeting that Stan and others in the community came to re-

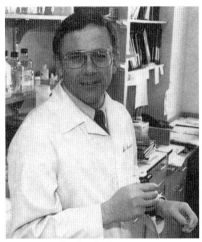

Stanley J. Korsmeyer
1950–2005

alize that chromosomal translocations might represent oncogenic events that could be molecularly characterized. Stan started working on this problem as a postdoctoral fellow in the laboratories of Phil Leder and Tom Waldman. Armed with that training, he joined the faculty at Washington University in St. Louis as an assistant professor. Stan did not start out as a central figure in the outstanding hematology and oncology faculty assembled there by Stuart Kornfield. Stan stood at the edge of that group, bridging it to molecular biology. However, even then, Stan was quickly moving to the center of our community. By characterizing chromosomal translocations, Stan's laboratory was one of the groups that cloned the oncogenes Bcl-2 and MLL. By the time of the 1994 CSHL Symposium on Cancer, Stan's work led many of us to consider the role of apoptosis in cancer. That was the first meeting where we started to discuss whether the regulation of programmed cell death played a critical role in the pathogenesis of cancer. Stan believed understanding apoptosis might contribute to new therapies for cancer.

Stan's work over the next few years brought him to the leading edge of biology. His groundbreaking work defining the Bcl-2 family members as interactive partners controlling the rheostat of apoptosis moved him to center stage. In 1998, Stan was recruited to Harvard University to nucleate a research program in apoptosis. With his positive and interactive personality, he quickly became a leader at the Dana-Farber Cancer Center.

At every scientific meeting, Stan was the one asking the probing questions and suggesting collaborations that would lead to the answers to those questions. Stan had that unique capability of organizing people, focusing them on the activity at hand, and, even though they'd never done it before, giving them the skills to go out and do research on the murky waters of cancer biology.

In closing, we remember him as a friend, colleague, and a real leader in this community, and for the positive interactions that he spurred within the cancer biology community. It is in that spirit that CSHL dedicates this volume to his memory.

Craig B. Thompson

Foreword

During the past quarter century or so, much effort has been devoted toward the understanding of the molecular basis of cancer. We now understand that cancer is primarily a genetic disease of mutations in the tumor genome acquired over a lifetime. The products of oncogenes and tumor suppressor genes have been placed into pathways of gene networks that are altered in tumor cells compared to normal cells in tissue. Furthermore, we also understand that tumors function as abnormal organs, forming an architecture of a number of different cell types and recruiting a blood supply, albeit an irregular one. There have been many Symposia in this series that dealt with cancer directly, and even more that focused on basic biology that contributed greatly to understanding cancer.

As a result of some interesting developments in cancer diagnosis and therapy over the past five years, it was appropriate that a Symposium be devoted for the first time to molecular approaches to cancer therapy. Several examples now exist of targeted therapy that works in patients that have been profiled based on genetic diagnosis of the patient's tumor. Additionally, therapies targeting the tumor as an organ, such as anti-angiogenic therapy, are now used in the clinic with modest success. The hope is that this type of molecular approach to cancer therapy will accelerate and become more effective in the future.

In organizing this Symposium with help from Terri Grodzicker, we relied on the assistance of a number of colleagues for suggestions for speakers. They included David Livingston, Craig Thompson, and Scott Lowe, and we thank them for their valuable advice. We also thank the first evening speakers, Dennis Slamon, Harold Varmus, Mina Bissell, and Jim Allison, for providing an overview of the areas to be covered. This year's Reginald Harris Lecture was delivered by Titia de Lange on telomere biology and genomic stability. We particularly thank Tyler Jacks for delivering a thoughtful and realistic summary of where we are in relation to our goal. Charles Sawyers, who conveyed the excitement which many of us feel knowing that some inroads into treating cancer will be made by targeted therapies, presented the Dorcas Cummings Lecture to the local community and the attending scientists. The effort put into the Dorcas Cummings Lecture by Charles and the summary by Tyler resulted in highlights of the meeting.

This Symposium was attended by 515 scientists and clinicians, and the program included 71 oral presentations and 241 poster presentations. Bruce Alberts chaired a discussion of the proposal to analyze the genomes of all major human cancers to advance cancer diagnosis and therapy approaches.

Essential funds to run this meeting were obtained from the National Cancer Institute, a branch of the National Institutes of Health. In addition, financial help from the corporate benefactors, sponsors, affiliates, and contributors of our meetings program is essential for these Symposia to remain a success, and we are most grateful for their continued support.

We thank Val Pakaluk and Mary Smith in the Meetings and Courses office for their efficient help in organizing the Symposium. Joan Ebert, Patricia Barker, and Susan Schaefer in the Cold Spring Harbor Laboratory Press, headed by John Inglis, ensured that this volume would be produced. We thank them for their dedication to producing high-quality publications.

Bruce Stillman
David Stewart
April 2006

Sponsors

This meeting was funded in part by the **National Cancer Institute,** a branch of the **National Institutes of Health.**

Contributions from the following companies provide core support for the Cold Spring Harbor meetings program.

Corporate Benefactors

Amgen, Inc.
Bristol-Myers Squibb Company

GlaxoSmithKline
Novartis Institutes for BioMedical Research

Corporate Sponsors

Applied Biosystems
AstraZeneca
BioVentures, Inc.
Diagnostic Products Corporation
Forest Laboratories, Inc.
Genentech, Inc.
Hoffmann-La Roche, Inc.
Johnson & Johnson Pharmaceutical
   Research & Development, L.L.C.

Kyowa Hakko Kogyo Co., Ltd.
Lexicon Genetics, Inc.
Merck Research Laboratories
New England BioLabs, Inc.
OSI Pharmaceuticals, Inc.
Pall Corporation
Schering-Plough Research Institute
Wyeth Genetics Institute

Plant Corporate Associates

ArborGen
Monsanto Company

Corporate Affiliates

Affymetrix, Inc.
Agencourt Biosciences

Corporate Contributors

Aviva Systems Biology
Biogen, Inc.
EMD Bioscience

Illumina
IRx Therapeutics, Inc.
Qiagen

Foundations

Albert B. Sabin Vaccine Institute, Inc.
Hudson Alpha Institute for Biotechnology

Contents

Symposium Participants   v
Dedication   xxiii
Foreword   xxv

Cancer Genetics and Genomes

Oncogenes Come of Age *H. Varmus, W. Pao, K. Politi, K. Podsypanina, and Y.-C.N. Du*   1
Common and Contrasting Genomic Profiles among the Major Human Lung Cancer Subtypes
    G. Tonon, C. Brennan, A. Protopopov, G. Maulik, B. Feng, Y. Zhang, D.B. Khatry, M.J. You,
    A.J. Aguirre, E.S. Martin, Z. Yang, H. Ji, L. Chin, K.-K. Wong, and R.A. DePinho   11
"Lineage Addiction" in Human Cancer: Lessons from Integrated Genomics *L.A. Garraway,*
    B.A. Weir, X. Zhao, H. Widlund, R. Beroukhim, A. Berger, D. Rimm, M.A. Rubin, D.E. Fisher,
    M.L. Meyerson, and W.R. Sellers   25
Polygenic Inherited Predisposition to Breast Cancer *B.A.J. Ponder, A. Antoniou, A. Dunning,*
    D.F. Easton, and P.D.P. Pharoah   35
Somatic Mutations in Human Cancer: Insights from Resequencing the Protein Kinase Gene Family
    P.A. Futreal, R. Wooster, and M.R. Stratton   43
High-Resolution ROMA CGH and FISH Analysis of Aneuploid and Diploid Breast Tumors
    J. Hicks, L. Muthuswamy, A. Krasnitz, N. Navin, M. Riggs, V. Grubor, D. Esposito,
    J. Alexander, J. Troge, M. Wigler, S. Maner, P. Lundin, and A. Zetterberg   51
Ductal Pancreatic Cancer in Humans and Mice *D.A. Tuveson and S.R. Hingorani*   65
Detection of Oncogenic Mutations in the EGFR Gene in Lung Adenocarcinoma with Differential
    Sensitivity to EGFR Tyrosine Kinase Inhibitors *R.K. Thomas, H. Greulich, Y. Yuza, J.C. Lee,*
    T. Tengs, W. Feng, T.-H. Chen, E. Nickerson, J. Simons, M. Egholm, J.M. Rothberg,
    W.R. Sellers, and M.L. Meyerson   73
Two Decades of Cancer Genetics: From Specificity to Pleiotropic Networks *S. Grisendi*
    and P.P. Pandolfi   83

DNA Damage Response

Abnormalities of the Inactive X Chromosome Are a Common Feature of BRCA1 Mutant and
    Sporadic Basal-like Breast Cancer *S. Ganesan, A.L. Richardson, Z.C. Wang, J.D. Iglehart,*
    A. Miron, J. Feunteun, D. Silver, and D.M. Livingston   93
The ATM-dependent DNA Damage Signaling Pathway *R. Kitagawa and M.B. Kastan*   99
Single-Nucleotide Polymorphisms in the p53 Pathway *S.L. Harris, G. Gil, W. Hu, H. Robins,*
    E. Bond, K. Hirshfield, Z. Feng, X. Yu, A.K. Teresky, G. Bond, and A.J. Levine   111
Transcriptional Regulation by p53 and p73 *M. Lokshin, T. Tanaka, and C. Prives*   121
p53-Dependent and -Independent Functions of the Arf Tumor Suppressor *C.J. Sherr, D. Bertwistle,*
    W. den Besten, M.-L. Kuo, M. Sugimoto, K. Tago, R.T. Williams, F. Zindy, and M.F. Roussel   129
Exploiting the DNA Repair Defect in BRCA Mutant Cells in the Design of New Therapeutic
    Strategies for Cancer *A.N.J. Tutt, C.J. Lord, N. McCabe, H. Farmer, N. Turner, N.M. Martin,*
    S.P. Jackson, G.C.M. Smith, and A. Ashworth   139

Cancer Biology and Stem Cells

Identifying Site-specific Metastasis Genes and Functions *G.P. Gupta, A.J. Minn, Y. Kang,*
    P.M. Siegel, I. Serganova, C. Cordón-Cardo, A.B. Olshen, W.L. Gerald, and J. Massagué   149
The von Hippel-Lindau Tumor Suppressor Protein: Roles in Cancer and Oxygen Sensing
    W.G. Kaelin, Jr.   159
The Src Substrate Tks5, Podosomes (Invadopodia), and Cancer Cell Invasion *S.A. Courtneidge,*
    E.F. Azucena, Jr., I. Pass, D.F. Seals, and L. Tesfay   167

CONTENTS

Modeling Neurofibromatosis Type 1 Tumors in the Mouse for Therapeutic Intervention
L.F. Parada, C.-H. Kwon, and Y. Zhu   173

Stem Cell Self-Renewal and Cancer Cell Proliferation Are Regulated by Common Networks
That Balance the Activation of Proto-oncogenes and Tumor Suppressors *R. Pardal,
A.V. Molofsky, S. He, and S.J. Morrison*   177

Prostate Stem Cells and Prostate Cancer *D.A. Lawson, L. Xin, R. Lukacs, Q. Xu, D. Cheng, and
O.N. Witte*   187

Telomeres, Senescence, and Aging

Telomere-related Genome Instability in Cancer *T. de Lange*   197

Telomerase and Cancer Stem Cells *M. Armanios and C.W. Greider*   205

Regulation of Telomerase by Human Papillomaviruses *D.A. Galloway, L.C. Gewin, H. Myers,
W. Luo, C. Grandori, R.A. Katzenellenbogen, and J.K. McDougall*   209

Animal Models for Cancer

Genomic Progression in Mouse Models for Liver Tumors *A.D. Tward, K.D. Jones, S. Yant,
M.A. Kay, R. Wang, and J.M. Bishop*   217

Genotype–Phenotype Relationships in a Mouse Model for Human Small-Cell Lung Cancer *J. Calbó,
R. Meuwissen, E. van Montfort, O. van Tellingen, and A. Berns*   225

Cell Cycle and Cancer: Genetic Analysis of the Role of Cyclin-dependent Kinases *M. Barbacid,
S. Ortega, R. Sotillo, J. Odajima, A. Martín, D. Santamaría, P. Dubus, and M. Malumbres*   233

Mouse Models of Human Non-Small-Cell Lung Cancer: Raising the Bar *C.F.B. Kim, E.L. Jackson,
D.G. Kirsch, J. Grimm, A.T. Shaw, K. Lane, J. Kissil, K.P. Olive, A. Sweet-Cordero,
R. Weissleder, and T. Jacks*   241

Generation and Analysis of Genetically Defined Liver Carcinomas Derived from Bipotential
Liver Progenitors *L. Zender, W. Xue, C. Cordón-Cardo, G.J. Hannon, R. Lucito, S. Powers,
P. Flemming, M.S. Spector, and S.W. Lowe*   251

Oncogene-dependent Tumor Suppression: Using the Dark Side of the Force for Cancer Therapy
*G.I. Evan, M. Christophorou, E.A. Lawlor, I. Ringshausen, J. Prescott, T. Dansen, A. Finch,
C. Martins, and D. Murphy*   263

Chromosomal Translocation Engineering to Recapitulate Primary Events of Human Cancer
*A. Forster, R. Pannell, L. Drynan, F. Cano, N. Chan, R. Codrington, A. Daser, N. Lobato,
M. Metzler, C.-H. Nam, S. Rodriguez, T. Tanaka, and T. Rabbitts*   275

Deciphering Cancer Complexities in Genetically Engineered Mice *K. Simin, R. Hill, Y. Song,
Q. Zhang, R. Bash, R.D. Cardiff, C. Yin, A. Xiao, K. McCarthy, and T. Van Dyke*   283

Gene Expression and Cancer

The Evolving Portrait of Cancer Metastasis *P.B. Gupta, S. Mani, J. Yang, K. Hartwell, and
R.A. Weinberg*   291

Genomic Binding and Transcriptional Regulation by the *Drosophila* Myc and Mnt Transcription
Factors *A. Orian, S.S. Grewal, P.S. Knoepfler, B.A. Edgar, S.M. Parkhurst, and R.N. Eisenman*   299

Regulation of the *Arf/p53* Tumor Surveillance Network by E2F *P.J. Iaquinta, A. Aslanian, and
J.A. Lees*   309

Genetic and Epigenetic Changes in Mammary Epithelial Cells Identify a Subpopulation of Cells
Involved in Early Carcinogenesis *H. Berman, J. Zhang, Y.G. Crawford, M.L. Gauthier,
C.A. Fordyce, K. McDermott, M. Sigaroudinia, K. Kozakiewicz, and T.D. Tlsty*   317

Epigenetic Changes in Cancer and Preneoplasia *J.G. Herman*   329

A Genetic Approach to Cancer Epigenetics *A.P. Feinberg*   335

Tumor Responses to Microenvironment

Microenvironmental Regulators of Tissue Structure and Function Also Regulate Tumor Induction
and Progression: The Role of Extracellular Matrix and Its Degrading Enzymes *M.J. Bissell,
P.A. Kenny, and D.C. Radisky*   343

How Do Cancer Cells Acquire the Fuel Needed to Support Cell Growth? *C.B. Thompson,*
  D.E. Bauer, J.J. Lum, G. Hatzivassiliou, W.-X. Zong, D. Ditsworth, F. Zhao, M. Buzzai, and
  T. Lindsten   357
Mitochondria and Cancer: Warburg Addressed *D.C. Wallace*   363
Inductions of Complete Regressions of Oncogene-induced Breast Tumors in Mice *R. Benezra,*
  E. Henke, A. Ciarrocchi, M. Ruzinova, D. Solit, N. Rosen, D. Nolan, V. Mittal, and
  P. de Candia   375
The Fibroblastic Coconspirator in Cancer Progression *M. Egeblad, L.E. Littlepage, and Z. Werb* 383

Angiogenesis

Is Oncogene Addiction Angiogenesis-dependent? *J. Folkman and S. Ryeom*   389
Structural Basis for the Functions of Endogenous Angiogenesis Inhibitors *M.A. Grant and*
  R. Kalluri   399
VEGF Trap as a Novel Antiangiogenic Treatment Currently in Clinical Trials for Cancer and
  Eye Diseases, and VelociGene-based Discovery of the Next Generation of Angiogenesis
  Targets *J.S. Rudge, G. Thurston, S. Davis, N. Papadopoulos, N. Gale, S.J. Wiegand, and*
  G.D. Yancopoulos   411

Discovering Cancer Targets

Molecular Targeted Therapy of Lung Cancer: EGFR Mutations and Response to EGFR Inhibitors
  D.A. Haber, D.W. Bell, R. Sordella, E.L. Kwak, N. Godin-Heymann, S.V. Sharma, T.J. Lynch,
  and J. Settleman   419
Aberrant Gene Silencing in Tumor Progression: Implications for Control of Cancer *S.B. Baylin*
  and W.Y. Chen   427
Dissecting Cancer Pathways and Vulnerabilities with RNAi *T.F. Westbrook, F. Stegmeier, and*
  S.J. Elledge   435
Emerging Approaches in Molecular Profiling Affecting Oncology Drug Discovery *S.H. Friend* 445
Screens Using RNAi and cDNA Expression as Surrogates for Genetics in Mammalian Tissue
  Culture Cells *J. Pearlberg, S. Degot, W. Endege, J. Park, J. Davies, E. Gelfand, J. Sawyer,*
  A. Conery, J. Doench, W. Li, L. Gonzalez, F.M. Boyce, L. Brizuela, J. LaBaer, D. Grueneberg,
  and E. Harlow   449
Cancer Targets in the Ras Pathway *P. Rodriguez-Viciana, O. Tetsu, K. Oda, J. Okada, K. Rauen,*
  and F. McCormick   461

Therapeutic Approaches

Subversion of the Bcl-2 Life/Death Switch in Cancer Development and Therapy *J.M. Adams,*
  D.C.S. Huang, A. Strasser, S. Willis, L. Chen, A. Wei, M. Van Delft, J.I. Fletcher,
  H. Puthalakath, J. Kuroda, E.M. Michalak, P.N. Kelly, P. Bouillet, A. Villunger, L. O'Reilly,
  M.L. Bath, D.P. Smith, A. Egle, A.W. Harris, M. Hinds, P. Colman, and S. Cory 469
Making Progress through Molecular Attacks on Cancer *C.L. Sawyers*   479
Predicting Clinical Benefit in Non-Small-Cell Lung Cancer Patients Treated with Epidermal
  Growth Factor Tyrosine Kinase Inhibitors *L.C. Amler, A.D. Goddard, and K.J. Hillan* 483
Exploiting the p53 Pathway for the Diagnosis and Therapy of Human Cancer *D.P. Lane* 489
Drugging the Cancer Kinome: Progress and Challenges in Developing Personalized Molecular
  Cancer Therapeutics *P. Workman*   499
Modeling of Protein Signaling Networks in Clinical Proteomics *D.H. Geho, E.F. Petricoin,*
  L.A. Liotta, and R.P. Araujo   517
Summary: The Beginning of the End of Frustration *T. Jacks*   525

Author Index   529

Subject Index   531

Oncogenes Come of Age

H. VARMUS, W. PAO,* K. POLITI, K. PODSYPANINA, AND Y.-C.N. DU

Program in Cancer Biology and Genetics, Sloan-Kettering Institute,
Memorial Sloan-Kettering Cancer Center, New York, New York 10021

Mutations of proto-oncogenes are common events in the pathogenesis of cancers, as shown in a wide range of studies during the 30 years since the discovery of these genes. The benefits of novel therapies that target the products of mutant alleles in human cancers, and the demonstrated dependence of cancers in mouse models on continued expression of initiating oncogenes, are especially promising signs that revolutionary improvements in cancer care are possible. Full realization of the promise of targeted therapies, however, will require better definitions of the genotypes of human cancers, new approaches to interrupt the biochemical consequences of oncogenic mutations, and a greater understanding of drug resistance and tumor progression. In this paper, we summarize recent efforts toward these goals in our laboratory and others.

It is now about 30 years since the cellular progenitors of retroviral oncogenes, the first proto-oncogenes, were identified in vertebrate genomes (Stehelin et al. 1976; Rosenberg and Jolicoeur 1997), and over 20 years since mutant versions of such genes were first discovered in human cancers. In the past two decades, the list of mutant proto-oncogenes in human tumors has grown dramatically; many genes belonging to at least two other categories—tumor suppressors and governors of genomic integrity—have been implicated in carcinogenesis, and the proteins encoded by such genes have been extensively characterized. These developments have set the stage for more rational approaches to the detection, diagnosis, classification, treatment, and prevention of human cancers. Yet the most common and most lethal of these diseases are still inadequately controlled with traditional methods (chemotherapy and radiation), which do not take advantage of our new understanding of cancer at the molecular level.

In this survey of recent work from our laboratory and many others, we emphasize evidence that encourages the belief that therapies targeted against the specific genetic damage present in each cancer, especially therapies affecting proteins encoded by mutant proto-oncogenes, are likely to have increasingly prominent roles in future efforts to control cancer. Reaching this objective will require a fuller description of cancer genotypes through a nationally coordinated effort; a better understanding of signaling pathways altered by oncogenic mutations; a deeper picture of interactions among the multiple cancer genes in a single tumor; more drugs and antibodies that counter the effects of such mutations, in part to prevent the emergence of drug resistance; and a more refined description of how tumors progress as a consequence of changes within cancer cells and the microenvironment.

We address these issues by considering mutant proto-oncogenes in several mouse models of human cancers

and, in at least one case, a human disease, adenocarcinoma of the lung. One overriding notion that we stress is the idea that oncogenes are not required simply to initiate and maintain tumor growth; in several contexts, continued expression of mutant oncogenes is required to maintain the viability of the cancer cell. Such "oncogene dependence" provides an important vulnerability that some drugs already in clinical use—most obviously imatinib (Gleevec) and other inhibitors of protein-tyrosine kinases—effectively exploit. Since different types of tumors can be dependent on the same or similar oncogenes, and, conversely, histologically indistinguishable tumors from the same organ often depend on different oncogenes, it is essential that tumor genotypes be precisely and fully determined. We contend that much of contemporary cancer research should now be directed toward defining the molecular targets and therapeutic agents that show promise of producing "imatinib equivalents" for all forms of human cancer.

ONCOGENE DEPENDENCE IN CANCER

Viral Mutants

The idea that cancers are dependent on continued production of an oncogenic protein has its most explicit origin in classic studies of a temperature-sensitive mutant of the *src* gene of Rous sarcoma virus (RSV) (Martin 1970). These experiments not only clearly separated the oncogenic from the replicative functions (genes) of RSV; they also showed that the viral oncogene (v-*src*) was required to maintain as well as to initiate the transformed state.

Transgenic Mice with Inducible Oncogenes

More recent studies with transgenic mice that express oncogenes under the control of regulated promoters have made a dramatic point: After the oncogenes are turned on and tumors emerge, extinction of expression often leads to rapid disappearance of the tumor, as a result of apopto-

---

*Present address: Human Oncology and Pathogenesis Program, Memorial Sloan-Kettering Cancer Center, New York, New York 10021.

Table 1. Examples of Tumor Maintenance in Mouse Models

Tumor type	Oncogene	Mechanism of regression	Reference
Melanoma	*H-ras*	Ink4a/Arf and VEGF independent; apoptosis in tumor cells and host-derived endothelial cells; decreased proliferation; not immune-related	Chin et al. (1999)
T-cell lymphoma/acute myeloid leukemia	*Myc*	differentiation, proliferative arrest, and apoptosis in tumor cells	Felsher and Bishop (1999)
Osteosarcoma	*Myc*	differentiation in tumor cells	Jain et al. (2002)
Mammary	*Myc*	unknown	D'Cruz et al. (2001)
Mammary	*Neu*	apoptosis and decreased proliferation in tumor cells	Moody et al. (2002)
Mammary	*Wnt*	unknown; p53 independent	Gunther et al. (2003)
Pancreatic beta-cell	*Myc*	apoptosis, redifferentiation, decreased proliferation in tumor cells and vascular degeneration; occurs despite presence of Bcl-x$_L$; p19Arf and p53 independent	Pelengaris et al. (2002); G.I. Evans (unpubl.)
Non-small-cell lung cancer	*K-ras*	apoptosis (Ink4A/Arf and p53 independent) and decreased proliferation in tumor cells	Fisher et al. (2001)
Non-small-cell lung cancer	*EGFR*	unknown	K. Politi et al. (in prep.)
Sarcoma	*K-ras*	apoptosis and decreased proliferation in tumor cells; p53 independent; T-cell independent	Pao et al. (2003)
Leukemia	*Bcr-abl*	apoptosis in tumor cells	Huettner et al. (2000)
Skin	*Myc*	growth arrest and irreversible differentiation	Flores et al. (2004)
Hepatocellular carcinoma	*Myc*	differentiation	Shachaf et al. (2004)
Hepatocellular carcinoma	*Met*	apoptosis and decreased proliferation in tumor cells	Wang et al. (2001)

sis, differentiation of the cancer cells, or disappearance of vascular endothelial cells (Table 1). For example, about 5 years ago, our group constructed mice in which a mutant transgenic form of the Kirsten *Ras* gene (*K-Ras*^{G12D}) is regulated by a tetracycline-dependent transcription factor encoded by a second lung-specific transgene (Fisher et al. 2001). Using this system *K-Ras*^{G12D} is expressed in the lung at levels similar to the endogenous normal *K-Ras* gene, when a tetracycline analog, doxycycline, is provided in the diet. Lungs from such animals appear normal, and the mutant transgene is silent in the absence of the antibiotic. If the mice are maintained on doxycycline, foci of hyperplastic cells appear throughout the lung fields after about a month; by 2–3 months of doxycycline adminstration, adenomas and adenocarcinomas appear at multiple sites. If, however, doxycycline is then withdrawn, levels of mutant *K-Ras* RNA (and presumably protein) fall precipitously, and the tumor cells display signs of programmed cell death; as a result, the tumors disappear within 3–7 days, as judged by magnetic resonance imaging or by histopathology, and do not recur in the absence of drug (Fig. 1A).

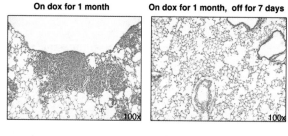

A WT background

On dox for 2 months   On dox for 2 months, off for 7 days

B Ink4a/Arf-/- background

On dox for 1 month   On dox for 1 month, off for 7 days

Bitransgenic *TetO-Kras*^{G12D}*/CCSP-rtTA* Mice

Figure 1. Oncogenic *K-ras* is required for lung tumor maintenance with or without loss of tumor suppressor genes. Samples of lung tissue, stained with hematoxylin and eosin, after exposure to doxycycline for 1 or 2 months and after withdrawal for 7 days are shown (Fisher et al. 2001). Withdrawal of doxycycline leads to rapid tumor regression in bi-transgenic *CCSP-rtTA/TetOKras*^{G12D} in a wild-type (WT) background (*A*) and in an *Ink4A/Arf*-deficient background (*B*). Similar results were obtained in a *p53*-deficient background (Fisher et al. 2001). Magnification, 100x.

To ask whether this apparent oncogene dependence occurs only in the absence of other oncogenic mutations, we repeated the experiments in mice known to be deficient in the tumor suppressor genes *p53* or *Ink4a/Arf*. Under these conditions, adenocarcinomas appeared more rapidly, usually within a month after doxycycline induction, but again quickly regressed by an apoptotic mechanism when the doxycycline was withdrawn (Fig. 1B). Thus, dependence of the mouse lung adenocarcinomas on the initiating *K-Ras* oncogene is not relieved by additional mutations in important tumor suppressor genes.

Our *K-Ras*-dependent lung cancer model and many of the other doxycycline-inducible mouse models listed in Table 1 prompt a general comment about oncogene dependence. It seems from these studies that cells that were at one time fully viable in the absence of the product of each inducible oncogene have become "imbalanced" in some way, so that sudden deprivation of the oncogene product now triggers an event—apoptosis, differentiation, or loss of angiogenic signals—that leads to tumor regression. Understanding such imbalances and their consequences could offer new ways to interfere with signaling downstream of an oncogenic activity. Particularly in the case of *RAS* genes, which are mutant in about a third of human tumors but for which no effective targeted inhibitor has been found, such insights might be an important step toward improving therapies of common human cancers.

Cancer Therapies in Patients

An example of dramatically improved therapy for a human cancer underscores the importance of the concept of oncogene dependence. As discussed elsewhere (see Sawyers, this volume), the use of imatinib—a potent inhibitor of at least three protein-tyrosine kinases, including ABL (and its mutant form BCR-ABL)—for the treatment of chronic myeloid leukemia (CML), a leading form of adult leukemia, rapidly reverses the hematological and symptomatic manifestations of the disease and maintains remissions for up to 5 years and more, especially when therapy is begun during early stages of the disease (for review, see Deininger et al. 2005). The appearance of second-site mutations in the kinase domain of BCR-ABL that confer imatinib resistance (Gorre et al. 2001) constitutes powerful evidence that the drug response is indeed due to the dependence of the leukemic cells on mutant ABL kinase activity. Strategies based on these mutations are now being pursued to prevent or overcome drug resistance (Shah et al. 2004; Burgess et al. 2005; Carter et al. 2005; Gumireddy et al. 2005; Sawyers, this volume).

Several other human cancers, including solid tumors, bearing changes in *ABL*—or mutations in the other two genes, *CKIT* and *PDGFR-A*, encoding kinases known to be inhibited by imatinib—also respond to this drug. This strengthens the argument that oncogene dependence is a general phenomenon, affecting solid and liquid cancers. Thus, therapeutic responses in human patients, not just regulated expression of transgenes in mice or temperature-sensitive mutant oncogenes in cell culture, provide important evidence for oncogene dependence.

EVIDENCE FOR *EGFR* ONCOGENE DEPENDENCE IN HUMAN LUNG ADENOCARCINOMA

Two small chemical inhibitors of the EGFR tyrosine kinase, gefitinib (Iressa) and erlotinib (Tarceva), were tested for efficacy in human lung cancer for several years (Fukuoka et al. 2003; Kris et al. 2003) before it was recognized that some lung cancers carry dominantly acting mutations in the *EGFR* gene (Lynch et al. 2004; Paez et al. 2004; Pao et al. 2004). The recent discovery of such *EGFR* mutations offers a striking example of how drug responses in patients can reveal dependence of cancers on a mutant oncogene.

Non-small-cell lung cancer (NSCLC) is the leading cause of cancer death worldwide (Parkin et al. 2005). In about 10% of patients in the U.S. and Europe with adenocarcinoma of the lung, the most common form of NSCLC, rapid partial remissions occur when these drugs are used, even late in the course of metastatic disease, and in parts of Asia the response rate is significantly higher (Fukuoka et al. 2003; Kris et al. 2003). Sometimes (as shown in Fig. 2A) the response is dramatic, resembling the tumor regression seen in our *K-Ras*-based mouse model of lung cancer when doxycycline is withdrawn (Fisher et al. 2001).

Observations like these suggested that the two tyrosine kinase inhibitors (TKIs) might be inactivating mutant kinases, either the known target for these drugs, EGFR, or some other unsuspected protein-tyrosine kinase among the 90 encoded in the human genome (Manning et al. 2002). Sequencing of the coding exons of *EGFR* genes in tumors that showed radiographic responses to the TKIs revealed that sensitivity to gefitinib and erlotinib were highly associated with mutations in the *EGFR* kinase domain (Lynch et al. 2004; Paez et al. 2004; Pao et al. 2004; see Thomas et al.; Haber et al.; both this volume). (For an example, see the computerized tomography scans in Fig. 2B.) Surprisingly, these mutations are highly idiosyncratic: Nearly 90% are either point mutations that change leucine at position 858 to arginine (L858R) or three- to seven-codon deletions affecting the highly conserved sequence, LREA, that is positioned close to the ATP-binding site in the kinase domain (for review, see Pao and Miller 2005).

The biochemical, physiological, and structural consequences of these mutations and several other substitution mutations that have been associated with TKI responsiveness are still under study (Sordella et al. 2004; Tracy et al. 2004; Amann et al. 2005; Engelman et al. 2005; Greulich et al. 2005; Chen et al. 2006), but several observations support the idea that this subset of lung adenocarcinomas is dependent on the mutant EGFR kinase. The mutations are strongly associated with a measurable radiological response to the TKIs; such responses are rarely observed in tumors without detectable *EGFR* mutations, including the 20–30% of tumors with mutations in *KRAS* (Eberhard et al. 2005; Pao et al. 2005b), the product of which acts "downstream" of EGFR. In addition, second-site mutations in one of the exons encoding the EGFR kinase domain are observed in about half of drug-resistant tumors that resume growth during treatment with the

A Radiograms of patient with adenoCA

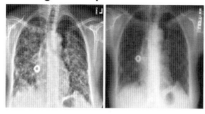

Before gefitinib   After 4 days on gefitinib

B CT scans of patient with adenoCA with an EGFR del L747–E749;A750P mutation

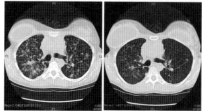

Before erlotinib   After 4 months on erlotinib

C MRI scans of a bitransgenic *TetO-EGFR^{L858R}/CCSP-rtTA* mouse

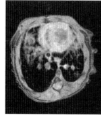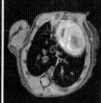

On dox for 10 weeks   On dox for 10.5 weeks +Erlotinib for 4 days

Figure 2. Lung tumors with *EGFR* mutations respond dramatically to treatment with tyrosine kinase inhibitors. Chest radiographs (*A*) and chest computerized tomography-generated images (*B*) showing a tumor response to gefitinib (*A*) after 4 days of treatment and erlotinib (*B*) after 4 months of treatment in two patients, one of which is known to have a tumor with an *EGFR* mutation. (*C*) Magnetic resonance images of lungs from a mouse expressing the EGFR L858R mutant before (*left panel*) and after 4 days (*right panel*) of erlotinib treatment.

TKIs (Kobayashi et al. 2005; Pao et al. 2005a).

Strikingly, these resistance-inducing secondary *EGFR* mutations all encode the same change, threonine to methionine at position 790, a change that is strictly analogous to one of the mutations observed in imatinib-resistant forms of *BCR-ABL*, *CKIT*, and *PDGFR-A* in various types of tumors treated with imatinib (Gorre et al. 2001; Cools et al. 2003; Tamborini et al. 2004; see Sawyers, this volume). The introduction of a bulky side chain in the methionine residue is likely to interfere with drug binding; screening of additional TKIs for their ability to bind to or inhibit the doubly mutant kinases have already identified agents that are effective in the presence of T790M and analogous mutations (Carter et al. 2005; Kwak et al. 2005); such drugs might be used after primary resistance occurs or in combination with the first TKI to prevent the emergence of resistance.

As described elsewhere (see Hillan et al., this volume), long-term outcomes of gefitinib or erlotinib treatment of *EGFR*-mutant tumors, as measured by survival or by time to tumor progression, are not as good as those observed in the treatment of CML with imatinib. Although a full explanation of these disappointing results is not yet at hand, the emergence of drug resistance, generally within a year

of commencing therapy, is likely to be part of the problem and may be alleviated by the use of additional TKIs. The relatively modest effects of TKIs on survival may also reflect the use of these drugs relatively late in the course of the disease, a phase more akin to the blast crisis than the early stages of CML, so that other oncogenic mutations may dampen the therapeutic efficacy. Consistent with this idea, partial rather than complete radiographic responses to the TKIs are commonly seen in patients with metastatic NSCLC. From this perspective, treatment of early-stage disease (e.g., adjuvant therapy with TKIs at the time of surgery) or first-line treatment of advanced disease with TKIs might have more potent effects on survival.

Some tumors with increased copy numbers of wild-type *EGFR*, as determined by fluorescent in situ hybridization, appear to be sensitive to treatment with gefitinib, since at least one group has reported a stronger correlation of the outcome, especially survival, with *EGFR* gene amplification than with *EGFR* mutation (Cappuzzo et al. 2005). Similar results have been described with erlotinib (Tsao et al. 2005). It will be important to confirm these findings in additional, larger studies and, if they prove valid, to understand how TKIs produce benefit in this situation.

MOUSE MODELS OF EGFR-DEPENDENT LUNG CANCER

Building mouse models of lung cancer is a useful means to characterize the dependence of lung adenocarcinomas on mutant *EGFR*, to study the mechanism of tumor induction and regression, to test candidate therapies, and to investigate mechanisms of drug resistance. To those ends, we have produced a series of transgenic mice that encode wild-type *EGFR*, L858R *EGFR*, and an LREA deletion form of *EGFR* under the control of a doxycycline-responsive regulatory system (K. Politi et al., in prep.). Induction of the L858R mutant form of EGFR leads to development of diffuse lung tumors comprising cells expressing markers of type II pneumocytes and highly reminiscent of human bronchioalveolar carcinoma, followed by the appearance of multifocal adenocarcinomas. The tumors rapidly regress, as observed by magnetic resonance imaging or histopathology, when the animals are deprived of doxycycline or when they are treated with erlotinib (Fig. 2C), demonstrating that the tumors are dependent on continued production or activity of the mutant *EGFR*. A detailed description of these lines and others, and their responses to induction and de-induction of *EGFR* and to drugs, will be published elsewhere (K. Politi et al., in prep.).

WHAT IS LIMITING THE IMPACT OF THE MOLECULAR UNDERSTANDING OF CANCER ON PATIENT CARE?

The widespread evidence for oncogene dependence in mouse models and human tumors and the results of treatment of some human cancers with TKIs, especially imatinib, provide strong grounds for optimism about controlling cancer more effectively in the future. Yet the outcomes of most efforts to treat the common cancers have not changed significantly over the past several decades. Why is this? And what is impeding more dramatic change?

Defining Cancer Genotypes

Despite the remarkable growth of knowledge about genes that have been implicated in carcinogenesis, we still have a very meager picture of the genotype of most of the 50 or more types of human cancer. For many cancer types, some proto-oncogene or tumor suppressor gene is known to be aberrant (subtly mutated, deleted, rearranged, amplified, or epigenetically modified). However, when studied intensively, most tumors appear to have multiple altered cancer genes. Furthermore, tumors that are histologically indistinguishable are often genetically different, and important elements in the clinical history, such as occupational exposures or never smoking, sometimes correlate more strongly than histology with the tumor genotype.

Consider, for example, the situation with lung adenocarcinoma, one of most common and lethal human cancers. About a quarter of such tumors have a mutant copy of *KRAS*, and this occurs nearly exclusively in smokers (Ahrendt et al. 2001). Similarly, we now know that about 10% have a mutant copy of *EGFR*, mainly in "never smokers" (Pao et al. 2004). In addition, small numbers of tumors have mutations in genes that encode other components of the growth factor signaling network: *ERBB2, BRAF*, and *PIK3CA* (see Fig. 3) (Brose et al. 2002; Naoki et al. 2002; Samuels et al. 2004; Stephens et al. 2004; Shigematsu et al. 2005). Interestingly, mutations in more than one of these genes are rarely encountered in a single tumor, implying that no further selective advantage is conferred by additional lesions affecting this signaling network. However, the combined percentage of tumors known to have even a single mutation in this network is relatively small; thus, a mutant oncogene that might provide a therapeutic target has not been identified in the majority of lung adenocarcinomas (Fig. 3). Furthermore, although loss of tumor suppressor genes, especially *P53* and *INK4A/ARF*, is known to occur at high frequency in such tumors (for review, see Forgacs et al. 2001), the influence of tumor suppressor deficiencies on treatment outcomes in the context of specific oncogenic mutations is not known, nor is the effect of mutations in additional proto-oncogenes, as discussed further below.

The development of high-throughput methods for assessing mutations, changes in DNA copy number, and even epigenetic changes provides an opportunity to repair, at least partially, our deficient knowledge of tumor genotypes. The National Institutes of Health is now considering a coordinated, long-term effort to find many of

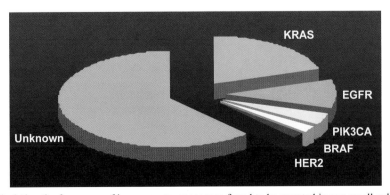

Figure 3. Pie chart depicting the frequency of known proto-oncogenes found to be mutated in non-small-cell lung cancers. As discussed in the text, these genes all encode components of the EGFR signaling network.

the genotypic changes that occur with at least 5% frequency in the 50 or so major types of human cancer (the NCAB Report can be found at http://www.genome.gov/Pages/About/NACHGR/May2005NACHGRAgenda/ReportoftheWorkingGrouponBiomedicalTechnology.pdf). Preliminary efforts at several centers to determine genotypes, mainly by re-sequencing the coding exons of genes encoding kinases, have yielded interesting results (Bardelli et al. 2003; Samuels et al. 2004; Davies et al. 2005; Parsons et al. 2005; Stephens et al. 2005; see Futreal et al., this volume), but the findings are not yet on a scale adequate to describe the molecular basis of human cancer in the way that will be required for major therapeutic advances.

Finding Novel Inhibitors of Mutant Oncogenes

A second obstacle to greater clinical impact of molecular oncology is the relative paucity of tools that affect potential therapeutic targets other than protein-tyrosine kinases (mostly inhibited by small compounds) or transmembrane proteins and their ligands (mostly blocked by monoclonal antibodies). As noted earlier, this deficiency is especially acute in relation to *RAS* mutants, but applies also to a wide range of oncogenic proteins. Thus far, nearly all beneficial therapies have been targeted against the products of mutant genes, but it seems reasonable to assume that nonmutated components of affected signaling pathways—for example, proteins phosphorylated by tyrosine kinases—will also prove to be vulnerable to attack.

It also seems likely to be important to understand the alterations that are responsible for the "imbalance" in cell signaling responsible for the phenomenon of oncogene dependence. For example, the apoptotic response that is observed when oncogenes are down-regulated in mouse models is presumably blocked in cancer cells expressing oncogenes by proteins induced by the oncogenes. Such proteins might be attractive therapeutic targets, especially when the mutant oncoprotein itself is refractory to inhibition by small molecules.

Minimizing Resistance to Targeted Cancer Therapies

Just as drug resistance is a problem in conventional chemotherapy and in treating infectious diseases, it is already apparent that cancer therapies targeted against known proteins will eventually encounter significant resistance. The encouraging news is that such resistance is usually attributable to secondary mutations affecting the target protein—a situation that permits rational approaches to overcoming resistance through drug screens and protein design. The goal is to develop combination therapies, not unlike those now in wide use for the treatment of HIV/AIDS, which greatly diminish the probability that resistant clones of cancer cells will emerge by genetic selection.

Coping with Mutations in Multiple Proto-oncogenes

Most human cancers, if not all, are the products of multiple genetic changes, but we do not yet have a full account

of the impact of additional oncogenic mutations on a tumor's dependence on any single oncogene. Recent studies of mouse tumor models from Lewis Chodosh and his colleagues indicate that oncogene dependence (for instance, dependence of a mouse mammary tumor on a *Myc* transgene) can be abrogated by secondary mutations in other genes, such as endogenous *Ras* genes (D'Cruz et al. 2001).

These observations have stimulated us to seek secondary spontaneous mutations in mammary tumors arising in tumor-prone transgenic mice. One attractive feature of these experiments is that the detection of a secondary mutation by DNA sequencing implies that it has conferred a selective growth advantage, otherwise it would not be present in a large enough percentage of tumor cells to permit detection by sequencing of unfractionated tumor DNA. In this way, we have shown that secondary mutations in *H-Ras* are encountered in about half of breast tumors induced by an MMTV-*Wnt1* transgene (Podsypanina et al. 2004). Such mutations are not found in tumors induced by an MMTV-*Neu/ERBB2* transgene; this is presumably so because Ras proteins act in the same growth factor signaling pathway, and thus, mutants would confer no growth advantage. *Ras* mutations are also not found in the tumors that rapidly appear in bi-transgenic mice, expressing both *Wnt-1* and *Neu/ERBB2*. Unexpectedly, however, the *Wnt1* transgene removes the selective pressure for the secondary mutations in the *Neu/ERBB2* gene that commonly enhance kinase activity in tumors arising in mono-transgenic mice (Siegel et al. 1994; Podsypanina et al. 2004). Also unexpectedly, *Ras* mutations do not occur in MMTV-*Wnt1* tumors when they are induced in *p53*-deficient mice. An understanding of these genetic interactions could help to predict which mutant cancer genes are likely to coexist in tumors and which might be the best targets for therapeutic intervention.

Additional insight into the interactions among mutant cancer genes can be obtained by expressing two or more transgenic oncogenes, at least one of which can be transcriptionally controlled. For example, we have built transgenic mice that express *Myc* and mutant *H-Ras* in mammary epithelium, with one or the other under the control of doxycycline, in order to determine whether oncogene dependence of ensuing tumors pertains to one gene, both, or neither with this genetic combination (K. Podsypanina et al., unpubl.).

Assessing Tumor Progression

Approaches to targeted therapy remain limited by a poor understanding of metastasis, invasion, and angiogenesis—the aspects of tumor progression that are responsible for the lethal effects of most tumors. Several papers address these issues (see Egeblad et al.; Bissell et al.; Courtneidge et al.; G.P. Gupta et al.; all this volume; D. Hanahan; J.S. Brugge; both unpubl.). We have developed a novel experimental system in which the progression of phenotypes in a well-characterized model of pancreatic islet cell tumors (Hanahan 1985) can be used to measure the effects of genes (or inhibitory RNAs) that have been introduced into islet cells by cell-specific infection with retroviral vectors. In this strategy, bi-transgenic mice in which the rat insulin promoter drives production of the SV40 T antigen (RIP-Tag) and the avian retrovirus subgroup A receptor (RIP-TVA) are infected with avian RCAS vectors encoding a variety of factors that might influence tumor progression. Early results suggest that two suspected progression factors, an anti-apoptotic protein (Bcl-xL) and a dominant-negative version of E-cadherin (Naik et al. 1996; Perl et al. 1998), each accelerate the formation of islet cell tumors with invasive properties (Y.-C.N. Du et al., unpubl.).

CONCLUSIONS

As demonstrated in many papers in this volume, cancer research has progressed rapidly over the past three decades and is now well-positioned to contribute powerfully to the control of human cancer. However, the long-anticipated benefits for patients have appeared only recently and in limited sectors of clinical oncology. A more deliberate effort to catalog and comprehend the mutations that afflict all the common human cancers, and more innovative approaches to therapeutic development will now be required to achieve the long-range goals of molecular oncology.

ACKNOWLEDGMENTS

We thank Jennifer Doherty for expert technical assistance, Maureen Zakowski for pathological evaluation of the murine lung tumors, and Jason Koutcher and Carl Le for magnetic resonance imaging of mice. This work was supported in part by a Mouse Models of Human Cancer Consortium Grant (to H. Varmus), P01 CA94060-02 (to H. Varmus), funds from the Martel Foundation (to H. Varmus) and the Carmel Hill Fund (to H. Varmus). K. Politi received support from the Labrecque Foundation and the American Cancer Society (PF-05-078-01-MGO); K. Podsypanina was supported by a Cancer Research Institute award; W. Pao received support from the CHEST and LUNGevity Foundations.

REFERENCES

Ahrendt S.A., Decker P.A., Alawi E.A., Zhu Y.R., Sanchez-Cespedes M., Yang S.C., Haasler G.B., Kajdacsy-Balla A., Demeure M.J., and Sidransky D. 2001. Cigarette smoking is strongly associated with mutation of the K-ras gene in patients with primary adenocarcinoma of the lung. *Cancer* **92:** 1525.

Amann J., Kalyankrishna S., Massion P.P., Ohm J.E., Girard L., Shigematsu H., Peyton M., Juroske D., Huang Y., Stuart Salmon J., Kim Y.H., Pollack J.R., Yanagisawa K., Gazdar A., Minna J.D., Kurie J.M., and Carbone D.P. 2005. Aberrant epidermal growth factor receptor signaling and enhanced sensitivity to EGFR inhibitors in lung cancer. *Cancer Res.* **65:** 226.

Bardelli A., Parsons D.W., Silliman N., Ptak J., Szabo S., Saha S., Markowitz S., Willson J.K., Parmigiani G., Kinzler K.W., Vogelstein B., and Velculescu V.E. 2003. Mutational analysis of the tyrosine kinome in colorectal cancers. *Science* **300:** 949.

Brose M.S., Volpe P., Feldman M., Kumar M., Rishi I., Gerrero R., Einhorn E., Herlyn M., Minna J., Nicholson A., Roth J.A., Albelda S.M., Davies H., Cox C., Brignell G., Stephens P., Futreal P.A., Wooster R., Stratton M.R., and Weber B.L. 2002. BRAF and RAS mutations in human lung cancer and melanoma. *Cancer Res.* **62:** 6997.

Burgess M.R., Skaggs B.J., Shah N.P., Lee F.Y., and Sawyers C.L. 2005. Comparative analysis of two clinically active BCR-ABL kinase inhibitors reveals the role of conformation-specific binding in resistance. *Proc. Natl. Acad. Sci.* **102:** 3395.

Cappuzzo F., Hirsch F.R., Rossi E., Bartolini S., Ceresoli G.L., Bemis L., Haney J., Witta S., Danenberg K., Domenichini I., Ludovini V., Magrini E., Gregorc V., Doglioni C., Sidoni A., Tonato M., Franklin W.A., Crino L., Bunn P.A., Jr., and Varella-Garcia M. 2005. Epidermal growth factor receptor gene and protein and gefitinib sensitivity in non-small-cell lung cancer. *J. Natl. Cancer Inst.* **97:** 643.

Carter T.A., Wodicka L.M., Shah N.P., Velasco A.M., Fabian M.A., Treiber D.K., Milanov Z.V., Atteridge C.E., Biggs W.H., III, Edeen P.T., Floyd M., Ford J.M., Grotzfeld R.M., Herrgard S., Insko D.E., Mehta S.A., Patel H.K., Pao W., Sawyers C.L., Varmus H., Zarrinkar P.P., and Lockhart D.J. 2005. Inhibition of drug-resistant mutants of ABL, KIT, and EGF receptor kinases. *Proc. Natl. Acad. Sci.* **102:** 11011.

Chen Y.R., Fu Y.N., Lin C.H., Yang S.T., Hu S.F., Chen Y.T., Tsai S.F., and Huang S.F. 2006. Distinctive activation patterns in constitutively active and gefitinib-sensitive EGFR mutants. *Oncogene* **25:** 1205.

Chin L., Tam A., Pomerantz J., Wong M., Holash J., Bardeesy N., Shen Q., O'Hagan R., Pantginis J., Zhou H., Horner J.W., 2nd, Cordon-Cardo C., Yancopoulos G.D., and DePinho R.A. 1999. Essential role for oncogenic Ras in tumour maintenance. *Nature* **400:** 468.

Cools J., DeAngelo D.J., Gotlib J., Stover E.H., Legare R.D., Cortes J., Kutok J., Clark J., Galinsky I., Griffin J.D., Cross N.C., Tefferi A., Malone J., Alam R., Schrier S.L., Schmid J., Rose M., Vandenberghe P., Verhoef G., Boogaerts M., Wlodarska I., Kantarjian H., Marynen P., Coutre S.E., Stone R., and Gilliland D.G. 2003. A tyrosine kinase created by fusion of the PDGFRA and FIP1L1 genes as a therapeutic target of imatinib in idiopathic hypereosinophilic syndrome. *N. Engl. J. Med.* **348:** 1201.

Davies H., Hunter C., Smith R., Stephens P., Greenman C., Bignell G., Teague J., Butler A., Edkins S., Stevens C., Parker A., O'Meara S., Avis T., Barthorpe S., Brackenbury L., Buck G., Clements J., Cole J., Dicks E., Edwards K., Forbes S., Gorton M., Gray K., Halliday K., Harrison R., Hills K., Hinton J., Jones D., Kosmidou V., Laman R., Lugg R., Menzies A., Perry J., Petty R., Raine K., Shepherd R., Small A., Solomon H., Stephens Y., Tofts C., Varian J., Webb A., West S., Widaa S., Yates A., Brasseur F., Cooper C.S., Flanagan A.M., Green A., Knowles M., Leung S.Y., Looijenga L.H., Malkowicz B., Pierotti M.A., Teh B.T., Yuen S.T., Lakhani S.R., Easton D.F., Weber B.L., Goldstraw P., Nicholson A.G., Wooster R., Stratton M.R., and Futreal P.A. 2005. Somatic mutations of the protein kinase gene family in human lung cancer. *Cancer Res.* **65:** 7591.

D'Cruz C.M., Gunther E.J., Boxer R.B., Hartman J.L., Sintasath L., Moody S.E., Cox J.D., Ha S.I., Belka G.K., Golant A., Cardiff R.D., and Chodosh L.A. 2001. c-MYC induces mammary tumorigenesis by means of a preferred pathway involving spontaneous Kras2 mutations. *Nat. Med.* **7:** 235.

Deininger M., Buchdunger E., and Druker B.J. 2005. The development of imatinib as a therapeutic agent for chronic myeloid leukemia. *Blood* **105:** 2640.

Eberhard D.A., Johnson B.E., Amler L.C., Goddard A.D., Heldens S.L., Herbst R.S., Ince W.L., Janne P.A., Januario T., Johnson D.H., Klein P., Miller V.A., Ostland M.A., Ramies D.A., Sebisanovic D., Stinson J.A., Zhang Y.R., Seshagiri S., and Hillan K.J. 2005. Mutations in the epidermal growth factor receptor and in KRAS are predictive and prognostic indicators in patients with non-small-cell lung cancer treated with chemotherapy alone and in combination with erlotinib. *J. Clin. Oncol.* **23:** 5900.

Engelman J.A., Janne P.A., Mermel C., Pearlberg J., Mokuhara T., Fleet C., Cichowski K., Johnson B.E., and Cantley L.C. 2005. ErbB-3 mediates phosphoinositide 3-kinase activity in gefitinib-sensitive non-small cell lung cancer cell lines. *Proc. Natl. Acad. Sci.* **102:** 3788.

Felsher D.W. and Bishop J.M. 1999. Reversible tumorigenesis by MYC in hematopoietic lineages. *Mol. Cell* **4:** 199.

Fisher G.H., Wellen S.L., Klimstra D., Lenczowski J.M., Tichelaar J.W., Lizak M.J., Whitsett J.A., Koretsky A., and Varmus H.E. 2001. Induction and apoptotic regression of lung adenocarcinomas by regulation of a K-Ras transgene in the presence and absence of tumor suppressor genes. *Genes Dev.* **15:** 3249.

Flores I., Murphy D.J., Swigart L.B., Knies U., and Evan G.I. 2004. Defining the temporal requirements for Myc in the progression and maintenance of skin neoplasia. *Oncogene* **23:** 5923.

Forgacs E., Zochbauer-Muller S., Olah E., and Minna J.D. 2001. Molecular genetic abnormalities in the pathogenesis of human lung cancer. *Pathol. Oncol. Res.* **7:** 6.

Fukuoka M., Yano S., Giaccone G., Tamura T., Nakagawa K., Douillard J.Y., Nishiwaki Y., Vansteenkiste J., Kudoh S., Rischin D., Eek R., Horai T., Noda K., Takata I., Smit E., Averbuch S., Macleod A., Feyereislova A., Dong R.P., and Baselga J. 2003. Multi-institutional randomized phase II trial of gefitinib for previously treated patients with advanced non-small-cell lung cancer. *J. Clin. Oncol.* **21:** 2237.

Gorre M.E., Mohammed M., Ellwood K., Hsu N., Paquette R., Rao P.N., and Sawyers C.L. 2001. Clinical resistance to STI-571 cancer therapy caused by BCR-ABL gene mutation or amplification. *Science* **293:** 876.

Greulich H., Chen T.H., Feng W., Janne P.A., Alvarez J.V., Zappaterra M., Bulmer S.E., Frank D.A., Hahn W.C., Sellers W.R., and Meyerson M. 2005. Oncogenic transformation by inhibitor-sensitive and -resistant EGFR mutants. *PLoS Med.* **2:** e313.

Gumireddy K., Baker S.J., Cosenza S.C., John P., Kang A.D., Robell K.A., Reddy M.V., and Reddy E.P. 2005. A non-ATP-competitive inhibitor of BCR-ABL overrides imatinib resistance. *Proc. Natl. Acad. Sci.* **102:** 1992.

Gunther E.J., Moody S.E., Belka G.K., Hahn K.T., Innocent N., Dugan K.D., Cardiff R.D., and Chodosh L.A. 2003. Impact of p53 loss on reversal and recurrence of conditional Wnt-induced tumorigenesis. *Genes Dev.* **17:** 488.

Hanahan D. 1985. Heritable formation of pancreatic beta-cell tumours in transgenic mice expressing recombinant insulin/simian virus 40 oncogenes. *Nature* **315:** 115.

Huettner C.S., Zhang P., Van Etten R.A., and Tenen D.G. 2000. Reversibility of acute B-cell leukaemia induced by BCR-ABL1. *Nat. Genet.* **24:** 57-60.

Jain M., Arvanitis C., Chu K., Dewey W., Leonhardt E., Trinh M., Sundberg C.D., Bishop J.M., and Felsher D.W. 2002. Sustained loss of a neoplastic phenotype by brief inactivation of MYC. *Science* **297:** 102.

Kobayashi S., Boggon T.J., Dayaram T., Janne P.A., Kocher O., Meyerson M., Johnson B.E., Eck M.J., Tenen D.G., and Halmos B. 2005. EGFR mutation and resistance of non-small-cell lung cancer to gefitinib. *N. Engl. J. Med.* **352:** 786.

Kris M., Natale R.B., Herbst R., Lynch T., Jr., Prager D., Belani C.P., Schiller J.H., Kelly K., Spiridonidis H., Sandler A., Albain K., Cella D., Wolf M., Averbuch S., Ochs J., and Kay A. 2003. Efficacy of gefitinib, an inhibitor of the epidermal growth factor receptor tyrosine kinase, in symptomatic patients with non-small cell lung cancer. *J. Am. Med. Assoc.* **290:** 2149.

Kwak E.L., Sordella R., Bell D.W., Godin-Heymann N., Okimoto R.A., Brannigan B.W., Harris P.L., Driscoll D.R., Fidias P., Lynch T.J., Rabindran S.K., McGinnis J.P., Wissner A., Sharma S.V., Isselbacher K.J., Settleman J., and Haber D.A. 2005. Irreversible inhibitors of the EGF receptor may circumvent acquired resistance to gefitinib. *Proc. Natl. Acad. Sci.* **102:** 7665.

Lynch T.J., Bell D.W., Sordella R., Gurubhagavatula S., Okimoto R.A., Brannigan B.W., Harris P.L., Haserlat S.M.,

Supko J.G., Haluska F.G., Louis D.N., Christiani D.C., Settleman J., and Haber D.A. 2004. Activating mutations in the epidermal growth factor receptor underlying responsiveness of non-small-cell lung cancer to gefitinib. *N. Engl. J. Med.* **350:** 2129.

Manning G., Whyte D.B., Martinez R., Hunter T., and Sudarsanam S. 2002. The protein kinase complement of the human genome. *Science* **298:** 1912.

Martin G.S. 1970. Rous sarcoma virus: A function required for the maintenance of the transformed state. *Nature* **227:** 1021.

Moody S.E., Sarkisian C.J., Hahn K.T., Gunther E.J., Pickup S., Dugan K.D., Innocent N., Cardiff R.D., Schnall M.D., and Chodosh L.A. 2002. Conditional activation of Neu in the mammary epithelium of transgenic mice results in reversible pulmonary metastasis. *Cancer Cell* **2:** 451.

Naik P., Karrim J., and Hanahan D. 1996. The rise and fall of apoptosis during multistage tumorigenesis: Down-modulation contributes to tumor progression from angiogenic progenitors. *Genes Dev.* **10:** 2105.

Naoki K., Chen T.H., Richards W.G., Sugarbaker D.J., and Meyerson M. 2002. Missense mutations of the BRAF gene in human lung adenocarcinoma. *Cancer Res.* **62:** 7001.

Paez J.G., Janne P.A., Lee J.C., Tracy S., Greulich H., Gabriel S., Herman P., Kaye F.J., Lindeman N., Boggon T.J., Naoki K., Sasaki H., Fujii Y., Eck M.J., Sellers W.R., Johnson B.E., and Meyerson M. 2004. *EGFR* mutations in lung cancer: Correlation with clinical response to gefitinib therapy. *Science* **304:** 1497.

Pao W. and Miller V.A. 2005. *EGFR* mutations, small molecule kinase inhibitors, and non-small cell lung cancer: Current knowledge and future directions. *J. Clin. Oncol.* **23:** 2556.

Pao W., Klimstra D.S., Fisher G.H., and Varmus H.E. 2003. Use of avian retroviral vectors to introduce transcriptional regulators into mammalian cells for analyses of tumor maintenance. *Proc. Natl. Acad. Sci.* **100:** 8764.

Pao W., Miller V.A., Politi K.A., Riely G.J., Somwar R., Zakowski M.F., Kris M.G., and Varmus H. 2005a. Acquired resistance of lung adenocarcinomas to gefitinib or erlotinib is associated with a second mutation in the EGFR kinase domain. *PLoS Med.* **2:** e73.

Pao W., Wang T.Y., Riely G.J., Miller V.A., Pan Q., Landanyi M., Zakowski M.F., Heelan R.T., Kris M.G., and Varmus H.E. 2005b. *KRAS* mutations and primary resistance of lung adenocarcinomas to gefitinib or erlotinib. *PLoS Med.* **2:** e17.

Pao W., Miller V., Zakowski M., Doherty J., Politi K., Sarkaria I., Singh B., Heelan R., Rusch V., Fulton L., Mardis E., Kupfer D., Wilson R., Kris M., and Varmus H. 2004. EGF receptor gene mutations are common in lung cancers from "never smokers" and are associated with sensitivity of tumors to gefitinib and erlotinib. *Proc. Natl. Acad. Sci.* **101:** 13306.

Parkin D.M., Bray F., and Pisani P. 2005. Global cancer statistics, 2002. *CA Cancer J. Clin.* **55:** 74.

Parsons D.W., Wang T.L., Samuels Y., Bardelli A., Cummins J.M., DeLong L., Silliman N., Ptak J., Szabo S., Willson J.K., Markowitz S., Kinzler K.W., Vogelstein B., Lengauer C., and Velculescu V.E. 2005. Colorectal cancer: Mutations in a signalling pathway. *Nature* **436:** 792.

Pelengaris S., Khan M., and Evan G.I. 2002. Suppression of Myc-induced apoptosis in beta cells exposes multiple oncogenic properties of Myc and triggers carcinogenic progression. *Cell* **109:** 321.

Perl A.K., Wilgenbus P., Dahl U., Semb H., and Christofori G. 1998. A causal role for E-cadherin in the transition from adenoma to carcinoma. *Nature* **392:** 190.

Podsypanina K., Li Y., and Varmus H.E. 2004. Evolution of somatic mutations in mammary tumors in transgenic mice is influenced by the inherited genotype. *BMC Med.* **2:** 24.

Rosenberg N. and Jolicoeur P. 1997. Retroviral pathogenesis. In *Retroviruses* (ed. J.M. Coffin et al.), p. 475. Cold Spring Harbor Laboratory Press, Cold Spring Harbor, New York.

Samuels Y., Wang Z., Bardelli A., Silliman N., Ptak J., Szabo S., Yan H., Gazdar A., Powell S.M., Riggins G.J., Willson J.K., Markowitz S., Kinzler K.W., Vogelstein B., and Velculescu

V.E. 2004. High frequency of mutations of the PIK3CA gene in human cancers. *Science* **304:** 554.

Shachaf C.M., Kopelman A.M., Arvanitis C., Karlsson A., Beer S., Mandl S., Bachmann M.H., Borowsky A.D., Ruebner B., Cardiff R.D., Yang Q., Bishop J.M., Contag C.H., and Felsher D.W. 2004. MYC inactivation uncovers pluripotent differentiation and tumour dormancy in hepatocellular cancer. *Nature* **431:** 1112.

Shah N.P., Tran C., Lee F.Y., Chen P., Norris D., and Sawyers C.L. 2004. Overriding imatinib resistance with a novel ABL kinase inhibitor. *Science* **305:** 399.

Shigematsu H., Takahashi T., Nomura M., Majmudar K., Suzuki M., Lee H., Wistuba I.I., Fong K.M., Toyooka S., Shimizu N., Fujisawa T., Minna J.D., and Gazdar A.F. 2005. Somatic mutations of the *HER2* kinase domain in lung adenocarcinomas. *Cancer Res.* **65:** 1642.

Siegel P.M., Dankort D.L., Hardy W.R., and Muller W.J. 1994. Novel activating mutations in the neu proto-oncogene involved in induction of mammary tumors. *Mol. Cell. Biol.* **14:** 7068.

Sordella R., Bell D.W., Haber D.A., and Settleman J. 2004. Gefitinib-sensitizing EGFR mutations in lung cancer activate anti-apoptotic pathways. *Science* **305:** 1163.

Stehelin D., Varmus H.E., Bishop J.M., and Vogt P.K. 1976. DNA related to the transforming gene(s) of avian sarcoma viruses is present in normal avian DNA. *Nature* **260:** 170.

Stephens P., Hunter C., Bignell G., Edkins S., Davies H., Teague J., Stevens C., O'Meara S., Smith R., Parker A., Barthorpe A., Blow M., Brackenbury L., Butler A., Clarke O., Cole J., Dicks E., Dike A., Drozd A., Edwards K., Forbes S., Foster R., Gray K., Greenman C., Halliday K., Hills K., Kosmidou V., Lugg R., Menzies A., Perry J., Petty R., Raine K., Ratford L., Shepherd R., Small A., Stephens Y., Tofts C., Varian J., West S., Widaa S., Yates A., Brasseur F., Cooper C.S., Flanagan A.M., Knowles M., Leung S.Y., Louis D.N., Looijenga L.H., Malkowicz B., Pierotti M.A., Teh B., Chenevix-Trench G., Weber B.L., Yuen S.T., Harris G., Goldstraw P., Nicholson A.G., Futreal P.A., Wooster R., and Stratton M.R. 2004. Lung cancer: Intragenic ERBB2 kinase mutations in tumours. *Nature* **431:** 525.

Stephens P., Edkins S., Davies H., Greenman C., Cox C., Hunter C., Bignell G., Teague J., Smith R., Stevens C., O'Meara S., Parker A., Tarpey P., Avis T., Barthorpe A., Brackenbury L., Buck G., Butler A., Clements J., Cole J., Dicks E., Edwards K., Forbes S., Gorton M., Gray K., Halliday K., Harrison R., Hills K., Hinton J., Jones D., Kosmidou V., Laman R., Lugg R., Menzies A., Perry J., Petty R., Raine K., Shepherd R., Small A., Solomon H., Stephens Y., Tofts C., Varian J., Webb A., West S., Widaa S., Yates A., Brasseur F., Cooper C.S., Flanagan A.M., Green A., Knowles M., Leung S.Y., Looijenga L.H., Malkowicz B., Pierotti M.A., Teh B., Yuen S.T., Nicholson A.G., Lakhani S., Easton D.F., Weber B.L., Stratton M.R., Futreal P.A., and Wooster R. 2005. A screen of the complete protein kinase gene family identifies diverse patterns of somatic mutations in human breast cancer. *Nat. Genet.* **37:** 590.

Tamborini E., Bonadiman L., Greco A., Albertini V., Negri T., Gronchi A., Bertulli R., Colecchia M., Casali P.G., Pierotti M.A., and Pilotti S. 2004. A new mutation in the KIT ATP pocket causes acquired resistance to imatinib in a gastrointestinal stromal tumor patient. *Gastroenterology* **127:** 294.

Tracy S., Mukohara T., Hansen M., Meyerson M., Johnson B.E., and Janne P.A. 2004. Gefitinib induces apoptosis in the EGFRL858R non-small-cell lung cancer cell line H3255. *Cancer Res.* **64:** 7241.

Tsao M.S., Sakurada A., Cutz J.C., Zhu C.Q., Kamel-Reid S., Squire J., Lorimer I., Zhang T., Liu N., Daneshmand M., Marrano P., da Cunha Santos G., Lagarde A., Richardson F., Seymour L., Whitehead M., Ding K., Pater J., and Shepherd F.A. 2005. Erlotinib in lung cancer: Molecular and clinical predictors of outcome. *N. Engl. J. Med.* **353:** 133.

Wang R., Ferrell L.D., Faouzi S., Maher J.J., and Bishop J.M. 2001. Activation of the Met receptor by cell attachment induces and sustains hepatocellular carcinomas in transgenic mice. *J. Cell Biol.* **153:** 1023.

Common and Contrasting Genomic Profiles among the Major Human Lung Cancer Subtypes

G. Tonon,[§] C. Brennan,* A. Protopopov,[§] G. Maulik,* B. Feng,[§] Y. Zhang,[§]
D.B. Khatry,[§] M.J. You,[†] A.J. Aguirre,* E.S. Martin,* Z. Yang,* H. Ji,* L. Chin,[§‡]
K.-K. Wong,* and R.A. DePinho[§ ¶]

*Departments of Medical Oncology and [§]Center for Applied Cancer Science, Dana-Farber Cancer Institute;
[†]Department of Pathology, Brigham and Women's Hospital; [‡]Department of Dermatology, and
[¶]Department of Genetics and Medicine, Harvard Medical School, Boston, Massachusetts 02115

Lung cancer is the leading cause of cancer mortality worldwide. With the recent success of molecularly targeted therapies in this disease, a detailed knowledge of the spectrum of genetic lesions in lung cancer represents a critical step in the development of additional effective agents. An integrated high-resolution survey of regional amplifications and deletions and gene expression profiling of non-small-cell lung cancers (NSCLC) identified 93 focal high-confidence copy number alterations (CNAs), with 21 spanning less than 0.5 Mb with a median of five genes. Most CNAs were novel and included high-amplitude amplification and homozygous deletion events. Pathogenic relevance of these genomic alterations was further reinforced by their recurrence and overlap with focal alterations of other tumor types. Additionally, the comparison of the genomic profiles of the two major subtypes of NSCLC, adenocarcinoma (AC) and squamous cell carcinoma (SCC), showed an almost complete overlap with the exception of one amplified region on chromosome 3, specific for SCC. Among the few genes overexpressed within this amplicon was p63, a known regulator of squamous cell differentiation. These findings suggest that the AC and SCC subtypes may arise from a common cell of origin and they are driven to their distinct phenotypic end points by altered expression of a limited number of key genes such as p63.

Lung cancer is the leading cause of cancer-related mortality in the United States, accounting for more than one-fourth of all cancer fatalities in 2004. Distinctive clinical and pathobiological features serve to classify lung cancers into two major subtypes: small-cell lung cancer (SCLC) and non-small-cell lung cancer (NSCLC). NSCLC constitutes 75% of lung cancer cases and is subdivided further into three major histologically distinct subtypes, including adenocarcinoma (AC), squamous cell carcinoma (SCC), and large-cell carcinoma. Adenocarcinoma and squamous carcinoma subtypes represent over 85% of NSCLC cases. Whereas these NSCLC subtypes exhibit distinct clinical and pathological characteristics, the treatment approaches have remained generic and largely ineffective despite advances in cytotoxic drugs, radiotherapy, and clinical management. The cure rate for advanced NSCLC remains among the most dismal in oncology. For all stages of NSCLC, the 5-year survival rate has remained fixed at 15% for the last 15 years. The recent success of molecularly targeted therapies for a limited number of cases with specific cancer genotypes (Lynch et al. 2004; Paez et al. 2004) has solidified the view that a more detailed knowledge of the spectrum of genetic lesions in lung cancer will in turn lead to meaningful therapeutic progress.

To date, the majority of lung cancer genetic studies have cataloged mutations or promoter methylation status of known cancer genes, performed genome-wide loss-of-heterozygosity (LOH) surveys, and applied comparative genomic hybridization (CGH) to audit regional copy number alterations (CNAs) on metaphase chromosomes or small-scale BAC arrays. These concerted efforts have identified a core set of lesions including K-RAS activation mutations and loss-of-function mutations in the p53 and Rb pathways (Minna et al. 2002). At the same time, the observed high number of recurrent chromosomal aberrations, particularly amplifications and deletions, suggests that only a small fraction of the lung cancer genes has been identified to date.

Integrated CGH and expression profiling have emerged as a highly effective approach to cancer gene discovery, capable of providing a genome-wide view of the regional gains and losses throughout the cancer genome (Kallioniemi et al. 1994) and associated copy-number-driven changes in gene expression (Pollack et al. 1999, 2002; Aguirre et al. 2004). In the case of NSCLC, chromosomal CGH studies have revealed recurrent gains at 1q31, 3q25-27, 5p13-14, and 8q23-24 and deletions at 3p21, 8p22, 9p21-22, 13q22, and 17p12-13 (Petersen et al. 1997; Bjorkqvist et al. 1998a; Luk et al. 2001; Pei et al. 2001; Balsara and Testa 2002). A recent limited array CGH survey of known genes/loci possibly contributing to lung cancer has demonstrated the utility of this approach by confirming recurrent chromosome 3p deletions and 3q gains—and identified PIK3CA as a resident of chromosome 3q amplicon (Massion et al. 2002), a gene shown subsequently to harbor activating point mutations in some lung cancer cases (Samuels et al. 2004).

In the microarray format, the resolution of CGH is dictated by the number and quality of mapped probes positioned along the genome (Albertson and Pinkel 2003). In this study, high-density cDNA- and oligonucleotide-based arrays were used to conduct high-resolution surveys of CNAs present in a well-defined collection of pri-

12   TONON ET AL.

mary ACs and SCCs and in a panel of established NSCLC cell lines (Tonon et al. 2005). Zhao et al. (2005) have recently performed a similar analysis on NSCLC and SCLC cell lines and primary tumors, using single-nucleotide polymorphism arrays.

The application of novel custom bioinformatics tools, along with integration of expression profiles and public databases, has yielded a dramatic increase in the number of recurrent amplifications and deletions detectable in the NSCLC genome. The high degree of NSCLC genomic complexity, the recurrent nature of these lesions, and preliminary functional characterization of resident genes point to a large number of relevant oncogenic events, opening potential therapeutic and diagnostic opportunities.

RESULTS

Identification of Known and Novel CNAs in the NSCLC Genome

Genome-wide array-CGH (aCGH) profiling was performed on 44 tumors, 18 ACs, and 26 SCCs, presenting greater than 70% tumor cellularity. Additionally, 34 NSCLC cell lines were analyzed by CGH (Tonon et al. 2005). Expression profiling was also performed on most of the primary tumors and cell lines analyzed by CGH.

CGH profiles were generated to identify CNAs as described previously (Aguirre et al. 2004). To identify copy number changes above noise background, we applied a modified version of the circular binary segmentation method as described previously (Aguirre et al. 2004; Olshen et al. 2004). The most striking feature of the NSCLC data set was the large number of CNAs ($n = 319$) which,

along with the high degree of structural complexity for each CNA, prompted us to filter the data set through an algorithm proven effective in defining and prioritizing CNAs across large, highly complex aCGH data sets (Aguirre et al. 2004). Some of these CNAs were present across different samples, allowing the definition of a minimal common region (MCR) of gain/amplification or loss/deletion. To facilitate the identification of those MCRs that might have strong pathogenetic relevance (referred to as high-priority MCRs), we applied a set of criteria that includes the occurrence in at least one tumor sample and the presence of at least one high-amplitude event ($\log_2 0.8$) (Tonon et al. 2005). This algorithm yielded 93 so-called "high-confidence" MCRs (Table 1). Seventy-four of these high-priority MCRs were amplifications and 19 were deletions, with a median size of 1.5 Mb. Moreover, given that the parameters used by our automated MCR definition program are relatively conservative and that not all genes are represented by probes on these microarrays, real-time quantitative polymerase chain reaction (QPCR) measurement of gene dosage and fluorescence in situ hybridization (FISH) analysis can further refine and narrow the boundaries of an MCR, as illustrated by the 8p12-p11.2 amplicon (see Figs. 5 and 6), thereby presenting a large number of loci with a highly tractable number of candidate cancer genes for further analysis.

On first inspection, the data set contained all the regional gains and losses previously identified in NSCLC by chromosomal CGH and conventional genomic methods including the known gains at 1q31, 3q25-27, 5p13-14, and 8q23-24, as well as the known deletions at 3p21, 8p22, 9p21-22, 13q22, and 17p12-13 (Fig. 1). Furthermore, virtually all of the genes implicated in the patho-

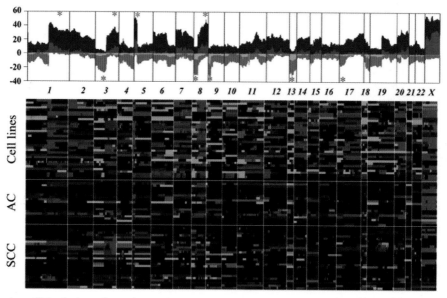

Figure 1. Genomic profiles of primary lung adeno and squamous carcinomas and lung cancer cell lines. (*Upper panel*) Recurrence of chromosomal alterations. Integer-value recurrence of CNAs in segmented data (*y* axis) is plotted for each probe evenly aligned along the *x* axis in chromosome order. Dark red or green bars denote gain or loss of chromosome material, bright red or green bars represent probes within regions of amplification or deletion. Asterisks identify the most frequent region of gains (*red*) and losses (*green*), as reported previously (Balsara et al. 2002). (*Lower panel*) Heat map plot showing discrete CNAs within all samples with the *x* axis representing probes ordered by genomic map positions and the *y* axis representing individual samples. Red represents chromosomal gain/amplification and green denotes chromosomal loss/deletion. (Reprinted, with permission, from Tonon et al. 2005 [©National Academy of Sciences].)

Table 1. High-Confidence MCRs in Lung AC and SCC Primary Tumors and Cell Lines

Cytogenetic band	Minimal common regions (MCRs)				MCR recurrence					Cancer-related genes	miRNA
	position (Mb)	size (Mb)	max/min value	# transcripts	gain/loss			amp/del			
					%	T	C	T	C		
Gain and amplification											
1p36.32-1p36.32	2.37-2.47	0.1	1.2	2	22	9	9	3	0		
1p36.21-1p36.12	15.29-20.69	5.4	1.32	86	20	8	9	1	1	SDHB, PAX7	
1p34.3-1p34.3	37.82-38.13	0.32	2.92	11	18	7	8	1	1		
1p34.2-1p34.1	41.65-44.9	3.26	2.35	50	19	6	10	3	2		
1q21.3-1q22	150.95-151.92	0.98	1.96	29	49	17	24	3	13		
1q31.2-1q32.1	189.28-197.57	8.29	1.22	35	40	16	17	1	4		hsa-mir-181b-1, hsa-mir-213
1q32.2-1q32.2	206.17-206.24	0.06	1.05	3	39	15	17	1	4		
2p16.3-2p14	49.1-64.73	15.63	1.11	54	40	13	21	1	3	BCL11A, REL	hsa-mir-217, hsa-mir-216
2q11.2-2q11.2	96.68-96.95	0.27	2.16	8	35	14	16	4	4		
2q14.1-2q14.2	118.58-120.16	1.57	0.88	11	28	9	14	1	2		
2q31.1-2q31.1	170.19-170.32	0.13	1.14	4	28	11	13	1	1		
3p12.1-3p11.1	87.07-88.45	1.38	1.32	8	17	6	8	1	1		
3q11.2-3q12.3	95.26-103.06	7.8	0.82	43	33	15	12	2	1	TFG	
3q21.3-3q25.32	130.02-159.3	29.28	0.85	182	45	21	17	6	4	GMPS	
3q29-3q29	195.34-196.56	1.22	1.06	12	36	16	14	6	3		
4q12-4q12	53.58-55	1.42	1.47	6	22	9	10	1	4	FIP1L1, CHIC2	
4q13.3-4q13.3	75.33-76.03	0.7	0.92	6	17	7	7	2	1		
4q21.1-4q21.1	77.09-78.06	0.97	0.85	13	14	5	7	1	1		
5p15.33-5p15.33 ♦	**0.53-0.92** ♦	0.38	2.67	5	60	27	24	6	15		
5p12-5p12	42.76-43.48	0.73	2.69	9	52	23	20	3	13		
5q31.3-5q31.3	140.55-140.66	0.12	1.99	11	19	6	10	2	4		
6p25.2-6p24.3	2.96-8.04	5.09	1.59	33	39	16	16	2	2		
6p22.3-6p22.3	17.87-20.56	2.69	1.59	9	36	15	15	2	3	DEK	
6p22.1-6p22.1	27.95-28.47	0.52	0.91	24	33	13	14	1	1		
6p12.3-6p12.2	49.91-52.16	2.25	1.21	6	35	13	16	2	2		hsa-mir-206, hsa-mir-133b
6p12.1-6p12.1	53.47-55.73	2.26	1.21	11	35	13	16	3	2		
6q24.3-6q25.1	145.99-149.77	3.79	1.16	11	17	6	8	2	1		
6q25.2-6q25.2	153.38-154.67	1.28	1.68	5	16	5	8	1	1		
7p11.2-7p11.2	54.41-55.94	1.53	3.62	15	36	13	18	2	7	EGFR	
7q21.3-7q21.3	93.2-95.37 ♦	2.17	1.96	13	40	11	22	2	7		
7q21.3-7q22.1	97.13-98.66 ♦	1.54	1.96	17	40	10	23	2	7		
7q31.2-7q31.2	**115.22-116.9**	1.68	2.15	10	34	10	18	2	7	MET	
8p12-8p11.22*	**38.24-38.45*** ♦	0.21	1.98	2	35	17	12	6	4	WHSC1L1, FGFR1	
8q11.21-8q22.1	48.86-97.23 ♦	48.37	1.42	192	52	19	24	5	11	NCOA2, NBS1, CBFA2T1	hsa-mir-124a-2
8q24.13-8q24.13	123.37-126.14 ♦	2.76	0.9	23	54	21	24	4	9		
8q24.21-8q24.21	128.5-129.02 ♦	0.52	4.36	3	59	22	27	4	14	MYC	
8q24.3-8q24.3	145.67-146.25	0.58	0.81	21	52	20	23	4	8	RECQL4	
10q24.1-10q24.1	97.62-98.11	0.49	1.15	8	16	3	10	1	1		
10q26.3-10q26.3	135.24-135.24	0.01	1.28	1	11	1	8	1	3		
11p14.2-11p14.1	26.54-28	1.46	0.95	13	20	7	10	1	1		
11p13-11p13	31.76-34.08	2.32	2.84	21	23	9	10	1	1	WT1, LMO2	
11q13.3-11q13.3	69.3-69.99	0.69	3.46	8	37	11	21	3	6		
11q22.1-11q22.2	**99.73-102.15**	2.41	0.94	16	27	9	13	1	3	BIRC3	
12p13.33-12p13.33	**0.17-0.81**	0.64	1.09	7	36	12	18	1	6		
12p13.2-12p12.3	12.37-16.6	4.22	1.16	39	29	11	13	2	5		
12p12.1-12p11.23	**24.61-26.95**	2.34	1.98	13	37	15	16	5	7	KRAS2	
12q12-12q13.11	43.74-46.42	2.68	2.68	14	31	11	15	2	6		
12q13.2-12q13.2	**54.72-54.84**	0.12	1.4	8	29	10	14	2	2	ERBB3	
12q15-12q15	67.42-67.95	0.53	1.82	5	34	14	14	5	4		
13q32.1-13q32.1	94.07-95.21	1.14	1.03	6	6	3	2	1	1		
13q34-13q34	111.77-112.97 ♦	1.2	1.21	16	14	4	8	2	5		
13q34-13q34	113.25-114.11	0.86	1.12	10	14	4	8	1	5		
14q13.2-14q13.3	**34.64-36.22** ♦	1.58	2.23	20	29	9	15	2	4		
14q22.2-14q22.3	53.49-55.15	1.66	1.41	22	30	8	17	1	6		
14q32.13-14q32.13	93.66-94.03	0.37	1.1	9	29	6	18	1	4		
15q25.2-15q25.3	82.35-83.48	1.13	0.95	22	31	10	16	2	5		
16p12.1-16p12.1	23.68-27.37	3.69	0.89	21	18	6	9	1	2		
16q12.1-16q12.2	51.03-52.87	1.84	1.3	9	20	7	10	1	4		
16q22.2-16q22.2	69.62-69.87	0.26	1.08	2	18	6	9	1	4		
16q24.2-16q24.3	86.43-87.23	0.81	1.7	9	18	5	10	2	3		
17p11.2-17p11.2	17.09-18.86	1.77	0.84	40	20	7	10	1	1		
18p11.32-18p11.32	0.2-0.9	0.7	1.7	9	25	13	9	4	1		

(Continued on following page.)

Table 1. High-Confidence MCRs in Lung AC and SCC Primary Tumors and Cell Lines (*Continued*)

Cytogenetic band	Minimal common regions (MCRs) position (Mb)	size (Mb)	max/min value	# transcripts	MCR recurrence gain/loss %	T	C	amp/del T	C	Cancer-related genes	miRNA
18q11.2-18q11.2	18.25-20.9 ♦	2.65	0.96	15	20	8	9	2	0		
18q12.1-18q12.1	26.83-27.31	0.48	1.55	6	19	9	7	2	1		
18q12.3-18q21.1	**37.92-46.03**	8.12	1.41	33	23	11	8	1	1		
19p13.12-19p13.12	14.8-16.01	1.22	1.53	39	11	5	4	1	1	BRD4	
19q12-19q12	35.01-35.73	0.73	1.91	4	31	13	13	2	5		
19q13.33-19q13.33	55.52-55.68 ♦	0.16	1.01	8	17	5	9	1	1		
20p12.3-20p12.2	7.91-10.57	2.66	0.85	12	31	13	14	1	3		
20q11.21-20q11.21	**29.66-29.88** ♦	0.22	3.85	5	42	13	23	1	8		
20q13.32-20q13.33	**57.04-60.21** ♦	3.17	1.61	19	41	12	23	1	11	SS18L1	
21q11.2-21q21.1	14.52-18.56	4.04	1.14	13	17	7	7	2	0		hsa-mir-99a, hsa-let-7c, hsa-mir-125b-2
22q11.21-22q11.21	19.09-20.3	1.22	1.02	28	25	11	10	1	3		
Loss and deletion											
1p22.1-1p22.1	**92.45-94.07**	1.62	-0.89	15	18	9	7	1	1		
2q34-2q35	209.15-217.17	8.02	-0.83	25	11	6	3	1	1	ATIC	
2q36.1-2q37.1	223.74-230.87	7.12	-1.03	28	8	5	2	1	1		
3p26.3-3p26.2	0.43-3.09	2.66	-0.87	4	23	11	9	1	3		
3p11.2-3p11.1	87.39-88.45	1.07	-0.92	6	24	14	7	3	1		
4p15.32-4p15.32	15.84-17.48	1.64	-0.88	8	14	8	5	2	0		
6p21.32-6p21.32	32.47-33.01	0.54	-1.05	17	11	3	6	2	1		
6q21-6q22.33	**111.4-128.94** ♦	17.55	-1	72	23	8	11	1	4		
7p22.3-7p22.3	1.36-2.05	0.69	-1.21	7	10	5	3	1	1		
7q34-7q34	142.28-142.44	0.16	-1.39	4	13	7	4	2	1		
8p21.1-8p12	28.74-33.48 ♦	4.74	-1.28	22	36	15	16	1	8	WRN	
9p21.3-9p21.3	**21.47-22** ♦	0.53	-4.81	4	43	16	21	1	18	CDKN2A	hsa-mir-31
11q11-11q11^	55.1-55.18^	0.08	-4.06	2	23	13	6	7	1		
11q24.3-11q24.3	128.13-129.24	1.11	-0.84	9	16	5	8	1	4		
12q12-12q13.11	42.41-44.87 ♦	2.46	-1.94	13	7	2	4	1	2		
13q12.11-13q12.11	**19.14-19.56**	0.41	-3.51	5	34	14	14	1	7		
13q14.13-13q21.1	**45.82-57.2**	11.38	-1.35	60	35	16	13	1	8	RB1	hsa-mir-16-1, hsa-mir-15a
13q32.2-13q32.2	**97.47-97.9**	0.42	-3.25	3	29	13	11	1	8		
18q21.33-18q22.2	58.4-65.82 ♦	7.43	-1.26	26	29	10	14	1	5		
21p11.2-21p11.1	**9.93-10.08** ♦	0.15	-1.33	3	17	9	6	1	1		

The numbers of primary tumors (T) or cell lines (C) with gain or loss, and amplification or deletion, are listed, respectively. For other definitions, see text and Tonon et al. (2005). MCR recurrence is denoted as percentage of the total data set. In bold, the MCRs verified by RT-PCR and FISH (Figs. 5 and 6; data not shown). Number of transcripts is based on build 35, NCBI. Only the known genes within the boundaries have been included. The list of cancer-related genes was derived from Futreal et al. (2004). The short arm of chromosome 3 was consistently lost across several primary tumors and cell lines (Figs. 1 and 2). Three smaller regions within the short arm of chromosome 3 were identified by the automated locus definition program, based on the presence and recurrence of deletions in a subset of samples (Fig. 2, bright green bars). (Reprinted, with permission, from Tonon et al. 2005 [©National Academy of Sciences].)

(♦) High-priority MCRs that are common with the PDAC data set (Aguirre et al. 2004).

(*) MCR in 8p, which was subject to further fine mapping (Figs. 5 and 6, and see text).

(^) The MCR at 11q11 has recently been shown by Sebat et al. (2004) to be a copy number polymorphism (ORF5I1, chromosome 11q11).

genesis of NSCLC were contained within the high-confidence MCRs, including p16^INK4A and RB1 tumor suppressor genes and MYC, EGFR, and KRAS2 oncogenes (Table 1). Additionally, most of the altered regions identified in a recent study using single-nucleotide polymorphism arrays on NSCLC and SCLC samples (Zhao et al. 2005) were included among the high-confidence MCRs in the present study.

The whole short arm of chromosome 3 was consistently lost, as described previously (Zabarovsky et al. 2002; Protopopov et al. 2003; Kashuba et al. 2004), with a peak recurrence at around 50 Mb, corresponding to 3p21.1 (29 of 79 samples, 36%). Segmentation did not identify obvious homozygous deletions that would point to a specific target in this recurrently deleted region of 3p; however, this region contains RASSF1, TUSC2,

SEMA3B, HYAL2, and FHIT, genes that have shown LOH in NSCLC (Figs. 1 and 2) (Lerman and Minna 2000; Balsara and Testa 2002; Danilkovitch-Miagkova et al. 2003; Imreh et al. 2003).

The most notable feature of the high-priority MCR data set was a subset (21 of 93) of highly focal MCRs that spanned less than 0.5 Mb with a median number of only 5 genes (Table 2). From a total of 120 genes (of 139 genes in these 0.5-Mb MCRs) represented on the Affymetrix Plus 2.0 microarray platform, 53 (~40%) demonstrated copy-number-driven expression. Among this subset of genes, some already have an established role in cancer (e.g., ERBB3) or are homologous to known cancer genes (a PTEN-related molecule that is in a region of deletion). Additionally, three members of the cyclin family were present in two different MCRs (cyclin M3, M4, and cy-

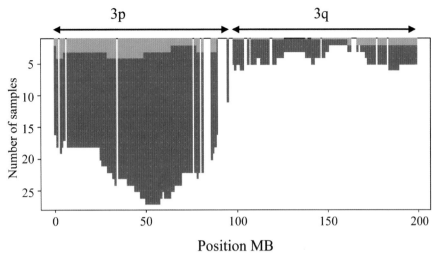

Figure 2. Recurrence of chromosome 3 alterations. Integer-value recurrence of CNAs in segmented data (*y* axis) is plotted for each probe aligned along the *x* axis in chromosome order. Dark green bars denote loss of chromosome material, bright green bars represent probes within regions of deletion. White spaces represent gaps between probes. (Reprinted, with permission, from Tonon et al. 2005 [©National Academy of Sciences].)

Table 2. High-Confidence MCRs in Lung ACs and SCCs, Spanning Less Than 0.5 Mb

| | Minimal common regions (MCRs) | | | | MCR recurrence | | | | | |
| | position | size | max/min | # | gain/loss | | | amp/del | | |
Cytogenetic band	(Mb)	(Mb)	value	transcripts	%	T	C	T	C	Candidates
	Gains/amplification									
1p36.32-1p36.32	2.37-2.47	0.10	2.92	2	22	9	9	3	0	PEX10, RER1
1p34.3-1p34.3	37.82-38.13	0.32	2.16	11	18	7	8	1	1	FLJ31434, YRDC, FLJ45459
1q32.2-1q32.2	206.17-206.24	0.06	1.14	3	39	15	17	1	4	LAMB3
2q11.2-2q11.2	96.68-96.95	0.27	1.39	8	35	14	16	4	4	CNNM3, CNNM4, SEMA4C
2q31.1-2q31.1	170.19-170.32	0.13	2.67	4	28	11	13	1	1	PPIG
5p15.33-5p15.33	**0.53-0.92**	0.38	1.99	5	60	27	24	6	15	BRD9
5q31.3-5q31.3	140.55-140.66	0.12	1.59	11	19	6	10	2	4	PCDHB11, PCDHB12, PCDHB13
8p12-8p11.22*	**38.24-38.45***	0.21	1.98	2	35	17	12	6	4	FGFR1, WHSC1L1, LETM2
10q24.1-10q24.1	97.62-98.11	0.49	1.96	8	16	3	10	1	1	CCNJ
10q26.3-10q26.3	135.24-135.24	0.01	1.04	1	11	1	8	1	3	C10orf94
12q13.2-12q13.2	**54.72-54.84**	0.12	1.98	8	29	10	14	2	2	ERBB3
14q32.13-14q32.13	93.66-94.03	0.37	1.15	9	29	6	18	1	4	KIAA1622
16q22.2-16q22.2	69.62-69.87	0.26	1.4	2	18	6	9	1	4	Hs.368781
18q12.1-18q12.1	26.83-27.31	0.48	1.1	6	19	9	7	2	1	DSC1, DSC2, DSG2
19q13.33-19q13.33	55.52-55.68	0.16	0.73	8	17	5	9	1	1	SPIB
20q11.21-20q11.21	**29.66-29.88**	0.22	1.08	5	42	13	23	1	8	BCL2L1, TPX2
	Loss /deletion									
7q34-7q34	142.28-142.44	0.16	−1.39	4	13	7	4	2	1	LOC154761
11q11-11q11^	55.1-55.18	0.08	−4.06	6	23	13	6	7	1	OR4C11, OR4C6, OR4V1P^
13q12.11-13q12.11	**19.14-19.56**	0.41	−3.51	2	34	14	14	1	7	HSMPP8, PSPC1
13q32.2-13q32.2	**97.47-97.9**	0.42	−3.25	6	29	13	11	1	8	FARP1
21p11.2-21p11.1	**9.93-10.08**	0.15	−1.33	5	17	9	6	1	1	TPTE

The numbers of primary tumors (T) or cell lines (C) with gain or loss, and amplification or deletion, are listed, respectively. See text for other definitions. MCR recurrence is denoted as percentage of the total data set. Number of transcripts is based on build 35, NCBI. Only the known genes within the boundaries have been included. In bold the MCRs verified by RT-PCR and/or FISH (Figs. 5 and 6; data not shown). The genes listed are among the subset of genes within the MCRs showing copy-number-driven expression in the Affymetrix 2.0 Plus. (Reprinted, with permission, from Tonon et al. 2005 [©National Academy of Sciences].)

(*) MCR in 8p, which was subject to further fine mapping (see text).

(^) The MCR at 11q11 has recently been shown by Sebat et al. (2004) to be a copy number polymorphism (ORF5I1, chromosome 11q11).

clin J), and BRD9, a bromodomain gene with potential functional relatedness to BRD4, a gene located within the high-priority MCRs and involved in virus-induced cellular transformation (Table 1; and see Discussion), was also present in one highly focal MCR. These findings highlight the potential for focused and high-yield cancer gene discovery.

Several of the known microRNAs were located within the MCRs (Table 1). The role of microRNA in cancer has been recently established, and the presence of miRNAs within MCRs will require additional study to see whether these genetic elements participate in the development of these lung cancers (Calin et al. 2004a,b; Metzler et al. 2004; He et al. 2005; Lu et al. 2005; O'Donnell et al. 2005).

Common and Distinct Genomic Features in AC and SCC

Next, we sought to determine the common and distinguishing features of the AC and SCC subtypes on the genome level. A comparison of overall copy number variation across the genomes of AC and SCC subtypes revealed a higher degree of genomic complexity in the SCC subtype (Fig. 3). Here, complexity is inferred from the number and size of copy number aberrations detected by an objective change-point or segmentation analysis (Olshen et al. 2004). In this analysis, each contiguous genomic region of uniform copy number is delineated as a segment: Each segment contains a copy number different from its neighboring segments. Borders between adjacent segments mark transition in copy number. The number of segments and the size of these segments are indicators of frequency of CNA across the genome. By comparing the incidences of segmentation within each profile, it is clear that the SCC subtype harbors higher overall segment numbers, particularly of the smaller segment sizes (Fig. 3).

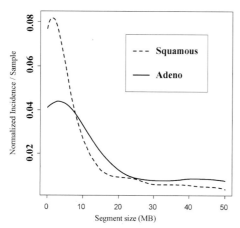

Figure 3. Chromosomal segment length distribution. The incidence of segmentation per sample (*y* axis) is shown as a function of segment size (*x* axis) for squamous (*dashed line*) and adenocarcinoma (*solid line*) samples. Only aberrations of Log2 ratio greater than +0.4 or less than –0.4 are counted. Because segment boundaries are determined by discrete changes in copy number, the number and length of segments within a sample profile are indices of copy number aberration and thus genomic disruption. Note that squamous cell carcinoma samples show a higher incidence of CNA, particularly events less than 2.5 Mb.

Taking a global view of the profiles, however, the comparison of overall copy number variation for high-intensity events across the genomes of these two subtypes revealed near complete overlap, including gains/amplifications at 1q, 5p, and 20q and losses/deletions at 3p and 9p (data not shown). Previous reports using chromosomal CGH and low-resolution array CGH BAC arrays have suggested that the only genomic aberration consistently differentiating SCC from the AC subtype is 3q gain/amplification (Petersen et al. 1997; Bjorkqvist et al. 1998b; Luk et al. 2001; Pei et al. 2001; Balsara and Testa 2002; Massion et al. 2002). We reasoned that with our higher-resolution platform capable of detecting previously unrecognized focal CNAs we might be able to determine whether there exist additional genomic events that are characteristic of either SCC or AC. To determine whether there are recurrent regional gains/amplifications or losses/deletions that might be distinct between these subtypes, the incidence of events in each primary tumor group was compared and significance was estimated by permutation test (Tonon et al. 2005). There were no genomic losses/deletions that could differentiate AC and SCC subtypes. Similarly, there were no gains/amplifications that were unique for the AC subtype. However, one region of gain/amplification on the long arm of chromosome 3, from 180 Mb to 199 Mb, corresponding to 3q26 to 3q29, was significantly targeted in the SSCs (Fig. 4A)—a finding in line with previous reports (Petersen et al. 1997; Bjorkqvist et al. 1998b; Luk et al. 2001; Pei et al. 2001; Balsara and Testa 2002; Massion et al. 2002). Therefore, despite completely distinct histological presentations, SCC and AC are remarkably similar on the genomic level and are likely driven by many of the same oncogenes and tumor suppressor gene mutations.

Given these common and distinct CNA profiles of the NSCLC subsets, we next sought to correlate specific CNAs with expression profile data of the same samples and available expression data sets (Bhattacharjee et al. 2001). In particular, these integrated analyses assessed the extent to which the 3q might drive the subtype-specific expression patterns. As a corollary, by linked subtype expression patterns and copy number gains, it might be possible to identify subtype diagnostics with more direct linkage to disease pathogenesis. We analyzed the global expression profile data for the same NSCLC samples using SAM (Significant Analysis for Microarray Data; Tusher et al. 2001). A total of 297 probes were significantly different between SCCs and ACs, based on a q-value (false discovery rate, FDR) cutoff of 0.05 (Storey and Tibshirani 2003). Upon mapping of these genes to their genomic positions, we used a 10-Mb moving-window analysis across the genome and then applied a Fisher's exact test to identify the genomic regions significantly enriched for differentially expressed probes (Tonon et al. 2005). As shown in Figure 4B, this global analysis again identified 3q 180-199MB as the genomic region whose resident genes were most significantly enriched among the list of differentially expressed genes between AC and SCC. We performed a similar analysis with another recently published lung cancer expression profiling data set (Bhattacharjee et al. 2001), and again, only probes mapping 180-199MB 3q showed a statisti-

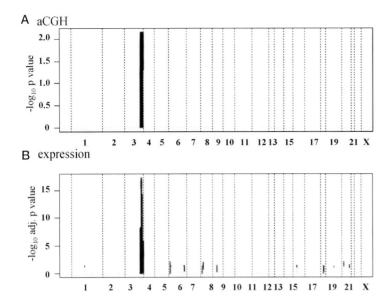

Figure 4. Chromosome 3q, from 180 Mb to 199 Mb, is the only genomic region that shows significant difference between AC and SCC by both aCGH and expression profiling. On both plots, *x*-axis coordinates represent probes ordered by genomic map positions, from chromosome 1 to chromosome X. (*A*) Probes significantly gained/amplified comparing SCC and AC primary tumors, on array-CGH. *y* axis represents the $-\log_{10} p$ value of the permutation test. Probes presenting a $p<0.05$ are plotted in black, probes with a $p>0.05$ in gray. No probes were significantly lost/deleted after comparison between SCC and AC primary tumors. (*B*) Genomic regions significantly enriched for differentially expressed probes comparing SCC and AC primary tumors. *y* axis represents the $-\log_{10}$ adjusted *p* values of Fisher's exact test for enrichment. Black lines highlight regions with an adjusted $p<0.05$ adjusted for multiple testing, probes with an adjusted $p>0.05$ are in gray. (Reprinted, with permission, from Tonon et al. 2005 [©National Academy of Sciences].)

cally significant enrichment (data not shown). These findings suggest that genes residing within this region on chromosome 3 often show copy-number-driven expression in SCCs.

Gain/amplification of 3q is present in many, but not all, cases of SCC, 54% in our samples and between 50% and 85% in the literature (Petersen et al. 1997; Bjorkqvist et al. 1998b; Luk et al. 2001; Pei et al. 2001; Balsara and Testa 2002; Massion et al. 2002). Given the certain importance of this locus in SCC pathogenesis, we sought to determine whether a subset of probes residing within the 3q180-Mb to 199-Mb region would exhibit robust expression via mechanisms other than gain/amplification consistent with their key role in SCC development. To this end, a one-way ANOVA and a post-hoc Bonferroni test using all the Affymetrix Plus 2.0 probes ($n = 166$, corresponding to 106 genes) residing within the 180-Mb to 199-Mb boundaries on 3q identified a subset of genes showing significant overexpression in SCCs versus ACs, even in the absence of gene copy number gains on 3q in SCCs: p63, Claudin 1, Phosphatidylinositol glycan, class X, and discs large homolog 1. The p63 gene is most notable, given its seminal role in squamous tissue development and its links to squamous cancer subtypes (Massion et al. 2003; Koster et al. 2004; McKeon 2004; Westfall and Pietenpol 2004). In conclusion, based on the given level of resolution, our integrated aCGH and expression analyses strongly implicate a limited number of genes residing within 3q as key potential drivers of the SCC histopathological phenotype.

Cross Tumor Type Genomic Comparisons

The large number of MCRs prompted us to merge the NSCLC data set with another high-resolution pancreatic ductal adenocarcinoma (PDAC) data set (64 MCRs identified in Aguirre et al. 2004) in an effort to identify loci of prime relevance to epithelial carcinogenesis. Comparison of NSCLC and PDAC was motivated by their common

epithelial origin, similar clinical aggressiveness, commonality in signature mutations (KRAS, c-Myc, p53, INK4a/ARF, among others), and extreme genomic complexity. As expected, these comparisons identified several loci that are known to be commonly targeted in these cancers including KRAS, c-MYC, and INK4a/ARF loci (data not shown), as well as other novel loci. Among these novel loci were two focal amplicons—one at 8p12-p11.2 (position 37.84-39.72) encompassing FGFR1 and another at 20q11 (position 29.66-29.88 MB).

The presence of FGFR1, a cancer-relevant gene not previously implicated in lung cancer, prompted a detailed mapping of the 8p12-p11.2 amplicon. Real-time quantitative PCR (QPCR) and FISH on all eight samples (two cell lines and six primary tumors) confirmed the presence of a high-copy-number amplicon at 8p (Figs. 5 and 6). Based on two informative primary tumor cases, PT3 and PT5, this analysis defined the MCR as 0.14 Mb in size and containing only two annotated genes: WHSC1L1 and LETM2 (Fig. 5A). As QPCR analysis clearly positioned the FGFR1 gene outside of the telomeric boundary of this MCR, and previous studies have implicated FGFR1 as the prime target of 8p amplicon in other cancer types (Simon et al. 2001; Edwards et al. 2003; Mao et al. 2003), interphase FISH was used to verify the amplicon boundaries in several informative samples. Consistent with QPCR data, FISH with a BAC outside of the MCR and including FGFR1 on PT3 revealed only two copies (Fig. 6B), providing clear evidence that FGFR1 is not amplified in this sample.

Since CNAs are believed to be one of the mechanisms for altered gene expression, integration of DNA copy number and RNA expression data can serve as an effective early filter for culling bystanders from true targets (Pollack et al. 2002). To this end, we assessed the expression pattern of genes residing within this MCR both by gene expression profiling and by directed RT-QPCR (Fig. 7). The expression patterns of the MCR resident genes (WHSC1L1 and LETM2) and neighboring genes

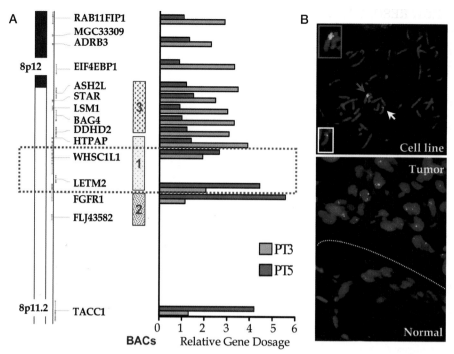

Figure 5. Verification and boundary delimitation of the 8p12-p11.2 amplicon. (*A*) Real-time PCR verification of the 8p amplicon and its boundaries. Two primary tumors were used to delimit the boundaries, PT3 and PT5. The dotted blue square includes the genes involved in the amplicon. (*B*) (*Upper panel*) Metaphase FISH analysis of the cell line NCI-H1703 showing multiple green signals on one derivative chromosome (*red arrow* and *top inset*; *green signal*, BAC#2). A normal copy of chromosome 8 is also evident (*white arrow* and *bottom inset*) showing two signals for BAC#2 (*green*) and two signals for the control BAC (RP11-138J2, *red* signal). (*Lower panel*) Interphase FISH analysis on a section from the primary tumor PT3, comparing adjacent normal and tumor tissues. Note multiple, high-intensity signals with BAC#1 (*green*) in the tumor part and single or double signals with BAC#1 in the normal part of the section. Control BAC, RP11-138J2, red signal. (Reprinted, with permission, from Tonon et al. 2005 [©National Academy of Sciences].)

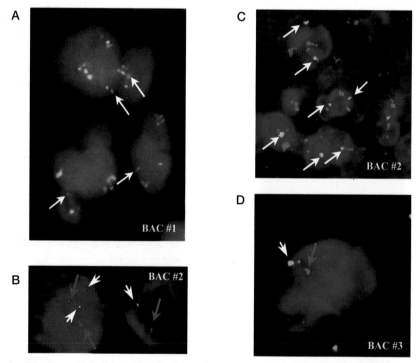

Figure 6. FISH analysis of the 8p amplicon in a section from the primary tumor PT3 and PT5 to define the boundaries of the amplicon. (*A*) Interphase FISH analysis on a tissue section from the primary tumor PT3, showing multiple high-intensity signals when using BAC#1 (*green*). (*White arrow*) Control BAC (RP11-138J2, *red signal*). (*B*) Interphase FISH analysis on a tissue section from the primary tumor PT3, showing two signals per cell, for both BAC#2 (*red signal, red arrow*) and control BAC (RP11-138J2, *green signal, white arrow*). (*C*) Interphase FISH analysis on a tissue section from the primary tumor PT5, showing multiple high-intensity signals when using BAC#2 (*red signal*). (*White arrow*) Control BAC (RP11-138J2, *green signal*). (*D*) Interphase FISH analysis on a tissue section from the primary tumor PT5, showing two signals per cell, for both BAC#3 (*red signal, red arrow*) and control BAC (RP11-138J2, *green signal, white arrow*). (Reprinted, with permission, from Tonon et al. 2005 [©National Academy of Sciences].)

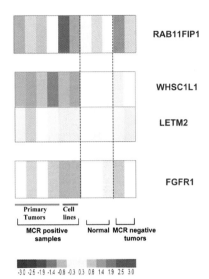

Primary   Cell
Tumors   lines

MCR positive   Normal MCR negative
samples   tumors

-3.0 -2.5 -1.9 -1.4 -0.8 -0.3 0.3 0.8 1.4 1.9 2.5 3.0

Figure 7. Expression analyses of genes residing in the chromosome 8p amplicon. Heat map representation of the expression level of each of the genes in the amplicon from Affymetrix analysis. When multiple Affymetrix probes for a gene were present, the median value among the probes was used. Each column represents an individual sample, and each row represents a gene. The color intensity on the heat map correlates with the intensity of the expression, red representing overexpression and blue indicating reduced expression. The MCR-positive samples include four of six SCC primary tumors demonstrating the 8p amplicon and NCI-H1703 and NCI-H520, two lung cancer cell lines with the 8p amplicon. Normal represents three independent normal RNA references, isolated from adjacent histologically normal lung tissues; MCR-negative tumors are two primary tumors not showing amplification at 8p. (Reprinted, with permission, from Tonon et al. 2005 [©National Academy of Sciences].)

(RAB11FIP1 and FGFR1, positioned external to the telomeric and centromeric boundaries of the MCR, respectively) were assessed. As shown in Figure 7, only WHSC1L1 exhibited robust expression in those samples harboring the amplicon, whereas LETM2 showed low and inconsistent expression in the presence or absence of amplification. FGFR1 showed an expression pattern that was consistent with placement outside the amplicon MCR.

To evaluate further the relevance of WHSC1L1 relative to FGFR1 in lung cancer, the biological impact of siRNA-mediated knockdown of each target was assessed in cell lines with and without 8p amplification (NCI-H1703 and NCI-H1395, respectively). For all genes, RT-QPCR documented >70% knockdown following SMART siRNA pool transduction (data not shown). In soft agar assays with NCI-H1703, siRNA-mediated knockdown of WHSC1L1 resulted in 50% reduction in the number of H1703 soft agar colonies, whereas near complete FGFR1 depletion had no impact on colony formation in soft agar. As expected, knockdown of these two genes had no effect on NCI-H1395 colony formation. The copy-number-driven expression data, coupled with knockdown studies, argue against a role for FGFR1 in lung cancers harboring an 8p amplicon and point to another gene, WHSC1L1, as the potential target of the amplification event.

Another amplicon present in both NSCLC and PDAC mapped to 20q11.2 and was detected in one primary lung AC, one adenosquamous cell line, one SCC cell line, and 2 AC cell lines. These samples together delimited the MCR to 220 kb, spanning position 29.66 to 29.88 Mb and containing five genes: ID1, COX4I2, BCL2L1, TPX2, and MYLK2. Although BCL2L1, a known oncogene implicated in multiple cancer types, indeed exhibited modestly elevated expression, another gene in the amplicon, TPX2, showed high-level expression in most lung cell lines and primary tumors tested, even in the absence of amplification, when compared with RNA derived from normal lung (Fig. 8). These findings suggest that, in addition to a known oncogene BCL2L1, TPX2 is a potential candidate oncogene targeted for amplification in both lung and pancreas cancers.

DISCUSSION

This study has revealed a highly complex and rearranged NSCLC genome with many previously unrecognized regions of amplification and deletion with potential pathogenetic relevance to this lethal disease. In particular, we have identified and defined 93 high-confidence

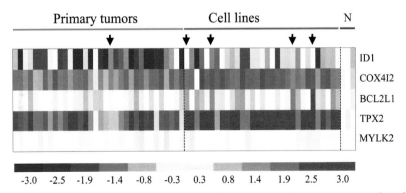

-3.0   -2.5   -1.9   -1.4   -0.8   -0.3   0.3   0.8   1.4   1.9   2.5   3.0

Figure 8. Expression analyses of genes residing in the chromosome 20q11 amplicon. Heat map representation of the expression level of each of the five genes, ID1, COX4I2, BCL2L1, TPX2, and MYLK2, in the amplicon from Affymetrix analysis. When multiple Affymetrix probes for a gene were present, the median value among the probes was used. Each column represents an individual sample, and each row represents a gene. The color intensity on the heat map correlates with the intensity of the expression, red representing overexpression and blue indicating reduced expression. The arrows indicate the samples that present amplification. (Reprinted, with permission, from Tonon et al. 2005 [©National Academy of Sciences].)

CNAs. It is notable that 22% of these span less than 0.5 Mb with a median of five resident genes. The significance of these findings rests on the fact that, to date, only a limited number of genes have been shown to be critical for the pathogenesis and maintenance of non-small-cell lung cancer (Minna et al. 2002). The identification, based on integrated DNA–RNA analyses, of candidate targets with plausible or known links to cancers resident within these focal CNAs reinforces the validity of the approach employed in this study.

Upon analysis of the highly focal CNAs, a number of genes emerged as strong oncogene and tumor suppressor gene candidates. Most notable were two loci harboring genes with structural similarity to known cancer genes: TPTE, related to PTEN (Walker et al. 2001), and BRD9, a bromodomain protein, related to BRD4 (You et al. 2004). Indeed, BRD4 mapped to a high-confidence MCR spanning 1.2 Mb on chromosome 19 and showed high-level expression (Table 1). Other genes located within these small amplicons and showing a strong correlation with expression level included YRDC, a ribosome maturation factor, and Laminin Beta 3, which has been shown to be overexpressed in NSCLC cell lines (Manda et al. 2000). In addition, three recently described cyclins of unknown function—J, M3, and M4—resided in two different MCRs and all showed overexpression. Other notable genes residing in the focal MCRs included members of the semaphorin family, in two different amplicons, and proteins involved in the desmosome structure, as Desmocollin 1 and 2, and Desmoglein 2. ERBB3 was among the genes showing copy-number-driven expression, consistent with recent reports of ERBB3 overexpression in NSCLC (Amann et al. 2005; Muller-Tidow et al. 2005). Indeed, all of the above mentioned genes showed copy-number-driven expression, and further analysis through Oncomine (Rhodes et al. 2004) showed that most of these genes were significantly deregulated in other cancer types relative to normal tissue controls. Finally, it is worth emphasizing that, in a number of the cases cited above, highly related genes were targeted in distinct amplification and deletion events in different tumor samples, suggesting that these functionally related molecules are critical in the development of NSCLC.

Our high-resolution genome-wide analysis has also uncovered a difference in overall genomic complexity between the two major subtypes of NSCLC. Specifically, the SCC subtype harbors genomic features suggestive of a much higher degree of genomic instability compared to the AC subtype, consistent with previous reports (Massion et al. 2002). Yet, it is striking that despite these widespread genomic differences, only one chromosomal region, at 3q26-q29, is consistently different between these two histological phenotypes, as previously suggested (Petersen et al. 1997; Bjorkqvist et al. 1998b; Luk et al. 2001; Pei et al. 2001; Balsara and Testa 2002; Massion et al. 2002). Of potential significance is the observation that this region has been reported to be the most common and early genetic alteration in SCC of the head and neck, a group of tumors that share similar developmental, histological, and pathogenetic features with SCCs of the lung (Huang et al. 2002). One potential explanation for

this similarity is that these two histological subtypes of lung cancer are derived from the same lung stem/precursor cell and that only a few unique genetic alterations are sufficient to confer either an AC or a SCC phenotype. Indeed, there is some experimental evidence that the alveolar type II cell is a pluripotential stem cell involved in the genesis of both human AC and SCC (Ten Have-Opbroek et al. 1997). Our results suggest that, in a subset of lung SCCs, overexpression of genes residing within 3q, mediated either by amplification or by other mechanisms, could selectively induce a squamous cell phenotype against the backdrop of a genetic background that is otherwise common between ACs and SCCs. Interestingly, among the genes that did show overexpression in SCC samples irrespectively of copy number changes, there was p63. Overexpression of p63 has been reported in several squamous carcinomas (Massion et al. 2003; McKeon 2004), and mutations in p63 have been reported in human genetic disorders affecting ectodermal development (Westfall and Pietenpol 2004). In the mouse, p63 deficiency leads to profound defects or frank loss of the entire spectrum of epithelial tissues (McKeon 2004). Conditional transgenic mice expressing p63 isoforms in the epithelial lining of the bronchioles developed severe squamous metaplasia in the lung (Koster et al. 2004). These collective findings support the view that p63 exerts a critical role in maintaining the proliferative capacity of epidermal cell population as well as driving an epithelial stratification program (McKeon 2004). On the basis of our data and the prerogatives of the genes overexpressed in 3q, it is tempting to speculate that AC and SCC arise from a common cellular origin and are driven to a malignant end point by common genetic and biological mechanisms.

Despite this discovery advance, this very large number of amplifications in human lung cancer presents significant challenges in prioritizing those amplified oncogenes for in-depth validation and ultimate enlistment into drug discovery and development. Given the common and overlapping role of many bona fide oncogenes or tumor suppressor genes across multiple cancer types, we tested the assumption that the comparison with array-CGH data sets from other cancer types could identify common CNAs harboring highly important oncogenes or tumor suppressor genes. To this end, we compared the NSCLC genome with that of pancreatic ductal adenocarcinoma (PA) (Aguirre et al. 2004). These comparisons identified several loci that are known to be commonly targeted in these cancers, including KRAS, c-MYC, and INK4a/ARF loci, as well as other loci not described previously.

Although novel for NSCLC, the amplicon on chromosome 8p has been observed in several other cancer types, including breast, prostate, bladder carcinomas, and T-cell lymphomas (Dib et al. 1995; Simon et al. 2001; Edwards et al. 2003; Mao et al. 2003; Ray et al. 2004). Although FGFR1 resides within this larger CNA and has been considered the prime candidate target of this amplification, detailed QPCR and FISH mapping performed in this study defined both boundaries and narrowed the minimal common region that excludes the FGFR1 gene.

Gene dosage alterations represent a common mechanism of oncogene activation and tumor suppressor inactivation by modulating expression of their target genes. Thus, integration of DNA copy number with expression provides a powerful early filter for culling bystanders of CNAs. In other words, it seems reasonable to assume that the true target of a CNA would exhibit altered expression in a copy-number-driven manner. However, definition of over- or underexpressed levels is itself a major challenge, particularly in cases where the true cell of origin remains unknown, and thus a premalignant physiological frame of reference is not available. In this study, we utilized three independent normal RNA references, isolated from adjacent histologically normal lung tissues (data not shown). Using such as reference, one can tentatively eliminate LETM2 as a candidate for this amplicon based on its lack of overexpression despite increased copy number (Fig. 7). Correspondingly, expression analysis demonstrated that FGFR1 was not overexpressed in most of the samples harboring this amplicon, and sequence analysis of exons encoding the juxtamembrane and kinase domains of FGFR1 failed to reveal any mutations. These findings in lung cancer are consistent with recent studies in breast cancer showing that FGFR1 does not play a pathogenetic role in breast cancer cells harboring amplification of this 8p locus (Dib et al. 1995; Ray et al. 2004), thereby pointing to other resident gene(s) as the true target of this 8p12-p11.2.

The gene that appears to be the most likely candidate target for this amplicon is WHSC1L1, on the basis of the physical mapping data, copy-driven expression patterns, and functional assay results. Additionally, data from the literature strongly point to this gene as causally involved in hematological and solid tumors. WHSC1L1 is involved in a chromosomal translocation in acute myeloid leukemia, t(8;11)(p11.2;p15), that preserves all the domains in WHSC1L1 excluding one PWWP domain (Rosati et al. 2002). In addition, amplification of WHSC1L1 has been demonstrated in breast cancer (Angrand et al. 2001). Several members of the SET2 family of histone lysine methyltransferases, to which this gene belongs, have roles in cancer (Schneider et al. 2002). In particular, the two homologs of WHSC1L1, NSD1 and WHSC1, have been implicated in acute myeloid leukemia and multiple myeloma, respectively (Stec et al. 1998; Jaju et al. 2001). Together, these data provide a compelling case for WHSC1L1 as a novel lung cancer oncogene and as a prime target for amplification in NSCLC.

The chromosome 20 amplicon MCR contained five genes, and only BCL2L1 (known as BCL-xL) and TPX2 showed copy-number-driven expression. The identification of BCL2L1 suggests that gene amplification is one of the mechanisms driving BCL2L1 activation in NSCLC. The relevance of BCL2L1 amplification and overexpression in the development of NSCLC is strengthened by previous studies establishing a critical oncogenic role for BCL2L1 in PDAC (Bold et al. 2001; Xu et al. 2001; Trauzold et al. 2003). TPX2 is also a strong candidate target for amplification, and its frequent overexpression is observed in the presence or absence of amplification. TPX2 is required for targeting Aurora A kinase to the spindle

apparatus. Elevated expression of Aurora A has been reported in breast, bladder, colon, ovarian, and pancreatic cancers and correlates with chromosomal instability and clinically aggressive disease. Up to 62% of breast cancers overexpress Aurora A, even where gene amplification is not detected. Elevated Aurora A expression causes abnormalities in mitosis and chromosome segregation and ectopically expressed Aurora A can transform rodent cells (Bischoff et al. 1998; Miyoshi et al. 2001; Anand et al. 2003). However, no reports of specific amplification or overexpression of this gene have been reported so far in NSCLC, a finding consistent with the absence of Aurora Kinase A gene amplification in our data set. TPX2 activates Aurora Kinase A (Gruss et al. 2002) and when overexpressed, it induces accumulation of cells in G_2-M phase and polyploidization (Heidebrecht et al. 2003). Manda et al. (1999) have demonstrated that this gene is overexpressed in lung cancer tissue when compared with normal lung. TPX2 expression is tightly correlated with poor prognosis in patients with neuroblastoma (Krams et al. 2003). Additionally, using Oncomine (Rhodes et al. 2004), we compared the expression level of TPX2 in different cancer types to the corresponding levels in normal tissues. Lung SCCs and ACs, lung small-cell carcinomas (Bhattacharjee et al. 2001; Garber et al. 2001), as well as prostate (Dhanasekaran et al. 2001; LaTulippe et al. 2002) and hepatocellular carcinoma (Chen et al. 2002) showed significant overexpression of TPX2 when compared with the respective normal tissues. Intriguingly, in our expression data, a high correlation existed between TPX2 and Aurora Kinase A expression (r = 0.7801, $p<0.001$) and even more with many other genes involved in spindle formation and mitotic progression, as for example, Bub1 (r = 0.93, $p<0.001$), CDC20 (r = 0.93, $p<0.001$), Aurora Kinase B (r = 0.90, $p<0.001$). The amplification of TPX2 and the correlation of its expression with genes involved in spindle formation and progression through the cell cycle suggest a possible critical role for TPX2 in lung and pancreas carcinogenesis.

In conclusion, using gene-specific CGH platforms and novel custom bioinformatics tools, along with integration of expression profiles, we have identified many new recurrent amplifications and deletions in the NSCLC genome. The high degree of NSCLC genomic complexity, the recurrent nature of these lesions, and preliminary functional characterization of resident genes support the view that a large number of important oncogenes and tumor suppressor genes remain to be identified, opening potential therapeutic and diagnostic opportunities for this dismal disease.

ACKNOWLEDGMENTS

We are grateful to Drs. Ruben Carrasco, Elizabeth Maher, Ergun Sahin, Omar Kabbarah, Mariela Jaskelioff, and Aram Hezel for helpful discussions and manuscript revisions, and to Chris Leo, Melissa Donovan, and Ilana Perna for superb technical advice and support. Array-CGH profiles were performed at the Arthur and Rochelle Belfer Cancer Genomic Center at Dana-Farber Cancer Institute. G.T. is supported by a grant from The Fund to

Cure Myeloma and a SPORE Multiple Myeloma Career Development Award. K.K.W. is supported by a National Institutes of Health (NIH) grant K08AG 2400401, the Sidney Kimmel Foundation for Cancer Research, and the Joan Scarangello Foundation to Conquer Lung Cancer. L.C. is supported by NIH grants RO1 CA099041 and UO1 U01-CA084313-07. R.A.D. is an American Cancer Society Research Professor and an Ellison Medical Foundation Senior Scholar and is supported by grants from the American Cancer Society and the NIH (U01-CA084313-07 and R01 CA084628-12).

REFERENCES

Aguirre A.J., Brennan C., Bailey G., Sinha R., Feng B., Leo C., Zhang Y., Zhang J., Gans J.D., Bardeesy N., Cauwels C., Cordon-Cardo C., Redston M.S., DePinho R.A., and Chin L. 2004. High-resolution characterization of the pancreatic adenocarcinoma genome. *Proc. Natl. Acad. Sci.* **101:** 9067.

Albertson D.G. and Pinkel D. 2003. Genomic microarrays in human genetic disease and cancer. *Hum. Mol. Genet.* **12:** 145R.

Amann J., Kalyankrishna S., Massion P.P., Ohm J.E., Girard L., Shigematsu H., Peyton M., Juroske D., Huang Y., Stuart Salmon J., Kim Y.H., Pollack J.R., Yanagisawa K., Gazdar A., Minna J.D., Kurie J.M., and Carbone D.P. 2005. Aberrant epidermal growth factor receptor signaling and enhanced sensitivity to EGFR inhibitors in lung cancer. *Cancer Res.* **65:** 226.

Anand S., Penrhyn-Lowe S., and Venkitaraman A.R. 2003. AURORA-A amplification overrides the mitotic spindle assembly checkpoint, inducing resistance to Taxol. *Cancer Cell* **3:** 51.

Angrand P.O., Apiou F., Stewart A.F., Dutrillaux B., Losson R., and Chambon P. 2001. NSD3, a new SET domain-containing gene, maps to 8p12 and is amplified in human breast cancer cell lines. *Genomics* **74:** 79.

Balsara B.R. and Testa J.R. 2002. Chromosomal imbalances in human lung cancer. *Oncogene* **21:** 6877.

Bhattacharjee A., Richards W.G., Staunton J., Li C., Monti S., Vasa P., Ladd C., Beheshti J., Bueno R., Gillette M., Loda M., Weber G., Mark E.J., Lander E.S., Wong W., Johnson B.E., Golub T.R., Sugarbaker D.J., and Meyerson M. 2001. Classification of human lung carcinomas by mRNA expression profiling reveals distinct adenocarcinoma subclasses. *Proc. Natl. Acad. Sci.* **98:** 13790.

Bischoff J.R., Anderson L., Zhu Y., Mossie K., Ng L., Souza B., Schryver B., Flanagan P., Clairvoyant F., Ginther C., Chan C.S., Novotny M., Slamon D.J., and Plowman G.D. 1998. A homologue of *Drosophila* aurora kinase is oncogenic and amplified in human colorectal cancers. *EMBO J.* **17:** 3052.

Bjorkqvist A.M., Tammilehto L., Nordling S., Nurminen M., Anttila S., Mattson K., and Knuutila S. 1998a. Comparison of DNA copy number changes in malignant mesothelioma, adenocarcinoma and large-cell anaplastic carcinoma of the lung. *Br. J. Cancer* **77:** 260.

Bjorkqvist A.M., Husgafvel-Pursiainen K., Anttila S., Karjalainen A., Tammilehto L., Mattson K., Vainio H., and Knuutila S. 1998b. DNA gains in 3q occur frequently in squamous cell carcinoma of the lung, but not in adenocarcinoma. *Genes Chromosomes Cancer* **22:** 79.

Bold R.J., Virudachalam S., and McConkey D.J. 2001. BCL2 expression correlates with metastatic potential in pancreatic cancer cell lines. *Cancer* **92:** 1122.

Calin G.A., Sevignani C., Dumitru C.D., Hyslop T., Noch E., Yendamuri S., Shimizu M., Rattan S., Bullrich F., Negrini M., and Croce C.M. 2004a. Human microRNA genes are frequently located at fragile sites and genomic regions involved in cancers. *Proc. Natl. Acad. Sci.* **101:** 2999.

Calin G.A., Liu C.G., Sevignani C., Ferracin M., Felli N., Dumitru C.D., Shimizu M., Cimmino A., Zupo S., Dono M., Dell'Aquila M.L., Alder H., Rassenti L., Kipps T.J., Bullrich F., Negrini M., and Croce C.M. 2004b. MicroRNA profiling reveals distinct signatures in B cell chronic lymphocytic leukemias. *Proc. Natl. Acad. Sci.* **101:** 11755.

Chen X., Cheung S.T., So S., Fan S.T., Barry C., Higgins J., Lai K.M., Ji J., Dudoit S., Ng I.O., Van De Rijn M., Botstein D., and Brown P.O. 2002. Gene expression patterns in human liver cancers. *Mol. Biol. Cell* **13:** 1929.

Danilkovitch-Miagkova A., Duh F.M., Kuzmin I., Angeloni D., Liu S.L., Miller A.D., and Lerman M.I. 2003. Hyaluronidase 2 negatively regulates RON receptor tyrosine kinase and mediates transformation of epithelial cells by jaagsiekte sheep retrovirus. *Proc. Natl. Acad. Sci.* **100:** 4580.

Dhanasekaran S.M., Barrette T.R., Ghosh D., Shah R., Varambally S., Kurachi K., Pienta K.J., Rubin M.A., and Chinnaiyan A.M. 2001. Delineation of prognostic biomarkers in prostate cancer. *Nature* **412:** 822.

Dib A., Adelaide J., Chaffanet M., Imbert A., Le Paslier D., Jacquemier J., Gaudray P., Theillet C., Birnbaum D., and Pebusque M.J. 1995. Characterization of the region of the short arm of chromosome 8 amplified in breast carcinoma. *Oncogene* **10:** 995.

Edwards J., Krishna N.S., Witton C.J., and Bartlett J.M. 2003. Gene amplifications associated with the development of hormone-resistant prostate cancer. *Clin. Cancer Res.* **9:** 5271.

Futreal P.A., Coin L., Marshall M., Down T., Hubbard T., Wooster R., Rahman N., and Stratton M.R. 2004. A census of human cancer genes. *Nat. Rev. Cancer* **4:** 177.

Garber M.E., Troyanskaya O.G., Schluens K., Petersen S., Thaesler Z., Pacyna-Gengelbach M., van de Rijn M., Rosen G.D., Perou C.M., Whyte R.I., Altman R.B., Brown P.O., Botstein D., and Petersen I. 2001. Diversity of gene expression in adenocarcinoma of the lung. *Proc. Natl. Acad. Sci.* **98:** 13784.

Gruss O.J., Wittmann M., Yokoyama H., Pepperkok R., Kufer T., Sillje H., Karsenti E., Mattaj I.W., and Vernos I. 2002. Chromosome-induced microtubule assembly mediated by TPX2 is required for spindle formation in HeLa cells. *Nat. Cell Biol.* **4:** 871.

He L., Thomson J.M., Hemann M.T., Hernando-Monge E., Mu D., Goodson S., Powers S., Cordon-Cardo C., Lowe S.W., Hannon G.J., and Hammond S.M. 2005. A microRNA polycistron as a potential human oncogene. *Nature* **435:** 828.

Heidebrecht H.J., Adam-Klages S., Szczepanowski M., Pollmann M., Buck F., Endl E., Kruse M.L., Rudolph P., and Parwaresch R. 2003. repp86: A human protein associated with the progression of mitosis. *Mol. Cancer Res.* **1:** 271.

Huang Q., Yu G.P., McCormick S.A., Mo J., Datta B., Mahimkar M., Lazarus P., Schaffer A.A., Desper R., and Schantz S.P. 2002. Genetic differences detected by comparative genomic hybridization in head and neck squamous cell carcinomas from different tumor sites: Construction of oncogenetic trees for tumor progression. *Genes Chromosomes Cancer* **34:** 224.

Imreh S., Klein G., and Zabarovsky E.R. 2003. Search for unknown tumor-antagonizing genes. *Genes Chromosomes Cancer* **38:** 307.

Jaju R.J., Fidler C., Haas O.A., Strickson A.J., Watkins F., Clark K., Cross N.C., Cheng J.F., Aplan P.D., Kearney L., Boultwood J., and Wainscoat J.S. 2001. A novel gene, NSD1, is fused to NUP98 in the t(5;11)(q35;p15.5) in de novo childhood acute myeloid leukemia. *Blood* **98:** 1264.

Kallioniemi O.P., Kallioniemi A., Piper J., Isola J., Waldman F.M., Gray J.W., and Pinkel D. 1994. Optimizing comparative genomic hybridization for analysis of DNA sequence copy number changes in solid tumors. *Genes Chromosomes Cancer* **10:** 231.

Kashuba V.I., Li J., Wang F., Senchenko V.N., Protopopov A., Malyukova A., Kutsenko A.S., Kadyrova E., Zabarovska V.I., Muravenko O.V., Zelenin A.V., Kisselev L.L., Kuzmin I., Minna J.D., Winberg G., Ernberg I., Braga E., Lerman M.I., Klein G., and Zabarovsky E.R. 2004. RBSP3 (HYA22) is a tumor suppressor gene implicated in major epithelial malignancies. *Proc. Natl. Acad. Sci.* **101:** 4906.

Koster M.I., Kim S., Mills A.A., DeMayo F.J., and Roop D.R. 2004. p63 is the molecular switch for initiation of an epithelial stratification program. *Genes Dev.* **18:** 126.

Krams M., Heidebrecht H.J., Hero B., Berthold F., Harms D., Parwaresch R., and Rudolph P. 2003. Repp86 expression and outcome in patients with neuroblastoma. *J. Clin. Oncol.* **21:** 1810.

LaTulippe E., Satagopan J., Smith A., Scher H., Scardino P., Reuter V., and Gerald W.L. 2002. Comprehensive gene expression analysis of prostate cancer reveals distinct transcriptional programs associated with metastatic disease. *Cancer Res.* **62:** 4499.

Lerman M.I. and Minna J.D. 2000. The 630-kb lung cancer homozygous deletion region on human chromosome 3p21.3: Identification and evaluation of the resident candidate tumor suppressor genes. The International Lung Cancer Chromosome 3p21.3 Tumor Suppressor Gene Consortium. *Cancer Res.* **60:** 6116.

Lu J., Getz G., Miska E.A., Alvarez-Saavedra E., Lamb J., Peck D., Sweet-Cordero A., Ebert B.L., Mak R.H., Ferrando A.A., Downing J.R., Jacks T., Horvitz H.R., and Golub T.R. 2005. MicroRNA expression profiles classify human cancers. *Nature* **435:** 834.

Luk C., Tsao M.S., Bayani J., Shepherd F., and Squire J.A. 2001. Molecular cytogenetic analysis of non-small cell lung carcinoma by spectral karyotyping and comparative genomic hybridization. *Cancer Genet. Cytogenet.* **125:** 87.

Lynch T.J., Bell D.W., Sordella R., Gurubhagavatula S., Okimoto R.A., Brannigan B.W., Harris P.L., Haserlat S.M., Supko J.G., Haluska F.G., Louis D.N., Christiani D.C., Settleman J., and Haber D.A. 2004. Activating mutations in the epidermal growth factor receptor underlying responsiveness of non-small-cell lung cancer to gefitinib. *N. Engl. J. Med.* **350:** 2129.

Manda R., Kohno T., Matsuno Y., Takenoshita S., Kuwano H., and Yokota J. 1999. Identification of genes (SPON2 and C20orf2) differentially expressed between cancerous and noncancerous lung cells by mRNA differential display. *Genomics* **61:** 5.

Manda R., Kohno T., Niki T., Yamada T., Takenoshita S., Kuwano H., and Yokota J. 2000. Differential expression of the LAMB3 and LAMC2 genes between small cell and non-small cell lung carcinomas. *Biochem. Biophys. Res. Commun.* **275:** 440.

Mao X., Onadim Z., Price E.A., Child F., Lillington D.M., Russell-Jones R., Young B.D., and Whittaker S. 2003. Genomic alterations in blastic natural killer/extranodal natural killer-like T cell lymphoma with cutaneous involvement. *J. Invest. Dermatol.* **121:** 618.

Massion P.P., Taflan P.M., Jamshedur Rahman S.M., Yildiz P., Shyr Y., Edgerton M.E., Westfall M.D., Roberts J.R., Pietenpol J.A., Carbone D.P., and Gonzalez A.L. 2003. Significance of p63 amplification and overexpression in lung cancer development and prognosis. *Cancer Res.* **63:** 7113.

Massion P.P., Kuo W.L., Stokoe D., Olshen A.B., Treseler P.A., Chin K., Chen C., Polikoff D., Jain A.N., Pinkel D., Albertson D.G., Jablons D.M., and Gray J.W. 2002. Genomic copy number analysis of non-small cell lung cancer using array comparative genomic hybridization: Implications of the phosphatidylinositol 3-kinase pathway. *Cancer Res.* **62:** 3636.

McKeon F. 2004. p63 and the epithelial stem cell: More than status quo? *Genes Dev.* **18:** 465.

Metzler M., Wilda M., Busch K., Viehmann S., and Borkhardt A. 2004. High expression of precursor microRNA-155/BIC RNA in children with Burkitt lymphoma. *Genes Chromosomes Cancer* **39:** 167.

Minna J.D., Roth J.A., and Gazdar A.F. 2002. Focus on lung cancer. *Cancer Cell* **1:** 49.

Miyoshi Y., Iwao K., Egawa C., and Noguchi S. 2001. Association of centrosomal kinase STK15/BTAK mRNA expression with chromosomal instability in human breast cancers. *Int. J. Cancer* **92:** 370.

Muller-Tidow C., Diederichs S., Bulk E., Pohle T., Steffen B., Schwable J., Plewka S., Thomas M., Metzger R., Schneider P.M., Brandts C.H., Berdel W.E., and Serve H. 2005. Identification of metastasis-associated receptor tyrosine kinases in non-small cell lung cancer. *Cancer Res.* **65:** 1778.

O'Donnell K.A., Wentzel E.A., Zeller K.I., Dang C.V., and Mendell J.T. 2005. c-Myc-regulated microRNAs modulate E2F1 expression. *Nature* **435:** 839.

Olshen A.B., Venkatraman E.S., Lucito R., and Wigler M. 2004. Circular binary segmentation for the analysis of array-based DNA copy number data. *Biostatistics* **5:** 557.

Paez J.G., Janne P.A., Lee J.C., Tracy S., Greulich H., Gabriel S., Herman P., Kaye F.J., Lindeman N., Boggon T.J., Naoki K., Sasaki H., Fujii Y., Eck M.J., Sellers W.R., Johnson B.E., and Meyerson M. 2004. EGFR mutations in lung cancer: Correlation with clinical response to gefitinib therapy. *Science* **304:** 1497.

Pei J., Balsara B.R., Li W., Litwin S., Gabrielson E., Feder M., Jen J., and Testa J.R. 2001. Genomic imbalances in human lung adenocarcinomas and squamous cell carcinomas. *Genes Chromosomes Cancer* **31:** 282.

Petersen I., Bujard M., Petersen S., Wolf G., Goeze A., Schwendel A., Langreck H., Gellert K., Reichel M., Just K., du Manoir S., Cremer T., Dietel M., and Ried T. 1997. Patterns of chromosomal imbalances in adenocarcinoma and squamous cell carcinoma of the lung. *Cancer Res.* **57:** 2331.

Pollack J.R., Perou C.M., Alizadeh A.A., Eisen M.B., Pergamenschikov A., Williams C.F., Jeffrey S.S., Botstein D., and Brown P.O. 1999. Genome-wide analysis of DNA copy-number changes using cDNA microarrays. *Nat. Genet.* **23:** 41.

Pollack J.R., Sorlie T., Perou C.M., Rees C.A., Jeffrey S.S., Lonning P.E., Tibshirani R., Botstein D., Borresen-Dale A.L., and Brown P.O. 2002. Microarray analysis reveals a major direct role of DNA copy number alteration in the transcriptional program of human breast tumors. *Proc. Natl. Acad. Sci.* **99:** 12963.

Protopopov A., Kashuba V., Zabarovska V.I., Muravenko O.V., Lerman M.I., Klein G., and Zabarovsky E.R. 2003. An integrated physical and gene map of the 3.5-Mb chromosome 3p21.3 (AP20) region implicated in major human epithelial malignancies. *Cancer Res.* **63:** 404.

Ray M.E., Yang Z.Q., Albertson D., Kleer C.G., Washburn J.G., Macoska J.A., and Ethier S.P. 2004. Genomic and expression analysis of the 8p11-12 amplicon in human breast cancer cell lines. *Cancer Res.* **64:** 40.

Rhodes D.R., Yu J., Shanker K., Deshpande N., Varambally R., Ghosh D., Barrette T., Pandey A., and Chinnaiyan A.M. 2004. ONCOMINE: A cancer microarray database and integrated data-mining platform. *Neoplasia* **6:** 1.

Rosati R., La Starza R., Veronese A., Aventin A., Schwienbacher C., Vallespi T., Negrini M., Martelli M.F., and Mecucci C. 2002. NUP98 is fused to the NSD3 gene in acute myeloid leukemia associated with t(8;11)(p11.2;p15). *Blood* **99:** 3857.

Samuels Y., Wang Z., Bardelli A., Silliman N., Ptak J., Szabo S., Yan H., Gazdar A., Powell S.M., Riggins G.J., Willson J.K., Markowitz S., Kinzler K.W., Vogelstein B., and Velculescu V.E. 2004. High frequency of mutations of the PIK3CA gene in human cancers. *Science* **304:** 554.

Schneider R., Bannister A.J., and Kouzarides T. 2002. Unsafe SETs: Histone lysine methyltransferases and cancer. *Trends Biochem. Sci.* **27:** 396.

Sebat J., Lakshmi B., Troge J., Alexander J., Young J., Lundin P., Maner S., Massa H., Walker M., Chi M., Navin N., Lucito R., Healy J., Hicks J., Ye K., Reiner A., Gilliam T.C., Trask B., Patterson N., Zetterberg A., and Wigler M. 2004. Large-scale copy number polymorphism in the human genome. *Science* **305:** 525.

Simon R., Richter J., Wagner U., Fijan A., Bruderer J., Schmid U., Ackermann D., Maurer R., Alund G., Knonagel H., Rist M., Wilber K., Anabitarte M., Hering F., Hardmeier T., Schonenberger A., Flury R., Jager P., Fehr J.L., Schraml P., Moch H., Mihatsch M.J., Gasser T., and Sauter G. 2001. High-throughput tissue microarray analysis of 3p25 (RAF1) and 8p12 (FGFR1) copy number alterations in urinary bladder cancer. *Cancer Res.* **61:** 4514.

Stec I., Wright T.J., van Ommen G.J., de Boer P.A., van Haeringen A., Moorman A.F., Altherr M.R., and den Dunnen J.T.

1998. WHSC1, a 90 kb SET domain-containing gene, expressed in early development and homologous to a *Drosophila* dysmorphy gene maps in the Wolf-Hirschhorn syndrome critical region and is fused to IgH in t(4;14) multiple myeloma. *Hum. Mol. Genet.* **7:** 1071.

Storey J.D. and Tibshirani R. 2003. Statistical significance for genomewide studies. *Proc. Natl. Acad. Sci.* **100:** 9440.

Ten Have-Opbroek A.A., Benfield J.R., van Krieken J.H., and Dijkman J.H. 1997. The alveolar type II cell is a pluripotential stem cell in the genesis of human adenocarcinomas and squamous cell carcinomas. *Histol. Histopathol.* **12:** 319.

Tonon G., Wong K.K., Maulik G., Brennan C., Feng B., Zhang Y., Khatry D.B., Protopopov A., You M.J., Aguirre A.J., Martin E.S., Yang Z., Ji H., Chin L., and Depinho R.A. 2005. High-resolution genomic profiles of human lung cancer. *Proc. Natl. Acad. Sci.* **102:** 9625.

Trauzold A., Schmiedel S., Roder C., Tams C., Christgen M., Oestern S., Arlt A., Westphal S., Kapischke M., Ungefroren H., and Kalthoff H. 2003. Multiple and synergistic deregulations of apoptosis-controlling genes in pancreatic carcinoma cells. *Br. J. Cancer* **89:** 1714.

Tusher V.G., Tibshirani R., and Chu G. 2001. Significance analysis of microarrays applied to the ionizing radiation response.

Proc. Natl. Acad. Sci. **98:** 5116.

Walker S.M., Downes C.P., and Leslie N.R. 2001. TPIP: A novel phosphoinositide 3-phosphatase. *Biochem. J.* **360:** 277.

Westfall M.D. and Pietenpol J.A. 2004. p63: Molecular complexity in development and cancer. *Carcinogenesis* **25:** 857.

Xu Z., Friess H., Solioz M., Aebi S., Korc M., Kleeff J., and Buchler M.W. 2001. Bcl-x(L) antisense oligonucleotides induce apoptosis and increase sensitivity of pancreatic cancer cells to gemcitabine. *Int. J. Cancer* **94:** 268.

You J., Croyle J.L., Nishimura A., Ozato K., and Howley P.M. 2004. Interaction of the bovine papillomavirus E2 protein with Brd4 tethers the viral DNA to host mitotic chromosomes. *Cell* **117:** 349.

Zabarovsky E.R., Lerman M.I., and Minna J.D. 2002. Tumor suppressor genes on chromosome 3p involved in the pathogenesis of lung and other cancers. *Oncogene* **21:** 6915.

Zhao X., Weir B.A., LaFramboise T., Lin M., Beroukhim R., Garraway L., Beheshti J., Lee J.C., Naoki K., Richards W.G., Sugarbaker D., Chen F., Rubin M.A., Janne P.A., Girard L., Minna J., Christiani D., Li C., Sellers W.R., and Meyerson M. 2005. Homozygous deletions and chromosome amplifications in human lung carcinomas revealed by single nucleotide polymorphism array analysis. *Cancer Res.* **65:** 5561.

"Lineage Addiction" in Human Cancer: Lessons from Integrated Genomics

L.A. Garraway,[*†‡**] B.A. Weir,[* **] X. Zhao,[*] H. Widlund,[†] R. Beroukhim,[*‡**] A. Berger,[§]
D. Rimm,[§] M.A. Rubin,[‡¶] D.E. Fisher,[*†‡] M.L. Meyerson,[*¶**] AND W.R. Sellers[*‡**]

*Department of Medical Oncology and †Melanoma Program in Medical Oncology, Dana-Farber Cancer Institute,
Boston, Massachusetts 02115; ‡Department of Medicine and ¶Departments of Pathology, Brigham and
Women's Hospital and Harvard Medical School, Boston, Massachusetts 02115; §Department of Pathology,
Yale University School of Medicine, New Haven, Connecticut 06510; **The Broad Institute
of Harvard and MIT, Cambridge, Massachusetts 02141

Genome-era advances in the field of oncology endorse the notion that many tumors may prove vulnerable to targeted therapeutic avenues once their salient molecular alterations are elucidated. Accomplishing this requires both detailed genomic
characterization and the ability to identify in situ the critical dependencies operant within individual tumors. To this end,
DNA microarray platforms such as high-density single-nucleotide polymorphism (SNP) arrays enable large-scale cancer
genome characterization, including copy number and loss-of-heterozygosity analyses at high resolution. Clustering analyses
of SNP array data from a large collection of tumor samples and cell lines suggest that certain copy number alterations correlate strongly with the tissue of origin. Such lineage-restricted alterations may harbor novel cancer genes directing genesis or
progression of tumors from distinct tissue types. We have explored this notion through combined analysis of genome-scale
data sets from the NCI60 cancer cell line collection. Here, several melanoma cell lines clustered on the basis of increased
dosage at a region of chromosome 3p containing the master melanocyte regulator *MITF*. Combined analysis of gene expression data and additional functional studies established *MITF* as an amplified oncogene in melanoma. MITF may therefore
represent a nodal point within a critical lineage survival pathway operant in a subset of melanomas. These findings suggest
that, like oncogene addiction, "lineage addiction" may represent a fundamental tumor survival mechanism with important
therapeutic implications.

Cancer results from a diseased genome. Each tumor contains a collection of genomic aberrations that activate oncogenes and inactivate tumor suppressor genes. A recent survey of the scientific literature identified 229 oncogenes (or "dominant" cancer genes) and 62 tumor suppressors ("recessive" cancer genes), suggesting that more than 1% of the human genome may contribute directly to carcinogenesis and/or tumor progression (Futreal 2004). Since many tumor mechanisms likely remain undiscovered, these numbers may underestimate the full spectrum of human cancer genes. Moreover, the path to cancer may require at least 5–10 genetic mutations (Hahn and Weinberg 2002). Theoretically, then, the total number of different genetic combinations possible across all human cancers exceeds ten trillion and may even reach 10^{18}. These estimates imply that a comprehensive genomic approach to cancer therapeutics may be exceedingly difficult to achieve.

Recent insights, however, suggest a more favorable conclusion: The enormous complexity possible in theory may indeed prove both functionally reducible and therapeutically tractable in practice. Among these is the recognition that most human cancers derive from perturbations within a finite number of fundamental physiological processes directing cellular proliferation, survival, angiogenesis, and invasion/metastasis (Hanahan and Weinberg 2000). By itself, this conceptual framework does not completely resolve the challenge of tumor complexity, because many diverse genetic players and mutation chronologies may affect each of these properties.

Nonetheless, the notion that cancer involves definable biological hallmarks suggests that, ultimately, logic and order may be discerned from the immense genomic diversity characteristic of human cancer once the appropriate molecular contexts are more fully understood.

Consistent with this viewpoint is the recognition that cancer genomic aberrations, although complex, do not occur randomly. Instead, a relatively small number of cancer genes tend to undergo alterations at high frequencies. The fact that cellular pathways involving RAS, p53, and pRb (among others) undergo genetic mutations so commonly (Vogelstein and Kinzler 2004) not only endorses the "hallmarks of cancer" model, but also suggests that cancers tend to employ the same genomic alterations to enact these processes. Thus, despite the inevitable complexity, an increased knowledge of cancer genomic alterations should contribute markedly to the elaboration of essential and broadly applicable tumor mechanisms.

ONCOGENE ADDICTION AND TUMOR DEPENDENCY

Another pivotal insight pertaining to deconvolution of cancer genomic complexity derives from the recent observation that some tumors require continued activity of a single activated oncogene for survival (Weinstein 2002). Termed "oncogene addiction," this phenomenon was first demonstrated in transgenic mouse models that enabled conditional overexpression of oncogenes such as *myc*, *ras*, and *bcr-abl* (Chin et al. 1999; Felsher and Bishop

1999; Huettner et al. 2000; Jain et al. 2002; Pelengaris et al. 2002). In these models, induction of the relevant oncogene triggered cancer formation; however, subsequent loss of oncogene expression resulted in regression and apoptosis of tumor cells. The presence of oncogene addiction in human malignancies was first demonstrated in chronic myelogenous leukemia (CML), which harbors the BCR-ABL translocation; and in gastrointestinal stromal tumors (GIST), which contain oncogenic mutations in the c-kit gene. Targeting the tyrosine kinase activity of these oncogenes with the small-molecule inhibitor imatinib was sufficient to induce complete remissions in the great majority of patients (Druker et al. 2001; Demetri et al. 2002; Kantarjian et al. 2002). More recently, oncogene addiction was also demonstrated in a subset of lung cancers that contain base mutations or small deletions in the epidermal growth factor receptor (EGFR) gene; these alterations confer sensitivity to EGFR inhibitors such as gefitinib or erlotinib (Lynch et al. 2004; Paez et al. 2004). Thus, a single oncogenic lesion may play a decisive role in tumor maintenance, even when many additional genetic alterations have also accrued (Kaelin 2004).

A synthesis of the oncogene addiction and "hallmarks of cancer" models offers a framework wherein massive apparent genetic complexity may be underpinned by a much smaller collection of critical "dependencies" operant in human tumors. By this view, the predicted tumor-promoting effects of many genomic perturbations may converge onto a finite number of physiological processes, which in turn exhibit an even smaller set of limiting

"nodes" or "bottlenecks" within key cellular pathways directing carcinogenesis. At the same time, these dependencies will likely be caused by or associated with identifiable genetic lesions. Thus, such concordant genomic events may allow tumor dependencies to be pinpointed in situ within individual tumor samples (Fig. 1). Such an approach would markedly enhance efforts toward targeted therapeutic interdiction; however, most critical tumor dependencies remain either undiscovered or invisible to current molecular pathological tools.

GENOMIC APPROACHES TO CANCER CHARACTERIZATION

The tumor dependency framework and the genomic basis of cancer suggest that in the future, targeted cancer therapeutic avenues will depend primarily on rigorous genetic definition (Weber 2002). Recent years have therefore witnessed numerous efforts toward comprehensive characterization of tumor genomic alterations. The most popular large-scale approaches to cancer characterization utilize DNA microarrays to profile the expressed genes within tumor samples (Ramaswamy and Golub 2002). Accordingly, gene expression studies of many tumor types have identified molecular subclasses based on unique mRNA signatures, suggesting that the goal of a complete "molecular taxonomy" of human cancer is achievable (Golub 2004).

In principle, elaborating this molecular taxonomy should also clarify salient tumor dependencies and

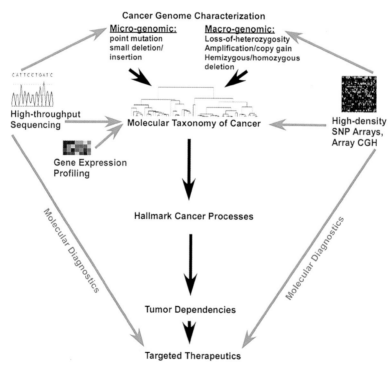

Figure 1. Cancer genomics and enabling technologies. The goal of high-resolution cancer genome mapping is the comprehensive identification of molecularly defined tumor types. Optimally, these subtypes will also clarify hallmark biological process and tumor dependencies that guide future targeted therapeutic avenues. High-throughput sequencing and microarray-based tools for RNA and DNA analysis (e.g., gene expression profiling, SNP arrays, and array CGH) represent important technologies for cancer genomic analyses.

thereby identify targetable cellular pathways directing tumor survival (Fig. 1). DNA microarrays have proved tremendously successful in identifying mRNA signatures predictive of a wide range of biological and clinical phenotypes. However, the explanatory power of these signatures with regard to the underlying biology remains variable. Instead, factors such as the degree of stromal/inflammatory infiltration within tumor samples and lineage-specific transcriptional programs may heavily influence the composition of microarray-derived signatures. In particular, cell lineage effects on gene expression often dominate the output of unsupervised analytical techniques such as hierarchical clustering or self-organizing maps (Ross et al. 2000; Ramaswamy et al. 2001) unless these studies are confined to samples from a single lineage.

A complementary approach to molecular cancer classification involves the systematic global analysis of tumor DNA. This avenue offers conceptual appeal given the genomic origins of human tumors. The structural alterations characteristic of cancer genomes are more refractory to technical variables (tissue hypoxia, media conditions, etc.) and agnostic to lineage- or differentiation-dependent transcriptional programs. Moreover, prevalent tumor DNA alterations tend to harbor oncogenes or tumor suppressors, and therefore, in combination with expression profiling, may speed the identification of critical tumor growth or survival mechanisms on a genome scale.

Enabling technologies such as high-throughput sequencing and DNA microarrays have propelled recent efforts at DNA-based cancer genomic analysis (Weber 2002). Large-scale sequencing provides detailed characterization of "micro-genomic" alterations (e.g., base mutations or small deletions/insertion events) (Weir et al. 2004), whereas microarray-based tools such as oligonucleotide comparative genomic hybridization (CGH) have facilitated studies of "macro-genomic" alterations (translocations, copy gains or losses spanning many kilobases) (Mantripragada et al. 2004; Garraway and Sellers 2005).

Recently, high-density DNA microarrays that perform massively parallel genotyping of single-nucleotide polymorphisms have become available (Cutler et al. 2001). Although these SNP arrays (Affymetrix) were designed for large-scale association studies in medical or population genetics, they have proved robust and versatile tools for cancer genome analysis. SNP arrays contain oligonucleotide probes tiled to detect the two alleles of a given SNP locus. The current generation SNP array contains probe densities capable of genotyping >100,000 SNPs simultaneously, providing a median intermarker distance of 8.5 kb. This high array marker density enables the inference of tumor loss-of-heterozygosity (LOH) events, even in the absence of matched normal samples (R. Beroukhim et al., in prep.). Moreover, analysis of the signal intensities that result from genomic DNA hybridization, and comparison to corresponding signal data from normal genomes, allow determination of copy number changes present within tumor samples at high resolution, as shown in Figure 2 (Bignell et al. 2004; Zhao et al. 2004).

LINEAGE-RESTRICTED DNA ALTERATIONS IN HUMAN TUMORS

To explore the utility of global cancer genome analysis using high-density SNP arrays, we applied an unsupervised learning algorithm to DNA copy number information derived from SNP array studies (Garraway et al. 2005). Here, we used 100K array data from the NCI60 cancer cell line collection as a model system (Stinson et al. 1992). This panel includes 59 cell lines from nine different tumor types accrued by the National Cancer Institute (NCI). NCI-sponsored studies of these lines have also generated pharmacological data for nearly 100,000 compounds (data from >40,000 compounds are publicly available through the NCI Web site at http://dtp.nci.nih.gov). Additional large-scale data sets available for this collection—including several gene expression microarray surveys (Ross et al. 2000), spectral karyotyping (SKY)

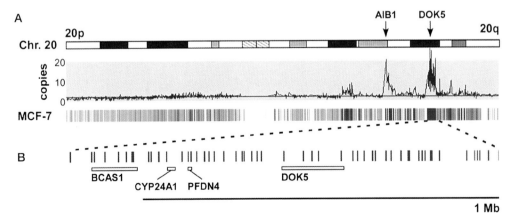

Figure 2. High-density SNP arrays for copy number analysis. (*A*) A SNP array-derived copy number plot (*middle*) of the MCF-7 breast cancer cell line is shown alongside the cytoband map of chromosome 20 (*top*). Marker density and signal intensities are indicated by the white-red colorgram (*bottom*). AIB1 and DOK5 are genes present within two high-level amplicons. (*B*) Expanded view of a 20q amplicon shows the 100K array marker density and a map of several genes located therein (*bottom*). (Reprinted, with permission, from Garraway and Sellers 2005 [©Elsevier].)

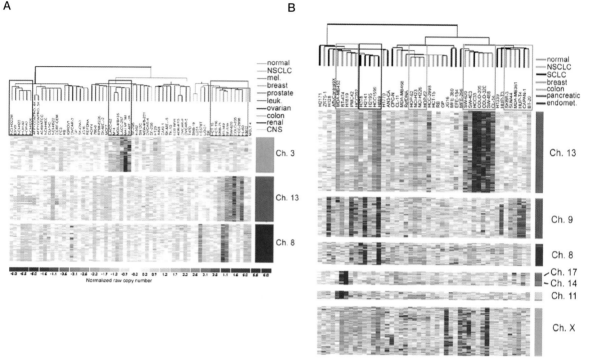

Figure 3. Copy number clustering of cancer cell lines. (*A*) Hierarchical clustering was applied to SNP array-based copy number data from 64 NCI60 cell lines and controls. (*B*) Dendrogram and associated SNP probe clusters from an independent cancer cell line set (several NCI60 cell lines were also included for confirmation). For both *A* and *B*, the resulting dendrograms (*top*), along with SNP probe clusters from correlated genomic regions (*bottom*), are shown. Columns represent cell lines, and each row (pixel) represents an individual SNP marker. Terminal branches are color-coded according to tissue type (*legend at right*). Pixel color represents copy number data (*red* = increased copy number and *blue* = decreased copy number). Lineage-enriched cell line subclusters are outlined by colored rectangles. (*A*, Reprinted, with permission, from Garroway et al. 2005 [©Nature Publishing Group].)

(Roschke et al. 2003), and proteomic profiles (Nishizuka et al. 2003)—make the NCI60 panel an attractive system in which to integrate large, orthogonal data sets and to query their respective biological importance.

When hierarchical clustering (Eisen et al. 1998) was used to group the NCI60 collection based on copy number alterations, the resulting cell line dendrogram contained three major branches, each consisting of samples from several different tumor types (Fig. 3A) (Garraway et al. 2005). Surprisingly, closer inspection of these branches revealed terminal subclusters where the cell lines appeared to segregate according to tissue of origin (e.g., non-small-cell lung cancer, melanoma, and colon cancer lines; Fig. 3A). These results suggested that despite the marked ploidy variances known to exist within these cell lines, their genomes might nonetheless harbor lineage-associated aberrations discernible by the unsupervised learning algorithms in common use.

To confirm this observation while also excluding a spurious phenomenon attributable to experimental batch effects, we carried out an independent SNP array hybridization that included a subset of NCI60 samples alongside 35 non-NCI60 cancer cell line DNAs within a single experimental batch. The resulting copy number information was also subjected to hierarchical clustering as described above. Lineage-restricted cell line subclusters were again observed, in this case consisting of breast, colon, small-cell, or non-small-cell lung cancer lines

(Fig. 3B). Together, these data raised the possibility that tissue lineage may exert a significant effect on patterns of copy number alterations in cells from many different tumor types.

To investigate the in vivo relevance of the lineage-restricted patterns observed in cell lines, we also examined the copy number patterns of a large collection of lung tumor DNAs analyzed by 100K SNP arrays (Zhao et al. 2005). Since these samples were processed and hybridized to arrays in several batches, the raw copy number values at each SNP locus were first converted to integer values by a hidden Markov model. Next, a prevalence threshold for amplifications and deletions was calculated by taking the mean frequencies plus one standard deviation of all SNPs having inferred copy number ≥ 4 and ≥ 1, respectively. SNP loci exceeding either threshold were filtered using dChipSNP software and subjected to hierarchical clustering. These manipulations effectively removed the "batch effects" that may confound clustering analysis of "raw" copy number data, while enriching for the genomic regions most likely to denote tumor subtypes.

The lung cancer samples organized into three discernible aggregates following hierarchical clustering of the regions described above, as shown in Figure 4. Interestingly, the lung cancer cell lines formed a cluster that was distinct from those of the tumor samples. This finding resembled prior observations from gene expression studies (Ross et al. 2000) and suggested that distinctive

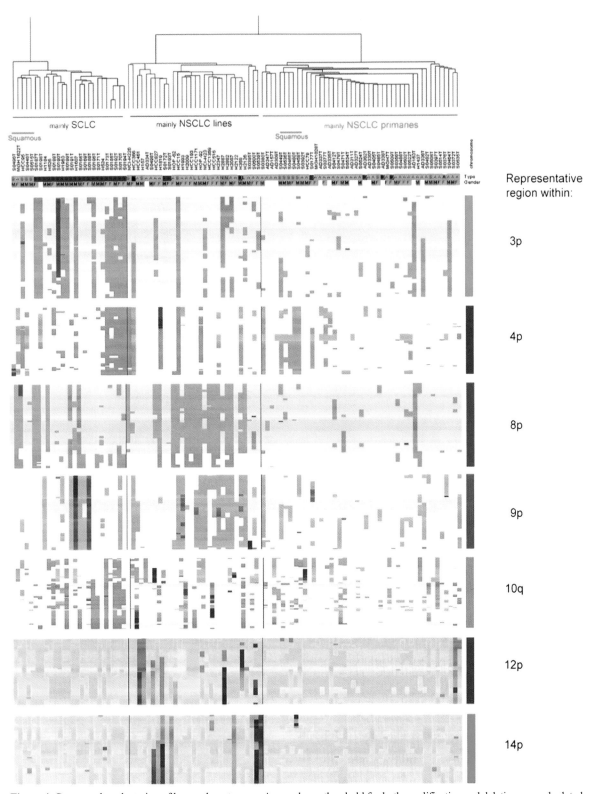

Figure 4. Copy number clustering of human lung tumors. A prevalence threshold for both amplification and deletion was calculated; SNP loci exceeding either threshold were filtered and used for inferred copy number clustering. The resulting dendrogram and selected SNP clusters from correlated chromosomal regions are illustrated. White areas represent mean copy number (copy number values for each SNP were standardized to have a mean of 0 and standard deviation of 1), blue areas represent copy number below the mean, and red areas represent copy number above the mean.

copy number alterations may either accompany or result from established in vitro cultivation. Nonetheless, lineage-restricted patterns were again apparent: The small-

cell lung cancer (SCLC) samples segregated mostly within a single cluster, whereas the non-small-cell lung cancers (NSCLC; mostly adenocarcinomas) formed a separate cluster. Although the squamous cell carcinoma samples did not form their own branch, they did comprise two terminal subclusters discernible within the larger SCLC or NSCLC clusters (Fig. 4). In general, these findings accord well with a recent meta-analysis of comparative genomic hybridization studies performed across many tumor types (Greshock et al. 2005) and suggest that cell or tissue lineage may exert a profound influence on the patterns of chromosomal aberrations observed within human tumors.

INTEGRATED GENOMIC ANALYSES IDENTIFY A LINEAGE-DEPENDENT MELANOMA ONCOGENE

Hierarchical, copy-number-based clustering algorithms applied to cancer cell lines were two-dimensional; as such, they also grouped SNPs deriving from the same chromosomal regions (Figs. 3,4). Inspection of these SNP clustering patterns identified specific genomic loci whose copy number alterations appeared to drive the terminal cell line subclusters. For example, the colon cancer cluster was largely based on copy number gain within chromosome 13 in both experiments (Fig. 3A,B), whereas the melanoma group reflected copy gain within chromosome 3 (Fig. 3A; *note:* no melanoma cell lines were included in the sample batch depicted in Fig. 3B).

The lung tumor clustering analysis also identified candidate genomic regions. For example, distinct SCLC subsets were associated with losses at chromosomes 3p, 4p, and 10q, consistent with prior studies (Fig. 4) (Levin 1995; Petersen 1998; Sattler and Salgia 2003). In contrast, NSCLC cell lines more commonly exhibited losses at chromosomes 8p and 9p (Fig. 4). Interestingly, additional tumor subsets appeared to cluster on the basis of alterations not previously described in lung cancer, such as a region of gain at chromosome 4p associated with a squamous carcinoma subset (Fig. 4). Presumably, genomic regions correlated with the lineage-restricted copy number clusters may harbor cancer genes directing key mechanisms governing tumor growth in these subtypes.

Cancer cell lines exhibiting lineage-dependent copy number alterations provide experimentally tractable model systems for the characterization of associated oncogenes or tumor suppressor genes. However, in most cases the aberrations identified by hierarchical clustering were too large for detailed functional studies. Even the smallest minimal common regions so identified were several megabases in length, and some cases exhibited low-level (e.g., single-copy) gain or loss involving much of a chromosome arm (polysomy).

We therefore applied an integrated genomic approach to identify candidate cancer genes located in these regions (Garraway et al. 2005). Here, we reasoned that the oncogene target of a genetic amplification event present in a set of samples might exhibit significantly increased steady-state gene expression when compared to samples lacking this amplicon. This rationale derived from several predicted properties of amplified oncogenes: (1) preferential (over)expression in tumor cells; (2) enrichment by clonal selection relative to bystander genes; and (3)

deregulation, e.g., increased refractoriness to negative feedback/regulatory mechanisms that might otherwise suppress a gene dosage effect. Since gene expression data from several groups are publicly available for the NCI60 cell lines, as noted above, this sample collection provided a convenient platform for an integrated approach.

To combine gene expression and copy number information in this way, we adapted supervised learning methods commonly utilized for microarray-based tumor classification (Golub et al. 1999). NCI60 samples were separated into two classes based on the presence or absence of a genomic lesion linked to lineage-restricted subsets identified by copy number clustering. Next, NCI60 gene expression data (generated on the Affymetrix U95 platform by the Genomics Institute of the Novartis Foundation) were organized according to these class distinctions to identify genes with significantly increased expression in association with the amplified class. Finally, highly expressed genes within the "amplicon" (or copy gain) class were mapped to their genomic locations to determine whether any also resided within the amplified segments.

As noted above, one of the NCI60 subsets identified by copy number clustering consisted exclusively of melanoma cell lines (Fig. 3A). This cluster correlated best with DNA copy gain at chromosome 3p14-3p13. When we applied the integrated genomic approach to the class distinction 3p-amplified versus non-amplified, only one gene was both significantly up-regulated in association with the amplified class (following Bonferroni correction) and located within the common region of copy gain that defined this class (Fig. 5A). This gene, *MITF*, belongs to the MiT family of helix-loop-helix/leucine-zipper transcription factors and effects critical functions in the development and survival of the melanocyte lineage (Goding 2000; Widlund and Fisher 2003). Although *MITF* itself was not previously shown to be altered in cancer, it had been implicated as a transcriptional regulator of the antiapoptotic *BCL2* oncogene in melanoma cells (McGill et al. 2002). Moreover, other bHLH-LZ and MiT transcription factors undergo genetic alterations causally implicated in several human malignancies; these include *MYC*, the prototype amplified oncogene; *NMYC*, amplified in 50% of pediatric neuroblastomas and associated with adverse outcome (Maris and Matthay 1999); and both *TFE3*, and TFEB, the targets of translocation-mediated gene fusions with *PRCC* or other partners in papillary renal cancer and soft-tissue sarcomas (Weterman et al. 1996; Ladanyi et al. 2001; Davis et al. 2003). In light of these observations, our genomic analysis suggested that *MITF* might function as a lineage-specific melanoma oncogene.

Several lines of experimental evidence have since confirmed the oncogenic function of MITF in human melanoma (Garraway et al. 2005). Quantitative genomic PCR performed on a series of DNAs derived from primary and metastatic melanomas demonstrated *MITF* copy gain (to ≥4 copies) in 10% of primary and more than 20% of metastatic specimens. Analysis of a melanoma tissue array by fluorescence in situ hybridization (FISH) revealed similar findings (Fig. 5B) and also enabled a

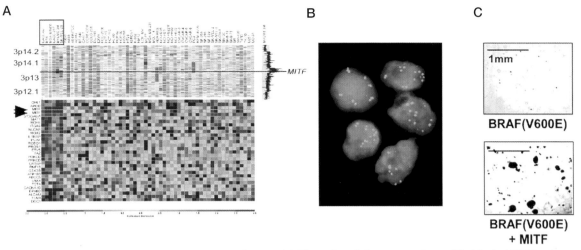

Figure 5. MITF as a lineage survival oncogene in melanoma. (*A*) The region of chromosome 3p amplified in the NCI60 melanoma subcluster was used in a supervised analysis of NCI60 gene expression data (see text for details). (*Top*) Colorgram shows high (*red*) and low (*blue*) copy number at 3p14-3p12; the location of MITF within chromosome 3p is indicated. (*Bottom*) A second colorgram depicts genes from chromosome 3 whose mRNA expression patterns correlated significantly with the 3p amplicon class. Arrows indicate *MITF* probe sets. (*B*) A digoxin-labeled probe (*green*) was used to detect the MITF locus, and a SpectrumOrange control probe (Vysis; *red*) detected the chromosome 3 centromere by FISH in a melanoma tissue microarray. A case of *MITF* amplification is shown. (*C*) Soft agar assays following BRAF(V600E) (*top*) or BRAF(V600E)+MITF retroviral transduction of immortalized melanocytes. Colonies were photographed after 8 weeks (Magnification, 32x). (All panels adapted, with permission, from Garraway et al. 2005 [©Nature Publishing Group].)

Kaplan-Meier analysis. Here, *MITF* amplification associated significantly with adverse patient overall survival. On the tissue array, *MITF* amplification was also associated with significantly increased MITF protein as measured by automated fluorescence analysis (AQUA) (Camp et al. 2003). Together, these data presented compelling genetic evidence that *MITF* might mediate an oncogenic function in melanoma.

We also examined the oncogenicity of MITF directly by ectopic expression within melanocytes that had been immortalized by serial retroviral transduction of telomerase (hTERT), CDK4(R24C) (an INK-resistant variant), and p53DD (a dominant-negative p53 protein) (Garraway et al. 2005). Although retrovirally transduced MITF was not oncogenic in these melanocytes when overexpressed by itself, it transformed these melanocytes in cooperation with the BRAF(V600E) mutant protein, as assayed by growth factor independence and soft agar experiments (Fig. 5C). Conversely, introduction of a dominant-negative MITF construct into melanoma cell lines resulted in growth inhibition. These findings strongly suggested a critical role for MITF in melanoma genesis and survival, particularly in the setting of cell cycle deregulation and excess BRAF-mediated MAP kinase activation.

LINEAGE ADDICTION AND TUMOR DEPENDENCY IN MELANOMA

To a first approximation, the tumor-promoting function of MITF may resemble oncogene addiction: A subset of melanomas exhibits deregulation of MITF (through increased gene dosage or by other mechanisms as yet undetermined), and this deregulation may be essential to melanoma cell survival. However, MITF action differs importantly from oncogene addiction in that it does not seem to involve a specific gain-of-function event that is absent in nontransformed melanocytes. Rather, it may represent the persistence in melanoma of a master survival function also operant in cells of the melanocytic lineage during development and differentiation. In this regard, MITF function constitutes a novel oncogenic mechanism, which we term lineage addiction or lineage survival. In hindsight, other well-characterized oncogenes may provide analogous lineage survival functions in their native cell types, such as the androgen receptor (prostate), FLT3 (myeloid), and cyclin D1 (breast). Thus, lineage addiction may represent a tumor dependency mechanism exploited by many cancer types through lineage-restricted genomic alterations.

In melanoma, this lineage addiction mechanism also pinpoints MITF as a nodal point within a key genetic dependency already recognized to offer therapeutic promise (Fig. 6). Here, the relevant tumor-promoting alteration (MITF amplification) converges on a fundamental lineage survival process, which itself depends crucially on a single cellular pathway centered around—but not restricted to—MITF. Indeed, this dependency is predicted to co-occur with other genetic alterations that activate MAP kinase signaling and inactivate the p16/Rb pathway. Aberrant MAP kinase pathway activation is commonly observed in melanoma, but MAP kinase triggers ERK- and RSK-dependent phosphorylation events that lead to tightly coupled activation and degradation of MITF under normal circumstances (Hemesath et al. 1998; Price et al. 1998; Wu et al. 2000). Presumably, melanomas that exploit a MITF-dependent lineage survival mechanism avert this degradatory MAP kinase effect by deregulating MITF through amplification or other mechanisms. Inactivation of the p16/Rb pathway should also be required because MITF has been shown to induce

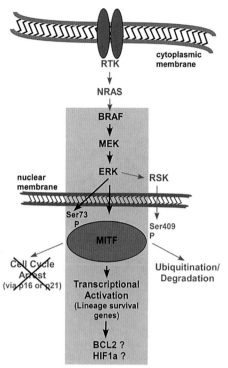

Figure 6. A lineage addiction pathway in melanoma. Deregulation of MITF activity may mediate a critical lineage dependency operant within a subset of melanomas. This dependency may also be characterized by aberrant MAP kinase pathway activation (e.g., through BRAF mutation) and cell cycle deregulation (e.g., through p16/CDK/pRB pathway inactivation). Transcriptional activation of lineage survival genes by MITF (possibly including the antiapoptotic BCL-2 oncogene and the proangiogenic HIF1a gene) may contribute to melanoma genesis and progression.

pathway regulation, a common melanoma occurrence that may cooperate with the MITF lineage survival mechanism (as described above), leads to increased cyclin D/CDK4 activity and cell cycle progression. Several CDK inhibitors are also in clinical or preclinical development (Dai and Grant 2003; Shapiro 2004); conceivably, these could be implemented along with MAP kinase and/or BCL-2 inhibitors in a combinatorial therapeutic cocktail tailored to the genetic makeup of a defined and clinically identifiable melanoma subtype.

CONCLUSIONS

The success of targeted cancer therapeutics depends heavily on the ability to define molecular tumor subtypes and the salient dependencies underlying their genesis and progression. Tools of the genome era offer tremendous promise in this regard; already, the application of DNA microarray platforms to cancer genome characterization has resulted in the discovery of novel tumor subsets as well as the cancer genes directing their biology. The discovery that MITF acts as a melanoma oncogene constitutes an informative example in this regard; its putative function in melanoma also illustrates a newly recognized lineage addiction mechanism that may prove both operant and therapeutically tractable in other cancer types. The broad application of genomic approaches to characterize human tumors and their counterpart model systems (cell lines, short-term cultures, xenografts, etc.) should enable a productive and integrated avenue that improves biological understanding and therapeutic application.

ACKNOWLEDGMENTS

This work was supported by grants from the National Institutes of Health (L.A.G., M.A.R., D.L.R., and D.E.F.), the American Cancer Society (M.L.M.), the Flight Attendant Medical Research Institute (M.L.M.), the Doris Duke Foundation (D.E.F.), the Tisch Family Foundation (W.R.S.), and the Damon Runyon Cancer Research Foundation (W.R.S.).

melanocyte growth arrest when this pathway is intact (Loercher et al. 2005). In support of this model, our data suggest that MITF may require both loss of p16/Rb function and aberrant MAP kinase signaling (e.g., through cooperation with mutated *BRAF*) to act as an oncogene. Moreover, these findings suggest that molecular probes interrogating the MITF locus, MAP kinase pathway activation, and p16/Rb pathway status may prove capable of identifying this dependency in situ at the time of melanoma diagnosis.

To this end, the MAP kinase/MITF dependency is also notable in that several putative effector proteins represent the targets of small molecules at various stages of clinical development. For example, BRAF undergoes an activating V600E mutation in a large percentage of melanomas (Davies et al. 2002); this enhanced activity appears to be required for melanoma cell survival (Hingorani et al. 2003). Accordingly, several companies have developed compounds that inhibit B-Raf or MEK, key MAP kinase effector proteins (Bollag et al. 2003; Sebolt-Leopold 2004; Wilhelm et al. 2004). Transcription factors such as MITF have historically been considered less "drug-able"; however, the MITF target gene BCL-2 has been targeted by antisense compounds in advanced clinical development (Manion and Hockenbery 2003). Loss of p16/Rb

REFERENCES

Bignell G.R., Huang J., Greshock J., Watt S., Butler A., West S., Grigorova M., Jones K.W., Wei W., Stratton M.R., Futreal P.A., Weber B., Shapero M.H., and Wooster R. 2004. High-resolution analysis of DNA copy number using oligonucleotide microarrays. *Genome Res.* **14:** 287.

Bollag G., Freeman S., Lyons J.F., and Post L.E. 2003. Raf pathway inhibitors in oncology. *Curr. Opin. Investig. Drugs* **4:** 1436.

Camp R.L., Dolled-Filhart M., King B.L., and Rimm D.L. 2003. Quantitative analysis of breast cancer tissue microarrays shows that both high and normal levels of HER2 expression are associated with poor outcome. *Cancer Res.* **63:** 1445.

Chin L., Tam A., Pomerantz J., Wong M., Holash J., Bardeesy N., Shen Q., O'Hagan R., Pantginis J., Zhou H., Horner J.W., 2nd, Cordon-Cardo C., Yancopoulos G.D., and DePinho R.A. 1999. Essential role for oncogenic Ras in tumour maintenance. *Nature* **400:** 468.

Cutler D.J., Zwick M.E., Carrasquillo M.M., Yohn C.T., Tobin K.P., Kashuk C., Mathews D.J., Shah N.A., Eichler E.E., Warrington J.A., and Chakravarti A. 2001. High-throughput variation detection and genotyping using microarrays. *Genome Res.* **11**: 1913.

Dai Y. and Grant S. 2003. Cyclin-dependent kinase inhibitors. *Curr. Opin. Pharmacol.* **3**: 362.

Davies H., Bignell G.R., Cox C., Stephens P., Edkins S., Clegg S., Teague J., Woffendin H., Garnett M.J., Bottomley W., Davis N., Dicks E., Ewing R., Floyd Y., Gray K., Hall S., Hawes R., Hughes J., Kosmidou V., Menzies A., Mould C., Parker A., Stevens C., Watt S., Hooper S., Wilson R., Jayatilake H., Gusterson B.A., Cooper C., Shipley J., Hargrave D., Pritchard-Jones K., Maitland N., Chenevix-Trench G., Riggins G.J., Bigner D.D., Palmieri G., Cossu A., Flanagan A., Nicholson A., Ho J.W., Leung S.Y., Yuen S.T., Weber B.L., Seigler H.F., Darrow T.L., Paterson H., Marais R., Marshall C.J., Wooster R., Stratton M.R., and Futreal P.A. 2002. Mutations of the BRAF gene in human cancer. *Nature* **417**: 949.

Davis I.J., Hsi B.L., Arroyo J.D., Vargas S.O., Yeh Y.A., Motyckova G., Valencia P., Perez-Atayde A.R., Argani P., Ladanyi M., Fletcher J.A., and Fisher D.E. 2003. Cloning of an Alpha-TFEB fusion in renal tumors harboring the t(6;11)(p21;q13) chromosome translocation. *Proc. Natl. Acad. Sci.* **100**: 6051.

Demetri G.D., von Mehren M., Blanke C.D., Van den Abbeele A.D., Eisenberg B., Roberts P.J., Heinrich M.C., Tuveson D.A., Singer S., Janicek M., Fletcher J.A., Silverman S.G., Silberman S.L., Capdeville R., Kiese B., Peng B., Dimitrijevic S., Druker B.J., Corless C., Fletcher C.D., and Joensuu H. 2002. Efficacy and safety of imatinib mesylate in advanced gastrointestinal stromal tumors. *N. Engl. J. Med.* **347**: 472.

Druker B.J., Talpaz M., Resta D.J., Peng B., Buchdunger E., Ford J.M., Lydon N.B., Kantarjian H., Capdeville R., Ohno-Jones S., and Sawyers C.L. 2001. Efficacy and safety of a specific inhibitor of the BCR-ABL tyrosine kinase in chronic myeloid leukemia. *N. Engl. J. Med.* **344**: 1031.

Eisen M.B., Spellman P.T., Brown P.O., and Botstein D. 1998. Cluster analysis and display of genome-wide expression patterns. *Proc. Natl. Acad. Sci.* **95**: 14863.

Felsher D.W. and Bishop J.M. 1999. Reversible tumorigenesis by MYC in hematopoietic lineages. *Mol. Cell* **4**: 199.

Futreal P.A., Coin L., Marshall M., Down T., Hubbard T., Wooster R., Rahman N., and Stratton M.R. 2004. A census of human cancer genes. *Nat. Rev. Cancer* **4**: 177.

Garraway L.A. and Sellers W.R. 2005. Array-based approaches to cancer genome analysis. *Drug Discov. Today: Disease Mechanisms* **2**: 171.

Garraway L.A., Widlund H.R., Rubin M.A., Getz G., Berger A.J., Ramaswamy S., Beroukhim R., Milner D.A., Granter S.R., Du J., Lee C., Wagner S.N., Li C., Golub T.R., Rimm D.L., Meyerson M.L., Fisher D.E., and Sellers W.R. 2005. Integrative genomic analyses identify MITF as a lineage survival oncogene amplified in malignant melanoma. *Nature* **436**: 117.

Goding C.R. 2000. Mitf from neural crest to melanoma: Signal transduction and transcription in the melanocyte lineage. *Genes Dev.* **14**: 1712.

Golub T.R. 2004. Toward a functional taxonomy of cancer. *Cancer Cell* **6**: 107.

Golub T.R., Slonim D.K., Tamayo P., Huard C., Gaasenbeek M., Mesirov J.P., Coller H., Loh M.L., Downing J.R., Caligiuri M.A., Bloomfield C.D., and Lander E.S. 1999. Molecular classification of cancer: Class discovery and class prediction by gene expression monitoring. *Science* **286**: 531.

Greshock J., Naylor T.L., Mosse Y., Brose M., Fakharzadeh S., Martin A., Athenasiadis G., Ward R., Medina A., Diskin S., Hegde P., Birkeland M., Ellis C., Paulazzo G., Zaks T., Brown J., Maris J., and Weber B. 2005. Measurement of genetic similarity in 10 common human tumor types using genome copy number data. In *Conference on Oncogenomics, 2005, San Diego, California*, B33. American Association for Cancer Research.

Hahn W.C. and Weinberg R.A. 2002. Rules for making human tumor cells. *N. Engl. J. Med.* **347**: 1593.

Hanahan D. and Weinberg R.A. 2000. The hallmarks of cancer. *Cell* **100**: 57.

Hemesath T.J., Price E.R., Takemoto C., Badalian T., and Fisher D.E. 1998. MAP kinase links the transcription factor Microphthalmia to c-Kit signalling in melanocytes. *Nature* **391**: 298.

Hingorani S.R., Jacobetz M.A., Robertson G.P., Herlyn M., and Tuveson D.A. 2003. Suppression of BRAF(V599E) in human melanoma abrogates transformation. *Cancer Res.* **63**: 5198.

Huettner C.S., Zhang P., Van Etten R.A., and Tenen D.G. 2000. Reversibility of acute B-cell leukaemia induced by BCR-ABL1. *Nat. Genet.* **24**: 57.

Jain M., Arvanitis C., Chu K., Dewey W., Leonhardt E., Trinh M., Sundberg C.D., Bishop J.M., and Felsher D.W. 2002. Sustained loss of a neoplastic phenotype by brief inactivation of MYC. *Science* **297**: 102.

Kaelin W.G., Jr. 2004. Gleevec: Prototype or outlier? *Sci. STKE* **2004**: pe12.

Kantarjian H., Sawyers C., Hochhaus A., Guilhot F., Schiffer C., Gambacorti-Passerini C., Niederwieser D., Resta D., Capdeville R., Zoellner U., Talpaz M., Druker B., Goldman J., O'Brien S.G., Russell N., Fischer T., Ottmann O., Cony-Makhoul P., Facon T., Stone R., Miller C., Tallman M., Brown R., Schuster M., Loughran T., Gratwohl A., Mandelli F., Saglio G., Lazzarino M., Russo D., Baccarani M., and Morra E. 2002. Hematologic and cytogenetic responses to imatinib mesylate in chronic myelogenous leukemia. *N. Engl. J. Med.* **346**: 645.

Ladanyi M., Lui M.Y., Antonescu C.R., Krause-Boehm A., Meindl A., Argani P., Healey J.H., Ueda T., Yoshikawa H., Meloni-Ehrig A., Sorensen P.H., Mertens F., Mandahl N., van den Berghe H., Sciot R., Cin P.D., and Bridge J. 2001. The der(17)t(X;17)(p11;q25) of human alveolar soft part sarcoma fuses the TFE3 transcription factor gene to ASPL, a novel gene at 17q25. *Oncogene* **20**: 48.

Levin N.A., Brzoska P.M., Warnock M.L., Gray J.W., and Christman M.F. 1995. Identification of novel regions of altered DNA copy number in small cell lung tumors. *Genes Chromosomes Cancer* **13**: 175.

Loercher A.E., Tank E.M., Delston R.B., and Harbour J.W. 2005. MITF links differentiation with cell cycle arrest in melanocytes by transcriptional activation of INK4A. *J. Cell Biol.* **168**: 35.

Lynch T.J., Bell D.W., Sordella R., Gurubhagavatula S., Okimoto R.A., Brannigan B.W., Harris P.L., Haserlat S.M., Supko J.G., Haluska F.G., Louis D.N., Christiani D.C., Settleman J., and Haber D.A. 2004. Activating mutations in the epidermal growth factor receptor underlying responsiveness of non-small-cell lung cancer to gefitinib. *N. Engl. J. Med.* **350**: 2129.

Manion M.K. and Hockenbery D.M. 2003. Targeting BCL-2-related proteins in cancer therapy. *Cancer Biol. Ther.* **2**: S105.

Mantripragada K.K., Buckley P.G., de Stahl T.D., and Dumanski J.P. 2004. Genomic microarrays in the spotlight. *Trends Genet.* **20**: 87.

Maris J.M. and Matthay K.K. 1999. Molecular biology of neuroblastoma. *J. Clin. Oncol.* **17**: 2264.

McGill G.G., Horstmann M., Widlund H.R., Du J., Motyckova G., Nishimura E.K., Lin Y.L., Ramaswamy S., Avery W., Ding H.F., Jordan S.A., Jackson I.J., Korsmeyer S.J., Golub T.R., and Fisher D.E. 2002. Bcl2 regulation by the melanocyte master regulator Mitf modulates lineage survival and melanoma cell viability. *Cell* **109**: 707.

Nishizuka S., Charboneau L., Young L., Major S., Reinhold W.C., Waltham M., Kouros-Mehr H., Bussey K.J., Lee J.K., Espina V., Munson P.J., Petricoin E., III, Liotta L.A., and Weinstein J.N. 2003. Proteomic profiling of the NCI-60 cancer cell lines using new high-density reverse-phase lysate microarrays. *Proc. Natl. Acad. Sci.* **100**: 14229.

Paez J.G., Janne P.A., Lee J.C., Tracy S., Greulich H., Gabriel S., Herman P., Kaye F.J., Lindeman N., Boggon T.J., Naoki K., Sasaki H., Fujii Y., Eck M.J., Sellers W.R., Johnson B.E., and Meyerson M. 2004. EGFR mutations in lung cancer: Correlation with clinical response to gefitinib therapy. *Science* **304**: 1497.

Pelengaris S., Khan M., and Evan G.I. 2002. Suppression of Myc-induced apoptosis in beta cells exposes multiple oncogenic properties of Myc and triggers carcinogenic progression. *Cell* **109**: 321.

Petersen S., Wolf G., Bockmuhl U., Gellert K., Dietel M., and Petersen I. 1998. Allelic loss on chromosome 10q in human lung cancer: Association with tumour progression and metastatic phenotype. *Br. J. Cancer* **77**: 270.

Price E.R., Ding H.F., Badalian T., Bhattacharya S., Takemoto C., Yao T.P., Hemesath T.J., and Fisher D.E. 1998. Lineage-specific signaling in melanocytes. C-kit stimulation recruits p300/CBP to microphthalmia. *J. Biol. Chem.* **273**: 17983.

Ramaswamy S. and Golub T.R. 2002. DNA microarrays in clinical oncology. *J. Clin. Oncol.* **20**: 1932.

Ramaswamy S., Tamayo P., Rifkin R., Mukherjee S., Yeang C.H., Angelo M., Ladd C., Reich M., Latulippe E., Mesirov J.P., Poggio T., Gerald W., Loda M., Lander E.S., and Golub T.R. 2001. Multiclass cancer diagnosis using tumor gene expression signatures. *Proc. Natl. Acad. Sci.* **98**: 15149.

Roschke A.V., Tonon G., Gehlhaus K.S., McTyre N., Bussey K.J., Lababidi S., Scudiero D.A., Weinstein J.N., and Kirsch I.R. 2003. Karyotypic complexity of the NCI-60 drug-screening panel. *Cancer Res.* **63**: 8634.

Ross D.T., Scherf U., Eisen M.B., Perou C.M., Rees C., Spellman P., Iyer V., Jeffrey S.S., Van de Rijn M., Waltham M., Pergamenschikov A., Lee J.C., Lashkari D., Shalon D., Myers T.G., Weinstein J.N., Botstein D., and Brown P.O. 2000. Systematic variation in gene expression patterns in human cancer cell lines. *Nat. Genet.* **24**: 227.

Sattler M. and Salgia R. 2003. Molecular and cellular biology of small cell lung cancer. *Semin. Oncol.* **30**: 57.

Sebolt-Leopold J.S. 2004. MEK inhibitors: A therapeutic approach to targeting the Ras-MAP kinase pathway in tumors. *Curr. Pharm. Des.* **10**: 1907.

Shapiro G.I. 2004. Preclinical and clinical development of the cyclin-dependent kinase inhibitor flavopiridol. *Clin. Cancer Res.* **10**: 4270s.

Stinson S.F., Alley M.C., Kopp W.C., Fiebig H.H., Mullendore L.A., Pittman A.F., Kenney S., Keller J., and Boyd M.R. 1992. Morphological and immunocytochemical characteristics of human tumor cell lines for use in a disease-oriented anticancer drug screen. *Anticancer Res.* **12**: 1035.

Vogelstein B. and Kinzler K.W. 2004. Cancer genes and the pathways they control. *Nat. Med.* **10**: 789.

Weber B.L. 2002. Cancer genomics. *Cancer Cell* **1**: 37.

Weinstein I.B. 2002. Cancer. Addiction to oncogenes—The Achilles heal of cancer. *Science* **297**: 63.

Weir B., Zhao X., and Meyerson M. 2004. Somatic alterations in the human cancer genome. *Cancer Cell* **6**: 433.

Weterman M.A., Wilbrink M., and Geurts van Kessel A. 1996. Fusion of the transcription factor TFE3 gene to a novel gene, PRCC, in t(X;1)(p11;q21)-positive papillary renal cell carcinomas. *Proc. Natl. Acad. Sci.* **93**: 15294.

Widlund H.R. and Fisher D.E. 2003. Microphthalamia-associated transcription factor: A critical regulator of pigment cell development and survival. *Oncogene* **22**: 3035.

Wilhelm S.M., Carter C., Tang L., Wilkie D., McNabola A., Rong H., Chen C., Zhang X., Vincent P., McHugh M., Cao Y., Shujath J., Gawlak S., Eveleigh D., Rowley B., Liu L., Adnane L., Lynch M., Auclair D., Taylor I., Gedrich R., Voznesensky A., Riedl B., Post L.E., Bollag G., and Trail P.A. 2004. BAY 43-9006 exhibits broad spectrum oral antitumor activity and targets the RAF/MEK/ERK pathway and receptor tyrosine kinases involved in tumor progression and angiogenesis. *Cancer Res.* **64**: 7099.

Wu M., Hemesath T.J., Takemoto C.M., Horstmann M.A., Wells A.G., Price E.R., Fisher D.Z., and Fisher D.E. 2000. c-Kit triggers dual phosphorylations, which couple activation and degradation of the essential melanocyte factor Mi. *Genes Dev.* **14**: 301.

Zhao X., Li C., Paez J.G., Chin K., Janne P.A., Chen T.H., Girard L., Minna J., Christiani D., Leo C., Gray J.W., Sellers W.R., and Meyerson M. 2004. An integrated view of copy number and allelic alterations in the cancer genome using single nucleotide polymorphism arrays. *Cancer Res.* **64**: 3060.

Zhao X., Weir B.A., LaFramboise T., Lin M., Beroukhim R., Garraway L., Beheshti J., Lee J.C., Naoki K., Richards W.G., Sugarbaker D., Chen F., Rubin M.A., Janne P.A., Girard L., Minna J., Christiani D., Li C., Sellers W.R., and Meyerson M. 2005. Homozygous deletions and chromosome amplifications in human lung carcinomas revealed by single nucleotide polymorphism array analysis. *Cancer Res.* **65**: 5561.

Polygenic Inherited Predisposition to Breast Cancer

B.A.J. PONDER, A. ANTONIOU, A. DUNNING, D.F. EASTON, AND P.D.P. PHAROAH

Departments of Oncology & Public Health & Cancer Research UK Genetic Epidemiology Unit, Strangeways Research Laboratories, University of Cambridge, Cambridge CB1 8RN, United Kingdom

The known breast cancer predisposing genes account for only about 20% of inherited susceptibility. Epidemiological analyses suggest that much of the remaining 80% is explained by the combined effect of many individually weak genetic variants, rather than by further rare, highly penetrant mutations. In the near term, identification of variants may indicate new pathways or mechanisms in breast cancer development. The polygenic model implies a wide distribution of risk in the population. In the longer term, it may be possible to construct individual risk profiles to guide public health interventions. The search for genetic variants has so far proved difficult. A key unanswered question is the "genetic architecture" of predisposition—that is, strong or weak alleles, common or rare. We describe a genome-wide scan designed to provide a first-pass answer to this question.

Our aim is to identify the genes that contribute to susceptibility to breast cancer. There are two potential applications. The first is to cancer biology. The demonstration that a particular gene contributes to susceptibility provides genetic evidence to confirm the importance of genes or pathways whose role in cancer development is already suspected, or it can highlight new genes and new pathways. The second is to defining individual risks. The polygenic model for susceptibility outlined below suggests a wide range of risk within the population. Knowledge of individual genetic makeup may allow prediction of risk and thus inform choices about screening and prevention.

Two predisposing genes are already well known: BRCA1 and BRCA2. Rare, strongly predisposing mutations in those genes give rise to multiple-case families, allowing the identification of the genes by linkage and positional cloning. Subsequently, knowledge of the genes has indeed led to new insights into cancer biology (see, e.g., Venkitaraman 2002), culminating recently in proposals for new therapeutic targets (Farmer et al. 2005), and to gene-based estimates of risk that guide clinical management (Antoniou et al. 2003).

Although important, mutations in BRCA1 and 2 account for only a small part of inherited susceptibility to breast cancer. The size of the total inherited contribution can be inferred from the extent of familial clustering. On average, the risk of breast cancer to the mother or sister of a case is about 1.8-fold higher than the risk across the population. Twin studies suggest that most of this family clustering is due to inheritance rather than shared environment (Lichtenstein et al. 2000). The contribution of BRCA1 and 2 can be estimated by taking a large population-based series of breast cancer cases with details of family history—and thus of the familial excess of breast cancers—and measuring the fraction of the familial excess that is accounted for by families in which there is a BRCA1 or 2 mutation. Such studies indicate a contribution of 15–20% (Easton 1999; Peto et al. 1999; Anglian Breast Study Group 2000). Mutations in other genes, including chk-2, ATM, PTEN, and p53, account for well under a further 5%. The question we seek to address is, What genes account for the remaining 80%?

POSSIBLE GENETIC MODELS

In principle, the remaining susceptibility could be due to single genes with rare, strongly predisposing alleles, similar to BRCA1 and 2. At the other extreme, predisposition could be polygenic: the result of the combined effects of weakly predisposing alleles in many genes. Each allele contributes a certain proportion of the overall genetic effect (that is, a percentage of the observed excess familial clustering) depending on its frequency and its strength in terms of risk. Thus, at one end of the spectrum, four BRCA-like genes with mutant allele frequency of 1 in 500 and an average risk of 10-fold would account for the total effect. At the polygenic end, large numbers of alleles in many genes will be required, the number depending on the allele frequency, the risks, and the genetic model (additive, multiplicative) by which their effects combine (Fig. 1).

Two points arise from this figure: (1) The strategy to search for the genes depends on the model. Linkage is appropriate for BRCA-like genes, but not for polygenes (Risch and Merikangas 1996; Risch 2000); association studies are appropriate for common polygenes but not for rare strong genes. (2) If the polygenic model is chosen, the "genetic architecture" will also be critical. One can hope to detect common alleles of moderate effect; but weak, and especially rare, alleles will be difficult. This is discussed further below.

THE POLYGENIC MODEL

The evidence for this model in breast cancer comes from population-based epidemiological studies. Most of the excess familial clustering of breast cancer is found to be distributed across many families, each with small numbers of cases, rather than in a few very extensive fam-

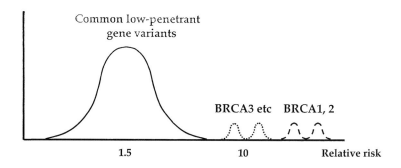

Allele freq.	(%) X^{s}FRR explained	Number	Allele freq.	(%) X^{s}FRR explained	Number
1%	.25	350	0.2%	16	5
10%	2.3	35			
30%	5.3	16			

Figure 1. The numbers and types of alleles that might account for the familial risk of breast cancer. Assuming a relative risk of 10 and a population frequency of 0.2%, four more BRCA-like genes would be needed to account for the component of susceptibility not explained by BRCA1 and 2. Alternatively, assuming an average relative risk of 1.5 and a dominant mode of action with multiplicative effects, as few as 10–20 common genetic variants, or several hundred rare variants, would be needed.

ilies (see, e.g., Cui et al. 2001; Antoniou et al. 2002). This is the pattern expected with a substantial contribution from a polygenic mode of predisposition, where the excess risk decays rapidly with increasing distance of relationship. A Mendelian BRCA-like model of a single mutant gene with strong effects, in contrast, would result in concentration of the excess cases in a few multiple-case families. We have therefore based our gene finding strategy on the polygenic model.

The polygenic model has important implications for the distribution of risk in the population (Pharoah et al. 2002). Risk is normally distributed, and the width of the distribution—which determines the magnitude of the difference in risk between the high- and low-risk groups—is related to the size of the overall genetic effect. For breast cancer, our model derived from a population-based series of cases from the East Anglian region of the UK suggests a 30- to 40-fold difference between women in the highest and lowest 20% of the population. This translates, for example, into the 12% of women most at risk accounting for half of all breast cancers, while the 50% at lowest risk account for only 12%. The public health implications, if individuals could be placed on the spectrum, are clear.

SEARCHING FOR THE GENES UNDER A POLYGENIC MODEL

Provided certain conditions (outlined below) are met, association studies are the most efficient design. In an association study, DNA sequence variants (generally in the form of single-nucleotide polymorphisms [SNPs]) in a series of candidate genes are compared for frequency in a set of cases and of controls, which should be as closely matched for genetic background as possible (Cardon and Bell 2001). The straightforward case is where the variant to be tested is functionally active and thought to be directly causally relevant to the disease. In this case, a consistent finding that the variant occurs at a higher frequency in cases than in controls is presumptive evidence

of cause. Usually, however, no clear candidate causative variant is known. In this case, the common variants in the gene (those with minor allele frequency greater than 5–10%) are identified as completely as possible by resequencing, and a subset is chosen, on the basis of allele frequency and linkage disequilibrium relationships, that will most efficiently report on the others. These are "tagging SNPs" (for more detailed discussion, see Chapman et al. 2003; Carlson et al. 2004; Wang et al. 2005). The intention is that one or more of the tagging SNPs, or a haplotype defined by them, will act as a surrogate for the putative but unknown disease allele.

For this strategy to succeed, even if the right candidate genes have been selected, several conditions must be fulfilled. These relate to the genetic architecture of disease predisposition, and they lie at the heart of the problem of finding these genes. First, the effect of any allele must be large enough for the association to be detected within the power of the study. It is usual to express the size of effect in terms of the relative risk of disease conferred by the allele, but of course, the allele frequency is an important determinant of its effect as well. We therefore prefer to use as our measure the percentage of the excess familial risk (the genetic variance) that is explained. Because this combines the effects of allele frequency and relative risk, power is fairly stable across a range of allele frequencies (Fig. 2). Note that even in the most easily detected plausible (dominant, or additive [co-dominant]) models, sample sizes of several thousands are needed to obtain significance values that provide some confidence of true association for common alleles that account for 1% of the genetic variance (Antoniou and Easton 2003; Pharoah et al. 2004). Given the practicalities of assembling and testing very large case/control sets, this indicates the constraints on the size of effect that can be searched for.

Second, for good power in such a study, the disease alleles must also be common, with minor allele frequencies ideally of at least 5–10%, and comparable to those of the "tagging" variants used to report them. Statistical power

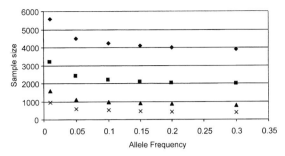

Figure 2. Power in association studies. Sample sizes (numbers of cases and numbers of controls) needed for 90% power at $p = 10^{-4}$ to detect dominant alleles of different frequencies that account for ◆ 1%, ■ 2%, ▲ 5%, and × 10% of the total genetic variance of breast cancer. These calculations assume that the SNP that is assayed reports perfectly on the disease allele. If the frequencies of reporting SNP and disease alleles are different, power will be less and the sample size needed will be greater. (Adapted from Antoniou & Easton 2003.)

is lost if the tagging variants are at a markedly different frequency from the alleles they are to tag. Current association studies are therefore based on common tagging variants, because the search is predicated on the existence of similarly common disease alleles, and because the search for rare alleles has very low statistical power.

Third, the tagging variant and the disease allele should have arisen only once in the history of the population. Variants that have arisen more than once probably have occurred on different chromosomes, which will destroy the co-inheritance of the tag and disease alleles (see Fig. 3).

In summary, the association study strategy is based on the "common variant:common disease" hypothesis, which states that a substantial component of predisposition is attributable to common variants which are likely to be ancient in the population, rather than to multiple individually rare variants recently arisen from new mutation. The likely validity of this hypothesis, and thus of the association-study-based search for common disease genes, has been the subject of a great deal of argument (Reich and Lander 2001; Wright and Hastie 2001; Pritchard and Cox 2002; Smith and Lusis 2002; Botstein and Risch 2003; Lohmueller et al. 2003), none of it conclusive. Probably,

some disease alleles are common and ancient, and others are rare and new. A reasonable way to find out the situation in breast cancer would seem to be: Do the experiment.

RESULTS

We have based our studies of breast cancer over the past 5 years on a variety of candidate genes and pathways, including steroid hormone metabolism and signaling, DNA repair, cell cycle and checkpoints, growth factors, carcinogen metabolism, tumor microenvironment, methylation, and candidate genes from mouse and rat models. To date, we have examined 525 SNPs in 110 genes, tagged with increasing efficiency as both experimental design and information on SNP variants have improved. The case/control set we have studied comprises 4,600 cases of invasive breast cancer diagnosed below age 70 ascertained through the Anglian Cancer Registry from the East Anglian region of the UK, and 4,600 controls from the EPIC cohort study based in the same region (Day et al. 1999). Simple epidemiological and clinical data are available for all cases, along with paraffin blocks of tumors from a large subset; the EPIC controls have extensive epidemiological data, frozen serum, and a range of phenotypes including mammographic data and levels of serum hormones and growth factors.

Our strategy has been to aim for 90% power at $p = 10^{-4}$ to detect common variants that account for 1% of the genetic variance. For economy, we have used a 2-stage genotyping strategy in which all SNPs are tested in a first set of 2,300 cases and controls, and those that meet specified statistical criteria ($p < 0.1$ in a test of genotype distribution or a test for trend) are tested in a second similar-sized case/control set drawn from the same sampling frame.

To date, we have found no SNP in any gene that gives us $p < 10^{-4}$ for association with breast cancer, or which accounts for 1% of the genetic variance. Of the first 500 SNPs analyzed, 36 gave a p value for association with breast cancer at $p \leq 0.05$, and 9 at $p \leq 0.01$, using the 2 df test for genotype distribution, compared to 25 and 5 expected by chance. Similar, but slightly different, results were obtained using a test for trend.

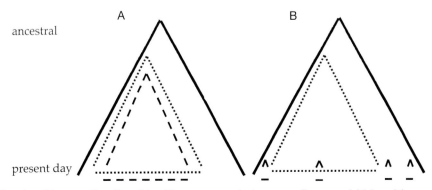

Figure 3. Genetic architecture of predisposition. The common variant:common disease model (*A*), and the rare variant model (*B*). The large solid triangles represent the expansion of the population over its history. The smaller triangles represent the distribution in the population of a tagging variant SNP (·······) and of a disease allele (— — —) on which it is to report. If the tagging SNP and disease allele have arisen only once in the history of the population and are present at roughly the same frequency (e.g., because they arose at roughly the same time), the tagging SNP will report effectively on the disease allele (*A*). This is not the case with a disease allele that has arisen on multiple occasions, or with an allele that has arisen only on one occasion but which is very different in frequency in the population from the marker allele (*B*).

No individual result at these levels of significance can be relied upon as a true positive rather than a chance result. Given the prior probability that any given variant might contribute to susceptibility, and setting aside the argument that particular genes are, a priori, more likely candidates, a p value of 0.001 in our studies has something like a 50:50 probability of representing a "true" result (Pharoah et al. 2004). We have therefore asked whether, taking the results in aggregate, we can reject the possibility that there is no effect—that is, that none of our tested candidates contributes to breast cancer risk. To address this, we have ranked the p values we have obtained, calculated a cumulative p value as each successive result is added, and used permutation testing (because of the incomplete independence of the individual SNPs) to compare these values with those expected under the hypothesis of no genetic effect. In addition to the global analysis, we have modeled different combinations of numbers, frequency, and relative risks of susceptibility alleles, and asked what power we would have had to detect these effects in the global permutation test. The details are not presented here: In summary, even with our case/control set, which is large in comparison to those that are usually reported, our power proves to be quite poor to detect the presence of genetic effects involving a few alleles that each contribute around 0.5–1% of the total variance, under a variety of plausible scenarios. We therefore remain uncertain whether, and to what extent, our results provide evidence for the presence of susceptibility alleles in our population. We are investigating further statistical methods to address this question.

HOW TO EVALUATE THE RESULTS?

The above analysis leaves open the possibility that, among the candidate genes we have tested, there may be some in which common variants do contribute to susceptibility, but that these effects are too weak for us to have detected them. Support for this possibility comes from the clearly positive results with serum hormones and growth factors as "intermediate phenotypes," described below. Probably none of these genes individually contributes as much as 1% of the genetic variance, and in aggregate, they probably account for less than 3%.

We may have missed alleles of larger effect because of shortcomings in our analysis and study design. Thus, we have not incorporated the possibility of gene interactions into the analyses (Marchini et al. 2005) but have concentrated on main effects, thereby possibly missing larger effects in a subset of individuals. Similarly, we have used a single dichotomous phenotype—breast cancer—whereas breast cancer is heterogeneous in molecular terms and probably in genetic etiology. Quantitative phenotypes, such as serum hormone levels or mammographic density, have greater statistical power. This is illustrated by our results with variants in the CYP19 gene, which is involved in the conversion of testosterone to estradiol, and their effects on serum levels of estradiol and of testosterone (Dunning et al. 2004). We found a highly significant association of the variants in CYP19 with hormone levels, but epidemiological data indicate that these effects on hormone levels would be predicted to correspond to a very small effect on breast cancer risk, consistent with our failure to detect an association of the same CYP19 variants with breast cancer (Fig. 4A,B).

The main argument that there may be undiscovered genes of larger effect is that we have tested as candidates only about 100 genes of the 30,000 that are possible; moreover, we have tested those incompletely, especially with respect to putative regulatory variants. Theoretical arguments, as well as empirical data from man and other organisms (for review, see Mackay 2001), suggest that the distribution of sizes of effect for alleles that modify phenotypes or influence susceptibility will be roughly exponential—that is, there will be some alleles of moderate effect, and a "tail" of many alleles of smaller effect. Some alleles of moderate effect have indeed been identified to contribute to susceptibility to other diseases (Lohmueller et al. 2003); in a model system such as *Drosophila* bristle number where a more complete analysis is possible, a range of effect sizes is seen (Long et al. 2000). To search efficiently for the few alleles with larger effects that may exist, we need to move from a candidate gene approach to an empirical genome-wide scan for association.

A GENOME-WIDE SCAN

The aim is to use a set of SNPs that will report as completely as possible on common disease alleles across the entire genome. Some have argued that for reasons of cost and practicality, a genome scan should be targeted at

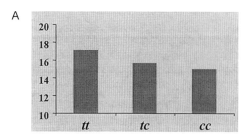
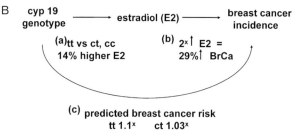

Figure 4. Intermediate phenotypes and prediction of breast cancer risk. Panel *A* shows levels of serum estradiol (in pmole/liter) in control women, corresponding to genotypes for the t-c polymorphism (rs 10046) in the 3′ UTR of CYP19. There is a significant correlation of hormone level with genotype (p for homogeneity = 0.0006). Panel *B* shows (*a*) the predicted effect, from the data in panel *A*, of CYP19 genotype on estradiol levels, (*b*) the predicted effect, from published studies, of a twofold increase in estradiol level on breast cancer risk, and (*c*) derived from these, the predicted effect of CYP19 genotype on breast cancer risk. Risks of this magnitude would require analysis of 34,000 cases and 34,000 controls to demonstrate with 50% power at $p = 10^{-4}$ the association between CYP19 genotype and breast cancer risk. (Data from Dunning et al. 2004.)

common nonsynonymous variants in known coding regions, since these are the most likely to be relevant. However, given the emerging data on interindividual variation in levels of gene expression, the evidence that many of the phenotypic differences between inbred strains of mice are regulatory in origin, and the data both on structural variations in the genome (Sebat et al. 2004) and on the existence of highly conserved extragenic regions with possible regulatory functions (Woolfe et al. 2005), we have thought it better to adopt a completely unbiased approach and to aim for as wide coverage of the genome as possible, with sufficient power to test the hypothesis that there are at least some alleles of moderate effect.

Over 6 million SNPs have been described across the genome, but it is not, of course, necessary to test them all. Many will be tightly associated with one or several others, which will then be mutually redundant. The first task is to assemble the set of tagging SNPs that is the best compromise between power and cost in reporting on the remainder of the common variation in the genome. The power of one SNP to report on another is expressed as the r^2 value; an r^2 of 1 means perfect power, whereas an r^2 of 0.5 means that the sample size to be tested must be doubled to obtain power equivalent to a SNP with r^2 of 1. The distribution of maximum r^2 values with which a set of tagging SNPs reports on all other known common variants provides an expression of the power of the proposed scan with these SNPs (Carlson et al. 2004).

Perlegen Sciences have identified over 2 million SNPs and typed them in single human chromosomes isolated in somatic cell hybrids, thus obtaining unequivocal haplotypes. From these, they defined in 2004 a subset of 266,000 SNPs that they showed empirically would report with r^2 0.8 or greater on an estimated 73% of all common SNPs in 152 genes for which resequencing data were available (Hinds et al. 2005). The process of SNP discovery of this set is described in detail in Patil et al. (2001) and Zhang et al. (2002). A substantially larger set of SNPs would have provided some increase in coverage, but at correspondingly greater cost.

Using these data, we designed what we believed to be the most cost-effective experiment available at the time, which was to use the 266,000 SNP set to search for any breast cancer susceptibility allele that would account for 2% or more of the total genetic variance. We estimated the power to detect such variants to be 80%. This estimate allows for loss of power from incomplete linkage disequilibrium and allele frequency differences. We analyzed only invasive breast cancer and treated breast cancer as a single diagnosis, not attempting to define subsets to recognize heterogeneity.

To attain this power, we needed to analyze several thousand breast cancer cases and controls; but with 266,000 SNPs in a single experiment, this would amount to well over a billion genotypes, and therefore would be too expensive. Pooling of samples (for example, in sets of 100) has been proposed as one means to reduce costs, but we rejected this. The unavoidable errors arising in the construction of the pools and from the effects of PCR amplification on the representation of individual alleles would, in our estimate, result in a level of noise that could

make effects of the size we thought might be important—relative risks of 1.3—difficult to detect reliably. We used instead a 2-stage strategy (Satagopan 2004) similar to that we had used for our previous candidate gene studies (Antoniou and Easton 2003). In the first stage, all 266,000 SNPs were tested against a small set of 400 breast cancer cases and controls, the cases genetically enriched by having a strong family history, but with no evidence of BRCA1 or 2 mutation. If our genetic models (Antoniou and Easton 2003) are correct, these 400 familial cases should be equivalent to about 1,600 unselected cases. The 400 controls taken from the EPIC cohort also provide substantial additional phenotypic data that can be used for genotypic analysis. The 12,000 or so SNPs with the most significant results from the first stage were then to be analyzed in a further, population-based, set of 4,600 cases and of 4,600 EPIC controls not overlapping with the first set. The best SNPs at this stage would be further analyzed as a third stage in a set of over 20,000 cases and controls currently being assembled through an International Consortium. These numbers should provide convincing statistical evidence to identify alleles associated with effects down to 1% of the overall genetic variance; but as for all association studies, the final identification of the functional allele, rather than simply the variant showing association with it, may require much more work.

The first-stage genotyping was completed in mid-summer 2005. The results provide encouragement that technical aspects of the experiment are satisfactory. 84% of the SNPs were scoreable in greater than 70% of individuals; for those SNPs, 95% of all the possible genotypes were obtained, with duplicate genotype reproducibility of 99.9%. There were no systematic differences in results obtained with DNA from each of the 4 UK centers that provided familial cases. Moreover, the distribution of p values for association that we observed was closely similar to that expected if there were no genetic effect, and with no highly positive outliers at the extreme—which suggests that there are no gross artefacts within the system. The results of the second stage should be available early in 2006.

RARE AND WEAK ALLELES

If the genome scan identifies some alleles of moderate effect, further analysis of these and their interactions should enlarge our knowledge of the genetic architecture of the disease. There will still be the question of common, weak alleles and of rare alleles which the association study is not powerful to detect.

The search for common weak alleles requires increased power. This will come from some combination of the following: larger studies; improved phenotyping of breast cancer, probably through molecular profiling of tumors; more sophisticated analysis of gene interactions; and possibly the use of quantitative intermediate phenotypes. With the tumor profiling data, it may, incidentally, be possible to address the interesting question of the relationship between germ-line genetic variation and the somatic genetic profile of the tumor: To what extent is the behavior and natural history of a neoplasm determined or constrained by the germ-line genetic environment? If there is a strong relationship, this may be particularly relevant to predicting the behavior of the preinvasive lesions that will be detected by the screening. This will be one consequence of the genetic definition of high-risk groups.

Rare alleles will require a different approach, presumably based on resequencing. Unless there are very clear functional data, the first evidence for the possible pathological significance of a given rare allele is likely to come, as with the association study, from the finding of a consistent and significantly greater frequency in cases and controls.

Again, the genetic architecture of rare variants and rare disease alleles in the population is unclear but will likely determine the most cost-effective approach. Questions include the numbers of rare sequence variants that will be found, the proportion of these that have pathological significance, and the confidence with which these can be recognized; the extent of allelic heterogeneity; and whether susceptibility alleles are concentrated in rather few genes (suggested by theoretical arguments and the example of the ABC A1 gene and plasma HDL levels; Cohen et al. 2004) or are widely dispersed. Until affordable genome-wide sequencing becomes available, a candidate gene approach might be based on rare variant discovery by resequencing in a few hundred "genetically enriched" individuals, followed by case/control comparisons using allele-specific assays. The choice of a quantifiable intermediate phenotype for which there are good candidate genes, such as some aspect of DNA repair function, combined with a search for rare variants across the candidate gene set, might provide a better-defined first step to investigate allelic architecture than the study of a cancer phenotype for which the candidate genes are uncertain.

CONCLUSIONS

Despite the growing recognition of the importance of polygenic susceptibility in cancer and in other diseases such as diabetes and hypertension, the search for the predisposing genes has so far been less successful than was hoped (Lohmueller et al. 2003). This disappointment stems in large part from a failure to appreciate the difficulties. Critical determinants of success are likely to include the following:

1. The genetic architecture of susceptibility. How much is due to alleles of sufficiently large effect that we can hope to identify them in the human population?

2. The resolution of phenotypic heterogeneity. In cancer, there are many ways to slice this cake, and we don't know which are best. If, as many believe, the cases to be included in association studies should be subclassified at the outset by molecular features of their tumor, the assembly of sufficiently large sets of cases with this information represents a formidable challenge.

3. The analysis of interactions. Although it can be argued that most predisposing alleles of sufficient impact to be of interest should be detectable by main effects, this is not always so—for example, in the case of interaction involving a rare allele. New statistical methods and, probably, better understanding of biology will

also be needed to tackle the problems of higher-dimensional interactions.

4. The extent to which the search is focused—for cost-effectiveness—on non-synonymous coding variants to the exclusion of regulatory variants including structural variations in extragenic regions (Morley et al. 2004; Sebat et al. 2004; Woolfe et al. 2005), mitochondrial (Taylor and Turnbull 2005) and possible epigenetic effects. All possibilities are still to be considered.

Progress over the next few years is likely to come from four directions: larger, and better defined, sample collections; improved genotyping and sequencing technologies; increasing databases of human genetic variation; and new statistical methods in complex genetics. Of these, possibly the most critical are the sample collections. These are expensive to set up and maintain, and funders need to understand their importance. The recent investments in large population cohorts in several countries may ultimately—in 10 or 20 years and more—provide valuable resources for the study of complex genetics and gene-environment interaction, but should not be a reason to neglect funding for the targeted case/control collections that are needed now to initiate gene discovery. The size of case/control sets that is needed will require international consortia and an ethos of sharing and collaboration perhaps rather different from the competitive days of Mendelian gene discovery.

When the genes are found, the first applications will almost certainly be to cancer biology: indications of new pathways, or genetic evidence to support the relevance of those already implicated. It is possible that a single common allele might contribute a sufficient fraction of disease incidence as to be itself a target for prevention (Fig. 5). The construction of individual risk profiles from multiple genotypes is potentially an important goal, but in breast cancer at least, still a distant prospect.

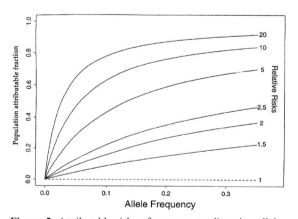

Figure 5. Attributable risks of common predisposing alleles. The vertical axis shows the population-attributable fraction—that is, the fraction of disease incidence that would be avoided if the predisposing allele were neutralized or removed from the population—for different combinations of frequency and relative risk of a dominant susceptibility allele. Thus, an allele with frequency 20% and a modest relative risk of around 1.5 has an attributable fraction of 15–20%. Note, for comparison, that the strongly predisposing mutant alleles of BRCA1 and 2, with population frequency 0.2%, have very small attributable fractions because of their rarity.

ACKNOWLEDGMENTS

Work in the author's laboratory is funded by Cancer Research UK. B.A.J.P. is a Gibb Fellow, D.F.E. is a Principal Fellow, and P.D.P.P. is a Senior Clinical Fellow of Cancer Research UK.

REFERENCES

Anglian Breast Cancer Study Group. 2000. Prevalence and penetrance of BRCA1 and BRCA2 mutations in a population-based series of breast cancer cases. *Br. J. Cancer* **83:** 1301.

Antoniou A.C. and Easton D.F. 2003. Polygenic inheritance of breast cancer: Implications for design of association studies. *Genet. Epidemiol.* **25:** 190.

Antoniou A.C., Pharoah P.D., McMullan G., Day N.E., Stratton M.R., Peto J., Ponder B.J., and Easton D.F. 2002. A comprehensive model for familial breast cancer incorporating BRCA1, BRCA2 and other genes. *Br. J. Cancer* **86:** 76.

Antoniou A., Pharoah P.D.P., Narod S., Risch H.A., Eyfjord J.E., Hopper J.L., Loman N., Olsson H., Johannsson O., Borg A., Pasini B., Radice P., Manoukian S., Eccles D.M., Tang N., Olah E., Anton-Culver H., Warner E., Lubinski J., Gronwald J., Gorski B., Tulinius H., Thorlacius S., Eerola H., Nevalinna H., Syrjakoski K., Kallioniemi O.P., Thompson D., Evans C., Peto J., Lalloo F., Evans D.G., and Easton D.F. 2003. Average risks of breast and ovarian cancer associated with BRCA1 or BRCA2 mutations detected in case series unselected for family history: A combined analysis of 22 studies. *Am. J. Hum. Genet.* **72:** 1117.

Botstein D. and Risch N. 2003. Discovering genotypes underlying human phenotypes: Past successes for Mendelian disease; future approaches for complex disease. *Nature Genet.* (suppl.) **33:** 228.

Cardon L.R. and Bell J.I. 2001. Association study designs for complex diseases. *Nat. Rev. Genet.* **2:** 91.

Carlson C.S., Eberle M.A., Rieder M.J., Yi Q., Kruglyak L., and Nickerson D.A. 2004. Selecting a maximally informative set of single-nucleotide polymorphisms for association analyses using linkage disequilibrium. *Am. J. Hum. Genet.* **74:** 106.

Chapman J.M., Cooper J.D., Todd J.A., and Clayton D.G. 2003. Detecting disease associations due to linkage disequilibrium using haplotype tags: A class of tests and the determinants of statistical power. *Hum. Hered.* **56:** 18.

Cohen J.C., Kiss R.S., Pertsemlidis A., Marcel Y.L., McPherson R., and Hobbs H.H. 2004. Multiple rare alleles contribute to low plasma levels of HDL cholesterol. *Science* **305:** 869.

Cui J., Antoniou A.C., Dite G.S., Southey M.C., Venter D.J., Easton D.F., Giles G.G., McCredie M.R., and Hopper J.L. 2001. After BRCA1 and BRCA2—what next? Multifactorial segregation analyses of three-generation, population-based Australian families affected by female breast cancer. *Am. J. Hum. Genet.* **68:** 420.

Day N., Oakes S., Luben R., Khaw K.T., Bingham S., Welch A., and Wareham N. 1999. EPIC-Norfolk: Study design and characteristics of the cohort. *Br. J. Cancer* (suppl. 1) **80:** 95.

Dunning A.M., Dowsett M., Healey C.S., Tee L., Luben R.N., Folkerd E., Novik K.L., Kelemen L., Ogata S., Pharoah P.D.P., Easton D.F., Day N.E., and Ponder B.A.J. 2004. Polymorphisms associated with circulating sex hormone levels in postmenopausal women. *J. Natl. Cancer Inst.* **96:** 936.

Easton D.F. 1999. How many more breast cancer predisposition genes are there? *Breast Cancer Res.* **1:** 14.

Farmer H., McCabe N., Lord C.J., Tutt A.N., Johnson D.A., Richardson T.B., Santarosa M., Dillon K.J., Hickson I., Knights C., Martin N.M., Jackson S.P., Smith G.C., and Ashworth A. 2005. Targeting the DNA repair defect in BRCA mutant cells as a therapeutic strategy. *Nature* **434:** 917.

Hinds D.A., Sture L.L., Nilsen G.B., Halperin E., Eskin E., Bellinger D.G., Frazer K.A., and Cox D.R. 2005. Whole genome patterns of common DNA variation in three human populations. *Science* **307:** 1072.

Lichtenstein P., Holm N.V., Verkasalo P.K., Iliadou A., Kaprio J., Koskenvuo M., Pukkala E., Skythe A., and Hemminki K. 2000. Environmental and heritable factors in the causation of cancer-analyses of cohorts of twins from Sweden, Denmark and Finland. *N. Engl. J. Med.* **343:** 78.

Lohmueller K.E., Pearce C.L., Pike M., Lander E.S., and Hirschhorn J.N. 2003. Meta-analysis of genetic association studies supports a contribution of common variants to susceptibility to common disease. *Nat. Genet.* **33:** 179.

Long A.D., Lyman R.F., Morgan A.H., Langley C.H., and Mackay T.F.C. 2000. Both naturally occurring insertions of transposable elements and intermediate frequency polymorphisms at the *achaete-scute* complex are associated with variation in bristle number in *Drosophila melanogaster*. *Genetics* **154:** 1255.

Mackay T.F.C. 2001. The genetic architecture of quantitiave traits. *Annu. Rev. Genet.* **35:** 303.

Marchini J., Donnelly P., and Cardon L.R. 2005. Genome-wide strategies for detecting multiple loci that influence complex diseases. *Nat. Genet.* **37:** 413.

Morley M., Moloney C.M., Weber T.M., Devlin J.L., Evans K.G., Spielman R.S., and Cheung V.G. 2004. Genetic analysis of genome wide variation in human gene expression. *Nature* **430:** 743.

Patil N., Berno A.J., Hinds D.A., Barrett W.A., Doshi J.M., Hacker C.R., Kautzer C.R., Lee D.H., Marjoribanks C., McDonough D.P., Nguyen B.T.N., Norris M.C., Sheehan J.B., Shen N., Stern D., Stokowski R.P., Thomas D.J., Trulson M.O., Vyas K.R., Frazer K.A., Fodor S.P., and Cox D.R. 2001. Blocks of limited haplotype diversity revealed by high-resolution scanning of human chromosome 21. *Science* **294:** 1719.

Peto J., Collins N., Barfoot R., Seal S., Warren W., Rahman N., Easton D.F., Evans C., Deacon J., and Stratton M.R. 1999. Prevalence of BRCA1 and BRCA2 gene mutations in patients with early onset breast cancer. *J. Natl. Cancer Inst.* **91:** 943.

Pharoah P.D.P., Dunning A.M., Ponder B.A.J., and Easton D.P. 2004. Association studies for finding cancer-susceptibility genetic variants. *Nat. Rev. Cancer* **4:** 850.

Pharoah P.D., Antoniou A., Bobrow M., Zimmern R.L., Easton D.F., and Ponder B.A. 2002. Polygenic susceptibility to breast cancer and implications for prevention. *Nat. Genet.* **31:** 33.

Pritchard J.K. and Cox N.J. 2002. The allelic architecture of human disease genes: Common disease-common variant ... or not? *Hum. Mol. Genet.* **11:** 2417.

Reich D.E. and Lander E.S. 2001. On the allelic spectrum of human disease. *Trends Genet.* **17:** 502.

Risch N. 2000. Searching for genetic determinants in the new millennium. *Nature* **405:** 847.

Risch N. and Merikangas K. 1996. The future of genetic studies of complex diseases. *Science* **273:** 1516.

Satagopan J.M., Venkatraman E.S., and Begg C.B. 2004. Two stage designs for gene-disease association studies with sample size constraints. *Biometrics* **60:** 589.

Sebat J., Lakshmi B., Troge J., Alexander J., Young J., Lundin P., Maner S., Massa H., Walker M., Chi M., Navin N., Lucito R., Healy J., Hicks J., Ye K., Reiner A., Gilliam T.C., Trask B., Patterson N., Zetterberg A., and Wigler M. 2004. Large-scale copy number polymorphism in the human genome. *Science* **305:** 525.

Smith D.J. and Lusis A.J. 2002. The allelic structure of common disease. *Hum. Mol. Genet.* **11:** 2455.

Taylor R.W. and Turnbull D.M. 2005. Mitochondrial DNA mutations in human disease. *Nat. Rev. Genet.* **6:** 389.

Venkitaraman A.R. 2002. Cancer susceptibility and the functions of BRCA1 and BRCA2. *Cell* **108:** 171.

Wang W.Y.S., Barratt B.J., Clayton D.G., and Todd J.A. 2005. Genome-wide association studies: Theoretical and practical concerns. *Nat. Rev. Genet.* **6:** 109.

Woolfe A., Goodson M., Goode D.K., Snell P., McEwen G.K., Vavouri T., Smith S.F., North P., Callaway H., Kelly K., Walter K., Abnizova I., Gilks W., Edwards Y.J.K., Cooke J.E., and Elgar G. 2005. Highly conserved non-coding sequences are associated with vertebrate development. *PLoS Biol.* **3:** e7.

Wright A.F. and Hastie N.D. 2001. Complex genetic diseases: Controversy over the Croesus code. *Genome Biol.* **2:** 1.

Zhang K., Deng M., Chen T., Waterman M.S., and Sun F. 2002. A dynamic programming algorithm for haplotype block partitioning. *Proc. Natl. Acad. Sci.* **99:** 7335.

Somatic Mutations in Human Cancer: Insights from Resequencing the Protein Kinase Gene Family

P.A. FUTREAL, R. WOOSTER, AND M.R. STRATTON

Cancer Genome Project, Wellcome Trust Sanger Institute, Hinxton, CB10 1SA, United Kingdom

All cancers arise due to the accumulation of mutations in critical target genes that, when altered, give rise to selective advantage in the cell and its progeny that harbor them. Knowledge of these mutations is key in understanding the biology of cancer initiation and progression, as well as the development of more targeted therapeutic strategies. We have undertaken a systematic screen of all annotated protein kinases in the human genome for mutations in a series of cancers including breast, non-small-cell lung, and testicular cancer. Our results show a wide diversity in mutation prevalence within and between tumor types. We have identified a mutator phenotype in human breast previously undescribed. The results presented from sequencing the same 1.3 million base pairs through several tumor types suggest that most of the observed mutations are likely to be passenger events rather than causally implicated in oncogenesis. However, this work does provide evidence for the likely existence of multiple, infrequently mutated kinases.

Cancer is a disease of DNA. All cancers arise due to the accumulation of mutations in DNA sequence. These sequence alterations give rise to mutations in critical target genes that ultimately provide a selective growth advantage for the cells harboring them, leading to the clinical manifestations of cancer. The identification of mutated genes in human cancer has been a major focus of cancer research for the past three decades. Identification of these mutations and the cellular pathways that are subverted holds the promise of better diagnostics and more targeted therapies. As well, a more general understanding of mutation prevalence and pattern in cancers will inform on both extrinsic and intrinsic erosive processes that buffet the genome, leading to oncogenesis as well as potential deficits in handling DNA damage.

Mutations in cancer can take the form of chromosomal-scale events such as rearrangements and translocations; subchromosomal alterations in the form of deletions and amplifications; and smaller-scale events comprising insertions, deletions, and base-pair substitutions. As well, the state of DNA methylation can be altered in cancers, providing an epigenetic means for gene deregulation.

Perhaps the least well investigated category of DNA alterations in cancer is that of point mutations—small insertions/deletions and substitutions. Genes primarily targeted by this class of mutation may leave few other positional clues (such as translocation, amplification, germ-line susceptibility alleles) to expedite their identification. Evidence from our recent census of cancer genes suggests that point-mutated genes are underrepresented, particularly in the solid tumors which comprise the bulk of the cancer burden in the population (Futreal et al. 2004). We have undertaken a systematic resequencing approach to ascertain those genes with mutations in this class with the hope of identifying important target genes and to begin to investigate the patterns of somatic mutation in a variety of human cancers.

WHY START WITH PROTEIN KINASES?

We have chosen the family of protein kinases as a first set of genes for resequencing efforts. Genes containing a protein kinase encoding domain are the most frequently mutated in human cancer. Kinases function as key molecular controllers of virtually all cellular processes including cell growth, division and apoptosis—all frequently aberrant in human cancer. As well, kinases have proven to be the most tractable class of proteins for the development of targeted therapeutics in cancer to date. Targeted inhibition of amplified *ERBB2/HER2-neu* receptor in metastatic breast cancer with trastuzumab (Herceptin) (a humanized monoclonal antibody) is the first example of targeted exploitation of a kinase target in cancer therapy (Slamon et al. 2001). The clinical efficacy of imatinib (Gleevec), a small-molecule inhibitor of rearranged and mutated *ABL, KIT,* and *PDGFRA/B* kinases, in chronic myelogenous leukemia (CML), gastrointestinal stromal tumors, and idiopathic hypereosinophilic syndrome has established the paradigm for small-molecule-inhibitor-based therapeutics in cancer (Sawyers 2004). Intragenic activating mutations in the *EFGR* gene have been shown to be important mediators of significant response to small-molecule EGFR inhibitors in stage III–IV adenocarcinoma of the lung (Lynch et al. 2004; Paez et al. 2004; Pao et al. 2004), thus extending the imatinib model into an adult epithelial cancer with undoubtedly more complex genetic alterations. Although the responses in lung cancer patients to two EGFR inhibitors, gefitinib (Iressa) and erlotinib (Tarceva), are not as dramatic or durable as those seen in CML with imatinib, they nevertheless show that targeted molecular therapeutics are active in an epithelial cancer which is otherwise refractory to treatment. This potential therapeutic vulnerability of cancers when treated with agents directed at specific mutated genes has been referred to as "oncogene addiction." In this model, a cancer becomes dependent on (addicted to) a particular oncogenically (mutationally) activated pathway for its survival, thus making that pathway particularly attractive for therapeutic intervention (Weinstein 2002).

More recently, the development of clinical resistance to both imatinib in CML and gefitinib in lung adenocarcinoma has been shown to be due to specific point mutations within the kinase domain binding site for the drug, further illustrating the critical role of the target gene in treatment efficacy (Gorre et al. 2001; Kobayashi et al. 2005). Certainly the success of exploiting mutated kinase targets and, conversely, the emergence of clinical resistance when targeting kinases with small-molecule inhibitors, suggest that further identification of mutated kinases in human cancer will provide an important opportunity for both the development of de novo therapeutics and the beginnings of poly-molecular therapy for cancer.

RESEQUENCING THE PROTEIN KINASES— OVERALL RESULTS

The protein kinase family comprises 518 genes (Manning et al. 2002). We have resequenced the coding exons plus splice junctions of the entire family (~1.3 million base pairs [Mb]/sample) in a series of 25 breast cancers, 33 non small-cell lung cancers (NSCLC), and 13 testicular germ-cell tumors (TGCT) (Table 1). In total, 92 Mb of sequence were generated from the 71 samples analyzed, providing the most in-depth analysis of somatic mutations in human cancer undertaken to date.

In each case studied there was a matching DNA sample from normal tissue (usually peripheral blood) from the same individual to verify the somatic nature of the observed mutations. Each coding exon including splice junctions was amplified and sequenced bidirectionally from tumor DNA. Any amplicon containing a sequence variant that was not an obvious single-nucleotide polymorphism (SNP) (present in dbSNP http://www.ncbi.nlm.nih.gov/SNP/ or previously observed to be a germline polymorphism in in-house sequencing efforts) was then amplified from matching normal DNA for the particular case. If the variant was not present in the germ-line DNA, indicating the mutation to be of somatic origin, both tumor and normal were reamplified and sequenced to confirm the somatic mutation. For a subset of genes with somatic mutations, a follow-up study in an independent set of cancers of roughly twice the size of the original screen was undertaken to investigate prevalence.

In total, we identified 279 somatic mutations distributed among 78 genes in the 71 sample (92 megabases) screens under discussion; 185 missense, 25 nonsense, 6 frameshift, 3 in-frame deletion, 12 consensus splice site, and 48 silent mutations were identified (http://www.sanger.ac.uk/genetics/CGP/Kinases/) (Bignell et al. 2005; Davies et al. 2005; Stephens et al. 2005). Of note, the rate of silent mutations (unlikely to be under selective pressure) reflects the minimum rate of somatic mutation "noise" to be dealt with in any such large-scale resequencing endeavor.

The most frequently mutated gene was *TTN*, encoding the Titin giant sarcomeric protein, with 15 somatic muta-

tions. Monte Carlo simulation analysis of mutation distribution by coding "footprint" size showed that mutations were not found any more often than predicted by chance when size of coding sequence was taken into account, suggesting that numbers of mutations per se was not a reliable indicator of presumptive oncogenic potential. Additional analyses included manual scrutiny for clustering in genes, for occurrence at conserved positions that are known to be mutated in other kinases, and for tumor type clustering.

To assess potential selection for coding (nonsynonymous) mutations, each nucleotide of the 1.3-Mb coding footprint of the protein kinases was mutated in silico to each of the other three bases (correcting for the observed mutational spectrum and sequence context of mutations), the resulting sequence was translated, and the mutations were classified into missense, nonsense, and silent (synonymous) changes. A higher than expected ratio of nonsynonymous:synonymous (nonsyn:syn) changes (which varies from 2:1 to 3:1 depending on the mutational spectrum) suggests that mutations which change the coding sequence are being selected and, hence, that a proportion of mutations detected may be implicated in cancer causation. For both the breast and lung screens, there was evidence for an excess of nonsynonymous changes, suggesting that proportion of mutations identified are likely contributory to oncogenesis, although any one was only mutated at low frequency. Even so, our data suggest that the majority of somatic mutations identified are passenger events and, as such, are significant confounders in trying to identify rare oncogenic mutations. Overall, the screens have not identified a frequently mutated protein kinase in the tumor types examined. However, given the small sample numbers and likely impact of tumor heterogeneity, additional screens are warranted.

The overall distribution of mutations among the samples examined is shown in Figure 1. Most striking is the diversity of mutation prevalence among and between tumor types examined. In general, NSCLC had the most mutations/sample examined, followed by breast cancer, then TGCT. Cancer cell lines tended to have more mutations than the primary cancers examined, but this trend was not particularly exaggerated in the NSCLC. For breast cancers, the cell lines comprised a select subset of breast cancers. All were TP53 mutant, and all but one were derived from a premenopausal breast cancer. However, there was one cell line that had no mutations. For primary tumors, each screen yielded a subset that had no detectable somatic mutations. This was most striking in TGCT, where 12 out of 13 cases had no detectable mutations. Within NSCLC, no carcinoid (n = 6) had a somatic mutation. Likewise, the majority of breast cancer primaries (12/16) had no mutations.

TGCT was included in these initial screens due to its unique clinical behavior. It is the only solid tumor curable with chemotherapy in the metastatic setting, despite being markedly aneuploid in nearly all cases (Oosterhuis and Looijenga 2005). We detected only a single somatic point mutation in over 15 Mb of sequence in this tumor type, giving it perhaps the lowest mutation prevalence yet observed. Such evidence is supportive of a model of chemosensitivity where there is demonstrable DNA re-

Table 1. Samples Screened for Somatic Mutations in the Protein Kinases

Sample	Study	Histology	Age at diagnosis	Sex	Smoking status
PD0025a	breast	IDC	83	female	ND
PD0062a	breast	IDC	37	female	ND
PD0091a	breast	IDC	83	female	ND
PD0118a	breast	IDC	78	female	ND
PD0119a	breast	pleomorphic lobular	84	female	ND
PD0127a	breast	IDC	81	female	ND
PD0128a	breast	IDC	85	female	ND
PD1232a	breast	mucinous	85	female	ND
PD1233a	breast	IDC	38	female	ND
PD1234a	breast	IDC	43	female	ND
PD1235a	breast	IDC	38	female	ND
PD1236a	breast	IDC	47	female	ND
PD1237a	breast	IDC	55	female	ND
PD1238a	breast	IDC	36	female	ND
PD1239a	breast	IDC	73	female	ND
PD1241a	breast	IDC	45	female	ND
HCC38	breast	IDC	50	female	ND
HCC1143	breast	IDC	52	female	ND
HCC1187	breast	IDC	41	female	ND
HCC1395	breast	IDC	43	female	ND
HCC1599	breast	IDC	44	female	ND
HCC1937	breast	IDC	23	female	ND
HCC1954	breast	IDC	61	female	ND
HCC2157	breast	IDC	48	female	ND
HCC2218	breast	IDC	38	female	ND
PD0248a	NSCLC	SCC	57	male	previous smoker
PD0250a	NSCLC	carcinoid	61	female	nonsmoker
PD0251a	NSCLC	SCC	57	male	current
PD0252a	NSCLC	BAC	83	male	previous smoker
PD0253a	NSCLC	adeno	60	male	current
PD0263a	NSCLC	LC	81	male	previous smoker
PD0269a	NSCLC	SCC	52	male	current
PD0276a	NSCLC	LC	71	male	previous smoker
PD1240	NSCLC	SCC	69	male	unknown
PD1339a	NSCLC	adeno	65	male	previous smoker
PD1345a	NSCLC	adeno	65	male	current
PD1351a	NSCLC	adeno	67	male	unknown
PD1352a	NSCLC	adeno	58	male	current
PD1353a	NSCLC	adeno	65	male	previous smoker
PD1354a	NSCLC	carcinoid	71	female	nonsmoker
PD1355a	NSCLC	carcinoid	40	male	previous smoker
PD1356a	NSCLC	carcinoid	60	female	previous smoker
PD1359a	NSCLC	carcinoid	52	female	previous smoker
PD1360a	NSCLC	carcinoid	34	female	nonsmoker
PD1362a	NSCLC	LC	64	male	previous smoker
PD1364a	NSCLC	LC	57	female	previous smoker
PD1365a	NSCLC	LC	61	female	nonsmoker
PD1367a	NSCLC	LC	53	male	previous smoker
PD1370a	NSCLC	SCC	68	male	previous smoker
PD1373a	NSCLC	SCC	60	female	previous smoker
PD1379a	NSCLC	SCC	76	male	current
NCI-H1395	NSCLC	adeno	55	female	current
NCI-H1437	NSCLC	adeno	60	male	current
NCI-H1770	NSCLC	adeno	57	male	nonsmoker
NCI-H2009	NSCLC	adeno	68	female	current
NCI-H2087	NSCLC	adeno	69	male	current
NCI-H2122	NSCLC	adeno	46	female	current
NCI-H2126	NSCLC	adeno	65	male	unknown
PD1381a	testis	SGCT	29	male	ND
PD1382a	testis	SGCT	31	male	ND
PD1383a	testis	SGCT	50	male	ND
PD1384a	testis	SGCT	72	male	ND
PD1385a	testis	SGCT	28	male	ND
PD1386a	testis	SGCT	31	male	ND
PD1388a	testis	SGCT	22	male	ND
PD1389a	testis	NSGCT (EC TE YST)	26	male	ND
PD1391a	testis	NSGCT (EC TE YST)	37	male	ND
PD1392a	testis	NSGCT (TE YST)	30	male	ND
PD1394a	testis	NSGCT (EC YST TE)	31	male	ND
PD1395a	testis	NSGCT (YST)	32	male	ND
PD1396a	testis	NSGCT (EC YST TE)	26	male	ND

(NSCLC) Non-small-cell lung cancer; (IDC) infiltrating ductal carcinoma; (SCC) squamous cell carcinoma; (BAC) bronchoalveolar carcinoma; (adeno) adenocarcinoma; (LC) large cell carcinoma; (SGCT) seminomatous germ-cell tumor; (NSGCT) non-seminomatous germ-cell tumor; (EC) embryonal carcinoma; (TE) teratoma; (YST) yolk sac tumor; (ND) no data. PD numbered samples are primary tumors.

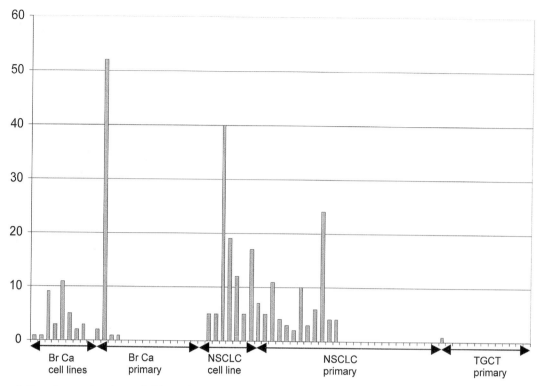

Figure 1. Somatic mutations in protein kinases by tumor type. Numbers of somatic mutations detected in resequencing the protein kinase gene are shown for each sample type. Y axis indicates the numbers of somatic mutation in each sample. Arrow brackets are provided to delineate specific sample subsets.

pair deficiency coupled with highly active apoptotic responses such that cells which accrue DNA damage are efficiently killed. Resequencing efforts will begin to provide more data to explore the relationship of somatic mutation prevalence, DNA repair competence, and response to therapy.

These screens allow more precise estimation of the absolute frequency of somatic mutations in cancer genomes as a whole. On the assumption that the 1.3-Mb protein kinase coding sequence is, to some extent, a representative sample of the genome, we can estimate the numbers of somatic mutations in each cancer genome and the numbers of consequent "bystander" amino acid changes. Some individual cancers have as many as 100,000 somatic mutations in their genomes, encoding approximately 1,000 amino acid changes (in 1:30 genes). In contrast, it appears that most breast and testis cancers have fewer than 2,000 somatic point mutations and fewer than 20 bystander amino acid changes.

RESEQUENCING THE PROTEIN KINASES–A NEW BREAST CANCER MUTATOR PHENOTYPE

Our analyses have demonstrated substantial diversity of mutation number and pattern in individual breast cancers. Particularly striking was primary tumor PD0119a (a pleomorphic lobular carcinoma occurring in an 84-year-old woman), which had 52 somatic mutations, more than all other breast cancer samples combined. The cancer was ER[+], ERRB2[−], TP53 mutation-negative, and negative for

E-cadherin staining, consistent with a luminal-ductal origin. The mutation spectrum in the cancer is characterized by a high frequency of C:G>G:C transversions occurring at TpC(GpA) dinucleotides (Fig. 2). Inactivating mutations in *BRCA1* or *BRCA2* are not associated with this mutational spectrum, and it is not obviously similar to any reported eukaryotic repair defect. The data suggest the characterization of a novel mutator phenotype in human breast cancer, although formally, the results could be due to a massive exposure. Of note, at least one breast cancer cell line appears to have a similar phenotype, derived from a ductal carcinoma in a 38-year-old (Fig. 2). This observation supports the existence of mutator phenotype in breast cancer. It is important to note that the only way currently to identify and characterize such phenotypes is through in-depth sequencing.

RESEQUENCING THE PROTEIN KINASES—MUTATED GENES

Several genes with somatic mutations identified in the screens are worth highlighting. We detected a single in-frame insertion in the kinase domain of *ERBB2* of a NSCLC primary sample, prompting a further screen of this gene in a larger series of cancers. Data from a larger series of primary NSCLC showed that *ERBB2* mutations are present in about 10% of lung adenocarcinoma (Stephens et al. 2004). This was the first report of intragenic mutation in this well-studied cancer gene. Mutations were found in the kinase domain affecting the α C-helix region, similar to the deletion mutations found in

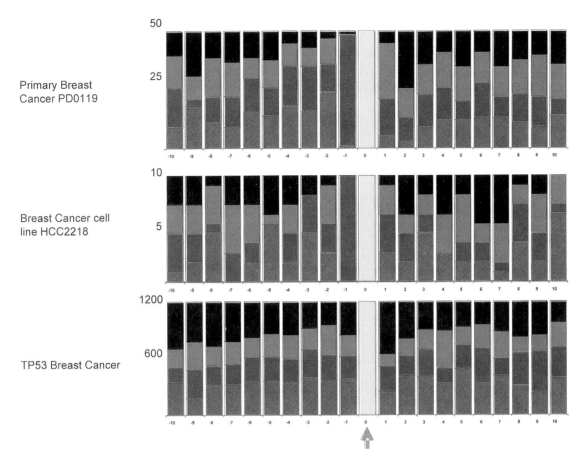

Figure 2. Sequence context specificity for the mutator phenotype breast cancer. Arrow and yellow bar indicate the position of C:G>G:C transversion mutations identified. Numbering is relative to the position of the mutation. All mutations were regularized to the "C" strand for this analysis. Note the almost complete predominance of a T residue before the mutated C. The sequence of TP53 C:G>G:C transversion mutations in breast cancer is shown for comparison. Red = T, green = A, blue = C, black = G. TP53 data from http://www-p53.iarc.fr/

EFGR (Lynch et al. 2004; Paez et al. 2004; Pao et al. 2004). Mutant *ERBB2* was neither overexpressed nor amplified in the cases examined. We found no obvious correlation with smoking history or sex, unlike subsequent studies (Shigematsu et al. 2005). Additional rare *ERBB2* mutations were found in cases of gastric cancer, ovarian cancer, and glioblastoma. Subsequent studies have reported low-frequency mutations (Sasaki et al. 2005), suggesting that *ERBB2* mutations, like those found in *EGFR*, may be restricted to specific subsets of NSCLC. Further work is needed to more clearly delineate the characteristics of this cohort to investigate the potential for the treatment of this subset of patients with anti-ERBB2 therapies.

Activating germ-line mutations of the fibroblast growth factor receptors, *FGFR1*, *FGFR2,* and *FGFR3*, have been reported in skeletal dysplasias (Wilkie et al. 2002). Somatic mutations of *FGFR3* found in papillary transitional-cell bladder cancer affect identical positions to germ-line mutations predisposing to thanatophoric dwarfism (Cappellen et al. 1999). Analogous to these data, we identified a somatic mutation in *FGFR1* (pP252T) in a bronchoalveolar NSCLC affecting a key codon known to have mutated in the skeletal dysplasia Pfeiffer syndrome (Human Gene Mutation Database,

http://archive.uwcm.ac.uk/uwcm/mg/hgmd0.html). Likewise, a somatic mutation was identified in *FGFR2* (pW290C) in a squamous cell lung carcinoma at an identical position reported for germ-line mutations in the skeletal dysplasias, craniosynostosis, Crouzon, and Pfeiffer syndromes. *FGFR2* point mutations have been previously described only in gastric cancer—again at residues analogous to germ-line mutations. These results strongly suggest that mutations in *FGFR1* and *FGFR2* are likely to play a role, albeit uncommonly, in lung carcinogenesis. Further work is needed to determine the rates and subtype distributions of *FGFR* mutations and the possible role of FGFR kinase inhibitors in lung cancer therapy.

Somatic mutations within the catalytic loop (pR678Q, pH677Y) and activation segment (pR721F) in *NTRK3*, encoding a neurotrophic growth factor receptor tyrosine kinase, were detected in breast and NSCLC. Mutations in *NTRK3* were also detected in a screen of the tyrosine kinases in colorectal cancers (Bardelli et al. 2003). The clustering of somatic mutations in key highly conserved residues and between tumor types suggests that *NTRK3* mutations are likely contributory to oncogenesis. Likewise, kinase domain mutations in both the primary and follow-up screen of NSCLC were detected in *AURKC* (*STK13*) encoding the aurora kinase C chromosomal passenger protein implicated in centrosome/spindle regulation during mitosis. The aurora kinases are the target for several inhibitors in clinical development (Andrews 2005). The extent of *AURKC* involvement in breast and lung cancers needs to be further investigated to potentially leverage these new therapeutics for these cancers.

CONCLUSIONS

Our resequencing efforts to date have provided evidence for multiple, infrequently mutated kinases in human cancer. Indeed, commonly mutated protein kinases such as *BRAF*, previously identified in a pilot screen in our laboratory (Davies et al. 2002), may well be the exception rather than the rule. Mutation screening of the protein kinases published for colorectal cancer are in agreement with the data presented here (Bardelli et al. 2003; Parsons et al. 2005). Taken together, the data paint a picture of increasing complexity of human cancer with any number of infrequently mutated protein kinases playing a role in oncogenesis. If such is the case, much larger studies will be needed to garner the statistical genetic support for discriminating between rare oncogenic and passenger mutations. New approaches for functional characterization involving high-throughput cell biological assays will be needed to further investigate the effects of these mutations. Newly developed animal model systems for introduction of multiple mutant alleles into specific tissues of the mouse, such as the Sleeping Beauty transposon system (Collier et al. 2005), will need to be exploited. The development of targeted therapeutics becomes more challenging if multiple small-molecule inhibitors are required to make a major impact on a given cancer type.

The data presented here represent the most in-depth look at the state of cancer genomes at the sequence level published to date. It is hoped that this work will help to inform future large-scale efforts such that we can begin to affect treatment of this complex set of diseases at pace and begin to deliver on the promise of the human genome sequence.

ACKNOWLEDGMENTS

We are indebted to all of the patients who participated in the studies described here, our collaborators, and all members of the Cancer Genome Project, past and present. This work was supported by the Wellcome Trust.

REFERENCES

Andrews P.D. 2005. Aurora kinases: Shining lights on the therapeutic horizon? *Oncogene* **24:** 5005.

Bardelli A., Parsons D.W., Silliman N., Ptak J., Szabo S., Saha S., Markowitz S., Willson J.K.V., Parmigiani G., Kinzler K.W., Vogelstein B., and Velculescu V.E. 2003. Mutational analysis of the tyrosine kinome in colorectal cancers. *Science* **300:** 949.

Bignell G., Smith R., Hunter C., Stephens P., Davies H., Greenman C., Teague J., Butler A., Edkins S., Stevens C., O'Meara S., Parker A., Avis T., Barthorpe S., Brackenbury L., Buck G., Clements J., Cole J., Dicks E., Edwards K., Forbes S., Gorton M., Gray K., Halliday K., Harrison R., Hills K., Hinton J., Jones D., Kosmidou V., Laman R., Lugg R., Menzies A., Perry J., Petty R., Raine K., Shepherd R., Small A., Solomon H., Stephens Y., Tofts C., Varian J., Webb A., West S., Widaa S., Yates A., Gillis A.J.M., Stoop H.J., Gurp R.J.H.L.M.v., Oosterhuis J.W., Looijenga L.H., Futreal P.A., Wooster R., and Stratton M.R. 2005. Sequence analysis of the protein kinase gene family in human testicular germ-cell tumours of adolescents and adults. *Genes Chromosomes Cancer.* **45:** 42.

Cappellen D., De Oliveira C., Ricol D., de Medina S., Bourdin J., Sastre-Garau X., Chopin D., Thiery J., and Radvanyi F. 1999. Frequent activating mutations of FGFR3 in human bladder and cervix carcinomas. *Nat. Genet.* **23:** 18.

Collier L.S., Carlson C.M., Ravimohan S., Dupuy A.J., and Largaespada D.A. 2005. Cancer gene discovery in solid tumours using transposon-based somatic mutagenesis in the mouse. *Nature* **436:** 272.

Davies H., Bignell G.R., Cox C., Stephens P., Edkins S., Clegg S., Teague J., Woffendin H., Garnett M.J., Bottomley W., Davis N., Dicks E., Ewing R., Floyd Y., Gray K., Hall S., Hawes R., Hughes J., Kosmidou V., Menzies A., Mould C., Parker A., Stevens C., Watt S., Hooper S., Wilson R., Jayatilake H., Gusterson B.A., Cooper C., Shipley J., Hargrave D., Pritchard-Jones K., Maitland N., Chenevix-Trench G., Riggins G.J., Bigner D.D., Palmieri G., Cossu A., Flanagan A., Nicholson A., Ho J.W., Leung S.Y., Yuen S.T., Weber B.L., Seigler H.F., Darrow T.L., Paterson H., Marais R., Marshall C.J., Wooster R., Stratton M.R., and Futreal P.A. 2002. Mutations of the BRAF gene in human cancer. *Nature* **417:** 949.

Davies H., Hunter C., Smith R., Stephens P., Greenman C., Bignell G., Teague J., Butler A., Edkins S., Stevens C., Parker A., O'Meara S., Avis T., Barthorpe S., Brackenbury L., Buck G., Clements J., Cole J., Dicks E., Edwards K., Forbes S., Gorton M., Gray K., Halliday K., Harrison R., Hills K., Hinton J., Jones D., Kosmidou V., Laman R., Lugg R., Menzies A., Perry J., Petty R., Raine K., Shepherd R., Small A., Solomon H., Stephens Y., Tofts C., Varian J., Webb A., West S., Widaa S., Yates A., Brasseur F., Cooper C.S., Flanagan A.M., Green A., Knowles M., Leung S.Y., Looijenga L.H.J., Malkowicz B., Pierotti M.A., Teh B.T., Yuen S.T., Lakhani S.R., Easton D.F., Weber B.L., Goldstraw P., Nicholson A.G., Wooster R., Stratton M.R., and Futreal P.A. 2005. Somatic mutations of the protein kinase gene family in human lung cancer. *Cancer Res.* **65:** 7591.

Futreal P.A., Coin L., Marshall M., Down T., Hubbard T., Wooster R., Rahman N., and Stratton M.R. 2004. A census of human cancer genes. *Nat. Rev. Cancer* **4:** 177.

Gorre M.E., Mohammed M., Ellwood K., Hsu N., Paquette R., Rao P.N., and Sawyers C.L. 2001. Clinical resistance to STI-571 cancer therapy caused by BCR-ABL gene mutation or amplification. *Science* **293:** 876.

Kobayashi S., Boggon T.J., Dayaram T., Janne P.A., Kocher O., Meyerson M., Johnson B.E., Eck M.J., Tenen D.G., and Halmos B. 2005. EGFR mutation and resistance of non-cell-cell lung cancer to gefitinib. *N. Engl. J. Med.* **352:** 786.

Lynch T.J., Bell D.W., Sordella R., Gurubhagavatula S., Okimoto R.A., Brannigan B.W., Harris P.L., Haserlat S.M., Supko J.G., Haluska F.G., Louis D.N., Christiani D.C., Settleman J., and Haber D.A. 2004. Activating mutations in the epidermal growth factor receptor underlying responsiveness of non-small-cell lung cancer to gefitinib. *N. Engl. J. Med.* **350:** 2129.

Manning G., Whyte D.B., Martinez R., Hunter T., and Sudarsanam S. 2002. The protein kinase complement of the human genome. *Science* **298:** 1912.

Oosterhuis J.W. and Looijenga L.H.J. 2005. Testicular germ-cell tumours in a broader perspective. *Nat. Rev. Cancer* **5:** 210.

Paez J.G., Janne P.A., Lee J.C., Tracy S., Greulich H., Gabriel S., Herman P., Kaye F.J., Lindeman N., Boggon T.J., Naoki K., Sasaki H., Fujii Y., Eck M.J., Sellers W.R., Johnson B.E., and Meyerson M. 2004. EGFR mutations in lung cancer: Correlation with clinical response to gefitinib therapy. *Science* **304:** 1497.

Pao W., Miller V., Zakowski M., Doherty J., Politi K., Sarkaria I., Singh B., Heelan R., Rusch V., Fulton L., Mardis E., Kupfer D., Wilson R., Kris M., and Varmus H. 2004. EGF receptor gene mutations are common in lung cancers from "never smokers" and are associated with sensitivity of tumors to gefitinib and erlotinib. *Proc. Natl. Acad. Sci.* **101:** 13306.

Parsons D.W., Wang T.-L., Samuels Y., Bardelli A., Cummins J.M., DeLong L., Silliman N., Ptak J., Szabo S., Willson J.K.V., Markowitz S., Kinzler K.W., Vogelstein B., Lengauer C., and Velculescu V.E. 2005. Colorectal cancer mutations in a signalling pathway. *Nature* **436:** 792.

Sasaki H., Shimizu S., Endo K., Takada M., Kawahara M., Tanaka H., Matsumura A., Iuchi K., Haneda H., Suzuki E., Kobayashi Y., Yano M., and Fujii Y. 2005. EGFR and erbB2 mutation status in Japanese lung cancer patients. *Int. J. Cancer* **118:** 180.

Sawyers C. 2004. Targeted cancer therapy. *Nature* **432:** 294.

Shigematsu H., Takahashi T., Nomura M., Majmudar K., Suzuki M., Lee H., Wistuba I.I., Fong K.M., Toyooka S., Shimizu N., Fujisawa T., Minna J.D., and Gazdar A.F. 2005. Somatic mutations of the HER2 kinase domain in lung adenocarcinomas. *Cancer Res.* **65:** 1642.

Slamon D.J., Leyland-Jones B., Shak S., Fuchs H., Paton V., Bajamonde A., Fleming T., Eiermann W., Wolter J., Pegram M., Baselga J., and Norton L. 2001. Use of chemotherapy plus a monoclonal antibody against HER2 for metastatic breast cancer that overexpresses HER2. *N. Engl. J. Med.* **344:** 783.

Stephens P., Hunter C., Bignell G., Edkins S., Davies H., Teague J., Stevens C., O'Meara S., Smith R., Parker A., Barthorpe A., Blow M., Brackenbury L., Butler A., Clarke O., Cole J., Dicks E., Dike A., Drozd A., Edwards K., Forbes S., Foster R., Gray K., Greenman C., Halliday K., Hills K., Kosmidou V., Lugg R., Menzies A., Perry J., Petty R., Raine K., Ratford L., Shepherd R., Small A., Stephens Y., Tofts C., Varian J., West S., Widaa S., Yates A., Brasseur F., Cooper C.S., Flanagan A.M., Knowles M., Leung S.Y., Louis D.N., Looijenga L.H.J., Malkowicz B., Pierotti M.A., Teh B., Chenevix-Trench G., Weber B.L., Yuen S.T., Harris G., Goldstraw P., Nicholson A.G., Futreal P.A., Wooster R., and Stratton M.R. 2004. Lung cancer: Intragenic ERBB2 kinase mutations in tumours. *Nature* **431:** 525.

Stephens P., Edkins S., Davies H., Greenman C., Cox C., Hunter C., Bignell G., Teague J., Smith R., Stevens C., O'Meara S., Parker A., Tarpey P., Avis T., Barthorpe A., Brackenbury L., Buck G., Butler A., Clements J., Cole J., Dicks E., Edwards K., Forbes S., Gorton M., Gray K., Halliday K., Harrison R., Hills K., Hinton J., Jones D., Kosmidou V., Laman R., Lugg R., Menzies A., Perry J., Petty R., Raine K., Shepherd R., Small A., Solomon H., Stephens Y., Tofts C., Varian J., Webb A., West S., Widaa S., Yates A., Brasseur F., Cooper C.S., Flanagan A.M., Green A., Knowles M., Leung S.Y., Looijenga L.H.J., Malkowicz B., Pierotti M.A., Teh B., Yuen S.T., Nicholson A.G., Lakhani S., Easton D.F., Weber B.L., Stratton M.R., Futreal P.A., and Wooster R. 2005. A screen of the complete protein kinase gene family identifies diverse patterns of somatic mutations in human breast cancer. *Nat. Genet.* **37:** 590.

Weinstein I.B. 2002. Cancer. Addiction to oncogenes—The Achilles heal of cancer. *Science* **297:** 63.

Wilkie A., Patey S., Kan S., van den Ouweland A., and Hamel B. 2002. FGFs, their receptors, and human limb malformations: Clinical and molecular correlations. *Am. J. Med. Genet.* **112:** 266.

High-Resolution ROMA CGH and FISH Analysis of Aneuploid and Diploid Breast Tumors

J. Hicks,* L. Muthuswamy,* A. Krasnitz,* N. Navin,*[†] M. Riggs,*
V. Grubor,* D. Esposito,* J. Alexander,* J. Troge,* M. Wigler,*
S. Maner,[‡] P. Lundin,[‡] and A. Zetterberg[‡]

*Cold Spring Harbor Laboratory, [†]Watson School of Biological Sciences,
Cold Spring Harbor, New York 11724; [‡]Karolinska Institutet, Department of Oncology-Pathology,
Cancer Center Karolinska, 171 76 Stockholm, Sweden

Combining representational oligonucleotide microarray analysis (ROMA) of tumor DNA with fluorescence in situ hybridization (FISH) of individual tumor cells provides the opportunity to detect and validate a wide range of amplifications, deletions, and rearrangements directly in frozen tumor samples. We have used these combined techniques to examine 101 aneuploid and diploid breast tumors for which long-term follow-up and detailed clinical information were available. We have determined that ROMA provides accurate and sensitive detection of duplications, amplifications, and deletions and yields defined boundaries for these events with a resolution of <50 kbp in most cases. We find that diploid tumors exhibit fewer rearrangements on average than aneuploids, but rearrangements occur at the same locations in both types. Diploid tumors reflect at least three consistent patterns of rearrangement. The reproducibility and frequency of these events, especially in very early stage tumors, provide insight into the earliest chromosomal events in breast cancer. We have also identified correlations between certain sets of rearrangement events and clinically relevant parameters such as long-term survival. These correlations may enable novel prognostic indicators for breast and other cancers as more samples are analyzed.

Alterations in chromosome organization and structure are a hallmark of many human cancers (Balmain et al. 2003; DePinho and Polyak 2004), reflecting the evolution of the tumor and its ability to proliferate and spread within the host. Breast tumors in particular exhibit a wide range of karyotypic changes including duplication or loss of multiple chromosome arms or entire chromosomes, along with a variety of segmental deletions and amplifications.

The first global studies capable of resolving deletions and amplifications combined comparative genomic hybridization (CGH) and cytogenetics (A. Kallioniemi et al. 1992a,b; O.P. Kallioniemi et al. 1992), and this approach has been applied to breast tumors (Kallioniemi et al. 1994; Ried et al. 1997; Tirkkonen et al. 1998). Subsequently, microarray methods employing CGH have increased resolution and reproducibility, and have improved throughput (Ried et al. 1995; Pollack et al. 2002; Albertson 2003; Lage et al. 2003). These published microarray studies have largely validated the results of cytogenetic CGH, but have not had sufficient resolution to significantly improve our knowledge of the role of genetic events in the etiology of disease, nor assist in the treatment of the patient. On the other hand, knowledge of specific genetic events, like amplification of c-ErbB2, as studied by fluorescence in situ hybridization (FISH) or quantitative PCR, has been clinically useful (van de Vijver et al. 1987; Slamon et al. 1989; Menard et al. 2001). Representational oligonucleotide microarray analysis (ROMA) provides an extra measure of resolution in genomic analysis that might be useful in clinical evaluation, as well as delineating loci important in disease evolution.

We have therefore begun a long-term genomic study on a clinically defined set of cancer patients that will combine FISH analysis of specific sites with an ultrahigh resolution microarray CGH technique called ROMA (Lucito et al. 2003) capable of detecting chromosomal events at a resolution approaching 35 kbp. This study is intended to determine whether a detailed knowledge of the events observable in various tumor stage and patient outcomes can elucidate the progression of chromosomal events in breast cancer and provide a means for more accurately directing therapy on the basis of a genomic biopsy.

Both FISH and ROMA can reproducibly detect deletions, duplications, and higher-order amplifications in tissue samples, yet the two techniques have specific differences with valuable and complementary features. Interphase FISH has the advantage of revealing the absolute copy number of a specific genomic sequence or locus complementary to the hybridization probe in each cell examined. Therefore, FISH can distinguish tumor cells with aberrant copy numbers distributed among normal cells in a tumor or biopsy sample. It can likewise detect the presence of subpopulations or subclones of cells within a tumor sample that exhibit different copy numbers for a given probe. The disadvantage of FISH is that the technique depends on some foreknowledge of loci likely to be of interest and examined and is limited to only a few different probes for each experiment, usually fewer than ten. It is therefore highly advantageous to couple FISH with a technology that will survey the entire genome for copy number alterations at the highest possible resolution.

ROMA CGH (Lucito et al. 2003) has the advantage of "seeing" the complete genome in each experiment at a resolution that depends on the number of unique features arrayed on the chip. The microarray chip used in this study has nearly 85,000 features spaced at roughly <50-kbp intervals throughout the genome. Like all microarray-based methods, the copy number that is reported reflects an average of all cells in the sample. The presence of normal cells in a tumor sample or biopsy will therefore proportionally depress the signal resulting from a rearrangement associated with tumor cells. In addition, although our FISH results confirm all ROMA signals in nearly all tumor cells, some fraction of tumor cells in a sample may not be identical with respect to amplification or deletion at each locus. It is thus possible that tumor heterogeneity may contribute some loss of signal.

The first phase of this breast cancer survey project is being carried out on frozen tumor tissue collected from 140 breast cancer patients at the Karolinska Institute, Stockholm, Sweden. These tumors represent a wide range of size, clinical stage, and outcome, and all samples carry extensive clinical information. In this paper, we present an outline of our combined ROMA/FISH analysis of a subset of these tumors.

Each of the tumors in this study was initially categorized as aneuploid or diploid based on flow cytometry and was then examined by two-color FISH to determine copy number of 12 critical loci known to be frequently amplified in breast tumors. The amplification profiles obtained by FISH were then compared with profiles obtained by ROMA carried out on DNA isolated from the tumor blocks. ROMA data confirmed all of the events identified by FISH in each sample but, as expected, also revealed many more copy number alterations at additional loci, including deletions as well as amplifications. We then produced hybridization probes for a subset of these loci and carried out FISH on cells from the tumor blocks in order to cross-confirm the ROMA results.

These results confirm that ROMA profiles proportionally reflect the copy number of each microarray feature as measured by two-color FISH, and that ROMA can be used to identify the boundaries of deletions, duplications, and amplifications. By compiling data from a large number of samples, we have begun to identify specific types of overall genomic patterns in breast cancer and to relate them to clinical status and eventual patient outcome. The goal of these studies is to identify useful prognostic and therapeutic markers that will eventually help direct therapy in a clinical setting.

MATERIALS AND METHODS

Patient samples. A total of 140 frozen tumor specimens was selected from archives at the Cancer Center of the Karolinska Institute, Stockholm, Sweden. Samples in this particular data set were selected to represent several distinct diagnostic categories in order to populate groups for comparison by FISH and ROMA.

Clinical parameters. Status of the estrogen and progesterone receptors (ER, PR) was determined by ligand binding with a threshold value of >0.05 fg/μg protein for classification as receptor positive.

ROMA DNA microarray analysis. ROMA was performed on a high-density oligonucleotide array containing approximately 85,000 features, manufactured by NimbleGen (Reykjavik, Iceland). Hybridization conditions and statistical analysis have been described previously (Lucito et al. 2003).

Sample preparation, microarray hybridization, and image analysis. The preparation of genomic representations, labeling, and hybridization were performed as described previously (Lucito et al. 2003). Briefly, the complexity of the samples was reduced by making BglII genomic representations, consisting of small (200–1200 bp) fragments amplified by adapter-mediated PCR of genomic DNA. For each experiment, two different samples were prepared in parallel. DNA samples (10 μg) were then labeled differentially with Cy5-dCTP or Cy3-dCTP using Amersham-Pharmacia Megaprime Labeling Kit and hybridized in comparison to each other. Each experiment was hybridized in duplicate, where in one replicate, the Cy5 and Cy3 dyes were swapped (i.e., color reversal). Hybridizations consisted of 25 μl of hybridization solution (50% formamide, 5x SSC, and 0.1% SDS) and 10 μl of labeled DNA. Samples were denatured in an MJ Research Tetrad at 95°C for 5 minutes, and then preannealed at 37°C for 30 minutes. This solution was then applied to the microarray and hybridized under a coverslip at 42°C for 14–16 hours. After hybridization, slides were washed 1 minute in 0.2% SDS/0.2x SSC, 30 seconds in 0.2x SSC, and 30 seconds in 0.05x SSC. Slides were dried by centrifugation and scanned immediately. An Axon GenePix 4000B scanner was used, setting the pixel size to 5 μm. GenePix Pro 4.0 software was used for quantitation of intensity for the arrays.

Data processing. Array data were imported into S-PLUS for further analysis. Measured intensities without background subtraction were used to calculate ratios. Data were normalized using an intensity-based lowess curve-fitting algorithm similar to that described in Yang et al. (2002). Log ratio values obtained from color-reversal experiments were averaged and displayed as presented in the figures.

Segmentation algorithm. Segmentation views the probe ratio distribution as an ordered series of probe log ratios, placed in genome order, and breaks it into intervals each with a mean and a standard deviation. At the end of this process, the probe data, in genome order, are divided into segments (long and certain intervals), each segment and feature with its own mean and standard deviation, and each feature associated with a likelihood that the feature is not the result of chance clustering of probes with deviant ratios.

The ratio data are processed in three phases. In the first phase, we iteratively segment the log ratio data by minimizing variance, then test the segment boundaries, and move them slightly if needed, by setting a very stringent Kolmogorov-Smirnov (K-S) p-value statistic for each segment relative to its neighboring segment ($p = 10^{-5}$). No segment smaller than six probes in length is considered. In the second phase, we compute the "residual string" of segmented log ratio data, adjusting the mean and standard deviation of each segment so that the residual string has a mean of 0 and a standard deviation of 1.

"Outliers" are defined based on deviance within the population, and features are defined as clusters of outliers (at least two). In the third phase, the features are assigned likelihood. We determine a "deviance measure" for each feature that reflects its deviance from the remainder of the data string. We then, in effect, either randomize or model randomization of the residual string (i.e., look at the residual data in a randomized order) many times, and collect deviance measures of all features generated by purely random processes. After binning the features by their length and their deviance measure, we can determine the likelihood that a given feature with a given length and deviance measure would have been generated by random processes if the probe data were noise.

Fluorescence in situ hybridization. FISH analysis was performed using interphase cells, and probes were either prepared from bacterial artificial chromosomes (BACs) or amplified from specific genomic regions by PCR. Based on the human genome sequence, primers (1–2 kb in length) were designed from the repeat-masked sequence of each copy number polymorphism (CNP) interval, and limited to an interval no larger than 100 kb. For each probe, a total of 20–25 different fragments were amplified, then pooled, and purified by ethanol precipitation. Probe DNA was then labeled by nick translation with SpectrumOrange™ or SpectrumGreen™ (Vysis Inc., Downers Grove, Illinois). Denaturation of probe and target DNA was performed at 90°C for 5 minutes, followed by hybridization in a humidity chamber at 47°C overnight. The coverglasses were then removed and the slides were washed in 2x SSC for 10 minutes at 72°C, and slides were dehydrated in graded alcohol. The slides were mounted with anti-fade mounting medium containing DAPI (4′, 6-diamino-2-phenylindole; Vectashield) as a counterstain for the nuclei. Evaluation of signals was carried out in an epifluorescence microscope. Selected cells were photographed in a Zeiss Axioplan 2 microscope equipped with Axio Cam MRM CCD camera and Axio Vision software.

Probe design for FISH. Hybridization probes for FISH were constructed by one of two methods. For the interdigitation analysis, probes were created from BACs selected using the University of California, Santa Cruz, genome browser. For the determination of copy number in the deletions and amplifications of the aneuploid tumors, probes were made by PCR amplification of primers identified through the PROBER algorithm designed in this laboratory. Genomic sequences of 100 kb containing target amplifications were tiled with 50 probes (800–1400 bp) selected with PROBER Probe Design Software created in our laboratory. PROBER uses a distributed annotated sequence retrieval request (Dowell et al. 2001) to request a genomic sequence and the Mer-Engine (Healy et al. 2003) to mask the sequence for repeats. Mer lengths of 18 that occur more than twice in the human genome (UCSC Goldenpath Apr. 10, 2004) with a geometric mean greater than 2 were masked with (N). Probes were selected from the remaining unmasked regions according to an algorithm to be published elsewhere.

Oligonucleotide primers were ordered in 96-well plates from Sigma Genosys and resuspended to 25 μM. Probes were amplified with the PCR Mastermix kit from Eppendorf (Cat. 0032002.447) from EBV-immortalized cell line DNA (Chp-Skn-1) DNA (100 ng) with 55°C annealing, 72°C extension, 2-minute extension time, and 23 cycles. Probes were purified with Qiagen PCR purification columns (Cat. 28104) and combined into a single probe cocktail (10–25 μg total probes) for dye labeling and metaphase/interphase FISH.

Measurement of DNA content. The ploidy of each tumor was determined by measurement of DNA content using Feulgen photocytometry (Forsslund and Zetterberg 1990; Forsslund et al. 1996). The optical densities of the nuclei in a sample were measured, and a DNA index was calculated and displayed as a histogram (Kronenwett et al. 2004). Normal cells and diploid tumors display a major peak at 2c DNA content with a smaller peak of G_2 phase replicating cells that corresponds to the mitotic index. Highly aneuploid tumors display broad peaks that often center on 4c copy number but may include cells from 2c to 6c or above.

Patient consent and institutional review board (IRB) approvals. KI samples were collected from patients undergoing radical mastectomy at the Karolinska Institute between 1984 and 1991. Patient consent for research use was specified under clinical research approvals from the IRB of the Karolinska Hospital, Stockholm, Sweden. Work at Cold Spring Harbor Laboratory was carried out under approval by the CSHL IRB on October 17, 2005 for a project entitled "Quantitative determination of gene amplification in breast tumors."

RESULTS

A subset of 140 frozen tumor specimens was selected from archives at the Cancer Center of the Karolinska Institute. Samples in this particular data set were selected to represent several distinct diagnostic categories in order to populate groups for comparison by FISH and ROMA. Most important, these samples are from patients for whom complete clinical data have been kept and for whom long-term outcome data (15–18 years) are available. The clinical characteristics of this sample set are shown in Table 1.

Each of the tumors in this study was initially categorized as aneuploid or diploid based on flow cytometry (see Materials and Methods) and then examined by two-color FISH to determine copy number of several loci known to be frequently amplified in breast tumors. The amplification profiles obtained by FISH were then compared with profiles obtained by ROMA carried out on DNA isolated from the frozen tumor blocks. ROMA was run by using 85K BglII Version 4 chip design manufactured to our specifications by NimbleGen, Inc. (Reykjavik, Iceland) which displays 82,972 separate features, each consisting of single-stranded DNA, 60 bases in length, as described previously (Lucito et al. 2003; Sebat

Table 1. Distribution of Patients and Clinical Parameters in the Swedish and Norwegian Data Sets

Karolinska Inst. Sweden	Total	Node (pos/neg)	Median age at diagnosis	Grade I/II/III	Size (mm) <20/>20	PR* (+/–)	ER* (+/–)	ERBB2[+] amp/norm
Diploid (Survival >7 yr)	60	28/31	52	8/11/33	19/41	41/9	43/7	3/57
	39	14/25	57	3/12/16	11/25	20/13	24/8	9/30
Diploid (Survival <7 yr)								
Aneuploid	41	28/13	49	0/2/22	21/20	14/19	25/10	15/26

Numbers will not add up exactly because of partial information on certain individual cases. *Progesterone (PR) and estrogen (ER) receptors measured by ligand binding; (pos) >0.5 fg/μg protein. [+]ERBB2 amplification scored by ROMA as segmented ratio greater than 0.1 above baseline.

et al. 2004). After hybridization and fluorescent scanning, the data consist of ratios calculated by taking the geometric mean of normalized hybridization data from two separate color-reversed chips, each comparing a tumor sample to the laboratory standard male fibroblast cell line. Typical results are shown for sample WZ1 in Figure 1.

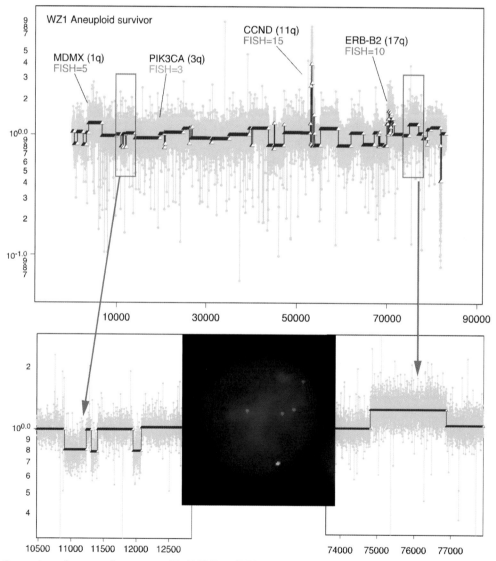

Figure 1. Comparison of copy number as assayed by ROMA and FISH. Tumor WZ1 is aneuploid with an average genome copy number of 3n by FACS analysis. The results of FISH probes for various loci are indicated in the top graph. The bottom panels show enlarged views of small deletions and duplications picked to demonstrate the correspondence between FISH and ROMA. The photograph shows a two-color FISH experiment using probes for the deletion and duplication, respectively, depicting loss and gain, respectively, of the two probes relative to the nominal genome copy number. PIK3CA on chromosome 3q yields a value of 1.0 by ROMA and 3 copies by FISH. MDMX on 1q yields a copy number of 5 by FISH, consistent with a near doubling of the copy number of the entire 1q arm as shown by ROMA.

Figure 1 depicts the typical ROMA profile used for all of the breast cancer samples presented in this study, with genomes arranged in chromosome order from left to right. The figure shows the normalized data, known as the "geomean ratio" (Lucito et al. 2003), for each probe, in gray. These "raw" geometric mean ratio data must be further refined in order to reliably identify specific amplifications, duplications, and deletions and to determine their amplitudes and, most importantly, their boundaries. This refinement is achieved through a series of statistical methods that comprise the Bridge 5 segmentation algorithm, described in Sebat et al. (2004) and in Materials and Methods. Segmentation provides a consistent and reliable method for interpretation of data by associating each data feature with a likelihood measure that the feature is not the result of the chance clustering of random noise in probe ratios. The geomean ratio data in Figure 1 are overlaid with the results of the segmentation algorithm in red. The expected ratio differences for the X and Y chromosomes for female versus male DNA are clearly visible.

It is clear from the profile of WZ1 in Figure 1 that there are at least two major classes of events: large segmental deletions and duplications of one or two copies of chromosome arms and narrow, high-copy-number amplifications, both of which have been observed previously by other CGH microarray methods (Ried et al. 1997; Pollack et al. 2002; Albertson 2003; Lage et al. 2003). The values predicted by ROMA and the observed values measured by FISH are shown above representative loci. As shown for this one example, ROMA data were consistent with all of the amplifications identified by FISH in each sample but also revealed copy number alterations at additional loci, including deletions as well as amplifications. We then produced hybridization probes for a subset of these loci, and carried out FISH on cells from the tumor blocks in order to confirm the ROMA results.

The three small panels in Figure 1 are an example of the probes made specifically for this tumor using the PROBER software (Materials and Methods) to regions that had undergone less obvious events. The image shows a two-color FISH result for probes made to the two regions of deletion and duplication identified in the flanking panels. The result clearly shows that this tumor, with a genomic equivalent of 3c, has lost at least two copies of the chromosome 2 locus and gained one copy of the chromosome 20 locus. Similar results from 10 different tumors (not shown here) provide confidence that ROMA profiles proportionally reflect the copy number of each microarray feature as measured by two-color FISH, and that ROMA can be used to identify the boundaries of deletions, duplications, and amplifications. Furthermore, we can use ROMA to define a mathematical parameter that reflects the degree to which a population of tumor cells differs from a normal euploid genome.

We note that the segmented mean value for the X chromosome in a typical diploid female/diploid male experiment ranges from 1.3 to 1.5. We have established a theoretical peak broad mean value for the X chromosome at 1.65. This is significantly higher than values reported for an expected 2:1 ratio in non-representational microarray CGH methods (Pollack et al. 2002), but still less than the expected value of 2. This ratio, which averages about 1.45 in our experiments, sets a rough benchmark for other events, particularly duplications or deletions of chromosome arms or segments. Most other broad events, particularly in diploids, show amplitudes less than that of the X as would be expected since tumor samples generally contain a certain fraction of normal cells. Additionally, because all chromosomal events may not have occurred at the same time in the development of the tumor, the segmentation value of later events would have a characteristic fractional representation in the ROMA profile. Using FISH to confirm copy numbers, we have determined that whereas ROMA values underestimate copy number, they are very sensitive to the existence of events and can accurately detect events with a deviation from the baseline segmentation of as little as ± 0.1.

Aneuploids Versus Diploids

Because of the complexity of data accumulated in CGH experiments, it is usually necessary to process multiple experiments together and to analyze the aggregate by statistical methods. The drawback of such methods is that they obscure the potential for identifying unique patterns and phenotypes among individual tumors. We therefore present in Figure 2A a representative set of ROMA profiles for tumors to demonstrate the variety of forms that samples in this study can take.

As in Figure 1, breast cancer profiles provide a rough internal calibration for copy number based on having 2:1 copy number for X and complete lack (equivalent to a homozygous loss) of the Y. One important point to note is that this expectation has limitations because ROMA measures the average copy number of cells in tumors, and some tumor cells have lost one of their X chromosomes. Furthermore, the presence of a variable number of normal cells in any tumor cells complicates the estimates of copy number based purely on ROMA.

It is clear from inspection that diploids, in general, exhibit fewer events than aneuploids, and with the exception of the certain clustered amplifications described below, the events are most often gains or losses of whole chromosome arms. Aneuploids average 42 events, whereas diploids average 16, and it is only logical to assume that aneuploids, having multiple copies of most chromosomes, have more degrees of freedom to gain or lose copies without deleterious effects on proliferation that might be caused by wholesale gene imbalances, as would be the case in diploids. Yet, on a case-by-case basis, diploid tumors can exhibit the same pathogenic potential for proliferation and for local and distant metastasis as aneuploids. In fact, the locations of the events for diploids and aneuploids are comparable, as shown in Figure 2B, but the frequency of these events in aneuploids is higher, as expected.

The combination of fewer overall events coupled with the frequent narrow, high-copy-number amplicons makes it particularly advantageous to focus on diploid tumors for CGH analysis in general. In particular, exercises in

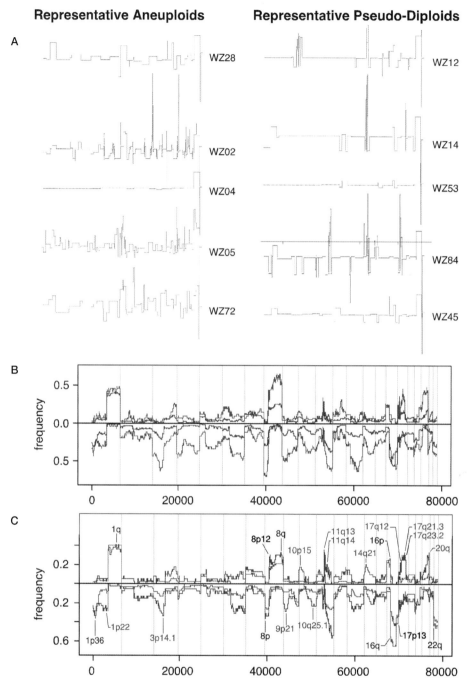

Figure 2. Examples of aneuploid and pseudo-diploid tumors. (*A*) Representative ROMA profiles showing that aneuploid tumors in general exhibit an overall greater frequency of chromosome rearrangements than do pseudo-diploid tumors. (*B*) Comparative frequency plots of amplification (up) and deletion (down) in various data sets. Frequency calculated on normalized, segmented ROMA profiles using a minimum of six consecutive probes identifying a segment with a minimum mean of 0.1 above (amplification) or below (deletion) baseline. Frequencies are plotted only for chromosomes 1–22. (*C*)The Swedish diploid subset (*blue*) is compared to the total Swedish aneuploid subset (*red*). Comparative frequency plots of Swedish diploid subset >7-year survivors (*red*) and <7-year non-survivors (*blue*).

novel oncogene and tumor suppressor discovery may be facilitated by the lower frequency of observable events in diploids. It is likely that diploids may exhibit less background "chatter" from unselected events that might occur randomly in the more permissive aneuploid environment, thus reducing the number of events and loci that must be screened. Likewise, the apparent restriction on gain or loss in diploids leads to the generation of smaller, more discrete events, particularly amplifications that can point directly to oncogenes. The insights gained from the increased resolution of ROMA combined with FISH for both of these aspects of CGH are described below.

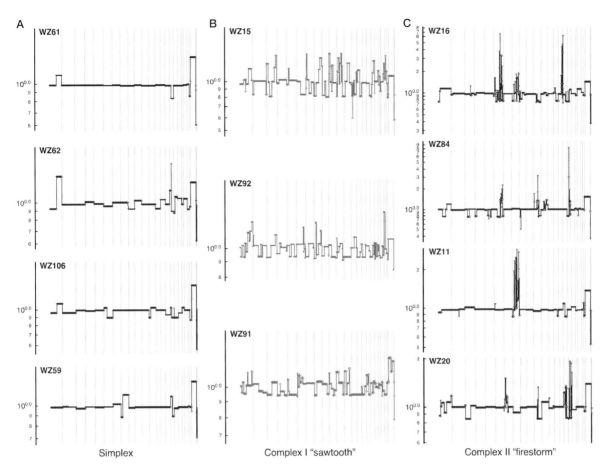

Figure 3. Major types of tumor genomic profiles. Segmentation profiles for individual tumors representing each category: (*A*) simplex; (*B*) complex type I or "sawtooth"; (*C*) complex type II or "firestorm." Scored events consist of a minimum of six consecutive probes in the same state. Y-axis displays the geometric mean value of two experiments on log scale. Note that the scale of the amplifications in panel *C* is compressed relative to panels *A* and *B* due to the high levels of amplification in firestorms. Chromosomes 1–22 plus X and Y are displayed in order from left to right according to probe position.

Patterns of Diploid Genome Profiles

Visual inspection of segmented diploid profiles suggests those with rearrangements comprise three basic profile types. The first profile pattern (Fig. 3A), which we call "simplex," has broad segments of duplication and deletion, usually comprising entire chromosomes or chromosome arms, with occasional isolated narrow peaks of amplifications. This type represents 60% of the diploid tumors in this sample. In the second type, "sawtooth" (Fig. 3B), the cancer cells have many sub-arm-length segments of amplification and deletions, often alternating, more or less affecting all the chromosomes. Little of the genome remains at normal copy number in this type, which makes up less than 5% of this selected data set. Sawtooth patterns apparently result from a genome-wide loss of mitotic segregation control that eventually becomes clonal.

The third pattern (Fig. 3C) resembles the simplex type except that the cancers contain at least one localized region of clustered peaks of amplification, each cluster confined to a single chromosome arm, which we call "firestorms." In contrast to the sawtooth pattern, the clusters of amplifications in these tumors are clearly due to repeated recombination/rearrangement events that result from a structural change, such as telomere loss, that affects the stability of that arm alone. We cannot distinguish all profiles with this system, but the fundamental difference in the patterns may represent genomic lesions resulting from different mechanisms, and more than one mechanism may be operant to varying degrees within any given cancer.

A fourth type is the "flat" profile, cancer cells in which we observe no clear amplifications or deletions other than CNPs (Sebat et al. 2004) and single probe events, as discussed above, and the difference in the sex chromosomes. These profiles may represent either a sample with few tumor cells relative to the surrounding stroma, or a cancer that has no genomic rearrangements. Flat profiles such as WZ04 in Figure 2A represent less than 10% of the samples we have analyzed.

Characterization of Firestorm Instability

In ROMA profiles, firestorms display dramatic multiple segmental amplifications grouped on one arm, or occasionally, on both arms. The individual amplicons in these firestorms are often separated by segments that do not appear to be amplified, yielding a pattern of interdigitated amplification as shown for chromosome 8 in tumor WZ11 (shown graphically in Fig. 3C). In cases where this pattern of amplification is observed, the interdigitated amplification pattern is limited to one or a few chromosome arms, and amplicons are clearly not randomly distributed throughout the genome (Figs. 2A and 3B, C). We infer from this observation that the phenomenon is a result of aberrant replication/recombination events that occur on a particular chromosome arm rather than a general induction of amplification functions operating throughout the genome.

Firestorms have been observed at least once on most chromosomes in the tumors we have analyzed, but certain arms undergo this process more frequently. In particular, chromosomes 6, 8, 11, 17, and 20 are often affected, with 11q and 17q being the most frequently subject to these dramatic rearrangements. Notably, within the latter, the loci containing cyclin D1 on 11q and ERBB2 on 17q are most frequently amplified and may "drive" the selection of the events. Chromosomes 6, 8, and 20 have comparable frequency of firestorms, but the "drivers" for these events are less obvious.

The prediction that the amplification events were taking place on a chromosome arm was tested by a series of FISH experiments. We selected BACs or made primer-based probes from each narrow amplicon and each of the "spacer" regions in between. Two-color FISH experiments were performed on touch preparations made from a section of tumor samples WZ11 (presented here) and others to be published elsewhere. The results of the FISH experiments showed complete correspondence with the ROMA profile shown in Figure 4B. Probes from each amplicon yielded 8–15 spots in the FISH exposures, whereas probes for the intervening regions showed only the 2 spots expected for a diploid genome. Moreover, as shown previously for the aneuploid amplicons in WZ1, the spots corresponding to amplicons were clustered, suggesting that they colocalized on a single chromosome arm rather than being distributed throughout the genome as is the case for supernumerary or double minute chromosomes that are sometimes observed in cell culture. More notable, however, was the observation that when cells were exposed to probes from two different amplified peaks from the same firestorm in a two-color FISH experiment, the resulting sets of spots were colocalized in a single cluster. Figure 4B shows two examples using one pair of probes corresponding to MYC and CKS1 and another pair carrying FGFR1/BAG4 on the p arm of chromosome 8 and an unknown locus AK096200 on the 8q arm. These results suggest that, at least for the firestorm in WZ11, all of the amplified DNA regions are being carried on the same region of a single chromosome, as would be expected if the chromosome had entered into break-fusion-bridge (BFB) (McClintock 1938, 1941; Coquelle et al. 1997; Gisselsson et al. 2000) or break-induced replication (BIR) (Difilippantonio et al. 2002) models that have been invoked to explain chromosome instability in cancer cell lines, and by inference, in tumors themselves.

We have also been able to test the localization of the amplicons from two different multiply amplified chromosome arms occurring in the same tumor sample. A chromosome localization model would predict that the spots from amplicons on different chromosomes would cluster separately from each other. This is what was observed in two-color FISH experiments using probes for ERBB2 on 17p and CCND (cyclin D1) on 11q in three tumor samples where both genes had been previously shown to be amplified by both FISH and ROMA. An example of this result is shown in Figure 4C using cells from sample WZ20 where earlier FISH experiments had shown ERBB2 to be present in more than 15 copies per cell and cyclin D1 to be present in 6 copies per cell. Two separate clusters are clearly visible, one containing only the red spots corresponding to cyclin D1 and the large cluster of green spots corresponding to ERBB2. Similar results were obtained using samples WZ1 (Fig. 1),WZ2 (Fig. 2A), and WZ17.

Prognostic Potential of Chromosome Rearrangement Patterns

One of the fundamental targets of this initial study is the comparison of whole-genome ROMA profiles from different clinical groups to evaluate the potential for ROMA as a prognostic tool. In this heuristic example, we analyzed all of the diploid samples in this collection by comparing subsets of patients grouped according to tumor grade, tumor size, node condition, and outcome (7-year survival). Due to the small numbers in this preliminary analysis, the samples were not sorted according to postoperative treatment. Two graphical methods for visualizing the aggregate data sets were frequency plots and mean amplitude plots. The frequency plot method reflects the fraction of samples in the subset for which each data point rises above (amplification) or below (deletion) a threshold value determined by the noise level in the experiments. The frequency plot method gives frequency of amplification or deletion of a given region, but it does not provide any indication of the degree of amplification, a factor that may often correlate with importance of a given locus in breast cancer.

The mean amplitude method sums the mean segmentation values for each probe over multiple experiments and divides by the total number of experiments. The rationale behind the mean amplitude plot is to provide an indication of the potential at any site for high-level amplification, while maintaining the ability to visualize deletions, which are generally limited in negative amplitude to the value of a hemizygous loss. Regions of hemizygous loss would be expected to yield ratios of 0.5, but operationally yield an intermediate value approaching 0.75 at most. Amplification, on the other hand, can yield very strong peaks (comparative ratios of sample to control approaching 5.0) reflecting up to 30 copies of a given locus in the tumor as measured by FISH. Based on the ubiquity of amplification in breast tumors, it is logical to assume that copy number is related to phenotype

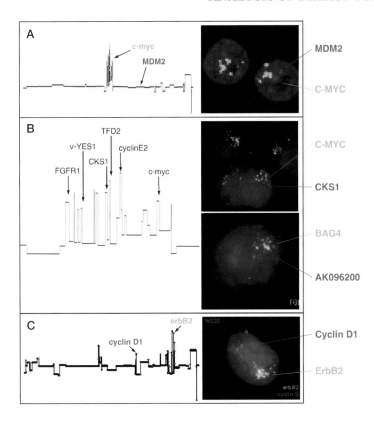

Figure 4. FISH analysis of multiply amplified regions. Photographs show two-color FISH images of loci labeled in the ROMA profiles. (*A*) Tumor WZ11 showing a firestorm of amplification on chromosome 8 and cluster of spots compared to single-copy MDM2 on chromosome 12. (*B*) Enlarged view of chromosome 8 showing location of amplicons and putative oncogenes. FISH images show results of probing two separate pairs of amplicons within the same region. (*C*) Tumor WZ20 where amplicons appear on different chromosomes. FISH image shows that the repeated loci occupy separate regions of the nucleus.

in some way and, therefore, that peak height must be considered in comparative studies. The mean amplitude method takes into account both frequency and amplitude of a given locus, but peak height clearly can be driven by high values in a small fraction of the experiments.

The mean amplitude method also yields more information than a simple frequency plot when comparing deletions. Hemizygous deletions would be expected to give similar values on a cell-by-cell basis, but a deletion that has only recently appeared in a tumor will be less well represented in the ROMA profile than one that occurred earlier and is carried by a larger percentage of tumor cells. Therefore, the mean amplitude of the deletions shown in Figure 4C may be less than the frequency, where each event gets a unit value.

The data plotted in Figure 5 result from combining segmented data from 19 diploid, Grade III non-survivors (<7 years) and comparing them to 16 long-term diploid survivors matched for tumor size and grade. Clearly, designating a patient as a "survivor" or "non-survivor" at a specific time after surgery is not accurate in terms of the real progression of the disease. However, it is useful for understanding the relationship of disease progression to molecular events.

It is clear from Figure 5, A and B, and Figure 5, C and D, that, on average, tumors from non-survivors have suffered more genomic rearrangement than comparable survivors. This is consistent with accepted models for the relationship between genome instability and aggres-siveness in breast cancer. What is perhaps surprising is that both the differences and the similarities between the survivor and non-survivor plots by either plotting method are nonrandom. The black arrows in each panel denote places where the activity as measured by frequency or amplitude is very similar between the two data sets and can be easily seen in individual tumors. These regions include duplications of 16p, deletion of 16q and 11q, and the duplication of 1q, as well as deletion of all of chromosome 22. With the possible exception of the frequency of chromosome 22 deletion, the frequencies of these events are nearly identical between the two data sets. That identity makes the differences, denoted by red arrows, at 8p, chromosome 6 amplification and deletion, 3p deletion, 11q amplification, 15q amplification, and 17q amplification. Although these data sets are too small to draw clear conclusions regarding prognosis, they do point to genomic regions that may well harbor such markers.

Nonetheless, the degree of similarity observed between the two analytical methods is striking. This means that important regions tend to be frequently affected by a high-amplitude genomic event. As described in subsequent sections, these amplicons are often parts of multiple amplification events on the same chromosome arm and are often very narrow. We have observed known oncogenes and tumor suppressors in breast cancer using these two methods. They have also pointed to regions that have not been previously identified as important in breast cancer.

Rearrangements in Low-Grade Tumors

Grade I diploid tumors in which the cells maintain their differentiation are generally considered to be less aggressive and have a very good prognosis irrespective of migration to the lymph nodes. Ten examples of Grade I tumors were examined in the current study, including four in which one or more nodes were affected. All were medium to large tumors between 20 mm and 30 mm in size. Although the number of samples is small, the similarity in ROMA profiles among the eight samples depicted in Figure 6 is dramatic and may provide insight into some of the earliest events leading to invasive breast cancer. Two of the ten Grade I samples yielded no detectable events and were not included in the figure. Six of eight tumors with any detectable events showed a characteristic rearrangement in chromosome 16 along with either a similar rearrangement of the arms of chromosome 8 or a duplication of the q arm of chromosome 1. All three of these events are seen in more highly rearranged breast cancer genomes such as those in Figure 6, and in fact, are among the most common events by frequency in all samples (see Fig. 2B). We believe that these low-grade tumors with little rearrangement in the genome provide an ideal opportunity to study the importance of these frequent events. Moreover, it is tempting to infer that these events are very likely among the earliest events taking place in a large fraction of tumors.

DISCUSSION

Microarry CGH and FISH Are Complementary Methods for Analyzing Genomic Change

The progression of cancer cells from their original normal state to uncontrolled growth, invasion, and metastasis clearly involves multiple genetic changes and may occur through a multiplicity of distinct pathways. Microarray CGH and FISH provide complementary tools for examining those events that involve gene copy number and nonreciprocal chromosome rearrangements. Microarray methods allow examination of the whole genome in one experiment, but by necessity, the data reflect an average of all of the genomes in all of the cells present in the original sample, both normal and cancerous. On the other hand, FISH reveals the exact number of copies of a given locus in each individual nucleus and can therefore detect and quantify the cancer-related events in tumor cells even when they are mixed with a significant fraction of normal cells, as is the case in most biopsy or surgical samples. Interphase FISH can also provide limited but important information concerning the structures of rearranged loci in a tumor cell population, as demonstrated by the "clustering" phenomenon observed in this work that bolsters (but does not prove) our firestorm interpretation. By itself, however, FISH is limited to testing only a few genes in each

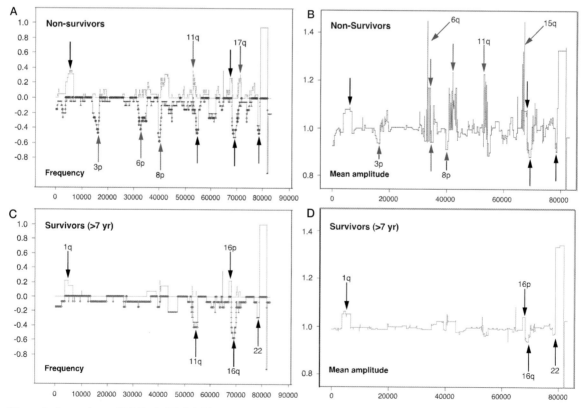

Figure 5. Comparison of 35 Grade III diploid tumors from eventual survivors vs. non-survivors. Survival longer or shorter than 7 years as shown in Fig. 2C. (A and B) Frequency plots; (C and D) mean amplitude plots. Black arrows indicate events common to both classes. Red arrows indicate events enriched in the non-survivor class.

experiment. We have used a combined approach, using ROMA CGH to survey the genome and subsequent FISH to examine individual loci. Among the various microarray CGH methods, ROMA provides the highest resolution and sensitivity through the combination of reduced target complexity and the high density of features available from our proprietary version of the NimbleGen feature array.

Firestorms and Sawtooth Patterns

The complex genome profiles seen in highly rearranged breast tumors by ROMA CGH appear to represent different paths that cells may take in acquiring the altered gene expression that leads first to tumorigenesis and ultimately to metastasis. We have gone to some lengths to validate these patterns in view of their potential use in both prognosis and oncogene discovery. First, we have shown by interphase FISH studies on firestorm tumors that narrow peaks resolved by ROMA represent separate amplicons and are not simply the result of any noise in the system. Furthermore, we have shown that the multiple amplifications seen by ROMA CGH most often occur in the same cell and therefore represent an accumulation of events in a clonal population. Finally, we have learned that firestorms occur at preferred sites that are correlated with the genomic locations associated with higher risk, based on frequency plots of survivors and non-survivors.

Additional work is under way using a combined FISH and ROMA approach to understand the mechanisms that induce global sawtooth patterns of rearrangement and the chromosome-limited rearrangements characteristic of firestorms. Multiple head-to-tail and head-to-head repeating amplicons have been observed in cancer cell lines (Coquelle et al. 1997; Gisselsson et al. 2000). Likewise, the

telltale anaphase bridges characteristic of breakage-fusion-bridge cycles (McClintock 1938, 1941) are also frequently seen in cancer mitotic figures, leading to the suggestion that telomere fusion of chromatids is the major mechanism for high levels of amplification as observed in firestorms. Clearly, the process requires some structural characteristic of the recombining chromosome arms. Whether the key to that process resides in telomere loss or in recombination at short inverted repeats (Tanaka et al. 2002) or through a related mechanism, break-induced replication, where segments are copied from internal chromosome breaks (Difilippantonio et al. 2002), is as yet an open question. It will be most interesting to determine whether a component of that peculiar cancer-related process can be blocked, thus providing another target for anticancer therapy.

A Possible Pattern to Progression

Another intriguing possibility that stems from studies of genomic rearrangement is the possibility of dissecting the pathways leading from noninvasive to invasive to metastatic cancer by tracking the events that occur in the most highly differentiated (least evolved) breast tumors. Certain specific chromosome arm gains and losses appear to be unexpectedly frequent in those tumors that show less than five total events. These lesions, all of which have been reported elsewhere at various times in different contexts (Kallioniemi et al. 1994; Ried et al. 1995; Tirkkonen et al. 1998; Pollack et al. 2002; Nessling et al. 2005), are duplication of 1q, 8q, and 16p, and deletion of 8p, 16q, and 22q. Not all of the events occur together in the same tumor, and there are not enough data as yet to test whether there is any intrinsic order to the timing of their appearance. We do note, however, that the frequency of these specific changes remains constant when we compare tumors from surviving

Common Origins in Low Grade Breast Tumors

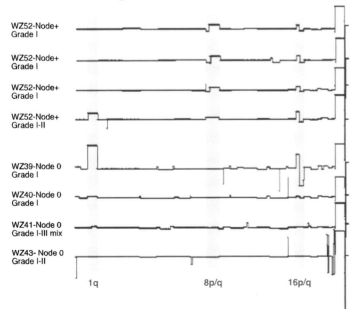

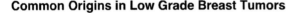

Figure 6. Comparison of Grade I/II diploid tumors by ROMA. A total of 10 low-grade tumors were included in the data set. The two samples not shown exhibited no detectable events. Regions of common chromosomal rearrangements are shaded. All of the shaded areas are among the most common sites of rearrangement in all breast tumors collectively shown in Fig. 5.

patients (or those with few events) (Fig. 6B) with subsets of tumors that have poor survival (and many more total events) (Fig. 6A). One interpretation of these results is that in the early stages of tumor development, cells undergo a subset of these specific gain or loss events as they give rise to proliferating clones. Subsequently, as these clones become less differentiated and gain potential to spread in the host, additional events accumulate. Thus, it is reasonable to speculate that there are early and late genomic events that can be separated according to the degree of progression exhibited by the cancer and that there is likely to be a genetic pathway, albeit a complex one, at work in the evolution of tumors.

This work, along with our previous published results (Lucito et al. 2003), confirms that ROMA profiles proportionally reflect the copy number of each microarray feature as measured by two-color FISH and that ROMA can be used to identify the boundaries of deletions, duplications, and amplifications. By compiling data from a large number of samples, we have begun to identify specific types of overall genomic patterns in breast cancer and relate them to clinical status and eventual patient outcome. The goal of these studies is to identify useful prognostic and therapeutic markers that will eventually help direct therapy in a clinical setting. We are confident that as the number of clinically annotated samples grows, prognostic information regarding clinical outcome as well as information regarding preferred treatment modalities can and will be derived.

ACKNOWLEDGMENTS

This work was supported by grants to M.W. from the National Institutes of Health (5R01-CA078544-07); the Department of the Army (W81XWH04-1-0477; W81XWH-05-1-0068; W81XWH-04-0905); The Simons Foundation; Miracle Foundation; Breast Cancer Research Foundation; Long Islanders Against Breast Cancer; West Islip Breast Cancer Foundation; Long Island Breast Cancer (1 in 9); Elizabeth McFarland Breast Cancer Research Grant; and Breast Cancer Help Inc. M.W. is an American Cancer Society Research Professor. This work was supported by grants to A.Z. from the Swedish Cancer Society (grant number 0046-B04-38XAC) and from the Stockholm Cancer Society (03:171 and 02:144). The authors thank Dr. James Feramisco for careful review and helpful comments on the manuscript.

REFERENCES

Albertson D.G. 2003. Profiling breast cancer by array CGH. *Breast Cancer Res. Treat.* **78:** 289.
Balmain A., Gray J., and Ponder B. 2003. The genetics and genomics of cancer. *Nat. Genet.* (suppl.) **33:** 238.
Coquelle A., Pipiras E., Toledo F., Buttin G., and Debatisse M. 1997. Expression of fragile sites triggers intrachromosomal mammalian gene amplification and sets boundaries to early amplicons. *Cell* **89:** 215.
DePinho R.A. and Polyak K. 2004. Cancer chromosomes in crisis. *Nat. Genet.* **36:** 932.
Difilippantonio M.J., Petersen S., Chen H.T., Johnson R., Jasin M., Kanaar R., Ried T., and Nussenzweig A. 2002. Evidence for replicative repair of DNA double-strand breaks leading to oncogenic translocation and gene amplification. *J. Exp. Med.* **196:** 469.
Dowell R.D., Jokerst R.M., Day A., Eddy S.R., and Stein L. 2001. The distributed annotation system. *BMC Bioinformatics* **2:** 7.
Forsslund G. and Zetterberg A. 1990. Ploidy level determinations in high-grade and low-grade malignant variants of prostatic carcinoma. *Cancer Res.* **50:** 4281.
Forsslund G., Nilsson B., and Zetterberg A. 1996. Near tetraploid prostate carcinoma. Methodologic and prognostic aspects. *Cancer* **78:** 1748.
Gisselsson D., Pettersson L., Hoglund M., Heidenblad M., Gorunova L., Wiegant J., Mertens F., Dal Cin P., Mitelman F., and Mandahl N. 2000. Chromosomal breakage-fusion-bridge events cause genetic intratumor heterogeneity. *Proc. Natl. Acad. Sci.* **97:** 5357.
Healy J., Thomas E.E., Schwartz J.T., and Wigler M. 2003. Annotating large genomes with exact word matches. *Genome Res.* **13:** 2306.
Kallioniemi A., Kallioniemi O.P., Sudar D., Rutovitz D., Gray J.W., Waldman F., and Pinkel D. 1992a. Comparative genomic hybridization for molecular cytogenetic analysis of solid tumors. *Science* **258:** 818.
Kallioniemi A., Kallioniemi O.P., Waldman F.M., Chen L.C., Yu L.C., Fung Y.K., Smith H.S., Pinkel D., and Gray J.W. 1992b. Detection of retinoblastoma gene copy number in metaphase chromosomes and interphase nuclei by fluorescence in situ hybridization. *Cytogenet. Cell Genet.* **60:** 190.
Kallioniemi A., Kallioniemi O.P., Piper J., Tanner M., Stokke T., Chen L., Smith H.S., Pinkel D., Gray J.W., and Waldman F.M. 1994. Detection and mapping of amplified DNA sequences in breast cancer by comparative genomic hybridization. *Proc. Natl. Acad. Sci.* **91:** 2156.
Kallioniemi O.P., Kallioniemi A., Kurisu W., Thor A., Chen L.C., Smith H.S., Waldman F.M., Pinkel D., and Gray J.W. 1992. ERBB2 amplification in breast cancer analyzed by fluorescence in situ hybridization. *Proc. Natl. Acad. Sci.* **89:** 5321.
Kronenwett U., Huwendiek S., Ostring C., Portwood N., Roblick U.J., Pawitan Y., Alaiya A., Sennerstam R., Zetterberg A., and Auer G. 2004. Improved grading of breast adenocarcinomas based on genomic instability. *Cancer Res.* **64:** 904.
Lage J.M., Leamon J.H., Pejovic T., Hamann S., Lacey M., Dillon D., Segraves R., Vossbrinck B., Gonzalez A., Pinkel D., Albertson D.G., Costa J., and Lizardi P.M. 2003. Whole genome analysis of genetic alterations in small DNA samples using hyperbranched strand displacement amplification and array-CGH. *Genome Res.* **13:** 294.
Lucito R., Healy J., Alexander J., Reiner A., Esposito D., Chi M., Rodgers L., Brady A., Sebat J., Troge J., West J.A., Rostan S., Nguyen K.C.Q., Powers S., Ye K.Q., Olshen A., Venkatraman E., Norton L., and Wigler M. 2003. Representational oligonucleotide microarray analysis: A high-resolution method to detect genome copy number variation. *Genome Res.* **13:** 2291.
McClintock B. 1938. The production of homozygous deficient tissues with mutant characteristics by means of the aberrant mitotic behavior of ring-shaped chromosomes. *Genetics* **23:** 315.
———. 1941. The stability of broken ends of chromosomes in *Zea mays. Genetics* **26:** 234.
Menard S., Fortis S., Castiglioni F., Agresti R., and Balsari A. 2001. HER2 as a prognostic factor in breast cancer. *Oncology* **61:** 67.
Nessling M., Richter K., Schwaenen C., Roerig P., Wrobel G., Wessendorf S., Fritz B., Bentz M., Sinn H.-P., Radwimmer B., and Lichter P. 2005. Candidate genes in breast cancer revealed by microarray-based comparative genomic hybridization of archived tissue. *Cancer Res.* **65:** 439.
Pollack J.R., Sorlie T., Perou C.M., Rees C.A., Jeffrey S.S., Lonning P.E., Tibshirani R., Botstein D., Borresen-Dale A.L., and Brown P.O. 2002. Microarray analysis reveals a major direct role of DNA copy number alteration in the transcriptional

program of human breast tumors. *Proc. Natl. Acad. Sci.* **99:** 12963.

Ried T., Liyanage M., du Manoir S., Heselmeyer K., Auer G., Macville M., and Schröck E. 1997. Tumor cytogenetics revisited: Comparative genomic hybridization and spectral karyotyping. *J. Mol. Med.* **75:** 801.

Ried T., Just K.E., Holgreve-Grez H., du Manoir S., Speicher M.R., Schröck E., Latham C., Blegen H., Zetterberg A., Cremer T., and Auer G. 1995. Comparative genomic hybridization of formalin-fixed, paraffin-enbedded breast tumors reveals different patterns of chromosomal gains and losses in fibroadenomas and diploid and aneuploid carcinomas. *Cancer Res.* **55:** 5415.

Sebat J., Lakshmi B., Troge J., Alexander J., Young J., Lundin P., Maner S., Massa H., Walker M., Chi M., Navin N., Lucito R., Healy J., Hicks J., Ye K., Reiner A., Gilliam T.C., Trask B., Patterson N., Zetterberg A., and Wigler M. 2004. Large-scale copy number polymorphism in the human genome. *Science* **305:** 525.

Slamon D.J., Godolphin W., Jones L.A., Holt J.A., Wong S.G., Keith D.E., Levin W.J., Stuart S.G., Udove J., and Ullrich A., et al. 1989. Studies of the HER-2/neu proto-oncogene in human breast and ovarian cancer. *Science* **244:** 707.

Tanaka H., Tapscott S.J., Trask B.J., and Yao M.-C. 2002. Short inverted repeats initiate gene amplification through the formation of a large DNA palindrome in mammalian cells. *Proc. Natl. Acad. Sci.* **99:** 8772.

Tirkkonen M., Tanner M., Karhu R., Kallioniemi A., Isola J., and Kallioniemi O.P. 1998. Molecular cytogenetics of primary breast cancer by CGH. *Genes Chromosomes Cancer* **21:** 177.

van de Vijver M.J., van de Bersselaar R., Devilee P., Cornelisse C., Peterse J., and Nusse R. 1987. Amplification of the neu (c-erbB-2) oncogene in human mammmary tumors is relatively frequent and is often accompanied by amplification of the linked c-erbA oncogene. *Mol. Cell. Biol.* **7:** 2019.

Yang Y.H., Dudoit S., Luu P., Lin D.M., Peng V., Ngai J., and Speed T.P. 2002. Normalization of cDNA microarray data: A robust composite method addressing single and multiple slide sytematic variation. *Nucleic Acids Res.* **30:** e15.

Ductal Pancreatic Cancer in Humans and Mice

D.A. Tuveson[*] and S.R. Hingorani[†]

[*]*Department of Medicine, Abramson Family Cancer Research Institute,*
Abramson Cancer Center at the University of Pennsylvania, Philadelphia, Pennsylvania 19104;
[†]*Fred Hutchinson Cancer Research Center, Seattle, Washington 98109*

Pancreatic ductal adenocarcinoma (PDA) eludes early detection and resists current therapies, earning its distinction as the most lethal malignancy by organ site in the western world. This dire reality prompted extensive yet generally disappointing efforts to generate transgenic mouse models of this malignancy. Recently, mutant mice that develop pancreatic intraepithelial neoplasms (PanIN), the presumed preinvasive stage of PDA, were produced by conditionally expressing an endogenous oncogenic *Kras* allele in the developing murine pancreas. Mice with PanIN demonstrated promise in the pursuit of biomarkers of early pancreatic cancer, and, importantly, such mice eventually developed and succumbed to PDA after a long latency, establishing PanINs as true precursors to the invasive disease. Furthermore, the incorporation of conditional mutations in tumor suppressor alleles known to be altered in human PDA synergized with oncogenic Kras to produce advanced PDA with a short latency, recapitulating central pathophysiological events in human PDA. These models facilitate a variety of biological and clinical investigations such as explorations of the cellular origins of PDA and the development of treatment strategies for advanced PanIN and PDA. In addition, lessons from modeling PDA may be applicable to other tumor types and illuminate general principles of carcinogenesis.

Animal models of cognate human conditions permit the rigorous exploration of mechanisms of disease pathogenesis and provide systems to devise and test therapeutic and detection strategies. Although inbred mouse strains offer many advantages over other animals for investigations of malignant disease, mice unfortunately do not develop PDA spontaneously or even following carcinogen treatment. Recent technological developments in conditional gene targeting have enabled the generation of mutant mouse cancer models of PanIN and PDA that closely mimic human pancreatic cancer and are thus suitable for investigations of the human disease process. In this paper, we summarize the knowledge of the human disease that has informed the ability to generate accurate mouse models of pancreatic cancer and describe potential biological and clinical applications.

EPIDEMIOLOGY OF PANCREATIC CANCER

Epithelial carcinomas account for the majority of cancer deaths in the United States, and among them, pancreatic cancer is the fourth most common with the highest case–fatality ratio. Pancreatic ductal adenocarcinomas (PDA) comprise more than 90% of pancreatic cancer cases and are its most lethal form among an assortment of additional histological subtypes including cystic neoplasms, acinar carcinomas, and islet cell endocrine tumors. Risk factors associated with the development of PDA include increased age, tobacco usage (Silverman et al. 1994), African heritage (Ahlgren 1996), and a family history of pancreatic cancer (Lynch et al. 1996). Despite the relatively large numbers of patients stricken with PDA, estimated at 32,180 for 2005, our expanding knowledge of critical aspects of this disease remains terribly inadequate and undoubtedly contributes to our inability to intervene meaningfully. The impetus to investigate the biological underpinnings of PDA is further motivated by the predicted doubling in PDA incidence over the next two decades as the population ages (Hruban et al. 2006a). Nonetheless, the public investment in pancreatic cancer research is woefully inadequate relative to other malignancies, and consequently, the number of investigators pursuing PDA is unfortunately restricted.

GENETICS OF PDA AND PanIN

PDA is thought to evolve from a preinvasive precursor state termed pancreatic intraepithelial neoplasms (PanINs) because PanINs demonstrate cytological and genetic changes that reflect those evident in invasive PDA. PanINs are divided into three stages characterized by increasing degrees of cellular and architectural atypia. PanIN-1A lesions are flat and contain tall columnar ductal cells in distinction to the short cuboidal cells that line normal pancreatic ducts; PanIN-1B lesions additionally demonstrate mild papillary architecture in the ducts but no nuclear atypia; the PanIN-2 stage signifies cells with moderate nuclear atypia and loss of cellular polarity; PanIN-3s represent the carcinoma-in-situ stage of pancreatic cancer, characterized by marked atypia, dysregulated growth, cribriform structures, and pinched-off clusters of epithelial cells within the ductal lumen. Molecular studies from a limited number of resected human PanIN specimens demonstrate oncogenic *KRAS* mutations in PanIN-1A/B (35–43%) that increase to the majority of PanIN-3 examined (86%) (Klimstra and Longnecker 1994; Moskaluk et al. 1997; van Heek et al. 2002), followed by *p16INK4a/ARF* loss in PanIN-2 (55%) (Wilentz et al. 1998), and finally, *p53* mutation and loss of *DPC4/SMAD4/MADH4* and *BRCA2* in a minority of PanIN-3s (21–31%) (DiGiuseppe et al. 1994; Goggins et al. 2000; Wilentz et al. 2000). These mutational frequencies approach those in advanced PDA tissue samples and cell lines, including activating mutations in *KRAS* (>90% samples) and inactivating mutations in the tumor suppressor genes *p16INK4a* (>95%), *p53* (50–75%), *DPC4/SMAD4/MADH4* (55%), and *BRCA2* (5–10%) (Jaffee et al. 2002). Less frequent mutated genes include *LKB1* (5%), *TGFβ* and Activin receptors (4%), *MKK4* (4%), *FANCC* and *FANCG* (<5%), *AKT2* (10–20%), and *MYB* (10%) (Hansel et al. 2003; Rogers et al. 2004). Of course, these findings do not establish unequivocally that PanINs progress to invasive ductal carcinomas, nor do they exclude the possibility of other pathways to such cancers. Indeed, extensive genetic heterogeneity often exists among similar PanINs found within a given specimen (Rozenblum et al. 1997). Finally, although PanIN-1As are commonly identified in autopsy studies from the general population (Kern 2000), PanIN-3 specimens are difficult to obtain, and thus, our knowledge of the molecular events critical for the progression from PanIN to PDA remains quite limited.

Interestingly, many of the genes mutated in PanIN and invasive pancreatic cancer are present as germ-line mutations in several familial cancer syndromes with a predisposition to pancreatic cancer, including familial atypical multiple mole and melanoma (FAMMM) syndrome, Peutz-Jeghers syndrome (PJS), the breast cancer and ovarian cancer syndrome type II (BRCA2), and hereditary nonpolyposis colon cancer (HNPCC). These syndromes are associated with monoallelic germ-line mutations of the tumor suppressor genes *p16INK4a* (Goldstein et al. 1995), *LKB1/STK11* (Su et al. 1999), *BRCA2* (Goggins et al. 1996; Thorlacius et al. 1996), and *hMLH1/hMSH2/hMSH6* (Lynch et al. 1985), respectively. Finally, patients with hereditary pancreatitis are also at a substantial risk for developing PDA (Lowenfels et al. 1997). Unfortunately, little is known about the role of these mutant genes in the development of sporadic and familial pancreatic cancer, due in part to the lack of identifiable early-stage patients. Furthermore, it is hypothesized that the major cause(s) of inherited susceptibility to pancreatic cancer remains to be identified (see, e.g., Eberle et al. 2002).

CLINICAL CONSIDERATIONS IN PANCREATIC CANCER

The poor outcome of patients with PDA has been attributed to the advanced stage of disease at diagnosis, the poor response to systemic and local therapies, and the aggressive biological nature of the disease. Early pancreatic cancer goes undiagnosed for a number of reasons, including anatomical location, nonlocalizing symptoms, and a lack of adequately sensitive and specific biomarkers of disease (Konner and O'Reilly 2002). Patients oftentimes develop a clinical prodrome that can include vague upper gastrointestinal symptoms, jaundice, adult-onset diabetes, unexplained pancreatitis, back pain, and weight loss. Initial evaluation includes radiologic assessment with transabdominal and/or endoscopic ultrasound (EUS), computed tomography (CT), and/or magnetic resonance imaging (MRI) to identify suspicious pancreatic masses in a patient, followed by definitive diagnosis established by

direct biopsy of a pancreatic mass. Notably, approximately 80% of patients present with radiographically evident unresectable pancreatic cancer at the time of initial diagnosis (Warshaw and Fernandez-del Castillo 1992a).

Efforts to improve the early detection of PDA include surveillance EUS in patients at high risk for the development of PDA (Canto et al. 2004) and the development of molecular markers of early disease. Serum CA (carbohydrate antigen) 19-9 and, less commonly, CEA (carcinoembryonic antigen) are tumor markers that can be used to follow response to therapy and disease recurrence in patients who present with elevated levels at diagnosis. However, neither marker is adequate for primary detection. Many of the genetic events described above, most notably *KRAS* activating mutations, have been investigated in potential disease-detection strategies. *KRAS* mutations have been searched for in serum (Tada et al. 1993; Maire et al. 2002), pancreatic secretions (Berthelemy et al. 1995; Queneau et al. 2001), fine-needle aspirates (Villanueva et al. 1996; Mora et al. 1998), duct brushings (Van Laethem et al. 1995), and stool specimens (Caldas et al. 1994). However, none of these tests demonstrated the requisite sensitivity and specificity to be useful as a general screening tool. The same is unfortunately true of a number of other potential targets, including *hTert* (telomerase catalytic subunit) (Uehara et al. 1999), matrix metalloproteinase-2 (MMP-2) (Yokoyama et al. 2002), and, more recently, aberrantly methylated promoter CpG islands of key genes (see, e.g., Fukushima et al. 2002). Novel labeling and fractionation methods for pancreatic tissue (Chen et al. 2005), serum proteins (Yu et al. 2005), and secreted proteins (Gronborg et al. 2006) coupled with tandem mass spectrometry have suggested additional candidate markers which await validation. Although these techniques continue to evolve in sophistication, to date, no marker or method has proved adequately robust, or able to detect sufficiently early disease, to significantly affect overall patient survival.

Surgical resection of a localized pancreatic tumor is currently the only hope for cure, with multi-modality therapies offering only limited palliative benefit to patients with advanced disease. Despite treatment, less than 20% of all patients will be alive 1 year after diagnosis, and less than 5% at 5 years (Warshaw and Fernandez-del Castillo 1992a). Even among the carefully selected 5–15% of patients who present with resectable disease and undergo surgery, the 5-year survival is still approximately 20% (Warshaw and Fernandez-del Castillo 1992b). For the small subset of patients with diploid DNA content, disease-free lymph nodes, and small primaries (less than 1 cm), an elevated 5-year survival is observed (Crist et al. 1987; Trede et al. 1990; Allison et al. 1998). Importantly, however, many of even these highly selected patients still succumb from recurrent and metastatic disease (Allison et al. 1998; Trede et al. 2001). The chemotherapeutic agent gemcitabine has been the mainstay for the treatment of advanced pancreatic cancer for the past decade, due to a modest increase in median survival when compared to 5-fluorouracil (5-FU) (5.6 months vs. 4.4 months) and a measurable increase in a patient's quality of life index

(Burris et al. 1997). Radiotherapy is offered in combination with 5-FU as an adjuvant therapy for patients with resected PDA and in some patients with locally advanced and unresectable PDA, although the precise benefit of radiotherapy is still under evaluation. Immunotherapeutic (Jaffee et al. 2001; Laheru and Jaffee 2005) and immunomodulatory (Picozzi et al. 2003; Picozzi and Traverso 2004) approaches are also being explored as a means to prevent recurrence in resected PDA patients.

Molecular therapies that target the autonomous or non-cell-autonomous compartments of PDA may improve upon the limited efficacy of gemcitabine for advanced pancreatic cancer patients. The most logical therapeutic agents for PDA would appear to be oncogenic KRAS inhibitors (Brummelkamp et al. 2002); however, none currently exists, and KRAS is unfortunately considered an intractable drug target. Nevertheless, signaling pathways downstream of oncogenic KRAS, such as the MAP kinase and the PI3-kinase cascades, may serve as suitable surrogates for oncogenic KRAS; suitable agents that inhibit these pathways are currently or will shortly be evaluated in patients. Additionally, preclinical and clinical investigations are under way with agents designed to interrupt a number of signaling pathways in PDA including PDGFR, VEGFR, EGFR, Her-2/Neu (Hansel et al. 2003), Hedgehog (Berman et al. 2003; Thayer et al. 2003), and Notch (Miyamoto et al. 2003). Indeed, the epidermal growth factor receptor antagonist erlotinib was recently approved by the FDA for administration in combination with gemcitabine in advanced pancreatic cancer patients after demonstrating a modest increase in median survival and prolonged survival in a subpopulation of patients (Tang et al. 2006; M. Moore, unpubl.). The rapid progression of PDA permits most patients only one opportunity to enroll in an investigational study and, thus, methods that would reliably predict efficacy of specific therapeutic agents for specific patients are sorely needed.

MODELS OF MURINE PanIN AND PDA

Several early attempts to produce a genetically engineered murine model of PanIN and PDA were unsuccessful. For example, "knockout" mice harboring constitutive or conditional mutations of *DPC4/SMAD4/MADH4* (Sirard et al. 1998; Yang et al. 2002), *BRCA2* (Suzuki et al. 1997), *p16INK4a/ARF* (Serrano et al. 1996), and *Trp53* (Donehower et al. 1992) did not develop PanIN or PDA, suggesting that tumor suppressor gene loss alone does not initiate pancreatic cancer. Alternatively, a number of transgenic "oncomouse" strains were described as developing murine exocrine pancreatic cancer, but none faithfully recapitulated the cardinal features of PanIN or PDA. The majority of the published transgenic models involved the expression of oncogenes or growth factors from heterologous promoters that were most active in acinar cells of the pancreas. These models generally demonstrated diffuse acinar metaplasia and acinar carcinoma (Quaife et al. 1987). Several models reported pancreatic "acinar-tubular-ductal" transdifferentiation, and neoplasms found in these mice share some properties with human pancre-

atic serous cystadenocarcinoma (Bardeesy et al. 2001) and ductal carcinomas (Wagner et al. 2001). However, the relevance of acinar-tubular-ductal transdifferentiation in human ductal pancreatic cancer remains speculative, with the direct transformation of ductal epithelial cells or pancreatic stem cells serving as an alternative model (Reya et al. 2001). For example, two strains of genetically engineered mice that directed expression of oncogenic *Kras* alleles from promoters predominantly active in mature acinar cells, *MIST1* (Tuveson et al. 2006) and *Elastase* (Grippo et al. 2003), have been described. As expected, most $MIST1\text{-}Kras4B^{G12D}$ and $Elastase\text{-}Kras^{G12V}$ mice developed acinar hyperplasia and neoplasia, although $MIST1\text{-}Kras4B^{G12D}$ animals additionally developed a mixed histological spectrum that included cystadenocarcinoma and preinvasive cancer with ductal features but without classic PanIN. Intriguingly, the direct expression of oncogenic $Kras^{G12V}$ in the mature ductal compartment by virtue of a transgenic Cytokeratin 19 promoter also failed to generate PanIN or PDA, although occasional ductal hyperplasia was noted (Brembeck et al. 2003). Finally, mice bearing a latent oncogenic $Kras^{G12D}$ allele that becomes active somatically following a stochastic recombination event succumb to lung cancer and do not demonstrate any pancreatic neoplasia (Johnson et al. 2001). Perhaps not surprisingly, there was no evidence that the recombination event required to activate the latent $Kras^{G12D}$ allele had ever occurred in the pancreata of these mice. These findings notwithstanding, *KRAS* mutations can be identified at high frequency in PanIN-1A in vivo, and in the absence of other obvious genetic mutations, suggesting that they do indeed participate in the initiation of tumorigenesis (Hruban et al. 1993; Yanagisawa et al. 1993; Caldas et al. 1994; Tada et al. 1996; Moskaluk et al. 1997; Terhune et al. 1998; Luttges et al. 1999). Another possible explanation for the lack of effective *Kras*-dependent murine pancreatic cancer models is that oncogenic *RAS*, when ectopically expressed at supraphysiological levels in primary cells, induces cellular senescence rather than proliferation (Serrano et al. 1997). Indeed, activating endogenous expression from a conditional targeted "Lox-Stop-Lox" (LSL)-$Kras^{G12D}$ allele caused immortalization and proliferation of primary fibroblast cultures, as opposed to senescence (Jackson et al. 2001; Tuveson et al. 2004). Physiological expression of this conditional $LSL\text{-}Kras^{G12D}$ allele alone and in combination with endogenous mutations in pertinent tumor suppressor genes ultimately led to the development of faithful models of PanIN and PDA.

The first murine model of PanIN was generated by directing the conditional expression of an endogenous $LSL\text{-}Kras^{G12D}$ allele to pancreatic progenitor cells with either a Pdx1-Cre or P48-Cre allele (Hingorani et al. 2003). The entire spectrum of PanINs occurred in compound mutant mice with complete penetrance, and murine PanINs (mPanINs) were histologically indistinguishable from human PanINs, including the presence of an abundant stromal reaction in advanced PanIN (Fig. 1). Analyses of aged cohorts of mice demonstrated that mPanINs progress temporally and, furthermore, older mice harbor-

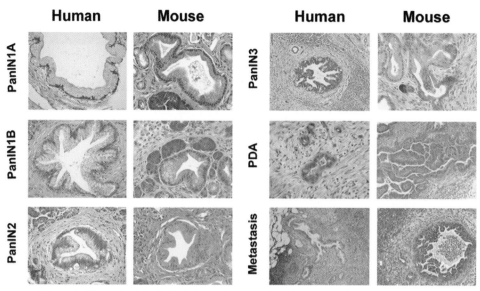

Figure 1. Histological similarity between human and murine pancreatic cancer progression.

ing mPanINs spontaneously developed PDA after a prolonged latency, supporting the premise that mPanINs were truly preinvasive neoplasms. The slow progression of mPanIN to PDA also meant that this mouse model offered the unique opportunity to identify biomarkers of PanIN. Indeed, experiments analyzing the low-molecular-weight serum proteome suggested that specific patterns of biomolecules could distinguish mPanIN mice from controls, although individual biomarkers await definitive identification. This finding was reproduced in a limited fashion by others expressing an endogenous *LSL-Kras$^{G12V-IRES-\beta Geo}$* allele in the pancreas, in which PanIN-1A-like lesions were described (Guerra et al. 2003). Thus, the murine model of PanIN was successfully produced by expressing an endogenous allele of oncogenic *Kras^{G12D}* at physiological levels in the developing pancreas, clarifying the gatekeeper role of *Kras* mutation as the initiating event in PanIN and PDA.

The mouse PanIN model also served as an ideal platform to generate models of advanced PDA by incorporating conditional tumor suppressor gene mutations in the pancreas while concomitantly expressing *Kras^{G12D}*. Indeed, the conditional biallelic deletion of the *Ink4a/ARF* locus (Aguirre et al. 2003), or the heterozygous expression of *Trp53^{R172H}* (Hingorani et al. 2005), cooperated with *Kras^{G12D}* to produce lethal and metastatic PDA with a significantly shortened latency. Metastatic sites included the liver, lung, mesentery, adrenal glands, celiac plexus, and diaphragm, closely resembling the patterns of disease spread observed in patients (Fig. 2). Furthermore, mice with advanced disease oftentimes presented with significant cachexia and hemorrhagic ascites, mimicking the systemic effects observed in patients. These models of advanced PDA confirmed the importance of the tumor suppressor genes previously implicated in human pancreatic cancer and

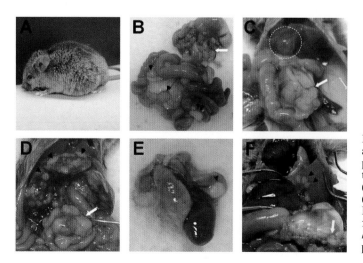

Figure 2. Clinical and pathological sequelae of advanced and metastatic PDA in mice. (*A*) Photograph of mouse presenting with cachexia, lethargy, and abdominal distention. (*B*) Primary PDA at the head of the pancreas (*white arrow*) and mesenteric metastases (*arrowheads*). (*C*) Gall bladder distention (*dotted circle*) due to primary PDA tumor (*arrow*). (*D*) Liver metastases (*arrowheads*) from primary PDA (*arrow*). (*E*) Lung metastasis (*arrowhead*). (*F*) Diaphragmatic metastases (*arrowheads*) and primary PDA (*arrow*).

Figure 3. Comparison between human and murine PDA. Histological, pathological, pathophysiological, molecular, and clinical aspects of human and murine PDA. (*) Mouse PDA is detected by ultrasound; (**) under investigation.

	HUMAN	MOUSE
	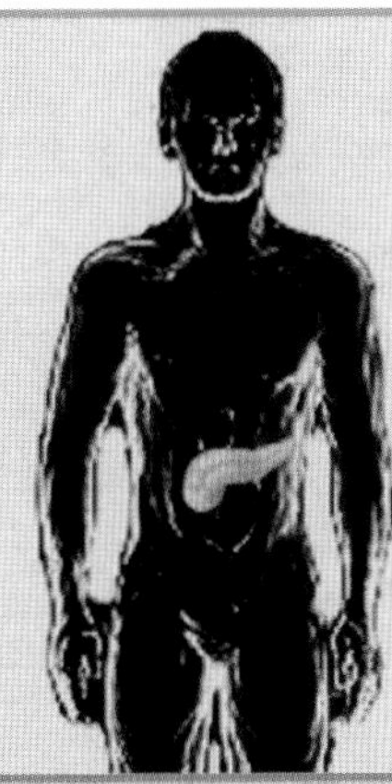	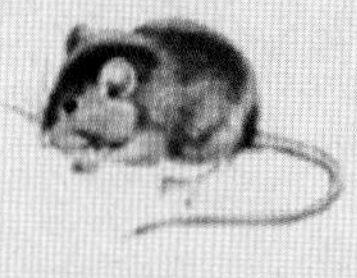 Pdx1-cre;LSL-Kras^{G12D}; Trp53^{R172H}
Histology		
Pre-invasive	PanIN	mPanIN
Invasive	PDA-Predominantly Glandular	PDA-Predominantly Glandular
Pathology		
Primary Tumor Predominant Location	Head of Pancreas	Head of Pancreas
Metastatic Sites	Lymph Nodes Liver Lung Pleura Peritoneum Celiac Plexus Adrenal Glands	Lymph Nodes Liver Lung Pleura Peritoneum Celiac Plexus Adrenal Glands
Pathophysiology		
Signs	Cachexia, Jaundice, Fatigue, Abdominal Pain	Cachexia, Ascites, Lethargy, Bowel Obstruction
Median Survival after Detection	4-6 months	1 month*
Lethality	99%	100%
Molecular		
Signaling Pathways	EGFR, Her2/neu, Notch Hedgehog, Cox2	EGFR, Her2/neu, Notch Hedgehog, Cox2
Genetic Mutations	KRAS, Tp53, p16 INK4a SMAD4, BRCA2, LKB1	Kras, Trp53, p16 Ink4a Smad4?, Brca2?, Lkb1?
Genomic Alterations	CIN	CIN
Clinical		
BioMarkers	**	**
Therapies — Local Disease	Surgery	**
Therapies — Advanced Disease	Palliative (Chemo + Radiation)	**

supported the relevance of the PanIN model for the study of human PDA.

The murine PanIN and PDA models were further vali-

dated by the elevated expression of several potential therapeutic targets previously identified in human PanIN and PDA, including EGFR, Her-2/neu, Sonic Hedgehog ligand, Cox-2, matrix metalloproteinase 7, and an activated Notch signaling pathway. However, the expression of several of these targets was not uniform throughout tumors from the *Pdx1-cre*; *Kras^{G12D}*; *Trp53^{R172H}* mice, suggesting a profound underlying molecular heterogeneity. Primary cell lines prepared from these mice uniformly demonstrated the loss of the remaining wild-type *Trp53* allele, but no mutations in the *p16Ink4a*, *Cdk4* or *Smad4/Dpc4/Madh4* gene. Notably, the isolated cell lines displayed impressive centrosome amplification, and karyotypic analysis revealed a widespread chromosomal instability that is uncommon in mouse tumor models but is a hallmark feature of human PDA and is thought to contribute to the molecular complexity of human epithelial cancers. Thus, these mouse models of PanIN and PDA faithfully recapitulated the central features of the cognate human condition at the clinical, histopathological, biochemical, genetic, and genomic levels (Fig. 3).

CONCLUSION

Murine models of PanIN and PDA have now been established and should serve as important components of the preclinical tool box for pancreatic cancer researchers (Hruban et al. 2006b). Much optimism exists that such models will serve an important role in the development of early detection methods and the assessment of potential therapeutic strategies. Furthermore, mouse models of PanIN and PDA should enable biological investigations into the cellular origins and molecular pathways required for pancreatic cancer development and maintenance, including topics as diverse as metastasis and chromosomal instability.

ACKNOWLEDGMENTS

The authors thank current and past Tuveson and Hingorani lab members and our outside collaborators who have contributed to this research. Particularly, we thank Dr. Ralph Hruban for photomicrographs of human PanIN and PDA, and Mike Jacobetz and Chelsea Combs for figure preparation. Funding is acknowledged from the AACR-PanCAN Career Development Award (S.R.H.), National Institutes of Health grants R01 CA101973 and U01 CA084291 (D.A.T.). D.A.T. is a Rita Allen Foundation Scholar.

REFERENCES

Aguirre A.J., Bardeesy N., Sinha M., Lopez L., Tuveson D.A., Horner J., Redston M.S., and DePinho R.A. 2003. Activated Kras and Ink4a/Arf deficiency cooperate to produce metastatic pancreatic ductal adenocarcinoma. *Genes Dev.* **17:** 3112.

Ahlgren J.D. 1996. Epidemiology and risk factors in pancreatic cancer. *Semin. Oncol.* **23:** 241.

Allison D.C., Piantadosi S., Hruban R.H., Dooley W.C., Fishman E.K., Yeo C.J., Lillemoe K.D., Pitt H.A., Lin P., and Cameron J.L. 1998. DNA content and other factors associated with ten-year survival after resection of pancreatic carcinoma. *J. Surg. Oncol.* **67:** 151.

Bardeesy N., Sharpless N.E., DePinho R.A., and Merlino G. 2001. The genetics of pancreatic adenocarcinoma: A roadmap for a mouse model. *Semin. Cancer Biol.* **11:** 201.

Berman D.M., Karhadkar S.S., Maitra A., Montes De Oca R., Gerstenblith M.R., Briggs K., Parker A.R., Shimada Y., Eshleman J.R., Watkins D.N., and Beachy P.A. 2003. Widespread requirement for Hedgehog ligand stimulation in growth of digestive tract tumours. *Nature* **425:** 846.

Berthelemy P., Bouisson M., Escourrou J., Vaysse N., Rumeau J.L., and Pradayrol L. 1995. Identification of K-ras mutations in pancreatic juice in the early diagnosis of pancreatic cancer. *Ann. Intern. Med.* **123:** 188.

Brembeck F.H., Schreiber F.S., Deramaudt T.B., Craig L., Rhoades B., Swain G., Grippo P., Stoffers D.A., Silberg D.G., and Rustgi A.K. 2003. The mutant K-ras oncogene causes pancreatic periductal lymphocytic infiltration and gastric mucous neck cell hyperplasia in transgenic mice. *Cancer Res.* **63:** 2005.

Brummelkamp T.R., Bernards R., and Agami R. 2002. Stable suppression of tumorigenicity by virus-mediated RNA interference. *Cancer Cell* **2:** 243.

Burris H.A., III, Moore M.J., Andersen J., Green M.R., Rothenberg M.L., Modiano M.R., Cripps M.C., Portenoy R.K., Storniolo A.M., Tarassoff P., Nelson R., Dorr F.A., Stephens C.D., and Von Hoff D.D. 1997. Improvements in survival and clinical benefit with gemcitabine as first-line therapy for patients with advanced pancreas cancer: A randomized trial. *J. Clin. Oncol.* **15:** 2403.

Caldas C., Hahn S.A., Hruban R.H., Redston M.S., Yeo C.J., and Kern S.E. 1994. Detection of K-ras mutations in the stool of patients with pancreatic adenocarcinoma and pancreatic ductal hyperplasia. *Cancer Res.* **54:** 3568.

Canto M.I., Goggins M., Yeo C.J., Griffin C., Axilbund J.E., Brune K., Ali S.Z., Jagannath S., Petersen G.M., Fishman E.K., Piantadosi S., Giardiello F.M., and Hruban R.H. 2004. Screening for pancreatic neoplasia in high-risk individuals: An EUS-based approach. *Clin. Gastroenterol. Hepatol.* **2:** 606.

Chen R., Yi E.C., Donohoe S., Pan S., Eng J., Cooke K., Crispin D.A., Lane Z., Goodlett D.R., Bronner M.P., Aebersold R., and Brentnall T.A. 2005. Pancreatic cancer proteome: The proteins that underlie invasion, metastasis, and immunologic escape. *Gastroenterology* **129:** 1187.

Crist D.W., Sitzmann J.V., and Cameron J.L. 1987. Improved hospital morbidity, mortality, and survival after the Whipple procedure. *Ann. Surg.* **206:** 358.

DiGiuseppe J.A., Hruban R.H., Goodman S.N., Polak M., van den Berg F.M., Allison D.C., Cameron J.L., and Offerhaus G.J. 1994. Overexpression of p53 protein in adenocarcinoma of the pancreas. *Am. J. Clin. Pathol.* **101:** 684.

Donehower L.A., Harvey M., Slagle B.L., McArthur M.J., Montgomery C.A., Jr., Butel J.S., and Bradley A. 1992. Mice deficient for p53 are developmentally normal but susceptible to spontaneous tumours. *Nature* **356:** 215.

Eberle M.A., Pfutzer R., Pogue-Geile K.L., Bronner M.P., Crispin D., Kimmey M.B., Duerr R.H., Kruglyak L., Whitcomb D.C., and Brentnall T.A. 2002. A new susceptibility locus for autosomal dominant pancreatic cancer maps to chromosome 4q32-34. *Am. J. Hum. Genet.* **70:** 1044.

Fukushima N., Sato N., Ueki T., Rosty C., Walter K.M., Wilentz R.E., Yeo C.J., Hruban R.H., and Goggins M. 2002. Aberrant methylation of preproenkephalin and p16 genes in pancreatic intraepithelial neoplasia and pancreatic ductal adenocarcinoma. *Am. J. Pathol.* **160:** 1573.

Goggins M., Hruban R.H., and Kern S.E. 2000. BRCA2 is inactivated late in the development of pancreatic intraepithelial neoplasia: Evidence and implications. *Am. J. Pathol.* **156:** 1767.

Goggins M., Schutte M., Lu J., Moskaluk C.A., Weinstein C.L., Petersen G.M., Yeo C.J., Jackson C.E., Lynch H.T., Hruban R.H., and Kern S.E. 1996. Germline BRCA2 gene mutations in patients with apparently sporadic pancreatic carcinomas. *Cancer Res.* **56:** 5360.

Goldstein A.M., Fraser M.C., Struewing J.P., Hussussian C.J., Ranade K., Zametkin D.P., Fontaine L.S., Organic S.M., Dracopoli N.C., and Clark W.H., Jr. 1995. Increased risk of pancreatic cancer in melanoma-prone kindreds with p16INK4 mutations (comments). *N. Engl. J. Med.* **333:** 970.

Grippo P.J., Nowlin P.S., Demeure M.J., Longnecker D.S., and Sandgren E.P. 2003. Preinvasive pancreatic neoplasia of ductal phenotype induced by acinar cell targeting of mutant Kras in transgenic mice. *Cancer Res.* **63:** 2016.

Gronborg M., Kristiansen T.Z., Iwahori A., Chang R., Reddy R., Sato N., Molina H., Jensen O.N., Hruban R.H., Goggins M.G., Maitra A., and Pandey A. 2006. Biomarker discovery from pancreatic cancer secretome using a differential proteomic approach. *Mol. Cell. Proteomics* **5:** 157.

Guerra C., Mijimolle N., Dhawahir A., Dubus P., Barradas M., Serrano M., Campuzano V., and Barbacid M. 2003. Tumor induction by an endogenous K-ras oncogene is highly dependent on cellular context. *Cancer Cell* **4:** 111.

Hansel D.E., Kern S.E., and Hruban R.H. 2003. Molecular pathogenesis of pancreatic cancer. *Annu. Rev. Genomics Hum. Genet.* **4:** 237.

Hingorani S.R., Wang L., Multani A.S., Combs C., Deramaudt T.B., Hruban R.H., Rustgi A.K., Chang S., and Tuveson D.A. 2005. Trp53R172H and KrasG12D cooperate to promote chromosomal instability and widely metastatic pancreatic ductal adenocarcinoma in mice. *Cancer Cell* **7:** 469.

Hingorani S.R., Petricoin E.F., Maitra A., Rajapakse V., King C., Jacobetz M.A., Ross S., Conrads T.P., Veenstra T.D., Hitt B.A., Kawaguchi Y., Johann D., Liotta L.A., Crawford H.C., Putt M.E., Jacks T., Wright C.V., Hruban R.H., Lowy A.M., and Tuveson D.A. 2003. Preinvasive and invasive ductal pancreatic cancer and its early detection in the mouse. *Cancer Cell* **4:** 437.

Hruban R.H., Rustgi A.K., Brentnall T.A., Tempero M.A., Wright C.V., and Tuveson D.A. 2006a. Pancreatic cancer in mice and man: The Penn Workshop 2004. *Cancer Res.* **66:** 14.

Hruban R.H., van Mansfeld A.D., Offerhaus G.J., van Weering D.H., Allison D.C., Goodman S.N., Kensler T.W., Bose K.K., Cameron J.L., and Bos J.L. 1993. K-ras oncogene activation in adenocarcinoma of the human pancreas. A study of 82 carcinomas using a combination of mutant-enriched polymerase chain reaction analysis and allele-specific oligonucleotide hybridization. *Am. J. Pathol.* **143:** 545.

Hruban R.H., Adsay N.V., Albores-Saavedra J., Anver M.R., Biankin A.V., Boivin G.P., Furth E.E., Furukawa T., Klein A., Klimstra D.S., Kloppel G., Lauwers G.Y., Longnecker D.S., Luttges J., Maitra A., Offerhaus G.J., Perez-Gallego L., Redston M., and Tuveson D.A. 2006b. Pathology of genetically engineered mouse models of pancreatic exocrine cancer: Consensus report and recommendations. *Cancer Res.* **66:** 95.

Jackson E.L., Willis N., Mercer K., Bronson R.T., Crowley D., Montoya R., Jacks T., and Tuveson D.A. 2001. Analysis of lung tumor initiation and progression using conditional expression of oncogenic K-ras. *Genes Dev.* **15:** 3243.

Jaffee E.M., Hruban R.H., Canto M., and Kern S.E. 2002. Focus on pancreas cancer. *Cancer Cell* **2:** 25.

Jaffee E.M., Hruban R.H., Biedrzycki B., Laheru D., Schepers K., Sauter P.R., Goemann M., Coleman J., Grochow L., Donehower R.C., Lillemoe K.D., O'Reilly S., Abrams R.A., Pardoll D.M., Cameron J.L., and Yeo C.J. 2001. Novel allogeneic granulocyte-macrophage colony-stimulating factor-secreting tumor vaccine for pancreatic cancer: A phase I trial of safety and immune activation. *J. Clin. Oncol.* **19:** 145.

Johnson L., Mercer K., Greenbaum D., Bronson R.T., Crowley D., Tuveson D.A., and Jacks T. 2001. Somatic activation of the K-ras oncogene causes early onset lung cancer in mice (comments). *Nature* **410:** 1111.

Kern S.E. 2000. Molecular genetic alterations in ductal pancreatic adenocarcinomas. *Med. Clin. N. Am.* **84:** 691.

Klimstra D.S. and Longnecker D.S. 1994. K-ras mutations in pancreatic ductal proliferative lesions. *Am. J. Pathol.* **145:** 1547.

Konner J. and O'Reilly E. 2002. Pancreatic cancer: Epidemiology, genetics, and approaches to screening. *Oncology* **16:** 1615.

Laheru D. and Jaffee E.M. 2005. Immunotherapy for pancreatic cancer: Science driving clinical progress. *Nat. Rev. Cancer* **5:** 459.

Lowenfels A.B., Maisonneuve P., DiMagno E.P., Elitsur Y.,

Gates L.K., Jr., Perrault J., and Whitcomb D.C. 1997. Hereditary pancreatitis and the risk of pancreatic cancer. International Hereditary Pancreatitis Study Group. *J. Natl. Cancer Inst.* **89:** 442.

Luttges J., Schlehe B., Menke M.A., Vogel I., Henne-Bruns D., and Kloppel G. 1999. The K-ras mutation pattern in pancreatic ductal adenocarcinoma usually is identical to that in associated normal, hyperplastic, and metaplastic ductal epithelium. *Cancer* **85:** 1703.

Lynch H.T., Voorhees G.J., Lanspa S.J., McGreevy P.S., and Lynch J.F. 1985. Pancreatic carcinoma and hereditary nonpolyposis colorectal cancer: A family study. *Br. J. Cancer* **52:** 271.

Lynch H.T., Smyrk T., Kern S.E., Hruban R.H., Lightdale C.J., Lemon S.J., Lynch J.F., Fusaro L.R., Fusaro R.M., and Ghadirian P. 1996. Familial pancreatic cancer: A review. *Semin. Oncol.* **23:** 251.

Maire F., Micard S., Hammel P., Voitot H., Levy P., Cugnenc P.H., Ruszniewski P., and Puig P.L. 2002. Differential diagnosis between chronic pancreatitis and pancreatic cancer: Value of the detection of KRAS2 mutations in circulating DNA. *Br. J. Cancer* **87:** 551.

Miyamoto Y., Maitra A., Ghosh B., Zechner U., Argani P., Iacobuzio-Donahue C.A., Sriuranpong V., Iso T., Meszoely I.M., Wolfe M.S., Hruban R.H., Ball D.W., Schmid R.M., and Leach S.D. 2003. Notch mediates TGF alpha-induced changes in epithelial differentiation during pancreatic tumorigenesis. *Cancer Cell* **3:** 565.

Mora J., Puig P., Boadas J., Urgell E., Montserrat E., Lerma E., Gonzalez-Sastre F., Lluis F., Farre A., and Capella G. 1998. K-ras gene mutations in the diagnosis of fine-needle aspirates of pancreatic masses: Prospective study using two techniques with different detection limits. *Clin. Chem.* **44:** 2243.

Moskaluk C.A., Hruban R.H., and Kern S.E. 1997. p16 and K-ras gene mutations in the intraductal precursors of human pancreatic adenocarcinoma. *Cancer Res.* **57:** 2140.

Picozzi V.J. and Traverso L.W. 2004. The Virginia Mason approach to localized pancreatic cancer. *Surg. Oncol. Clin. N. Am.* **13:** 663.

Picozzi V.J., Kozarek R.A., and Traverso L.W. 2003. Interferon-based adjuvant chemoradiation therapy after pancreaticoduodenectomy for pancreatic adenocarcinoma. *Am. J. Surg.* **185:** 476.

Quaife C.J., Pinkert C.A., Ornitz D.M., Palmiter R.D., and Brinster R.L. 1987. Pancreatic neoplasia induced by ras expression in acinar cells of transgenic mice. *Cell* **48:** 1023.

Queneau P.E., Adessi G.L., Thibault P., Cleau D., Heyd B., Mantion G., and Carayon P. 2001. Early detection of pancreatic cancer in patients with chronic pancreatitis: Diagnostic utility of a K-ras point mutation in the pancreatic juice. *Am. J. Gastroenterol.* **96:** 700.

Reya T., Morrison S.J., Clarke M.F., and Weissman I.L. 2001. Stem cells, cancer, and cancer stem cells. *Nature* **414:** 105.

Rogers C.D., Van Der Heijden M.S., Brune K., Yeo C.J., Hruban R.H., Kern S.E., and Goggins M. 2004. The genetics of FANCC and FANCG in familial pancreatic cancer. *Cancer Biol. Ther.* **3:** 167.

Rozenblum E., Schutte M., Goggins M., Hahn S.A., Panzer S., Zahurak M., Goodman S.N., Sohn T.A., Hruban R.H., Yeo C.J., and Kern S.E. 1997. Tumor-suppressive pathways in pancreatic carcinoma. *Cancer Res.* **57:** 1731.

Serrano M., Lin A.W., McCurrach M.E., Beach D., and Lowe S.W. 1997. Oncogenic ras provokes premature cell senescence associated with accumulation of p53 and p16INK4a. *Cell* **88:** 593.

Serrano M., Lee H., Chin L., Cordon-Cardo C., Beach D., and DePinho R.A. 1996. Role of the INK4a locus in tumor suppression and cell mortality. *Cell* **85:** 27.

Silverman D.T., Dunn J.A., Hoover R.N., Schiffman M., Lillemoe K.D., Schoenberg J.B., Brown L.M., Greenberg R.S., Hayes R.B., and Swanson G.M., et al. 1994. Cigarette smoking and pancreas cancer: A case-control study based on direct interviews. *J. Natl. Cancer Inst.* **86:** 1510.

Sirard C., de la Pompa J.L., Elia A., Itie A., Mirtsos C., Cheung A., Hahn S., Wakeham A., Schwartz L., Kern S.E., Rossant J., and Mak T.W. 1998. The tumor suppressor gene Smad4/Dpc4 is required for gastrulation and later for anterior development of the mouse embryo. *Genes Dev.* **12:** 107.

Su G.H., Hruban R.H., Bansal R.K., Bova G.S., Tang D.J., Shekher M.C., Westerman A.M., Entius M.M., Goggins M., Yeo C.J., and Kern S.E. 1999. Germline and somatic mutations of the STK11/LKB1 Peutz-Jeghers gene in pancreatic and biliary cancers. *Am. J. Pathol.* **154:** 1835.

Suzuki A., de la Pompa J.L., Hakem R., Elia A., Yoshida R., Mo R., Nishina H., Chuang T., Wakeham A., Itie A., Koo W., Billia P., Ho A., Fukumoto M., Hui C.C., and Mak T.W. 1997. Brca2 is required for embryonic cellular proliferation in the mouse. *Genes Dev.* **11:** 1242.

Tada M., Omata M., Kawai S., Saisho H., Ohto M., Saiki R.K., and Sninsky J.J. 1993. Detection of ras gene mutations in pancreatic juice and peripheral blood of patients with pancreatic adenocarcinoma. *Cancer Res.* **53:** 2472.

Tada M., Ohashi M., Shiratori Y., Okudaira T., Komatsu Y., Kawabe T., Yoshida H., Machinami R., Kishi K., and Omata M. 1996. Analysis of K-ras gene mutation in hyperplastic duct cells of the pancreas without pancreatic disease (comments). *Gastroenterology* **110:** 227.

Tang P.A., Tsao M.S., and Moore M.J. 2006. A review of erlotinib and its clinical use. *Expert Opin. Pharmacother.* **7:** 177.

Terhune P.G., Phifer D.M., Tosteson T.D., and Longnecker D.S. 1998. K-ras mutation in focal proliferative lesions of human pancreas. *Cancer Epidemiol. Biomark. Prev.* **7:** 515.

Thayer S.P., di Magliano M.P., Heiser P.W., Nielsen C.M., Roberts D.J., Lauwers G.Y., Qi Y.P., Gysin S., Fernandez-del Castillo C., Yajnik V., Antoniu B., McMahon M., Warshaw A.L., and Hebrok M. 2003. Hedgehog is an early and late mediator of pancreatic cancer tumorigenesis. *Nature* **425:** 851.

Thorlacius S., Olafsdottir G., Tryggvadottir L., Neuhausen S., Jonasson J.G., Tavtigian S.V., Tulinius H., Ogmundsdottir H.M., and Eyfjord J.E. 1996. A single BRCA2 mutation in male and female breast cancer families from Iceland with varied cancer phenotypes (comments). *Nat. Genet.* **13:** 117.

Trede M., Richter A., and Wendl K. 2001. Personal observations, opinions, and approaches to cancer of the pancreas and the periampullary area. *Surg. Clin. N. Am.* **81:** 595.

Trede M., Schwall G., and Saeger H.D. 1990. Survival after pancreatoduodenectomy. 118 consecutive resections without an operative mortality. *Ann. Surg.* **211:** 447.

Tuveson D.A., Zhu L., Gopinathan A., Willis N.A., Kachatrian L., Grochow R., Pin C.L., Mitin N.Y., Taparowsky E.J., Gimotty P.A., Hruban R.H., Jacks T., and Konieczny S.F. 2006. Mist1-KrasG12D knock-in mice develop mixed differentiation metastatic exocrine pancreatic carcinoma and hepatocellular carcinoma. *Cancer Res.* **66:** 242.

Tuveson D.A., Shaw A.T., Willis N.A., Silver D.P., Jackson E.L., Chang S., Mercer K.L., Grochow R., Hock H., Crowley D., Hingorani S.R., Zaks T., King C., Jacobetz M.A., Wang L., Bronson R.T., Orkin S.H., DePinho R.A., and Jacks T.

2004. Endogenous oncogenic K-ras(G12D) stimulates proliferation and widespread neoplastic and developmental defects. *Cancer Cell* **5:** 375.

Uehara H., Nakaizumi A., Tatsuta M., Baba M., Takenaka A., Uedo N., Sakai N., Yano H., Iishi H., Ohigashi H., Ishikawa O., Okada S., and Kakizoe T. 1999. Diagnosis of pancreatic cancer by detecting telomerase activity in pancreatic juice: Comparison with K-ras mutations. *Am. J. Gastroenterol.* **94:** 2513.

van Heek N.T., Meeker A.K., Kern S.E., Yeo C.J., Lillemoe K.D., Cameron J.L., Offerhaus G.J., Hicks J.L., Wilentz R.E., Goggins M.G., De Marzo A.M., Hruban R.H., and Maitra A. 2002. Telomere shortening is nearly universal in pancreatic intraepithelial neoplasia. *Am. J. Pathol.* **161:** 1541.

Van Laethem J.L., Vertongen P., Deviere J., Van Rampelbergh J., Rickaert F., Cremer M., and Robberecht P. 1995. Detection of c-Ki-ras gene mutation from pancreatic duct brushings in the diagnosis of pancreatic tumours. *Gut* **36:** 781.

Villanueva A., Reyes G., Cuatrecasas M., Martinez A., Erill N., Lerma E., Farre A., Lluis F., and Capella G. 1996. Diagnostic utility of K-ras mutations in fine-needle aspirates of pancreatic masses. *Gastroenterology* **110:** 1587.

Wagner M., Greten F.R., Weber C.K., Koschnick S., Mattfeldt T., Deppert W., Kern H., Adler G., and Schmid R.M. 2001. A murine tumor progression model for pancreatic cancer recapitulating the genetic alterations of the human disease. *Genes Dev.* **15:** 286.

Warshaw A.L. and Fernandez-del Castillo C. 1992a. Pancreatic carcinoma. *N. Engl. J. Med.* **326:** 455.

———. 1992b. Pancreatic carcinoma. *N. Engl. J. Med.* **326:** 455.

Wilentz R.E., Iacobuzio-Donahue C.A., Argani P., McCarthy D.M., Parsons J.L., Yeo C.J., Kern S.E., and Hruban R.H. 2000. Loss of expression of Dpc4 in pancreatic intraepithelial neoplasia: Evidence that DPC4 inactivation occurs late in neoplastic progression. *Cancer Res.* **60:** 2002.

Wilentz R.E., Geradts J., Maynard R., Offerhaus G.J., Kang M., Goggins M., Yeo C.J., Kern S.E., and Hruban R.H. 1998. Inactivation of the p16 (INK4A) tumor-suppressor gene in pancreatic duct lesions: Loss of intranuclear expression. *Cancer Res.* **58:** 4740.

Yanagisawa A., Ohtake K., Ohashi K., Hori M., Kitagawa T., Sugano H., and Kato Y. 1993. Frequent c-Ki-ras oncogene activation in mucous cell hyperplasias of pancreas suffering from chronic inflammation. *Cancer Res.* **53:** 953.

Yang X., Li C., Herrera P.L., and Deng C.X. 2002. Generation of Smad4/Dpc4 conditional knockout mice. *Genesis* **32:** 80.

Yokoyama M., Ochi K., Ichimura M., Mizushima T., Shinji T., Koide N., Tsurumi T., Hasuoka H., and Harada M. 2002. Matrix metalloproteinase-2 in pancreatic juice for diagnosis of pancreatic cancer. *Pancreas* **24:** 344.

Yu K.H., Rustgi A.K., and Blair I.A. 2005. Characterization of proteins in human pancreatic cancer serum using differential gel electrophoresis and tandem mass spectrometry. *J. Proteome Res.* **4:** 1742.

Detection of Oncogenic Mutations in the EGFR Gene in Lung Adenocarcinoma with Differential Sensitivity to EGFR Tyrosine Kinase Inhibitors

R.K. Thomas,[*†] H. Greulich,[*†] Y. Yuza,[*] J.C. Lee,[*†] T. Tengs,[*†] W. Feng,[*†] T.-H. Chen,[*†] E. Nickerson,[‡] J. Simons,[‡] M. Egholm,[‡] J.M. Rothberg,[‡] W.R. Sellers,[*†] and M.L. Meyerson[*†¶]

*Department of Medical Oncology, Dana-Farber Cancer Institute, Harvard Medical School, Boston, Massachusetts 02115; †The Broad Institute of MIT and Harvard, Cambridge, Massachusetts 02141; ‡ 454 Life Sciences, Branford, Connecticut 06405; ¶Department of Pathology, Harvard Medical School, Boston, Massachusetts 02115

The complete sequencing of the human genome and the development of molecularly targeted cancer therapy have promoted efforts to identify systematically the genetic alterations in human cancer. By high-throughput sequencing of tyrosine kinase genes in human non-small-cell lung cancer, we identified somatic mutations in the kinase domain of the epidermal growth factor receptor tyrosine kinase gene (*EGFR*) that are correlated with clinical response to EGFR tyrosine kinase inhibitors (TKIs). We have shown that these mutant forms of *EGFR* induce oncogenic transformation in different cellular systems. Cells whose growth depends on *EGFR* with mutations in exons 19 and 21 are sensitive to EGFR-TKIs, whereas cells expressing insertion mutations in exon 20 or the T790M point mutant, found in tumor biopsies from patients that relapsed after an initial response to EGFR-TKIs, are resistant. Furthermore, by applying a novel, massively parallel sequencing technology, we have shown that clinically relevant oncogene mutations can be detected in clinical specimens with very low tumor content, thereby enabling optimal patient selection for mutation-directed therapy. In summary, by applying high-throughput genomic resequencing, we have identified a novel therapeutic target, mutant EGFR, in lung cancer and evaluated its role in predicting response to targeted therapy.

Lung cancer is the major cause of cancer-related deaths in the western world. In 2005, an estimated 163,510 Americans have died from lung cancer (Jemal et al. 2005). Although numerous novel drugs have been introduced, overall lung-cancer-specific survival for all patients has only increased by 5% in the last 30 years, supporting the notion that chemotherapy is largely ineffective against this cancer type. After 5 years, less than 15% of patients with lung cancer are still alive (Jemal et al. 2005). Lung cancer is generally subcategorized into small-cell lung cancer (SCLC, ~15% of cases) and non-small-cell lung cancer (NSCLC, ~85% of cases) comprising adenocarcinoma, squamous-cell carcinoma, large-cell carcinoma, and undifferentiated carcinoma (Brambilla et al. 2001). Adenocarcinoma is the most frequent subtype, followed by squamous-cell carcinoma.

The efforts to determine novel cancer-causing gene mutations in lung cancer were inspired by the clinical success of small-molecule inhibitors of tyrosine kinases. Almost all patients with chronic myeloid leukemia (CML) achieve complete remission by administration of imatinib, an inhibitor that is active against the BCR-ABL kinase—the fusion protein resulting from the translocation causing CML. This observation has created a paradigm that is the basis for many cancer genomics projects: Find a genetic lesion and find the agent that is active against the lesion (Druker et al. 1996, 2001a,b). This

paradigm has been strengthened by the detection of mutations in genes encoding kinases that were strongly associated with clinical response to inhibitors targeting the respective kinase (Hirota et al. 1998, 2003; Demetri et al. 2002; Cools et al. 2003; Heinrich et al. 2003; Fiedler et al. 2005; Stone et al. 2005). The development of mutation-targeted therapy has necessitated systematic gene resequencing efforts in cancer. The complete sequencing of the human genome and the concurrent development of technologies that allow high-throughput generation of genomic data have opened avenues for such systematic resequencing approaches (Risch 2000; Lander et al. 2001; Venter et al. 2001).

In lung cancer, systematic resequencing efforts led to the discovery of mutations in the BRAF gene in approximately 2% of primary lung adenocarcinomas (Brose et al. 2002; Davies et al. 2002; Naoki et al. 2002; Tuveson et al. 2003) and in PIK3CA, the gene encoding the p110α subunit of the phosphoinositol-3 kinase (Samuels et al. 2004). Further analysis of the most frequent PIK3CA mutants, among them the E545K, revealed that these mutations are in fact oncogenic in vitro (Kang et al. 2005).

Recently, small-molecule inhibitors targeting the epidermal growth factor receptor (EGFR) tyrosine kinase were introduced for second-line treatment of NSCLC. These inhibitors (further referred to as EGFR TKIs), erlotinib and gefitinib, specifically target the EGFR tyrosine kinase (Wakeling et al. 2002; Grunwald and Hidalgo 2003), with estimated 100-fold lower activity against other kinases. The introduction of EGFR TKIs was mainly based on the detection of recurrent overexpression of the EGFR protein in NSCLC (Rusch et al. 1993). In fact, results from phase II clinical trials showed responses in 10% of Caucasian and approximately 30–40% of Japanese patients treated with EGFR TKIs (Fukuoka et al. 2003; Kris et al. 2003; Soulieres et al. 2004). However, responses were not correlated with EGFR expression status because EGFR is overexpressed in almost all patients with NSCLC (Hirsch et al. 2003), indicating that the target of EGFR TKIs in the patients with responses was not the overexpressed EGFR protein. In contrast, clinical responses were mostly seen in Asian patients, in patients with adenocarcinoma, in women, and in never-smokers (Fukuoka et al. 2003; Kris et al. 2003; Miller et al. 2004). Despite the fact that several hundred thousand patients had been treated throughout the world by 2004, the actual target of EGFR TKIs remained elusive.

DETECTION OF EGFR KINASE DOMAIN MUTATIONS IN LUNG CANCER BY SYSTEMATIC KINASE GENE RESEQUENCING

When we systematically resequenced the juxtamembrane domains and the activation loops within the kinase domains of all receptor tyrosine kinases in NSCLC, we detected heterozygous mutations in the EGFR kinase domain in 16 of 119 unselected NSCLC samples (Paez et al. 2004). Included were 58 samples of Japanese origin and 61 samples of U.S. origin; 70 of the 119 samples were adenocarcinomas. We detected a mutation in the glycine-rich nucleotide triphosphate-binding P loop encoded by exon 18 leading to substitution of glycine 719 with serine (G719S), small heterozygous in-frame deletion mutations in exon 19 affecting the residues ELREA and nearby residues, and a heterozygous mutation leading to substitution of leucine 858 located directly adjacent to the DFG motif of the activation loop, with arginine (L858R). Interestingly, all types of mutations that we detected were located around the active site of the kinase, suggesting that they might affect catalytic activity. The residues affected by substitution mutations were all highly conserved within the protein kinases, also pointing toward a role in malignant transformation. Furthermore, all mutations were somatic, because they were detected only in the tumors and not in the corresponding normal DNA. These results imply that somatic mutations in the EGFR gene underlie malignant transformation in a subset of NSCLC patients. Numerous other reports have added to these initial findings and the distribution of different EGFR mutations. Approximately 45% of all EGFR mutations are exon 19 deletions, 40% are L858R mutations, 10% are in-frame duplications/insertions in exon 20, and 5% are other mutations (including G719S) (Huang et al. 2004; Kosaka et al. 2004; Marchetti et al. 2005; Shigematsu et al. 2005). In addition, the mutation frequencies vary significantly depending on ethnicity;

whereas the frequency of EGFR gene mutations appears to be roughly 10% in Caucasian patient populations, in East Asian patients this number is about 30% (Jänne et al. 2005; Shigematsu et al. 2005). The reason for these differences remains elusive. It is conceivable that differences in exposure to environmental factors may act in concert with polymorphisms inherent to different genetic backgrounds.

Mutations were more frequent in adenocarcinomas, in women, in never-smokers, and in patients with East Asian ethnicity (Jänne et al. 2005). Interestingly, these features match those of patients who responded to EGFR TKI treatment in initial phase II trials (Fukuoka et al. 2003; Kris et al. 2003; Miller et al. 2004; Perez-Soler et al. 2004). We therefore sequenced the EGFR kinase domain in patients showing dramatic responses to gefitinib and in non-responders. Importantly, we detected mutations in 5/5 responders, but in none of 4 non-responders ($p = 0.0027$) (Paez et al. 2004). These results indicate that patients whose tumors harbor a mutation in the EGFR kinase domain have a high chance of experiencing at least a partial response (reduction of the tumor volume of at least 50%). Findings reported from other groups investigating EGFR gene mutations in EGFR TKI responders are in line with our findings, as they also found mutations in responders but not in non-responders (Lynch et al. 2004; Pao et al. 2004). Although the patients analyzed in these studies were highly selected (i.e., patients showing progressive disease were analyzed in the control group but no patients experiencing disease stabilization), results from several other studies are supporting these initial findings (Huang et al. 2004; Han et al. 2005; Mitsudomi et al. 2005; Tokumo et al. 2005).

Most recently, it was found that EGFR copy number changes as determined by fluorescence in situ hybridization (FISH) and even EGFR protein expression may be better predictors of survival (Cappuzzo et al. 2005). Several factors should be taken into consideration when examining these data: A survival advantage may also exist for the patients experiencing stable disease, whereas EGFR mutations were found in patients experiencing major, occasionally dramatic, responses. Additionally, it was found that EGFR copy number changes are correlated with the presence of mutations (Tracy et al. 2004; Amann et al. 2005; Cappuzzo et al. 2005). Thus, the cases with amplification in the EGFR gene might also harbor yet unidentified mutations. Conversely, it might also be the wild-type allele that is amplified followed by subsequent mutation, and, thus, the mutant allele might have escaped detection due to the limited sensitivity of Sanger dideoxy sequencing. Finally, in most cases, sequencing is being performed on paraffin-embedded archival specimens. Because in most studies EGFR TKIs have been used at a very late clinical stage, the question remains whether these analyses actually represent the tumor cell clone that is being treated. Future prospective studies will help to determine which molecular alteration is most stringently associated with response to EGFR TKIs.

RELAPSE TO EGFR TKIs IS ASSOCIATED WITH A SECOND-SITE MUTATION IN THE EGFR GENE

Unfortunately, all NSCLC patients treated with the EGFR TKIs gefitinib or erlotinib will eventually relapse and succumb to their tumor. In CML, acquired resistance to Gleevec was found to be mainly caused by the emergence of secondary resistance mutations in the BCR-ABL kinase domain (Gorre et al. 2001; Shah et al. 2002). In some cases, these mutations were existent prior to treatment, indicating that they contribute to malignant growth and implying that continuous molecular monitoring of a patient's tumor cell clone should help guide the optimal therapy. The resistance mutations in CML fall into three major classes: mutations that impair binding of the inhibitor in the nucleotide-binding pocket of the kinase domain, mutations that impair acquisition of an inactive state (a prerequisite for binding of Gleevec), and mutations that lead to autonomous signaling. Interestingly, one of the residues frequently mutated in CML, T315, is conserved in EGFR (T790) and was shown crystallographically to bind erlotinib via a bridging water molecule (Stamos et al. 2002). When an EGFR expression construct harboring the mutation, T790M, which is analogous to the T315I mutation in CML, was introduced into CHO-K1 cells, they became resistant to EGFR TKI treatment (Blencke et al. 2003). Moreover, Kobayashi and colleagues, in collaboration with our group, sequenced the EGFR kinase domain in a patient who had relapsed after a complete response to gefitinib that lasted for 24 months. Whereas sequencing of the pre-therapy sample revealed the presence of a heterozygous exon 19 deletion (delL747-S752), sequencing of the sample obtained at relapse showed the presence of the T790M resistance mutation in addition to delL747-S752. These results indicated that the T790M is in fact a clinically meaningful resistance mutation (Kobayashi et al. 2005). In this study, too, the T790M resistance mutation rendered transfected cells resistant to gefitinib, underlining the initial findings by Blencke et al. Similar results were also reported by another group which found the T790M mutation in 3/6 pa-

tients who suffered acquired or primary resistance to gefitinib or erlotinib (Pao et al. 2005). We have introduced the T790M mutation into murine Ba/F3 cells in combination with a variety of lung cancer-derived *EGFR* mutations, including the various substitution mutations as well as various deletions, to determine the effect on sensitivity to EGFR TKIs (Fig. 1 and data not shown). Figure 1 shows the impact of the T790M mutation on EGFR TKI sensitivity of cells carrying the L858R mutation. Whereas L858R-only cells (dotted lines) were exquisitely sensitive to gefitinib (Fig. 1A) and erlotinib (Fig. 1B), cells harboring both the L858R and the T790M mutations (solid lines) were completely resistant to both inhibitors.

However, treatment with irreversible inhibitors of the EGFR kinase at concentrations that might be achievable in patients effectively killed cells carrying the T790M resistance mutation (Kobayashi et al. 2005; Kwak et al. 2005). One of these inhibitors, HKI-272, is currently in clinical trials.

ONCOGENIC TRANSFORMATION BY INHIBITOR-SENSITIZING EGFR MUTANTS WITH DIFFERENTIAL RESPONSE TO EGFR TKI

We have asked whether the EGFR mutations observed in lung tumor samples were oncogenic, capable of contributing to tumor development (Greulich et al. 2005). A representative mutation from each of the four major categories of EGFR mutations (exon 18 missense substitution, exon 19 deletion, exon 20 insertion, and exon 21 missense substitution) was recreated in the wild-type EGFR cDNA by site-directed mutagenesis and expressed in NIH-3T3 cells. Expression of these four mutants, G719S, L747_E749del A750P, D770_N771insNPG, and L858R, affected cell morphology and supported anchorage-independent growth, focus formation, and tumor formation in immunocompromised mice (Greulich et al. 2005). Anchorage-independent growth was also observed upon expression of the mutant EGFR in the more physiologically relevant human tracheobronchial epithelial cells. The mutant EGFR were shown to be constitutively active and lig-

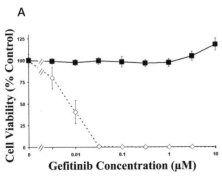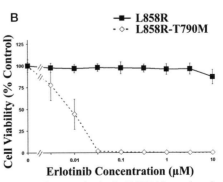

Figure 1. Resistance to EGFR tyrosine kinase inhibitors caused by a second-site mutation in the EGFR kinase domain. The sensitivity of EGFR-transformed Ba/F3 cells to EGFR inhibitors in the absence of IL-3 was assayed using the MTS assay. Percentage of cell viability, as assayed by MTS assay, is shown relative to untreated controls. Results are indicated as mean ± standard deviation. (A,B) The L858R-T790M double mutant EGFR (IC$_{50}$ >10 μM) showed very strong resistance to both gefitinib (A) and erlotinib (B), whereas the L858R mutant EGFR was highly sensitive to both TKIs (IC$_{50}$ ~10 nM).

and-independent, to associate with endogenous Shc, and to constitutively activate the Stat3 and Akt signaling pathways. We have more recently confirmed that other exon 19 deletions and exon 20 insertions, including E746_A750del, L747_S752del,E746V, S752_I759del, V769_D770insASV, and H773_V774insH also support anchorage-independent growth in the murine fibroblast model (Fig. 2 and data not shown).

The sensitivity of transformation to EGFR inhibitors was determined by treating the NIH-3T3 cells with gefitinib, erlotinib, and the irreversible inhibitor CL-387,785. Addition of exogenous EGF to cells expressing the wild-type EGFR causes these cells to become transformed. However, transformation of cells expressing the L858R mutant EGFR was more sensitive to gefitinib treatment than the EGF-stimulated wild-type EGFR-expressing cells (Greulich et al. 2005). Whereas NIH-3T3 cells expressing G719S and L747_E749del A750P behaved similarly to cells expressing L858R EGFR, cells expressing the exon 20 insertion mutant D770_N771insNPG were surprisingly relatively resistant to reversion of transformation by gefitinib and erlotinib (Fig. 3) (Greulich et al. 2005). However, the irreversible inhibitor CL-387,785 was significantly more effective against the insertion mutant than gefitinib and erlotinib, similar to the situation with the previously described T790M resistance mutation, also in exon 20 (Fig. 4) (Greulich et al. 2005).

The sensitivity of lung adenocarcinoma cell lines to gefitinib has also been extensively studied. Functional experiments showed that the H3255 adenocarcinoma cell line harboring the L858R mutation was extremely sensitive to treatment with gefitinib, with an IC_{50} of only 40 nM compared to wild-type cell lines that were growth-inhibited only at concentrations that were 100-fold higher (Paez et al. 2004). Additionally, levels of phosphorylated EGFR, ERK1/2, and Akt were strongly reduced by gefitinib treatment in H3255 cells but not in wild-type cells, implying a role for these proteins in mutant EGFR-dependent cell survival. Similar enhanced apoptosis results were reported for treatment of HCC827, a NSCLC cell line expressing mutant EGFR encoding an exon 19 deletion, with the EGFR-targeted monoclonal antibody cetuximab (Amann et al. 2005). Cos-7 cells genetically engineered to express one of the deletion mutations or the L858R mutation exhibited enhanced EGFR phosphorylation only upon addition of EGF, and this autophosphory-

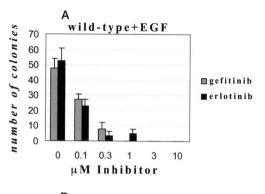

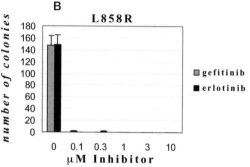

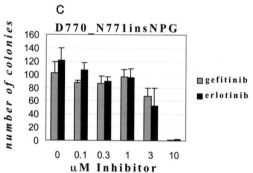

Figure 3. NIH-3T3 expressing L858R EGFR are sensitized to inhibition of transformation by gefitinib or erlotinib, whereas NIH-3T3 expressing an exon 20 insertion mutant are resistant to gefitinib or erlotinib. Panels A–C show numbers of colonies of different EGFR mutants following treatment with EGFR tyrosine kinase inhibitors gefitinib and erlotinib. Cells were treated with inhibitors and suspended in soft agar as described previously (Greulich et al. 2005). (A) EGF-stimulated cells expressing wild-type EGFR (unstimulated cells expressing the wild-type EGFR are not transformed and do not form colonies in soft agar). (B) Unstimulated cells expressing L858R EGFR. (C) Unstimulated cells expressing the exon 20 insertion mutant D770_N771insNPG.

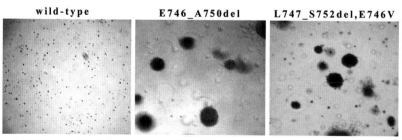

Figure 2. Expression of EGFR exon 19 deletion mutants in NIH-3T3 cells enables cells to grow in an anchorage-independent manner. Wild-type or mutant EGFR was stably expressed in NIH-3T3 cells by retrovirus-mediated gene transfer and suspended in soft agar as described previously (Greulich et al. 2005). Shown are images from soft agar colonies after 14 days of culture.

μM Inhibitor: 0   0.1   0.3   1   3   10

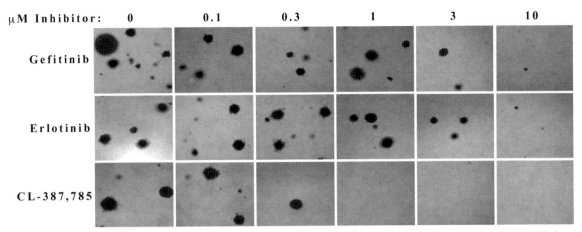

Figure 4. Transformation induced by the exon 20 insertion mutant is more sensitive to the irreversible inhibitor CL-387,785 than to gefitinib or erlotinib. Cells were treated with inhibitors and suspended in soft agar as described previously (Greulich et al. 2005). Shown are images of NIH-3T3 cells engineered to carry the exon 20 insertion mutant after 14 days of culture.

lation was 10-fold more sensitive to gefitinib than EGF-stimulated phosphorylation of the wild-type receptor (Lynch et al. 2004). In a subsequent analysis, Sordella and colleagues showed that lung-cancer-derived EGFR mutations activate the antiapoptotic Akt and STAT pathways, providing a link between these mutations and sensitivity of cell survival to EGFR inhibition (Sordella et al. 2004). This activation of the PI3K/Akt pathway appears to be mediated by ErbB3, a heterodimerization partner of EGFR in NSCLC cell lines (Engelman et al. 2005). Furthermore, by specifically silencing the mutant EGFR allele using RNA interference, Sordella and colleagues demonstrated induction of apoptosis in EGFR mutant but not wild-type cells and, thus, a dependency of NSCLC cells harboring EGFR mutations on this oncogene. It is still an unresolved issue whether the mechanism by which the mutations confer response to EGFR TKIs involves changing the biochemical properties of the kinase, or exploiting oncogene addiction, or some combination of these two mechanisms.

DETECTION OF HIDDEN EGFR MUTATIONS BY MASSIVELY PARALLEL SEQUENCING FROM CLONALLY AMPLIFIED SINGLE MOLECULES

Given the low sensitivity of Sanger sequencing in detecting mutations in clinical samples with low tumor content, other technologies that are capable of interrogating a locus of interest with greater depth are essential. We therefore used a novel ultradeep, massively parallel technology (further on referred to as "picotiter plate sequencing") to search for mutations in the EGFR kinase domain in patients with NSCLC. Picotiter sequencing involves the following steps (Margulies et al. 2005): clonal PCR amplification of single DNA molecules on beads in a water-in-oil emulsion; deposition of the beads into high-density picotiter plates together with enzymes required for pyrophosphate-dependent chemiluminescence signal generation; sequencing-by-synthesis dependent on flow-

cell addition of individual nucleotide triphosphates, with concomitant generation of pyrophosphate upon nucleotide incorporation; and detection of the resultant chemiluminescence with a charge-coupled device. Since in excess of 200,000 high-quality reads can be generated during one round of sequencing from one sequencing plate, it is possible to cover a single locus of interest to a depth that allows statistically significant low-level mutation detection. Moreover, given the fact that each sequencing read represents a single template, analyzing complex mutations such as heterozygous deletions could easily be performed.

PCR products were generated covering the EGFR kinase domain from 22 patients with known mutational status. The mutations in this sample set comprised the substitution mutations G719S ($n = 1$) and L858R ($n = 2$), a 15-bp deletion (E746_A750del, $n = 5$), and a 24-bp deletion mutation (S752_I759del, $n = 1$). Traces were generated using 454 sequencing, and sequence variants were scored as real when they appeared in sequencing reads from both directions, when they were present in overlapping amplicons, and when they did not appear in the matched normal. All mutations that we had previously detected by Sanger sequencing could reliably be called by 454 sequencing. In addition to the known mutations, we were also able to detect three mutations that had not been detected by Sanger sequencing. All three mutations appeared at a relative allele frequency of less than 15%. One mutation was an E709A mutation in a sample with a known G719S mutation. Interestingly, this mutation was located on the same allele as the G719S. The other mutations were a 15-bp deletion and a trinucleotide insertion mutation. Analysis of the original Sanger traces revealed a low-level peak in the case of E709A that had been missed by the analysis software in combination with manual scoring and peaks that appeared as noise at the site of the deleted or inserted nucleotides in the case of the 15-bp deletion or the insertion, respectively.

These results encouraged us to search for EGFR kinase domain mutations in clinical specimens with low tumor content that had been extracted from the pleural effusion of patients with relapse to EGFR TKI. Since many cancer patients present with pleural effusion at time of relapse, and since drainage of the fluid often becomes necessary to assist the patients' vital functions, such material is frequently available without the possibility of sophisticated molecular analysis. The first patient that we tested, a 47-year-old male Caucasian, never-smoker, was originally diagnosed with lung adenocarcinoma in December 2003. He initially responded strongly to erlotinib with more than 50% of his original tumor burden disappearing. This response lasted for 12 months. In April 2005, the patient presented with massive pleural effusion. Drainage of the fluid and pathological examination of the cells in the fluid revealed relapse of lung adenocarcinoma. DNA was extracted from this specimen. A pathology report on this specimen confirmed the rare presence of scattered tumor cells. Using picotiter plate sequencing on this sample, we detected an 18-bp deletion mutation (L747-752del_P753S) in exon 19 at a frequency of approximately 3%. We had originally detected this mutation in a patient responding to gefitinib (Paez et al. 2004), suggesting that this mutation had rendered the patient's tumor cells sensitive to EGFR TKI treatment. Furthermore, picotiter plate sequencing revealed a T790M mutation in exon 20 occurring at a frequency of 2% (Fig. 5). This mutation has been found in tumors explanted from patients experiencing relapse to EGFR TKI (Kobayashi et al. 2005; Pao et al. 2005) suggesting that in the patient studied here, too, this mutation had led to resistance to treatment and to the occurrence of relapse. Importantly, attempts to detect the two mutations by conventional Sanger sequencing failed.

It has now been shown, both from in vitro experiments and from analysis of clinical samples, that the various exon 19 deletion mutations predict response to EGFR TKI whereas the emergence of the T790M mutation leads to acquired resistance to these drugs. Thus, using picotiter plate sequencing, we were able to recapitulate, on a molecular level, the clinical course of a patient who initially responded to EGFR TKI and then relapsed. More importantly, this monitoring was performed on clinical samples with a very low tumor percentage and, in the case of the pre-therapy sample, on a paraffin-embedded sample with extremely low tumor content. These results show that cancer gene mutation detection for both clinical and research purposes may now be feasible without the need for sample purification. Thus, picotiter plate sequencing could significantly help to guide patient selection for tailored treatment on a molecular basis in the near future.

CONCLUSIONS

The discovery of mutations in the EGFR gene in lung adenocarcinoma is a significant advance in this disease. These mutations are oncogenic and are associated with differential clinical response to EGFR TKI. Whereas most of the kinase domain mutations, including exon 19 deletion mutations and the L858R mutation, are associated with responsiveness to EGFR TKIs in vitro and in vivo, one insertion mutation in exon 20 was found to render genetically engineered cells resistant to EGFR TKIs. Another mutation, T790M, was found to emerge during therapy with EGFR TKIs and to lead to resistance. Importantly, irreversible inhibitors of the EGFR kinase were able to overcome resistance by T790M and the insertion mutant. By making use of a novel, extremely sensitive high-throughput sequencing technology, we were able to detect clinically meaningful EGFR kinase domain mutation in samples with very low tumor content. These latter results demonstrate that clinical sequencing is feasible in low-tumor-content samples without the need for sample purification. Thus, the clinical course of lung cancer patients treated with TKIs may now be predicted and monitored using picotiter plate sequencing.

Taken together, our findings have an impact on the understanding of the molecular biology of lung cancer as well as on clinical decision-making. The fact that lung tumors carrying particular EGFR mutations are exquisitely sensitive to EGFR inhibitory strategies (EGFR TKIs and RNAi) suggests that this subset of tumors represents a biologically distinct subentity where mutant EGFR is the

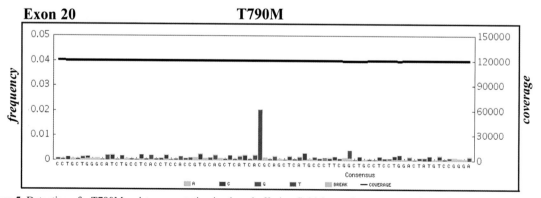

Figure 5. Detection of a T790M resistance mutation in pleural effusion fluid from a lung cancer patient who relapsed after a 1-year response to erlotinib. Shown is a variation plot analysis of a picotiter plate sequencing run of EGFR exon 20 amplified from DNA extracted at the time of relapse from a pleural effusion specimen with low tumor content. Nucleotide reads deviating from the reference signal appear as bars with the height indicating the relative frequency of the variant alleles (left Y-axis). The black bar indicates the coverage at the position of each nucleotide (right Y-axis).

driving oncogene. Apparently, these mutations occur in a specific context (women, non-smokers, adenocarcinomas, etc.), indicating that differential exposure to carcinogens might act in concert with a particular genetic context inherent to certain ethnicities. This observation emphasizes the need to broaden ongoing cancer-genome resequencing efforts to take into account patient ethnicity. Furthermore, EGFR and KRAS mutations were found to occur in a mutually exclusive fashion in lung cancer, suggesting that the net effect on activation of central downstream signaling elements might be equivalent. This might be of importance when considering gene families for resequencing efforts since genetic lesions (e.g., gene mutations, copy number changes) might be present in other, yet unidentified members of the EGFR/KRAS signaling pathway. Clinically, our results suggest that patient selection based on the presence of EGFR mutations might help to increase response rates and overall survival in a subgroup of NSCLC patients. A clinical trial is currently under way at the DFCI/Harvard Cancer Center that aims at prospectively assessing the predictive value of EGFR mutations for response and overall survival in patients with NSCLC treated with EGFR TKIs. Additionally, patients might be monitored on a molecular level to detect the occurrence of resistance mutations at an early time point. The development of a massively parallel sequencing technology, picotiter plate sequencing, that allows in-depth analysis of clinical specimens with low tumor content might help to guide cancer patient selection based on the presence or absence of certain mutations. We anticipate that this technology will permit clinical sequencing not only of lung cancer patients, but also of patients with other tumors that are known to harbor mutations associated with clinical response. We envision that treating a cancer patient based on the genetic makeup of his tumor and switching his treatment to other (e.g., irreversible) inhibitors upon the occurrence of resistance mutations detected early by ultradeep sequencing will become a clinical reality soon.

However, despite these encouraging findings, the overall response rates to these inhibitors are generally low. Thus, other targeted strategies are needed to improve outcome of NSCLC patients. We believe that among the most promising strategies to achieving this goal are genomic approaches such as SNP array-based genome-wide analyses of copy number changes as well as endeavors aiming at resequencing entire cancer genomes in the most common cancer subtypes, including NSCLC. These efforts may lead to identification of more "druggable" mutations in lung cancer. Finally, one even more inspiring conclusion from these findings might be that the discovery of EGFR mutations causing clinical responses to EGFR TKIs, second-site mutations such as T790M causing relapse, and, finally, irreversible kinase inhibitors overcoming resistance are an impressive example of how high-throughput genomic technologies can be successfully applied in collaborative projects involving clinicians, genome biologists, and basic scientists, finally leading to improvement in lung cancer patient care.

ACKNOWLEDGMENTS

Roman Thomas holds a Dr. Mildred Scheel Fellowship for Cancer Research from the Deutsche Krebshilfe. Our own work cited in this paper was supported by the Claudia-Adams Barr Foundation and the Novartis Foundation.

REFERENCES

Amann J., Kalyankrishna S., Massion P.P., Ohm J.E., Girard L., Shigematsu H., Peyton M., Juroske D., Huang Y., Stuart Salmon J., Kim Y.H., Pollack J.R., Yanagisawa K., Gazdar A., Minna J.D., Kurie J.M., and Carbone D.P. 2005. Aberrant epidermal growth factor receptor signaling and enhanced sensitivity to EGFR inhibitors in lung cancer. *Cancer Res.* **65:** 226.

Blencke S., Ullrich A., and Daub H. 2003. Mutation of threonine 766 in the epidermal growth factor receptor reveals a hotspot for resistance formation against selective tyrosine kinase inhibitors. *J. Biol. Chem.* **278:** 15435.

Brambilla E., Travis W.D., Colby T.V., Corrin B., and Shimosato Y. 2001. The new World Health Organization classification of lung tumours. *Eur. Respir. J.* **18:** 1059.

Brose M.S., Volpe P., Feldman M., Kumar M., Rishi I., Gerrero R., Einhorn E., Herlyn M., Minna J., Nicholson A., Roth J.A., Albelda S.M., Davies H., Cox C., Brignell G., Stephens P., Futreal P.A., Wooster R., Stratton M.R., and Weber B.L. 2002. BRAF and RAS mutations in human lung cancer and melanoma. *Cancer Res.* **62:** 6997.

Cappuzzo F., Hirsch F.R., Rossi E., Bartolini S., Ceresoli G.L., Bemis L., Haney J., Witta S., Danenberg K., Domenichini I., Ludovini V., Magrini E., Gregorc V., Doglioni C., Sidoni A., Tonato M., Franklin W.A., Crino L., Bunn P.A., Jr., and Varella-Garcia M. 2005. Epidermal growth factor receptor gene and protein and gefitinib sensitivity in non-small-cell lung cancer. *J. Natl. Cancer Inst.* **97:** 643.

Cools J., DeAngelo D.J., Gotlib J., Stover E.H., Legare R.D., Cortes J., Kutok J., Clark J., Galinsky I., Griffin J.D., Cross N.C., Tefferi A., Malone J., Alam R., Schrier S.L., Schmid J., Rose M., Vandenberghe P., Verhoef G., Boogaerts M., Wlodarska I., Kantarjian H., Marynen P., Coutre S.E., Stone R., and Gilliland D.G. 2003. A tyrosine kinase created by fusion of the PDGFRA and FIP1L1 genes as a therapeutic target of imatinib in idiopathic hypereosinophilic syndrome. *N. Engl. J. Med.* **348:** 1201.

Davies H., Bignell G.R., Cox C., Stephens P., Edkins S., Clegg S., Teague J., Woffendin H., Garnett M.J., Bottomley W., Davis N., Dicks E., Ewing R., Floyd Y., Gray K., Hall S., Hawes R., Hughes J., Kosmidou V., Menzies A., Mould C., Parker A., Stevens C., Watt S., and Hooper S., et al. 2002. Mutations of the BRAF gene in human cancer. *Nature* **417:** 949.

Demetri G.D., von Mehren M., Blanke C.D., Van den Abbeele A.D., Eisenberg B., Roberts P.J., Heinrich M.C., Tuveson D.A., Singer S., Janicek M., Fletcher J.A., Silverman S.G., Silberman S.L., Capdeville R., Kiese B., Peng B., Dimitrijevic S., Druker B.J., Corless C., Fletcher C.D., and Joensuu H. 2002. Efficacy and safety of imatinib mesylate in advanced gastrointestinal stromal tumors. *N. Engl. J. Med.* **347:** 472.

Druker B.J., Sawyers C.L., Kantarjian H., Resta D.J., Reese S.F., Ford J.M., Capdeville R., and Talpaz M. 2001a. Activity of a specific inhibitor of the BCR-ABL tyrosine kinase in the blast crisis of chronic myeloid leukemia and acute lymphoblastic leukemia with the Philadelphia chromosome. *N. Engl. J. Med.* **344:** 1038.

Druker B.J., Tamura S., Buchdunger E., Ohno S., Segal G.M., Fanning S., Zimmermann J., and Lydon N.B. 1996. Effects of a selective inhibitor of the Abl tyrosine kinase on the growth of Bcr-Abl positive cells. *Nat. Med.* **2:** 561.

Druker B.J., Talpaz M., Resta D.J., Peng B., Buchdunger E., Ford J.M., Lydon N.B., Kantarjian H., Capdeville R., Ohno-Jones S., and Sawyers C.L. 2001b. Efficacy and safety of a specific inhibitor of the BCR-ABL tyrosine kinase in chronic myeloid leukemia. *N. Engl. J. Med.* **344:** 1031.

Engelman J.A., Janne P.A., Mermel C., Pearlberg J., Mukohara T., Fleet C., Cichowski K., Johnson B.E., and Cantley L.C. 2005. ErbB-3 mediates phosphoinositide 3-kinase activity in gefitinib-sensitive non-small cell lung cancer cell lines. *Proc. Natl. Acad. Sci.* **102:** 3788.

Fiedler W., Serve H., Dohner H., Schwittay M., Ottmann O.G., O'Farrell A.M., Bello C.L., Allred R., Manning W.C., Cherrington J.M., Louie S.G., Hong W., Brega N.M., Massimini G., Scigalla P., Berdel W.E., and Hossfeld D.K. 2005. A phase 1 study of SU11248 in the treatment of patients with refractory or resistant acute myeloid leukemia (AML) or not amenable to conventional therapy for the disease. *Blood* **105:** 986.

Fukuoka M., Yano S., Giaccone G., Tamura T., Nakagawa K., Douillard J.Y., Nishiwaki Y., Vansteenkiste J., Kudoh S., Rischin D., Eek R., Horai T., Noda K., Takata I., Smit E., Averbuch S., Macleod A., Feyereislova A., Dong R.P., and Baselga J. 2003. Multi-institutional randomized phase II trial of gefitinib for previously treated patients with advanced non-small-cell lung cancer. *J. Clin. Oncol.* **21:** 2237.

Gorre M.E., Mohammed M., Ellwood K., Hsu N., Paquette R., Rao P.N., and Sawyers C.L. 2001. Clinical resistance to STI-571 cancer therapy caused by BCR-ABL gene mutation or amplification. *Science* **293:** 876.

Greulich H., Chen T.-H., Feng W., Jänne P.A., Alvarez J.V., Zappaterra M., Frank D.A., Hahn W.C., Sellers W.R., and Meyerson M. 2005. Oncogenic transformation by inhibitor-sensitive and -resistant EGFR mutants. *PLoS Med.* **2:** e313.

Grunwald V. and Hidalgo M. 2003. Development of the epidermal growth factor receptor inhibitor OSI-774. *Semin. Oncol.* **30:** 23.

Han S.W., Kim T.Y., Hwang P.G., Jeong S., Kim J., Choi I.S., Oh D.Y., Kim J.H., Kim D.W., Chung D.H., Im S.A., Kim Y.T., Lee J.S., Heo D.S., Bang Y.J., and Kim N.K. 2005. Predictive and prognostic impact of epidermal growth factor receptor mutation in non-small-cell lung cancer patients treated with gefitinib. *J. Clin. Oncol.* **23:** 2493.

Heinrich M.C., Corless C.L., Duensing A., McGreevey L., Chen C.J., Joseph N., Singer S., Griffith D.J., Haley A., Town A., Demetri G.D., Fletcher C.D., and Fletcher J.A. 2003. PDGFRA activating mutations in gastrointestinal stromal tumors. *Science* **299:** 708.

Hirota S., Ohashi A., Nishida T., Isozaki K., Kinoshita K., Shinomura Y., and Kitamura Y. 2003. Gain-of-function mutations of platelet-derived growth factor receptor alpha gene in gastrointestinal stromal tumors. *Gastroenterology* **125:** 660.

Hirota S., Isozaki K., Moriyama Y., Hashimoto K., Nishida T., Ishiguro S., Kawano K., Hanada M., Kurata A., Takeda M., Muhammad Tunio G., Matsuzawa Y., Kanakura Y., Shinomura Y., and Kitamura Y. 1998. Gain-of-function mutations of c-kit in human gastrointestinal stromal tumors. *Science* **279:** 577.

Hirsch F.R., Varella-Garcia M., Bunn P.A., Jr., Di Maria M.V., Veve R., Bremmes R.M., Baron A.E., Zeng C., and Franklin W.A. 2003. Epidermal growth factor receptor in non-small-cell lung carcinomas: Correlation between gene copy number and protein expression and impact on prognosis. *J. Clin. Oncol.* **21:** 3798.

Huang S.F., Liu H.P., Li L.H., Ku Y.C., Fu Y.N., Tsai H.Y., Chen Y.T., Lin Y.F., Chang W.C., Kuo H.P., Wu Y.C., Chen Y.R., and Tsai S.F. 2004. High frequency of epidermal growth factor receptor mutations with complex patterns in non-small cell lung cancers related to gefitinib responsiveness in Taiwan. *Clin. Cancer Res.* **10:** 8195.

Jänne P.A., Engelman J.A., and Johnson B.E. 2005. Epidermal growth factor receptor mutations in non-small-cell lung cancer: Implications for treatment and tumor biology. *J. Clin. Oncol.* **23:** 3227.

Jemal A., Murray T., Ward E., Samuels A., Tiwari R.C., Ghafoor A., Feuer E.J., and Thun M.J. 2005. Cancer statistics, 2005. *CA Cancer J. Clin.* **55:** 10.

Kang S., Bader A.G., and Vogt P.K. 2005. Phosphatidylinositol 3-kinase mutations identified in human cancer are oncogenic.

Proc. Natl. Acad. Sci. **102:** 802.

Kobayashi S., Boggon T.J., Dayaram T., Janne P.A., Kocher O., Meyerson M., Johnson B.E., Eck M.J., Tenen D.G., and Halmos B. 2005. EGFR mutation and resistance of non-small-cell lung cancer to gefitinib. *N. Engl. J. Med.* **352:** 786.

Kosaka T., Yatabe Y., Endoh H., Kuwano H., Takahashi T., and Mitsudomi T. 2004. Mutations of the epidermal growth factor receptor gene in lung cancer: Biological and clinical implications. *Cancer Res.* **64:** 8919.

Kris M.G., Natale R.B., Herbst R.S., Lynch T.J., Jr., Prager D., Belani C.P., Schiller J.H., Kelly K., Spiridonidis H., Sandler A., Albain K.S., Cella D., Wolf M.K., Averbuch S.D., Ochs J.J., and Kay A.C. 2003. Efficacy of gefitinib, an inhibitor of the epidermal growth factor receptor tyrosine kinase, in symptomatic patients with non-small cell lung cancer: A randomized trial. *J. Am. Med. Assoc.* **290:** 2149.

Kwak E.L., Sordella R., Bell D.W., Godin-Heymann N., Okimoto R.A., Brannigan B.W., Harris P.L., Driscoll D.R., Fidias P., Lynch T.J., Rabindran S.K., McGinnis J.P., Wissner A., Sharma S.V., Isselbacher K.J., Settleman J., and Haber D.A. 2005. Irreversible inhibitors of the EGF receptor may circumvent acquired resistance to gefitinib. *Proc. Natl. Acad. Sci.* **102:** 7665.

Lander E.S., Linton L.M., Birren B., Nusbaum C., Zody M.C., Baldwin J., Devon K., Dewar K., Doyle M., FitzHugh W., Funke R., Gage D., Harris K., Heaford A., Howland J., Kann L., Lehoczky J., LeVine R., McEwan P., McKernan K., Meldrim J., Mesirov J.P., Miranda C., Morris W., and Naylor J., et al. (International Human Genome Sequencing Consortium). 2001. Initial sequencing and analysis of the human genome. *Nature* **409:** 860.

Lynch T.J., Bell D.W., Sordella R., Gurubhagavatula S., Okimoto R.A., Brannigan B.W., Harris P.L., Haserlat S.M., Supko J.G., Haluska F.G., Louis D.N., Christiani D.C., Settleman J., and Haber D.A. 2004. Activating mutations in the epidermal growth factor receptor underlying responsiveness of non-small-cell lung cancer to gefitinib. *N. Engl. J. Med.* **350:** 2129.

Marchetti A., Martella C., Felicioni L., Barassi F., Salvatore S., Chella A., Camplese P.P., Iarussi T., Mucilli F., Mezzetti A., Cuccurullo F., Sacco R., and Buttitta F. 2005. EGFR mutations in non-small-cell lung cancer: Analysis of a large series of cases and development of a rapid and sensitive method for diagnostic screening with potential implications on pharmacologic treatment. *J. Clin. Oncol.* **23:** 857.

Margulies M., Egholm, M., Altman W.E., Attiya S., Bader J.S., Bemben L.A., Berka J., Braverman M.S., Chen Y.J., Chen Z., Dewell S.B., Du L., Fierro J.M., Gomes X.V., Godwin B.C., He W., Helgesen S., Ho C.H., Irzyk G.P., Jando S.C., Alenquer M.L., Jarvie T.P., Jirage K.B., Kim J.B., and Knight J.R., et al. 2005. Genome sequencing in microfabricated high-density picolitre reactors. *Nature* **437:** 376.

Miller V.A., Kris M.G., Shah N., Patel J., Azzoli C., Gomez J., Krug L.M., Pao W., Rizvi N., Pizzo B., Tyson L., Venkatraman E., Ben-Porat L., Memoli N., Zakowski M., Rusch V., and Heelan R.T. 2004. Bronchioloalveolar pathologic subtype and smoking history predict sensitivity to gefitinib in advanced non-small-cell lung cancer. *J. Clin. Oncol.* **22:** 1103.

Mitsudomi T., Kosaka T., Endoh H., Horio Y., Hida T., Mori S., Hatooka S., Shinoda M., Takahashi T., and Yatabe Y. 2005. Mutations of the epidermal growth factor receptor gene predict prolonged survival after gefitinib treatment in patients with non-small-cell lung cancer with postoperative recurrence. *J. Clin. Oncol.* **23:** 2513.

Naoki K., Chen T.H., Richards W.G., Sugarbaker D.J., and Meyerson M. 2002. Missense mutations of the BRAF gene in human lung adenocarcinoma. *Cancer Res.* **62:** 7001.

Paez J.G., Janne P.A., Lee J.C., Tracy S., Greulich H., Gabriel S., Herman P., Kaye F.J., Lindeman N., Boggon T.J., Naoki K., Sasaki H., Fujii Y., Eck M.J., Sellers W.R., Johnson B.E., and Meyerson M. 2004. EGFR mutations in lung cancer: Correlation with clinical response to gefitinib therapy. *Science* **304:** 1497.

Pao W., Miller V.A., Politi K.A., Riely G.J., Somwar R., Zakowski M.F., Kris M.G., and Varmus H. 2005. Acquired resistance of lung adenocarcinomas to gefitinib or erlotinib is associated with a second mutation in the EGFR kinase domain. *PLoS Med.* **2:** e73.

Pao W., Miller V., Zakowski M., Doherty J., Politi K., Sarkaria I., Singh B., Heelan R., Rusch V., Fulton L., Mardis E., Kupfer D., Wilson R., Kris M., and Varmus H. 2004. EGF receptor gene mutations are common in lung cancers from "never smokers" and are associated with sensitivity of tumors to gefitinib and erlotinib. *Proc. Natl. Acad. Sci.* **101:** 13306.

Perez-Soler R., Chachoua A., Hammond L.A., Rowinsky E.K., Huberman M., Karp D., Rigas J., Clark G.M., Santabarbara P., and Bonomi P. 2004. Determinants of tumor response and survival with erlotinib in patients with non-small-cell lung cancer. *J. Clin. Oncol.* **22:** 3238.

Risch N.J. 2000. Searching for genetic determinants in the new millennium. *Nature* **405:** 847.

Rusch V., Baselga J., Cordon-Cardo C., Orazem J., Zaman M., Hoda S., McIntosh J., Kurie J., and Dmitrovsky E. 1993. Differential expression of the epidermal growth factor receptor and its ligands in primary non-small cell lung cancers and adjacent benign lung. *Cancer Res.* **53:** 2379.

Samuels Y., Wang Z., Bardelli A., Silliman N., Ptak J., Szabo S., Yan H., Gazdar A., Powell S.M., Riggins G.J., Willson J.K., Markowitz S., Kinzler K.W., Vogelstein B., and Velculescu V.E. 2004. High frequency of mutations of the PIK3CA gene in human cancers. *Science* **304:** 554.

Shah N.P., Nicoll J.M., Nagar B., Gorre M.E., Paquette R.L., Kuriyan J., and Sawyers C.L. 2002. Multiple BCR-ABL kinase domain mutations confer polyclonal resistance to the tyrosine kinase inhibitor imatinib (STI571) in chronic phase and blast crisis chronic myeloid leukemia. *Cancer Cell* **2:** 117.

Shigematsu H., Lin L., Takahashi T., Nomura M., Suzuki M., Wistuba, II, Fong K.M., Lee H., Toyooka S., Shimizu N., Fujisawa T., Feng Z., Roth J.A., Herz J., Minna J.D., and Gazdar A.F. 2005. Clinical and biological features associated with epidermal growth factor receptor gene mutations in lung cancers. *J. Natl. Cancer Inst.* **97:** 339.

Sordella R., Bell D.W., Haber D.A., and Settleman J. 2004. Gefitinib-sensitizing EGFR mutations in lung cancer activate anti-apoptotic pathways. *Science* **305:** 1163.

Soulieres D., Senzer N.N., Vokes E.E., Hidalgo M., Agarwala S.S., and Siu L.L. 2004. Multicenter phase II study of erlotinib, an oral epidermal growth factor receptor tyrosine kinase inhibitor, in patients with recurrent or metastatic squamous cell cancer of the head and neck. *J. Clin. Oncol.* **22:** 77.

Stamos J., Sliwkowski M.X., and Eigenbrot C. 2002. Structure of the epidermal growth factor receptor kinase domain alone and in complex with a 4-anilinoquinazoline inhibitor. *J. Biol. Chem.* **277:** 46265.

Stone R.M., DeAngelo D.J., Klimek V., Galinsky I., Estey E., Nimer S.D., Grandin W., Lebwohl D., Wang Y., Cohen P., Fox E.A., Neuberg D., Clark J., Gilliland D.G., and Griffin J.D. 2005. Patients with acute myeloid leukemia and an activating mutation in FLT3 respond to a small-molecule FLT3 tyrosine kinase inhibitor, PKC412. *Blood* **105:** 54.

Tokumo M., Toyooka S., Kiura K., Shigematsu H., Tomii K., Aoe M., Ichimura K., Tsuda T., Yano M., Tsukuda K., Tabata M., Ueoka H., Tanimoto M., Date H., Gazdar A.F., and Shimizu N. 2005. The relationship between epidermal growth factor receptor mutations and clinicopathologic features in non-small cell lung cancers. *Clin. Cancer Res.* **11:** 1167.

Tracy S., Mukohara T., Hansen M., Meyerson M., Johnson B.E., and Janne P.A. 2004. Gefitinib induces apoptosis in the EGFRL858R non-small-cell lung cancer cell line H3255. *Cancer Res.* **64:** 7241.

Tuveson D.A., Weber B.L., and Herlyn M. 2003. BRAF as a potential therapeutic target in melanoma and other malignancies. *Cancer Cell* **4:** 95.

Venter J.C., Adams M.D., Myers E.W., Li P.W., Mural R.J., Sutton G.G., Smith H.O., Yandell M., Evans C.A., Holt R.A., Gocayne J.D., Amanatides P., Ballew R.M., Huson D.H., Wortman J.R., Zhang Q., Kodira C.D., Zheng X.H., Chen L., Skupski M., Subramanian G., Thomas P.D., Zhang J., Gabor Miklos G.L., and Nelson C., et al. 2001. The sequence of the human genome. *Science* **291:** 1304.

Wakeling A.E., Guy S.P., Woodburn J.R., Ashton S.E., Curry B.J., Barker A.J., and Gibson K.H. 2002. ZD1839 (Iressa): An orally active inhibitor of epidermal growth factor signaling with potential for cancer therapy. *Cancer Res.* **62:** 5749.

Two Decades of Cancer Genetics: From Specificity to Pleiotropic Networks

S. Grisendi and P.P. Pandolfi

Cancer Biology & Genetics Program, Department of Pathology, Sloan-Kettering Institute,
Memorial Sloan-Kettering Cancer Center, New York, New York 10021

Modeling cancer in mice has reached an even greater relevance in the field of hematological malignances, due to the already advanced characterization of the molecular basis of many hematological disorders. These mouse models have often allowed us to achieve insight into the pathogenesis of the human disease as well as to test novel therapeutic modalities in preclinical studies. However, one of the most rewarding cultural shifts triggered by these modeling efforts stems from what was originally perceived as background noise or modeling inaccuracy. Manipulation of the involved genes often triggered cancer susceptibility in cell types other than the hematopoietic lineages. This prompted us to challenge a fundamental misconception in cancer genetics that the approximately 200 genes directly involved in chromosomal translocations associated with hematopoietic malignancies are specifically and functionally restricted to leukemia/lymphoma pathogenesis only. The genetics underlying the pathogenesis of leukemia and lymphoma have historically been regarded as distinct from those underlying the pathogenesis of solid tumors because hematopoietic malignancies are often associated with characteristic chromosomal translocations that are leukemia- or lymphoma-specific. In this paper, we discuss how leukemia/lymphoma genes indeed participate in fundamental proto-oncogenic and growth-suppressive networks and may play a wider role in cancer pathogenesis. We focus on paradigmatic examples such as c-myc and PML, as well as on more recent findings from our laboratory concerning the role of NPM in tumorigenesis.

In this review paper, we discuss how recent findings in our laboratory have allowed us to challenge a self-inflicted dogma in cancer genetics whereby the genes involved in the pathogenesis of hematopoietic malignances would be "specific" to these disorders. Although this belief is clearly wrong, as is probably obvious to the majority of the people reading this paper, it still surprisingly permeates the imagination of a vast number of people involved in cancer research and, importantly, in the clinical practice of cancer management and therapy. This misconception has in turn led to a dangerous conceptual drift and important implications both investigational and practical. First of all, very few laboratories are actively studying the possible direct involvement of leukemia/lymphoma genes in the pathogenesis of non-hematopoietic cancers; second, on the basis of this tenet, the motivation of pharmaceutical companies to embark on drug discovery efforts for "leukemia/lymphoma genes" is often low, as many hematopoietic malignances are extremely rare, therefore not constituting a sufficient justification for a business enterprise.

As mentioned above, the "dogma" is self-inflicted, and it is in fact the outcome of 20 years, or more, of dramatic progress in elucidating the molecular genetics underlying hematopoietic malignances. This has led to a novel molecular reclassification of these malignances on the basis of distinctive genetic lesions (often chromosomal translocations either leading to the generation of fusion genes as frequently observed in myelogenous leukemia, or to the deregulated expression of proto-oncogenes as is many times the case in lymphomas) (Fig. 1). Although these advances have certainly had a tremendous impact on our ability to better diagnose these diseases and to tailor therapeutic intervention modalities, the enthusiasm that ensued led to the misleading notion that the genes involved in these translocations are "specifically" involved in the pathogenesis of hematopoietic malignances, even though their expression pattern is often very broad and dynamic. The notion of specificity has been further exacerbated by two facts: (1) Chromosomal translocations are thought to be extremely rare in non-hematopoietic tumors with few notable exceptions, e.g., Ewing's sarcoma (possibly another key misconception, as a very recent study describing the identification of recurrent chromosomal translocations in a very high percentage of prostate cancers strongly suggests [Tomlins et al. 2005]); (2) hematopoietic-associated chromosomal translocations are specifically associated with distinct subtypes of leukemia and lymphoma (e.g., chromosomal translocations involving the *RARα* gene specifically associated with acute promyelocytic leukemia [APL], as we discuss in this review). However, the caveat is, as it clearly turns out when analyzing the published literature, that in very few instances these genes have been thoroughly analyzed in non-hematopoietic neoplasms, and a systematic analysis has never been undertaken, despite numerous high-throughput searches for cancer genes involved in solid tumor pathogenesis.

In our laboratory, we have decided to undertake a systematic study to learn whether leukemia/lymphoma genes are indeed implicated in solid tumor pathogenesis. This "inside out" cultural shift is proving extremely rewarding and has already led to unexpected and exciting outcomes that we discuss here.

BREAKING THE DOGMA AT THE ONSET: c-*myc* AS A GENERAL PROTO-ONCOGENE

A compelling example of the broad function of genes first identified as associated with hematological malignan-

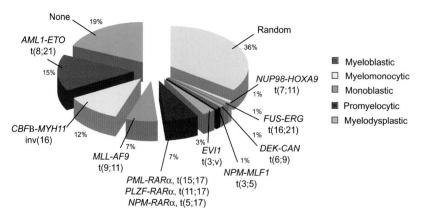

Figure 1. Aberrant transcription in AML. Mostly recurrent chromosomal translocations associated with acute myeloid leukemia (AML) and their relative distribution (adapted from T. Look). Such structural abnormalities represent cytological and molecular markers for the diagnosis and prognosis of the disease. In many cases, the genetic basis of the disease has been firmly established, and many translocations and mutations are recognized as critical in the leukemia pathogenesis. In the majority of cases, genetic alterations in AML affect transcription factors that have an important role in normal hematopoiesis, as in the case of the retinoic acid receptor gene (*RARα*), which translocates to several different partner genes (*PML, PLZF, NPM1,* etc.) in acute promyelocytic leukemia (APL).

cies is represented by the proto-oncogene c-*myc*. This powerful oncogene was one of the first proto-oncogenes to be identified as a mammalian homolog of the viral transforming oncogene, v-*myc*, responsible for avian myelocytomatosis, and soon recognized as a crucial causative agent in the pathogenesis of human lymphoma, where it is activated through chromosomal translocations (Dalla-Favera et al. 1982; Vennstrom et al. 1982). Virtually every case of Burkitt's lymphoma (BL) involves the juxtaposition of c-*myc*, located on chromosome 8, with regulatory elements of the immunoglobulin μ heavy chain or λ and κ light chains located on chromosome 14, 22, or 2, respectively (for review, see Spencer and Groudine 1991). Although the positions of the chromosomal breakpoints relative to the c-*myc* gene may vary considerably in individual cases of BL, the consequence of the translocations is invariably the same—deregulation of c-*myc* expression—leading to uncontrolled cellular proliferation.

c-*myc* was also one of the earliest oncogenes demonstrated to induce tumorigenesis in animal models: In one of the first and most popular transgenic models developed 20 years ago, it was shown in fact that transgenic c-*myc* under control of the immunoglobulin heavy-chain Eμ enhancer predictably caused malignant B-cell tumors in mice (Adams et al. 1985). The Eμ-*myc* model had a large impact on the field of B-cell neoplasms and lymphomagenesis. This mouse model gave rise to countless studies concerning myc-dependent apoptosis, cooperative tumorigenesis allowing the identification of oncogenes and tumor suppressor genes that collaborate with c-*myc* in neoplastic development, the identification of cellular pathways that determine the susceptibility or resistance of myc-driven tumors to chemotherapeutic agents, and many other aspects of myc biology.

Over the last two decades, the understanding of the function of c-myc in normal cells and in cancer cells has significantly progressed. It is now clear that uncoupling of myc expression from cell cycle and cellular environmental controls is crucial for myc-mediated cellular transformation and subsequent tumorigenesis. Even more

significantly, it is now clear that c-*myc* oncogenic activation occurs through different mechanisms and, importantly, that c-myc plays a direct role not only in a variety of hematological tumors but also in a large fraction of solid cancers (for review, see Oster et al. 2002). Numerous studies have established that the c-*myc* gene is in fact constitutively expressed or mutated in approximately 30% of human cancers (breast, prostate, colon, small-cell lung cancer, and melanoma; for review, see Nesbit et al. 1999). Whereas constitutive or deregulated expression of c-*myc* (which may be affected in *cis* by signaling pathways that converge at the myc promoter, or in *trans* by genomic rearrangements that juxtapose the gene to ectopic enhancers or gene amplification) results in elevated myc expression levels, mutations in the protein encoding region may diminish myc degradation in the ubiquitin-proteasome pathway and therefore leads to stabilization and up-regulation of the oncoprotein.

All these observations have been accompanied by compelling evidence that c-myc plays a role in the pathogenesis of cancer at large from the use of mouse models. A multitude of transgenic models have been generated demonstrating that myc overexpression can induce tumorigenesis in most tissues (for review, see Morgenbesser and DePinho 1994). Importantly, recently generated conditional transgenic models have been used to demonstrate that even a brief inactivation of myc can reverse tumorigenesis (for review, see Arvanitis and Felsher 2005). Thus, the universal deregulation of c-myc expression in cancer makes it an attractive target for therapeutic intervention, and its important role in tumor maintenance suggests that its functional inactivation may constitute an effective treatment for many types of cancer.

LEUKEMIA GENE SPECIFICITY: THE DOGMA STILL PERSISTS

In the years following the cloning of the Burkitt's lymphoma-associated chromosomal translocation and the identification of c-myc, the idea that the molecular genetics of leukemia and lymphoma could be somewhat distinct from that of other tumors carved its way in the perception of many, and for compelling reasons. First of all, as mentioned above, leukemias and lymphomas are associated with specific chromosomal translocations that mediate activation of proto-oncogenes by their juxtaposition with promoter sequences (e.g., c-myc) or generate fusion of genes, whereas chromosomal translocations are rarely observed in solid tumors. Second, as both oncogene products and fusion proteins are often transcription factors or chimeric transcription factors, deregulated transcriptional control was thought to be the crucial and etiologically relevant force underlying hematopoietic malignancies, as opposed to solid tumors where aberrant signaling would be the most common underlying mechanism (once again an obvious misconception, as the examples of the Rb and p53 tumor suppressors clearly demonstrate). Third, the dramatic acceleration that our understanding of the molecular genetics of leukemia and lymphoma experienced in the 1990s (more than 200 genes have been directly implicated to date) has further corroborated the notion of the genetic uniqueness of hematopoietic malignancies. Although it is tremendously useful and conceptually rewarding to be able to diagnose one AML or lymphoma subtype almost in real time by utilizing convenient and affordable molecular tools such as RT-PCR, this perception of specificity slowly but surely insinuated that perhaps these genes of hematopoietic malignancies would not be perturbed in other tumor types. Although proto-oncogenic receptor tyrosine kinases and classic tumor suppressor genes (e.g., Rb, p53, PTEN) are also mutated/lost in hematopoietic malignancies, experimental evidence that the converse is true for the 200 or so leukemia/lymphoma genes is still lacking. To date, in only a few instances have alterations in AML-related genes been firmly associated with the pathogenesis of other tumor types (e.g., RUNX3, an AML1 family member, in gastric carcinomas [Li et al. 2002] or C/EBPα, which is down-regulated in a significant percentage of non-small-cell lung cancers [Halmos et al. 2002]).

We advocate here that the role of the vast majority of these leukemia/lymphoma genes in tumorigenesis at

large has not yet been thoroughly investigated and that a systematic analysis is in fact warranted, discussing specific examples directly stemming from our own work.

THE APL PARADIGM AND PROMYELOCYTIC LEUKEMIA

Acute promyelocytic leukemia (APL), the M3 subtype in the FAB classification of AML, represents the perfect example of a form of leukemia where the molecular genetics currently informs the diagnosis, the prognosis, the management, and the treatment of the disease, and where the knowledge of the molecular basis had a direct and major impact on the development of targeted therapeutic modalities (Melnick and Licht 1999; Piazza et al. 2001). APL was considered invariably fatal only 20 years ago, whereas the current cure rate approximates 90%, representing a genuine triumph of contemporary molecular medicine. Yet, these dramatic progresses have made leukemias such as APL or chronic myelogenous leukemia (CML) the archetypes on which the misconception of "hematopoietic specificity" rests: distinct AML subtype, specific molecular basis, specific treatment, and specific genes.

Indeed, the molecular genetics of APL is extremely specific to this AML subtype. APL is invariably associated with chromosomal translocations where the retinoic acid receptor (RARα) gene fuses with variable partner genes (referred to as X genes/proteins). RARα fuses to the PML gene in the vast majority of APL cases (> 95%), and in the remaining cases to the PLZF, NPM1, NuMA, and STAT5 genes (for review, see Piazza et al. 2001). As a consequence, X-RARα and RARα-X fusion genes are generated encoding aberrant fusion proteins that can interfere with RARα and/or the X protein function (Fig. 2). Since the RARα portion of the fusion protein is able to mediate heterodimerization with RXRs as well as DNA and ligand binding through the DNA and retinoic acid (RA) binding domains of RARα, respectively, X-RARα fusion products always retain the ability to interfere with the RAR/RXR pathway at the transcription level. The various X-RARα proteins also invariably display the

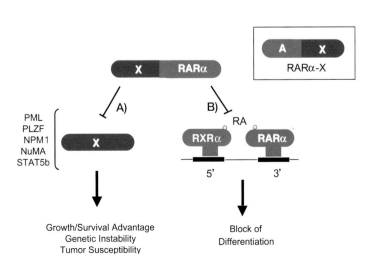

Figure 2. Fusion proteins in the pathogenesis of APL. APL is associated with specific chromosomal translocations where *RARα* fuses with variable partner genes (X genes): *PML, PLZF, NPM1, NuMA,* and *STAT5.* As a consequence, X-RARα and RARα-X fusion genes are generated, which encode aberrant fusion proteins capable of interfering with (*A*) the product of the remaining allele of the X gene (already reduced to heterozygosity as a consequence of the translocation), and (*B*) the transcriptional activity of the RARα/RXRα heterodimeric complex.

ability of heterodimerizing with the respective product of the remaining X allele (e.g., PML-RARα with PML, PLZF-RARα with PLZF, etc.), suggesting that X-RARα could simultaneously interfere with both X and RARα pathways. Moreover, as a consequence of the transloca- tion, the leukemia cell becomes heterozygous for both X and the RARα genes. On the basis of these facts and—as soon as we cloned the PML gene—of preliminary obser- vations that PML overexpression induced growth arrest and/or apoptosis depending on the cellular context, we originally proposed a working model by which the X genes could be regarded as leukemia suppressor genes whose function is interfered with by the APL fusion pro- teins. In vivo genetic testing of this hypothesis—initially studying PML and subsequently the other partners of RARα—has on the one hand provided ample support to this notion, but on the other hand clearly revealed how the role of these APL genes in tumor suppression goes be- yond the pathogenesis of this subtype of leukemia.

PML Is a Pleiotropic Tumor Suppressor

The ability of the APL-associated fusion products to interfere with the function of the X genes in a dominant negative fashion has been clearly demonstrated in the case of PML-RARα. PML is typically found in multipro- tein speckled subnuclear structures termed PML nuclear bodies (PML-NBs) (Zhong et al. 2000a; Jensen et al. 2001; and references therein). In *Pml*[-/-] mouse primary cells, PML-NB components acquire an aberrant nuclear localization pattern that can be restored to normal when PML is added back (Zhong et al. 2000b). Thus, PML is essential for the formation and stability of PML-NB. With the use of antibodies against PML, it has been demonstrated that in the APL blasts PML-RARα delo- calizes PML into microspeckled nuclear structures through physical association, in turn causing the disrup- tion of the PML-NBs (Melnick and Licht 1999; Zhong et al. 2000b). These observations lead then to the conclusion that PML may regulate the nuclear-body-associated func- tions of multiple nuclear body components (more than 50 proteins including p53, Rb, Daxx, and CBP), and that these functions may be impaired in the APL blast or in cells lacking PML function.

In fact, PML can modulate a number of tumor suppres- sive pathways (Salomoni and Pandolfi 2002). For in- stance, PML acts as a transcriptional coactivator of p53 and its family members p73 and p63 (Guo et al. 2000; Bernassola et al. 2004, 2005). It is also required for p53- dependent induction of apoptosis and cellular senescence upon exposure to ionizing radiation and oncogenic trans- formation (Guo et al. 2000; Pearson et al. 2000). More- over, *Pml*[-/-] mice and cells are protected from multiple caspase-dependent pro-apoptotic stimuli, such as Fas, tu- mor necrosis factor, ceramide, and interferon treatment (Wang et al. 1998). More recently, we have shown that PML is also an essential modulator of transforming growth factor beta (TGF-β) signaling, a pluripotent cy- tokine that controls key tumor suppressive functions (Lin et al. 2004). Therefore, PML is implicated in the modula- tion of cellular functions such as apoptosis, growth sup-

pression, and cellular senescence, that are essential for tu- mor suppression (Salomoni and Pandolfi 2002). On this basis, it was perhaps not surprising that *Pml* inactivation in knockout (KO) mutants would induce a dramatic accel- eration of the leukemic phenotype in mouse models of APL (Rego et al. 2001). However, PML—like many other leukemia/lymphoma-specific genes and the other genes of APL—is also dynamically expressed in non-hematopoi- etic cells. It was therefore tempting to hypothesize and test whether PML loss may participate in the pathogenesis of non-hematopoietic tumors as well. Indeed, using a high- throughput approach, we have recently demonstrated that PML expression is frequently lost in a number of epithe- lial tumor types such as, for instance, prostate cancer (Gurrieri et al. 2004). Importantly, PML loss correlated with tumor progression and grade (Gurrieri et al. 2004). The relevance of these findings is further corroborated by additional data obtained from *Pml* null mice, which in- deed demonstrated to be prone to spontaneously develop epithelial cancers (L.C. Trotman et al., in prep.). Taken to- gether, this comprehensive analysis of the PML status in human cancers provides compelling evidence that leukemia genes may participate in the pathogenesis of ma- lignancies other than APL, in this case through modula- tion of critical tumor suppressive pathways.

THE NUCLEOPHOSMIN PARADIGM

Nucleophosmin Is Often Aberrant in Human Cancer

Although a role for PML-RARα as dominant negative over PML function is apparent and led to the discovery of PML as a pleiotropic tumor suppressor gene in human cancer, the same concept seemed at first difficult to apply to the *NPM1* gene (another partner of RARα in APL) and the correspondent fusion product NPM-RARα. In fact, nucleophosmin (NPM) has been traditionally regarded as a tumor marker and a putative proto-oncogene rather than a putative tumor suppressor gene, in view of the fact that its expression is typically up-regulated by mitogenic sig- nals and correlates with cell proliferation and survival. Indeed, malignant and actively dividing cells express el- evated levels of NPM, and cells expressing large amounts of NPM are resistant to apoptosis induced by either UV damage or hypoxia (Wu et al. 2002; Li et al. 2004). On the other hand, the *NPM1* gene (genetic locus 5q35) is found translocated to other fusion partner genes beside RARα (Redner et al. 1996) in a number of human hematopoietic malignancies: It rearranges with the *ALK* gene in anaplastic large cell lymphomas (ALCL) (Morris et al. 1994) and with the *MLF1* gene in AML, CML, and myelodysplastic syndrome (MDS) (Yoneda-Kato et al. 1996). In addition, NPM has been recently found mutated and aberrantly localized in a high proportion of AML pa- tients (Falini et al. 2005; Grisendi and Pandolfi 2005a). Although these observations strongly implicate NPM in the pathogenesis of human cancer, they make it difficult to visualize it as a putative oncogene or tumor suppressor gene exclusively.

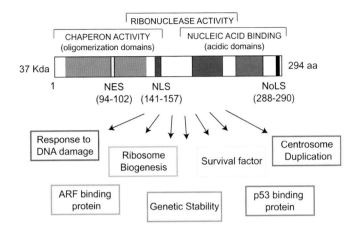

Figure 3. NPM is a multifunctional protein, composed of distinct functional domains which mediate diverse biochemical activities. In addition, NPM subcellular localization is tightly regulated by different localization signals: nuclear export signal (NES), nuclear localization signal (NLS), and nucleolar localization signal (NoLS). NPM participates in a number of biological processes: ribosome biogenesis, response to stress stimuli and DNA damage, control of centrosome duplication and genetic stability, and binding and stability control of key tumor suppressor genes such as p19^{Arf} and p53.

The Complexity of NPM Biology

As the involvement of NPM in human cancer is compelling but complex, the picture is further complicated by the multifaceted nature of this protein and its direct involvement in both proto-oncogenic and anti-oncogenic pathways. NPM is in fact a multifunctional protein (Fig. 3), which has been originally recognized as a nucleolar factor implicated in ribosome biogenesis and transport (Savkur and Olson 1998; Hingorani et al. 2000). Proliferating cells express higher NPM levels, and levels of expression of this protein seem to play an important role in protecting cells from apoptosis in different cell types (Pang et al. 2003; Ahn et al. 2005).

However, NPM also has been shown to associate to the centrosome and to inhibit its duplication in a cell-cycle-dependent manner controlled by phosphorylation by the CDK2–cyclin E complex (Okuda et al. 2000) and to be the target of mitotic kinases such as Nek2 and Plk1 (Yao et al. 2004; Zhang et al. 2004), involved in the control of proper cell division.

NPM has been proposed to modulate both positively and negatively the activity of major tumor suppressor genes such as p53 and p19^{Arf}. Although it seemingly stabilizes p53 upon overexpression in primary cells (Colombo et al. 2002), and protects p53 from HDM2-mediated degradation in response to UV irradiation (Kurki et al. 2004), NPM is also proposed to down-regulate p53 stability and antagonizes stress-induced apoptosis in human normal and malignant hematopoietic cells (Li et al. 2005). A comparable level of complexity applies to the recently discovered functional link between NPM and p19^{Arf} tumor suppressor. Whereas p19^{Arf} has been described to induce NPM degradation and protein synthesis inhibition (Itahana et al. 2003) and to impede NPM shuttling in an Mdm2-sensitive pathway (Brady et al. 2004), NPM seems to play a role in both favoring p19^{Arf} stability within high-molecular-weight protein complexes (Bertwistle et al. 2004) and inhibiting p19^{Arf} cytoplasmic function by sequestering it inside the nucleolus (Korgaonkar et al. 2005). Thus, the literature is complex, and it is difficult to discern to which extent what is reported is the result of cell line- and overexpression-related artifacts.

In this laboratory, we have historically dissected the molecular genetics underlying APL and human cancer in the mouse through the use of a direct genetic approach in transgenic and KO models. Thus, in order to disentangle the complexity underlying the role of NPM in tumorigenesis, we generated not solely KO mutants, but rather a whole hypomorphic *Npm* mutant series [$Npm^{+/-} < Npm^{hy/hy} < Npm^{-/-}$] in the mouse (Grisendi et al. 2005). To this end, we created a null allele by replacing 5 exons within the gene with a GFP coding sequence, as well as a hypomorphic allele by knocking the Neomycin cassette into an intronic region of the gene with the aim to interfere with the transcriptional activity of *Npm*.

A Role for Npm in the Regulation of the Centrosome Cycle

The first important information we obtained from this approach is that total abrogation (null) or even a strong reduction (hypomorphic) in Npm expression results in embryonic lethality on average around embryonic day 11.5–16.5, depending on the residual expression levels of the gene. Detailed analysis of the mutant embryos revealed that Npm is an essential developmental regulator that exerts functions specifically required for proper forebrain and blood development (Grisendi et al. 2005). Collectively, these observations led to two surprising conclusions: First, although ultimately crucial for survival, Npm is unexpectedly dispensable for embryonic life up to mid-gestation, different from what is observed for other genes firmly involved in ribosome biogenesis. This suggests either that Npm is redundant in this function, at least up to mid-gestation, or that the extent of the defect in ribosome biogenesis caused by Npm inactivation is still compatible with cell proliferation. Second, Npm controls embryogenesis and organogenesis in a specific manner.

Npm$^{-/-}$ embryos also showed high degrees of apoptosis. This was not totally unexpected since NPM has been described to be an important player in the apoptotic response and to protect cells from programmed cell death stimuli (see above). This increased apoptosis was accompanied by a robust p53 up-regulation, in spite of the fact that NPM has been described to act as a positive regulator of p53 stabilization upon overexpression (Colombo et al. 2002) and in response to stress stimuli (Kurki et al. 2004). This p53 response was also observed in embryonic fibroblasts (MEFs), where it takes place along with a concomitant up-regulation of p21[Wafl/Cip1], resulting in a premature senescence phenotype. We therefore went in search of a possible explanation for this p53 response. DNA damage and genomic instability are known to trigger a p53 response (Levine 1997). An increase in apoptosis accompanied by p53 up-regulation is observed in mutants such as Brca1-deficient embryos, whose cells suffer from genetic instability (Xu et al. 1999, 2001). Interestingly, we observed that *Npm*-deficient cells consistently underwent cell cycle arrest and exhibit a 4N DNA content. Polyploidy was detectable by cell cycle and DNA content analysis, suggesting that Npm loss or hypomorphism triggered a p53-dependent postmitotic tetraploid cell cycle arrest, as previously described in MEFs subjected to mitotic spindle disruption (Lanni and Jacks 1998). This reasoning is supported by the aforementioned increased expression of p21[Wafl/Cip1], typically known to mediate cell cycle arrest in G_1 phase, and lack of up-regulation of G_2-M markers (e.g., phospho-histone H3 and cyclin B). We therefore investigated the status of mitotic spindles in $Npm^{-/-}$ cells and, to our surprise, we found significant numbers of aberrant mitotic figures characterized by the presence of multipolar spindles as well as multiple functional centrosomes. $Npm^{-/-}$ interphase MEFs display centrosome amplification (3 or more centrosomes per cell) in up to 30% of the cell population. Furthermore, blood precursor cells isolated from the yolk sac of $Npm^{-/-}$ mutant embryos also show a massive increase in the number of centrosomes detectable in large multinucleated cells with up to 4 nuclei. Taken together, these findings suggest that Npm loss of function may lead to inappropriate centrosome duplication (Fig. 4). This in turn may cause centrosome amplification accompanied by aberrant cell division, and these effects ultimately contribute to the developmental defects observed in the Npm mutant embryos.

Npm Can Act as a Bona Fide Tumor Suppressor

Although less drastically affected, early-passage $Npm^{+/-}$ also displayed decreased cell proliferation rates and supernumerary centrosomes. Moreover, chromosome FISH analysis revealed significant levels of tetraploidy and aneuploidy not only in *Npm* null and hypomorphic cells, but also in heterozygous MEFs in a dose-dependent manner. Because the *NPM1* gene dosage is reduced by half in cancer cells harboring chromosomal rearrangements/deletions at the *NPM1* locus, we hypothesized that *Npm* could be haploinsufficient in the control of centrosome duplication and genomic stability and, hence, behave as a haploinsufficient tumor suppressor. We tested this possibility both in vitro using once again MEFs, and in vivo. In contrast to $Npm^{-/-}$ and hypomorphic MEFs, which eventually stop proliferating and undergo irreversible senescence, $Npm^{+/-}$ and wild-type cells could be maintained in culture for a comparable number of passages. This is likely due to the fact that in $Npm^{+/-}$

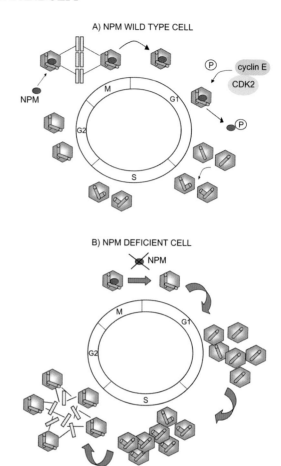

Figure 4. NPM loss of function causes centrosome amplification. (*A*) In the normal condition, NPM localizes to the centrosome during mitosis and the early G_1 phase of the cell's cycle. During the G_1-S phase transition, NPM is phosphorylated by the CDK2–cyclin E complex and dissociates from the centrosome. This allows centriole separation, and the centrosome duplicates. NPM is kept phosphorylated and separated from the centrosome until the end of the G_2 phase, when it re-associates to the centrosome at mitosis. (*B*) A reduction in NPM expression results in untimely and/or unrestricted centrosome duplication, leading to the formation of additional centrosomes and multipolar spindles. Aberrant mitosis in turn results in unbalanced chromosome segregation and, eventually, aneuploidy.

cells the defects observed are milder, still allowing the cells to survive and proliferate, although at a different rate. We therefore used $Npm^{+/-}$ cells to investigate whether the observed genetic instability arising from centrosome defects would affect the ability of these cells to immortalize in culture and their susceptibility toward cellular immortalization and transformation. In a stringent 3T9 protocol, at early passages, the proliferation rates of $Npm^{+/-}$ MEFs were lower, but, upon immortalization, the same cells acquired considerably higher proliferation rates compared to wild-type controls. This was accompanied by higher aneuploidy and a greater ability to efficiently form transformation foci in low-density seeding assays. In addition, upon immortalization, $Npm^{+/-}$ MEFs also display a higher susceptibility to transformation induced by acute expression of known oncogenes, such as

Ras^{V12} or c-myc. Taken together, these observations suggest that the *Npm* gene dosage is a critical determinant in maintaining proper centrosome numbers and chromosomal stability, and that the underlying genetic instability exhibited by *Npm*-deficient cells is a driving force toward faster acquisition of additional genetic mutations required initially for immortalization and then for transformation.

This working model is further supported by what we observed in vivo in *Npm*$^{+/-}$/Eμ-myc transgenic compound mice, which we generated in order to determine whether *Npm* heterozygous inactivation increases susceptibility to lymphomagenesis. Not only was the onset of lymphoma in *Npm*$^{+/-}$; Eμ-myc compound mice significantly accelerated in comparison with the Eμ-myc cohort, but, importantly, the karyology of these lymphomas was profoundly affected by the heterozygous loss of *Npm*. Whereas tumors from *Npm*$^{+/-}$; Eμ-myc mice displayed mostly numerical abnormalities, in contrast, in tumors from the Eμ-myc cohort we observed mostly structural abnormalities, as previously reported.

Npm plays a role in hematopoiesis during embryonic development as hematopoietic precursors in the yolk sac are drastically reduced in number and differentiation ability. Since Npm proved to be haploinsufficient in the control of cellular ploidy, we asked whether this would translate into an overt phenotype in the hematopoiesis of *Npm*$^{+/-}$ mutants. Remarkably, *Npm*$^{+/-}$ mice displayed features resembling some of those identified in the human MDS, such as, for instance, signs of dyserythropoiesis in the bone marrow, with a high proportion of dysplastic and bi-nucleated erythroid cells, as well as hypercellularity of red blood cell precursors. These observations are particularly relevant in view of the fact that deletion of variable portions of the long arm of chromosome 5 (5q) or of the whole chromosome 5 is frequently observed in patients with de novo and therapy-related MDS (for review, see Olney and Le Beau 2002). The deleted fragment (often located between bands 5q13 and 5q35) is variable in size and breakpoint localization, and it can be either the sole genetic anomaly or it can be accompanied by additional structural and numerical chromosomal changes. MDS is therefore regarded as a genetically and clinically heterogeneous condition where more than one gene may contribute to the final pathological outcome, although to date no gene has been firmly linked to the pathogenesis of these syndromes. Our findings indicate *NPM1* heterozygous loss as one of the genetic events that, in combination with loss of other genes located in the deleted region, could cooperate in the pathogenesis of full-blown human MDS.

Importantly, loss of 5q35, the genetic region where *NPM1* resides, is frequently observed in non-hematopoietic tumors. For instance, it is a frequent event in non-small-cell lung carcinoma (Mendes-da-Silva et al. 2000). Loss of 5q and consequent NPM haploinsufficiency could therefore constitute an engine toward genomic instability in these tumors, in turn favoring tumor progression. Taken together, these observations once again indicate that the role of NPM in tumorigenesis might not be solely confined to hematopoietic malignancies.

Oncogene or Tumor Suppressor: Is the Answer in the Dose?

We found that Npm is required to maintain genomic integrity through the regulation of centrosome duplication and cellular ploidy. NPM is haploinsufficient for this function since *Npm* heterozygous cells display a significant degree of genomic instability, which results in increased susceptibility to oncogenic transformation both in vitro and in vivo. The acquisition of genetic mutations is a crucial driving force during tumorigenesis, in both solid and hematopoietic malignancies. The importance of this aspect is underlined by the fact that the maintenance of genetic stability is a tightly regulated biological function, and that crucial and pleiotropic tumor suppressor genes are strictly involved in the growth arrest/apoptotic response to DNA damage insults and aneuploidy (e.g., p53). Alteration in NPM function might therefore have a larger impact on tumorigenesis, not only restricted to the field of hematopoietic disorders. This is especially relevant in view of the fact that not only is NPM translocated in a number of leukemia/lymphomas—determining a heterozygous state—and deleted in a proportion of cases of MDS, but it is also frequently lost in solid tumors (Mendes-da-Silva et al. 2000). However, NPM is also found overexpressed in a number of human cancers (both solid tumors and hematopoietic disorders). Thus, NPM could fall in a novel category of genes that act both as oncogene and tumor suppressor gene, depending on expression levels and gene dosage. Either a partial functional loss or an aberrant overexpression of this type of cancer gene would lead to neoplastic transformation through distinct mechanisms (Fig. 5).

CONCLUSIONS

We have discussed here representative examples in support of a more global role for "leukemia/lymphoma" genes in the pathogenesis of human cancer. Many of these genes in fact participate in the control of fundamental oncogenic and tumor suppressive networks that are shared by several cell types rather than being unique to hematopoietic malignancies. Even though a deregulated function of leukemia- or lymphoma-related genes may have differential outcomes and varying degrees of penetrance depending on the tissue/cell context, a systematic analysis of their status in human cancer is warranted. It would be wise to take advantage of the dramatic progress made in the last 20 years in determining the molecular genetics of most hematological malignancies and to apply this detailed knowledge to the analysis of other tumors whose genetic bases are still poorly understood. Thus, if we are to embark on a cancer genome anatomy project enterprise, we ought to pay particular attention to this specific subset of genes already directly implicated in the pathogenesis of human cancer. More in general, it could be very insightful to determine in detail the status of these genes in any given tumor type, address their function (if any) in the corresponding normal cell/type, and relate these functions to known oncogenic and tumor suppressive pathways in a systematic fashion.

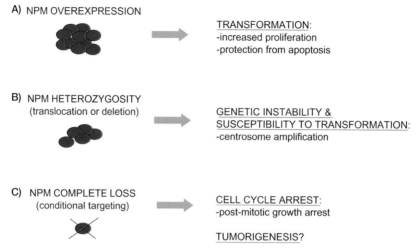

Figure 5. The dose of NPM in tumorigenesis. The dose of the NPM gene dictates distinct outcomes in tumorigenesis: Whereas NPM overexpression may promote the growth of cancerous cells due to increased cell proliferation and inhibition of the apoptotic response (*A*), NPM heterozygosity (or further dose reduction of NPM below 50%) renders the cells genetically unstable and susceptible to transformation (*B*). As the complete loss in NPM expression induces cell cycle arrest and cellular senescence (*C*), it remains to be determined whether complete somatic loss of the NPM gene would be compatible and selected for by the transformed cell.

ACKNOWLEDGMENTS

We thank all past and present members of the Pandolfi laboratory, and Linda DiSantis for editing of the manuscript.

REFERENCES

Adams J.M., Harris A.W., Pinkert C.A., Corcoran L.M., Alexander W.S., Cory S., Palmiter R.D., and Brinster R.L. 1985. The c-myc oncogene driven by immunoglobulin enhancers induces lymphoid malignancy in transgenic mice. *Nature* **318:** 533.

Ahn J.Y., Liu X., Cheng D., Peng J., Chan P.K., Wade P.A., and Ye K. 2005. Nucleophosmin/B23, a nuclear PI(3,4,5)P(3) receptor, mediates the anti-apoptotic actions of NGF by inhibiting CAD. *Mol. Cell* **18:** 435.

Arvanitis C. and Felsher D.W. 2005. Conditionally MYC: Insights from novel transgenic models. *Cancer Lett.* **226:** 95.

Bernassola F., Oberst A., Melino G., and Pandolfi P.P. 2005. The promyelocytic leukaemia protein tumour suppressor functions as a transcriptional regulator of p63. *Oncogene* **24:** 6982.

Bernassola F., Salomoni P., Oberst A., Di Como C.J., Pagano M., Melino G., and Pandolfi P.P. 2004. Ubiquitin-dependent degradation of p73 is inhibited by PML. *J. Exp. Med.* **199:** 1545.

Bertwistle D., Sugimoto M., and Sherr C.J. 2004. Physical and functional interactions of the Arf tumor suppressor protein with nucleophosmin/B23. *Mol. Cell. Biol.* **24:** 985.

Brady S.N., Yu Y., Maggi L.B., Jr., and Weber J.D. 2004. ARF impedes NPM/B23 shuttling in an Mdm2-sensitive tumor suppressor pathway. *Mol. Cell. Biol.* **24:** 9327.

Colombo E., Marine J.C., Danovi D., Falini B., and Pelicci P.G. 2002. Nucleophosmin regulates the stability and transcriptional activity of p53. *Nat. Cell Biol.* **4:** 529.

Dalla-Favera R., Bregni M., Erikson J., Patterson D., Gallo R.C., and Croce C.M. 1982. Human c-myc oncogene is located on the region of chromosome 8 that is translocated in Burkitt lymphoma cells. *Proc. Natl. Acad. Sci.* **79:** 7824.

Falini B., Mecucci C., Tiacci E., Alcalay M., Rosati R., Pasqualucci L., La Starza R., Diverio D., Colombo E., Santucci A., Bigerna B., Pacini R., Pucciarini A., Liso A., Vignetti M., Fazi P., Meani N., Pettirossi V., Saglio G., Mandelli

F., Lo-Coco F., Pelicci P.G., and Martelli M.F. 2005. Cytoplasmic nucleophosmin in acute myelogenous leukemia with a normal karyotype. *N. Engl. J. Med.* **352:** 254.

Grisendi S. and Pandolfi P.P. 2005. NPM mutations in acute myelogenous leukemia. *N. Engl. J. Med.* **352:** 291.

Grisendi S., Bernardi R., Rossi M., Cheng K., Khandker L., Manova K., and Pandolfi P.P. 2005. Role of nucleophosmin in embryonic development and tumorigenesis. *Nature* **437:** 147.

Guo A., Salomoni P., Luo J., Shih A., Zhong S., Gu W., and Pandolfi P.P. 2000. The function of PML in p53-dependent apoptosis. *Nat. Cell Biol.* **2:** 730.

Gurrieri C., Capodieci P., Bernardi R., Scaglioni P.P., Nafa K., Rush L.J., Verbel D.A., Cordon-Cardo C., and Pandolfi P.P. 2004. Loss of the tumor suppressor PML in human cancers of multiple histologic origins. *J. Natl. Cancer Inst.* **96:** 269.

Halmos B., Huettner C.S., Kocher O., Ferenczi K., Karp D.D., and Tenen D.G. 2002. Down-regulation and antiproliferative role of C/EBPalpha in lung cancer. *Cancer Res.* **62:** 528.

Hingorani K., Szebeni A., and Olson M.O. 2000. Mapping the functional domains of nucleolar protein B23. *J. Biol. Chem.* **275:** 24451.

Itahana K., Bhat K.P., Jin A., Itahana Y., Hawke D., Kobayashi R., and Zhang Y. 2003. Tumor suppressor ARF degrades B23, a nucleolar protein involved in ribosome biogenesis and cell proliferation. *Mol. Cell* **12:** 1151.

Jensen K., Shiels C., and Freemont P.S. 2001. PML protein isoforms and the RBCC/TRIM motif. *Oncogene* **20:** 7223.

Korgaonkar C., Hagen J., Tompkins V., Frazier A.A., Allamargot C., Quelle F.W., and Quelle D.E. 2005. Nucleophosmin (B23) targets ARF to nucleoli and inhibits its function. *Mol. Cell. Biol.* **25:** 1258.

Kurki S., Peltonen K., Latonen L., Kiviharju T.M., Ojala P.M., Meek D., and Laiho M. 2004. Nucleolar protein NPM interacts with HDM2 and protects tumor suppressor protein p53 from HDM2-mediated degradation. *Cancer Cell* **5:** 465.

Lanni J.S. and Jacks T. 1998. Characterization of the p53-dependent postmitotic checkpoint following spindle disruption. *Mol. Cell. Biol.* **18:** 1055.

Levine A.J. 1997. p53, the cellular gatekeeper for growth and division. *Cell* **88:** 323.

Li J., Zhang X., Sejas D.P., and Pang Q. 2005. Negative regulation of p53 by nucleophosmin antagonizes stress-induced apoptosis in human normal and malignant hematopoietic cells. *Leuk. Res.* **29:** 1415.

Li J., Zhang X., Sejas D.P., Bagby G.C., and Pang Q. 2004. Hypoxia-induced nucleophosmin protects cell death through inhibition of p53. *J. Biol. Chem.* **279:** 41275.

Li Q.L., Ito K., Sakakura C., Fukamachi H., Inoue K., Chi X.Z., Lee K.Y., Nomura S., Lee C.W., Han S.B., Kim H.M., Kim W.J., Yamamoto H., Yamashita N., Yano T., Ikeda T., Itohara S., Inazawa J., Abe T., Hagiwara A., Yamagishi H., Ooe A., Kaneda A., Sugimura T., Ushijima T., Bae S.C., and Ito Y. 2002. Causal relationship between the loss of RUNX3 expression and gastric cancer. *Cell* **5:** 113.

Lin H.K., Bergmann S., and Pandolfi P.P. 2004. Cytoplasmic PML function in TGF-beta signalling. *Nature* **431:** 205.

Melnick A. and Licht J.D. 1999. Deconstructing a disease: RARα, its fusion partners, and their roles in the pathogenesis of acute promyelocytic leukemia. *Blood* **93:** 3167.

Mendes-da-Silva P., Moreira A., Duro-da-Costa J., Matias D., and Monteiro C. 2000. Frequent loss of heterozygosity on chromosome 5 in non-small cell lung carcinoma. *Mol. Pathol.* **53:** 184.

Morgenbesser S.D. and DePinho R.A. 1994. Use of transgenic mice to study myc family gene function in normal mammalian development and in cancer. *Semin. Cancer Biol.* **5:** 21.

Morris S.W., Kirstein M.N., Valentine M.B., Dittmer K.G., Shapiro D.N., Saltman D.L., and Look A.T. 1994. Fusion of a kinase gene, ALK, to a nucleolar protein gene, NPM, in non-Hodgkin's lymphoma. *Science* **263:** 1281.

Nesbit C.E., Tersak J.M., and Prochownik E.V. 1999. MYC oncogenes and human neoplastic disease. *Oncogene* **18:** 3004.

Okuda M., Horn H.F., Tarapore P., Tokuyama Y., Smulian A.G., Chan P.K., Knudsen E.S., Hofmann I.A., Snyder J.D., Bove K.E., and Fukasawa K. 2000. Nucleophosmin/B23 is a target of CDK2/cyclin E in centrosome duplication. *Cell* **103:** 127.

Olney H.J. and Le Beau M.M. 2002. The cytogenetics and molecular biology of the myelodysplastic syndromes. In *The myelodysplastic syndromes, pathobiology and clinical management* (ed. J.M. Bennet), p. 89. Marcel Dekker, New York.

Oster S.K., Ho C.S.W., Soucie E.L., and Penn L.Z. 2002. The *myc* oncogene: Marvelously complex. *Adv. Cancer Res.* **84:** 81.

Pang Q., Christianson T.A., Koretsky T., Carlson H., David L., Keeble W., Faulkner G.R., Speckhart A., and Bagby G.C. 2003. Nucleophosmin interacts with and inhibits the catalytic function of eukaryotic initiation factor 2 kinase PKR. *J. Biol. Chem.* **278:** 417091.

Pearson M., Carbone R., Sebastiani C., Cioce M., Fagioli M, Saito S., Higashimoto Y., Appella E., Minucci S., Pandolfi P.P., and Pelicci P.G. 2000. PML regulates p53 acetylation and premature senescence induced by oncogenic Ras. *Nature* **406:** 207.

Piazza F., Gurrieri C., and Pandolfi P.P. 2001. The theory of APL. *Oncogene* **20:** 7216.

Redner R.L., Rush E.A., Faas S., Rudert W.A., and Corey S. J. 1996. The t(5;17) variant of acute promyelocytic leukemia expresses a nucleophosmin-retinoic acid receptor fusion. *Blood* **87:** 882.

Rego E.M., Wang Z.G., Peruzzi D., He L.Z., Cordon-Cardo C., and Pandolfi P.P. 2001. Role of promyelocytic leukemia (PML) protein in tumor suppression. *J. Exp. Med.* **193:** 521.

Salomoni P. and Pandolfi P.P. 2002. The role of PML in tumor suppression. *Cell* **108:** 165.

Savkur R.S. and Olson M.O. 1998. Preferential cleavage in pre-ribosomal RNA by protein B23 endoribonuclease. *Nucleic Acids Res.* **26:** 4508.

Spencer C.A. and Groudine M. 1991. Control of c-myc regulation in normal and neoplastic cells. *Adv. Cancer Res.* **56:** 1.

Tomlins S.A., Rhodes D.R., Perner S., Dhanasekaran S.M., Mehra R., Sun X., Varambally S., Cao X., Tchinda J., Kuefer R., Lee C., Montie J.E., Shah R.B., Pienta K.J., Rubin M.A., and Chinnaiyan A.M. 2005. Recurrent fusion of *TMPRSS2* and ETS transcription factor genes in prostate cancer. *Science* **310:** 644.

Vennstrom B., Sheiness D., Zabielski J., and Bishop J.M. 1982. Isolation and characterization of c-myc, a cellular homolog of the oncogene (v-myc) of avian myelocytomatosis virus strain 29. *J. Virol.* **42:** 773.

Wang Z.G., Ruggero D., Ronchetti S., Zhong S., Gaboli M., Rivi R., and Pandolfi P.P. 1998. PML is essential for multiple apoptotic pathways. *Nat. Genet.* **20:** 266.

Wu M.H., Chang J.H., and Yung B.Y.M. 2002. Resistance to UV-induced cell-killing in nucleophosmin/B23 over-expressed NIH3T3 fibroblasts: Enhancement of DNA repair and up-regulation of PCNA in association with nucleophosmin/B23 over-expression. *Carcinogenesis* **23:** 93.

Xu X., Qiao W., Linke S.P., Cao L., Li W.M., Furth P.A., Harris C.C., and Deng C.X. 2001. Genetic interactions between tumor suppressor Brca1 and p53 in apoptosis, cell cycle and tumorigenesis. *Nat. Genet.* **28:** 266.

Xu X., Weaver Z., Linke S.P., Li C., Gotay J., Wang X.W., Harris C.C., Ried T., and Deng C.X. 1999. Centrosome amplification and defective G2-M cell cycle check-point induce genetic instability in BRCA1 exon 11 isoform-deficient cells. *Mol. Cell* **3:** 389.

Yao J., Fu C., Ding X., Guo Z., Zenreski A., Chen Y., Ahmed K., Liao J., Dou Z., and Yao X. 2004. Nek2A kinase regulates the localization of numatrin to centrosome in mitosis. *FEBS Lett.* **575:** 112.

Yoneda-Kato N., Look A.T., Kirstein M.N., Valentine M.B., Raimondi S.C., Cohen K.J., Carroll A.J., and Morris S.W. 1996. The t(3;5)(q25.1;q34) of myelodysplastic syndrome and acute myeloid leukemia produces a novel fusion gene, NPM-MLF1. *Oncogene* **12:** 265.

Zhang H., Shi X., Paddon H., Hampong M., Dai W., and Pelech S. 2004. B23/nucleophosmin serine 4 phosphorylation mediates mitotic functions of polo-like kinase 1. *J. Biol. Chem.* **279:** 35726.

Zhong S., Salomoni P. ,and Pandolfi P.P. 2000a. The transcriptional role of PML and the nuclear body. *Nat. Cell Biol.* **2:** E85.

Zhong S., Muller S., Ronchetti S., Freemont P.S., Dejean A., and Pandolfi P.P. 2000b. Role of SUMO-1 modified PML in nuclear body formation. *Blood* **95:** 2748.

Abnormalities of the Inactive X Chromosome Are a Common Feature of BRCA1 Mutant and Sporadic Basal-like Breast Cancer

S. Ganesan,[*][†] A.L. Richardson,[†] Z.C. Wang, J.D. Iglehart, A. Miron, J. Feunteun,[‡] D. Silver, and D.M. Livingston

Dana-Farber Cancer Institute, Brigham and Women's Hospital, and Harvard Medical School, Boston, Massachusetts 02115; and [‡]Institut Gustav Roussy, Villejuif, France

As a clinical entity, breast cancer appears to be a series of subforms, each with a relatively specific molecular phenotype. Among the characteristics that differentiate these subforms are sex hormone receptor expression, HER2 expression, p53 mutation, high-grade histopathology, and particular gene expression array patterns. Sporadic basal-like breast cancer is one such form. It is a relatively common, high-grade, hormone receptor and HER2-expression-negative, p53 mutation-bearing tumor and is particularly lethal. Although wild type for BRCA1, it is a sporadic phenocopy of most cases of BRCA1[−/−] breast cancer. Not only do the cells of the two tumors resemble one another with respect to the above-noted characteristics, they also share a defect in the maintenance of an intact, inactive X chromosome (Xi). Other high-grade and most low-grade tumors are rarely defective at Xi. This evidence suggests that an Xi defect contributes to the evolution of both sporadic and BRCA1[−/−] basal-like breast tumors.

Breast cancer, once believed to constitute a single pathological entity, is actually a family of disorders, each with a distinctive molecular and biological signature. Each of these disease subtypes is composed of cells that constitute a subset of the mammary epithelium, a complex and internally diverse entity in its own right. Analysis of a combination of histopathological, immunocytochemical, genetic, direct genomic, and gene array expression characteristics is beginning to provide growing insight into the distinctive nature of each of the various forms of the disease that have been detected.

A small minority of patients with the disease carry a germ-line, loss-of-function mutation in a gene that substantially elevates their risk of developing the disease. The best-known and most prevalent of these genes are BRCA1 and BRCA2. These loci map to different chromosomes (chr. 17 and 13, respectively) and encode large, nuclear proteins that bear no similarity to one another. However, they each provide a major contribution to cellular genome integrity control and do so, in part, by interacting physically with one another and with a sizable number of other DNA repair and checkpoint control proteins. Indeed, both BRCA proteins promote efficient repair of double-strand DNA breaks (DSBRs) and contribute to multiple forms of cell cycle checkpoint control (Venkitaraman 2002; Narod and Foulkes 2004; Scully et al. 2004).

BRCA1 and BRCA2 are not alone among the genes that, when mutated in the germ line, elevate the risk of developing breast cancer. Three others, ATM, p53, and CHK2, are also known to do so, and, importantly, like BRCA1 and BRCA2, they, too, provide key contributions to proper DNA damage responses (Venkitaraman 2003; Narod and Foulkes 2004). Given these observations, it has been widely hypothesized that a breakdown in DSBRs and elements of checkpoint control are pathophysiological forces with a tendency to elicit a neoplastic phenotype in the human mammary epithelium (Venkitaraman 2003; Narod and Foulkes 2004).

Surprisingly, although germ-line mutations in these DNA damage response genes are powerful triggers of the disease, sporadic breast cancer rarely, if ever, is a product of somatic mutations in BRCA1, BRCA2, ATM, or CHK2. The circumstance is different in other relatively common and certain uncommon epithelial tumors where germ-line and somatic mutations in the same gene contribute, respectively, to the inherited and acquired forms of the same tumor. Whether the mammary epithelium commonly develops loss-of-function mutations in genes that operate in the same pathways served by the BRCA1, BRCA2, CHK2, and/or ATM loci or experiences failure of epigenetic controls that compromise, indirectly, the functions of one or more of these genes are major, unanswered questions.

In this regard, there is growing evidence pointing to the existence of a particular subform of sporadic breast cancer, basal-like breast cancer (BLC), that appears to be a pathophysiological phenocopy of the most prevalent form of inherited, BRCA1 mutation-bearing tumors (Lakhani et al. 2000, 2005; Foulkes et al. 2003, 2004; Sorlie et al. 2003; N. Turner et al. 2004b; Laakso et al. 2005; Palacios et al. 2005). It is the subject of this paper.

*Present address: Cancer Institute of New Jersey, UMDNJ-RWJMS, New Brunswick, New Jersey.

[†]These authors contributed equally to this work.

SPORADIC BASAL-LIKE AND BRCA1$^{-/-}$ BREAST CANCERS

BLC constitutes approximately 15% of the cases of sporadic breast cancer detected in the U.S. and Europe each year. They are, typically, aggressive lesions that do not produce sex hormone receptors (Perou et al. 2000; Sorlie et al. 2001). In addition, most synthesize cytokeratins that are normally detected in the basal cell layer of mammary epithelium, a component of which are myoepithelial cells. In addition, BLC lesions rarely overproduce HER2, frequently carry somatic p53 mutation, and are highly proliferative (see Fig. 1).

BLC maintains a gene expression array signature that separates them from the other relatively common subsets of sporadic breast cancer (Perou et al. 2000). Importantly, much, if not all, of this signature is shared with BRCA1 tumors (Sorlie et al. 2003). These findings suggest that both tumor subsets—one sporadic and the other inherited—affect the same species of mammary epithelial cell(s). Sporadic BLC and BLC arising in BRCA1 mutation-bearing women share additional characteristics. Both are clinically aggressive, commonly carry p53 mutations, fail to overproduce HER2, and are particularly aneuploid. Taken together, one wonders whether both tumor types are products of a common—or at least a closely related—pathophysiological mechanism.

BRCA1 FUNCTION AFFECTS THE HETEROCHROMATINIZATION OF THE INACTIVE Xi CHROMOSOME

Previously, it was shown that the p220 BRCA1 protein can be detected by immunofluorescence microscopy to decorate the XY body in murine spermatocytes (Ganesan et al. 2002; J.M. Turner et al. 2004). Because the X is transcriptionally silenced in this meiotic structure, the question of whether it also decorates the Xi chromosome in female somatic cells was posed. The data show that BRCA1 does, indeed, colocalize with Xi in both primary and certain immortalized human tumor cells in culture, although colocalization is a transient phenomenon during the cell cycle, leaving most cells undecorated in asynchronous cultures (Ganesan et al. 2002). Others have observed Xi decoration by BRCA1 during a subset of S phase (Chadwick and Lane 2005). It has not been detected during other cell-cycle intervals, despite the almost constant presence of a readily detected Xi in G_0, G_1, S, and G_2. Therefore, any direct communication between BRCA1 (and its p220 subform, in particular) and Xi is likely to be transient.

Further investigation showed that BRCA1 function and the ability of a cell to maintain a fully heterochromatinized Xi superstructure were linked. In particular, it was shown that most cells depleted of BRCA1 p220 by RNAi lacked an Xi fully decorated by XIST RNA or macrohis-

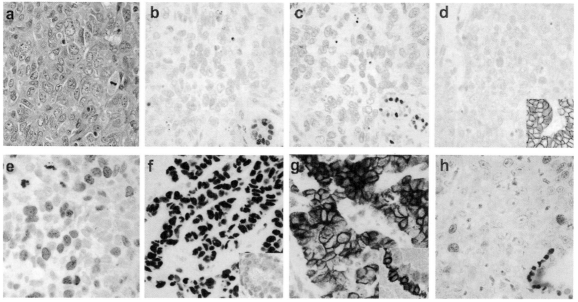

Figure 1. Histology and immunophenotype of representative BLC to demonstrate commonly occurring patterns. *a–h*, magnification, 51x. (*a*) H&E-stained section demonstrating high nuclear grade and lack of tubule formation in this tumor. (*b*) Immunohistochemistry (IHC) for estrogen receptor demonstrating negativity in the tumor cells. Inset shows positive immunoreactivity in normal breast epithelium (internal positive control). (*c*) IHC for progesterone receptor, showing negative staining in tumor cells and positive staining in normal breast cells (*inset*). (*d*) IHC for HER2/neu, demonstrating lack of overexpression in tumor cells. Inset shows positive control staining of a HER2- amplified tumor. (*e*) IHC for Ki67 demonstrating a high proportion of proliferative cells in BLC. (*f*) IHC for p53 demonstrating aberrant accumulation of p53 protein typically associated with p53 mutation. Inset shows negative staining in adjacent normal breast tissue. (*g*) IHC for cytokeratin 14 (CK14) demonstrating positive reactivity for this basal keratin in tumor cells. The inset depicts the normal pattern of CK14 positivity in basally located normal breast epithelium. (*h*) IHC for p63 demonstrating focal nuclear immunoreactivity in tumor cells. The inset shows a normal pattern of p63 staining of basally located myoepithelial cells in adjacent normal breast tissue.

tone H2A 1.2. Both are established components of the Xi heterochromatin superstructure. Similarly, frozen sections of all clinically isolated, BRCA1$^{-/-}$ human tumors analyzed to date by us also lacked XIST/Xi staining (Ganesan et al. 2002).

Similarly, the human tumor cell line, HCC 1937, which is derived from a BRCA1$^{-/-}$ breast cancer, was shown to contain two X chromosomes, but no nuclear concentration of XIST RNA, macrohistone H2A 1.2, or histone H3 meK27, all signatures of a normal Xi. However, after being reconstituted with physiological concentrations of p220 by retroviral BRCA1 cDNA infection, these cells reacquired detectable focal nuclear XIST RNA (Ganesan et al. 2002). Similarly, when these cells were stably transfected with a tetracycline-inducible wild-type BRCA1 allele, they reacquired XIST/Xi staining in cells that produced wild-type p220 protein (Fig. 2) (Ganesan et al. 2002). In addition, when ectopically encoded p220 was synthesized in HCC 1937 cells, there was no change in the abundance of XIST in these cells (Ganesan et al. 2002). Taken together, the above-noted results imply that p220 operates, in part, by promoting the maintenance of proper Xi heterochromatinization, possibly by supporting—directly or indirectly—the stable localization of XIST on Xi. However, it remains possible that p220 also affects the synthesis and/or stability of this RNA species. Clearly, additional experiments that investigate these

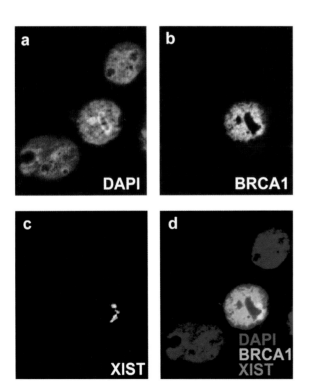

Figure 2. Images of HCC1937 cells (BRCA1$^{-/-}$) stably transfected with a tetracycline-inducible wild-type BRCA1 allele and induced with doxycycline (2 mcg/ml for 24 hours). (*a*) DAPI staining of nuclei. (*b*) Immunofluorescence with a monoclonal antibody directed against human BRCA1 p220. (*c*) RNA FISH for XIST. (*d*) Merged image for DAPI (*blue*), BRCA1 (*green*), and XIST (*red*).

possibilities in other cell species need to be undertaken.

What remains to be answered is the question of whether this new heterochromatinization function of p220 is in any way related to its ability to perform its DNA damage response and its breast cancer suppression function. Viewed in a slightly different manner, it seems reasonable to ask whether the defect in Xi heterochromatinization observed in BRCA1$^{-/-}$ tumor cells contributes to the emergence of BRCA1 breast cancer. The data, described in synopsis form above, do not speak to this question.

BLC, LIKE MOST BRCA1 BREAST CANCERS, ALSO DISPLAYS A MAJOR DEFECT IN Xi

During the course of analyzing a sizable collection of frozen human breast cancer samples for BRCA1 protein, we have analyzed a recently obtained collection of clinically annotated, sporadic BLC samples (Richardson et al. 2006). To assign them to the sporadic BLC category, several criteria had to be met. They included negative staining by immunohistochemistry for ER/PR/HER2; high-grade histology; and a characteristic gene expression array signature of BLC (Perou et al. 2000; Sorlie et al. 2001; Wang et al. 2004). A series of 17 such tumors were selected for further analysis along with 20 high-grade non-BLC lesions (which served as controls in this experiment; Richardson et al. 2006).

Among the BLC tumor set, all were analyzed by BRCA1 IF, employing a monoclonal antibody to p220. Of 17 BLC (and all controls), 16 were composed of tumor cells that displayed BRCA1 nuclear dots, a signature of the existence of biologically active p220 during S phase. Heteroduplex-based sequence analysis demonstrated the presence of at least one wild-type copy of BRCA1 in 5/5 BLC tested (Richardson et al. 2006). Because nuclear dots in cells that have not undergone purposeful DNA damage correlate closely with the existence of a wild-type BRCA1 genotype, these data, along with the direct sequence analysis results noted above, strongly suggest that this collection of BLC lesions was, in all likelihood, uniformly wild type for BRCA1.

Next, each BLC sample was scored for Xi by XIST RNA fluorescence in situ hybridization (FISH), and 14 of 17 proved to be negative, like BRCA1$^{-/-}$ tumors (Ganesan et al. 2002; Richardson et al. 2006). Normal stromal cells in each BLC specimen revealed clearly detectable Xi structures, serving as positive controls in these analyses. Furthermore, when the 17 BLC tumors were analyzed for X copy number by X DNA FISH and/or quantitative SNP array analysis, all but one contained two copies. The remaining tumor was X trisomic. Had it contained two Xi structures, both would have been expected to stain positively for XIST and H3meK27. However, this BLC revealed only monofocal H3meK27 and XIST, consistent with its having two active X chromosomes and one Xi (Richardson et al. 2006).

Such a defect was seen only in 2/20 control, high-grade non-BLC tumors that were also analyzed in this effort. Most revealed a single, classic Xi structure. Where X trisomy was encountered, two Xi structures—which co-stained for XIST and H3meK27—were detected. Taken together, this evidence points to a highly prevalent defect in Xi maintenance in a significant collection of sporadic BLC tumor cells that is not shared with a similar-size cohort of high-grade non-BLC (Richardson et al. 2006).

CONCLUSIONS

Although data acquired before the above-noted, clinically oriented studies were performed point to a highly prevalent defect in X heterochromatinization in BRCA1$^{-/-}$ tumors (Ganesan et al. 2002), they did not address the question of whether such a defect is material to BRCA1$^{-/-}$ tumor development. Here, we describe the analysis of a set of sporadic BLC, a disease with pathological, clinical, immunohistophenotyping, and functional genomic characteristics similar to those of BRCA1$^{-/-}$ tumors. What was surprising was the finding that, whereas all of the BLC analyzed were wild type for BRCA1, they were largely defective at Xi. Either there was no classic Xi structure or, in the few cases where an intact Xi was retained, there was gain of active X chromosome territory involving either the whole X chromosome or parts of Xp. Therefore, all sporadic BLC, like all BRCA1$^{-/-}$ tumors analyzed, revealed an Xi-related defect.

Among sporadic and BRCA1$^{-/-}$ BLC, certain common characteristics were already known prior to this study. What is new are the findings that the former (1) are, where tested, wild type for BRCA1, (2) express a nuclear p220 species that can localize in dot structures—a sign of intact p220 subnuclear localization—and yet (3) lack a clear Xi structure. In keeping with the last finding, we now know that approximately 25% of these lesions contained biparental X chromosomes—one from each parent—whereas ~60% contain two X chromosomes, both from the same parent (Richardson et al. 2006). Thus, failure to sustain a proper, inactivated X chromosome—whether a product of the duplication of what is assumed to be the active X and loss of the inactive one or of failure to heterochromatinize what was once Xi—appears to be a generic characteristic of BLC. The uniform finding of apparent misbehavior at Xi in these BRCA1 wild-type lesions as well as in BRCA1$^{-/-}$ tumors strongly suggests that this form of molecular pathology contributes to BLC development, whether sporadic or inherited. Thus, these data provide new insight into the question of whether an Xi defect contributes to breast cancer development and constitutes part of the BRCA1 cancer suppression mechanism (Richardson et al. 2006).

It is worth noting that the vast majority of patients who carry germ-line BRCA1 mutations and develop cancer are female. If misbehavior at Xi is a powerful contributor to BLC development, it would be missing in male cells. One wonders whether this concept underlies, at least in part, the female-tropic nature of BRCA1 cancer.

Finally, how the absence of Xi heterochromatinization contributes in a mechanistic sense to tumor development is a mystery. In the simplest scenario, failure to silence one or more genes that are normally silenced on Xi might be part of the story. Conceivably, overexpression of certain X-linked genes, by even a small increment over normal, elicits cellular effects destined to evoke a neoplastic outcome. Alternatively, one might imagine that, as in BRCA1$^{-/-}$ tumors where a defined set of defects in DSBR and checkpoint control can be detected, a similar situation pertains to sporadic BLC. In that case, one wonders whether the lack of Xi heterochromatinization heightens the risk of at least one X chromosome acquiring certain forms of DNA damage during proliferation of BLC precursor (?stem) cells and/or of such a cell responding abnormally to such damage.

Whatever the case, much work remains to be done before the essence of the molecular BLC disease mechanism comes to light. In its absence, one can, nonetheless, hypothesize that sporadic BLC and a common subset of BRCA1$^{-/-}$ tumors are, on multiple levels, phenocopies of one another and, thus, are driven by certain common mechanistic forces. One such force is associated with a gross epigenetic defect at Xi, at least in those BLC cases bearing biparental X chromosomes. In those that have undergone X chromosome isodisomy, the mechanism is unclear, although one wonders whether loss of Xi in these tumors is a product of persistent DNA damage directed at that chromosome accompanied by selection for a duplicated, active X chromosome.

ACKNOWLEDGMENTS

We thank all members of the Livingston, Richardson, and Iglehart laboratories for encouragement and numerous helpful conversations. This work was, in part, supported by funds provided by the National Cancer Institute SPORE grant in breast cancer at Dana-Farber/Harvard Cancer Center, by other grants from the National Cancer Institute, by the Women's Cancer Program of Dana-Farber Cancer Institute, and by Deborah and Robert First.

REFERENCES

Chadwick B.P. and Lane T.F. 2005. BRCA1 associates with the inactive X chromosome in late S-phase, coupled with transient H2AX phosphorylation. *Chromosoma* **114:** 432.

Foulkes W.D., Stefansson I.M., Chappuis P.O., Begin L.R., Goffin J.R., Wong N., Trudel M., and Akslen L.A. 2003. Germline BRCA1 mutations and a basal epithelial phenotype in breast cancer. *J. Natl. Cancer Inst.* **95:** 1482.

Foulkes W.D., Brunet J.S., Stefansson I.M., Straume O., Chappuis P.O., Begin L.R., Hamel N., Goffin J.R., Wong N., Trudel M., Kapusta L., Porter P., and Akslen L.A. 2004. The prognostic implication of the basal-like (cyclin E high/p27 low/p53+/glomeruloid-microvascular-proliferation+) phenotype of BRCA1-related breast cancer. *Cancer. Res.* **64:** 830.

Ganesan S., Silver D.P., Greenberg R.A., Avni D., Drapkin R., Miron A., Mok S.C., Randrianarison V., Brodie S., Salstrom J., Rasmussen T.P., Klimke A., Marrese C., Marahrens Y., Deng C.X., Feunteun J., and Livingston D.M. 2002. BRCA1 supports XIST RNA concentration on the inactive X chromosome. *Cell* **111:** 393.

Laakso M., Loman N., Borg A., and Isola J. 2005. Cytokeratin 5/14-positive breast cancer: True basal phenotype confined to BRCA1 tumors. *Mod. Pathol* **18:** 1321.

Lakhani S.R., Gusterson B.A., Jacquemier J., Sloane J.P., Anderson T.J., van de Vijver M.J., Venter D., Freeman A., Antoniou A., McGuffog L., Smyth E., Steel C.M., Haites N., Scott R.J., Goldgar D., Neuhausen S., Daly P.A., Ormiston

W., McManus R., Scherneck S., Ponder B.A., Futreal P.A., Peto J., Stoppa-Lyonnet D., Bignon Y.J., and Stratton M.R. 2000. The pathology of familial breast cancer: Histological features of cancers in families not attributable to mutations in BRCA1 or BRCA2. *Clin. Cancer Res.* **6:** 782.

Lakhani S.R., Reis-Filho J.S., Fulford L., Penault-Llorca F., van der Vijver M., Parry S., Bishop T., Benitez J., Rivas C., Bignon Y.J., Chang-Claude J., Hamann U., Cornelisse C.J., Devilee P., Beckmann M.W., Nestle-Kramling C., Daly P.A., Haites N., Varley J., Lalloo F., Evans G., Maugard C., Meijers-Heijboer H., Klijn J.G., Olah E., Gusterson B.A., Pilotti S., Radice P., Scherneck S., Sobol H., Jacquemier J., Wagner T., Peto J., Stratton M.R., McGuffog L., and Easton D.F. 2005. Prediction of BRCA1 status in patients with breast cancer using estrogen receptor and basal phenotype. *Clin. Cancer Res.* **11:** 5175.

Narod S.A. and Foulkes W.D. 2004. BRCA1 and BRCA2: 1994 and beyond. *Nat. Rev. Cancer* **4:** 665.

Palacios J., Honrado E., Osorio A., Cazorla A., Sarrio D., Barroso A., Rodriguez S., Cigudosa J.C., Diez O., Alonso C., Lerma E., Dopazo J., Rivas C., and Benitez J. 2005. Phenotypic characterization of BRCA1 and BRCA2 tumors based in a tissue microarray study with 37 immunohistochemical markers. *Breast Cancer Res. Treat.* **90:** 5.

Perou C.M., Sorlie T., Eisen M.B., van de Rijn M., Jeffrey S.S., Rees C.A., Pollack J.R., Ross D.T., Johnsen H., Akslen L.A.F., O., Pergamenschikov A., Williams C., Zhu S.X., Lonning P.E., Borresen Dale A.L., Brown P.O., and Botstein D. 2000. Molecular portraits of human breast tumours. *Nature* **406:** 747.

Richardson A.L., Wang Z.C., De Nicolo A., Lu X., Brown M., Miron A., Liao X., Iglehart J.D., Livingston D.M., and Ganesan S. 2006. X chromosomal abnormalities in basal-like, human breast cancer. *Cancer Cell* **9:** 121.

Scully R., Xie A., and Nagaraju G. 2004. Molecular functions of BRCA1 in the DNA damage response. *Cancer Biol. Ther.* **3:** 521.

Sorlie T., Tibshirani R., Parker J., Hastie T., Marron J.S., Nobel A., Deng S., Johnsen H., Pesich R., Geisler S., Demeter J., Perou C.M., Lonning P.E., Brown P.O., Borresen-Dale A.L., and Botstein D. 2003. Repeated observation of breast tumor subtypes in independent gene expression data sets. *Proc. Natl. Acad. Sci.* **100:** 8418.

Sorlie T., Perou C.M., Tibshirani R., Aas T., Geisler S., Johnsen H., Hastie T., Eisen M.B., van de Rijn M., Jeffrey S.S., Thorsen T., Quist H., Matese J.C., Brown P.O., Botstein D., Eystein Lonning P., and Borresen-Dale A.L. 2001. Gene expression patterns of breast carcinomas distinguish tumor subclasses with clinical implications. *Proc. Natl. Acad. Sci.* **98:** 10869.

Turner J.M., Aprelikova O., Xu X., Wang R., Kim S., Chandramouli G.V.R., Barrett J.C., Burgoyne P.S., and Deng C.X. 2004. BRCA1, histone H2AX phosphorylation, and male meiotic sex chromosome inactivation. *Curr. Biol.* **14:** 2135.

Turner N., Tutt A., and Ashworth A. 2004. Hallmarks of 'BRCAness' in sporadic cancers. Nat. Rev. *Cancer* **4:** 814.

Venkitaraman A.R. 2002. Cancer susceptibility and the functions of BRCA1 and BRCA2. *Cell* **108:** 171.

———. 2003. A growing network of cancer-susceptibility genes. *N. Engl. J. Med.* **348:** 1917.

Wang Z.C., Lin M., Wei L.J., Li C., Miron A., Lodeiro G., Harris L., Ramaswamy S., Tanenbaum D.M., Meyerson M., Iglehart J.D., and Richardson A. 2004. Loss of heterozygosity and its correlation with expression profiles in subclasses of invasive breast cancers. *Cancer Res.* **64:** 64.

The ATM-dependent DNA Damage Signaling Pathway

R. KITAGAWA* AND M.B. KASTAN

*Department of Hematology-Oncology, St. Jude Children's Research Hospital,
Memphis, Tennessee 38105*

Many of the insights that we have gained into the mechanisms involved in cellular DNA damage response pathways have come from studies of human cancer susceptibility syndromes that are altered in DNA damage responses. ATM, the gene mutated in the disorder, ataxia-telangiectasia, is a protein kinase that is a central mediator of responses to DNA double-strand breaks in cells. Recent studies have elucidated the mechanism by which DNA damage activates the ATM kinase and initiates these critical cellular signaling pathways. The SMC1 protein appears to be a particularly important target of the ATM kinase, playing critical roles in controlling DNA replication forks and DNA repair after the damage. A major role for the NBS1 and BRCA1 proteins appears to be in the recruitment of an activated ATM kinase molecule to the sites of DNA breaks so that ATM can phosphorylate SMC1. Generation of mice and cells that are unable to phosphorylate SMC1 demonstrated the importance of SMC1 phosphorylation in the DNA-damage-induced S-phase checkpoint, in determining rates of repair of chromosomal breaks, and in determining cell survival after DNA damage. Focusing on ATM and SMC1, the molecular controls of these pathways is discussed.

Cells from patients with the cancer-prone disorder, ataxia telangiectasia, exhibit many abnormalities in cellular DNA damage responses. For example, these cells have defective G_1, intra-S-phase, and G_2/M checkpoints and exhibit decreased survival and increased chromosomal breakage in response to ionizing irradiation (IR). These observations suggest that the gene product that is defective in this disorder, ATM (ataxia telangiectasia, mutated), is an important component of cellular responses to DNA damage. Results from numerous laboratories generated over the past decade since the gene was cloned have shed light on the central role that the ATM protein plays in DNA damage responses (Shiloh and Kastan 2001). In this paper, we discuss what is known about the molecular mechanisms by which the ATM protein kinase is activated by DNA damage, then follow with an overview of the substrates of ATM that have been implicated in cellular responses to DNA damage including a more extensive discussion of one particular substrate, SMC1, that appears to be involved in influencing cell cycle progression, cell survival, and genetic integrity following DNA damage.

ACTIVATION OF THE ATM PROTEIN KINASE

Identification of the ATM gene by Shiloh and colleagues (Savitsky et al. 1995) revealed a very large gene that coded for a protein containing a phosphoinositide 3 (PI3) kinase-like sequence in its carboxyl terminus. Once it became technically feasible to generate wild-type and mutant full-length recombinant cDNAs and protein, we demonstrated that ATM was a bona fide protein kinase

with no detectable lipid kinase activity (Canman et al. 1998). Following exposure of human cells to IR, the cellular activity of ATM increases (Banin et al. 1998; Canman et al. 1998). The observation that ATM itself was a phosphoprotein whose phosphorylation increased while performing in vitro kinase reaction assays (Canman et al. 1998) focused our attention on ATM phosphorylation as a potential contributor to its increased cellular activity during DNA damage responses. A site of DNA-damage-induced phosphorylation in this 3056-amino acid protein was found to be Ser-1981 by incubating cells with [^{32}P]orthophosphate, immunoprecipitating ATM protein, identifying one primary phosphopeptide during two-dimensional gel analysis after proteolytic degradation, followed by manual Edman degradation of proteolyzed peptides (Bakkenist and Kastan 2003). Ser-1981 is located in the amino terminus of the FAT domain (a domain shared by FRAP, ATM, and TRRAP) of ATM (Fig. 1A). The FAT domain is a region of approximately 500 amino acids that has some conservation among members of the PI3 kinase family of proteins (Bosotti et al. 2000).

We generated a rabbit polyclonal antibody specific for phosphorylated Ser-1981 in order to begin characterization of the functional role of this phosphorylation event. The kinetics and quantitation of the phosphorylation turned out to be quite extraordinary (Bakkenist and Kastan 2003). More than 50% of all cellular ATM is phosphorylated on Ser-1981 in less than 5 minutes after exposure to doses of IR as low as 0.5 Gy (Fig. 1B). The presence of phosphorylated ATM could be detected at doses as low as 0.1 Gy, which should theoretically induce approximately four DNA strand breaks per cellular genome on average. Since ATM phosphorylation was also induced by the introduction of DNA strand breaks following transfection of the restriction enzyme I-*Sce1*, ATM was responding to DNA breakage rather than to some other effect of irradiation on cells. Thus, ATM

*Present address: Department of Molecular Pharmacology, St. Jude Children's Research Hospital, 322 N. Lauderdale Street, Memphis, Tennessee 38105.

A

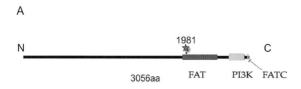

B

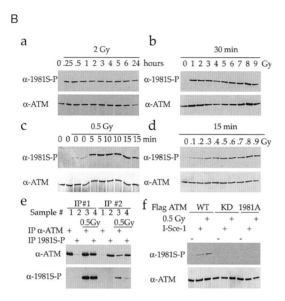

Figure 1. Autophosphorylation of the ATM kinase. (*A*) Schematic representation of the domains of ATM illustrating the approximate location of the Ser-1981 with the star. (*B*) Kinetics, stoichiometry, and detection sensitivity of ATM phosphorylation. (*a,b*) Phosphorylation of Ser-1981 is maximal within 5 min after exposure to IR. Exponentially growing primary fibroblasts were exposed to 0.5 or 2 Gy IR. ATM immunoprecipitation was performed at the times indicated, and the levels of phosphorylation at Ser-1981 and total immunoprecipitated ATM were assessed by immunoblotting. (*c,d*) Phosphorylation of Ser-1981 is maximal at about 0.4 Gy of IR. ATM was immunoprecipitated from exponentially growing primary fibroblasts 30 min after various doses of IR, and the levels of phosphorylation at Ser-1981 and total ATM were determined by immunoblotting. (*e*) Over 50% of ATM is phosphorylated within 15 min following irradiation at 0.5 Gy. Exponentially growing primary fibroblasts were exposed to 0 or 0.5 Gy IR, and lysates were subjected to sequential immunoprecipitation with conventional anti-ATM or anti-ATMS1981p antibody followed by conventional anti-ATM antibody. The amount of ATM immunoprecipitated was determined by anti-ATM immunoblotting, and the specificity and completeness of ATMS1981p immunoprecipitation were confirmed by anti-ATMS1981p immunoblotting. (*f*) The anti-ATMS1981p antibody can detect the presence of a few DNA breaks in the human genome. Constructs expressing Flag-tagged wild-type ATM, ATMkd, or ATMS1981A were cotransfected with a construct encoding the restriction enzyme I-*Sce1* into GM00637 cells that had integrated two copies of a plasmid containing the sequence cut by I-*Sce1*. As a control, ATM was immunoprecipitated from irradiated cells (0.5 Gy for 30 min). Phosphorylation of Ser-1981 and total ATM were assessed by immunoblotting with anti-ATMS1981p or anti-Flag. (Reprinted, with permission, from Bakkenist and Kastan 2003 [© Nature Publishing Group].)

phosphorylation after DNA damage was extraordinarily rapid, extensive, and sensitive.

The next question to ask was what kinase phosphorylated ATM following IR. Although an unbiased schema

was used to identify the phosphorylation site, the Ser-1981 site was a perfect ATM kinase consensus target (Kim et al. 1999). Thus, it was likely that ATM was either phosphorylated by a family member, such as ATR or DNA-PK, with similar target recognition, or we were observing an autophosphorylation event. Using a variety of approaches, we were able to show that the IR-induced phosphorylation required ATM kinase activity and that this was indeed an autophosphorylation event (Bakkenist and Kastan 2003).

To determine the physiological role of ATM S1981 phosphorylation, we generated an ATM mutant in which the Ser-1981 residue was replaced with alanine (ATMS1981A) so that IR-induced phosphorylation could not occur. Initially, we observed that the ATMS1981A mutant had normal in vitro kinase activity (Bakkenist and Kastan 2003), a result that seemed disappointing since it suggested that this phosphorylation event was not involved in the activation of the ATM kinase following IR. However, the ATMS1981A mutant had no activity in cells, since it failed to complement AT cells and had dominant-inhibitory effects in irradiated cells containing normal endogenous ATM. The reason for this apparent discrepancy between the in vitro and in vivo activities of the ATM S19181A mutant became clear when we observed that an isolated ATM kinase domain bound tightly to a fragment of ATM containing the ATM autophosphorylation site (amino acid residues 1961–2046) in *Escherichia coli*. If S1981 was mutated to alanine, the kinase domain still bound to this fragment, but if this serine was mutated to phosphorylation-mimic mutants such as aspartic acid or glutamic acid, the kinase domain could no longer bind to the S1981 domain. These observations led to a model where the kinase domain of ATM binds to this internal domain of ATM containing Ser-1981, but only when the serine residue is not phosphorylated. This could occur either because ATM exists in the cell as a homodimer or because the kinase domain folds over and binds to the S1981 domain in the same ATM molecule. We went on to demonstrate that ATM is present in unirradiated cells as a homodimer and that exposure of cells to IR resulted in a dissociation of this dimer. If one molecule of the dimer could not be phosphorylated on S1981, either because one molecule was mutated to be kinase-dead or because the S1981 site was mutated to alanine, then IR did not cause a dissociation of the dimer. This observation, combined with the autophosphorylation results, led to a model in which ATM is inactive in unstressed cells because the kinase domain is blocked by its binding to the internal S1981 domain and IR induces an intermolecular autophosphorylation event that causes dissociation of the ATM homodimer and release of an active ATM kinase.

Although the mechanism by which cellular ATM activity was increased following DNA damage was explained by this model, it remained unclear why intermolecular autophosphorylation of ATM was initiated following the introduction of DNA strand breaks. We reasoned that ATM might not need to go to the DNA strand break itself in order to be activated. This concept arose from the fact that ATM was activated so rapidly and

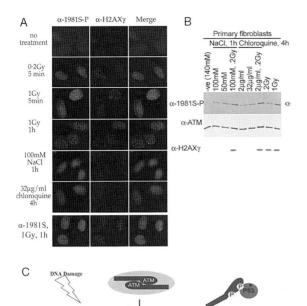

Figure 2. Activation of the ATM kinase independent of binding to DNA DSBs. (*A*) Primary fibroblasts grown on glass slides were irradiated (0.2 or 1 Gy) and allowed to recover for 5 min or 1 hr, incubated in hypotonic buffer containing 100 mM for 1 hr, or treated with chloroquine for 4 hr. Cells were fixed, and immunofluorescence for H2AXγ, ATMS1981p, and ATM(S1981) was assessed. (*B*) Exponentially growing fibroblasts were incubated in hypotonic (100 mM or 50 mM NaCl) buffer for 1 hr or in chloroquine for 4 hr. ATM was immunoprecipitated, and the levels of phosphorylated ATM, total ATM, and H2AXγ were determined by immunoblotting. No cell death was observed in chloroquine or in the hypotonic conditions, and all cells recovered when returned to isotonic conditions. (*C*) Schematic model of ATM activation after irradiation. DNA strand breaks lead to an alteration of chromatin structures that induce intermolecular autophosphorylations of an ATM dimer on Ser-1981, and dissociation of the previously inert dimer. Active ATM monomers are then free to migrate to and phosphorylate substrates such as Nbs1 and p53. (Reprinted, with permission, from Bakkenist and Kastan 2003 [© Nature Publishing Group].)

so completely after the introduction of so few DNA breaks. We postulated that one way in which ATM intermolecular autophosphorylation could be responding to DNA breaks at a distance was that the breaks were causing a change in higher-order chromatin structure through release of structural constraints by breaking the phosphodiester backbone. It was challenging to design experiments to test the hypothesis that ATM can be activated by alterations in higher-order chromatin structures, but we found that treatment of cells with either the topoisomerase inhibitor chloroquine or hypotonic buffer, both of which alter chromatin structure without generating detectable DNA breaks, induced phosphorylation of ATM at Ser-1981 (Fig. 2A,B) (Bakkenist and Kastan 2003).

More recently, we have observed that treatment of non-replicating G0 fibroblasts with the topoisomerase I poison, camptothecin, also results in ATM activation (C.J. Bakkenist and M.B. Kastan, unpubl.). In the absence of DNA replication, this drug treatment induces no DNA strand breaks, thus providing another example of ATM activation in the absence of DNA breakage. Immunofluorescence assays using the anti-S1981 phosphoantibody were also consistent with the model of ATM activation not requiring binding to DNA breaks. Following IR, immunostaining reveals a diffuse distribution of phospho-ATM in the first few minutes after IR and then accumulation in foci, presumably at the sites of DNA breaks. However, following the hypotonic swelling or chloroquine treatments, phosphorylated ATM remains diffusely distributed throughout the nucleus, and no foci are ever seen. These results are all consistent with a model in which ATM activation is not dependent on direct binding of ATM to DNA double-strand breaks (DSBs) but instead results from changes in the structure of chromatin. Our current model of IR-induced ATM activation proposes that DNA breaks cause an alteration in some aspect of higher-order chromatin structure which in turn induces a conformational change in ATM that causes intermolecular autophosphorylation of Ser-1981 in the ATM dimer and consequent dimer dissociation (Fig. 2C). Active ATM monomers are then free to interact with and phosphorylate downstream targets of the signaling pathway, such as Nbs1 and p53.

Interestingly, in addition to Nbs1 protein being a substrate of ATM, the Mre11/Rad50/Nbs1 (MRN) complex appears to be quantitatively important for ATM activation following IR (but not following many other cellular stresses) (Carson et al. 2003; Mochan et al. 2003; Uziel et al. 2003; Kitagawa et al. 2004). How the MRN complexes influence ATM activation after IR remains to be elucidated, but this observation by itself does not necessarily mean that the ATM dimer goes to DNA breaks to get activated; MRN could be influencing the chromatin structure changes that occur following IR and thus influence ATM activation directly. Once activated, it is clear that MRN is important for recruiting the activated ATM to the DNA break (Kitagawa et al. 2004). The fact that other stresses, such as hypotonic swelling, do not require MRN for ATM activation also demonstrates that binding of ATM dimers to DNA breaks is not required for ATM activation.

Lee and Paull (2005) recently developed an elegant in vitro assay to assess ATM activation. Using a gradient analysis, they confirmed our model and the work of Unsal-Kucmaz and Sancar (2004) by demonstrating that ATM exists as a dimer and that activation associated with S1981 phosphorylation results in dimer dissociation. The major distinction between our model and the results described using this in vitro assay is that they concluded that S1981 phosphorylation was not required for ATM activation because the S1981A mutant was already active in vitro. Since we found that the S1981 mutant was active in vitro but had no cellular activity, it seems more appropriate to draw the conclusion that their in vitro model for testing ATM activation, dissociation, and activity, although elegant, does not accurately reproduce the in vivo situation for initiating ATM activation. It is likely that this results from an artifactual dissociation of the ATM dimer under these in vitro conditions, even in the absence of S1981 phosphorylation. The fact that there was plenty of ATM monomer in their preparations of S1981A mutant ATM would be consistent with this conclusion.

PHOSPHORYLATION OF SUBSTRATES BY ATM

When cells are irradiated, ATM is quickly activated, and it phosphorylates many substrates (Kastan and Lim 2000). Phosphorylation of p53, mdm2, and Chk2 activates the G_1 checkpoint (Canman et al. 1998; Ahn et al. 2000; Matsuoka et al. 2000; Maya et al. 2001). Phosphorylation of Nbs1, FancD2, and Ser-1387 of Brca1 is required for the S-phase checkpoint (Lim et al. 2000; Taniguchi et al. 2002; Xu et al. 2002b), and phosphorylation of Rad17 and Ser-1423 of Brca1 is involved in the G_2 checkpoint (Bao et al. 2001; Xu et al. 2002b). Recently, we identified SMC1 (structural maintenance of chromosomes 1) as an ATM substrate. We also identified two ATM phosphorylation sites on SMC1 and found that the phosphorylation of this substrate by ATM is required for the proper activation of the S-phase checkpoint (Kim et al. 2002; Yazdi et al. 2002). To identify which checkpoint and which target are important for determining cellular radiosensitivity, we mutated selected phosphorylation sites in the various proteins and were somewhat surprised to be able to demonstrate that neither the G_1 checkpoint, intra-S-phase checkpoint, nor early G_2 checkpoint affected cellular survival after irradiation (Slichenmyer et al. 1993; Lim et al. 2000; Xu et al. 2002a,b). Interestingly, the only target of ATM in which mutation of the phosphorylation sites affected cellular radiosensitivity was SMC1 (Kim et al. 2002; Kitagawa et al. 2004). Subsequent comments focus just on the role of SMC1 and its phosphorylation in DNA damage responses.

SMC1 IS AN ATM SUBSTRATE AND PARTICIPATES IN CELLULAR RESPONSES TO DNA DAMAGE

SMC1 is a member of the structural maintenance of chromosomes family (Strunnikov and Jessberger 1999). It was originally identified in budding yeast as a component of the cohesin complex (Michaelis et al. 1997), where it exists as a heterodimer with Smc3 (Anderson et al. 2002; Haering et al. 2002). This SMC1–SMC3 heterodimer has also been identified in the RC-1 complex, which is a mammalian protein complex involved in DNA recombination (Jessberger et al. 1996; Stursberg et al. 1999). These findings provided the first suggestion that SMC1 might be involved in DNA recombination and DNA repair. Unexpectedly, we found that SMC1 was phosphorylated on two sites, Ser-957 and Ser-966, in response to IR in an ATM-dependent manner (Fig. 3A,B) (Kim et al. 2002; Yazdi et al. 2002). Both sites were also phosphorylated in response to ultraviolet (UV) light or

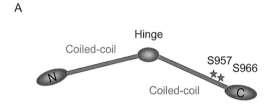

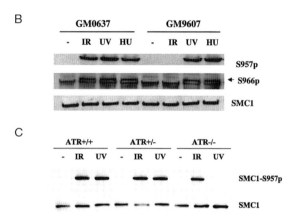

Figure 3. DNA damage-induced phosphorylation of Ser-957 and Ser-966 of SMC1. (*A*) Schematic representation of the domains of Smc1 illustrating the approximate location of the Ser-957 and Ser-966 sites with the stars. (*B*) ATM-dependent and -independent phosphorylation of SMC1 on Ser-957 and Ser-966. Immunoblot analyses using the two phosphoserine-specific antibodies (*top* and *middle*) or an anti-SMC1 antibody (K1; *bottom*) on SMC1 protein from normal (WT; GM0637) or A-T (GM9607) fibroblasts treated with ionizing irradiation (IR; 10 Gy, 2 hr), ultraviolet light (UV; 50 Jm-2, 2 hr) or hydroxyurea (HU; 1 mM, 24 hr). The arrow (*middle*) points to the band specifically recognized by the antiphosphoserine 966 antibody (note a nonspecific band runs just below the S966-p band). (*C*) ATR-dependent phosphorylation of S957 of SMC1. Immunoblot analyses using a phosphoserine-specific antibody against SMC1S957p or an anti-SMC1 antibody (K1; *bottom*) on SMC1 protein from ATR$^{+/+}$ (HCT116), ATR$^{+/}$ (HCT116 flox), or ATR$^{/}$ (HCT flox infected with AdCre virus) cells 30 min after treatment with 0.06 J/m2 UV radiation. (*B*, Reprinted with permission from Kim et al. 2002; *C*, reprinted, with permission, from Garg et al. 2004.)

hydroxyurea treatment in an ATM-independent manner (Kim et al. 2002); in this setting, the related kinase ATR was phosphorylating these same two serines (Fig. 3C) (Garg et al. 2004). Therefore, Ser-957 and Ser-966 are phosphorylated after virtually every type of DNA damage, suggesting that phosphorylation of SMC1 is important in many cellular stress responses.

Although we had previously investigated the functional significance of phosphorylation events in NBS1 or BRCA1 by complementing NBS1-deficient cells or BRCA1-deficient cells with phosphorylation-mutant constructs, we could not use this approach to study SMC1 phosphorylation because there are no SMC1-null cell lines available. To explore the physiological significance of SMC1 phosphorylation, we overexpressed recombi-

nant SMC1 cDNA constructs in which Ser-957 and Ser-966 were replaced with alanine residues such that DNA-damage-induced phosphorylation of those sites does not occur, and asked whether dominant-negative effects could be seen with overexpression of this ectopic mutant protein. Cells overexpressing mutant SMC1 exhibited increased radiosensitivity and an intra-S-phase checkpoint defect (Kim et al. 2002), thus implicating these phosphorylation events as determinants of these cellular endpoints.

SMC1 IS "DOWNSTREAM" IN THE ATM SIGNALING PATHWAY

We were surprised to find that radiation-induced phosphorylation of Ser-957 and Ser-966 in SMC1 did not occur in cells lacking full-length NBS1 or BRCA1 proteins and could be restored by complementation of these cells with full-length constructs of their respective mutant proteins (Kim et al. 2002). These effects did not result from a lack of ATM activation in the mutant cells, leading us to hypothesize that NBS1 and BRCA1 played a role in recruiting activated ATM to sites of DNA DSBs, and that once there, the activated ATM could phosphorylate SMC1. To test this theory, we analyzed the subcellular localization of phosphorylated ATM in cells lacking full-length NBS1 or full-length BRCA1. In the presence of full-length NBS1 and BRCA1, phosphorylated ATM localized at the sites of DNA strand breaks after IR, but in the absence of either full-length protein, ATM was activated but remained diffusely distributed throughout the nucleus and did not form foci (Kitagawa et al. 2004). These observations suggested that NBS1 and BRCA1 are required for efficient recruitment and/or retention of activated ATM to the sites of DNA breaks, where the activated ATM can then phosphorylate substrates at the break, such as SMC1, resulting in proper activation of the DNA-damage-induced signaling pathway. Consistent with this hypothesis, Lee and Paull (2004) demonstrated that the MRN complex stabilizes the binding of ATM to substrates in vitro and that the MRN complex is required for in vitro binding of purified ATM to linearized DNA molecules immobilized on beads (Lee and Paull 2005).

The only insights we had at this point about the functional role of SMC1 phosphorylation had come from the studies overexpressing the phospho-mutant SMC1 constructs. To more effectively study the functional role of SMC1 phosphorylation, we generated mice and cells that contained normally regulated SMC1, but where the SMC1 protein could not be phosphorylated because of mutation of the target serines. In mouse fibroblasts containing Smc1S957AS966A, IR-induced phosphorylation of Atm, p53, Nbs1, and Brca1 were all comparable to that seen in cells containing wild-type Smc1 (Fig. 4A) (Kitagawa et al. 2004). However, as expected, no phosphorylation of Smc1 was detectable (Fig. 4A). Despite the absence of phosphorylated Smc1 at the sites of DNA strand breaks, we easily detected foci containing activated (phosphorylated) Atm, H2AXγ, Nbs1, 53BP1, Chk2T68p, and Brca1 (Fig. 5). Thus, SMC1 phosphory-

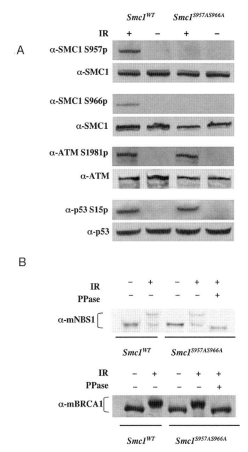

Figure 4. IR-induced phosphorylation of ATM and its target proteins in the absence of phosphorylation of SMC1. (*A*) Wild-type (*Smc1WT*) or *Smc1S957AS966A* immortalized mouse fibroblast cells were exposed to 0 Gy (IR–) or 10 Gy (IR+) of IR and cellular extracts were prepared 30 min later. Whole-cell lysates were subjected to immunoblotting with antibodies as indicated. (*B*) Thirty minutes after exposure to 0 (–) or 10 (+) Gy of IR, whole-cell lysates were prepared from wild-type, or mutant knock-in fibroblasts were immunoblotted with anti-mouse Nbs1 or Brca1 antibodies. Duplicate samples of cell lysates from irradiated knock-in cells were treated with protein phosphatase (PPase+) prior to electrophoresis. (Reprinted, with permission, from Kitagawa et al. 2004.)

lation was dependent on ATM, Nbs1, and Brca1, but nothing in the pathway appeared to be dependent on the phosphorylation of SMC1, thus placing SMC1 phosphorylation at the bottom of the ATM DNA damage response pathway characterized to date (Kitagawa et al. 2004).

However, if we were to conclude that SMC1 phosphorylation played any critical role in this DNA damage response pathway, we needed to demonstrate that the cells containing unphosphorylatable SMC1 had some defect in DNA damage responses. Consistent with results from studies using human cells overexpressing SMC1 mutant proteins, we found that the Smc1S957AS966A cells both lacked the IR-induced intra-S-phase checkpoint (Fig. 6A) and were hypersensitive to DNA damaging agents such as IR and methylmethane sulfonate (MMS) (Fig. 6B,C). Furthermore, we found that these "knock-in" cells exhibited decreased removal of chromosome gaps and breaks

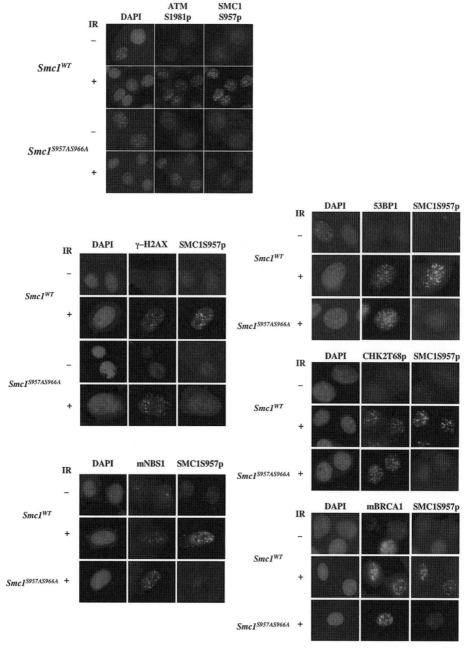

Figure 5. Smc1 phosphorylation is not required for IR-induced formation of foci containing phospho-Atm, H2AX, Nbs1, 53BP1, phosphorylated Chk2, or Brca1. Wild-type (*Smc1WT*) or *Smc1* phosphorylation mutant knockin (*Smc1S957AS966A*) fibroblast cells were fixed with 4% paraformaldehyde 30 min after 0 Gy (–) 10 Gy (+) of IR, then subjected to immunofluorescence microscopy. (*A*) Staining with antibodies recognizing phosphorylated Atm or Smc1. (*B*) Staining with antibodies recognizing H2AX, Nbs1, 53BP1, phosphorylated Chk2, Brca1, and phosphorylated Smc1. For costaining of phosphorylated Smc1 with Brca1, rabbit polyclonal anti-Ser957p antibody was used. (Reprinted, with permission, from Kitagawa et al. 2004.)

after IR, a phenotype shared with cells lacking ATM (Fig. 6D). This finding suggests that a DNA repair activity is reduced in Smc1S957AS966A cells, at least during the first hour after DNA breaks are introduced.

Phosphorylation of Smc1 at Ser-957 and Ser-966 thus appears to be a crucial downstream event in the DNA-damage-induced signaling pathway and may be required for proper activation of DNA repair activity to maintain optimal cell viability after DNA damage. As shown in the

model we propose (Fig. 7), an ordered dependency of events occurs after the initiation of the DNA-damage-induced signaling pathway. Ionizing radiation introduces DNA breaks into genomic DNA, resulting in some high-order structural changes in chromatin. (This aspect is admittedly speculative but is most consistent with our data.) The chromatin change generates a signal that induces intermolecular autophosphorylation of ATM. The phosphorylated ATM monomer is then released from its inac-

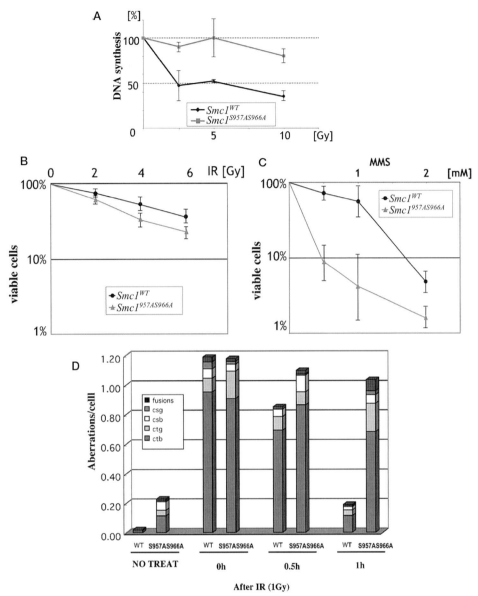

Figure 6. Radiation response abnormalities in *Smc1S957AS966A* cells. (*A*) Defect in the S-phase checkpoint. Mouse embryonic fibroblasts (MEFs) derived from wild-type (*Smc1WT*) or *Smc1S957AS966A* embryos were assessed for inhibition of DNA synthesis 30 min after exposure to indicated doses of IR. Error bars are average of triplicate samples. (*B*) Increased sensitivity to IR. Wild-type or *Smc1S957AS966A* immortalized mouse fibroblast cells were plated in 6-well culture dishes and irradiated with the indicated doses of IR. Cell viability was assessed 72 hr after treatment and is plotted as the percent viable cells relative to results for untreated control cultures. Each point represents the mean of three samples, with error bars showing standard deviation. (*C*) Increased sensitivity to alkylating agents. Wild-type or *Smc1* mutant knockin immortalized mouse fibroblast cells were plated in 6-well culture dishes, and treated with methylmethane sulfonate (MMS) for 1 hr. Cell viability was assessed 72 hr after treatment, and is plotted as the percent viable cells relative to results for untreated control cultures. Each point represents the mean of three samples, with error bars showing standard deviation. (*D*) Defect in chromosomal repair after IR. MEFs derived from wild-type or *Smc1S957AS966A* embryos were irradiated with 1 Gy of IR, then treated with colcemid at indicated times after irradiation. Chromosome aberrations were scored in 100 metaphase spreads of each sample, and numbers of chromosome gaps (csg), chromosome breaks (csb), chromatid gaps (ctg), and chromatid breaks (ctb) per cell were charted. (Reprinted, with permission, from Kitagawa et al. 2004.)

tive dimer complex and phosphorylates nucleoplasmic substrates such as p53. At the same time, proteins migrate in a highly ordered manner to the DSB sites to form foci of protein complexes that include SMC1. The recruitment of previously activated ATM to the DSBs depends on the presence of NBS1 and BRCA1. Once the activated ATM binds to the focus complex, the ATM substrates can be phosphorylated. Phosphorylation of these proteins is required for proper activation of the DNA repair pathway and the cell cycle checkpoint pathways, and phosphorylation of SMC1 is specifically critical for cell survival and maintenance of optimal chromosomal stability.

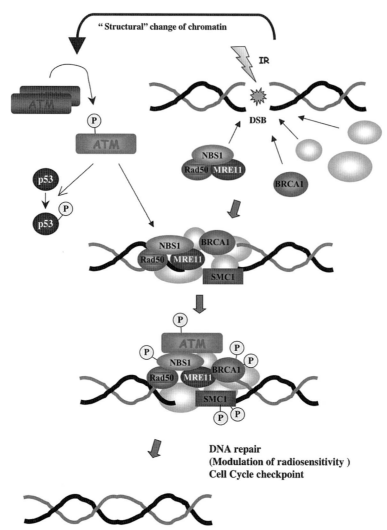

Figure 7. Proposed model for an IR-induced signaling pathway. Chromatin structure changes caused by DNA breakage or other mechanisms lead to intermolecular autophosphorylation of ATM dimers, resulting in release of phosphorylated and active ATM monomers. If DNA strand breaks are present, several proteins, including NBS1 and BRCA1, are recruited to the sites of the breaks independent of the ATM activation process. After activation, monomeric ATM can phosphorylate nucleoplasmic substrates, like p53, and if NBS1 and BRCA1 have localized to DNA breaks, activated ATM is recruited to the break. At the DNA break, activated ATM can phosphorylate substrates, including SMC1. The phosphorylation of SMC1 reduces chromosomal breakage and enhances cell survival. (Reprinted, with permission, from Kitagawa et al. 2004.)

SMC1 AND MECHANISMS OF DNA REPAIR

Although the results described above strongly implicate SMC1 and its phosphorylation in cellular responses to DNA damage and to DNA repair specifically, we have no insights yet as to the exact repair mechanisms that SMC1 might influence. Based on known repair mechanisms and characterized aspects of the cohesin complex, the following discussion speculates on potential roles for SMC1 in DNA repair processes. DNA DSBs can be repaired by either nonhomologous end-joining (NHEJ) or homologous recombination (HR). HR repair of DNA DSBs requires an intact DNA sequence homologous to the one needing repair to serve as a template. Because the sister chromatid would be the preferential template for repair, it has been suspected that the sister chromatid cohesin complex plays a role in efficient HR repair of DNA

DSBs, at least in yeast. Mutants of the cohesin proteins such as *scc1/rad21* in yeast are hypersensitive to γ-irradiation (Birkenbihl and Subramani 1992), and we showed that a hypomorphic mutation of *smc1* causes yeast to be sensitive to various types of DNA damage (Kim et al. 2002). Sjogren and Nasmyth (2001) demonstrated defective DSB repair activity of cohesin mutants including *scc1*, *scc2*, and *smc1* by using pulse-field gel electrophoresis to monitor induction and disappearance of DSBs in synchronized yeast cells. Their analysis revealed that cohesin proteins are specifically required for postreplicative HR repair of chromosomal DNA. In addition, two groups have demonstrated the recruitment of components of the cohesin complex to the sites of DNA DSBs generated by induction of HO endonuclease (Strom et al. 2004; Unal et al. 2004). Both groups used chromatin immunoprecipitation (ChIP) assays to show the accumulation of cohesin proteins at the single HO site when a break was introduced. The DNA-break-specific cohesin domain expanded to an approximately 100-kb chromosomal region around the lesion, and the formation of that domain required the phosphorylation of H2AXγ.

The efficiency of the DNA DSB repair pathway, which is distinct from the HR repair pathway, also depends on Smc1. Schar et al. (2004) demonstrated that the loss of functional Smc1 reduced the efficiency of NHEJ repair in episomal DSBs and substantially increased the frequency of errors in the remaining end-joining activity in yeast. The *smc1* hypomorphic mutant genetically interacted with *dnl4*, a factor involved in the NHEJ pathway, and *rad54*, a factor required for the HR pathway. Smc1 negatively regulates the inhibitory effects of Rad52 and Rad54 on NHEJ activity. These genetic findings suggest that Smc1 coordinates the appropriate balance between the HR and NHEJ repair pathways. However, whether the role of Smc1 is distinct from that of other cohesin proteins and whether Smc1 always forms a heterodimer with Smc3 or is always a component of the cohesin complex remain unknown. Thus, fully functional Smc1 is required for a proper DNA damage response in yeast, presumably as a component of the functional cohesin complex. Although the phosphorylation sites identified in human SMC1 are not conserved in budding yeast, a fundamental mechanism by which this ATM substrate contributes to the efficient repair of DNA DSBs could be conserved.

To study the molecular mechanism(s) underlying the phosphorylation events at Ser-957 and Ser-966 of human SMC1, it was important to determine whether phosphorylation at those sites affects the cohesion function of the sister chromatid. SMC proteins have globular domains at their amino and carboxyl termini, which are separated by two long stretches of coiled-coil domains. The coiled-coil domains are connected to the third globular domain, which is called the "hinge" due to its flexible feature (Fig. 3A). SMC proteins form V-shaped molecules by dimerizing via their central hinge domain. In eukaryotes, different SMC proteins heterodimerize in specific pairs: Smc1–Smc3, Smc2–Smc4, and Smc5–Smc6 (Hirano and Hirano 2002; Haering and Nasmyth 2003). In the cohesin complex, Smc1 and Smc3 associate with non-SMC subunits Scc1/Rad21 and Scc3 (in humans, SA1 and SA2 replace Scc3). Scc1/Rad21 binds to the head of Smc3 via its amino-terminal domain and to that of Smc1 via its carboxy-terminal domain (Haering et al. 2002). Scc3 associates with Smc1–Smc3 by interacting with the central domain of Scc1/Rad21. SMC1 phosphorylation sites, Ser-957 and Ser-966, are located at the carboxy-terminal end of the coiled-coil domain, near the carboxy-terminal globular domain (Fig. 3A). IR-induced phosphorylation of those sites does not affect the interaction of SMC1 with SMC3 or RAD21 (Kim et al. 2002; R. Kitagawa and M.B. Kastan, unpubl.). Consistent with the finding that the phosphorylation status of SMC1 did not affect the formation of the cohesin complex, mouse Smc1S957AS966A cells do not exhibit any noticeable cohesion defects (e.g., premature sister chromatid separation or mitotic-checkpoint-dependent delay of mitosis)

(R. Kitagawa and M.B. Kastan, unpubl.).

Although the phosphorylation of SMC1 has no noticeable effect on the formation of the cohesin complex, it may affect the association of cohesin with chromosomes. Based on a recent finding that TEV-protease-dependent cleavage of the Smc3 coiled-coil domain triggers the dissociation of cohesin from chromosomes, it has been proposed that cohesin forms a ring-like structure that encircles two sister chromatids (Gruber et al. 2003). The ATPase activity of the head domain in Smc proteins is required for its binding to Scc1/Rad21 and results in the formation of the cohesin ring, which enables cohesin to associate with chromosomes (Arumugam et al. 2003; Weitzer et al. 2003). The cohesin ring model in which the association of cohesin with chromosomes is possibly topological in nature rather than protein–DNA binding reasonably explains why the separase-mediated cleavage of Scc1/Rad21 at metaphase–anaphase transition is sufficient to trigger the dissociation of the cohesin complex from chromosomes. Furthermore, topological association of the cohesin ring with chromatin would allow cohesin considerable mobility. This flexibility in movement explains the instantaneous formation of DSB-specific cohesin complexes. Again, Smc1S957AS966A cells do not exhibit any noticeable cohesin defects during the normal cell cycle progression, a finding that suggests that the phosphorylation of SMC1 does not affect the association of the cohesin complex with chromosomes at the cohesions. However, assuming that the formation of DSB-specific cohesin complex is a common event in eukaryotic cells, phosphorylation status of SMC1 might specifically affect the establishment or stability of the complex at the sites of DSBs.

In addition to being a component of the cohesin complex, SMC1 is a DNA-binding protein (Akhmedov et al. 1998). Specific binding of the carboxy-terminal region of Smc1 to highly structured DNA (e.g., stem-loop-structured DNA or DNA-containing AT-rich sequences) has been demonstrated in vitro by using purified recombinant protein. As described above, SMC1 is phosphorylated at two serine residues in the carboxy-terminal end of the coiled-coil domain. Therefore, its phosphorylation status may affect the DNA-binding activity of SMC1 via its carboxy-terminal domain. Although the physiological role of this DNA-binding activity of SMC1 has not been elucidated, it may be required for the DNA damage response.

Zheng et al. (2000) showed that the DNA-binding activity of Smc1 affinity-purified from yeast cells was enhanced when human Hec1 and Rb protein were artificially expressed in yeast cells. Human SMC1 also coimmunoprecipitates with Rb and human Hec1 from human T24 cell lysate. Thus, the interaction between SMC1 and DNA is modulated by SMC1's association with non-cohesin proteins. Phosphorylation of SMC1 might affect the association of the cohesin complex with chromosomes by altering the interaction between the complex and other proteins such as Hec1.

Another attractive model for the mechanism by which phosphorylation of SMC1 plays a role in DNA damage

response is that phosphorylation affects the binding of
SMC1 to proteins required for DNA repair activities
(e.g., DNA-modifying enzymes) and plays a role in recruitment of those enzymes to the sites of DNA lesions.
Castano et al. (1996) identified Trf4, a member of DNA
polymerase sigma protein family, as an SMC1 interactor
and showed its role in DNA damage response. Trf4 exhibits DNA polymerase activity (Wang et al. 2000) and
RNA polyadenylase activity (Saitoh et al. 2002). Trf4
may be recruited to the sites of DNA damage via its interaction with Smc1, and that interaction may be regulated by the phosphorylation status of Smc1.

CONCLUSIONS

The Atm protein kinase is a central mediator of cellular
responses to aberrant introduction of DNA strand breaks.
When such breaks are introduced in cells, Atm is rapidly
activated by intermolecular phosphorylation at Ser-1981,
which causes dissociation of the Atm homodimer. The activated Atm is then free to circulate in the cell and phosphorylate substrates, such as p53 in the nucleoplasm. Full-
length Nbs1 and Brca1 proteins are required to attract or
retain the activated Atm at the site of the DNA break.
Once Atm is brought to the break, it can phosphorylate
substrates at the break, with SMC1 appearing to be a critical substrate for maximizing cell survival and minimizing
chromosomal aberrations. Although the phosphorylation
of SMC1 does not significantly affect the formation of the
cohesin complex, it may control the association of this
complex with a particular structure of chromosomes or
other repair proteins in cells after DNA damage is introduced. Identifying other proteins or DNA structures that
directly associate with SMC1 and analyzing whether the
phosphorylation status of SMC1 affects complex formation with those factors will help us further elucidate the
molecular mechanism by which phosphorylation of
SMC1 mediates the DNA repair pathway. The use of
Smc1S957AS966A cells will be a powerful and invaluable reagent in this pursuit.

REFERENCES

Ahn J.Y., Schwarz J.K., Piwnica-Worms H., and Canman C.E.
2000. Threonine 68 phosphorylation by ataxia telangiectasia
mutated is required for efficient activation of Chk2 in response to ionizing radiation. *Cancer Res.* **60:** 5934.
Akhmedov A.T., Frei C., Tsai-Pflugfelder M., Kemper B.,
Gasser S.M., and Jessberger R. 1998. Structural maintenance
of chromosomes protein C-terminal domains bind preferentially to DNA with secondary structure. *J. Biol. Chem.* **273:**
24088.
Anderson D.E., Losada A., Erickson H.P., and Hirano T. 2002.
Condensin and cohesin display different arm conformations
with characteristic hinge angles. *J. Cell Biol.* **156:** 419.
Arumugam P., Gruber S., Tanaka K., Haering C.H., Mechtler
K., and Nasmyth K. 2003. ATP hydrolysis is required for co-
hesin's association with chromosomes. *Curr. Biol.* **13:** 1941.
Bakkenist C.J. and Kastan M.B. 2003. DNA damage activates
ATM through intermolecular autophosphorylation and dimer
dissociation. *Nature* **421:** 499.
Banin S., Moyal L., Shieh S., Taya Y., Anderson C.W., Chessa
L., Smorodinsky N.I., Prives C., Reiss Y., Shiloh Y., and Ziv

Y. 1998. Enhanced phosphorylation of p53 by ATM in response to DNA damage. *Science* **281:** 1674.
Bao S., Tibbetts R.S., Brumbaugh K.M., Fang Y., Richardson
D.A., Ali A., Chen S.M., Abraham R.T., and Wang X.F.
2001. ATR/ATM-mediated phosphorylation of human Rad17
is required for genotoxic stress responses. *Nature* **411:** 969.
Birkenbihl R.P. and Subramani S. 1992. Cloning and characterization of rad21 an essential gene of *Schizosaccharomyces
pombe* involved in DNA double-strand-break repair. *Nucleic
Acids Res.* **20:** 6605.
Bosotti R., Isacchi A., and Sonnhammer E.L. 2000. FAT: A
novel domain in PIK-related kinases. *Trends Biochem. Sci.*
25: 225.
Canman C.E., Lim D.S., Cimprich K.A., Taya Y., Tamai K.,
Sakaguchi K., Appella E., Kastan M.B., and Siliciano J.D.
1998. Activation of the ATM kinase by ionizing radiation and
phosphorylation of p53. *Science* **281:** 1677.
Carson C.T., Schwartz R.A., Stracker T.H., Lilley C.E., Lee
D.V., and Weitzman M.D. 2003. The Mre11 complex is required for ATM activation and the G2/M checkpoint. *EMBO
J.* **22:** 6610.
Castano I.B., Brzoska P.M., Sadoff B.U., Chen H., and Christman M.F. 1996. Mitotic chromosome condensation in the
rDNA requires TRF4 and DNA topoisomerase I in *Saccharomyces cerevisiae. Genes Dev.* **10:** 2564.
Garg R., Callens S., Lim D.S., Canman C.E., Kastan M.B., and
Xu B. 2004. Chromatin association of rad17 is required for an
ataxia telangiectasia and rad-related kinase-mediated S-phase
checkpoint in response to low-dose ultraviolet radiation. *Mol.
Cancer Res.* **2:** 362.
Gruber S., Haering C.H., and Nasmyth K. 2003. Chromosomal
cohesin forms a ring. *Cell* **112:** 765.
Haering C.H. and Nasmyth K. 2003. Building and breaking
bridges between sister chromatids. *Bioessays* **25:** 1178.
Haering C.H., Lowe J., Hochwagen A., and Nasmyth K. 2002.
Molecular architecture of SMC proteins and the yeast cohesin
complex. *Mol. Cell* **9:** 773.
Hirano M. and Hirano T. 2002. Hinge-mediated dimerization of
SMC protein is essential for its dynamic interaction with
DNA. *EMBO J.* **21:** 5733.
Jessberger R., Riwar B., Baechtold H., and Akhmedov A.T.
1996. SMC proteins constitute two subunits of the mam-
malian recombination complex RC-1. *EMBO J.* **15:** 4061.
Kastan M.B. and Lim D.S. 2000. The many substrates and func-
tions of ATM. *Nat. Rev. Mol. Cell. Biol.* **1:** 179.
Kim S.T., Xu B., and Kastan M.B. 2002. Involvement of the co-
hesin protein, Smc1, in Atm-dependent and independent responses to DNA damage. *Genes Dev.* **16:** 560.
Kim S.T., Lim D.S., Canman C.E., and Kastan M.B. 1999. Substrate specificities and identification of putative substrates of
ATM kinase family members. *J. Biol. Chem.* **274:** 37538.
Kitagawa R., Bakkenist C.J., McKinnon P.J., and Kastan M.B.
2004. Phosphorylation of SMC1 is a critical downstream event
in the ATM-NBS1-BRCA1 pathway. *Genes Dev.* **18:** 1423.
Lee J.H. and Paull T.T. 2004. Direct activation of the ATM protein kinase by the Mre11/Rad50/Nbs1 complex. *Science* **304:**
93.
———. 2005. ATM activation by DNA double-strand breaks
through the Mre11-Rad50-Nbs1 complex. *Science* **308:** 551.
Lim D.S., Kim S.T., Xu B., Maser R.S., Lin J., Petrini J.H., and
Kastan M.B. 2000. ATM phosphorylates p95/nbs1 in an S-
phase checkpoint pathway. *Nature* **404:** 613.
Matsuoka S., Rotman G., Ogawa A., Shiloh Y., Tamai K., and
Elledge S.J. 2000. Ataxia telangiectasia-mutated phosphorylates Chk2 in vivo and in vitro. *Proc. Natl. Acad. Sci.* **97:**
10389.
Maya R., Balass M., Kim S.T., Shkedy D., Leal J.F., Shifman O.,
Moas M., Buschmann T., Ronai Z., Shiloh Y., Kastan M.B.,
Katzir E., and Oren M. 2001. ATM-dependent phosphoryla-
tion of Mdm2 on serine 395: Role in p53 activation by DNA
damage. *Genes Dev.* **15:** 1067.
Michaelis C., Ciosk R., and Nasmyth K. 1997. Cohesins: Chromosomal proteins that prevent premature separation of sister

chromatids. *Cell* **91**: 35.

Mochan T.A., Venere M., DiTullio R.A., Jr., and Halazonetis T.D. 2003. 53BP1 and NFBD1/MDC1-Nbs1 function in parallel interacting pathways activating ataxia-telangiectasia mutated (ATM) in response to DNA damage. *Cancer Res.* **63**: 8586.

Saitoh S., Chabes A., McDonald W.H., Thelander L., Yates J.R., and Russell P. 2002. Cid13 is a cytoplasmic poly(A) polymerase that regulates ribonucleotide reductase mRNA. *Cell* **109**: 563.

Savitsky K., Bar-Shira A., Gilad S., Rotman G., Ziv Y., Vanagaite L., Tagle D.A., Smith S., Uziel T., and Sfez S., et al. 1995. A single ataxia telangiectasia gene with a product similar to PI-3 kinase. *Science* **268**: 1749.

Schar P., Fasi M., and Jessberger R. 2004. SMC1 coordinates DNA double-strand break repair pathways. *Nucleic Acids Res.* **32**: 3921.

Shiloh Y. and Kastan M.B. 2001. ATM: Genome stability, neuronal development, and cancer cross paths. *Adv. Cancer Res.* **83**: 209.

Sjogren C. and Nasmyth K. 2001. Sister chromatid cohesion is required for postreplicative double-strand break repair in *Saccharomyces cerevisiae*. *Curr. Biol.* **11**: 991.

Slichenmyer W.J., Nelson W.G., Slebos R.J., and Kastan M.B. 1993. Loss of a p53-associated G1 checkpoint does not decrease cell survival following DNA damage. *Cancer Res.* **53**: 4164.

Strom L., Lindroos H.B., Shirahige K., and Sjogren C. 2004. Postreplicative recruitment of cohesin to double-strand breaks is required for DNA repair. *Mol. Cell* **16**: 1003.

Strunnikov A.V. and Jessberger R. 1999. Structural maintenance of chromosomes (SMC) proteins: Conserved molecular properties for multiple biological functions. *Eur. J. Biochem.* **263**: 6.

Stursberg S., Riwar B., and Jessberger R. 1999. Cloning and characterization of mammalian SMC1 and SMC3 genes and proteins, components of the DNA recombination complexes RC-1. *Gene* **228**: 1.

Taniguchi T., Garcia-Higuera I., Xu B., Andreassen P.R., Gregory R.C., Kim S.T., Lane W.S., Kastan M.B., and D'Andrea A.D. 2002. Convergence of the fanconi anemia and ataxia telangiectasia signaling pathways. *Cell* **109**: 459.

Unal E., Arbel-Eden A., Sattler U., Shroff R., Lichten M., Haber J.E., and Koshland D. 2004. DNA damage response pathway uses histone modification to assemble a double-strand break-specific cohesin domain. *Mol. Cell* **16**: 991.

Unsal-Kacmaz K. and Sancar A. 2004. Quaternary structure of ATR and effects of ATRIP and replication protein A on its DNA binding and kinase activities. *Mol. Cell. Biol.* **24**: 1292.

Uziel T., Lerenthal Y., Moyal L., Andegeko Y., Mittelman L., and Shiloh Y. 2003. Requirement of the MRN complex for ATM activation by DNA damage. *EMBO J.* **22**: 5612.

Wang Z., Castano I.B., De Las Penas A., Adams C., and Christman M.F. 2000. Pol kappa: A DNA polymerase required for sister chromatid cohesion. *Science* **289**: 774.

Weitzer S., Lehane C., and Uhlmann F. 2003. A model for ATP hydrolysis-dependent binding of cohesin to DNA. *Curr. Biol.* **13**: 1930.

Xu B., Kim S.T., Lim D.S., and Kastan M.B. 2002a. Two molecularly distinct G(2)/M checkpoints are induced by ionizing irradiation. *Mol. Cell. Biol.* **22**: 1049.

Xu B., O'Donnell A.H., Kim S.T., and Kastan M.B. 2002b. Phosphorylation of serine 1387 in Brca1 is specifically required for the Atm-mediated S-phase checkpoint after ionizing irradiation. *Cancer Res.* **62**: 4588.

Yazdi P.T., Wang Y., Zhao S., Patel N., Lee E.Y., and Qin J. 2002. SMC1 is a downstream effector in the ATM/NBS1 branch of the human S-phase checkpoint. *Genes Dev.* **16**: 571.

Zheng L., Chen Y., Riley D.J., Chen P.L., and Lee W.H. 2000. Retinoblastoma protein enhances the fidelity of chromosome segregation mediated by hsHec1p. *Mol. Cell. Biol.* **20**: 3529.

Single-Nucleotide Polymorphisms in the p53 Pathway

S.L. Harris,*[†] G. Gil,*[†] W. Hu,* H. Robins,[‡] E. Bond,* K. Hirshfield,* Z. Feng,* X. Yu,*
A.K. Teresky,* G. Bond,[‡] and A.J. Levine*[‡]

*The Cancer Institute of New Jersey, Robert Wood Johnson Medical School, New Brunswick, New Jersey 08903;
[‡]Institute for Advanced Study, School of Natural Sciences, Princeton, New Jersey 08540

A cell culture assay has been developed that detects and validates single-nucleotide polymorphisms (SNPs) in genes that populate the p53 pathway. One hundred thirteen EBV-transformed human B-lymphocyte cell lines obtained from a diverse population were employed to measure the apoptotic response to gamma radiation. Each cell line undergoes a reproducible, characteristic frequency of apoptosis, and the response of the population forms a normal distribution around a median of 35.5% apoptosis with a range from 12% to 58% apoptosis. Polymorphisms in the *AKT1* and *Perp* genes significantly affect the frequency of apoptosis. The assay can detect both racial and sexual dimorphisms in these genes and has the ability to demonstrate epistatic relationships within the p53 pathway. The cell lines used in this assay provide biological materials to explore the molecular basis of the polymorphisms.

The p53 protein and its signal transduction pathway respond to a wide variety of intrinsic and extrinsic cellular stresses. Among these stresses are DNA damage, telomere length shortening, hypoxia, reduction in ribonucleoside triphosphate pools and ribosomal biogenesis, spindle damage, and even mutational activation of oncogenes (Vogelstein et al. 2000). These stress signals are communicated to the p53 protein and its ubiquitin ligase, MDM2, via an extensive set of protein modifications that result in reduced expression or activity of the MDM2 protein, a negative regulator of p53 (Appella and Anderson 2001). In response to stress, the stability of p53 is increased and it becomes an active transcription factor. This in turn results in the transcription of a set of genes whose products bring about cell cycle arrest, senescence, or apoptosis. This provides time to either reverse the stress before cell duplication or kill the cell and its offspring that have duplicated under stressful conditions and made errors in that process. The replication of damaged DNA can increase the mutation rate by hundreds of fold. In this fashion, p53 and the signal transduction pathway it controls prevent errors in cell division that could give rise to mutations and changes in ploidy in a clone of cells. Several lines of evidence support this explanation; individuals that inherit a mutation in one of their *p53* alleles develop multiple cancers at a young age and at a high rate (Li 1990; Malkin et al. 1990), a set of phenotypes now known as Li-Fraumeni syndrome, and up to 50% of all cancers harbor somatic *p53* mutations that inactivate its function as a transcription factor (Soussi and Beroud 2001). Thus, there is a good deal of evidence that the p53 protein and its signal transduction pathway act in humans to suppress the development of tumors.

Several years ago, the sequencing of the human genome was completed, and it became clear that humans are a young species, with any two individuals being 99.8% identical (Lander et al. 2001; Venter et al. 2001). Among the differences between individuals are up to 10 million single-nucleotide polymorphisms (SNPs) distributed throughout the genome (Sachidanandam et al. 2001), and these differences may contribute to many of the individual traits that make us unique. This includes predispositions to diseases, responses to drugs or therapies, or even interactions with known mutations that predispose patients to diseases. Thus, we might anticipate that *p53*, and those genes which encode the proteins that make up the p53 pathway, would contain SNPs which would either enhance or decrease the ability of this network to suppress tumor development. Indeed, some of these SNPs have been identified. There are two common alleles of *p53* that encode different amino acids at codon 72, either proline or arginine, and allele frequencies within populations differ as one goes from the equator to northern latitudes (Beckman et al. 1994), suggesting selective forces play a role in maintaining both alleles. Indeed, the arginine form of p53 is associated with a stronger apoptotic response (Dumont et al. 2003), and the arginine-encoding allele of *p53* is preferentially mutated and maintained in squamous cell tumors (Marin et al. 2000). Recently, a SNP in the human *MDM2* gene was shown to influence the number of independent cancers developed by Li-Fraumeni patients and to lower the age of onset of both familial and sporadic soft-tissue sarcomas (Bond et al. 2004).

To identify SNPs populating the p53 pathway that affect cancers in humans, we have used the candidate signal transduction pathway approach. From the growing list of genes within the p53 pathway, we have selected 82 genes and have identified 1335 SNPs within these genes. Although it might be possible to choose from among these SNPs those with the highest probability of altering the efficiency or functions of the p53 pathway, it became clear that a cell-based assay to test for the efficiency of

---

[†]These authors contributed equally to this work.

p53 function should be developed which would permit an assessment of the impact of a SNP or gene upon the functions of the p53 pathway. This paper describes the development of an assay that, in addition to providing a method to demonstrate which SNPs alter the efficiency of the p53 pathway, provides cell lines that permit one to determine the molecular and cellular mechanism of the SNP. As the genotypes from multiple SNPs are determined within the same group of cell lines, this provides, for the first time, the chance to examine epistasis in the pathway and the combinatorial impact of several SNPs in the same cell. This assay has uncovered both sexual and racial dimorphisms in the p53 pathway.

The assay employed 113 EBV-transformed B-cell lines (LCLs) that were derived from unrelated, healthy volunteers. The input stress signal employed to activate the p53 protein was 5 Gy of gamma radiation (γ IR), and the output or phenotype measured was the percentage of cells that underwent apoptosis 24 hours after the radiation. The results demonstrate that the p53 pathway plays a central role in determining this phenotype. Interestingly, each cell line undergoes a reproducible frequency of apoptosis with a small standard error, whereas the population responds with a range of 12.3–58.9% apoptosis around a median of 35.5% apoptosis. The tails of this distribution (high and low ends) are two standard deviations from the mean, providing a statistically robust method to characterize the distributions of any SNP in this population of cell lines. This assay has uncovered SNPs or haplotypes in two genes in the p53 pathway (Jin and Levine 2001): *AKT1* and *Perp*, each of which alters the distribution of apoptotic response to irradiation. Because the cell lines are available to any investigator and have been previously classified for a phenotype (apoptosis after γ IR), other researchers can now test for the impact of a SNP (or haplotype) by genotyping the DNA samples obtained from this collection. Furthermore, this approach can be adapted to many other phenotypes that can be measured in B cells in culture.

MATERIALS AND METHODS

Response of EBV-transformed B cells to γ radiation. A total of 120 EBV-transformed lymphoblast cell lines (LCLs) derived from anonymous, unrelated healthy volunteers were purchased from the Coriell Institute for Medical Research (Camden, New Jersey). Cells were cultured in RPMI supplemented with L-glutamine and 15% FBS (Sigma). Cells were seeded into T25 flasks at a density of 2×10^5 cells/ml and were grown at 37°C at 5% CO_2 until the density reached 1×10^6 cells/ml (defined as one passage). Once the cultures reached a viability of 90% or greater, response to radiation was measured. For each cell line, two 10-ml cultures were seeded into T25 flasks at a density of 2×10^5 cells/ml and were grown for 48 hours. One culture was irradiated with 5 Gy radiation (CIS BioInternational IBL 437C^{137}Cs γ-radiation source), and the control culture was mock-irradiated. Cell death was measured in both cultures 24 hours post-radiation using a Guava Personal Cell Analysis flow cytome-

ter (Hayward, California). Guava Viacount reagent, which differentially stains viable and nonviable cells based on their permeability to two dyes, was used to measure apoptosis. Control experiments on four LCLs demonstrated that assays of multicaspase activation, TUNEL staining and nexin staining, gave very similar results to Viacount (data not shown). The radiation-induced percent apoptotic cell death for a culture was obtained by comparison of the irradiated to the mock-treated control culture. The average apoptotic response for each cell line was calculated from at least three measurements, each taken from a different passage. The total number of cell lines in our analysis was reduced to 113 after elimination of data from cell lines that never reached 90% viability, grew very slowly, underwent crisis during the experiment, or did not give reproducible results in the assay.

Genotyping. Genomic DNAs corresponding to the 113 LCLs were purchased from Coriell Institute (Camden, New Jersey). The five polymorphisms in *AKT1* (Emamian et al. 2004) (rs3803300, rs1130214, rs3730358, rs2498799, rs2494732) and the *Perp* polymorphism (rs2484067) were genotyped on an ABI Prism 7000 using Applied Biosystems (Foster City, California) allelic discrimination assays. All genotype frequencies were in Hardy-Weinberg equilibrium.

siRNA gene silencing. To prepare cells for transfection, LCLs were grown to a density of 1×10^6 cells/ml and then centrifuged at 300g for 10 minutes, and the medium was removed. Cells were resuspended at room temperature in Nucleofector solution included with the Nucleofector kit V (Amaxa, Maryland). A culture (100 μl) at a density of 4×10^6 to 5×10^6 cells/ml was mixed with siRNA and transferred to the provided cuvette and electroporated with an Amaxa Nucleofector device (Amaxa, Germany) set with the A-30 pulsing parameter, and cells were immediately transferred into a flask containing prewarmed (37°C) culture medium. Transfection efficiency was determined by fluorescent microscopy using Alexa Fluor 546 control nonsilencing duplex siRNAs (Qiagen). Typical transfection efficiency was 70–80%, and viability at 48 hours post-transfection was near 90%. *AKT1* siRNA Smartpool (Dharmacon) was used to silence *Akt1* expression. A *p53* siRNA Smartpool (Dharmacon) was used to reduce *p53* expression. *Lamin* A/C and control nonsilencing duplex siRNAs (Qiagen) were used at the same concentration as *AKT1* and *p53* siRNAs (600 picomoles). For radiation studies of siRNA-transfected cells, cells were irradiated (5 Gy) 24 hours post-transfection, and percent cell death was measured 24 hours after radiation by comparing irradiated and mock-irradiated transfected cultures. Subsequently, the cells were lysed, and protein levels were analyzed as described below.

Western analysis. Protein levels were analyzed from total cell extracts prepared by lysis in RIPA buffer (Sigma Aldrich) in the presence of a protease and phosphatase inhibitor cocktail (Sigma Aldrich). Protein concentration was measured using Bio-Rad's protein assay and spectrometry at 595 nm. Total protein (40 μg) was separated on a 4–20% Tris-glycine gel and transferred to a PVDF membrane. The AKT1 (2H10), Lamin A/C (#2032), and phospho-MDM2 Ser166 (#3521) antibodies were purchased from Cell Signaling Tech, α-Tubulin (DM1A) antibody was from Sigma Aldrich, the p53 (DO-1) and MDM2 (SMP14) antibodies were from Santa Cruz.

The proteins were visualized using HRP-conjugated secondary antibodies (Pierce Biotech) and SuperSignal West Fento (Pierce Biotech).

Determination of AKT1 protein concentration by ELISA. For each cell line, cultures were seeded into T25 flasks at a density of 2×10^5 cells/ml and were grown for 72 hours. Total cell protein extracts were prepared and quantitated as described above. AKT1 protein in each extract was determined using the PathScan Total AKT1 Sandwich ELISA kit from Cell Signaling Technology (Beverly, Massachusetts) according to the manufacturer's recommendations. The results of the ELISA assay were confirmed by western analysis (data not shown).

RNA analysis. To measure basal *Perp* mRNA levels, total RNA was isolated from cell pellets using Rneasy (Qiagen). cDNAs were made using TaqMan reverse transcription reagents from Applied Biosystems. Real-time PCR was carried out on an ABI Prism 7000 sequence detection system. Probe and primer sets were as follows: human *Perp* (catalog number Hs00751717_s1) and human GAPDH (catalog number Hs99999905_m1) (Applied Biosystems).

Statistical analysis. Means and standard deviations of total protein were compared by unpaired two-tailed *t*-tests. Means and standard deviations of apoptotic responses of cell lines were compared by unpaired *t*-tests, one- or two-tailed as indicated in the text, or by the Fisher's exact test when appropriate.

Determination of haplotype structure. Haplotypes were determined by Expectation Maximization using the SNPHAP software (www-gene.cimr.cam.as.uk/clayton).

RESULTS

The Response of LCLs to Radiation Is Heterogeneous

To measure the response of cells from different individuals to DNA damage, we chose to irradiate EBV-transformed B cells derived from those individuals. It has been demonstrated in both mice (Lowe et al. 1993) and humans (Camplejohn et al. 2000) that apoptotic responses in lymphocytes are significantly reduced by *p53* mutations. EBV-transformed B-cell lines were chosen to reduce the cell type heterogeneity and environmental variables that are observed when peripheral blood lymphocytes are taken directly from an individual and placed in culture (Camplejohn et al. 2003). In addition, the LCLs provide a permanent source of cells that can be tested multiple times for a given phenotype or phenotypes. Of the 113 LCLs included in the study, 77 are derived from females and 36 from males. To increase the genetic diversity, roughly half (58) of the LCLs are derived from African-American donors and half (55) are from Caucasian donors. Each cell line was irradiated with 5 Gy of gamma radiation (γ IR), and 24 hours later the percent of cells in the culture undergoing apoptotic cell death was measured. Radiation-induced apoptosis was measured at least three times for each LCL. The average standard error was 2.2% apoptosis and ranged from 0.2% to 5.3%. Thus, the response of each individual LCL was very reproducible. When the percent of apoptosis was measured at 48 hours, the frequency of apoptosis increased, but the relative order of responses of different LCLs remained substantially the same. In Figure 1, data for the 113 LCLs are plotted as the number of cell lines as a function of the frequency of apoptosis at 24 hours. Response varied with a range of 12.3–58.9% apoptosis forming a Gaussian distribution with an average apoptotic frequency of 34.9%, a median of 35.5%, and a standard deviation of 9.9%. On the basis of the standard error and the standard deviation, we chose to bin the responses into 10% intervals of apoptosis (Fig. 1). The midpoints of the highest (8 LCLs) and lowest (11 LCLs) bins of this distribution are two standard deviations removed from the median. This experiment demonstrates that heterogeneity exists in the response of individual B-cell lines to DNA damage induced by γ IR. In addition, these data suggest that it should be possible to identify, in a statistically valid fashion, individual traits or SNPs that generate some of this variation.

Although the presence of Epstein-Barr virus in these cells may alter some of their properties, it is unlikely that the distribution of apoptotic response is drastically altered. The results presented in Figure 1 are similar to those of Camplejohn (Camplejohn et al. 2003) and K. Onel and A.J. Levine (unpubl.), whereby peripheral blood lymphocytes, isolated directly from donors, were tested in a similar assay. Second, when an EBV-transformed LCL derived from a Li-Fraumeni patient (cell line 051-019) was tested in this assay, the frequency of apoptosis was only 13.3% (Fig. 2A), similar to that found using peripheral blood lymphocytes from Li-Fraumeni pa-

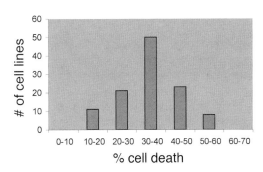

Figure 1. The response of LCLs to radiation is heterogeneous. 113 LCLs from unrelated individuals were irradiated with 5 Gy γ IR to induce DNA damage, and apoptosis was measured 24 hr later. Each cell line was measured at least three times; the average standard error for all cell lines was 2.2%. Each cell line was placed in a bin based on its average apoptotic response. The bin size of 10% represents one standard deviation (9.9%) for the population.

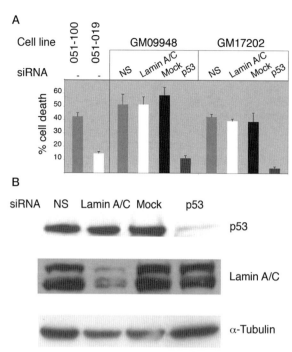

Figure 2. Reduction in p53 function results in reduced apoptotic response in LCLs. (*A*) An LCL (051-019) derived from a patient with Li-Fraumeni syndrome (*p53* mutant) and an LCL from an unrelated individual with wild-type *p53* alleles (051-100) were irradiated with 5 Gy γ IR to induce DNA damage; apoptotic cell death was measured 24 hr later. Each cell line was measured four times; the average cell death and standard error are shown. LCLs GM09948 and GM17202 were transfected with siRNAs specific for *p53*, *lamin A/C*, or a nonspecific siRNA (NS). Cells were treated with γ IR 24 hr after transfection with siRNAs, and cell death was measured 24 hr post-radiation. Shown are the mean and standard deviation from two separate experiments. (*B*) Shown are western blots of basal (no radiation) whole-cell extracts made from the GM09948 cell line 48 hr post-transfection with the indicated siRNAs.

tients (Camplejohn and Rutherford 2001) and markedly different from a second LCL (051-100) derived from a volunteer with wild-type *p53* that underwent considerable apoptosis (44%). To further demonstrate the central role of the p53 pathway in this assay, two LCLs with high apoptotic responses were transfected with *p53* siRNA to reduce the expression of *p53* and test whether this would affect the efficiency of apoptosis. As shown in Figure 2A, transfection of the GM09948 cell line, shown previously to have an apoptotic frequency of 53.6%, with a nonspecific siRNA or with a siRNA directed against *lamin*, resulted in no change in the response to γ IR. Transfection of the same cell line with a *p53* siRNA that lowered the amount of p53 expression (Fig. 2B) resulted in a reduction of apoptotic response to about 10% (Fig. 2A). A similar result was obtained with a second LCL, GM17202; *p53* siRNA reduced apoptosis from 44.4% to below 10% (Fig. 2A). It is clear from these experiments that this assay measures p53-mediated apoptosis in response to γ IR and that the efficiency of that response is quite heterogeneous in the population.

The Genetic Background of the LCLs Plays a Role in the Heterogeneity of Their Responses to DNA Damage

Of the 113 cell lines shown in Figure 1, 55 are derived from the B cells of self-identified Caucasians and 58 are derived from self-identified African-American donors. The LCLs were chosen this way to maximize the number of polymorphisms that would be present. The African and African-American populations have been shown to have a greater number of unique or population-specific polymorphisms compared to the European Caucasian population (Hinds et al. 2005). Figure 3 presents the 113 cell lines separated by the race of the donor as a function of apoptotic cell death. Both the Caucasian and the African-American LCLs produced a similar normal distribution of responses between 20% and 60% apoptosis, but all of the 11 LCLs exhibiting between 10% and 20% apoptosis were of Caucasian origin (*p* = 0.0002; Fisher's exact test, two-tailed). This significant overrepresentation of Caucasians in the lowest response group is seen for both female and male LCLs (*p* = 0.005 and 0.04, Fisher's exact, two-tailed, respectively). Since the culture conditions employed in this assay are relatively constant for all cell lines, these data support the idea that genetic factors are contributing to the heterogeneity of the p53 response to radiation damage.

A Haplotype in *AKT1* Affects Radiation-induced Cell Death

Recently, a haplotype composed of five SNPs in *AKT1* was reported to reduce the amount of AKT1 protein in lymphocytes and brain tissue of schizophrenic patients, and this haplotype was found in higher than expected frequencies in individuals with schizophrenia (Emamian et al. 2004). AKT1 is an antiapoptotic protein kinase (Bellacosa et al. 2004), and one of its substrates is the MDM2 protein (Mayo and Donner 2001; Zhou et al. 2001; Gottlieb et al. 2002; Ogawara et al. 2002). Phosphorylation of MDM2 by AKT1 at serine residues 166 and 188 inhibits MDM2 auto-ubiquitination leading to the stabilization of MDM2 (Ogawara et al. 2002; Feng et al. 2004). In some cells, phosphorylation also promotes the movement of MDM2 into the nucleus (Zhou et al. 2001) where it can act to destabilize p53 protein levels and lower apoptosis. Thus, *AKT1*

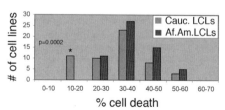

Figure 3. The response of LCLs to radiation is influenced by genetic factors. LCLs are grouped by average response to radiation and by the race of the donor. 55 LCLs are derived from self-identified Caucasian donors, and 58 are derived from self-identified African-American donors.

have markedly different apoptotic potential. *Nat. Genet.* **33:** 357.

Emamian E.S., Hall D., Birnbaum M.J., Karayiorgou M., and Gogos J.A. 2004. Convergent evidence for impaired AKT1-GSK3beta signaling in schizophrenia. *Nat. Genet.* **36:** 131.

Feng J., Tamaskovic R., Yang Z., Brazil D.P., Merlo A., Hess D., and Hemmings B.A. 2004. Stabilization of Mdm2 via decreased ubiquitination is mediated by protein kinase B/Akt-dependent phosphorylation. *J. Biol. Chem.* **279:** 35510.

Gottlieb T.M., Leal J.F., Seger R., Taya Y., and Oren M. 2002. Cross-talk between Akt, p53 and Mdm2: Possible implications for the regulation of apoptosis. *Oncogene* **21:** 1299.

Hinds D.A., Stuve L.L., Nilsen G.B., Halperin E., Eskin E., Ballinger D.G., Frazer K.A., and Cox D.R. 2005. Whole-genome patterns of common DNA variation in three human populations. *Science* **307:** 1072.

Hwang S.J., Lozano G., Amos C.I., and Strong L.C. 2003. Germline p53 mutations in a cohort with childhood sarcoma: Sex differences in cancer risk. *Am. J. Hum. Genet.* **72:** 975.

Ihrie R.A. and Attardi L.D. 2004. Perp-etrating p53-dependent apoptosis. *Cell Cycle* **3:** 267.

Ihrie R.A., Reczek E., Horner J.S., Khachatrian L., Sage J., Jacks T., and Attardi L.D. 2003. Perp is a mediator of p53-dependent apoptosis in diverse cell types. *Curr. Biol.* **13:** 1985.

Ihrie R.A., Marques M.R., Nguyen B.T., Horner J.S., Papazoglu C., Bronson R.T., Mills A.A., and Attardi L.D. 2005. Perp is a p63-regulated gene essential for epithelial integrity. *Cell* **120:** 843.

Jin S. and Levine A.J. 2001. The p53 functional circuit. *J. Cell Sci.* **114:** 4139.

Lander E.S., Linton L.M., Birren B., Nusbaum C., Zody M.C., Baldwin J., Devon K., Dewar K., Doyle M., FitzHugh W., Funke R., Gage D., Harris K., Heaford A., Howland J., Kann L., Lehoczky J., LeVine R., McEwan P., McKernan K., Meldrim J., Mesirov J.P., Miranda C., Morris W., and Naylor J., et al. (International Human Genome Sequencing Consortium). 2001. Initial sequencing and analysis of the human genome. *Nature* **409:** 860.

Li F.P. 1990. Familial cancer syndromes and clusters. *Curr. Probl. Cancer* **14:** 73.

Lowe S.W., Schmitt E.M., Smith S.W., Osborne B.A., and Jacks T. 1993. p53 is required for radiation-induced apoptosis in mouse thymocytes. *Nature* **362:** 847.

Malkin D., Li F.P., Strong L.C., Fraumeni J.F., Jr., Nelson C.E.,

Kim D.H., Kassel J., Gryka M.A., Bischoff F.Z., and Tainsky M.A., et al. 1990. Germ line p53 mutations in a familial syndrome of breast cancer, sarcomas, and other neoplasms. *Science* **250:** 1233-8.

Marin M.C., Jost C.A., Brooks L.A., Irwin M.S., O'Nions J., Tidy J.A., James N., McGregor J.M., Harwood C.A., Yulug I.G., Vousden K.H., Allday M.J., Gusterson B., Ikawa S., Hinds P.W., Crook T., and Kaelin W.G., Jr. 2000. A common polymorphism acts as an intragenic modifier of mutant p53 behaviour. *Nat. Genet.* **25:** 47.

Mayo L.D. and Donner D.B. 2001. A phosphatidylinositol 3-kinase/Akt pathway promotes translocation of Mdm2 from the cytoplasm to the nucleus. *Proc. Natl. Acad. Sci.* **98:** 11598.

Nowak M., Koster C., and Hammerschmidt M. 2005. Perp is required for tissue-specific cell survival during zebrafish development. *Cell Death Differ.* **12:** 52.

Ogawara Y., Kishishita S., Obata T., Isazawa Y., Suzuki T., Tanaka K., Masuyama N., and Gotoh Y. 2002. Akt enhances Mdm2-mediated ubiquitination and degradation of p53. *J. Biol. Chem.* **277:** 21843.

Sachidanandam R., Weissman D., Schmidt S.C., Kakol J.M., Stein L.D., Marth G., Sherry S., Mullikin J.C., Mortimore B.J., Willey D.L., Hunt S.E., Cole C.G., Coggill P.C., Rice C.M., Ning Z., Rogers J., Bentley D.R., Kwok P.Y., Mardis E.R., Yeh R.T., Schultz B., Cook L., Davenport R., Dante M., and Fulton L., et al. (International SNP Map Working Group). 2001. A map of human genome sequence variation containing 1.42 million single nucleotide polymorphisms. *Nature* **409:** 928.

Soussi T. and Beroud C. 2001. Assessing TP53 status in human tumours to evaluate clinical outcome. *Nat. Rev. Cancer* **1:** 233.

Venter J.C., Adams M.D., Myers E.W., Li P.W., Mural R.J., Sutton G.G., Smith H.O., Yandell M., Evans C.A., Holt R.A., Gocayne J.D., Amanatides P., Ballew R.M., Huson D.H., Wortman J.R., Zhang Q., Kodira C.D., Zheng X.H., Chen L., Skupski M., Subramanian G., Thomas P.D., Zhang J., Gabor Miklos G.L., and Nelson C., et al. 2001. The sequence of the human genome. *Science* **291:** 1304.

Vogelstein B., Lane D., and Levine A.J. 2000. Surfing the p53 network. *Nature* **408:** 307.

Zhou B.P., Liao Y., Xia W., Zou Y., Spohn B., and Hung M.C. 2001. HER-2/neu induces p53 ubiquitination via Akt-mediated MDM2 phosphorylation. *Nat. Cell Biol.* **3:** 973.

Transcriptional Regulation by p53 and p73

M. Lokshin,* T. Tanaka,* and C. Prives

Department of Biological Sciences, Columbia University, New York, New York 10027

The tumor suppressor p53 exerts its effect through transactivation of a wide variety of genes leading to outcomes such as cell cycle arrest or apoptosis. Both p53 protein levels and modification status are thought to play a role in its ability to discriminate between different target genes and, thereby, cell fate. Here, we have determined the contribution of p53 levels to promoter selectivity when ectopically expressed in H1299 cells. Interestingly, p53AIP1, a pro-apoptotic p53 target gene, requires a significantly higher threshold level of p53 for its activation than p21WAF1, a cell cycle arrest gene. We also found that whereas exogenous p73 exhibits similar transcriptional activity to p53 in H1299 cells, the endogenous p73 that accumulates upon DNA damage in HCT116 cells is unable to compensate for p53 function. Quantification of protein expression levels revealed that the basal expression of TAp73 in HCT116 cells is very low and, even after induction by DNA damage, it accumulates to levels that are lower than basal uninduced levels of p53. These results might partially explain why, unlike p53, p73 does not function as a major tumor suppressor.

The tumor suppressor p53, which is mutated in more than 50% of human cancer, is stabilized and activated in cells in response to genotoxic stresses or oncogenic stimuli and then initiates different cellular outcomes, including cell cycle arrest, apoptosis, or senescence (for review, see Ko and Prives 1996; Levine 1997; Bates and Vousden 1999; Prives and Hall 1999). The biological functions of p53 involve its activities as a sequence-specific transcription factor, and cellular outcomes following stress are determined through the transactivation of a wide variety of p53 target genes such as p21WAF1, MDM2, PIG3, BAX, PUMA, p53AIP1, and numerous others. Several models have been proposed to explain how the activity of p53 is regulated and how the promoter discrimination of p53 is achieved on the molecular level, leading, in some cases, to a decision between cell cycle arrest and apoptosis in response to distinct stimuli.

It has been proposed that the choice in response depends on the amount of p53 present in the cell as well as the modification state of p53 (Wang and Prives 1995; Gu and Roeder 1997; Sakaguchi et al. 1998; Oda et al. 2000; Appella and Anderson 2001). The stabilization of p53 after DNA damage is thought to occur largely through phosphorylation events that disrupt its interaction with its negative regulator, MDM2, although the literature reveals considerable complexity in that regard (Shieh et al. 1997; Prives and Hall 1999; Moll and Petrenko 2003; Poyurovsky and Prives 2006). Furthermore, some modifications, such as phosphorylation of Ser-46, may increase the affinity of p53 for a specific promoter independently of p53 expression level (Oda et al. 2000).

Analysis of target gene mRNA induction and chromatin immunoprecipitation (ChIP) assays has shown a difference in binding affinity and kinetics of p53's association with and transactivation of its target gene promoters (Szak et al. 2001; Kaeser and Iggo 2002). Although there are notable

exceptions (e.g., the PUMA gene), low-affinity sites are frequently found in pro-apoptotic genes, suggesting that the level of p53 expression can determine the threshold for promoter activation and cellular outcome in some experimental conditions (Chen et al. 1996; Ludwig et al. 1996). In situ, this might permit p53, when present at low levels, to induce cell cycle arrest, allowing time to repair the DNA damage, and at higher levels (perhaps following more extensive damage), to activate the apoptotic program. It has also been shown that some proteins, for example ASPP1/2 (Samuels-Lev et al. 2001), augment the p53-dependent transactivation of only the pro-apoptotic target genes. This suggests an initial weaker binding to some pro-apoptotic promoters that, in the case of severe enough DNA damage, is augmented by p53 modification and cofactors.

The p53 family member p73 was first identified in 1997 (Jost et al. 1997; Kaghad et al. 1997). Since then, much has been discovered about this protein, but many questions remain unanswered (Irwin and Kaelin 2001a,b; Yang et al. 2002; Moll and Slade 2004). The p73 gene contains 14 exons, which, through splicing, can produce seven TA full-length isoforms that differ in their carboxyl terminus (α–η) and the corresponding ΔN isoforms. The ΔN isoforms result from transcription from an alternative promoter and have a transactivation domain different from that of the full-length isoforms. In vivo, p73α and β are the most commonly found forms, in both the TA and ΔN varieties.

The p73 protein has approximately 65% homology with p53 in its DNA-binding domain, and some homology in the transactivation and oligomerization domains (20–30% and 35–45%, respectively.) Like p53, p73 functions as a transcription factor and has been shown to transactivate a number of p53 target genes, although each protein also transactivates its own unique class of downstream targets (for review, see Harms et al. 2004). Also like p53, p73 is up-regulated in the cell following DNA damage (Agami et al. 1999; Yuan et al. 1999), although

---

*These authors contributed equally to this work.

the mechanisms of its up-regulation are not fully understood. Finally, p73 can also exhibit modification-dependent target selectivity; for example, acetylation of p73 induces selective activation of apoptotic target genes (Costanzo et al. 2002).

Several lines of evidence challenge the role of p73 as a tumor suppressor. Whereas p53 is mutated or deleted in more than 50% of human tumors, p73 mutations in tumors are far rarer. It should be noted, however, that some tumors overexpress p73, and it is likely that it is the anti-

apoptotic ΔN isoforms which are overexpressed. There is also a significant difference in phenotype between p53 and p73 knockout mice: The former are highly susceptible to tumors (Donehower et al. 1992; Attardi and Jacks 1999), whereas the latter exhibit various neurological defects but no increased tumor susceptibility (Yang et al. 2000). It cannot be ruled out, however, that this is a defect in a very specific form of apoptosis. Nonetheless, even in cell lines that express TAp73, eliminating p53 expression has a profound effect on apoptosis, further questioning

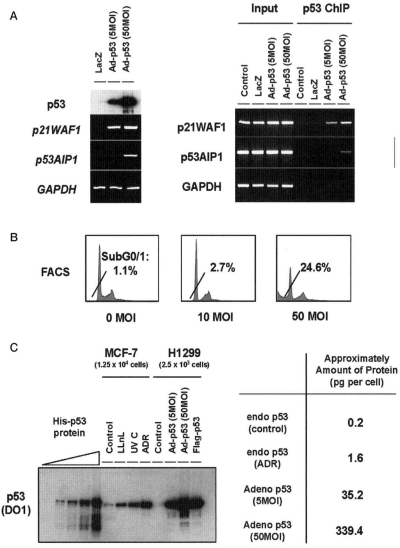

Figure 1. Differential regulation by p53 of induction of p53 target genes and binding to promoters in vivo. (*A*) Differential transactivation of p53 target genes after p53 adenovirus infection as detected by RT-PCR (*left*) and ChIP analysis (*right*). H1299 cells were transduced with p53- or LacZ-expressing adenoviruses at the indicated moi. After total mRNA was prepared, quantitative RT-PCR to detect p21, p53AIP1, and GAPDH was carried out (*left*). H1299 cells were transduced with p53 or LacZ-expressing adenoviruses at the indicated moi. Cells were treated or not with formaldehyde cross-linking. After cell lysis and sonication, p53-containing complexes were immunoprecipitated with p53 monoclonal antibodies Pab 1801 and DO-1. After reversal of cross-linking, input DNA and immunoprecipitates were determined by PCR to detect indicated promoter activity (*right*). (*B*) Differential induction of p53-dependent apoptosis by FACS analysis. H1299 cells were transduced with p53-expressing adenoviruses at the indicated moi, and collected and fixed with 70% ethanol in PBS after 36-hr infection. FACS analysis followed by PI staining was performed. (*C*) Estimation of expression level of endogenous and adeno-expressed p53 in cells. Either MCF-7 or H1299 cells were seeded at the same cell density in a 6-well plate (2.5×10^5 cells/well) and then treated with the different agents as indicated or infected with the p53 adenovirus. Cells were collected and lysed in SDS sample buffer directly and subjected to immunoblotting with p53 monoclonal antibodies (DO-1). First six lanes represent serial dilution of purified p53 recombinant protein.

the role of endogenous p73 as a tumor suppressor.

Here, we use adenoviral infection to assess whether the amount of p53 in a cell determines the protein's ability to transactivate "weaker" pro-apoptotic targets, and to determine the number of p53 molecules that are required per cell for transactivation of p21 or AIP1 promoters. Furthermore, to address the difference in apoptosis induced by endogenous p73 as compared to p53 in response to DNA damage, we have determined the levels of endogenous p73 and p53 proteins expressed in the HCT116 colorectal adenocarcinoma cell line following treatment with camptothecin.

RESULTS AND DISCUSSION

Different Levels of p53 Are Required to Transactivate Target Promoters

As mentioned above, several models have been proposed to explain how the promoter discrimination of p53 is regulated and why p53 induces cell cycle arrest under some conditions and apoptosis under others. One model postulates that p53 binds with high affinity to the promoters of cell cycle arrest genes and binds to the promoters of most pro-apoptotic genes with a low affinity. It has been shown, for example, that the p53-binding site in the p21 promoter is a much better match to the consensus sequence than the sites in some putative apoptotic target gene promoters and that the level of p53 expression determines the outcome in some experimental conditions (Chen et al. 1996; Ludwig et al. 1996).

To test whether DNA binding to select promoters is correlated with the levels of p53, we first examined both mRNA levels and chromatin binding upon expression of two different levels of p53 in H1299 cells by using different amounts (multiplicity of infection: moi) of recombinant adenovirus expressing p53 (Ad-p53). Induction of p21 and p53AIP1, a pro-apoptotic target gene, was compared by reverse-transcription polymerase chain reaction (RT-PCR) at various amounts of Ad-p53 (Fig. 1A, left panel). At a moi of 5, p53 induced p21 robustly but only barely induced AIP1, whereas at 50 moi, both p21 and AIP1 were well induced. The ChIP assay revealed that p53 at 50 moi bound both to the p21 and the AIP1 promoters, whereas at 5 moi only the p21 promoter was engaged by p53 (Fig. 1A, right panel). Consistent with these functional differences between p21 and p53AIP1, fluorescence-activated cell sorting (FACS) analysis showed that only at 50 moi of Ad-p53 was a significant level of apoptosis induced (Fig. 1B). Whereas apoptosis induced by high moi of adenovirally expressed p53 is not likely to be mediated exclusively by a single gene product, AIP1 represents a clear example of an apoptotic gene that requires a significantly higher threshold level of p53 for its activation than does a cell cycle p53 target promoter such as p21.

Next, to estimate the amount of endogenous and adenovirally expressed p53, immunoblotting was performed comparing serial dilutions of purified His-tagged human p53 recombinant protein from baculovirally infected insect SF9 cells as a standard p53

protein (Fig. 1C, left panel). In brief, either MCF-7 or H1299 cells were seeded at the same cell density (2.5×10^5 cells) and then treated with the different agents as indicated, or infected with the p53 adenovirus. Cells were lysed in SDS sample buffer directly and then subjected to immunoblotting using amounts that fall within linear range for quantification. As expected, the basal expression of endogenous p53 in MCF-7 cells was very low (~0.21 pg/cell), and p53 accumulated to 8-fold higher levels (~1.6 pg/cell) following adriamycin treatment in MCF-7 cells (Fig. 1B, right table). Interestingly, the p53 expression by Ad-p53 at 5 moi in H1299 cells was 22-fold (~35.2 pg/cell) higher than that of MCF-7 cells treated with adriamycin (Fig. 1B, right table). Adenovirally expressed p53 levels at 50 moi were 10-fold higher than at 5 moi (Fig. 1B, right table). Although we cannot exclude the possibility that posttranslational modifications of p53, such as phosphorylation and acetylation, are induced differentially at different moi, these results indicate that the levels of p53 expression determine the threshold of activation for at least some low-affinity pro-apoptotic promoters.

Comparison of Transcriptional Activities of p53 and p73

Although the DNA-binding domain of p73 interacts with the canonical p53 response element, and both p73 and p63 activate the expression of a number of p53 target genes and suppress cell growth when overexpressed, several lines of evidence indicate that although p53, p73, and p63 share structural and functional similarities and have overlapping functions, many target genes respond differentially to the different family members (Jost et al. 1997; Kaghad et al. 1997; Zhu et al. 1998; Lee and La Thangue 1999). It remains to be determined whether and how different stimuli selectively recruit one or more members of the p53 family to achieve specialized transcription responses in specific cellular contexts.

To accurately compare the transcriptional activity of p53 and p73, it is necessary to use a system where the expression levels of either p53, p73α, or p73β are normalized and regulated in the same cell line in the absence of cellular stress, since the stabilization and activation of p53 and p73 are regulated differentially after genotoxic stress through posttranslational modification, protein–protein interaction, and protein turnover. Previous work comparing the transcriptional activity of p53 and p73 is somewhat ambiguous, with some reports showing similar activity for p53 and p73β, some reporting weaker activity for p73β, and yet others showing that the difference in activity depends on the target gene. Most reports do agree that the ability of p73β to transactivate a variety of p53 target genes and to induce apoptosis is stronger than that of p73α (Lee and La Thangue 1999; Ueda et al. 1999), possibly due to the inhibitory effect of the SAM domain, located in the carboxy-terminal region specific to the alpha isoforms (Liu and Chen 2005). However, the reported difference in activity varies, with some data showing only a 2-fold difference in activity between exogenous p73α and p73β (Ozaki et al. 1999), and a 2-fold difference in ability to induce apoptosis (Zhu et al. 1998).

To determine the transcriptional activity of p53 and p73 in our system, we used tetracycline-regulated stable H1299 clones in which the induction of HA-p53, HA-p73α, and HA-p73β can be regulated precisely without any cellular stress, and the expression of p53 is close to physiological levels (Chen et al. 1996; Zhu et al. 1998). Indeed, when expressed to the same levels, HA-p53 and HA-p73β induced p21WAF1 expression similarly (Fig. 2A). p73α was able to induce p21, but the induction level was approximately 2.5-fold less than those of p53 and p73β, as had been reported previously (Fig. 2A). To gain further information about other target genes, RT-PCR was performed to detect p21, HDM2, PIG3, and PUMA, using p53- and p73β-expressing clones (Fig. 2B). The extent of transactivation was similar for all four target genes by p53 and p73β, even when their expression was down-regulated to low levels using tetracycline. These results suggest that p73 is likely to have transcriptional activity similar to that of p53 on several p53 target genes when the expression level is controlled without any cellular stresses.

Next, to examine and compare the transcriptional activity of endogenous p53 and p73, HCT116 cells which either express p53 (HCT-p53$^{+/+}$) or lack p53 (HCT-p53$^{-/-}$) were characterized. In both of these cell lines, as we have reported previously, the major p73 isoform expressed is TA-p73α, although TA-p73β has also been detected (Lin et al. 2004; Urist et al. 2004). Cells were treated with camptothecin (CPT), 5-fluorouracil (5-FU), or daunorubicin (Dauno) to induce p53 and p73 expression, and then western blot, RT-PCR, and FACS analyses were performed (Fig. 3). Both p53 and p73 were up-regulated following treatment with CPT and Dauno, whereas

only p53 levels were increased following 5-FU treatment, demonstrating that p53 and p73 are regulated in distinct ways upon different stimuli (Fig. 3A).

Although p21 mRNA and protein levels increased significantly following DNA damage in the p53$^{+/+}$ cells, no or little induction of p21 was observed after CPT or Dauno treatment in the p53$^{-/-}$ cells, even though there was a marked increase in detectable p73, suggesting either that levels of endogenous p73 induced by DNA damage were not enough to activate p21 in HCT116 cells lacking p53 or that p73 activity is somehow repressed in these cells. Furthermore, although both cell lines exhibited changes in cell cycle distribution following DNA damage, a significantly greater sub-G$_0$/G$_1$ population was observed in the p53$^{+/+}$ cells after CPT and 5-FU treatment (Fig. 3B). Consistent with the induction of p21, G$_1$ arrest was not observed after CPT or Dauno treatment in p53$^{-/-}$ cells (Fig. 3B, lower panel). In addition, the p53$^{-/-}$ cells did undergo G$_1$ arrest after 5-FU treatment but, because there was no p73 induction under these conditions, the p73 dependence of these cellular outcomes is questionable.

To confirm the binding ability of endogenous p73 to a target promoter in HCT116 cells, a p73 ChIP assay was performed using an anti-p73 monoclonal antibody. The endogenously expressed TA-p73α that accumulated after CPT treatment was associated with the p21WAF1 promoter in both HCT116$^{+/+}$ and HCT116$^{-/-}$ cells, suggesting that p73 is not functionally impaired in its ability to bind DNA in HCT116 cells (data not shown).

Taken together, our results indicate that whereas exogenous p73 exhibits similar transcriptional activity to p53, the endogenous p73 that accumulates upon DNA damage is unable to compensate for p53 function. Thus, the induction of endogenous p73 does not lead to cellular outcomes such as p21 induction, G$_1$ arrest, or apoptosis in HCT116 p53$^{-/-}$ cells.

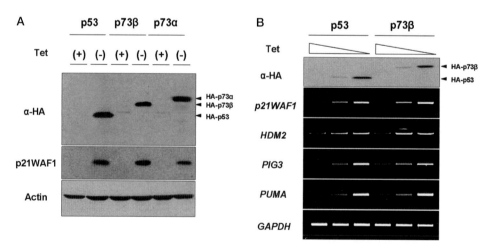

Figure 2. Induction of target genes by p53 and p73. (*A*) HA-p53, HA-p73α, or HA-p73β expression in tetracycline-regulated H1299 clones was induced by removal of tetracycline. To determine p21 protein induction by p53 and the p73 isoforms, HA-p53, HA-p73α, and HA-p73β levels were induced and detected by immunoblotting with anti-HA antibody. p21 expression was determined by anti-p21 monoclonal antibody (Oncogene Ab-1), and actin (Sigma) was used as loading control. (*B*) To assess the induction of several target genes by p53 and p73β, high and low protein expression level was regulated by tetracycline and visualized by immunoblotting (*top panel*). mRNA levels of p53 target genes, p21, HDM2, PIG3, PUMA, and as an internal control mRNA, GAPDH, were assessed by quantitative RT-PCR.

A

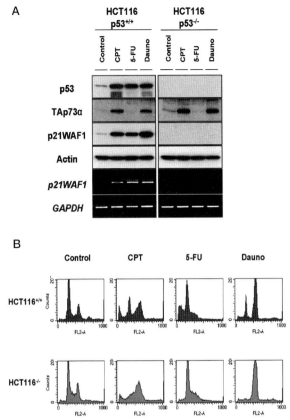

B

Figure 3. p73 in HCT116 cells does not detectably induce p21WAF1 expression or affect cell cycle distribution. (*A*) p53 and p73 expression was induced in p53$^{+/+}$ and p53$^{-/-}$ HCT116 cells by treatment with CPT (300 nM), 5-FU (488 μM), or Dauno (200 nM) for 24 hr (for immunoblotting or RT-PCR) or 48 hr (for flow cytometry). Western blotting was performed to detect p53 using DO-1, p73 using a TA-p73 polyclonal antibody, and p21WAF1 (Oncogene, Ab-1). As a loading control, actin was measured by anti-actin antibody (Sigma). Quantitative RT-PCR was then performed to assess the induction of p21WAF1 mRNA. (*B*) To determine the cell cycle profile, cells were collected and fixed with 70% ethanol 48 hr after drug treatment. After PI staining, FACS analysis was performed.

How Much p53 and p73 Protein Is Present in HCT116 Cells?

Returning to our findings that, whereas p73α and β induced several p53 target genes including p21 when expressed at comparable levels to p53 in H1299 cells, endogenous p73 could not induce p21WAF1 in HCT116$^{-/-}$ cells, we considered the possibility that there is a threshold amount of protein required to induce p53 target genes, and endogenous p73 levels after DNA damage were not enough to induce p21 in HCT116 cells. Therefore, we determined the amount of endogenous p53 and p73α protein in HCT116 cells. Because each antibody differs in its sensitivity in detecting its respective protein by immunoblotting, we used protein standards of purified HA-tagged p53 or p73α. To this end, HA-p53 and HA-p73α recombinant proteins were affinity-purified from baculovirally infected SF9 cells and then subjected to SDS-PAGE followed by silver staining (Fig. 4A, upper right

panel). Quantification was also performed using a bovine serum albumin (BSA) standard curve, and concentration of each stock solution is shown (Fig. 4A, left upper panel). Indeed, the signal intensity of these two proteins using anti-HA antibody (normalized by molar ratio) supports the quantification obtained by BSA standard in silver staining.

Next, to determine the amount of endogenous p53 and TA-p73α expressed in HCT116 cells, we made serial dilutions of the purified HA-p53 and HA-p73 proteins and compared them to the levels of endogenous protein induced following CPT treatment by immunoblotting using the anti-p53 monoclonal antibody (DO-1) and anti-p73 polyclonal antibody (TA-p73) (Fig. 4B). This allowed us to estimate the basal expression of endogenous p53 as ~5 × 10^{-4} pmole per microgram, whereas p53 levels reach 111.48 × 10^{-4} pmole per microgram of whole-cell extract (WCE) after CPT treatment (23 ng/μg of WCE). Thus, p53 accumulated 20-fold following DNA damage (Fig. 4B, left panel).

The basal expression of TA-p73α was too low to detect in this range of protein (probably less than 0.287 × 10^{-4} pmole per microgram of WCE; 2 ng/μg of WCE) (Fig. 4B; see table). In addition, the amount of endogenous TA-p73α expressed following DNA damage was in the range of that of uninduced p53, and about 30-fold lower than that of p53 following CPT treatment, suggesting that the endogenous p73α expression level is much lower than that of p53 in the presence or absence of DNA damage in HCT116 cells. Thus, it is possible that the inability of endogenous p73 to replace p53's function is, at least in part, due to the significantly lower levels of p73 in the cell.

Currently, it is thought that the choice between cell cycle arrest and apoptosis is determined in part by levels of p53 and in part by its modification status. In this work, we address this issue by using adenoviral infection to determine whether p53 levels in a cell correlate with its ability to transactivate pro-apoptotic targets. Indeed, the levels of p53 expression determined the threshold of activation for the low-affinity pro-apoptotic AIP1 promoter. Interestingly, a 10-fold difference in p53 levels could determine not only whether the pro-apoptotic AIP1 promoter was transactivated, but also whether binding at the AIP1, but not p21WAF1, promoter could be detected, suggesting a threshold at the level of DNA binding. Furthermore, we calculated the average number of p53 molecules that are required per cell for transactivation of p21 or AIP1 promoters. Interestingly, endogenous p53 is present in cells at levels below the apoptotic threshold calculated for adenovirally expressed p53, which raises a number of questions about the difference between endogenous and exogenous proteins and their ability to induce apoptosis. It should be noted as well that a number of experiments have indicated that endogenously expressed p73 is not inert. For example, siRNA knockdown of p73 in SW480 cells (Irwin et al. 2003) or H1299 cells (Urist et al. 2004) reduces the low level of apoptosis caused by some agents in the absence of p53. Perhaps HCT116 cells are particularly defective in responding to p73 induction. Nevertheless, ChIP analysis in these cell lines shows that endoge-

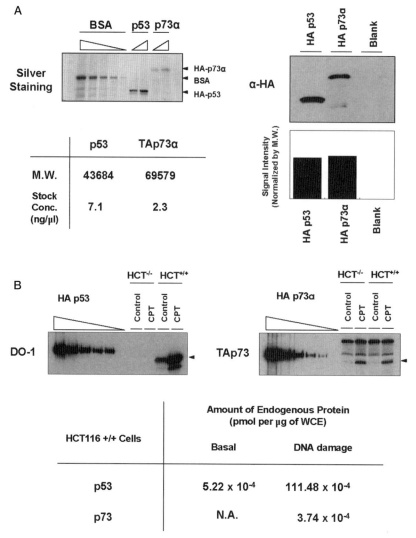

Figure 4. Quantification of expression levels of endogenous p73 and p53 after CPT treatment. (*A*) Purified p53 and p73 protein standard was obtained by affinity-purifying HA-p53 and HA-p73α baculovirally expressed in SF9 cells. To determine the nanogram amounts of each protein, a silver stain was performed, with BSA as control (*top left panel*). The quantification is presented in the bottom left panel. To assure the accuracy of our quantification, we performed a western blot using normalized amounts of the protein standards (*right top panel*). As shown in the bottom right panel, the p53 and p73 protein standards have similar amounts of protein. (*B*) To determine the amounts of endogenous p53 and p73 expressed in HCT116 cells, 80 μg of lysate from uninduced cells and cells treated with CPT was loaded onto an SDS-PAGE gel along with serial dilutions of the p53 or p73 protein standards. Immunoblotting was then performed using DO-1 antibody to detect p53 (*top right*) and TA-p73 polyclonal antibody to detect p73 (*top left*). The picogram and picomolar quantifications of p53 and p73 are presented in the bottom panel.

nous TA-p73α is bound to the p21 promoter, suggesting that this protein does have DNA-binding activity. Experiments with siRNA would be required to show whether the endogenous p73 has any transcriptional or pro-apoptotic activity, since, although unlikely, it is possible that this protein can bind promoters but cannot transactivate them in HCT116 cells. It would also be important to confirm whether ectopic p73 expression can induce p53 target genes and apoptosis in HCT116 cells.

The p53 family member p73, when first discovered, was postulated to be a tumor suppressor, largely based on the highly conserved functional activity between the two family members. However, data from both human tumors and p73 knockout mice brought the tumor suppressor function of this p53 family member into question. In screening a few cell lines for levels of p73, we have found that HCT116 cells are among those that are relatively more abundant in this protein. Therefore, our quantification of the levels of p73 present in these cells may at least partially explain the failure of cells to undergo significant arrest or apoptosis in the absence of p53.

Most published work shows that exogenous p53 and p73β have similar transcriptional activities, and p73α is somewhat weaker than p73β. We reproduced these findings using a tetracycline-regulated system where ectopic protein expression can be induced in the absence of DNA damage. Our data indicate that p53 and p73β do exhibit almost identical activity in initiating transcription of four canonical p53 target genes. We also found that p73α induced about three times less p21 protein expression than did p53 or p73β. Although we did not measure the effect of the overexpression of these proteins on cell cycle distribution, several lines of evidence suggest that the two family members can induce comparable levels of apoptosis. It is therefore likely that the inability of p73 to induce a p53-like cell cycle profile is because the levels to which p73 is expressed are insufficient. The quantification of p73 expressed in HCT116 cells compared to p53 shows that the levels of the former are almost 30 times lower than that of the latter. Such low levels of p73 (in addition to the already lower activity of the alpha isoform) could explain why this protein does not phenocopy p53. On the basis of these data, we would predict that if it were expressed at levels similar to p53, endogenous p73 should be able to transactivate target genes and induce cell cycle arrest and apoptosis to an extent similar to p53.

Considering that splicing variants of p73 display different transcriptional properties and biological functions, and that they are expressed differentially among normal human tissues and cell lines, further investigation using other cell lines will be required to examine the relation between the levels and activities of p73 or p53 and the threshold for target gene transactivation and induction of apoptosis. Taken together, although we cannot exclude the possibility of cell-type specificity and isoform-specific functions, our results indicate that compared to p53, TA-p73 is expressed at very low levels in cells, which may explain in part why p73 does not function as a tumor suppressor as does p53.

ACKNOWLEDGMENTS

Ella Freulich is thanked for expert technical assistance. We thank Yingchun Li and Christopher Neusch for discussions. This work was supported by National Cancer Institute grant CA87497.

REFERENCES

Agami R., Blandino G., Oren M., and Shaul Y. 1999. Interaction of c-Abl and p73α and their collaboration to induce apoptosis. *Nature* **399:** 809.

Appella E. and Anderson C.W. 2001. Post-translational modifications and activation of p53 by genotoxic stresses. *Eur. J. Biochem.* **268:** 2764.

Attardi L.D. and Jacks T. 1999. The role of p53 in tumour suppression: Lessons from mouse models. *Cell Mol. Life Sci.* **55:** 48.

Bates S. and Vousden K.H. 1999. Mechanisms of p-53-mediated apoptosis. *Cell Mol. Life Sci.* **55:** 28.

Chen X., Ko L.J., Jayaraman L., and Prives C. 1996. p53 levels, functional domains, and DNA damage determine the extent of the apoptotic response of tumor cells. *Genes Dev.* **10:** 2438.

Costanzo A., Merlo P., Pediconi N., Fulco M., Sartorelli V., Cole P.A., Fontemaggi G., Fanciulli M., Schiltz L., Blandino G., Balsano C., and Levrero M. 2002. DNA damage-dependent acetylation of p73 dictates the selective activation of apoptotic target genes. *Mol. Cell* **9:** 175.

Donehower L.A., Harvey M., Slagle B.L., McArthur M.J., Montgomery C.A., Jr., Butel J.S., and Bradley A. 1992. Mice deficient for p53 are developmentally normal but susceptible to spontaneous tumours. *Nature* **356:** 215.

Gu W. and Roeder R.G. 1997. Activation of p53 sequence-specific DNA binding by acetylation of the p53 C-terminal domain. *Cell* **90:** 595.

Harms K., Nozell S., and Chen X. 2004. The common and distinct target genes of the p53 family transcription factors. *Cell Mol. Life Sci.* **61:** 822.

Irwin M.S. and Kaelin W.G., Jr. 2001a. p53 family update: p73 and p63 develop their own identities. *Cell Growth Differ.* **12:** 337.

———. 2001b. Role of the newer p53 family proteins in malignancy. *Apoptosis* **6:** 17.

Irwin M.S., Kondo K., Marin M.C., Cheng L.S., Hahn W.C., and Kaelin W.G., Jr. 2003. Chemosensitivity linked to p73 function. *Cancer Cell* **3:** 403.

Jost C.A., Marin M.C., and Kaelin W.G., Jr. 1997. p73 is a simian [correction of human] p53-related protein that can induce apoptosis. *Nature* **389:** 191.

Kaeser M.D. and Iggo R.D. 2002. Chromatin immunoprecipitation analysis fails to support the latency model for regulation of p53 DNA binding activity in vivo. *Proc. Natl. Acad. Sci.* **99:** 95.

Kaghad M., Bonnet H., Yang A., Creancier L., Biscan J.C., Valent A., Minty A., Chalon P., Lelias J.M., Dumont X., Ferrara P., McKeon F., and Caput D. 1997. Monoallelically expressed gene related to p53 at 1p36, a region frequently deleted in neuroblastoma and other human cancers. *Cell* **90:** 809.

Ko L.J. and Prives C. 1996. p53: Puzzle and paradigm. *Genes Dev.* **10:** 1054.

Lee C.W. and La Thangue N.B. 1999. Promoter specificity and stability control of the p53-related protein p73. *Oncogene* **18:** 4171.

Levine A.J. 1997. p53, the cellular gatekeeper for growth and division. *Cell* **88:** 323.

Lin K.W., Nam S.Y., Toh W.H., Dulloo I., and Sabapathy K. 2004. Multiple stress signals induce p73β accumulation. *Neoplasia* **6:** 546.

Liu G. and Chen X. 2005. The C-terminal sterile alpha motif and the extreme C terminus regulate the transcriptional activity of the alpha isoform of p73. *J. Biol. Chem.* **280:** 20111.

Ludwig R.L., Bates S., and Vousden K.H. 1996. Differential activation of target cellular promoters by p53 mutants with impaired apoptotic function. *Mol. Cell. Biol.* **16:** 4952.

Moll U.M. and Petrenko O. 2003. The MDM2-p53 interaction. *Mol. Cancer Res.* **1:** 1001.

Moll U.M. and Slade N. 2004. p63 and p73: Roles in development and tumor formation. *Mol. Cancer Res.* **2:** 371.

Oda K., Arakawa H., Tanaka T., Matsuda K., Tanikawa C., Mori T., Nishimori H., Tamai K., Tokino T., Nakamura Y., and Taya Y. 2000. p53AIP1, a potential mediator of p53-dependent apoptosis, and its regulation by Ser-46-phosphorylated p53. *Cell* **102:** 849.

Ozaki T., Naka M., Takada N., Tada M., Sakiyama S., and Nakagawara A. 1999. Deletion of the COOH-terminal region of p73α enhances both its *trans*-activation function and DNA-binding activity but inhibits induction of apoptosis in mammalian cells. *Cancer Res.* **59:** 5902.

Poyurovsky M.V. and Prives C. 2006. Unleashing the power of p53: Lessons from mice and men. *Genes Dev.* **20:** 125. (11)

Prives C. and Hall P.A. 1999. The p53 pathway. *J. Pathol.* **187:** 112.

Sakaguchi K., Herrera J.E., Saito S., Miki T., Bustin M., Vassilev A., Anderson C.W., and Appella E. 1998. DNA damage activates p53 through a phosphorylation-acetylation cascade. *Genes Dev.* **12:** 2831.

Samuels-Lev Y., O'Connor D.J., Bergamaschi D., Trigiante G., Hsieh J.K., Zhong S., Campargue I., Naumovski L., Crook T., and Lu X. 2001. *Mol. Cell* **8:** 781.

Shieh S.Y., Ikeda M., Taya Y., and Prives C. 1997. DNA damage-induced phosphorylation of p53 alleviates inhibition by MDM2. *Cell* **91:** 325.

Szak S.T., Mays D., and Pietenpol J.A. 2001. Kinetics of p53 binding to promoter sites in vivo. *Mol. Cell. Biol.* **21:** 3375.

Ueda Y., Hijikata M., Takagi S., Chiba T., and Shimotohno K. 1999. New p73 variants with altered C-terminal structures have varied transcriptional activities. *Oncogene* **18:** 4993.

Urist M., Tanaka T., Poyurovsky M.V., and Prives C. 2004. p73 induction after DNA damage is regulated by checkpoint kinases Chk1 and Chk2. *Genes Dev.* **18:** 3041.

Wang Y. and Prives C. 1995. Increased and altered DNA binding of human p53 by S and G2/M but not G1 cyclin-dependent kinases. *Nature* **376:** 88.

Yang A., Kaghad M., Caput D., and McKeon F. 2002. On the shoulders of giants: p63, p73 and the rise of p53. *Trends Genet.* **18:** 90.

Yang A., Walker N., Bronson R., Kaghad M., Oosterwegel M., Bonnin J., Vagner C., Bonnet H., Dikkes P., Sharpe A., McKeon F., and Caput D. 2000. p73-deficient mice have neurological, pheromonal and inflammatory defects but lack spontaneous tumours. *Nature* **404:** 99.

Yuan Z.M., Shioya H., Ishiko T., Sun X., Gu J., Huang Y.Y., Lu H., Kharbanda S., Weichselbaum R., and Kufe D. 1999. p73 is regulated by tyrosine kinase c-Abl in the apoptotic response to DNA damage. *Nature* **399:** 814.

Zhu J., Jiang J., Zhou W., and Chen X. 1998. The potential tumor suppressor p73 differentially regulates cellular p53 target genes. *Cancer Res.* **58:** 5061.

p53-Dependent and -Independent Functions of the Arf Tumor Suppressor

C.J. Sherr,*[†] D. Bertwistle,*[†] W. den Besten,[†] M.-L. Kuo,*[†] M. Sugimoto,*[†] K. Tago,*[†] R.T. Williams,[†‡] F. Zindy,[†] and M.F. Roussel[†]

*Howard Hughes Medical Institute and Departments of [†]Genetics and Tumor Cell Biology and [‡]Hematology-Oncology, St. Jude Children's Research Hospital, Memphis, Tennessee 38105

The *Ink4a-Arf* locus encodes two closely wedded tumor suppressor proteins (p16[Ink4a] and p19[Arf]) that inhibit cell proliferation by activating Rb and p53, respectively. With few exceptions, the *Arf* gene is repressed during mouse embryonic development, thereby helping to limit p53 expression during organogenesis. However, in adult mice, sustained hyperproliferative signals conveyed by somatically activated oncogenes can induce *Arf* gene expression and trigger a p53 response that eliminates incipient cancer cells. Disruption of this tumor surveillance pathway predisposes to cancer, and inactivation of *INK4a-ARF* by deletion, silencing, or mutation has been frequently observed in many forms of human cancer. Although it is accepted that much of Arf's tumor-suppressive activity is mediated by p53, more recent genetic evidence has pointed to additional p53-independent functions of Arf, including its ability to inhibit gene expression by a number of other transcription factors. Surprisingly, the enforced expression of Arf in mammalian cells promotes the sumoylation of several Arf-interacting proteins, implying that Arf has an associated catalytic activity. We speculate that transcriptional down-regulation in response to Arf-induced sumoylation may account for Arf's p53-independent functions.

Mammalian INK4 proteins are specific polypeptide inhibitors of the cyclin D-dependent kinases (Cdk4 and Cdk6) whose expression helps to maintain proteins of the retinoblastoma family (RB, p107, and p130) in their active hypophosphorylated states. By doing so, the INK4 proteins enhance the growth-suppressive activities of RB and its relatives, thereby preventing cells from entering the DNA synthetic (S) phase of the cell division cycle and reinforcing RB-dependent transcriptional programs that regulate cell differentiation and senescence. The founding member of the *INK4* gene family, *INK4a* (Serrano et al. 1993), is one of four genes whose encoded products act in a biochemically similar manner to inhibit the Cdk4 and Cdk6 kinases (Roussel 1999; Ortega et al. 2002). In humans, *INK4a* and *INK4b* are closely linked on the short arm of chromosome 9, whereas the two other family members (*INK4c* and *INK4d*) reside on chromosomes 1 and 19, respectively. In the mouse, however, *Ink4a*, *Ink4b*, and *Ink4c* all map to chromosome 4 with *Ink4c* separated from the *Ink4a/Ink4b* cluster by 18 cM. The *Ink4c* and *Ink4d* genes are ubiquitously expressed in highly stereotypic patterns in the mouse embryo, and their loss of function can severely compromise the proper development of certain tissues. In contrast, neither *Ink4a* nor *Ink4b* is expressed during development or, at appreciable levels, in tissues of young mice (Zindy et al. 1997, 2003), and their inactivation in the germ line does not lead to obvious developmental anomalies (Serrano et al. 1996; Latres et al. 2000; Krimpenfort et al. 2001; Sharpless et al. 2001). Instead, their induction occurs in response to particular cellular stresses that can contribute to tumor formation (Lowe and Sherr 2003). At least three Ink4 proteins (p16[Ink4a], p15[Ink4b], and p18[Ink4c]) are tumor suppressors, but by far, the most frequently inactivated family member in human cancers is *INK4a* (Ruas and Peters 1998).

Remarkably, the mouse *Ink4a* locus was found to encode yet another tumor suppressor protein, p19[Arf] (p14[ARF] in humans) whose expression induces p53 (Quelle et al. 1995; Kamijo et al. 1997). The organization of the locus—now designated *Ink4a-Arf*—is unusual in the sense that the two protein products are encoded in part by alternative reading frames (from which *Arf* takes its name) within exon 2 (Fig. 1A). Because the *Ink4a* and *Arf* genes have alternative first exons and separate promoter elements, they can be independently regulated, mutated, and epigenetically silenced. Together, *INK4a*, *ARF*, *RB*, and *TP53* represent the most frequently inactivated tumor suppressors in human tumors, suggesting that their loss of function might be a necessary prerequisite for the transformation of normal cells into cancer cells. Here, we review *Arf*'s activities and discuss insights stemming from recent studies.

p19[Arf] INDUCES p53—THE ORIGINAL PARADIGM

Enforced expression of the p19[Arf] protein arrests cells in both the G_1 and G_2 phases of the cell division cycle (Quelle et al. 1995). Much of the growth-suppressive function of p19[Arf] depends on its ability to interfere with the p53 negative regulator Mdm2 (HDM2 in humans), which itself is a p53-responsive gene. Arf stabilizes p53 by blocking Mdm2's activity as an E3 ubiquitin protein ligase (Honda and Yasuda 1999). It can also relocalize Mdm2 into nucleoli, where the bulk of intracellular p19[Arf] resides (Weber et al. 1999), although this may not be necessary for p53 induction (Llanos et al. 2001). Whatever the exact mechanisms involved, growth arrest by p19[Arf] depends to a great extent on p53-dependent transcription, which up-regulates many antiproliferative

A.

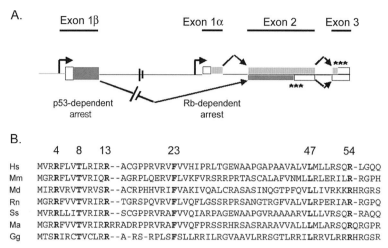

B.

```
              4   8   13          23                    47      54
    Hs   MVRRFLVTLRIRR--ACGPPRVRVFVVHIPRLTGEWAAPGAPAAVALVLMLLRSQR-LGQQ
    Mm   MGRRFLVTVRIQR--AGRPLQERVFLVKFVRSRRPRTASCALAFVNMLLRLERILR-RGPH
    Md   MIRRVRVTVRVSR--ACRPHHVRIFVAKIVQALCRASASINQGTPFQVLLIVRKKRHRGRS
    Rn   MGRRFVVTVRIRR--TGRSPQVRVFLVQFLGSSRPRSANGTRGFVALVLRPERIAR-RGPQ
    Ss   MVRRLLITVRIRR--SCGPPRVRAFVVQIARPAGEWAAPGVRAAAARVLLLVRSQR-RAQQ
    Ma   MGRRFVVTVRIRRRRADRPPRVRAFVVQFPRSSRHRSASRARAVVALLLMLARSQRQRGPR
    Gg   MTSRIRCTVCLRR--A-RS-RPLSFSLLRRILRGVAAVLRRSGTLRRILRRVLRRRHRGSR
```

Figure 1. Organization of the *Ink4a-Arf* locus and comparison of amino acid sequences encoded by *Arf* exon 1β in various species. (*A*) The *Ink4a* gene is composed of three exons (1α, 2, and 3 indicated by boxes). Coding segments are indicated by light gray shading above the horizontal line whereas noncoding segments are unshaded. The *Arf* gene is represented by exons 1β (~15 kb upstream), 2, and 3. Coding sequences (*dark gray shading*) in exon 2 are in an alternative reading frame from that which encodes p16^{Ink4a}. Arrows indicate the two promoters and splicing patterns. Asterisks denote the positions of termination codons. Strains of knockout (KO) mice include animals that lack both gene products (Serrano et al. 1996), *Arf* alone (Kamijo et al. 1997), and *Ink4a* alone (Krimpenfort et al. 2001; Sharpless et al. 2001). Sequences encoding GFP have also been knocked into (KI) the Arf locus replacing exon 1β (Zindy et al. 2003). (*B*). Amino-terminal sequences encoded by *Arf* exon 1(from *Homo sapiens* (Hs), *Mus musculus* (Mm), *Monodelphis domestica* (opossum) (Md), *Ratus norvegicus* (Rn), *Sus scrofa* (domestic pig) (Ss), *Mesocricetus auratus* (golden hamster) (Ma), and *Gallus gallus* (chicken) (Gg). The positions of six universally conserved residues are denoted by bold type and by numbers above the figure. (Adapted, with permission, from Sherr [1998] and Kuo et al. [2004].)

genes, such as the Cdk inhibitor p21^{Cip1} (El-Deiry et al. 1993), as well as a subset of genes that contribute to p53's pro-apoptotic functions (Vousden and Lu 2002). However, p19^{Arf} can arrest the division of cells lacking *Cip1* (Pantoja and Serrano 1999; Modestou et al. 2001) as well as those lacking *p53* alone or both *p53* and *Mdm2*, albeit much less efficiently than in cells that preserve p53 function (Carnero et al. 2000; Weber et al. 2000b). Thus, *Arf* has both p53-dependent and -independent activities.

Animals lacking *Arf* are highly tumor-prone, although spontaneous tumors occur with a rate and spectrum that differ from those of animals lacking *p53* (Jacks et al. 1994; Kamijo et al. 1999a). Whereas *p53*-null mice tend to develop lymphomas and die within 6 months of birth, the *Arf*-null animals live much longer (up to 15 months) and have a propensity to develop more sarcomas than lymphomas. In addition, about 25% of *Arf*-null animals develop gliomas and carcinomas, which rarely arise spontaneously in mice lacking *p53*. Although *Arf* is activated in response to various forms of stress (see below), it is not acutely induced in response to DNA double-strand breaks triggered by ionizing irradiation, although *Arf*'s absence can enhance Mdm2's ability to down-regulate p53 during the DNA damage response (Kamijo et al. 1997, 1999b). Triple knockout (TKO) mice lacking *Arf*, *Mdm2*, and *p53* rapidly develop many more tumors—and frequently, multiple tumors of different histological types per animal— than mice lacking both *Mdm2* and *p53* (Weber et al. 2000b). Indeed, most TKO animals die of various cancers before reaching breeding age. Although obtained with difficulty, TKO mouse embryonic fibroblasts (MEFs) can be growth-arrested when p19^{Arf} expression is reinforced. Together, these results underscore the ability of p19^{Arf} to interact with targets other than Mdm2 and p53.

Arf REGULATES REPLICATIVE SENESCENCE

Although *Arf* is expressed in the yolk sac and embryonic eye (see below), it is not appreciably expressed in other tissues within the mouse embryo, implying that the Arf–Mdm2–p53 pathway is generally shut off during development in utero (Zindy et al. 1997, 2003). However, explantation and passage of primary MEFs in tissue culture leads to *Arf* induction with a steady increase in its protein levels that correlates with the waning proliferative capacity of continuously propagated cells (Kamijo et al. 1997; Zindy et al. 1998). This seemingly spontaneous activation of p19^{Arf} in cultured MEFs results in their replicative senescence. Conversely, MEFs explanted from *Arf*-null animals not only proliferate faster than their wild-type counterparts in culture, but also do not senesce and behave like established mouse cell lines (Kamijo et al. 1997). Moreover, immortalized cell populations that arise stochastically as wild-type MEFs are continuously propagated in culture either acquire *p53* mutations (Harvey and Levine 1991) or sustain bi-allelic *Ink4a-Arf* deletions (Kamijo et al. 1997). These findings pointed to the idea that *Ink4a* and *Arf* are induced in response to the nonphysiological tissue culture milieu ("culture shock") (Sherr and DePinho 2001). The rate of *Arf* induction can be accelerated by introducing oncogenes such as activated Myc, Ras, or adenovirus E1A into primary cell strains (Zindy et al. 1998; De Stanchina et al. 1998; Palmero et al. 1998) or by subjecting MEFs to low but persistent levels of oxidative stress (Busuttil et al. 2003; Parrinello et al. 2003). *Ink4a* is also induced by many of the same stress stimuli that impinge upon *Arf*, but even though p16^{Ink4a} levels continue to rise to a maximum during continuous passage of MEFs in culture, *Ink4a* loss alone in MEFs does not bypass senescence (Krimpenfort et al. 2001; Sharpless et al. 2001). Still, the determinants of the senescence response of mouse cells are to some extent cell-type-specific. For example, bone-marrow-derived pre-B cells can be immortalized through *Arf* inactivation, whereas immortalization of bone-marrow-derived macrophages explanted from *Arf*-null animals depends on the inactivation of *Ink4a*, which undergoes epigenetic silencing (Randle et al. 2001).

The co-inactivation of *INK4a* and *ARF* (or co-elimination of both *RB* and *TP53*) endows human cells with an increased cellular life span in culture. However, these events are not sufficient to immortalize human cells in which replicative senescence is also triggered by telomere malfunction (Wright and Shay 2000). MEFs have considerably longer telomeres than those of human fibroblast strains, and they have a greater propensity to express telomerase and maintain telomere length. Engineered acute disruption of mouse telomere integrity activates the *Arf* checkpoint, whereas both *ARF* and *INK4a* respond in human cells (Smogorzewska and De Lange 2002). On the basis of these and other considerations, it has been suggested that *INK4a* may play a more significant role in governing the senescence of human versus mouse cells (Wright and Shay 2000). By genetically eliminating telomerase activity in the mouse germ line and interbreeding the progeny, later generations of telomerase-null mice that developed shorter telomeres were forced to confront the problem of telomere insufficiency (Blasco et al. 1997). Cells from these "humanized" mouse strains not only activated Rb- and p53-dependent checkpoints in response to telomere shortening but, in the absence of these checkpoints, manifested progressive telomere attrition and eventually entered "crisis" (Lee et al. 1998; Rudolph et al. 1999). The latter event is characterized by end-to-end chromosome fusions and fusion-bridge-breakage cycles that destabilize the genome and trigger mitotic catastrophe. Because cells from these mice cannot reactivate telomerase activity, they can only restabilize their telomeres through alternative recombination-based mechanisms. Mice lacking telomerase and intact checkpoint controls spontaneously develop a telling spectrum of tumors, the majority of which are carcinomas that are rarely observed in wild-type mice (Artandi et al. 2000). This response to checkpoint disruption and telomere attrition closely reflects the human cancer condition in which carcinomas predominate as we age.

ACTIVATING *Arf* GENE EXPRESSION

Abnormal hyperproliferative signals conveyed by oncogenes can remodel the otherwise insulated *Arf* promoter to enable its expression (Lowe and Sherr 2003). In turn, the ability of p19^{Arf} to activate p53 provides a safeguard that protects such cells from oncogenic challenge. In a Burkitt's lymphoma model in which a *Myc* transgene is driven by an immunoglobulin promoter-enhancer (Eμ-*Myc* mice) (Adams et al. 1985), *Arf* induction in *Myc*-expressing B cells limits Myc's pro-proliferative effects early in the course of disease. However, continued Myc

expression eventually selects for the appearance of cells that have sustained *p53* mutations or *Arf* deletions, thereby allowing lymphomas to arise (Eischen et al. 1999; Jacobs et al. 1999b; Schmitt et al. 1999). Eμ-*Myc*-induced lymphomagenesis is greatly accelerated in an *Arf*$^{+/-}$ genetic background where the wild-type *Arf* allele is rapidly inactivated; in an *Arf*$^{-/-}$ background, animals become moribund very soon after birth, and all die within 8 weeks of highly aggressive lympholeukemias with widespread visceral involvement (Eischen et al. 1999). Similar effects of *Arf* on tumor suppression have been observed in carcinogen-induced skin tumors where somatic mutation of Ras is the initiating step (Kelly-Spratt et al. 2004). Importantly, Myc or Ras signaling in normal cells, although important for their proliferative response to mitogens, is insufficient to activate *Arf*. Therefore, *Arf* acts as a fuse to monitor mitogenic "current" and to trigger a p53 response only when mitogenic signals are abnormally sustained and/or elevated above a potentially deleterious threshold level.

Strikingly, after replacement of Arf exon 1β genomic sequences with those encoding green fluorescent protein (GFP), tumors arising in functionally *Arf*-null *Arf*$^{GFP/GFP}$ homozygous mice were vividly fluorescent, whereas the non-tumor tissues in moribund mice did not express GFP (Fig. 2A,B,D) (Zindy et al. 2003). When the Eμ-*Myc* transgene was expressed in *Arf*$^{GFP/+}$ heterozygotes, the wild-type allele was lost and lymphomagenesis was accelerated relative to the rate of tumor formation in *Arf*$^{+/+}$

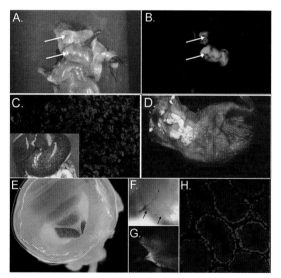

Figure 2. GFP expression in tissues of *Arf* GFP/GFP mice. (*A,B*) A green fluorescent fibrosarcoma in the neck region. (*C*) Macroscopic foci of GFP-positive lymphoma cells in the liver and a microscopic metastasis (*inset*) visualized by immunofluorescence (*red*) and counterstained with 4′,6-diamidino-2-phenylindole (*blue*). (*D*) Whole-body imaging of a shaved Arf$^{+/GFP}$ Eμ-*Myc* transgenic mouse with lymphoma. (*E*) Whole mount showing a funnel-shaped mass stretching from the lens (*top left*) toward the optic cup (*rear*). A closer view shows elements of the hyaloid vasculature (*F, arrows*) within the fluorescent mass (*G*). (*H*) Immunohistochemical staining of GFP (*red*) in the testis of an 8-month-old mouse. (Reprinted, with permission, from Zindy et al. 2003.)

littermates. Early in the course of disease, we detected GFP-positive cells in the bone marrow, spleen, and lymph nodes of Eμ-Myc transgenic Arf $^{GFP/+}$ mice, implying that Arf induction could be used to monitor precancerous lesions. In turn, once lymphomas arose, their metastatic spread was marked by the appearance of vividly fluorescent tumor nodules in various organs (Fig. 2C). Using a monoclonal antibody to p19^{Arf} that detects the endogenous protein in fixed lymphoid cells (Bertwistle et al. 2004b), we hope to determine how early in the course of Eμ-Myc-induced disease the endogenous Arf protein is induced.

Interestingly, with few exceptions, very few cells in young, normal Arf $^{GFP/GFP}$ homozygotes exhibited green fluorescence. However, Arf-null mice become blind soon after birth due to the formation of a cellular mass in the vitreous that disrupts the normal architecture of the lens and retina. Arf expression in the vitreous during the first week after birth is required for regression of the hyaloid vasculature system that nourishes the developing lens (McKeller et al. 2002). In newborn Arf-null mice, persistence of the hyaloid vasculature leads to an abnormal proliferation of perivascular cells that form a funnel-shaped mass in the vitreous (Fig. 2E,F). In Arf $^{GFP/GFP}$ animals, the retrolental mass included green fluorescent cells (Fig. 2G). Arf expression could also be observed in testicular tubules, in cells that most likely represent spermatogonia or leptotene spermatocytes at the earliest stages of meiosis I (Fig. 2H). Small pockets of green fluorescent cells could be seen in other ostensibly normal tissues, including the thymic medulla and lung alveoli, although such cells were rare and expressed only low levels of GFP detected by immunohistochemistry (Zindy et al. 2003).

Understanding how the Arf promoter distinguishes normal and abnormal signaling thresholds remains problematic. Arf is normally repressed by E2F complexes (Rowland et al. 2002), but unlike many E2F-responsive genes that govern DNA synthesis and replication, Arf is not periodically expressed when cells enter S phase. Yet, when Arf is induced by oncogenes, E2Fs 1, 2, and 3a replace repressive E2F complexes on the Arf promoter (Aslanian et al. 2004). Hence, other specificity factors must play a role in modulating this E2F response. An attractive candidate is the Dmp1 transcription factor, which binds adjacent to an E2F site in the proximal Arf promoter to activate the gene (Inoue et al. 1999). Several features suggest that Dmp1 plays a role in regulating Arf induction mediated by oncogenes: (1) Dmp1 is a Ras-responsive gene that is activated via the Raf–MEK–ERK pathway (Sreeramaneni et al. 2005); (2) Dmp1 overexpression in response to oncogenic Ras induces cell cycle arrest in primary MEFs in an Arf-dependent manner (Inoue et al. 1999); (3) conversely, Dmp1-null MEFs bypass senescence with relative ease and can be transformed even at early passage by oncogenic Ras at a detectable frequency (Inoue et al. 2000); (4) Dmp1$^{-/-}$ and Dmp1$^{+/-}$ mice, like Arf-null animals, are highly sensitive to Eμ-Myc- or carcinogen-induced lymphomagenesis, and in these settings, Dmp1 is haplo-insufficient for tumor suppression; (5) inactivation of Dmp1 reduces the frequency of Arf loss and p53 mutation during Eμ-Myc-induced lymphomagenesis, indicating that Dmp1

is a genetic modifier of the Arf–Mdm2–p53 signaling pathway (Inoue et al. 2001). It will be of interest to determine the status of various E2F complexes on the Arf promoter in cells lacking Dmp1 and in those reconstituted with wild-type and mutant Dmp1 alleles.

Arf is subject to repression by a variety of other proteins, including Bmi1, Tbx2 and Tbx3, Jun D, Twist, CBX7, and Pokemon (Jacobs et al. 1999b, 2000; Maestro et al. 1999; Weitzman et al. 2000; Lingbeek et al. 2002; Gil et al. 2004; Maeda et al. 2005). Some of these repressors are likely to be responsible for silencing the Arf locus during development. In particular, inactivation of Bmi1 results in inappropriate Ink4a-Arf expression in cerebellar granule neuron precursors and in adult hematopoietic stem cells, so that Bmi1-null animals exhibit defects in postnatal cerebellar development and die early in life from bone marrow aplasia. These defects are rescued on an Ink4a-Arf-null background, indicating that abnormal activation of the locus can interfere with these developmental processes (Jacobs et al. 1999a). In contrast, multiple embryonic defects arising in mice lacking Twist (W. den Besten, unpubl.) or yolk sac atresia occurring in homozygous Tbx3-null mice (Jerome-Majewska et al., in press) are not rescued in an Arf-null background.

THE p19^{Arf} PROTEIN: A CHALLENGE FOR BIOCHEMISTS

Arf proteins are highly basic (pI ~12) and contain ~20% arginine but only one (p19^{Arf}) or no (p14^{ARF}) lysines. Truncation of the mouse Arf gene near the exon 1β-exon 2 junction yielded a polypeptide of 64 amino acids that exhibited the growth-suppressing activity of the parental full-length molecule (Quelle et al. 1997). In this regard, chickens lack the Ink4a locus but have an Arf gene specifying a 7-kD protein encoded almost exclusively by exon 1β sequences (Fig. 1B) (Kim et al. 2003). Most recombinant p19^{Arf} protein expressed in bacteria is insoluble, and many arginyl codons are improperly translated. Reasoning that the more abundant species of bacterial arginyl tRNAs do not efficiently recognize a subset of mammalian arginine codons, we used synthetic oligonucleotides to construct an Arf minigene encoding the amino-terminal 62 amino acids of p19^{Arf}; in doing so, many codons were altered to improve translation in bacteria (Weber et al. 2000a). Although the correct product was produced, much of it remained insoluble and worthless for "test tube biochemistry" or for structural analysis.

Given the fact that Arf proteins must function at neutral pH, they must be highly buffered within living cells. Using tandem affinity-tagged p19^{Arf}, we purified Arf-associated proteins from mouse fibroblasts undergoing cell cycle arrest and identified them by mass spectroscopy. TAP-tagged Arf associated with many proteins, the most prominent being nucleophosmin (NPM/B23), an abundant and highly acidic nucleolar protein (Bertwistle et al. 2004a). Although only a small fraction of cellular NPM binds to p19^{Arf}, most of the Arf protein in cells is associated with NPM, and this interaction occurs equally well in primary cells lacking Mdm2 and p53. When p19^{Arf} expression is induced, it colocalizes with NPM in very high molecular weight complexes of 2–5 MD. The biological meaning of the Arf–NPM interaction remains unclear. One group of investigators suggested that p19^{Arf} can impede NPM nucleocytoplasmic shuttling (Brady et al. 2004), whereas others have argued that NPM helps to sequester p19^{Arf} in nucleoli (Korgaonkar et al. 2005). All agree that p19^{Arf} binds NPM through the same domains that mediate its binding to Mdm2, so that the latter two proteins can compete with one another for p19^{Arf} binding. When associated with NPM, p19^{Arf} is highly stable and turns over with a half-life of 6–8 hours (Kuo et al. 2004). Overexpression of NPM further slows p19^{Arf} turnover, whereas "knocking down" NPM with shRNA has the opposite effect. An Arf mutant lacking amino-terminal residues 2–14 or another in which alanines were substituted for all six conserved residues encoded by exon 1β (Fig. 1B) still localized to nucleoli but did not bind with high affinity to either Mdm2 or NPM and was handicapped in inducing growth arrest. These two mutant proteins turn over with half-lives of only 90–120 minutes (Kuo et al. 2004). Thus, the stoichiometric binding of p19^{Arf} to nucleolar NPM might enable Arf to fold into a stable conformation, whereas unbound p19^{Arf} mutants might be aberrantly folded and subject to more rapid degradation.

The absence of lysine residues in human p14^{ARF} implied that its turnover did not depend on ubiquitination. However, both mouse p19^{Arf} and human p14^{ARF} undergo amino-terminal ubiquitination and proteasomal degradation (Kuo et al. 2004). Most eukaryotic proteins are acetylated at their amino termini and are therefore not substrates for amino-terminal ubiquitination. N-acetylation is favored by the presence of amino-terminal methionine, which can be cleaved by methionine aminopeptidase when the penultimate amino acid has a small radius of gyration (Bradshaw et al. 1998). Proteolytic exposure of certain amino-terminal residues, such as serine, allows acetylation to proceed efficiently, whereas other amino acids, such as glycine, are poor substrates (Polevoda and Sherman 2003). In addition, penultimate acidic residues promote acetylation whereas basic residues inhibit it. The mouse p19^{Arf} amino-terminal tripeptide, Met-Gly-Arg, is processed by methionine aminopeptidase, and the resulting Gly-Arg dipeptide strongly blocks acetylation, allowing amino-terminal ubiquitination. Arf mutants that were engineered to contain more favorable amino-terminal consensus sequences for acetylation were more stable than wild-type p19^{Arf}, indicating that amino-terminal ubiquitination can regulate the rate of Arf protein turnover (Kuo et al. 2004). In high-molecular-mass complexes with NPM, p19^{Arf} may require ubiquitination for its unfolding and subsequent destruction, but unstable Arf mutants, although still subject to amino-terminal ubiquitination, may be less dependent on this process for their destruction.

p53-INDEPENDENT FUNCTIONS OF Arf

Despite cogent genetic arguments that p19^{Arf} has tumor suppressor activities that do not depend on Mdm2 and p53, the mechanism(s) underlying Arf's p53-independent functions remain unclear. Arf can physically or functionally interact with a variety of proteins, including

the transcription factors E2F-1, Myc, NF-κB, and HIF-1α, nucleolar proteins including NPM and nucleolin, topoisomerase I, the Werners helicase (WRN), cyclin G1, the adenovirus E1A-regulated transcriptional repressor p120^{E4F}, and the HIV Tat-binding protein (Eymin et al. 2001; Martelli et al. 2001; Rocha et al. 2003; Zhao et al. 2003; Ayrault et al. 2004; Bertwistle et al. 2004a; Datta et al. 2004; Qi et al. 2004; Woods et al. 2004; Rizos et al. 2005). Although these interactions are of great potential interest, there are many caveats in interpreting their biological relevance. Most of these protein–protein interactions have been uncovered through antibody-mediated coprecipitation, frequently of overexpressed proteins. Because Arf is so highly basic and has a strong propensity to nonspecifically bind to nucleic acids and acidic proteins, it is difficult to devise appropriate experimental controls for such analyses. In many cases, mutagenesis has been employed to pinpoint domains within Arf and its target proteins that govern these interactions. However, a common finding has been that multiple segments within Arf and its associated proteins seem to contribute, thereby negating the possibility of identifying discrete motifs that direct specific binding. These problems are further compounded by observations that Arf mutants lacking particular segments are highly unstable or localize aberrantly when expressed in cells (see above).

Despite these difficulties, however, certain emerging themes merit strong consideration. Induction of p19^{Arf} can inhibit the production of ribosomal RNA by affecting the processing of 47/45S and 32S precursors (Sugimoto et al. 2003). These effects are not strictly dependent on inhibition of rRNA transcription, do not require p53, and are not mimicked by cell cycle arrest per se. Hence, p19^{Arf} may play a distinct role within the nucleolus, possibly in coordinating ribosome synthesis and cell growth (mass) with p53-dependent proliferative arrest.

Arf has also been demonstrated to inhibit gene expression through functional interactions with various transcription factors, including E2F-1 (Eymin et al. 2001; Martelli et al. 2001), NF-κB (Rocha et al. 2003), and Myc (Datta et al. 2004; Qi et al. 2004). Again, none of these effects depends on p53. There is some evidence that p19^{Arf} can physically associate with E2F-1- and Myc-containing protein complexes (see above), but a direct interaction with NF-κB has not been reported. Overexpression of p19^{Arf} was found to accelerate E2F-1 degradation (Martelli et al. 2001), although this might potentially be due to an increase in E2F-1 turnover stemming from Arf-induced cell cycle arrest. In contrast, Arf has no apparent effect on Myc or NF-κB protein levels.

By repressing the transcriptional activity of NF-κB, ARF sensitizes cells to TNFα-induced apoptosis (Rocha et al. 2003). In human cells responding to a conditionally regulated ARF transgene, induction of p14^{ARF} was reported to trigger ATR- and Chk-1-dependent phosphorylation of the NF-κB RelA/p65 subunit on Thr-505, inhibiting its trans-activating function; ATR induction also resulted in p53 phosphorylation on Ser-15, a modification associated with p53 activation (Rocha et al. 2005). However, phosphorylation of RelA/p65, although dependent on ARF, ATR, and Chk1, was not observed when ATR and Chk1 were activated by UV irradiation, suggesting that p14[ARF] is somehow required to target Chk1 kinase activity to specific substrates. Although ARF might conceivably activate ATR by interfering with DNA replication, ARF-expressing cells accumulate in G_1 and G_2 with very few cells remaining in S phase, and analysis of arrested cells with an antibody to γ-H2AX revealed no increase in staining. The endogenous ATR protein was relocalized, together with BRCA1, to the nucleolus of ARF-expressing cells, and p14[ARF] and ATR cofractionated in high-molecular-weight (>1 MD) complexes. In cells sustaining DNA damage, RPA binds single-stranded DNA and interacts with ATRIP to recruit ATR to stalled replication forks, but no RPA foci were observed in nucleoli following p14[ARF] induction, again yielding no direct evidence for ARF-induced DNA damage. Hence, the manner by which p14[ARF] engages the ATR–Chk1 kinase cascade remains unknown. This is a crucial issue, particularly because a recent report has indicated that various oncogenes that, on the one hand, can induce *ARF* in precancerous lesions also induce DNA damage and activate the ATR/ATM and Chk kinases via ARF-independent signaling pathways (Bartkova et al. 2005).

Myc overexpression induces *Arf* (and can also damage DNA; Vafa et al. 2002), but, in turn, p19[Arf] can inhibit Myc function (Datta et al. 2004; Qi et al. 2004). One group of investigators reported that Myc binds directly to p19[Arf], relocalizing it from the nucleolus into the nucleoplasm (Qi et al. 2004). However, in other cell lines, p19[Arf] appeared to localize Myc to the nucleolus (Datta et al. 2004). This is reminiscent of the Mdm2–Arf interaction in which overexpression of Arf localized Mdm2 to the nucleolus (Weber et al. 1999), whereas the opposite occurred when Mdm2 expression was enforced at high levels (Zhang and Xiong 1999). Many genes are activated by Myc, and these include not only those transcribed by polymerase II, but also the pol-I-responsive rDNA clusters as well as the pol-III-driven genes encoding 5S RNA and tRNAs (Gomez-Roman et al. 2003; Orian et al. 2003; Grandori et al. 2005). Thus, Myc can be active within both the nucleoplasm and the nucleolus, and its relocalization between the two compartments in response to p19[Arf] may not simply reflect an artifact of protein overexpression. A very interesting finding is that p19[Arf] can associate with Myc–Max complexes, antagonizing their *trans*-activating functions on certain promoters without impairing their transrepression of others (Qi et al. 2004). Myc binding to these promoters occurs whether or not p19[Arf] (or p53) is present, so p19[Arf] plays no role in recruiting Myc to chromatin but instead inhibits Myc's activator function in situ. Again, the underlying mechanisms remain unclear.

Arf-INDUCED SUMOYLATION

Surprisingly, the enforced expression of p14[ARF] in human cells has been observed to promote the sumoylation of several cotransfected proteins, including Hdm2, the Werners helicase, E2F-1, and HIF-1α (Xirodimas et al. 2002; Chen and Chen 2003; Woods et al. 2004; Rizos et

al. 2005). Covalent addition of the small ubiquitin-like modifiers (SUMO 1, 2, and 3) to target proteins can generate diverse effects on protein transport, ubiquitination, DNA repair and chromatid adhesion, and on gene expression (usually, but not always, down-regulation) (Melchior 2000; Johnson 2004). Therefore, we speculate that the p53-independent activities of Arf might conceivably be due to this process.

Conjugation of SUMO to lysyl ε-amino groups in proteins occurs in a manner similar to ubiquitination (Johnson 2004). First, SUMO precursors must be cleaved by a protease to yield a carboxy-terminal diglycine motif. Processed SUMO is activated in an ATP-dependent manner by an E1 enzyme and transferred to a unique E2 conjugating enzyme (Ubc9), which can then affix SUMO to target proteins. The latter process can be accelerated by one of several E3 ligases that include the nucleoporin RanBP2 and a family of PIAS proteins (protein inhibitors of activated STATs) (Johnson and Gupta 2001; Sachdev et al. 2001; Pichler et al. 2002). SUMO-specific proteases assume a dual role in the cascade, being required for initial SUMO processing as well as the removal of SUMO from protein substrates (Hay 2001).

Sequences required for the efficient binding of p14[ARF] or p19[Arf] to (H)Mdm2, although differing between the human and mouse Arf proteins, are also necessary for sumoylation (Xirodimas et al. 2002; Tago et al. 2005). Endogenous NPM, to which Arf also binds, undergoes sumoylation in response to p19[Arf] induction, but Arf did not trigger sumoylation of other known SUMO substrates with which it did not physically interact (Fig. 3) (Tago et al. 2005). The induction and accumulation of p19[Arf] leads to increased sumoylation within nucleoli; however, an

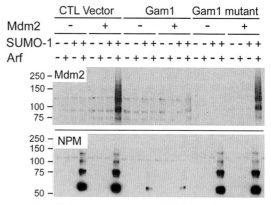

Figure 3. *Arf* induces sumoylation of Mdm2 and NPM. 293T cells were cotransfected with the combinations of expression vectors indicated at the top, which encoded Mdm2, His$_6$-tagged SUMO-1, p19[Arf], and either a control retroviral expression vector or vectors encoding wild-type Gam1 or a defective Gam1 mutant. Cellular proteins absorbed to nickel resin in the presence of 0.5 M NaCl and 8 M urea were eluted with imidazole and sodium dodecyl sulfate, electrophoretically separated on denaturing gels, and blotted with antibodies to Mdm2 (*upper panel*) or NPM (*lower panel*). The fastest-migrating species in the lower panel corresponds to the monosumoylated endogenous NPM protein, whereas slower-migrating forms are multisumoylated. (Reprinted, with permission, from Tago et al. 2005.)

Arf mutant that cannot efficiently enter nucleoli but still binds Mdm2 was defective in sumoylating it. Hence, Arf-induced sumoylation appears to depend on at least a transient association of p19^{Arf} with its targets, and this may preferentially occur within the nucleolus where the major pool of p19^{Arf} resides.

An avian adenoviral protein, Gam1, has the unique property of interfering with the SUMO E1 activating enzyme, a process that is accompanied by increased turnover of the SUMO E2, Ubc9 (Boggio et al. 2004). Either the introduction of Gam1 or shRNAs directed to Ubc9 can inhibit sumoylation within cells (Fig. 3). Although these manipulations ultimately prove toxic, inhibition of Arf-induced sumoylation of Mdm2 had no immediate effect on p53 stabilization or on the induction of canonical p53-responsive genes, such as *Cip1* or *Mdm2* itself (Tago et al. 2005). Therefore, sumoylation appears not to be needed for activation of the p53 transcriptional program per se, although we cannot preclude more subtle effects.

An attractive idea is that Arf is a component of a SUMO E3 ligase and acts as a specificity factor that bridges Ubc9 complexes to Arf-binding proteins. SUMO-1 conjugation of the WRN helicase triggered by the SUMO E1 and E2 enzymes in vitro could not be accelerated by recombinant p14^{ARF} (Woods et al. 2004). This may not be surprising, given the "sticky" binding properties of recombinant Arf proteins and their propensity to misfold, so a better approach might be to purify native Arf-containing complexes from cells and test them for an associated E3 ligase activity when recombined with potential substrates and other purified components of the SUMO cascade.

Mammalian transcription factors that control cell proliferation are sumoylated (Hilgarth et al. 2004; Johnson 2004) and Gam1 can increase promoter activation by several of them (Boggio et al. 2004). Gam1 reduces sumoylation of HDAC1 without affecting its enzymatic activity (Colombo et al. 2002), but its recruitment to promoters is enhanced when histone H4 is sumoylated (Shiio and Eisenman 2003). The fact that Arf can negatively regulate the transcriptional activities of E2F-1, NF-κB, and Myc raises the question of whether sumoylation mediates these effects. Because the key elements of the SUMO cascade are highly conserved among all eukaryotes, it is reasonable to expect that Arf might induce sumoylation-dependent phenotypes in other organisms that are more amenable to genetic dissection of this process.

CONCLUSIONS

From the time of its discovery, the properties of the Arf tumor suppressor have been surprising. The overlap of *Arf* and *Ink4a* gene sequences; the fact that the two gene products are both potent tumor suppressors that interact with p53 and Rb, respectively; the notion that Arf responds to a select subset of oncogenic signals that induce p53; the highly basic nature of Arf proteins and their localization to nucleoli; the amino-terminal ubiquitination of Arf; and recent results implicating Arf in the process of sumoylation were all unexpected. Illuminating the various activities of Arf, and particularly its p53-independent functions, still poses a significant challenge.

ACKNOWLEDGMENTS

We thank the other members of the Sherr/Roussel laboratory, both past and present, for their suggestions and criticisms throughout the course of these studies. This work was supported in part by Cancer Center CORE Grant CA21765, by P01-CA71907 (M.F.R.), and by AL-SAC of St. Jude Children's Research Hospital. C.J.S. is an investigator of the Howard Hughes Medical Institute.

REFERENCES

Adams J.M., Harris A.W., Pinkert C.A., Corcoran L.M., Alexander W.S., Cory S., Palmiter R.D., and Brinster R.L. 1985. The c-myc oncogene driven by immunoglobulin enhancers induces lymphoid malignancy in transgenic mice. *Nature* **318:** 533.

Artandi S.E., Chang S., Lee S.L., Alson S., Gottlieb G.J., Chin L., and DePinho R.A. 2000. Telomere dysfunction promotes non-reciprocal translocations and epithelial cancers in mice. *Nature* **406:** 573.

Aslanian A., Iaquinta P.J., Verona R., and Lees J.A. 2004. Repression of the Arf tumor suppressor by E2F3 is required for normal cell cycle kinetics. *Genes Dev.* **18:** 1413.

Ayrault O., Andrique L., Larsen C.J., and Seite P. 2004. Human Arf tumor suppressor specifically interacts with chromatin containing the promoter of rRNA genes. *Oncogene* **23:** 8097.

Bartkova J., Horejsi Z., Koed K., Kramer A., Tort F., Zieger K., Guldberg P., Sehested M., Nesland J.M, Lukas C., Orntoft T., Lukas J., and Bartek J. 2005. DNA damage response as a candidate anti-cancer barrier in early human tumorigenesis. *Nature* **434:** 864.

Bertwistle D., Sugimoto M., and Sherr C.J. 2004a. Physical and functional interactions of the Arf tumor suppressor protein with nucleophosmin/B23. *Mol. Cell. Biol.* **24:** 985.

Bertwistle D., Zindy F., Sherr C.J., and Roussel M.F. 2004b. Monoclonal antibodies to the mouse p19^{Arf} tumor suppressor protein. *Hybrid. Hybrid.* **23:** 293.

Blasco M.A., Lee H.-W., Hande M.P., Samper E., Lansdorp P.M., DePinho R.A, and Greider C.W. 1997. Telomere shortening and tumor formation by mouse cells lacking telomerase RNA. *Cell* **91:** 25.

Boggio R., Colombo R., Hay R.T., Draetta G.F., and Chiocca S. 2004. A mechanism for inhibiting the SUMO pathway. *Mol. Cell* **16:** 549.

Bradshaw R.A., Brickey W.W., and Walker K.W. 1998. N-terminal processing: The methionine aminopeptidase and N$^\alpha$-acetyl transferase families. *Trends Biochem. Sci.* **23:** 263.

Brady S.N., Yu Y., Maggi L.B., Jr., and Weber J.D. 2004. ARF impedes NPM/B23 shuttling in an Mdm2-sensitive tumor suppressor pathway. *Mol. Cell. Biol.* **24:** 9327.

Busuttil R.A., Rubio M., Dolle M.E., Campisi J., and Vijg J. 2003. Oxygen accelerates the accumulation of mutations during the senescence and immortalization of murine cells in culture. *Aging Cell* **2:** 287.

Carnero A., Hudson J.D., Price C.M., and Beach D.H. 2000. p16^{INK4a} and p19^{ARF} act in overlapping pathways in cellular immortalization. *Nat. Cell Biol.* **2:** 148.

Chen L. and Chen J. 2003. MDM2-ARF complex regulates p53 sumoylation. *Oncogene* **22:** 5348.

Colombo R., Boggio R., Seiser C., Draetta G.F., and Chiocca S. 2002. The adenovirus protein Gam1 interferes with sumoylation of histone deacetylase I. *EMBO Rep.* **3:** 1062.

Datta A., Nag A., Pan W., Hay N., Gartel A.L., Colamonici O., Mori Y., and Raychaudhuri P. 2004. Myc-ARF (alternative reading frame) interaction inhibits the functions of Myc. *J. Biol. Chem.* **279:** 36698.

De Stanchina E., McCurrach M.E., Zindy F., Shieh S.-Y., Ferbeyre G., Samuelson A.V., Prives C., Roussel M.F., Sherr C.J., and Lowe S.W. 1998. E1A signaling to p53 involves the p19^{ARF} tumor suppressor. *Genes Dev.* **12:** 2434.

Eischen C.M., Weber J.D., Roussel M.F., Sherr C.J., and Cleveland J.L. 1999. Disruption of the ARF-Mdm2-p53 tumor suppressor pathway in Myc-induced lymphomagenesis. *Genes Dev.* **13:** 2658.

El-Deiry W.S., Tokino T., Velculescu V.E., Levy D.B., Parsons R., Trent J.M., Lin D., Mercer E., Kinzler K.W., and Vogelstein B. 1993. WAF1, a potential mediator of p53 tumor suppression. *Cell* **75:** 817.

Eymin B., Karayan L., Seite P., Brambilla C., Brambilla E., Larsen C.J., and Gazzeri S. 2001. Human ARF binds E2F1 and inhibits its transcriptional activity. *Oncogene* **20:** 1033.

Gil J., Bernard D., Martinez D., and Beach D. 2004. Polycomb CBX7 has a unifying role in cellular lifespan. *Nat. Cell Biol.* **6:** 67.

Gomez-Roman N., Grandori C., Eisenman R.N., and White R.J. 2003. Direct activation of RNA polymerase III transcription by c-Myc. *Nature* **421:** 290.

Grandori C., Gomez-Roman N., Felton-Edkins Z.A., Ngouenet C., Galloway D.A., Eisenman R.N., and White R.J. 2005. c-Myc binds to human ribosomal DNA and stimulates transcription of rRNA genes by RNA polymerase I. *Nat. Cell Biol.* **7:** 311.

Harvey D.M. and Levine A.J. 1991. p53 alteration is a common event in the spontaneous immortalization of primary BALB/c murine embryo fibroblasts. *Genes Dev.* **5:** 2375.

Hay R.T. 2001. Protein modification by SUMO. *Trends Biochem. Sci.* **26:** 332.

Hilgarth R.S., Murphy L.A., Skaggs H.S., Wilkerson D.C., Xing H., and Sarge K.D. 2004. Regulation and function of SUMO modification. *J. Biol. Chem.* **279:** 53899.

Honda R. and Yasuda H. 1999. Association of p19^{ARF} with Mdm2 inhibits ubiquitin ligase activity of Mdm2 for tumor suppressor p53. *EMBO J.* **18:** 22.

Inoue K., Roussel M.F., and Sherr C.J. 1999. Induction of *ARF* tumor suppressor gene expression and cell cycle arrest by transcription factor DMP1. *Proc. Natl. Acad. Sci.* **96:** 3993.

Inoue K., Zindy F., Randle D.H., Rehg J.E., and Sherr C.J. 2001. *Dmp1* is haplo-insufficient for tumor suppression and modifies the frequencies of *Arf* and *p53* mutations in *Myc*-induced lymphomas. *Genes Dev.* **15:** 2934.

Inoue K., Wren R., Rehg J.E., Adachi M., Cleveland J.L., Roussel M.F., and Sherr C.J. 2000. Disruption of the *ARF* transcriptional activator *DMP1* facilitates cell immortalization, Ras transformation, and tumorigenesis. *Genes Dev.* **14:** 1797.

Jacks T., Remington L., Williams B.O., Schmitt E.M., Halachmi S., Bronson R.T., and Weinberg R.A. 1994. Tumor spectrum analysis in p53-mutant mice. *Curr. Biol.* **4:** 1.

Jacobs J.J.L., Kieboom K., Marino S., DePinho R.A., and van Lohuizen M. 1999a. The oncogene and Polycomb-group gene *bmi-1* regulates cell proliferation and senescence through the *ink4a* locus. *Nature* **397:** 164.

Jacobs J.J.L., Scheijen B., Vonchen J.-W., Kieboom K., Berns A., and van Lohuizen M. 1999b. Bmi-1 collaborates with c-Myc in tumorigenesis by inhibiting c-Myc induced apoptosis via INK4a/ARF. *Genes Dev.* **13:** 2678.

Jacobs J.J.L., Keblusek P., Robanus-Maandag E., Kristel P., Lingbeek M., Nederlof P.M., van Welsem T., van de Vijver M.J, Koh E.Y., Daley G.Q., and van Lohuizen M. 2000. Senescence bypass screen identifies TBX2, which represses *Cdkn2a* (*p19^{ARF}*) and is amplified in a subset of human breast cancers. *Nat. Genet.* **26:** 291.

Jerome-Majewska L.A., Jenkins G.P., Ernstoff E., Zindy F., Scherr C. J., and Papaioannou V.E. 2005. Tbx3, the ulnar-mammary syndrome gene, and Tbx2 interact in mammary gland development through a p19Arf/p53-independent pathway. *Dev. Dynamics* (in press).

Johnson E.S. 2004. Protein modification by SUMO. *Annu. Rev. Biochem.* **73:** 355.

Johnson E.S. and Gupta A.A. 2001. An E3-like factor that promotes SUMO conjugation to the yeast septins. *Cell* **106:** 735.

Kamijo T., Bodner S., van de Kamp E., Randle D.H., and Sherr C.J. 1999a. Tumor spectrum in ARF-deficient mice. *Cancer Res.* **59:** 2217.

Kamijo T., van de Kamp E., Chong M.J., Zindy F., Diehl A.J., Sherr C.J., and McKinnon P. 1999b. Loss of the ARF tumor suppressor reverses premature replicative arrest but not radiation hypersensitivity arising from disabled Atm function. *Cancer Res.* **59:** 2464.

Kamijo T., Zindy F., Roussel M.F., Quelle D.E., Downing J.R., Ashmun R.A., Grosveld G., and Sherr C.J. 1997. Tumor suppression at the mouse *INK4a* locus mediated by the alternative reading frame product p19^{ARF}. *Cell* **91:** 649.

Kelly-Spratt K.S., Gurley K.E., Yasui Y., and Kemp C.J. 2004. p19^{Arf} suppresses growth, progression, and metastasis of H-ras-driven carcinomas through p53-dependent and -independent pathways. *PLoS Biol.* **2:** 1138.

Kim S.H., Mitchell M., Fujii H., Llanos S., and Peters G. 2003. Absence of p16INK4a and truncation of ARF tumor suppressors in chickens. *Proc. Natl. Acad. Sci.* **100:** 211.

Korgaonkar C., Hagen J., Tompkins V., Frazier A.A., Allamargot C., Quelle F.W., and Quelle D.E. 2005. Nucleophosmin (B23) targets ARF to nucleoli and inhibits its function. *Mol. Cell. Biol.* **25:** 1258.

Krimpenfort P., Quon K.C., Mooi W.J., Loonstra A., and Berns A. 2001. Loss of *p16^{Ink4a}* confers susceptibility to metastatic melanoma in mice. *Nature* **413:** 83.

Kuo M.-L., den Besten W., Bertwistle D., Roussel M.F., and Sherr C.J. 2004. N-terminal polyubiquitination and degradation of the Arf tumor suppressor. *Genes Dev.* **18:** 1862.

Latres E., Malumbres M., Sotillo R., Martin J., Ortega S., Martin-Caballero J., Flores J.M., Cordon-Cardo C., and Barbacid M. 2000. Limited overlapping roles of P15(INK4b) and P18(INK4c) cell cycle inhibitors in proliferation and tumorigenesis. *EMBO J.* **19:** 3496.

Lee H.-W., Blasco M.A., Gottlieb G.J., Horber J.W., Greider C.W., and DePinho R.A. 1998. Essential role of mouse telomerase in highly proliferating organs. *Nature* **392:** 569.

Lingbeek T., Jacobs J.J., and van Lohuizen M. 2002. The T-box repressors TBX2 and TBX3 specifically regulate the tumor suppressor gene p14ARF via a variant T-site in the initiator. *J. Biol. Chem.* **277:** 26120.

Llanos S., Clark P.A., Rowe J., and Peters G. 2001. Stabilization of p53 by p14ARF without relocation of MDM2 to the nucleolus. *Nat. Cell Biol.* **3:** 445.

Lowe S.W. and Sherr C.J. 2003. Tumor suppression by *Ink4a-Arf*: Progress and puzzles. *Curr. Opin. Genet. Dev.* **13:** 77.

Maeda T., Hobbs R.M., Merghoub T., Guernah I., Zelent A., Cordon-Cardo C., Teruya-Feldstein J., and Pandolfi P.P. 2005. Role of the proto-oncogene Pokemon in cellular transformation and ARF repression. *Nature* **433:** 278.

Maestro R., Dei Tos A.P., Hamamori Y., Krasnokutsky S., Sartorelli V., Kedes L., Doglioni C., Beach D., and Hannon G.J. 1999. *Twist* is a potential oncogene that inhibits apoptosis. *Genes Dev.* **13:** 2207.

Martelli F., Hamilton T., Silver D.P., Sharpless N.E., Bardeesy N., Rokas M., DePinho R.A., Livingston D.M., and Grossman S.R. 2001. p19ARF targets certain E2F species for degradation. *Proc. Natl. Acad. Sci.* **98:** 4455.

McKeller R.N., Fowler J.L., Cunningham J.J., Warner N., Smeyne R.J., Zindy F., and Skapek S.X. 2002. The Arf tumor suppressor gene promotes hyaloid vascular regression during mouse eye development. *Proc. Natl. Acad. Sci.* **99:** 3848.

Melchior F. 2000. SUMO - Nonclassical ubiquitin. *Annu. Rev. Cell Dev. Biol.* **16:** 591.

Modestou M., Puig-Antich V., Korgaonkar C., Eapen A., and Quelle D.E. 2001. The alternative reading frame tumor suppressor inhibits growth through p21-dependent and p21-independent pathways. *Cancer Res.* **61:** 3145.

Orian A., van Steensel B., Delrow J., Bussemaker H.J., Li L., Sawado T., Williams E., Loo L.W., Cowley S.M., Yost C., Pierce S., Edgar B.A., Parkhurst S.M., and Eisenman R.N. 2003. Genomic binding by the *Drosophila* Myc, Max, Mad/Mnt transcription factor network. *Genes Dev.* **17:** 1101.

Ortega S., Malumbres M., and Barbacid M. 2002. Cyclin D-dependent kinases, INK4 inhibitors, and cancer. *Biochim. Bio-

phys. Acta **1602:** 73.

Palmero I., Pantoja C., and Serrano M. 1998. p19^ARF links the tumour suppressor p53 to Ras. *Nature* **395:** 125.

Pantoja C. and Serrano M. 1999. Murine fibroblasts lacking *p21* undergo senescence and are resistant to transformation by oncogenic Ras. *Oncogene* **18:** 4974.

Parrinello S., Samper E., Krtolica A., Goldstein J., Melov S., and Campisi J. 2003. Oxygen sensitivity severely limits the replicative lifespan of murine fibroblasts. *Nat. Cell Biol.* **5:** 741.

Pichler A., Gast A., Seeler J.S., Dejean A., and Melchior F. 2002. The nucleoporin RanBP2 has a SUMO1 E3 ligase activity. *Cell* **108:** 109.

Polevoda B. and Sherman F. 2003. N-terminal acetyltransferases and sequence requirements for N-terminal acetylation of eukaryotic proteins. *J. Mol. Biol.* **325:** 595.

Qi Y., Gregory M.A., Li Z., Brousal J.P., West K., and Hann S.R. 2004. p19ARF directly and differentially controls the functions of c-Myc independently of p53. *Nature* **431:** 712.

Quelle D.E., Cheng M., Ashmun R.A., and Sherr C.J. 1997. Cancer-associated mutations at the INK4a locus cancel cell cycle arrest by p16INK4a but not by the alternative reading frame protein p19ARF. *Proc. Natl. Acad. Sci.* **94:** 669.

Quelle, D.E., Zindy F., Ashmun R.A., and Sherr C.J. 1995. Alternative reading frames of the INK4a tumor suppressor gene encode two unrelated proteins capable of inducing cell cycle arrest. *Cell* **83:** 993.

Randle D.H., Zindy F., Sherr C.J., and Roussel M.F. 2001. Differential effects of p19^Arf and p16^Ink4a loss on senescence of murine bone marrow-derived pre-B cells and macrophages. *Proc. Natl. Acad. Sci.* **98:** 9654.

Rizos H., Woodruff S., and Kelford R.F. 2005. p14ARF interacts with the SUMO-conjugating enzyme Ubc9 and promotes the sumoylation of its binding partners. *Cell Cycle* **4:** e39.

Rocha S., Campbell K.J., and Perkins N.D. 2003. p53- and Mdm2-independent repression of NF-κB transactivation by the ARF tumor suppressor. *Mol. Cell* **12:** 15.

Rocha S., Garrett M.D., Campbell K.J., Schumm K., and Perkins N.D. 2005. Regulation of NF-κB and p53 through activation of ATR and Chk1 by the ARF tumour suppressor. *EMBO J.* **24:** 1157.

Roussel M.F. 1999. The INK4 family of cell cycle inhibitors in cancer. *Oncogene* **18:** 5311.

Rowland B.D., Denissov S.G., Douma S., Stunnenberg H.G., Bernards R., and Peepers D.S. 2002. E2F transcriptional repressor complexes are critical downstream targets of p19^ARF/p53-induced proliferative arrest. *Cancer Cell* **2:** 55.

Ruas M. and Peters G. 1998. The p16^INK4a/CDKN2A tumor suppressor and its relatives. *Biochim Biophys. Acta* **1378:** F115.

Rudolph K.L., Chang S., Lee H.W., Blasco M., Gottlieb G.J., Greider C., and DePinho R.A. 1999. Longevity, stress response, and cancer in aging telomerase-deficient mice. *Cell* **96:** 701.

Sachdev S., Bruhn L., Sieber H., Pichler A., Melchior F., and Grosschedl R. 2001. PIASy, a nuclear matrix-associated SUMO E3 ligase, represses LEF1 activity by sequestration into nuclear bodies. *Genes Dev.* **15:** 3088.

Schmitt C.A., McCurrach M.E., De Stanchina E., and Lowe S.W. 1999. INK4a/ARF mutations accelerate lymphomagenesis and promote chemoresistance by disabling p53. *Genes Dev.* **13:** 2670.

Serrano M., Hannon G.J., and Beach D. 1993. A new regulatory motif in cell cycle control causing specific inhibition of cyclin D/CDK4. *Nature* **366:** 704.

Serrano M., Lee H.-W., Chin L., Cordon-Cardo C., Beach D., and DePinho R.A. 1996. Role of the INK4a locus in tumor suppression and cell mortality. *Cell* **85:** 27.

Sharpless N.E., Bardeesy N., Lee K.-H., Carrasco D., Castrillon D.H., Aguirre A.J., Wu E.A., Horner J.W., and DePinho R.A. 2001. Loss of p16^Ink4a with retention of p19^Arf predisposes mice to tumorigenesis. *Nature* **413:** 86.

Sherr C.J. 1998. Tumor surveillance via the ARF-p53 pathway. *Genes Dev.* **12:** 2984.

Sherr C.J. and DePinho R.A. 2001. Cellular senescence: Mitotic clock or culture shock. *Cell* **102:** 407.

Shiio Y. and Eisenman R.N. 2003. Histone sumoylation is associated with transcriptional repression. *Proc. Natl. Acad. Sci.* **100:** 13118.

Smogorzewska A. and De Lange T. 2002. Different telomere damage signaling pathways in human and mouse cells. *EMBO J.* **21:** 4338.

Sreeramaneni R., Chaudhry A., McMahon M., Sherr C.J., and Inoue K. 2005. Ras-Raf-Arf signaling critically depends on the Dmp1 transcription factor. *Mol. Cell. Biol.* **25:** 220.

Sugimoto M., Kuo M.L., Roussel M.F., and Sherr C.J. 2003. Nucleolar Arf tumor suppressor inhibits ribosomal RNA processing. *Mol. Cell* **11:** 415.

Tago K., Chiocca S., and Sherr C.J. 2005. Sumoylation induced by the Arf tumor suppressor: A p53-independent function. *Proc. Natl. Acad. Sci.* **102:** 7689.

Vafa O., Wade M., Kern S., Beeche M., Pandita T.K., Hampton G.M., and Wahl G.M. 2002. c-Myc can induce DNA damage, increase reactive oxygen species, and mitigate p53 function: A mechanism for oncogene-induced genetic instability. *Mol. Cell* **9:** 1031.

Vousden K.H. and Lu X. 2002. Live or let die: The cell's response to p53. *Nat. Rev. Cancer* **2:** 594.

Weber J.D., Taylor L.J., Roussel M.F., Sherr C.J., and Bar-Sagi D. 1999. Nucleolar Arf sequesters Mdm2 and activates p53. *Nat. Cell Biol.* **1:** 20.

Weber J.D., Kuo M.-L., Bothner B., DiGiammarino E.L., Kriwacki R.W., Roussel M.F., and Sherr C.J. 2000a. Cooperative signals governing ARF-Mdm2 interaction and nucleolar localization of the complex. *Mol. Cell. Biol.* **20:** 2517.

Weber J.D., Jeffers J.R., Rehg J.E., Randle D.H., Lozano G., Roussel M.F., Sherr C.J., and Zambetti G.P. 2000b. p53-independent functions of the p19^ARF tumor suppressor. *Genes Dev.* **14:** 2358.

Weitzman J.B., Fiette L., Matsuo K., and Yaniv M. 2000. JunD protects cells from p53-dependent senescence and apoptosis. *Mol. Cell* **6:** 1109.

Woods Y.L., Xirodimas D.P., Prescott A.R., Sparks A., Lane D.P., and Saville M.K. 2004. p14ARF promotes small ubiquitin-like modifier conjugation of Werners helicase. *J. Biol. Chem.* **279:** 50157.

Wright W.E. and Shay J.W. 2000. Telomere dynamics in cancer progression and prevention: Fundamental differences in human and mouse telomere biology. *Nat. Med.* **6:** 849.

Xirodimas D.P., Chisholm J., Desterro J.M.S., Lane D.P., and Hay R.T. 2002. p14ARF promotes accumulation of SUMO-1 conjugated (H)Mdm2. *FEBS Lett.* **528:** 207.

Zhang Y. and Xiong Y. 1999. Mutations in human ARF exon 2 disrupt its nucleolar localization and impair its ability to block nuclear export of MDM2 and p53. *Mol. Cell* **3:** 579.

Zhao L., Samuels T., Winckler S., Korgaonkar C., Tompkins V., Horne M.C., and Quelle D.E. 2003. Cyclin G1 has growth inhibitory activity linked to the ARF-Mdm2-p53 and pRb tumor suppressor pathways. *Mol. Cancer Res.* **1:** 195.

Zindy F., Quelle D.E., Roussel M.F., and Sherr C.J. 1997. Expression of the p16^INK4a tumor suppressor versus other INK4 family members during mouse development and aging. *Oncogene* **15:** 203.

Zindy F., Eischen C.M., Randle D.H., Kamijo T., Cleveland J.L., Sherr C.J., and Roussel M.F. 1998. Myc signaling via the ARF tumor suppressor regulates p53-dependent apoptosis and immortalization. *Genes Dev.* **12:** 2424.

Zindy F., Williams R.T., Baudino T.A., Rehg J.E, Skapek S.X., Cleveland J.L., Roussel M.F., and Sherr C.J. 2003. *Arf* tumor suppressor promoter monitors latent oncogenic signals *in vivo*. *Proc. Natl. Acad. Sci.* **100:** 15930.

Exploiting the DNA Repair Defect in BRCA Mutant Cells in the Design of New Therapeutic Strategies for Cancer

A.N.J. Tutt,*† C.J. Lord,* N. McCabe,* H. Farmer,* N. Turner,* N.M. Martin,¶
S.P. Jackson,‡¶ G.C.M. Smith,¶ and A. Ashworth*

*The Breakthrough Breast Cancer Research Centre, Institute of Cancer Research, London SW3 6JB;
†Guy's Hospital, London SE1 9RT; ‡Wellcome Trust and Cancer Research UK, Gurdon Institute of Cancer
and Developmental Biology, and Department of Zoology, University of Cambridge, Cambridge CB2 1QN;
¶KuDOS Pharmaceuticals Ltd., Cambridge Science Park, Cambridge CB4 0WG, United Kingdom

Individuals harboring germ-line mutations in the *BRCA1* or *BRCA2* genes are at highly elevated risk of a variety of cancers. Ten years of research has revealed roles for BRCA1 and BRCA2 in a wide variety of cellular processes. However, it seems likely that the function of these proteins in DNA repair is critically important in maintaining genome stability. Despite this increasing knowledge of the defects present in BRCA-deficient cells, *BRCA* mutation carriers developing cancer are still treated similarly to sporadic cases. Here we describe our efforts, based on understanding the DNA repair defects in BRCA-deficient cells, to define the optimal existing treatment for cancers arising in *BRCA* mutation carriers and, additionally, the development of novel therapeutic approaches. Finally, we discuss how therapies developed to treat *BRCA* mutant tumors might be applied to some sporadic cancers sharing similar specific defects in DNA repair.

Carriers of germ-line heterozygous mutations in *BRCA1* or *BRCA2* are at highly elevated risk of developing breast, ovarian, and other cancers (Wooster and Weber 2003). Tumors arising as a result of a *BRCA* mutation generally show loss of the wild-type allele and retention of the mutated allele, suggesting that BRCA1 and BRCA2 deficiency is pathogenic. BRCA1 and BRCA2 are large proteins, yet have only a few structural features suggestive of their normal functions. Although many proteins have been described that associate with the two proteins, only in some cases is the functional significance of these interactions understood (Tutt and Ashworth 2002; Venkitaraman 2002). There are exceptions, however, where considerable indications of importance are available. In BRCA1, the RING domain has been implicated in ubiquitin-mediated protein degradation, and the pair of carboxy-terminal BRCT repeats comprise phosphopeptide-binding domains (Kerr and Ashworth 2001; Rodriguez et al. 2003). For BRCA2, the BRC repeats have been shown to bind the important DNA repair protein RAD51. A wide variety of functions have been proposed for the BRCA proteins in transcriptional regulation, DNA repair/recombination, cell cycle checkpoint control, and cytokinesis (Tutt and Ashworth 2002; Venkitaraman 2002; Daniels et al. 2004). However, it is still unclear which, if any, of these many functions are crucial for tumor suppression. The identification of the *BRCA1* and *BRCA2* genes, around 10 years ago, made genetic counseling of carriers possible (Wooster and Weber 2003). However, despite this knowledge of the defects present in BRCA-deficient cells, *BRCA* mutation carriers developing cancer are still treated similarly to sporadic cases (Couzin 2003; Narod and Foulkes 2004). Here we describe approaches, harnessing our understanding of the DNA repair defects in BRCA-deficient cells, to define the optimal existing treatment for cancers arising in *BRCA* mutation carriers and, in addition, the development of novel therapeutic approaches. We also discuss how these approaches might be used to treat a subset of sporadic cancers having similar specific defects in DNA repair pathways.

DEFICIENCY OF BRCA1 OR BRCA2 INDUCES A DEFECT IN HOMOLOGOUS RECOMBINATION

DNA double-strand breaks (DSBs) in mammalian cells are repaired by two principal mechanisms, non-homologous end joining (NHEJ) and homologous recombination (HR) (Hoejimakers 2001). NHEJ is the major route for DSB repair in the $G_{0/1}$ phases of the cell cycle and involves the alignment and ligation of DSB termini. Sequence changes that occur at the site of the DSB are generally not restored, and consequently, NHEJ can be mutagenic. Conversely, HR, which acts predominantly during S and G_2 phases, can be conservative (in the form of gene conversion) or nonconservative (in the form of single strand annealing). Gene conversion (GC) uses an identical sequence to copy and replace damaged DNA, namely the sister chromatid, whereas in single-stranded annealing (SSA), homologous sequences on either side of the DSB are aligned, followed by the deletion of the intermediate noncomplementary sequence (Fig. 1). HR is relatively suppressed in $G_{0/1}$, presumably to avoid potentially nonconservative recombination between autosomes, and mismatches in sequence are closely monitored by the mismatch repair surveillance complex to prevent erroneous selection of the target sequence (Elliott and Jasin 2001). Cells that lack BRCA1 or BRCA2 have a defect in the repair of DSBs by the conservative, potentially error-free, mechanism of HR by GC (Fig. 1) (Moynahan et al. 1999, 2001a,b; Tutt et al. 2001). This deficiency results in the re-

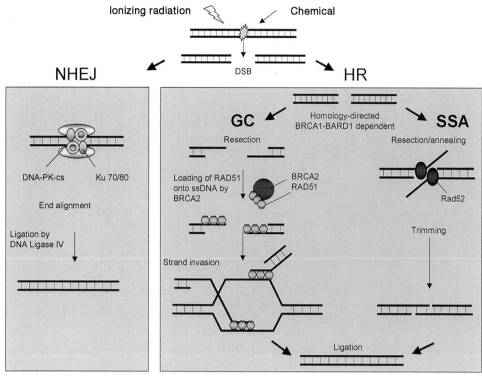

Figure 1. Role of BRCA1 and BRCA2 in DNA double-strand break repair. DSBs in DNA can arise spontaneously, frequently during replication, or be induced by exogenous or endogenous agents. DSBs are processed using two broad mechanisms of repair. The first mechanism, NHEJ, has no requirement for homologous sequences for repair, hence sequence changes at the site of DSBs are not restored. Homology-directed mechanisms use the presence of sequence homologous to that surrounding the DSB to act as a template for repair. In gene conversion, RAD51 forms a nucleoprotein filament, which searches for homologous sequences. An alternative, homology-directed, mechanism, SSA, involves alignment of the long 3′ single-stranded DNA tails at regions of complementary sequence on either side of the DSB followed by trimming of the intermediate noncomplementary sequence causing deletion. Hence, this SSA mechanism of repair, although homology-directed, is not conservative and may induce genome instability.

pair of these DNA lesions by the nonconservative, error-prone, and potentially mutagenic, mechanisms of NHEJ and SSA. This genomic instability probably underlies the cancer predisposition caused by loss-of-function mutations in *BRCA1* or *BRCA2* (Tutt et al. 2002).

BRCA1 appears to have a relatively early role in the regulation and promotion of HR. BRCA1 is phosphorylated in response to DNA DSBs by several kinases and likely acts in DNA damage signal transduction (Cortez et al. 1999; Lee et al. 2000; Tibbetts et al. 2000). Furthermore, BRCA1 is a component of large multiprotein complexes such as BASC (BRCA1-associated genome-surveillance complex) (Wang et al. 2000), where it may influence the choice of which repair pathway is utilized, depending on the type of DNA lesion. Moreover, BRCA1 has been shown to colocalize at sites of DNA damage with BASC-containing DNA repair signaling and repair factors in response to ionizing radiation. A specific role for BRCA1 in these complexes could be the regulation of initial DNA DSB processing by the MRE11/RAD50/NBS1 (MRN) complex (Zhong et al. 1999), allowing further progression down the HR pathway (Fig. 1). As a result, both HR-based gene conversion and deletional SSA are reduced in BRCA1-deficient cells (Stark et al. 2004). BRCA1 seems also to have an indirect role in marshaling a response to DNA damage by regulating the expression

of repair and cell cycle checkpoint proteins (Harkin et al. 1999). BRCA1, in complex with a heterodimeric partner BARD1, possesses E3 ubiquitin ligase activity (Kerr and Ashworth 2001). This activity may be involved in the regulation of the stability, activity, or stoichiometry of BRCA1-associated multiprotein complexes.

Compared to the more peripheral roles of BRCA1 in regulation of the core HR machinery, BRCA2 plays a more direct role via control of the RAD51 recombinase. BRCA2 binds to RAD51 through eight evolutionarily conserved RAD51-binding domains, the BRC repeats (Pellegrini et al. 2002). BRCA2 can also bind to single-stranded DNA via a domain toward the carboxyl terminus of the protein, the integrity of which is crucial to the ability of BRCA2 to promote recombination (Yang et al. 2002). Following DNA damage and initial DSB processing, BRCA2 relocalizes to the site of DNA damage (Yu et al. 2003). BRCA2 acts preferentially at the interface between double-stranded DNA and single-stranded 3′ overhangs that are generated by mechanisms that involve the MRN complex (Fig. 1), to displace RPA from the overhang and assist the loading of RAD51 (Yang et al. 2005). This process is dependent on the BRCA2-associated protein DSS1 (Gudmundsdottir et al. 2004). The RAD51 nucleoprotein filament then catalyzes the search for identical target sequences and strand invasion.

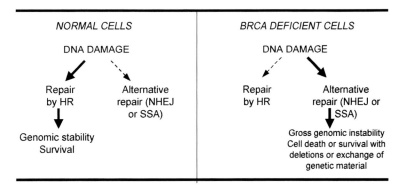

Figure 2. Alternative utilization of DSB DNA pathways in BRCA-deficient cells. DNA DSBs are repaired in normal cells, in part, by HR-based mechanisms. Functional BRCA1 and BRCA2 proteins are required for efficient repair by HR and genomic stability. In the absence of BRCA1 or BRCA2, alternative repair pathways, such as NHEJ and SSA, are utilized leading to cell death or survival with genomic damage.

OPTIMIZING TREATMENTS FOR CANCER IN *BRCA* MUTATION CARRIERS

Despite the demonstrated role of BRCA2 in DSB repair by gene conversion, no defect in overall DSB rejoining was noted in cells lacking wild-type *BRCA2* (Xia et al. 2001; A.N. Tutt, unpubl.). This implies that DNA DSB repair by gene conversion-independent mechanisms is proficient in *BRCA2* mutant cells. Indeed, experiments using repair constructs that can report repair by RAD51-independent forms of homology-directed repair have shown that, whereas BRCA2 deficiency affects the repair of chromosomal DSBs by GC, it also increases the use of the alternative nonconservative homology-directed DNA repair mechanism SSA (Tutt et al. 2001). This process is also up-regulated in yeast and mouse cells deficient in Rad51 function (Ivanov et al. 1996; Lambert and Lopez 2000) and in mouse ES cells lacking the *Rad54* gene (Dronkert et al. 2000). The increase in use of SSA (Tutt et al. 2001) and the demonstrated proficiency of the NHEJ mechanism in the absence of wild-type BRCA2 (Yu et al. 2000) indicate that the genomic instability apparent in otherwise isogenic *BRCA2*-mutant cell culture systems (Connor et al. 1997; Patel et al. 1998), and confirmed by in vivo mouse mutation reporter experiments (Tutt et al. 2002), is likely due to the alternative use of these error-prone mechanisms. The situation is slightly different in BRCA1 mutant cells in that both SSA and GC are decreased, suggesting that increased use of NHEJ is the source of the genomic instability (Fig. 2) (Snouwaert et al. 1999; Stark et al. 2004).

Cells deficient for BRCA2 have elevated sensitivity to mitomycin C, a phenotype known to be associated with abnormal HR (Yu et al. 2000; Tutt et al. 2001). Mitomycin C induces DNA interstrand cross-links that are repaired by a HR-dependent mechanism involving GC between sister chromatids and sister chromatid exchange (Sonoda et al. 1999). Furthermore, both *BRCA1* and *BRCA2* mutant cells show sensitivity to the commonly used chemotherapeutic agents cisplatin and carboplatin that also cross-link DNA (Fig. 3) (Overkamp et al. 1993; Bhattacharyya et al. 2000; Fedier et al. 2003). In principle, therefore, tumors arising in *BRCA1* or *2* mutation carriers that have lost the wild-type *BRCA* allele should be hypersensitive to this type of agent based on an inability to repair a specific class of DNA lesion. The normal tis-

sues in mutation carriers could also show elevated sensitivity to such agents because of loss of one copy of the relevant BRCA gene. However, there are currently few convincing data to support the existence of a haploinsufficiency phenomenon for *BRCA1* and *BRCA2* in humans (Santarosa and Ashworth 2004). The limited clinical data available from treatment of *BRCA* carriers for ovarian cancer with platinum-based chemotherapy support the notion of a widened therapeutic window in *BRCA*-associated cancers (Cass et al. 2003).

We have designed a mechanism-based randomized Phase II trial to prospectively test the hypothesis that the use of carboplatin chemotherapy is associated with a wider therapeutic ratio (greater tumor cell kill with no increase in normal tissue damage) in *BRCA1* or *BRCA2* carriers than previously noted in sporadic breast cancer (for further details, see www.Breakthroughcentre.org.uk). This is a multicenter international trial in confirmed *BRCA1* or *BRCA2* carriers with metastatic breast cancer. Patients will be randomly allocated to receive carboplatin chemotherapy followed by docetaxel at the time of progression or, alternatively, to docetaxel with carboplatin at progression. The trial will recruit 74 *BRCA1* and 74 *BRCA2* carriers. Given the challenge in recruiting this highly defined population, this randomized cross-over

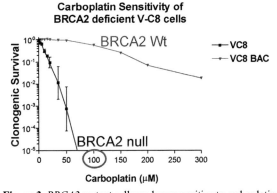

Figure 3. *BRCA2* mutant cells are hypersensitive to carboplatin. Clonogenic survival curves of VC-8 cells and VC-8 cells complemented with mouse BRCA2 BAC (VC-8-BAC) (Kraakman-van der Zwet et al. 2002) after one hour exposure to a range of concentrations of carboplatin. The cells were washed twice and after normal growth media was added were allowed to grow for 10 days.

design gives the opportunity to study carboplatin response and toxicity in all participants, while maintaining a standard therapy comparator arm. Tumor responses, normal tissue toxicity, and time to tumor progression will be the study end points. Results will be analyzed separately for each gene carrier group. The chief investigators for this study are James Mackay, Max Parmar, and Andrew Tutt, who may be contacted at brca@ctc.ucl.ac.uk.

COMBINATORIAL INHIBITION OF DNA REPAIR PATHWAYS

DNA is constantly damaged by exogenous agents (UV, IR, etc.) and endogenous activities (replication, free radical generation) that create different DNA lesions and forms of damage such as DSBs, single-strand breaks (SSBs), and intrastrand and interstrand cross links. These different forms of damage are repaired by different DNA repair pathways that are coordinated and act in concert to maintain the stability and integrity of the genome (Hoeijmakers 2001). We hypothesized, therefore, that cells harboring existing defects in DNA damage repair (such as those present in BRCA1- or BRCA2-deficient cells) would be more sensitive to the induced loss of other DNA damage repair mechanisms. Specifically, we hypothesized that inhibiting the base excision repair (BER) pathway would be selectively lethal in cells lacking wild-type *BRCA1* or *BRCA2* alleles, compared to their normal counterparts. The BER pathway is important for the repair of certain kinds of DNA base damage, DNA SSBs, and gaps (Dantzer et al. 2000; Hoeijmakers 2001).

To inhibit the BER pathway and test this concept of "synthetic lethality," we targeted the enzyme poly (ADP-ribose) polymerase-1 (PARP-1). PARP-1 plays a role in the BER pathway by rapidly binding to and "protecting" SSBs that are produced either directly by damage or indirectly by endonuclease action during the BER process (Dantzer et al. 2000; Hoeijmakers 2001). By rapidly binding to DNA breaks and covalently modifying itself and proteins, such as histones, in the proximity with poly (ADP-ribose) (PAR) polymers, PARP-1 instigates the BER process. The highly negatively charged PAR that is produced around the site of damage may also serve as an anti-recombinogenic factor preventing unwanted recombination. Deficiency of PARP-1 causes failure to repair such SSB lesions effectively but does not impede DSB repair (Noel et al. 2003). However, a persistent DNA SSB encountered by a DNA replication fork leads to the stalling of the fork and the potential formation of a DSB (Haber 1999; Arnaudeau et al. 2001; Symington 2005). Both of these outcomes can be resolved by GC. Interestingly, loss of PARP-1 function induces the formation of sister chromatid exchanges (SCEs) (Wang et al. 1997; Shall and de Murcia 2000), a product of Rad51-dependent GC. Loss of PARP-1 has also recently been shown to induce the formation of nuclear Rad51 foci as well as the formation of SCEs, but without increasing the activity of sister chromatid recombination as measured using a site-specific DNA DSB assay (Schultz et al. 2003). This suggested that loss of PARP-1 increases the formation of

DNA lesions that are repaired by GC without directly regulating GC itself. As loss of function of either BRCA1 or BRCA2 impairs GC (Moynahan et al. 1999, 2001a,b; Tutt et al. 2001), we hypothesized that loss of PARP-1 function in a BRCA1 or BRCA2 defective background might result in the generation of replication-associated DNA lesions normally repaired by SCE. If so, this increase in un-repaired or mis-repaired DNA damage might lead to cell cycle arrest and/or cell death. Therefore, inhibitors of PARP-1 might be selectively lethal to cells lacking wild-type BRCA1 or BRCA2 with minimal toxicity to normal cells.

BRCA1 AND BRCA2 MUTANT CELLS ARE VERY SENSITIVE TO INHIBITION OF PARP

To examine whether BRCA-deficient cells are selectively sensitive to loss of PARP function, we decreased Parp-1 expression levels using plasmid-based RNA interference. The depletion of Parp-1 caused a clear reduction in clonogenic survival of BRCA1- and BRCA2-deficient cells compared to wild-type cells (Farmer et al. 2005). This result suggested that chemical inhibitors of PARP activity might have similar effects. We used two novel and very potent small-molecule PARP inhibitors: KU0058684 (PARP-1 IC_{50} = 3.2 nM) and KU0058948 (PARP-1 IC_{50} = 3.4 nM) and a much less active but chemically related compound KU0051529 (PARP-1 IC_{50} = 730 nM) (Loh et al. 2005). These PARP inhibitors are based around a phthalazin-1-one core and are competitive inhibitors with respect to the PARP substrate NAD^+. KU0058684 and KU0058948 are potent and specific inhibitors of the poly (ADP-ribose) polymerase activity of the proteins PARP-1 and PARP-2, and exhibit between 1 and 3 orders of magnitude selectivity in comparison to other enzymes able to catalyze poly (ADP-ribose) polymerization such as PARP-3, vault PARP, and tankyrase (Farmer et al. 2005). Conversely, the chemically related compound KU0051529 is less effective by a factor of approximately 250 in the inhibition of these enzymes. To monitor inhibition of cellular poly(ADP-ribose) (PAR) formation by KU0058684 and KU0058948, a "whole-cell extract" assay for PAR was performed on HeLa cells that had been treated with the PARP inhibitors. Monitoring PAR formation, via an antibody specific for PAR demonstrated cellular IC_{50}s of 1 nM and 6 nM for KU0058684 and KU0058948, respectively (Farmer et al. 2005).

We used KU0058684, KU0058948, and KU0051529 to test the sensitivity of cells deficient in either Brca1 or Brca2 to the chemical inhibition of Parp activity. Clonogenic cell survival assays showed that ES cell lines lacking wild-type Brca1 or Brca2 were extremely sensitive to KU0058684 and KU0058948 compared to heterozygous mutant or wild-type cells (Fig. 4) (Farmer et al. 2005). Similar results were obtained with non-embryonic cells such as Chinese hamster ovary cells deficient in Brca2 (Kraakman-van der Zwet et al. 2002), which showed a greater than 1000-fold enhanced sensitivity compared to a Brca2-complemented derivative (Farmer et al. 2005).

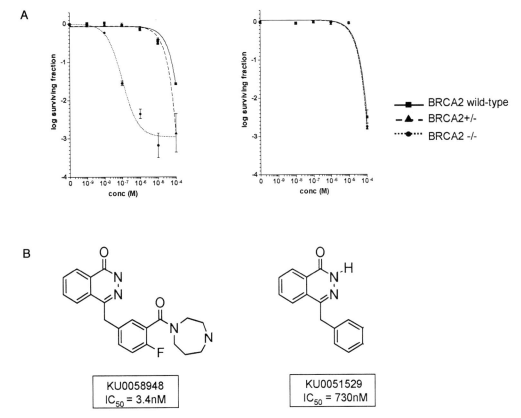

Figure 4. Inhibition of PARP activity selectively inhibits the survival of cells lacking wild-type Brca2. (*A*) Clonogenic survival curves of Brca2 wild-type, heterozygous, and deficient mouse ES cells after 10–12 days continuous exposure to a range of concentrations of chemical inhibitors (KU0058948 and KU0051529). (*B*) The PARP inhibitors are based around a phthalazin-1-one core and are competitive inhibitors with respect to the PARP substrate NAD^+ (Loh et al. 2005). KU0058948 is a potent and specific inhibitor of the poly (ADP-ribose) polymerase activity of the proteins PARP-1 and PARP-2, whereas KU0051529 is less effective by a factor of approximately 250 in the inhibition of these enzymes.

Likewise, depletion of *BRCA1* mRNA in MCF7 human breast cancer cells or of *BRCA2* mRNA in MCF7 or MDA-MB-231 cells induced hypersensitivity to PARP inhibition (Bryant et al. 2005; Farmer et al. 2005). In contrast, KU0051529, which does not effectively inhibit PARP-1 or PARP-2, had no selective effect on cells lacking wild-type Brca1 or Brca2. These results, in conjunction with our RNA interference data, demonstrate that the mechanism of sensitivity is specifically through inhibition of Parp (Farmer et al. 2005). Notably, none of the inhibitors had any selective effect on cells heterozygous for *Brca1* or *Brca2* mutations, which is important because non-tumor tissue in *BRCA* patients has only one copy of the relevant *BRCA* gene. As discussed above, Brca1- and Brca2-deficient cells are also selectively sensitive to the chemotherapeutic agents mitomycin C, cisplatin, and carboplatin, but this is to a much lesser degree than the effects of PARP inhibition (Farmer et al. 2005).

The mechanism of cell death in Brca1- or Brca2-deficient cells exposed to PARP inhibitors was characterized by cell cycle arrest in the G_2 phase 24 hours after the initial inhibitor treatment followed by apoptosis at 48 hours. Examination of those few Brca1- or Brca2-deficient cells that did pass through the G_2/M checkpoint showed in-

creased levels of chromosomal instability, illustrated by the presence of complex chromosome rearrangements (Fig. 5). These included chromatid breaks and more complex chromatid aberrations such as tri-radial and quadriradial chromosomes. Such aberrations were not increased in wild-type cells treated with the same doses of PARP inhibitor. These phenotypes are suggestive of a failure to repair DSBs by the conservative RAD51-dependent GC recombination pathway and the consequent use of alternative error-prone pathways such as SSA or NHEJ.

The in vivo efficacy of these PARP inhibitors in preventing the formation of BRCA2-deficient tumors was also tested. Existing tumor cell models of BRCA1 and BRCA2 deficiency are not very suitable for the rapid testing of the in vivo efficacy of small-molecule therapeutics. Therefore, the ability of ES cells to form teratocarcinomas after transplantation into athymic mice was exploited. This showed that small-molecule inhibitors of PARP can indeed selectively inhibit the formation of tumors derived from Brca2-deficient cells. In comparison, the growth of tumors derived from wild-type cells was completely unimpaired by these inhibitors (Farmer et al. 2005). However, these initial experiments only demonstrated that PARP inhibitors have the ability to prevent

A

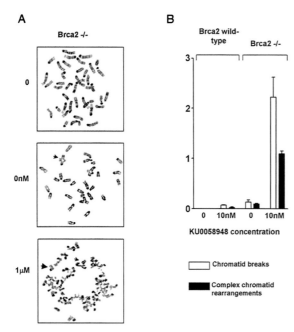

Figure 5. Inhibition of PARP results in chromatid breaks and complex rearrangements. (*A*) Chromosome analysis of ES cells lacking wild-type Brca2 exposed to KU0058948 or vehicle for 24 hours. The small arrows indicate complex chromatid rearrangements and the large arrow indicates a chromatid break. (*B*) Quantification of chromatid breaks and complex chromatid aberrations in Brca2 wild-type or deficient ES cells after PARP inhibition. Fifty metaphase spreads were quantified for three independent experiments. Error bars represent standard errors of the mean.

the formation of Brca2-deficient tumors and not to reduce the growth of existing tumors. We have now shown that this is also the case and that PARP inhibitors can significantly reduce the growth of established Brca2-deficient tumors in vivo while having no effect on wild-type tumors (C.J. Lord, unpubl.). Now that the in vivo efficacy of these small molecules is established in a relatively rapid xenograft model, it is important that these experiments are also corroborated by their use in more sophisticated animal models of BRCA tumorigenesis (Jonkers et al. 2001).

RATIONALE FOR THE SENSITIVITY OF BRCA MUTANT CELLS TO PARP INHIBITION

Why might BRCA1- and BRCA2-deficient cells exhibit extreme sensitivity to PARP inhibition? We suggest a model (Fig. 6) that arises from the observations that PARP is required for the efficient repair of DNA SSBs during BER (Dantzer et al. 2000; Hoeijmakers 2001) and that PARP inhibition leads to persistent single-strand gaps in DNA (Boulton et al. 1999). If these gaps are encountered by a replication fork, arrest would occur and the single-strand gaps may degenerate into DSBs (Haber 1999). Normally these DSBs can be repaired by RAD51-dependent GC (Arnaudeau et al. 2001), which, as detailed above, is a process in which both BRCA1 and BRCA2 are involved. In the absence of BRCA1 or BRCA2, the repli-

cation fork cannot be restarted and collapses (Lomonosov et al. 2003), causing persistent chromatid breaks. Repair of these by the alternative error-prone DSB repair mechanisms of SSA or NHEJ would induce large numbers of chromatid aberrations, leading to loss of cell viability (Fig. 6). This model suggests that it is the defect in GC that is being targeted in BRCA-deficient cells. This conjecture is supported by our demonstration that Rad54-deficient cells are also sensitive to PARP inhibition (N. McCabe, unpubl.). Rad54 is involved in HR and normally acts to stimulate the strand exchange activity of Rad51 (Hoeijmakers 2001). Therefore, this approach may be more widely applicable in the treatment of sporadic cancers with impairments of the HR pathway or "BRCA-ness" (Turner et al. 2004; and see below).

The results presented here suggest a potential new mechanism-based approach for the treatment of patients with *BRCA1*- and *BRCA2*-associated cancers. Tumors in carriers of *BRCA1* or *BRCA2* mutations lack wild-type BRCA1 or BRCA2, but normal tissues retain a single wild-type copy of the relevant gene. This difference provides the rationale for the inhibition of PARP to generate specific DNA lesions that require functional BRCA1 and BRCA2 for their repair. This approach is likely to be less toxic and more specific than standard cytotoxic chemotherapy, as PARP inhibitors are relatively nontoxic and do not directly damage DNA, and *Parp-1* knockout mice are viable (Wang et al. 1997).

DO A SUBSET OF SPORADIC CANCERS PHENOCOPY BRCA MUTATION AND SHOW "BRCA-NESS?"

Although germ-line mutations in *BRCA1* or *BRCA2* contribute to a substantial proportion of hereditary breast and ovarian cancer, inactivation of these genes by mutation occurs only rarely in sporadic cancers (Futreal et al. 1994; Merajver et al. 1995; Lancaster et al. 1996). This is, perhaps, surprising but an increasing amount of evidence suggests that these genes, or other components of the same biochemical pathways in which BRCA1 or BRCA2 act, may be inactivated by other means in sporadic tumors. If these cancers display "BRCA-ness" (Turner et al. 2004), that is, they share a DNA repair defect similar to BRCA1- and BRCA2-deficient cells, they may also be candidates for the treatment strategies outlined in this review.

BRCA1 hereditary tumors share many phenotypes with a subset of sporadic breast cancers called basal-like breast cancers (Fig. 7) (Foulkes et al. 2003). The similarity between basal-like breast cancers and BRCA1 hereditary tumors may suggest a common etiology, raising the possibility that basal-like cancers harbor an underlying defect in the BRCA1 pathway. Following anecdotal evidence of good responses of basal-like breast cancer to platinum chemotherapy-based regimens, a number of clinical trials have been designed to examine this issue. More direct evidence for inactivation of BRCA1 in sporadic cancers comes from the finding that 10–15% of sporadic breast and ovarian cancers have *BRCA1* promoter methylation (Catteau et al. 1999; Baldwin et al. 2000; Es-

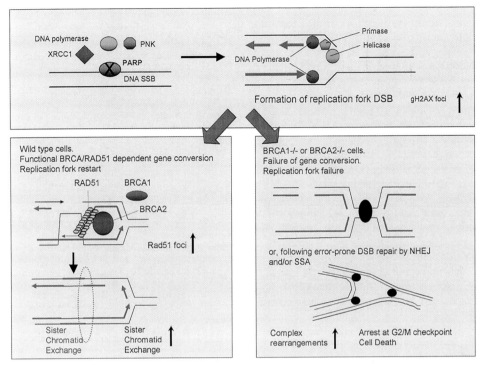

Figure 6. A model for the selective effects of PARP inhibition on cells lacking wild-type BRCA1 and BRCA2. (*A*) PARP is important for the repair of DNA lesions, including DNA SSBs, by BER. When PARP activity is impaired, DNA SSBs persist. When these are encountered by a DNA replication fork, fork arrest occurs, which may result in fork collapse or a DSB. (*B*) BRCA1 and BRCA2 are involved in the repair of such lesions by HR in association with RAD51. This allows restart of a collapsed replication fork. (*C*) The excess number of replication fork arrests associated with loss of PARP function leads to an increase in sister chromatid recombination events and sister chromatid exchanges. (*D*) In the absence of functional BRCA1 or BRCA2, sister chromatid recombination and the formation of RAD51 foci are severely impaired. This leads to the utilization of error-prone RAD51-independent mechanisms such as NHEJ or SSA, and complex chromatid rearrangements result. Cells harboring these rearrangements may permanently arrest or undergo apoptosis.

teller et al. 2000; Rice et al. 2000). In the majority of these tumors, BRCA1 expression is undetectable, suggesting complete gene silencing and loss of BRCA1 function.

Whether BRCA2 function can be disrupted in sporadic cancers is currently unclear. A gene for the novel BRCA2 interacting protein EMSY is found in a common breast cancer amplicon on chromosome 11q (Hughes-Davies et al. 2003). The resulting overexpression of EMSY may lead to inactivation of some of the functions of BRCA2, although further research is needed to clarify whether this includes the DNA repair function of BRCA2. Further possible mechanisms of inducing "BRCA-ness" include methylation of the promoter of *FANCF*, a Fanconi anemia gene, which has been reported in a number of sporadic cancers (Taniguchi et al. 2003), and ATM deficiency in approximately 30% of chronic lymphocytic leukemias (Boultwood 2001).

CONCLUSIONS

Although differences in the age of onset and pathology have been described for tumors in carriers of *BRCA* mutations (Lakhani et al. 2002; Couzin 2003), at the present time, treatment is the same as that for patients with sporadic disease (Couzin 2003). However, the specific genotype of a tumor is increasingly being targeted with mech-

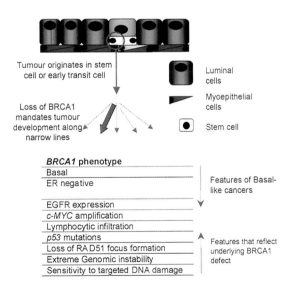

Figure 7. Phenotypes of BRCA1-related tumors. Breast cancers may arise in a common breast stem or progenitor cell. Loss of BRCA1 function leads to a phenotype that reflects development from this cell of origin down a basal-like pathway as well as resulting in phenotypes mandated directly by BRCA1 deficiency (Turner et al. 2004). Basal-like cancers resemble, in part, the basal/myoepithelial cells that line the normal breast duct and may harbor deficiencies in BRCA pathway(s) and display "BRCA-ness."

anism-based therapeutics such as Herceptin (Slamon et al. 2001). Tumors in carriers of *BRCA1* or *BRCA2* mutations lack wild-type BRCA1 or BRCA2, but normal tissues retain a single wild-type copy of the relevant gene. BRCA deficiency causes a specific defect in the repair of damaged DNA by GC. This provides the rationale for two new mechanism-based approaches to the treatment of patients with *BRCA1*- and *BRCA2*-associated cancers.

In the first approach, we are attempting to define the optimal treatment of these cancers with the existing chemotherapy drugs available. Laboratory results indicate that *BRCA* cancers will not be more sensitive than usual to the standard chemotherapies given for breast cancer. Rather, BRCA-deficient cells are much more sensitive to agents, such as carboplatin, which cross-link DNA. Therefore, we have established an international clinical trial, the BRCA Trial, to test this hypothesis. Clinical trials in genetically subdivided groups present significant problems in trial organization and management. However, given the heterogeneous and genetically determined response to several of the newer targeted cancer treatments, these problems will need to be addressed by the wider oncology community (Lynch et al. 2004). A critical point is that, if targeted treatments are to succeed in improving the therapeutic ratio, no common cancer can be regarded as one homogeneous disease.

The biochemical difference in capacity between the tumor and normal tissues, in a BRCA1 or BRCA2 carrier, to carry out specialized DNA repair also provides the rationale for our second approach. This involves using inhibitors of the DNA repair protein PARP to generate specific DNA lesions that require BRCA1 and BRCA2 specialized repair function(s) for their removal. Our preclinical data lead us to anticipate that tumors defective in wild-type BRCA1 or BRCA2 will be much more sensitive to PARP inhibition than unaffected heterozygous tissues, providing a potentially large therapeutic window. The safety and preliminary efficacy of this approach will shortly be tested in clinical trials.

Synthetic tumor lethality caused by combinatorial targeting of DNA repair pathways may have usefulness beyond that of familial breast cancer. The majority of solid tumors also exhibit genomic instability and aneuploidy. This suggests that pathways involved in the maintenance of genomic stability are dysfunctional in a significant proportion of neoplastic disorders (Vogelstein and Kinzler 2004). Understanding which specialized DNA damage response and repair pathways are abrogated in sporadic tumor subtypes may allow the development of therapies that target the residual repair pathways on which the cancer, but not normal tissue, is now completely dependent. This avenue may lead to that elusive goal in clinical oncology, therapies that significantly improve treatment response while causing fewer treatment-related toxicities.

ACKNOWLEDGMENTS

We thank Breakthrough Breast Cancer, Cancer Research UK, and the Mary-Jean Mitchell Green Foundation for generous financial support.

REFERENCES

Arnaudeau C., Lundin C., and Helleday T. 2001. DNA double-strand breaks associated with replication forks are predominantly repaired by homologous recombination involving an exchange mechanism in mammalian cells. *J. Mol. Biol.* **307:** 1235.

Baldwin R.L., Nemeth E., Tran H., Shvartsman H., Cass I., Narod S., and Karlan B.Y. 2000. BRCA1 promoter region hypermethylation in ovarian carcinoma: A population-based study. *Cancer Res.* **60:** 5329.

Bhattacharyya A., Ear U.S., Koller B.H., Weichselbaum R.R., and Bishop D.K. 2000. The breast cancer susceptibility gene BRCA1 is required for subnuclear assembly of Rad51 and survival following treatment with the DNA cross-linking agent cisplatin. *J. Biol. Chem.* **275:** 23899.

Boulton S., Kyle S., and Durkacz B.W. 1999. Interactive effects of inhibitors of polyADP-ribose polymerase and DNA-dependent protein kinase on cellular responses to DNA damage. *Carcinogenesis* **20:** 199.

Boultwood J. 2001. Ataxia telangiectasia gene mutations in leukemia and lymphoma. *J. Clin. Pathol.* **54:** 512.

Bryant H.E., Schultz N., Thomas H.D., Parker K.M., Flower D., Lopez E., Kyle S., Meuth M., Curtin N.J., and Helleday T. 2005. Specific killing of BRCA2-deficient tumours with inhibitors of polyADP-ribose polymerase. *Nature* **434:** 913.

Cass I., Baldwin R L., Varkey T., Moslehi R., Narod S.A., and Karlan B.Y. 2003. Improved survival in women with BRCA-associated ovarian carcinoma. *Cancer* **97:** 2187.

Catteau A., Harris W.H., Xu C.F., and Solomon E. 1999. Methylation of the BRCA1 promoter region in sporadic breast and ovarian cancer: Correlation with disease characteristics. *Oncogene* **18:** 1957.

Connor F., Bertwistle D., Mee P.J., Ross G.M., Swift S., Grigorieva E., Tybulewicz V.L., and Ashworth A. 1997. Tumorigenesis and a DNA repair defect in mice with a truncating Brca2 mutation. *Nat. Genet.* **17:** 423.

Cortez D., Wang Y., Qin J., and Elledge S.J. 1999. Requirement of ATM-dependent phosphorylation of brca1 in the DNA damage response to double-strand breaks. *Science* **286:** 1162.

Couzin J. 2003. Choices - and uncertainties - for women with BRCA mutations. *Science* **302:** 592.

Daniels M.J., Wang Y., Lee M., and Venkitaraman A.R. 2004. Abnormal cytokinesis in cells deficient in the breast cancer susceptibility protein BRCA2. *Science* **306:** 876.

Dantzer F., de La Rubia G., Menissier-De Murcia J., Hostomsky Z., de Murcia G., and Schreiber V. 2000. Base excision repair is impaired in mammalian cells lacking PolyADP-ribose polymerase-1. *Biochemistry* **39:** 7559.

Dronkert M.L., Beverloo H.B., Johnson R.D., Hoeijmakers J.H., Jasin M., and Kanaar R. 2000. Mouse RAD54 affects DNA double-strand break repair and sister chromatid exchange. *Mol. Cell. Biol.* **20:** 3147.

Elliott B. and Jasin M. 2001. Repair of double-strand breaks by homologous recombination in mismatch repair-defective mammalian cells. *Mol. Cell. Biol.* **21:** 2671.

Esteller M., Silva J.M., Dominguez G., Bonilla F., Matias-Guiu X., Lerma E., Bussaglia E., Prat J., Harkes I.C., Repasky E.A., Gabrielson E., Schutte M., Baylin S.B., and Herman J.G. 2000. Promoter hypermethylation and BRCA1 inactivation in sporadic breast and ovarian tumors. *J. Natl. Cancer Inst.* **92:** 564.

Farmer H., McCabe N., Lord C.J., Tutt A.N., Johnson D.A., Richardson T.B., Santarosa M., Dillon K.J., Hickson I., Knights C., Martin N.M., Jackson S.P., Smith G.C., and Ashworth A. 2005. Targeting the DNA repair defect in BRCA mutant cells as a therapeutic strategy. *Nature* **434:** 917.

Fedier A., Steiner R.A., Schwarz V.A., Lenherr L., Haller U., and Fink D. 2003. The effect of loss of Brca1 on the sensitivity to anticancer agents in p53-deficient cells. *Int. J. Oncol.* **22:** 1169.

Foulkes W.D., Stefansson I.M., Chappuis P.O., Begin L.R., Goffin J.R., Wong N., Trudel M., and Akslen L.A. 2003. Germline BRCA1 mutations and a basal epithelial phenotype in breast cancer. *J. Natl. Cancer Inst.* **95:** 1482.

Futreal P.A., Liu Q., Shattuck-Eidens D., Cochran C., Harshman K., Tavtigian S., Bennett L.M., Haugen-Strano A., Swensen J., and Miki Y., et al. 1994. BRCA1 mutations in primary breast and ovarian carcinomas. *Science* **266:** 120.

Gudmundsdottir K., Lord C.J., Witt E., Tutt A.N., and Ashworth A. 2004. DSS1 is required for RAD51 focus formation and genomic stability in mammalian cells. *EMBO Rep.* **5:** 989.

Haber J.E. 1999. DNA recombination: The replication connection. *Trends Biochem. Sci.* **24:** 271.

Harkin D.P., Bean J.M., Miklos D., Song Y.H., Truong V.B., Englert C., Christians F.C., Ellisen L.W., Maheswaran S., Oliner J.D., and Haber D.A. 1999. Induction of GADD45 and JNK/SAPK-dependent apoptosis following inducible expression of BRCA1. *Cell* **97:** 575.

Hoeijmakers J.H. 2001. Genome maintenance mechanisms for preventing cancer. *Nature* **411:** 366.

Hughes-Davies L., Huntsman D., Ruas M., Fuks F., Bye J., Chin S.F., Milner J., Brown L.A., Hsu F., Gilks B., Nielsen T., Schulzer M., Chia S., Ragaz J., Cahn A., Linger L., Ozdag H., Cattaneo E., Jordanova E.S., Schuuring E., Yu D.S., Venkitaraman A., Ponder B., Doherty A., Aparicio S., Bentley D., Theillet C., Ponting C.P., Caldas C., and Kouzarides T. 2003. EMSY links the BRCA2 pathway to sporadic breast and ovarian cancer. *Cell* **115:** 523.

Ivanov E.L., Sugawara N., Fishman-Lobell J., and Haber J.E. 1996. Genetic requirements for the single-strand annealing pathway of double-strand break repair in *Saccharomyces cerevisiae*. *Genetics* **142:** 693.

Jonkers J., Meuwissen R., van der Gulden H., Peterse H., van der Valk M., and Berns A. 2001. Synergistic tumor suppressor activity of BRCA2 and p53 in a conditional mouse model for breast cancer. *Nat. Genet.* **29:** 418.

Kerr P. and Ashworth A. 2001. New complexities for BRCA1 and BRCA2. *Curr. Biol.* **11:** R668.

Kraakman-van der Zwet M., Overkamp W.J., van Lange R.E., Essers J., van Duijn-Goedhart A., Wiggers I., Swaminathan S., van Buul P.P., Errami A., Tan R.T., Jaspers N.G., Sharan S.K., Kanaar R., and Zdzienicka M.Z. 2002. Brca2 XRCC11 deficiency results in radioresistant DNA synthesis and a higher frequency of spontaneous deletions. *Mol. Cell. Biol.* **22:** 669.

Lakhani S.R., Van De Vijver M.J., Jacquemier J., Anderson T.J., Osin P.P., McGuffog L., and Easton D.F. 2002. The pathology of familial breast cancer: Predictive value of immunohistochemical markers estrogen receptor, progesterone receptor, HER-2, and p53 in patients with mutations in BRCA1 and BRCA2. *J. Clin. Oncol.* **20:** 2310.

Lambert S. and Lopez B.S. 2000. Characterization of mammalian RAD51 double strand break repair using non-lethal dominant-negative forms. *EMBO J.* **19:** 3090.

Lancaster J.M., Wooster R., Mangion J., Phelan C.M., Cochran C., Gumbs C., Seal S., Barfoot R., Collins N., Bignell G., Patel S., Hamoudi R., Larsson C., Wiseman R.W., Berchuck A., Iglehart J.D., Marks J.R., Ashworth A., Stratton M.R., and Futreal P.A. 1996. BRCA2 mutations in primary breast and ovarian cancers. *Nat. Genet.* **13:** 238.

Lee J.S., Collins K.M., Brown A.L., Lee C.H., and Chung J.H. 2000. hCds1-mediated phosphorylation of BRCA1 regulates the DNA damage response. *Nature* **404:** 201.

Loh V.M., Jr., Cockcroft X.L., Dillon K.J., Dixon L., Drzewiecki J., Eversley P.J., Gomez S., Hoare J., Kerrigan F., Matthews I.T., Menear K.A., Martin N.M., Newton R.F., Paul J., Smith G.C., Vile J., and Whittle A.J. 2005. Phthalazinones. 1. The design and synthesis of a novel series of potent inhibitors of poly(ADP-ribose)polymerase. *Bioorg. Med. Chem. Lett.* **15:** 2235.

Lomonosov M., Anand S., Sangrithi M., Davies R., and Venkitaraman A.R. 2003. Stabilization of stalled DNA replication forks by the BRCA2 breast cancer susceptibility protein. *Genes Dev.* **17:** 3017.

Lynch T.J., Bell D.W., Sordella R., Gurubhagavatula S., Okimoto R.A., Brannigan B.W., Harris P.L., Haserlat S.M., Supko J.G., Haluska F.G., Louis D.N., Christiani D.C., Settleman J., and Haber D.A. 2004. Activating mutations in the epidermal growth factor receptor underlying responsiveness of non-small-cell lung cancer to gefitinib. *N. Engl. J. Med.* **350:** 2129.

Merajver S.D., Pham T.M., Caduff R.F., Chen M., Poy E.L., Cooney K.A., Weber B.L., Collins F.S., Johnston C., and Frank T.S. 1995. Somatic mutations in the BRCA1 gene in sporadic ovarian tumours. *Nat. Genet.* **9:** 439.

Moynahan M.E., Cui T.Y., and Jasin M. 2001a. Homology-directed dna repair, mitomycin-c resistance, and chromosome stability is restored with correction of a Brca1 mutation. *Cancer Res.* **61:** 4842.

Moynahan M.E., Pierce A.J., and Jasin M. 2001b. BRCA2 is required for homology-directed repair of chromosomal breaks. *Mol. Cell* **7:** 263.

Moynahan M.E., Chiu J.W., Koller B.H., and Jasin M. 1999. Brca1 controls homology-directed DNA repair. *Mol. Cell* **4:** 511.

Narod S.A. and Foulkes W.D. 2004. BRCA1 and BRCA2: 1994 and beyond. *Nat. Rev. Cancer* **4:** 665.

Noel G., Giocanti N., Fernet M., Megnin-Chanet F., and Favaudon V. 2003. PolyADP-ribose polymerase PARP-1 is not involved in DNA double-strand break recovery. *BMC Cell Biol.* **4:** 7.

Overkamp W.J., Rooimans M.A., Neuteboom I., Telleman P., Arwert F., and Zdzienicka M.Z. 1993. Genetic diversity of mitomycin C-hypersensitive Chinese hamster cell mutants: A new complementation group with chromosomal instability. *Somat. Cell Mol. Genet.* **19:** 431.

Patel K.J., Yu V.P., Lee H., Corcoran A., Thistlethwaite F.C., Evans M.J., Colledge W.H., Friedman L.S., Ponder B.A., and Venkitaraman A.R. 1998. Involvement of Brca2 in DNA repair. *Mol. Cell* **1:** 347.

Pellegrini L., Yu D.S., Lo T., Anand S., Lee M., Blundell T.L., and Venkitaraman A.R. 2002. Insights into DNA recombination from the structure of a RAD51-BRCA2 complex. *Nature* **420:** 287.

Rice J.C., Ozcelik H., Maxeiner P., Andrulis I., and Futscher B.W. 2000. Methylation of the BRCA1 promoter is associated with decreased BRCA1 mRNA levels in clinical breast cancer specimens. *Carcinogenesis* **21:** 1761.

Rodriguez M., Yu X., Chen J., and Songyang Z. 2003. Phosphopeptide binding specificities of BRCA1 COOH-terminal BRCT domains. *J. Biol. Chem.* **278:** 52914.

Santarosa M. and Ashworth A. 2004. Haploinsufficiency for tumour suppressor genes: When you don't need to go all the way. *Biochim. Biophys. Acta* **1654:** 105.

Schultz N., Lopez E., Saleh-Gohari N., and Helleday T. 2003. PolyADP-ribose polymerase PARP-1 has a controlling role in homologous recombination. *Nucleic Acids Res.* **31:** 4959.

Shall S. and de Murcia G. 2000. PolyADP-ribose polymerase-1: What have we learned from the deficient mouse model? *Mutat. Res.* **460:** 1.

Slamon D.J., Leyland-Jones B., Shak S., Fuchs H., Paton V., Bajamonde A., Fleming T., Eiermann W., Wolter J., Pegram M., Baselga J., and Norton L. 2001. Use of chemotherapy plus a monoclonal antibody against HER2 for metastatic breast cancer that overexpresses HER2. *N. Engl. J. Med.* **344:** 783.

Snouwaert J.N., Gowen L.C., Latour A.M., Mohn A.R., Xiao A., DiBiase L., and Koller B.H. 1999. BRCA1 deficient embryonic stem cells display a decreased homologous recombination frequency and an increased frequency of non-homologous recombination that is corrected by expression of a brca1 transgene. *Oncogene* **18:** 7900.

Sonoda E., Sasaki M.S., Morrison C., Yamaguchi-Iwai Y., Takata M., and Takeda S. 1999. Sister chromatid exchanges are mediated by homologous recombination in vertebrate cells. *Mol. Cell. Biol.* **19:** 5166.

Stark J.M., Pierce A.J., Oh J., Pastink A., and Jasin M. 2004. Genetic steps of mammalian homologous repair with distinct mutagenic consequences. *Mol. Cell. Biol.* **24:** 9305.

Symington L.S. 2005. Focus on recombinational DNA repair. *EMBO Rep.* **6:** 512.

Taniguchi T., Tischkowitz M., Ameziane N., Hodgson S.V.,

Mathew C.G., Joenje H., Mok S.C., and D'Andrea A.D. 2003. Disruption of the Fanconi anemia-BRCA pathway in cisplatin-sensitive ovarian tumors. *Nat. Med.* **9:** 568.

Tibbetts R.S., Cortez D., Brumbaugh K.M., Scully R., Livingston D., Elledge S.J., and Abraham R.T. 2000. Functional interactions between BRCA1 and the checkpoint kinase ATR during genotoxic stress. *Genes Dev.* **14:** 2989.

Turner N., Tutt A., and Ashworth A. 2004. Hallmarks of 'BRCAness' in sporadic cancers. *Nat. Rev. Cancer* **4:** 814.

Tutt A. and Ashworth A. 2002. The relationship between the roles of BRCA genes in DNA repair and cancer predisposition. *Trends Mol. Med.* **8:** 571.

Tutt A.N., van Oostrom C.T., Ross G.M., van Steeg H., and Ashworth A. 2002. Disruption of Brca2 increases the spontaneous mutation rate in vivo: Synergism with ionizing radiation. *EMBO Rep.* **3:** 255.

Tutt A., Bertwistle D., Valentine J., Gabriel A., Swift S., Ross G., Griffin C., Thacker J., and Ashworth A. 2001. Mutation in Brca2 stimulates error-prone homology-directed repair of DNA double-strand breaks occurring between repeated sequences. *EMBO J.* **20:** 4704.

Venkitaraman A.R. 2002. Cancer susceptibility and the functions of BRCA1 and BRCA2. *Cell* **108:** 171.

Vogelstein B. and Kinzler K.W. 2004. Cancer genes and the pathways they control. *Nat. Med.* **10:** 789.

Wang Y., Cortez D., Yazdi P., Neff N., Elledge S.J., and Qin J. 2000. BASC, a super complex of BRCA1-associated proteins involved in the recognition and repair of aberrant DNA structures. *Genes Dev.* **14:** 927.

Wang Z.Q., Stingl L., Morrison C., Jantsch M., Los M., Schulze-Osthoff K., and Wagner E.F. 1997. PARP is important for genomic stability but dispensable in apoptosis. *Genes Dev.* **11:** 2347.

Wooster R. and Weber B.L. 2003. Breast and ovarian cancer. *N. Engl. J. Med.* **348:** 2339.

Xia F., Taghian D.G., DeFrank J.S., Zeng Z.C., Willers H., Iliakis G., and Powell S.N. 2001. Deficiency of human BRCA2 leads to impaired homologous recombination but maintains normal nonhomologous end joining. *Proc. Natl. Acad. Sci.* **98:** 8644.

Yang H., Li Q., Fan J., Holloman W.K., and Pavletich N.P. 2005. The BRCA2 homologue Brh2 nucleates RAD51 filament formation at a dsDNA-ssDNA junction. *Nature* **433:** 653.

Yang H., Jeffrey P.D., Miller J., Kinnucan E., Sun Y., Thoma N.H., Zheng N., Chen P.L., Lee W.H. and Pavletich N.P. 2002. BRCA2 function in DNA binding and recombination from a BRCA2-DSS1-ssDNA structure. *Science* **297:** 1837.

Yu D.S., Sonoda E., Takeda S., Huang C.L., Pellegrini L., Blundell T.L., and Venkitaraman A.R. 2003. Dynamic control of Rad51 recombinase by self-association and interaction with BRCA2. *Mol. Cell* **12:** 1029.

Yu V.P., Koehler M., Steinlein C., Schmid M., Hanakahi L.A., van Gool A.J., West S.C., and Venkitaraman A.R. 2000. Gross chromosomal rearrangements and genetic exchange between nonhomologous chromosomes following BRCA2 inactivation. *Genes Dev.* **14:** 1400.

Zhong Q., Chen C.F., Li S., Chen Y., Wang C.C., Xiao J., Chen P.L., Sharp Z.D., and Lee W.H. 1999. Association of BRCA1 with the hRad50-hMre11-p95 complex and the DNA damage response. *Science* **285:** 747.

Identifying Site-specific Metastasis Genes and Functions

G.P. Gupta,* A.J. Minn,*§ Y. Kang,* ** P.M. Siegel,*# I. Serganova,[†]
C. Cordón-Cardo,[‡] A.B. Olshen,[¶] W.L. Gerald,[‡] and J. Massagué*

*Cancer Biology and Genetics Program and Howard Hughes Medical Institute, and Departments of [†]Neurology,
[‡]Pathology, and [¶]Biostatistics, Memorial Sloan-Kettering Cancer Center, New York, New York 10021

Metastasis is a multistep and multifunctional biological cascade that is the final and most life-threatening stage of cancer progression. Understanding the biological underpinnings of this complex process is of extreme clinical relevance and requires unbiased and comprehensive biological scrutiny. In recent years, we have utilized a xenograft model of breast cancer metastasis to discover genes that mediate organ-specific patterns of metastatic colonization. Examination of transcriptomic data from cohorts of primary breast cancers revealed a subset of site-specific metastasis genes that are selected for early in tumor progression. High expression of these genes predicts the propensity for lung metastasis independently of several classic markers of poor prognosis. These genes fulfill dual functions—enhanced primary tumorigenicity and augmented organ-specific metastatic activity. Other metastasis genes fulfill functions specialized for the microenvironment of the metastatic site and are consequently not selected for in primary tumors. These findings improve our understanding of metastatic progression, facilitate the interpretation of primary tumor gene expression data, and open several important possibilities for future clinical application.

Tumorigenesis involves the temporal acquisition of genetic and epigenetic alterations that ultimately enable a cell to divide without concern for the homeostatic constraints that limit the growth of normal tissues. As such, cancer is not a static phenomenon, but rather a dynamic process that evolves over the course of tumor initiation and progression, and can manifest with an impressively diverse array of phenotypic properties from one primary tumor to the next. One of these properties is the ability of cancerous cells from one organ to invade and thrive at another organ. Also known as metastasis, distant recurrence is the leading cause for mortality in patients with solid tumors of most organs. However, not all primary tumors acquire the metastatic phenotype in the course of disease progression, and prospectively identifying which patients are most (or least) likely to develop metastases is of immense clinical importance. Furthermore, understanding the mechanisms that drive the formation of metastases may identify novel targets for much-needed therapy against this deadly biological process (see Fig. 1).

From the perspective of an invasive cancer cell, not all potential sites for metastasis are created equal. Clinicians have observed for over a century that certain types of primary tumors are more likely to metastasize to specific organs (Fidler 2003). For example, advanced colon cancers frequently spread to liver, and breast cancers preferentially metastasize to bone and lung. On the basis of these clinical observations, Stephen Paget proposed in 1889 the "seed and soil hypothesis," which postulated that tumor cells (the seeds) will only grow in a distant organ if they are competent to thrive in that microenvironment (the

soil). This theory, which placed prime emphasis on the cross talk between metastatic tumor cells and their microenvironment, was contested by James Ewing in 1926, when he proposed that metastatic propensities are dictated primarily by circulatory patterns—i.e., cells will metastasize to the organ to which they have the greatest vascular access. Subsequent analyses of patterns of metastatic spread in patients as well as in experimental models concluded that although regional recurrences were highly dependent on the efficiency of vascular perfusion, distant metastatic recurrence for most tumors was truly non-random, with no correlation to anatomically defined patterns of hematogenous or lymphatic circulation. Thus, Paget's seed and soil hypothesis prevailed, although molecular determinants of this putative cross talk were still entirely unknown.

For a cell to successfully metastasize to a distant organ, it must resist cell death pathways while accomplishing several distinct biological steps, including intravasation, adhesion, extravasation, angiogenesis, and growth in a foreign tissue (Chambers et al. 2002). Presumably, there are molecular mediators of these various processes, and the seed and soil hypothesis would suggest that at least some of these mediators are tissue-specific (Fidler 2003). Because of these complexities, metastasis is considered an inefficient process. In fact, it is postulated that malignant tumors release many thousands of cells into circulation daily, yet several orders of magnitude fewer metastases are ever observed in patients. Mouse models of experimental metastasis also recapitulate this phenomenon, where only a fraction of cancer cells are able to generate macroscopic metastases. Cancer biologists have harnessed this highly selective feature of metastasis to discover genes that are specifically enriched (or depleted) in those tumorigenic cells that give rise to distant metastases in animal models.

How the multiple functions required for metastasis are selected for in the process of tumor progression is not

Present addresses: §Department of Radiation Oncology, University of Chicago, Chicago, Illinois 60637; **Department of Molecular Biology, Princeton University, Princeton, New Jersey 08544; #Departments of Medicine and Biochemistry, McGill University, Montreal, Quebec, Canada H34 1A4.

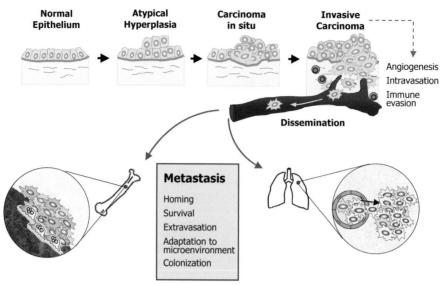

Figure 1. Steps in tumor progression and metastatic dissemination and growth. A schematic depicting the various pathologically defined stages of tumor progression, as well as various functions associated with metastatic spread. The functions related to dissemination are suspected to be more general mediators of metastasis. Subsequent functions required for metastatic colonization (*in purple box*) may be unique to the microenvironments of the different metastatic sites.

well understood, and is currently a subject for debate (Bernards and Weinberg 2002; Hynes 2003). Generally, it is agreed that the genomic and epigenomic instabilities known to exist in cancerous cells can spawn massive genetic heterogeneity within tumor cell populations. However, whether or not there are specific genetic events selected for during metastatic progression, and where and when this selection may be taking place, is still highly contentious. Conventional belief on this issue, largely from models of experimental metastasis, is that rare variants from primary tumor populations are selected for at the metastatic site based on an ability to survive and ultimately thrive at the distant site. However, why a cell with such unique abilities would be present with any prevalence in the primary tumor, coupled with the notion that metastasis itself is a physically inefficient process, makes it difficult to imagine why metastasis is not more rare than it actually is.

A breakthrough in this conundrum was revealed when microarray analysis was conducted on primary tumors from breast cancer patients. It was discovered by several laboratories that genes expressed in the bulk primary tumor population were sufficient to predict whether a patient would develop distant metastatic recurrence (van't Veer et al. 2002; Ramaswamy et al. 2003). These surprising findings demanded a reassessment of the prevailing models of metastasis. Some have interpreted from these results that primary tumors are, at a very early stage, destined to be either metastatic or non-metastatic, and that no further meaningful selection is necessary before cells from the primary tumor metastasize to a distant organ. However, whether any of the genes included in these poor prognosis signatures mediate metastasis remains an unanswered question. Additionally, the expression of poor prognosis genes in primary tumors does not explain the diversity of organ-specific metastasis patterns exhibited by advanced

breast cancers. It has more recently been appreciated that poor prognosis signatures derived from different cohorts of patients by different laboratories yield distinct genes with very little overlap (van de Vijver et al. 2002; Jenssen and Hovig 2005; Wang et al. 2005). Thus, the biological meaning, as well as the clinical utility, of poor prognosis genes in primary tumors remains to be unraveled.

In recent years, our laboratory has explored mechanisms of metastasis using a heterogeneous breast cancer cell line derived from the pleural effusion of a patient with widely metastatic breast cancer (Kang et al. 2003; Minn et al. 2005a,b). Through various techniques, we have identified subpopulations of cells within the parental cell line that exhibit distinct patterns of site-specific metastasis when inoculated into immunocompromised mice. We have demonstrated that these metastatic phenotypes can be linked to specific patterns of gene expression. By overexpressing candidate metastasis genes in weakly metastatic cells, or by knocking down their expression in aggressively metastatic cells, we have confirmed that many of these genes are mediators as well as markers of site-specific metastasis. Finally, we have applied these site-specific metastasis signatures to a cohort of primary breast cancers with known metastatic outcome, which has yielded significant insight into the biology driving this complex process. We present this body of work as a new methodological paradigm that couples experimental models of metastasis with the analysis of human breast tumors, in an attempt to discover clinically relevant mechanisms of breast cancer metastasis.

GENETIC HETEROGENEITY DETERMINES DIFFERENCES IN METASTATIC POTENTIAL

The MDA-MB-231 cell line is derived from the malignant pleural effusion of a patient with metastatic

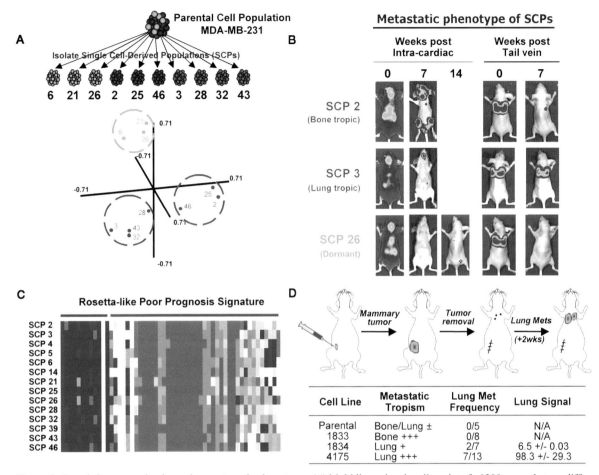

Figure 2. Genetic heterogeneity determines metastatic phenotypes. (*A*) Multidimensional scaling plot of ~1200 genes that are differentially expressed among SCPs derived from the parental MDA-MB-231 cell line. (*B*) Metastatic phenotypes after intracardiac and tail vein inoculation of representative SCPs. (*C*) Expression of a Rosetta-like poor prognosis signature by several SCPs derived from MDA-MB-231 cells. The Pearson correlation coefficient between the different SCPs is invariably greater than 0.95. (*D*) Orthotopic inoculation of different tumor cell populations and subsequent surgical resection and monitoring for emergent lung metastases. The table shows lung metastatic activity for parental MDA-MB-231 cells, highly bone metastatic 1833 cells, moderately lung metastatic 1834 cells, and aggressively lung metastatic 4175 (LM2) cells.

breast cancer (Cailleau et al. 1978). We postulated that this cell line might be composed of cells that are genetically heterogeneous. In fact, one may imagine that malignant cells in the pleural fluid of a patient with metastatic breast cancer may represent a demographic cross section of the circulating tumor cells that have been released from metastases in diverse organs. To test this hypothesis, we performed limiting dilution cloning of the parental cell line to derive several distinct populations of single cell-derived progeny, or SCPs. Transcriptomic analysis of these cells using Affymetrix HG-U133A microarrays revealed that over 1200 genes were differentially expressed among these different populations (Minn et al. 2005b). By representing these gene expression differences in three dimensions using multidimensional scaling, three distinct subgroups of SCPs were identified (Fig. 2A). These findings confirmed that cells within the MDA-MB-231 cell line were genetically heterogeneous and exhibited distinct patterns of gene expression.

We next sought to determine whether these genetic differences had implications for the metastatic potential of the different SCPs. Consequently, we xenografted the SCPs into either the left cardiac ventricle or the lateral tail vein of immunocompromised nude mice. To facilitate identification and monitoring of the emergent metastases, we engineered the SCPs to express a triple modality imaging vector encoding a fusion protein of thymidine kinase, GFP, and firefly luciferase (Ponomarev et al. 2004), and performed noninvasive bioluminescence imaging sequentially over time. To our surprise, the SCPs exhibited a diverse array of phenotypic patterns of metastatic spread (Fig. 2B). Some of the SCPs were robustly metastatic to the bones, yet displayed no metastatic activity to the lungs. Alternatively, some SCPs yielded aggressive metastases to the lungs and/or adrenal medulla, while being only mildly metastatic to the bones. A third group of SCPs exhibited dormant metastatic behavior, giving rise only to indolent growths that rarely developed into overt metastases. Gratifyingly, SCPs that were similar based on the multidimensional scaling plot of differentially expressed genes displayed similar metastatic behaviors. Thus, cells within the pleural effusion-derived MDA-MB-231 cell line were phenotypically diverse in their metastatic potential, and these differences correlated with distinct patterns of gene expression.

ORGAN-SPECIFIC METASTATIC POTENTIAL IS NOT RELATED TO DIFFERENCES IN A POOR PROGNOSIS SIGNATURE

By using supervised clustering of a cohort of primary breast cancers, van't Veer and colleagues (van't Veer et al. 2002) identified a 70-gene poor prognosis signature that classified breast cancers with a high likelihood of developing distant metastatic recurrence. This signature was validated on an independent cohort of 295 breast cancers and was shown to be an independent factor predicting patient prognosis (van de Vijver et al. 2002). We wanted to determine whether genes in this signature correlated with organ-specific patterns of metastasis. To this end, we confirmed that the parental MDA-MB-231 cell line expressed a Rosetta-type poor prognosis signature, containing 54 of the 70 poor prognosis genes identified by van't Veer et al. that are represented on the Affymetrix HG-U133A microarray platform. This subset of genes was validated by two methods. First, these 54 genes performed nearly as well as the original 70-gene signature in predicting patient prognosis of the 78-tumor cohort from which the gene set was derived. Second, Affymetrix probe sets corresponding to these 54 genes were able to segregate a subgroup of patients with a worse prognosis in an independent cohort of primary breast cancers with at least 5 years of follow-up obtained at our institution. Parental MDA-MB-231 cells expressed this Rosetta-type poor prognosis signature in a manner similar to primary breast cancers that fell into the poor prognosis classification. In contrast, MCF-10A cells (an immortalized nontumorigenic mammary epithelial cell line) did not express the poor prognosis signature.

All of the SCPs derived from MDA-MB-231 cells also expressed the poor prognosis signature. This was evident from a hierarchical clustering analysis of the SCPs combined with the MSKCC 82 primary breast cancer cohort. In addition, there was very little variation in the expression of the poor prognosis genes among the different SCPs (Fig. 2C, Pearson correlation coefficients greater than 0.95). Furthermore, none of the poor prognosis genes correlated with any of the organ-specific metastatic patterns exhibited by the different SCPs. Thus, although the poor prognosis genes may indicate whether a primary tumor is likely to develop distant metastatic recurrence, expression of these genes does not explain the diversity of metastatic patterns exhibited by advanced breast cancer cells. Interestingly, dormant SCPs that rarely gave rise to overt metastases also uniformly expressed the poor prognosis signature. This indicates that expression of these genes is not sufficient for metastasis and, consequently, that additional gene expression events must occur before cells gain a truly metastatic phenotype.

GENES THAT MEDIATE SITE-SPECIFIC METASTASIS

To identify genes that mediate organ-specific metastasis, we utilized in vivo selection of highly metastatic subpopulations from the weakly metastatic parental cell line by passaging it through immunocompromised mice. For bone metastasis assays we injected parental MDA-MB-231 cells into the left cardiac ventricle, and for lung metastasis we introduced weakly metastatic parental or 1834 cells (a bone metastasis isolate from the parental cell line that did not exhibit any enrichment in metastatic activity) into the lateral tail vein. By extracting metastatic lesions and reinoculating them into mice to assay for enrichment in metastatic activity, we were able to isolate aggressively bone metastatic sublines after one round of in vivo selection (denoted BM1), and highly lung metastatic populations after two rounds of in vivo selection (denoted LM2).

Transcriptomic analysis of these different in vivo selected subpopulations and the parental cell line enabled the elucidation of bone and lung metastasis gene expression signatures. The bone metastasis signature comprised 102 genes, of which 43 were overexpressed and 59 underexpressed in highly bone metastatic populations (Kang et al. 2003). Similarly, the lung metastasis signature contained 48 genes that were overexpressed and 47 genes that were underexpressed in aggressively lung metastatic LM2 populations (Minn et al. 2005a). Many of the genes in these signatures encoded secretory or cell-surface proteins, making them ideal candidates for enabling interactions between the metastatic tumor cells and their adopted microenvironments (see Fig. 3A,B). Interestingly, only 6 genes were concordantly expressed in both metastasis signatures.

There are likely to be many genes that facilitate general metastatic activity, such as those that promote intravasation from the primary tumor into the circulation. However, our experimental approach was in principle seeking no such genes, but genes that mediate metastatic events in the distant organs (see purple box in Fig. 1). First, our starting cell line was already derived from cells that had escaped from the patient's primary tumor and metastasized to the pleural cavity. In addition, our experimental metastasis assays involved direct inoculation into the circulation, thereby modeling the later steps of metastatic growth that are more likely to be site-specific. Nonetheless, the existence of distinct site-specific metastasis signatures expressed by subpopulations of cells from the same parental cell line confirmed the hypothesis that cells in malignant breast cancer pleural effusions are differentially genetically endowed to metastasize to various organs.

To distinguish genes that mediate metastasis from those that simply correlate with and serve as markers for metastatic potential, we performed functional assays (Kang et al. 2003). Overexpression of interleukin-11 (IL-11) and osteopontin (OPN) together, but neither alone, was sufficient to enhance the osteolytic bone metastatic activity of parental cells (Fig. 3C). Addition of either con-

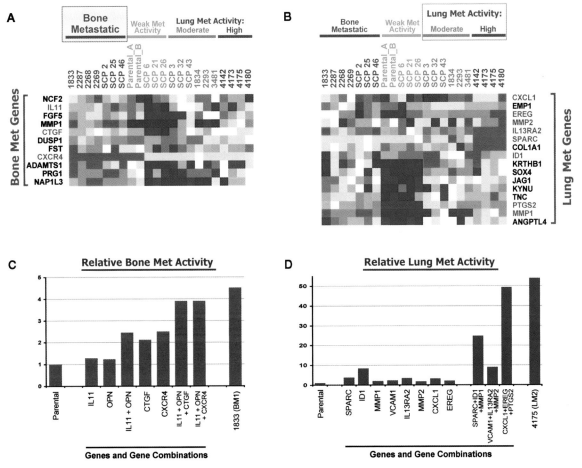

Figure 3. Cooperation between functional mediators of tissue-specific metastasis. (*A*) Expression patterns of several overexpressed bone metastasis genes. Populations listed include the two replicates of the parental MDA-MB-231 cells, in vivo selected subpopulations, and SCPs. Metastatic activity of the different populations is color-coded. (*B*) Heatmap showing expression of several lung metastasis genes overexpressed in lung metastatic populations. Lung metastatic SCPs expressed only a subset of lung metastasis genes. (*C*) Summary of overexpression experiments demonstrating the cooperative action of different bone metastasis mediators. Relative bone metastatic strength was calculated from the time until 50% of the bone metastatic events occurred and the total percentage of mice that developed bone metastasis for each cohort, both of which were normalized to the basal metastatic activity of parental MDA-MB-231 cells. (*D*) Relative lung metastatic activity after transducing parental cells with various genes and gene combinations. Lung metastatic activity was determined by bioluminescent imaging after approximately 7 weeks post-xenografting, normalized to parental cells transduced with a vector control.

nective tissue growth factor (CTGF) or chemokine (C-X-C motif) receptor 4 (CXCR4) to these genes increased the rate and frequency of bone metastasis (Fig. 3C). These observations supported the notion that metastasis is a multistep and multifunctional process and, as such, multiple genes may be required to see an enhancement in the metastatic rate. Based on the previously known biology of these gene products, we postulated that CXCR4 may facilitate homing to and survival in the bone microenvironment, that IL-11 and OPN may cooperate in the recruitment and activation of host osteoclasts, and that CTGF may modify the extracellular environment to facilitate angiogenesis. In this manner, metastasis genes may fulfill different aspects of the cross talk between the tumor cells and stromal cells that are necessary to enable metastatic growth.

Similar functional analysis identified nine lung metastasis genes that cooperated to promote aggressive lung metastatic growth (Minn et al. 2005a). Overexpression studies demonstrated that lung metastasis resulted from the cooperation of several extracellular modifiers, including the extracellular matrix molecule *SPARC*, the chemokine *CXCL1*, the mitogen *Epiregulin*, the matrix metalloproteinases *MMP1* and *MMP2*, the cell surface receptors *VCAM1* and *IL13RA2*, as well as intracellular modulators of gene expression and signaling including *ID1* and *COX2/PTGS2* (Fig. 3D). Importantly, overexpression of these genes had no effect on the bone metastatic activity of the parental cell line. RNAi-mediated knockdown of *ID1*, *VCAM1*, and *IL13RA2* resulted in a greater than 10-fold reduction in lung metastatic growth within 6 weeks after tail vein injection. These findings confirmed that many of the genes selected for during in vivo selection of highly lung metastatic subpopulations were mediators of aggressive lung metastasis. Furthermore, these genes cooperated to facilitate lung-specific functions necessary for aggressive lung metastatic growth.

SITE-SPECIFIC METASTASIS GENES ARE EXPRESSED BY A SUBSET OF CELLS IN THE PARENTAL CELL POPULATION

Although the site-specific metastasis signatures were generated by transcriptomic analysis of in vivo selected populations, they were also useful in identifying in vitro derived SCPs that were more or less metastatic to either bone or lung. Hierarchical clustering analysis of the SCPs with the bone metastasis signature identified a subgroup of SCPs that was genetically similar to the in vivo selected highly bone metastatic populations (Fig. 3A). Northern blot analysis of 46 SCPs from the parental MDA-MB-231 cell line for five of the most differentially expressed bone metastasis genes revealed SCPs that expressed a continuum of these genes, ranging from none of them to all five of them (Kang et al. 2003). The bone metastatic activity of these SCPs was directly correlated with the degree of expression of these genes, providing further evidence that these genes were mediators of osteolytic bone metastatic growth. By analyzing expression of bone metastasis genes in SCPs derived from in vivo selected populations, we noticed an approximately 5-fold enrichment in the proportion of cells expressing several bone metastasis genes. Thus, bone metastasis genes were expressed in a minority of cells in the malignant pleural effusion-derived parental cell line, and in vivo selection resulted in the enrichment of these preexisting highly bone metastatic cells.

Similarly, the in vivo selected lung metastasis signature was also able to segregate lung metastatic SCPs from those that were not metastatic to the lungs (Minn et al. 2005a). When compared to the LM2 lung metastatic populations obtained through three rounds of in vivo selection, the lung metastatic SCPs only expressed a partial lung metastasis signature (Fig. 3B). In accordance with this observation, lung metastatic SCPs were approximately 10-fold less metastatic than the in vivo selected populations upon injection into the lateral tail vein. An observation of interest was that the genes in the lung metastasis signature were naturally divided into two categories. We postulated that genes that were expressed by both the lung metastatic SCPs and the LM2 populations may facilitate a baseline level of lung metastatic activity, which we describe as "lung metastagenicity." Genes that were expressed exclusively by the most highly metastatic LM2 populations may confer functions enabling aggressive growth within the lung microenvironment, which we denote as "lung metastatic virulence." Lung metastagenicity genes included *ID1*, *COX2*, *CXCL1*, *MMP1*, and many others. Examples of lung metastatic virulence genes were *VCAM1*, *SPARC*, *IL13RA2*, and *MMP2*. Genes from both of these categories were shown to be mediators of lung metastasis in functional assays.

EXPRESSION OF SITE-SPECIFIC METASTASIS GENES IN PRIMARY BREAST CANCERS

Because of the recent discovery of poor prognosis signatures in primary breast cancers, we wanted to examine whether our organ-specific metastasis signatures may also be expressed at this early stage. To ask this question, we utilized a cohort of 82 primary breast tumors with at least 3 years of follow-up, and with known organ-specific metastatic outcome (hereby referred to as the MSKCC cohort). Direct hierarchical clustering of all 82 primary tumors with the bone metastasis signature did not identify a subgroup of tumors that expressed the signature in a manner resembling the BM1 populations (Minn et al. 2005b). When the analysis was restricted only to patients that were known to develop metastatic recurrence, the bone metastasis signature segregated patients that went on to develop primarily bone metastasis from those that developed metastasis to other sites. Thus, the experimentally derived bone metastasis signature was only marginally expressed by primary breast tumors, and partial expression of this signature could not be used to prospectively identify patients with an increased likelihood of developing bone metastatic recurrence.

Hierarchical clustering of this same primary tumor cohort with the lung metastasis signature yielded a dramatically different result (Minn et al. 2005a). A group of tumors in a highly reproducible branch of the dendrogram expressed the lung metastasis genes in a manner resembling the LM2 populations (Fig. 4A). This subset of tumors had molecular features of aggressive disease, including negative estrogen and progesterone receptor status, expression of a Rosetta-type poor prognosis signature, and a basaloid genotype. Examination of the metastatic outcome of these patients revealed a high prevalence of lung metastatic recurrence (Fig. 4A). This prompted us to examine these data in a statistically rigorous manner. First, univariate analysis of the lung metastasis signature identified expression of 12 genes that significantly correlated with tumors which gave rise to lung metastases. A classifier was generated by weighting the expression of lung metastasis genes according to the aforementioned univariate correlations, which identified patients that had a significantly higher likelihood of developing distant lung, but not bone, metastatic recurrence ($p = 0.0018$ for lung metastasis, and $p = 0.31$ [NS] for bone metastasis). In a separate analysis, weighting the expression of the lung metastasis genes according to the fold change exhibited by LM2 versus parental MDA-MB-231 populations also created a classifier that distinguished a subgroup of patients with a high risk of developing lung metastasis. Thus, an experimentally derived lung metastasis signature was at least partially expressed by a subset of primary breast cancers, and these patients were more likely to develop lung metastases in the course of their disease.

A biologically meaningful lung metastasis signature should be expressed by different cohorts of primary tumors transcriptomically profiled on different microarray platforms. We therefore validated our lung metastasis signature on the cohort of 78 primary breast cancers utilized by van't Veer et al. using dual color Agilent cDNA microarrays (Minn et al. 2005a). Hierarchical clustering revealed a group of tumors that coexpressed the lung metastasis signature in a manner resembling the LM2 in vivo selected populations. Of note, the 9 functionally validated lung metastasis genes were remarkably overex-

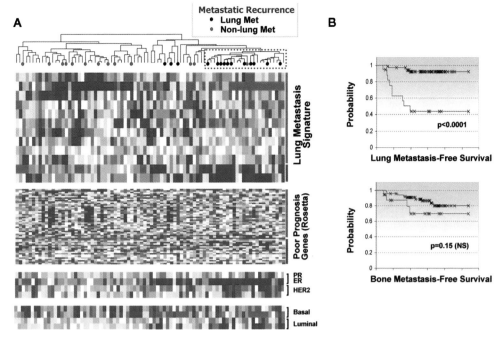

Figure 4. Expression of lung metastasis genes by primary breast cancers. (*A*) Unsupervised hierarchical clustering of the MSKCC cohort (82 tumors) with the 12 most univariately significant lung metastasis genes (correlation with lung metastatic outcome, $p<0.05$). Also shown are a Rosetta-like poor prognosis signature, ER, PR, and Her2 expression, as well as keratin markers of basal and luminal subtypes of breast cancer. Patients identified with a red dot developed metastases to sites other than the lung, whereas patients labeled with a black dot suffered from lung metastases. Highlighted in a light blue background is a robust branch of the dendrogram containing tumors that expressed the lung metastasis genes in a manner resembling the high lung metastatic populations derived from MDA-MB-231 cells. This group of tumors was enriched for those with a high likelihood of developing lung metastatic recurrence. (*B*) Lung (*top*) and bone (*bottom*) metastasis-free survival curves for patients that expressed the lung metastasis signature (*red*) and those that did not express the lung metastasis signature.

pressed in this group of tumors. Although organ-specific metastatic outcome is not publicly available for this cohort, time until distant metastatic recurrence and overall survival of these patients is known. The majority of primary breast cancers that expressed the lung metastasis signature in this cohort went on to develop distant metastatic recurrence and had a poor overall survival. We hypothesize that many of these patients may have suffered from lung metastasis.

Interestingly, not all of the genes in the experimentally derived lung metastasis signature were informative in predicting primary tumors that went on to develop lung metastasis. For this reason, training the signature on a primary tumor cohort to weight genes according to their robustness of expression among tumors that coexpress lung metastasis genes may engender a more accurate algorithm that is better suited to classify primary breast cancers. Because clinical outcome is not needed for algorithm training, the cohort studied by van't Veer et al. was used to generate a classifier that accurately segregated tumors which most resembled the LM2 populations (Minn et al. 2005a). Six of the nine functionally validated genes were among the most heavily weighted genes in this classifier. The remaining three genes were *SPARC*, *MMP2*, and *IL13RA2*, which were all lung metastasis virulence genes in MDA-MB-231 cells. This trained classifier was the most accurate predictor of lung metastatic recurrence in the MSKCC cohort (Fig. 4B), providing further evi-

dence that the lung metastasis signature is biologically relevant, reproducible, and informative in identifying breast cancer patients with a high likelihood of developing lung metastatic recurrence.

A SUBSET OF LUNG METASTASIS GENES, BUT NOT BONE METASTASIS GENES, FACILITATE PRIMARY TUMORIGENICITY

The selective pressure that encourages expression of metastasis genes in a subset of primary tumors is not apparent. One possibility is that some metastasis genes may facilitate growth of the primary tumor, thereby increasing the representation of cells expressing these genes in the cancerous population. This is supported by the clinical observation that larger breast cancers tend to have a poorer prognosis, with an increased likelihood of metastatic recurrence. According to this postulate, lung metastasis genes that were informatively expressed in primary tumors might encourage primary tumor growth, whereas lung metastasis genes that were not predictive in primary tumors, and all bone metastasis genes, might have no effect on primary tumorigenicity.

To test this hypothesis, we established an orthotopic model that mimicked breast cancer progression in patients (Fig. 2D). Injection of MDA-MB-231 populations in the mouse mammary fat pad gave rise to primary tumors. When these tumors were surgically resected, lung

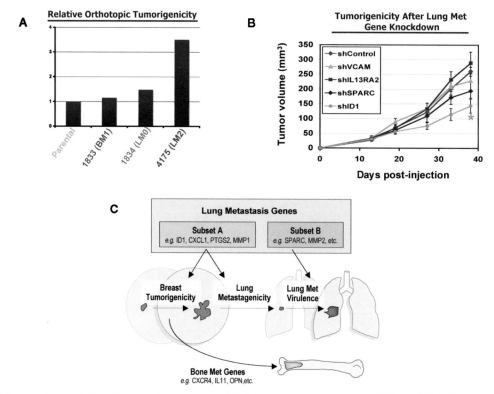

Figure 5. Lung metastagenicity and primary tumorigenicity. (*A*) Relative tumor growth rates of different MDA-MB-231 populations after orthotopic implantation into the mouse mammary fat pad. (*B*) Tumor growth rates after reducing the expression of various lung metastasis genes in the 4175 (LM2) population. (*C*) Model depicting different subsets of lung metastasis genes and the roles they play in primary tumorigenicity, lung metastagenicity, and lung metastatic virulence. Bone metastasis genes did not significantly affect primary tumor growth, and as such only have a role in bone metastatic growth.

metastases could be detected only in mice injected with cells that were selected for aggressive lung metastatic activity (Fig. 2D). We also noticed a difference in primary tumor growth rate upon orthotopic implantation of these populations. Although tumors formed by parental and bone metastatic populations grew at a similar rate in the mammary fat pad, the tumors formed by lung metastatic cell populations grew more rapidly in a manner proportional to their lung metastatic aggressiveness (Fig. 5A). This increase in primary tumor growth rate was not due to differences in the proliferative rate of the cells, because immunohistochemical analysis of cell division did not reveal significant disparities. Consequently, genes in the lung metastasis signature facilitated primary tumorigenicity, whereas bone metastasis genes had no effect on primary tumor growth rate.

To identify which of the lung metastasis genes were also facilitating primary tumorigenicity, we performed orthotopic injections of LM2 cells expressing RNAi vectors targeting *SPARC*, *IL13RA2*, *VCAM1*, or *ID1*. Whereas targeted inhibition of all of these genes had an effect on inhibiting lung metastasis both via tail vein assays and after surgical resection of primary mammary fat pad tumors, only *ID1* had a role in promoting primary tumorigenicity (Fig. 5B). Interestingly, *ID1* was the only lung metastagenicity gene among the four genes tested, and was among the 18 most heavily weighted genes in the lung metastasis classifier of primary breast cancers. Thus,

lung metastasis genes can be divided into two categories: those that facilitate both primary tumor formation and basal lung metastatic activity, and those that enable aggressive growth in the lung microenvironment without affecting growth in the primary tumor (Fig. 5C).

LESSONS LEARNED

By xenografting a malignant pleural effusion-derived breast cancer cell line into immunocompromised mice, we have learned several valuable lessons regarding principles governing metastasis. First, metastatic cells from the same primary tumor exhibit diverse metastatic tropisms, reflecting the genetic heterogeneity that pervades metastatic breast cancer populations. Second, genes that mediate metastasis to lung and bone are distinct, and encode many cell surface and secreted proteins that enable cross talk between the metastatic tumor cells and these two divergent organ microenvironments. Together, these gene products act in concert to facilitate the multifunctional task of metastasis.

The recent findings of others have identified poor prognosis genes that, when expressed in primary tumors, predict a poor prognosis for breast cancer patients. The organ-specific metastasis genes that we have identified are distinct from these poor prognosis signatures. In fact, analysis of SCPs from MDA-MB-231 cells revealed that expression of these poor prognosis genes is not sufficient to enable metastasis. Rather, malignant breast cancer cells become overtly metastatic only when organ-specific metastasis signatures are layered upon this predisposing genetic platform.

Analysis of organ-specific metastasis signatures in primary breast carcinomas has provided substantial biological insight into the mechanisms driving metastasis. Although bone metastasis genes were only weakly expressed in primary tumors that later disseminated to the bones, the lung metastasis signature was significantly expressed by a subset of breast cancers with a high likelihood of metastasizing to the lungs. This difference may be due to partial similarities between the breast and lung microenvironments that do not exist between breast and bone. In fact, cells expressing lung, but not bone, metastasis genes are significantly more tumorigenic when orthotopically inoculated into the mammary fat pad of immunocompromised mice. By selectively targeting different genetic mediators of lung metastasis, we exposed two distinct types of lung metastasis genes; one group that facilitated both primary tumorigenicity and lung metastatic ability, and another group that mediated aggressive growth exclusively in the lung microenvironment. Because none of the bone metastasis genes enhanced primary tumorigenicity, they are all examples of the latter category of metastasis genes (Fig. 5C).

FUTURE DIRECTIONS

Microarray analysis has unveiled a new era in the understanding of breast cancer. Examination of global differences in gene expression has confirmed the existence of distinct molecular subtypes of breast cancer with different clinical tendencies (Perou et al. 2000; Sorlie et al. 2003), a long-suspected postulate of breast cancer pathologists and clinicians. Microarray technology has also enabled the identification of gene expression signatures that indicate a poor prognosis for breast cancer patients (van de Vijver et al. 2002; Wang et al. 2005). However, the clinical utility of this application is hampered by concerns regarding the reproducibility and robustness of the correlations between these poor prognosis genes and clinical outcome, especially when tested on different patient populations using different microarray platforms (Jenssen and Hovig 2005). Indeed, clinical trials are currently ongoing to address some of these issues. Nonetheless, cancer biologists have, as yet, been unable to make a mechanistic link between the expression of these poor prognosis genes and the eventual clinical outcome that afflicts breast cancer patients. Consequently, improvements in the design of microarray-based experiments are necessary before the wealth of information provided by microarray analyses is harnessed for its true potential.

One way to extract biological meaning from microarrays of clinical samples may be to use an experimentally tractable model of cancer as a biological filter for the identification of functionally relevant metastasis genes. For example, a recent analysis of a "wound signature," derived by identifying serum-responsive genes in fibroblasts cultured in vitro, revealed that it classified tumors into good and poor prognosis categories almost as effectively as the van't Veer et al. poor prognosis signature (Chang et al. 2004, 2005). In contrast to the van't Veer et al. signature, the wound signature is based on biological principles and excites intriguing future experimental pursuits using both model systems and clinical specimens.

Our organ-specific metastasis signatures adopted the paradigm of functional derivation in a model system and subsequent validation using clinical samples. For this reason, we anticipate that the clinical correlations of the lung metastasis genes with lung metastatic outcome may be more reproducible across patient cohorts. Indeed, we have observed a subgroup of breast cancers expressing the lung metastasis signature in several other publicly available gene expression data sets derived from different microarray platforms. Whether these patients were also predisposed for developing lung metastasis is currently being investigated. In addition, we are developing quantitative RT-PCR methodology for the analysis of paraffin-extracted RNA (Cronin et al. 2004; Paik et al. 2004), which would enhance the validation potential of this signature as a clinically useful prognostic assay. It is our hope that because this signature is based on several experimentally validated mediators of lung metastasis, it may be more reproducible than other correlation-based gene expression signatures.

Our experimental approach could be applied to identify genes mediating metastasis to other clinically important sites such as the brain or the liver, or metastasis by other types of primary tumors. Furthermore, organ-specific metastasis signatures may have implications for cancer management and therapy. The prospective identification of subgroups of patients coexpressing sets of genes that collectively facilitate metastasis may aid in the selection of appropriate patient populations for the administration of novel or preexisting metastasis therapies. For example, patients with primary tumors that express the lung metastasis signature may be monitored more frequently by thoracic computed tomography (CT) scans, and treated more aggressively with conventional chemotherapies. Additionally, experimental drugs inhibiting specific biological pathways may be tested in a combinatorial fashion selectively in this high-risk group of patients. It is not difficult to imagine that targeted therapies which proved unsuccessful as single agents may be efficacious when rationally combined with other drugs. A thorough understanding of the biological mechanisms by which metastasis genes facilitate tumorigenicity and/or metastasis should drive the rational design of clinical trials to test new therapeutic strategies aimed at selectively targeting metastases, while being nontoxic to the patient.

Metastatic cancer remains, for the most part, a complex and incurable disease. In recent years, cancer biologists have accumulated a daunting array of technologies that facilitate the modeling, mechanistic dissection, and gene discovery of cancer progression. The next era in the fight against cancer has already begun, and it is founded upon the interdisciplinary efforts of engineers, biologists, biostatisticians, computer scientists, and clinicians. We are optimistic that this interdisciplinary communication will make the coming years among the most exciting in the war against cancer.

REFERENCES

Bernards R. and Weinberg R.A. 2002. A progression puzzle. *Nature* **418:** 823.

Cailleau R., Olive M., and Cruciger Q.V. 1978. Long-term human breast carcinoma cell lines of metastatic origin: Preliminary characterization. *In Vitro* **14:** 911.

Chambers A.F., Groom A.C., and MacDonald I.C. 2002. Dissemination and growth of cancer cells in metastatic sites. *Nat. Rev. Cancer* **2:** 563.

Chang H.Y., Sneddon J.B., Alizadeh A.A., Sood R., West R.B., Montgomery K., Chi J.T., van de Rijn M., Botstein D., and Brown P.O. 2004. Gene expression signature of fibroblast serum response predicts human cancer progression: Similarities between tumors and wounds. *PLoS Biol* **2:** E7.

Chang H.Y., Nuyten D.S., Sneddon J.B., Hastie T., Tibshirani R., Sorlie T., Dai H., He Y.D., van't Veer L.J., Bartelink H., van de Rijn M., Brown P.O., and van de Vijver M.J. 2005. Robustness, scalability, and integration of a wound-response gene expression signature in predicting breast cancer survival. *Proc. Natl. Acad. Sci.* **102:** 3738.

Cronin M., Pho M., Dutta D., Stephans J.C., Shak S., Kiefer M.C., Esteban J.M., and Baker J.B. 2004. Measurement of gene expression in archival paraffin-embedded tissues: Development and performance of a 92-gene reverse transcriptase-polymerase chain reaction assay. *Am. J. Pathol.* **164:** 35.

Fidler I.J. 2003. The pathogenesis of cancer metastasis: The 'seed and soil' hypothesis revisited. *Nat. Rev. Cancer* **3:** 453.

Hynes R.O. 2003. Metastatic potential: Generic predisposition of the primary tumor or rare, metastatic variants-or both? *Cell* **113:** 821.

Jenssen T.K. and Hovig E. 2005. Gene-expression profiling in breast cancer. *Lancet* **365:** 634.

Kang Y., Siegel P.M., Shu W., Drobnjak M., Kakonen S.M., Cordon-Cardo C., Guise T.A., and Massagué J. 2003. A multigenic program mediating breast cancer metastasis to bone. *Cancer Cell* **3:** 537.

Minn A.J., Gupta G.P., Siegel P.M., Bos P.D., Shu W., Giri D.D., Viale A., Olshen A.B., Gerald W.L., and Massagué J. 2005a. Genes that mediate breast cancer metastasis to lung. *Nature* **436:** 518.

Minn A.J., Kang Y., Serganova I., Gupta G.P., Giri D.D., Doubrovin M., Ponomarev V., Gerald W.L., Blasberg R., and Massagué J. 2005b. Distinct organ-specific metastatic potential of individual breast cancer cells and primary tumors. *J. Clin. Invest.* **115:** 44.

Paik S., Shak S., Tang G., Kim C., Baker J., Cronin M., Baehner F.L., Walker M.G., Watson D., Park T., Hiller W., Fisher E.R., Wickerham D.L., Bryant J., and Wolmark N. 2004. A multigene assay to predict recurrence of tamoxifen-treated, node-negative breast cancer. *N. Engl. J. Med.* **351:** 2817.

Perou C.M., Sorlie T., Eisen M.B., van de Rijn M., Jeffrey S.S., Rees C.A., Pollack J.R., Ross D.T., Johnsen H., Akslen L.A., Fluge O., Pergamenschikov A., Williams C., Zhu S.X., Lonning P.E., Borresen-Dale A.L., Brown P.O., and Botstein D. 2000. Molecular portraits of human breast tumours. *Nature* **406:** 747.

Ponomarev V., Doubrovin M., Serganova I., Vider J., Shavrin A., Beresten T., Ivanova A., Ageyeva L., Tourkova V., Balatoni J., Bornmann W., Blasberg R., and Gelovani Tjuvajev J. 2004. A novel triple-modality reporter gene for whole-body fluorescent, bioluminescent, and nuclear noninvasive imaging. *Eur. J. Nucl. Med. Mol. Imaging* **31:** 740.

Ramaswamy S., Ross K.N., Lander E.S., and Golub T.R. 2003. A molecular signature of metastasis in primary solid tumors. *Nat. Genet.* **33:** 49.

Sorlie T., Tibshirani R., Parker J., Hastie T., Marron J.S., Nobel A., Deng S., Johnsen H., Pesich R., Geisler S., Demeter J., Perou C.M., Lonning P.E., Brown P.O., Borresen-Dale A.L., and Botstein D. 2003. Repeated observation of breast tumor subtypes in independent gene expression data sets. *Proc. Natl. Acad. Sci.* **100:** 8418.

van de Vijver M.J., He Y.D., van't Veer L.J., Dai H., Hart A.A., Voskuil D.W., Schreiber G.J., Peterse J.L., Roberts C., Marton M.J., Parrish M., Atsma D., Witteveen A., Glas A., Delahaye L., van der Velde T., Bartelink H., Rodenhuis S., Rutgers E.T., Friend S.H., and Bernards R. 2002. A gene-expression signature as a predictor of survival in breast cancer. *N. Engl. J. Med.* **347:** 1999.

van't Veer L.J., Dai H., van de Vijver M.J., He Y.D., Hart A.A., Mao M., Peterse H.L., van der Kooy K., Marton M.J., Witteveen A.T., Schreiber G.J., Kerkhoven R.M., Roberts C., Linsley P.S., Bernards R., and Friend S.H. 2002. Gene expression profiling predicts clinical outcome of breast cancer. *Nature* **415:** 530.

Wang Y., Klijn J.G., Zhang Y., Sieuwerts A.M., Look M.P., Yang F., Talantov D., Timmermans M., Meijer-van Gelder M.E., Yu J., Jatkoe T., Berns E.M., Atkins D., and Foekens J.A. 2005. Gene-expression profiles to predict distant metastasis of lymph-node-negative primary breast cancer. *Lancet* **365:** 671.

The von Hippel-Lindau Tumor Suppressor Protein: Roles in Cancer and Oxygen Sensing

W.G. Kaelin, Jr.

Howard Hughes Medical Institute, Dana-Farber and Brigham and Women's Hospital,
Harvard Medical School, Boston, Massachusetts 02115

Biallelic inactivation of the von Hippel-Lindau (VHL) tumor suppressor gene is a common event in hereditary (von Hippel-Lindau disease) and sporadic hemangioblastomas and clear-cell renal carcinomas. Germ-line *VHL* mutations are also linked to some hereditary pheochromocytoma families. The *VHL* gene product, pVHL, interacts with a number of cellular proteins and is implicated in the control of angiogenesis, extracellular matrix formation, cell metabolism, and mitogenesis. The best understood function of pVHL relates to its role as the substrate recognition unit of an E3 ligase that targets the heterodimeric transcription factor HIF (hypoxia-inducible factor) for destruction in the presence of oxygen. Down-regulation of HIF appears to be both necessary and sufficient for renal tumor suppression by pVHL, and HIF is strongly suspected of contributing to hemangioblastoma development as well. Recent work suggests that pVHL's role in pheochromocytoma is not related to HIF but rather to the ability of pVHL to regulate neuronal apoptosis, which is mediated by c-Jun, when growth factors such as NGF become limiting. Loss of pVHL leads to up-regulation of JunB, which antagonizes c-Jun and blunts apoptosis.

Hereditary cancer syndromes are experiments of nature which, although devastating for the affected families, have helped to illuminate genes and pathways that are important for human carcinogenesis. von Hippel-Lindau disease is a hereditary cancer syndrome caused by inactivating mutations of the *VHL* tumor suppressor gene and is characterized by an increased risk of a number of different tumors, including central nervous system hemangioblastomas, clear-cell renal carcinomas, and pheochromocytomas (Kaelin 2002). Tumor development in this setting is due to inactivation or loss of the remaining wild-type *VHL* allele in a susceptible cell. In keeping with the Knudson 2-Hit model, biallelic *VHL* inactivation is also common in sporadic hemangioblastomas and clear-cell renal carcinomas (the most common form of kidney cancer) (Kim and Kaelin 2004). This review focuses on our current understanding of the functions of the *VHL* gene product, pVHL.

ISOLATION OF THE VHL GENE

Linkage studies performed in the 1980s revealed that the gene responsible for von Hippel-Lindau disease resides on chromosome 3p25, which is a region of the genome that is frequently altered in sporadic clear-cell renal carcinoma (Seizinger et al. 1988). The *VHL* gene, including a partial cDNA, was isolated in 1993 by a consortium led by Berton Zbar at the National Cancer Institute (Latif et al. 1993). This group also confirmed the presence of intragenic *VHL* mutations in affected individuals from VHL families (Latif et al. 1993). With state-of-the-art mutation detection methods, including semiquantitative Southern blot analysis (to detect the ~20% of VHL cases associated with loss of the entire *VHL* locus), *VHL* mutations can be detected in virtually every individual who carries a clinical diagnosis of VHL disease

(Stolle et al. 1998). Multiple groups have documented that *VHL* inactivation, due to either mutation or hypermethylation, is also common in sporadic clear-cell renal carcinomas and hemangioblastomas but rare in tumor types not seen in VHL disease (Kim and Kaelin 2004).

The *VHL* gene is ubiquitously expressed and gives rise to an ~4.5-kb mRNA (Iliopoulos et al. 1995; Renbaum et al. 1996). This mRNA encodes two protein isoforms as a result of alternative translation initiation from two inframe start codons (Iliopoulos et al. 1998; Schoenfeld et al. 1998; Blankenship et al. 1999). These two isoforms behave similarly in most biochemical and functional assays and so are often referred to generically as "pVHL".

THE VHL GENE PRODUCT, pVHL

pVHL is primarily cytosolic but shuttles to and from the nucleus in a transcription-dependent manner (Iliopoulos et al. 1995, 1998; Lee et al. 1996, 1999; Corless et al. 1997; Ye et al. 1998; Groulx and Lee 2002). Some pVHL can also be detected in association with the endoplasmic reticulum and with mitochondria (Ohh et al. 1998; Shiao et al. 2000; Schoenfeld et al. 2001). The best-understood function of pVHL relates to its role as a substrate adapter in a ubiquitin ligase complex that contains elongin B, elongin C, Cullin 2, and Rbx1 (Duan et al. 1995a,b; Kibel et al. 1995; Kishida et al. 1995; Pause et al. 1997, 1999; Lonergan et al. 1998; Kamura et al. 1999). In the presence of oxygen, pVHL binds directly to the α subunits of a heterodimeric transcription factor called HIF (hypoxia-inducible factor) and directs their polyubiquitination, which earmarks them for proteasomal degradation (Fig. 1) (Maxwell et al. 1999; Cockman et al. 2000; Kamura et al. 2000; Ohh et al. 2000; Tanimoto et al. 2000). pVHL contains two mutational hot spots (Stebbins et al. 1999). One, called the α domain, nucleates the elongin/Cul2/Rbx1

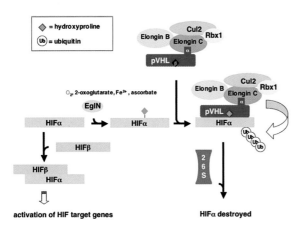

Figure 1. Control of HIF stability by pVHL. In the presence of oxygen and the indicated cofactors, HIFα subunits are hydroxylated on either (or both) of two specific proline residues by EglN family members (EglN1 is the main HIF prolyl hydroxylase under normal conditions). Hydroxylation of either site generates a binding site for a ubiquitin ligase complex containing pVHL, which targets HIFα for degradation by the 26S proteasome. Under low-oxygen conditions, or in the absence of pVHL, HIFα accumulates and forms a heterodimer with HIFβ that is capable of transcriptionally activating genes involved in acute or chronic adaptation to hypoxia.

complex (Kibel et al. 1995; Ohh et al. 1999). The other, called the β domain, binds directly to HIFα (Ohh et al. 2000).

Under low oxygen conditions, HIFα subunits accumulate, bind to specific DNA sequences (HIF-response elements or HREs) in a complex with a HIFβ subunit (such as HIF1β or ARNT), and activate the transcription of genes involved in acute or chronic adaptation to hypoxia, such as VEGF, PDGF B, and TGF-α (Semenza 2000). In cells lacking pVHL, however, HIFα accumulates to high levels irrespective of oxygen availability, leading to overexpression of these target genes (Gnarra et al. 1996; Iliopoulos et al. 1996; Siemeister et al. 1996; Stratmann et al. 1997; Maxwell et al. 1999; Krieg et al. 2000; Wykoff et al. 2000; Zatyka et al. 2002; Jiang et al. 2003). The interaction of pVHL with HIF is oxygen-dependent because HIFα must be hydroxylated on one of two prolyl residues by members of the EglN (EglN1, 2, or 3) family of dioxygenases before it can be recognized by pVHL (Bruick and McKnight 2001; Epstein et al. 2001; Ivan et al. 2001, 2002; Jaakkola et al. 2001; Masson et al. 2001; Yu et al. 2001). The crystal structure of pVHL bound to a HIF1α-derived peptide has been solved and shows that two hydrophobic residues within the pVHL β domain form critical contacts with the HIF prolyl hydroxyl group (Hon et al. 2002; Min et al. 2002).

The oxygen atom of the hydroxyl group is derived from molecular oxygen, and EglN-dependent HIF hydroxylation is sensitive to changes in oxygen over a physiologically relevant range (oxygen K_m ~200 μM) (Epstein et al. 2001; Hirsila et al. 2003). EglN1 (also called PHD2) appears to be the primary HIF prolyl hydroxylase under resting conditions (Berra et al. 2003), although other members of the family become important after prolonged

hypoxia. In fact, EglN3 (also called PHD3) is itself a HIF target (del Peso et al. 2003; Aprelikova et al. 2004; Marxsen et al. 2004). EglN-dependent prolyl hydroxylation requires several cofactors, including Fe^{2+}, 2-oxoglutarate, and ascorbate. Recent studies suggest that EglN activity is sensitive to changes in reactive oxygen species (ROS), perhaps through changes in iron oxidation (Gerald et al. 2004; Brunelle et al. 2005; Guzy et al. 2005; Mansfield et al. 2005). In addition, EglN protein abundance is regulated by members of the SIAH family, which polyubiquitinate EglN (Nakayama et al. 2004; Simon 2004).

A number of other pVHL-binding partners have been reported, including Sp1, atypical protein kinase C members (aPKC), the CCT chaperonin complex, FIH-1 (Factor Inhibiting HIF 1), specific RNA polymerase subunits, fibronectin, microtubules, and VDU1/2 (for review, see Czyzyk-Krzeska and Meller 2004). The functional relevance of many of these interactions is still under investigation. For example, pVHL-defective cells are defective with respect to extracellular fibronectin matrix assembly (Ohh et al. 1998), but whether and how this relates to pVHL's ability to bind to fibronectin remains unclear. A number of pVHL functions, including regulation of HIF-responsive enzymes that regulate matrix turnover (such as certain MMPs) (Koochekpour et al. 1999) and regulation of integrins (perhaps due to changes in aPKC activity) (Esteban-Barragan et al. 2002), might indirectly affect fibronectin matrix assembly. Regulation of aPKC by pVHL is discussed in greater detail below.

ANIMAL MODELS

VHL orthologs have been described in *Caenorhabditis elegans*, *Drosophila melanogaster*, and rodents (Duan et al. 1995a; Gao et al. 1995; Kessler et al. 1995; Gnarra et al. 1997; Adryan et al. 2000; Epstein et al. 2001; Bishop et al. 2004). Inactivation of *VHL* in *C. elegans* and *D. melanogaster* leads to increased HIF levels, as expected, and in the latter is associated with abnormal development of the tracheal system (Adryan et al. 2000; Epstein et al. 2001; Bishop et al. 2004). *VHL*[+/−] mice develop blood vessel tumors of the liver that resemble cavernous hemangiomas (Haase et al. 2001) (*VHL*[−/−] animals die during embryogenesis due to defective placentogenesis; Gnarra et al. 1997). Similar liver abnormalities are also observed in mice carrying conditional *VHL* alleles (*VHL* flox/flox) when crossed to mice expressing Cre recombinase under the liver-specific albumin promoter (Haase et al. 2001; Ma et al. 2003). Importantly, these lesions can be prevented by simultaneous inactivation of ARNT, suggesting that HIF dysregulation is *necessary* for the development of these lesions (Rankin et al. 2005). So far, tumors observed in human VHL disease (CNS hemangioblastomas, clear-cell renal carcinomas, pheochromocytomas) have not been seen in *VHL*[+/−] mice or in *VHL* flox/flox mice in which *VHL* has been inactivated in various tissues using Cre recombinase under the control of an actin promoter (Haase et al. 2001; Ma et al. 2003). This suggests that the mouse is not a permissive host for these lesions or that the right cell type has not yet been targeted at the right time.

pVHL AND HEMANGIOBLASTOMA

Hemangioblastomas are highly vascular tumors that consist of blood vessels (and hence endothelial cells and supporting pericytes) admixed with tumor cells of unclear embryological origins (Richard et al. 1998). Laser capture microdissection and immunohistochemistry studies have documented *VHL* inactivation in hemangioblastoma tumor cells leading to the overproduction of VEGF and PDGF, which support endothelial cells and pericytes, respectively, in a paracrine fashion, as well as EPO and TGF-α, which are suspected of acting as autocrine growth factors (Reifenberger et al. 1995; Wizigmann-Voos et al. 1995; Vortmeyer et al. 1997; Flamme et al. 1998; Chan et al. 1999). Anecdotal evidence suggests that inhibiting the VEGF receptor KDR can help to ameliorate symptoms in this disease but has not yet led to frank tumor regressions (Aiello et al. 2002; Girmens et al. 2003; Madhusudan et al. 2004). In mouse models of tumor angiogenesis, targeting VEGF alone is not sufficient to induce regression of established blood vessels, but instead dual blockade of both VEGF and PDGF (apparently to block survival signals provided to endothelial cells by surrounding pericytes) is needed (Benjamin et al. 1999; Bergers et al. 2003). It will be of interest to determine whether dual VEGF/PDGF blockade will cause regression of hemangioblastomas in man.

pVHL AND KIDNEY CANCER

pVHL inactivation can be demonstrated in preneoplastic renal cysts in VHL kidneys, suggesting that pVHL loss is an early step in renal carcinogenesis (Zhuang et al. 1995; Lubensky et al. 1996; Mandriota et al. 2002). As described above, biallelic *VHL* inactivation, due to mutation or hypermethylation, is common in sporadic clear-cell renal cancers. Moreover, restoration of pVHL function is sufficient to suppress tumor formation by $VHL^{-/-}$ clear-cell renal carcinoma lines established from sporadic tumors (Iliopoulos et al. 1995; Gnarra et al. 1996). Collectively, these observations suggest that *VHL* is a critical "gatekeeper" with respect to renal carcinogenesis. In contrast to many other tumor suppressor genes, restoration of pVHL function does not affect the growth of $VHL^{-/-}$ renal carcinoma lines in vitro under standard cell culture conditions. However, the growth-suppressive effects of pVHL can be revealed when cells are grown under low serum or as 3-dimensional spheroids (Lieubeau-Teillet et al. 1998; Pause et al. 1998; Davidowitz et al. 2001).

HIF-2α is a critical target of pVHL with respect to renal carcinogenesis. First, an apparent switch from HIF-1α to HIF-2α expression occurs in preneoplastic lesions arising in $VHL^{+/-}$ kidneys in association with increasing dysplasia and cellular atypia (Mandriota et al. 2002). Second, $VHL^{-/-}$ renal carcinoma lines either express both HIF-1α and HIF-2α or exclusively HIF-2α (Maxwell et al. 1999). Third, the ability of pVHL to suppress $VHL^{-/-}$

tumor growth in nude mouse xenograft assays can be abrogated by a HIF-2α variant that cannot be hydroxylated on proline, but not the corresponding HIF-1α variant (Kondo et al. 2002, 2003; Maranchie et al. 2002). Finally, eliminating HIF-2α in $VHL^{-/-}$ renal carcinoma lines using shRNA is sufficient to suppress tumor growth in vivo (Kondo et al. 2003; Zimmer et al. 2004). It is perhaps also noteworthy that a number of drugs that inhibit growth factors downstream of HIF (such as VEGF and PDGF B) demonstrate significant activity against human kidney cancer (Kaelin 2004).

VHL disease can be subdivided into Type 1 (low risk of pheochromocytoma) and Type 2 (high risk of pheochromocytoma). Type 2 can be subdivided into 2A (low risk of renal cancer), 2B (high risk of renal cancer), and 2C (pheochromocytoma only) (Kaelin 2002). The products of Type 1, 2A, and 2B are clearly defective with respect to HIF regulation and, in particular, differences in HIF regulation would not appear to explain the differential risk of renal carcinoma in Type 2A versus Type 2B families (Clifford et al. 2001; Hoffman et al. 2001). It is possible that a pVHL function unrelated to HIF is differentially affected by Type 2A and 2B *VHL* mutations and modifies the risk of renal carcinoma. Type 2C mutants retain the ability to regulate HIF, which was a clue that a HIF-independent pVHL function might be important for pheochromocytoma development.

pVHL AND PHEOCHROMOCYTOMA

Type 2 families almost always have missense mutations, whereas true null alleles cause Type 1 disease (Chen et al. 1995). This suggested to us either that pheochromocytoma development is due to a pVHL gain of function or that complete loss of pVHL is not tolerated in pheochromcytoma precursor cells. Moreover, *VHL* mutations are rare in sporadic pheochromocytomas (in contrast to sporadic renal carcinomas and hemangioblastomas) in the absence of an occult germ-line *VHL* mutation (Neumann et al. 2002). This suggested to us that *VHL* might play a specific role in the embryological development of primitive sympathetic neuronal precursor cells, which are the cells that give rise to pheochromocytoma.

In this regard, we recently discovered that inactivation of pVHL leads to up-regulation of JunB (Lee et al. 2005). This appears to be due, at least partly, to increased aPKC activity, which is known to enhance JunB transcription (Kieser et al. 1996). Multiple groups reported earlier that pVHL inhibits aPKC family members (Pal et al. 1997; Okuda et al. 1999, 2001). Every pVHL mutant we have tested so far, including those linked to Type 2C disease, fails to suppress JunB (Lee et al. 2005).

Many sympathetic neuronal progenitor cells normally die during development as they compete with one another for growth factors such as NGF (Deckwerth and Johnson 1993; Edwards and Tolkovsky 1994; Estus et al. 1994; Schlingensiepen et al. 1994; Ham et al. 1995). Death in this setting is the result of c-Jun-dependent apoptosis. JunB often antagonizes c-Jun. We showed that loss of pVHL (and increased JunB) leads to decreased apoptosis

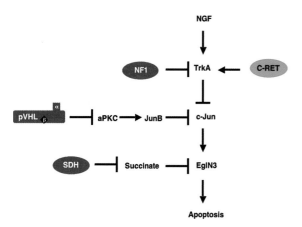

Figure 2. Control of neuronal apoptosis by familial pheochromocytoma genes. Pheochromocytomas are derived from the same cells that give rise to the sympathetic nervous system. These progenitors compete for growth factors such as NGF during development. NGF signals via TrkA, which suppresses the accumulation of c-Jun. Upon NGF withdrawal, c-Jun activity increases, leading to apoptosis. Gain-of-function *c-RET* mutations and loss-of-function *VHL*, *NF1*, and *SDH* (subunits B, C, or D) mutations have been linked to familial pheochromocytoma and the related tumor, paraganglioma. NF1 inhibits TrkA signaling, whereas activated c-RET stimulates TrkA activity. Loss of pVHL leads to increased JunB accumulation (in part due to aPKC dysregulation), which blunts c-Jun action. SDH inactivation leads to the accumulation of succinate, which inhibits the activity of EglN3. EglN3 acts downstream of c-Jun and induces neuronal apoptosis in a seemingly HIF-independent manner. Therefore, all known familial pheochromocytoma alleles would be predicted to attenuate developmental neuronal apoptosis.

of neuronal cells after NGF withdrawal, as does inactivation of NF-1 or activation of c-RET, both of which affect signaling by the NGF receptor TrkA and can, when mutated in the germ line, cause familial pheochromocytoma (Fig. 2) (Vogel et al. 1995; Maher and Eng 2002; Lee et al. 2005).

Another gene implicated in apoptosis after NGF withdrawal is SM-20/EglN3, which is a paralog of the primary HIF prolyl hydroxylase EglN1 (Lipscomb et al. 1999, 2001; Straub et al. 2003). We found that EglN3 acts downstream of c-Jun and is both necessary and sufficient for apoptosis after NGF withdrawal (Fig. 2) (Lee et al. 2005). Prolyl hydroxylation is coupled to the conversion of 2-oxoglutarate to succinate, which can then feedback-inhibit the hydroxylation reaction (Selak et al. 2005; Lee et al. 2005). Interestingly, germ-line mutations affecting succinate dehydrogenase (SDH) subunits B, C, and D have been linked to the development of familial pheochromocytoma (and the related tumor paraganglioma) (Maher and Eng 2002). We confirmed that *SDH* mutations lead to succinate accumulation and blunt EglN3-dependent neuronal apoptosis (Lee et al. 2005). Hence our findings place all of the known pheochromocytoma genes on the same pathway and suggest that failure of normal developmental culling of sympathetic neuronal precursors is the common feature of hereditary pheochromocytoma syndromes (Figs. 2 and 3). This could explain why mutations in these genes are linked to pheochromocytoma only if they are present in the germ line.

Developmental Culling and Cancer

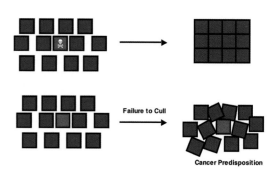

Figure 3. Developmental culling and familial pheochromocytoma. Many sympathetic neuronal precursor cells normally die (*red square, top*) during development as growth factors such as NGF become limiting. Familial pheochromocytoma alleles would be predicted to allow some of these cells to escape apoptosis (*red square, bottom*) (see also Fig. 2). These persistent cells might fail to form normal cell–cell or cell–matrix interactions. This, in conjunction with additional somatic mutations, is envisioned to result in pheochromocytoma.

EglN3, as described above, is a HIF target (Cioffi et al. 2003; del Peso et al. 2003; Aprelikova et al. 2004). Therefore, pVHL has both positive (via aPKC) and negative (via HIF) effects on EglN3 levels. We found that EglN3 levels are high in cells producing Type 1 pVHL mutants and low in Type 2 pVHL mutants (Lee et al. 2005). This potentially explains the distinction between Type 1 and Type 2 VHL disease. EglN1 does not induce neuronal apoptosis and EglN3-induced apoptosis, which requires that its catalytic domain be intact, is not blocked by nonhydroxylatable versions of HIF-1 or HIF-2α (Lee et al. 2005). This strongly argues that a hydroxylation target other than HIF links EglN3 to the induction of apoptosis.

CONCLUSIONS

The von Hippel-Lindau tumor suppressor protein is the substrate recognition unit of a ubiquitin ligase complex that targets HIF for degradation in the presence of oxygen. The interaction of pVHL with HIF is governed by prolyl hydroxylation of HIFα subunits by EglN family members. Inactivation of pVHL plays an important role in hereditary and sporadic hemangioblastomas and clear-cell renal carcinomas. Deregulation of HIF target genes contributes to tumorigenesis in these settings.

Germ-line *VHL* mutations can also give rise to pheochromocytomas, as can germ-line *NF1*, *c-RET*, and *SDH* mutations. Our recent work suggests that these mutations affect a common pathway involved in developmental culling of sympathetic neuronal precursor cells upon the withdrawal of growth factors such as NGF.

ACKNOWLEDGMENTS

I thank the past and present members of the Kaelin laboratory who have contributed to our current understanding of VHL disease. I am grateful for support from the Howard Hughes Medical Institute, the National Institutes of Health, and the Murray Foundation.

REFERENCES

Adryan B., Decker H.-J.H., Papas T.S., and Hsu T. 2000. Tracheal development and the von Hippel-Lindau tumor suppressor homolog in *Drosophila*. *Oncogene* **19:** 2803.

Aiello L.P., George D.J., Cahill M.T., Wong J.S., Cavallerano J., Hannah A.L., and Kaelin W.G., Jr. 2002. Rapid and durable recovery of visual function in a patient with von Hippel-Lindau syndrome after systemic therapy with vascular endothelial growth factor receptor inhibitor su5416. *Ophthalmology* **109:** 1745.

Aprelikova O., Chandramouli G.V., Wood M., Vasselli J.R., Riss J., Maranchie J.K., Linehan W.M., and Barrett J.C. 2004. Regulation of HIF prolyl hydroxylases by hypoxia-inducible factors. *J. Cell. Biochem.* **92:** 491.

Benjamin L.E., Golijanin D., Itin A., Pode D., and Keshet E. 1999. Selective ablation of immature blood vessels in established human tumors follows vascular endothelial growth factor withdrawal. *J. Clin. Invest.* **103:** 159.

Bergers G., Song S., Meyer-Morse N., Bergsland E., and Hanahan D. 2003. Benefits of targeting both pericytes and endothelial cells in the tumor vasculature with kinase inhibitors. *J. Clin. Invest.* **111:** 1287.

Berra E., Benizri E., Ginouves A., Volmat V., Roux D., and Pouyssegur J. 2003. HIF prolyl-hydroxylase 2 is the key oxygen sensor setting low steady-state levels of HIF-1α in normoxia. *EMBO J.* **22:** 4082.

Bishop T., Lau K.W., Epstein A.C., Kim S.K., Jiang M., O'Rourke D., Pugh C.W., Gleadle J.M., Taylor M.S., Hodgkin J., and Ratcliffe P.J. 2004. Genetic analysis of pathways regulated by the von Hippel-Lindau tumor suppressor in *Caenorhabditis elegans*. *PLoS Biol.* **2:** e289.

Blankenship C., Naglich J., Whaley J., Seizinger B., and Kley N. 1999. Alternate choice of initiation codon produces a biologically active product of the von Hippel Lindau gene with tumor suppressor activity. *Oncogene* **18:** 1529.

Bruick R. and McKnight S. 2001. A conserved family of prolyl-4-hydroxylases that modify HIF. *Science* **294:** 1337.

Brunelle J.K., Bell E.L., Quesada N.M., Vercauteren K., Tiranti V., Zeviani M., Scarpulla R.C., and Chandel N.S. 2005. Oxygen sensing requires mitochondrial ROS but not oxidative phosphorylation. *Cell Metab.* **1:** 409.

Chan C., Vortmeyer A., Chew E., Green W., Matteson D., Shen D., Linehan W., Lubensky I., and Zhuang Z. 1999. VHL gene deletion and enhanced VEGF gene expression detected in the stromal cells of retinal angioma. *Arch. Ophthalmol.* **117:** 625.

Chen F., Kishida T., Yao M., Hustad T., Glavac D., Dean M., Gnarra J.R., Orcutt M.L., Duh F.M., Glenn G., Green J., Hsia Y.E., Lamiell J., Ming H.W., Schmidt L., Kalman T., Kuzmin I., Stackhouse T., Latif F., Linehan W.M., Lerman M., and Zbar B. 1995. Germline mutations in the von Hippel-Lindau disease tumor suppressor gene: Correlations with phenotype. *Hum. Mutat.* **5:** 66.

Cioffi C.L., Liu X.Q., Kosinski P.A., and Bowen B.R. 2003. Differential regulation of HIF-1 alpha prolyl-4-hydroxylase genes by hypoxia in human cardiovascular cells. *Biochem. Biophys. Res. Commun.* **303:** 947.

Clifford S., Cockman M., Smallwood A., Mole D., Woodward E., Maxwell P., Ratcliffe P., and Maher E. 2001. Contrasting effects on HIF-1α regulation by disease-causing pVHL mutations correlate with patterns of tumourigenesis in von Hippel-Lindau disease. *Hum. Mol. Genet.* **10:** 1029.

Cockman M., Masson N., Mole D., Jaakkola P., Chang G., Clifford S., Maher E., Pugh C., Ratcliffe P., and Maxwell P. 2000. Hypoxia inducible factor-alpha binding and ubiquitylation by the von Hippel-Lindau tumor suppressor protein. *J. Biol. Chem.* **275:** 25733.

Corless C.L., Kibel A., Iliopoulos O., and Kaelin W.G., Jr. 1997. Immunostaining of the von Hippel-Lindau gene product (pVHL) in normal and neoplastic human tissues. *Hum. Pathol.* **28:** 459.

Czyzyk-Krzeska M.F. and Meller J. 2004. von Hippel-Lindau tumor suppressor: Not only HIF's executioner. *Trends Mol. Med.* **10:** 146.

Davidowitz E., Schoenfeld A., and Burk R. 2001. VHL induces renal cell differentiation and growth arrest through integration of cell-cell and cell-extracellular matrix signaling. *Mol. Cell. Biol.* **21:** 865.

Deckwerth T.L. and Johnson E.M., Jr. 1993. Temporal analysis of events associated with programmed cell death (apoptosis) of sympathetic neurons deprived of nerve growth factor. *J. Cell Biol.* **123:** 1207.

del Peso L., Castellanos M.C., Temes E., Martin-Puig S., Cuevas Y., Olmos G., and Landazuri M.O. 2003. The von Hippel Lindau/hypoxia-inducible factor (HIF) pathway regulates the transcription of the HIF-proline hydroxylase genes in response to low oxygen. *J. Biol. Chem.* **278:** 48690.

Duan D.R., Humphrey J.S., Chen D.Y.T., Weng Y., Sukegawa J., Lee S., Gnarra J.R., Linehan W.M., and Klausner R.D. 1995a. Characterization of the VHL tumor suppressor gene product: Localization, complex formation, and the effect of natural inactivating mutations. *Proc. Natl. Acad. Sci.* **92:** 6495.

Duan D.R., Pause A., Burgress W., Aso T., Chen D.Y.T., Garrett K.P., Conaway R.C., Conaway J.W., Linehan W.M., and R.D. Klausner R.D. 1995b. Inhibition of transcriptional elongation by the VHL tumor suppressor protein. *Science* **269:** 1402.

Edwards S.N. and Tolkovsky A.M. 1994. Characterization of apoptosis in cultured rat sympathetic neurons after nerve growth factor withdrawal. *J. Cell Biol.* **124:** 537.

Epstein A., Gleadle J., McNeill L., Hewitson K., O'Rourke J., Mole D., Mukherji M., Metzen E., Wilson M., Dhanda A., Tian Y., Masson N., Hamilton D., Jaakkola P., Barstead R., Hodgkin J., Maxwell P., Pugh C., Schofield C., and Ratcliffe P. 2001. *C. elegans* EGL-9 and mammalian homologs define a family of dioxygenases that regulate HIF by prolyl hydroxylation. *Cell* **107:** 43.

Esteban-Barragan M., Avila P., Alvarez-Tejado M., Gutierrez M., Garcia-Pardo A., Sanchez-Madrid F., and Landazuri M. 2002. Role of the von Hippel-Lindau tumor suppressor gene in the formation of beta1-integrin fibrillar adhesions. *Cancer Res.* **62:** 2929.

Estus S., Zaks W.J., Freeman R.S., Gruda M., Bravo R., and Johnson, E.M., Jr. 1994. Altered gene expression in neurons during programmed cell death: Identification of c-jun as necessary for neuronal apoptosis. *J. Cell Biol.* **127:** 1717.

Flamme I., Krieg M., and Plate K. 1998. Up-regulation of vascular endothelial growth factor in stromal cells of hemangioblastomas is correlated with up-regulation of the transcription factor HRF/HIF-2alpha. *Am. J. Pathol.* **153:** 25.

Gao J., Naglich J.G., Laidlaw J., Whaley J.M., Seizinger B.R., and Kley N. 1995. Cloning and characterization of a mouse gene with homology to the human von Hippel-Lindau disease tumor suppressor gene: Implications for the potential organization of the human von Hippel-Lindau disease gene. *Cancer Res.* **55:** 743.

Gerald D., Berra E., Frapart Y.M., Chan D.A., Giaccia A.J., Mansuy D., Pouyssegur J., Yaniv M., and Mechta-Grigoriou F. 2004. JunD reduces tumor angiogenesis by protecting cells from oxidative stress. *Cell* **118:** 781.

Girmens J.F., Erginay A., Massin P., Scigalla P., Gaudric A., and Richard S. 2003. Treatment of von Hippel-Lindau retinal hemangioblastoma by the vascular endothelial growth factor receptor inhibitor SU5416 is more effective for associated macular edema than for hemangioblastomas. *Am. J. Ophthalmol.* **136:** 194.

Gnarra J.R., Zhou S., Merrill M.J., Wagner J., Krumm A., Papavassiliou E., Oldfield E.H., Klausner R.D., and Linehan W.M. 1996. Post-transcriptional regulation of vascular endothelial growth factor mRNA by the VHL tumor suppressor gene product. *Proc. Natl. Acad. Sci.* **93:** 10589.

Gnarra J., Ward J., Porter F., Wagner J., Devor D., Grinberg A., Emmert-Buck M., Westphal H., Klausner R., and Linehan W. 1997. Defective placental vasculogenesis causes embryonic lethality in VHL-deficient mice. *Proc. Natl. Acad. Sci.* **94:** 9102.

Groulx I. and Lee S. 2002. Oxygen-dependent ubiquitination and degradation of hypoxia-inducible factor requires nuclear-cytoplasmic trafficking of the von Hippel-Lindau tumor suppressor protein. *Mol. Cell. Biol.* **22:** 5319.

Guzy R.D., Hoyos B., Robin E., Chen H., Liu L., Mansfield K.D., Simon M.C., Hammerling U., and Schumacker P.T. 2005. Mitochondrial complex III is required for hypoxia-induced ROS production and cellular oxygen sensing. *Cell Metab.* **1:** 401.

Haase V., Glickman J., Socolovsky M., and Jaenisch R. 2001. Vascular tumors in livers with targeted inactivation of the von Hippel-Lindau tumor suppressor. *Proc. Natl. Acad. Sci.* **98:** 1583.

Ham J., Babij C., Whitfield J., Pfarr C.M., Lallemand D., Yaniv M., and Rubin L.L. 1995. A c-Jun dominant negative mutant protects sympathetic neurons against programmed cell death. *Neuron* **14:** 927.

Hirsila M., Koivunen P., Gunzler V., Kivirikko K.I., and Myllyharju J. 2003. Characterization of the human prolyl 4-hydroxylases that modify the hypoxia-inducible factor. *J. Biol. Chem.* **278:** 30772.

Hoffman M., Ohh M., Yang H., Klco J., Ivan M., and Kaelin W.G., Jr. 2001. von Hippel-Lindau protein mutants linked to type 2C VHL disease preserve the ability to downregulate HIF. *Hum. Mol. Genet.* **10:** 1019.

Hon W.C., Wilson M.I., Harlos K., Claridge T.D., Schofield C.J., Pugh C.W., Maxwell P.H., Ratcliffe P.J., Stuart D.I., and Jones E.Y. 2002. Structural basis for the recognition of hydroxyproline in HIF-1alpha by pVHL. *Nature* **417:** 975.

Iliopoulos O., Ohh M., and Kaelin W. 1998. pVHL19 is a biologically active product of the von Hippel-Lindau gene arising from internal translation initiation. *Proc. Natl. Acad. Sci.* **95:** 11661.

Iliopoulos O., Kibel A., Gray S., and Kaelin W.G. 1995. Tumor suppression by the human von Hippel-Lindau gene product. *Nat. Med.* **1:** 822.

Iliopoulos O., Jiang C., Levy A.P., Kaelin W.G., and Goldberg M.A. 1996. Negative regulation of hypoxia-inducible genes by the von Hippel-Lindau protein. *Proc. Natl. Acad. Sci.* **93:** 10595.

Ivan M., Kondo K., Yang H., Kim W., Valiando J., Ohh M., Salic A., Asara J., Lane W., and Kaelin W.G., Jr. 2001. HIFα targeted for VHL-mediated destruction by proline hydroxylation: Implications for O2 sensing. *Science* **292:** 464.

Ivan M., Haberberger T., Gervasi D.C., Michelson K.S., Gunzler V., Kondo K., Yang H., Sorokina I., Conaway R.C., Conaway J.W., and Kaelin W.G., Jr. 2002. Biochemical purification and pharmacological inhibition of a mammalian prolyl hydroxylase acting on hypoxia-inducible factor. *Proc. Natl. Acad. Sci.* **99:** 13459.

Jaakkola P., Mole D., Tian Y., Wilson M., Gielbert J., Gaskell S., Kriegsheim A., Hebestreit H., Mukherji M., Schofield C., Maxwell P., Pugh C., and Ratcliffe P. 2001. Targeting of HIF-alpha to the von Hippel-Lindau ubiquitylation complex by O2-regulated prolyl hydroxylation. *Science* **292:** 468.

Jiang Y., Zhang W., Kondo K., Klco J.M., St. Martin T.B., Dufault M.R., Madden S.L., Kaelin W.G., Jr., and Nacht M. 2003. Gene expression profiling in a renal cell carcinoma cell line: Dissecting VHL and hypoxia-dependent pathways. *Mol. Cancer Res.* **1:** 453.

Kaelin W.G., Jr. 2002. Molecular basis of the VHL hereditary cancer syndrome. *Nat. Rev. Cancer* **2:** 673.

———. 2004. The von Hippel-Lindau tumor suppressor gene and kidney cancer. *Clin. Cancer Res.* **10:** 6290S.

Kamura T., Sato S., Iwain K., Czyzyk-Krzeska M., Conaway R.C., and Conaway J.W. 2000. Activation of HIF1α ubiquitination by a reconstituted von Hippel-Lindau tumor suppressor complex. *Proc. Natl. Acad. Sci.* **97:** 10430.

Kamura T., Koepp D.M., Conrad M.N., Skowyra D., Moreland R.J., Iliopoulos O., Lane W.S., Kaelin W.G., Jr., Elledge S.J., Conaway R.C., Harper J.W., and Conaway J.W. 1999. Rbx1, a component of the VHL tumor suppressor complex and SCF ubiquitin ligase. *Science* **284:** 657.

Kessler P., Vasavada S., Rackley R., Stackhouse T., Duh F., Latif F., Lerman M., Zbar B., and Williams B. 1995. Expression of the von Hippel-Lindau tumor-suppressor gene, VHL, in human fetal kidney and during mouse embryogenesis. *Mol. Med.* **1:** 457.

Kibel A., Iliopoulos O., DeCaprio J.D., and Kaelin W.G. 1995. Binding of the von Hippel-Lindau tumor suppressor protein to elongin B and C. *Science* **269:** 1444.

Kieser A., Seitz T., Adler H.S., Coffer P., Kremmer E., Crespo P., Gutkind J.S., Henderson D.W., Mushinski J.F., Kolch W., and Mischak H. 1996. Protein kinase C-zeta reverts v-raf transformation of NIH-3T3 cells. *Genes Dev.* **10:** 1455.

Kim W.Y. and Kaelin W.G. 2004. Role of VHL gene mutation in human cancer. *J. Clin. Oncol.* **22:** 4991.

Kishida T., Stackhouse T.M., Chen F., Lerman M.I., and Zbar B. 1995. Cellular proteins that bind the von Hippel-Lindau disease gene product: Mapping of binding domains and the effect of missense mutations. *Cancer Res.* **55:** 4544.

Kondo K., Kim W.Y., Lechpammer M., and Kaelin W.G., Jr. 2003. Inhibition of HIF2α is sufficient to suppress pVHL-defective tumor growth. *PLoS Biol.* **1:** E83.

Kondo K., Klco J., Nakamura E., Lechpammer M., and Kaelin W.G. 2002. Inhibition of HIF is necessary for tumor suppression by the von Hippel-Lindau protein. *Cancer Cell* **1:** 237.

Koochekpour S., Jeffers M., Wang P., Gong C., Taylor G., Roessler L., Stearman R., Vasselli J., Stetler-Stevenson W., Kaelin W.G., Jr., Linehan W., Klausner R., Gnarra J., and Vande Woude G. 1999. The von Hippel-Lindau tumor suppressor gene inhibits hepatocyte growth factor/scatter factor-induced invasion and branching morphogenesis in renal carcinoma cells. *Mol. Cell. Biol.* **19:** 5902.

Krieg M., Haas R., Brauch H., Acker T., Flamme I., and Plate K. 2000. Up-regulation of hypoxia-inducible factors HIF-1α and HIF-2α under normoxic conditions in renal carcinoma cells by von Hippel-Lindau tumor suppressor gene loss of function. *Oncogene* **19:** 5435.

Latif F., Tory K., Gnarra J., Yao M., Duh F.-M., Orcutt M.L., Stackhouse T., Kuzmin I., Modi W., Geil L., Schmidt L., Zhou F., Li H., Wei M.H., Chen F., Glenn G., Choyke P., Walther M.M., Weng Y., Duan D.-S.R., Dean M., Glavac D., Richards F.M., Crossey P.A., Ferguson-Smith M.A., Pasiler D.L., Chumakov I., Cohen D., Chinault A.C., Maher E.R., Linehan W.M., Zbar B., and Lerman M.I. 1993. Identification of the von Hippel-Lindau disease tumor suppressor gene. *Science* **260:** 1317.

Lee S., Chen D.Y.T., Humphrey J.S., Gnarra J.R., Linehan W.M., and Klausner R.D. 1996. Nuclear/cytoplasmic localization of the von Hippel-Lindau tumor suppressor gene product is determined by cell density. *Proc. Natl. Acad. Sci.* **93:** 1770.

Lee S., Neumann M., Stearman R., Stauber R., Pause A., Pavlakis G., and Klausner R. 1999. Transcription-dependent nuclear-cytoplasmic trafficking is required for the function of the von Hippel-Lindau tumor suppressor protein. *Mol. Cell. Biol.* **19:** 1486.

Lee S., Nakamura E., Yang H., Wei W., Linggi M., Sajan M., Farese R., Freeman R., Carter B., Kaelin W., and Schlisio S. 2005. Neuronal apoptosis linked to EglN3 prolyl hydroxylase and familial pheochromocytoma genes: Developmental culling and cancer. *Cancer Cell* (in press).

Lieubeau-Teillet B., Rak J., Jothy S., Iliopoulos O., Kaelin W., and Kerbel R. 1998. von Hippel-Lindau gene-mediated growth suppression and induction of differentiation in renal cell carcinoma cells grown as multicellular tumor spheroids. *Cancer Res.* **58:** 4957.

Lipscomb E.A., Sarmiere P.D., and Freeman R.S. 2001. SM-20 is a novel mitochondrial protein that causes caspase-dependent cell death in nerve growth factor-dependent neurons. *J. Biol. Chem.* **276:** 5085.

Lipscomb E., Sarmiere P., Crowder R., and Freeman R. 1999. Expression of the SM-20 gene promotes death in nerve growth factor-dependent sympathetic neurons. *J. Neurochem.* **73:** 429.

Lonergan K.M., Iliopoulos O., Ohh M., Kamura T., Conaway R.C., Conaway J.W., and Kaelin W.G. 1998. Regulation of hypoxia-inducible mRNAs by the von Hippel-Lindau protein requires binding to complexes containing elongins B/C and Cul2. *Mol. Cell. Biol.* **18:** 732.

Lubensky I.A., Gnarra J.R., Bertheau P., Walther M.M., Linehan W.M., and Zhuang Z. 1996. Allelic deletions of the VHL gene detected in multiple microscopic clear cell renal lesions in von Hippel-Lindau disease patients. *Am. J. Pathol.* **149:** 2089.

Ma W., Tessarollo L., Hong S.B., Baba M., Southon E., Back T.C., Spence S., Lobe C.G., Sharma N., Maher G.W., Pack S., Vortmeyer A.O., Guo C., Zbar B., and Schmidt L.S. 2003. Hepatic vascular tumors, angiectasis in multiple organs, and impaired spermatogenesis in mice with conditional inactivation of the VHL gene. *Cancer Res.* **63:** 5320.

Madhusudan S., Deplanque G., Braybrooke J.P., Cattell E., Taylor M., Price P., Tsaloumas M.D., Moore N., Huson S.M., Adams C., Frith P., Scigalla P., and Harris A.L. 2004. Antiangiogenic therapy for von Hippel-Lindau disease. *J. Am. Med. Assoc.* **291:** 943.

Maher E.R. and Eng C. 2002. The pressure rises: Update on the genetics of phaeochromocytoma. *Hum. Mol. Genet.* **11:** 2347.

Mandriota S.J., Turner K.J., Davies D.R., Murray P.G., Morgan N.V., Sowter H.M., Wykoff C.C., Maher E.R., Harris A.L., Ratcliffe P.J., and Maxwell P.H. 2002. HIF activation identifies early lesions in VHL kidneys: Evidence for site-specific tumor suppressor function in the nephron. *Cancer Cell* **1:** 459.

Mansfield K.D., Guzy R.D., Pan Y., Young R.M., Cash T.P., Schumacher P.T., and Simon M.C. 2005. Loss of cytochrome C impairs cellular oxygen sensing and hypoxic HIF-α activation. *Cell Metab.* **1:** 393.

Maranchie J.K., Vasselli J.R., Riss J., Bonifacino J.S., Linehan W.M., and Klausner R.D. 2002. The contribution of VHL substrate binding and HIF1-α to the phenotype of VHL loss in renal cell carcinoma. *Cancer Cell* **1:** 247.

Marxsen J.H., Stengel P., Doege K., Heikkinen P., Jokilehto T., Wagner T., Jelkmann W., Jaakkola P., and Metzen E. 2004. Hypoxia-inducible factor-1 (HIF-1) promotes its degradation by induction of HIF-α-prolyl-4-hydroxylases. *Biochem. J.* **381:** 761.

Masson N., Willam C., Maxwell P., Pugh C., and Ratcliffe P. 2001. Independent function of two destruction domains in hypoxia-inducible factor-α chains activated by prolyl hydroxylation. *EMBO J.* **20:** 5197.

Maxwell P., Weisner M., Chang G.-W., Clifford S., Vaux E., Pugh C., Maher E., and Ratcliffe P. 1999. The von Hippel-Lindau gene product is necessary for oxgyen-dependent proteolysis of hypoxia-inducible factor α subunits. *Nature* **399:** 271.

Min J.H., Yang H., Ivan M., Gertler F., Kaelin W.G., Jr., and Pavletich N.P. 2002. Structure of an HIF-1α-pVHL complex: Hydroxyproline recognition in signaling. *Science* **296:** 1886.

Nakayama K., Frew I.J., Hagensen M., Skals M., Habelhah H., Bhoumik A., Kadoya T., Erdjument-Bromage H., Tempst P., Frappell P.B., Bowtell D.D., and Ronai Z. 2004. Siah2 regulates stability of prolyl-hydroxylases, controls HIF1α abundance, and modulates physiological responses to hypoxia. *Cell* **117:** 941.

Neumann H., Bausch B., McWhinney S., Bender B., Gimm O., Franke G., Schipper J., Klisch J., Altehoefer C., Zerres K., Januszewicz A., Smith W., Munk R., Manz T., Glaesker S., Apel T., Treier M., Reineke M., Walz M., Hoang-Vu C., Brauckhoff M., Klein-Franke A., Klose P., Schmidt H., Maier-Woelfle M., Peczkowska M., Szmigielski C., Eng C., and the Freiburg-Warsaw-Columbus Pheochromocytoma Study Group. 2002. Germ-line mutations in nonsyndromic pheochromocytoma. *N. Engl. J. Med.* **343:** 1459.

Ohh M., Park C.W., Ivan M., Hoffman M.A., Kim T.-Y., Huang L.E., Chau V., and Kaelin W.G. 2000. Ubiquitination of HIF requires direct binding to the von Hippel-Lindau protein beta domain. *Nat. Cell Biol.* **2:** 423.

Ohh M., Takagi Y., Aso T., Stebbins C., Pavletich N., Zbar B., Conaway R., Conaway J., and Kaelin W.G., Jr. 1999. Synthetic peptides define critical contacts between elongin C, elongin B, and the von Hippel-Lindau protein. *J. Clin. Invest.* **104:** 1583.

Ohh M., Yauch R.L., Lonergan K.M., Whaley J.M., Stemmer-Rachamimov A.O., Louis D.N., Gavin B.J., Kley N., Kaelin W.G., Jr., and Iliopoulos O. 1998. The von Hippel-Lindau tumor suppressor protein is required for proper assembly of an extracellular fibronectin matrix. *Mol. Cell* **1:** 959.

Okuda H., Saitoh K., Hirai S., Iwai K., Takaki Y., Baba M., Minato N., Ohno S., and Shuin T. 2001. The von Hippel-Lindau tumor suppressor protein mediates ubiquitination of activated atypical protein kinase C. *J. Biol. Chem.* **276:** 43611.

Okuda H., Hirai S., Takaki Y., Kamada M., Baba M., Sakai N., Kishida T., Kaneko S., Yao M., Ohno S., and Shuin T. 1999. Direct interaction of the beta-domain of VHL tumor suppressor protein with the regulatory domain of atypical PKC isotypes. *Biochem. Biophys. Res. Commun.* **263:** 491.

Pal S., Claffey K., Dvorak H., and Mukhopadhyay D. 1997. The von Hippel-Lindau gene product inhibits vascular permeability factor/vascular endothelial growth factor expression in renal cell carcinoma by blocking protein kinase C pathways. *J. Biol. Chem.* **272:** 27509.

Pause A., Lee S., Lonergan K.M., and Klausner R.D. 1998. The von Hippel-Lindau tumor suppressor gene is required for cell cycle exit upon serum withdrawal. *Proc. Natl. Acad. Sci.* **95:** 993.

Pause A., Peterson B., Schaffar G., Stearman R., and Klausner R. 1999. Studying interactions of four proteins in the yeast two-hybrid system: Structural resemblance of the pVHL/elongin BC/hCUL-2 complex with the ubiquitin ligase complex SKP1/cullin/F-box protein. *Proc. Natl. Acad. Sci.* **96:** 9533.

Pause A., Lee S., Worrell R.A., Chen D.Y.T., Burgess W.H., Linehan W.M., and Klausner R.D. 1997. The von Hippel-Lindau tumor-suppressor gene product forms a stable complex with human CUL-2, a member of the Cdc53 family of proteins. *Proc. Natl. Acad. Sci.* **94:** 2156.

Rankin E.B., Higgins D.F., Walisser J.A., Johnson R.S., Bradfield C.A., and Haase V.H. 2005. Inactivation of the arylhydrocarbon receptor nuclear translocator (Arnt) suppresses von Hippel-Lindau disease-associated vascular tumors in mice. *Mol. Cell. Biol.* **25:** 3163.

Reifenberger G., Reifenberger J., Bilzer T., Wechsler W., and Collins V. 1995. Coexpression of transforming growth factor-alpha and epidermal growth factor receptor in capillary hemangioblastomas of the central nervous system. *Am. J. Pathol.* **147:** 245.

Renbaum P., Duh F.-M., Latif F., Zbar B., Lerman M., and Kuzmin I. 1996. Isolation and characterization of the full-length 3′ untranslated region of the human von Hippel-Lindau tumor suppressor gene. *Hum. Genet.* **98:** 666.

Richard S., Campello C., Taillandier L., Parker F., and Resche F. 1998. Haemangioblastoma of the central nervous system in von Hippel-Lindau disease. *J. Int. Med.* **243:** 547.

Schlingensiepen K.H., Wollnik F., Kunst M., Schlingensiepen R., Herdegen T., and Brysch W. 1994. The role of Jun transcription factor expression and phosphorylation in neuronal differentiation, neuronal cell death, and plastic adaptations in vivo. *Cell. Mol. Neurobiol.* **14:** 487.

Schoenfeld A., Davidowitz E., and Burk R. 1998. A second major native von Hippel-Lindau gene product, initiated from an internal translation start site, functions as a tumor suppressor. *Proc. Natl. Acad. Sci.* **95:** 8817.

———. 2001. Endoplasmic reticulum/cytosolic localization of von Hippel-Lindau gene products is mediated by a 64-amino acid region. *Int. J. Cancer* **91:** 457.

Seizinger B.R., Rouleau G.A., Ozelius L.J., Lane A.H., Farmer G.E., Lamiell J.M., Haines J., Yuen J.W.M., Collins D., Majoor-Krakauer D., Bonner T., Mathew C., Rubenstein A., Halperin J., McConkie-Rosell A., Green J.S., Trofatter J.A., Ponder B.A., Eierman L., Bowmer M.I., Schimke R., Oostra B., Aronin N., Smith D.I., Drabkin H., Waziri M.H., Hobbs W.J., Martuza R.L., Conneally P.M., Hsia Y.E., and Gusella J.F. 1988. von-Hippel-Lindau disease maps to the region of chromosome 3 associated with renal cell carcinoma. *Nature* **332:** 268.

Selak M.A., Armour S.M., Mackenzie E.D., Boulahbel H., Watson D.G., Mansfield K.D., Pan Y., Simon M.C., Thompson C.B., and Gottlieb E. 2005. Succinate links TCA cycle dysfunction to oncogenesis by inhibiting HIF-α prolyl hydroxylase. *Cancer Cell* **7:** 77.

Semenza G. 2000. HIF-1 and human disease: One highly involved factor. *Genes Dev.* **14:** 1983.

Shiao Y.H., Resau J.H., Nagashima K., Anderson L.M., and Ramakrishna G. 2000. The von Hippel-Lindau tumor suppressor targets to mitochondria. *Cancer Res.* **60:** 2816.

Siemeister G., Weindel K., Mohrs K., Barleon B., Martiny-Baron G., and Marme D. 1996. Reversion of deregulated expression of vascular endothelial growth factor in human renal carcinoma cells by von Hippel-Lindau tumor suppressor protein. *Cancer Res.* **56:** 2299.

Simon M.C. 2004. Siah proteins, HIF prolyl hydroxylases, and the physiological response to hypoxia. *Cell* **117:** 851-3.

Stebbins C.E., Kaelin W.G., Jr., and Pavletich N.P. 1999. Structure of the VHL-ElonginC-ElonginB complex: Implications for VHL tumor suppressor function. *Science* **284:** 455.

Stolle C., Glenn G., Zbar B., Humphrey J., Choyke P., Walther M., Pack S., Hurley K., Andrey C., Klausner R., and Linehan W. 1998. Improved detection of germline mutations in the von Hippel-Lindau disease tumor suppressor gene. *Hum. Mutat.* **12:** 417.

Stratmann R., Krieg M., Haas R., and Plate K. 1997. Putative control of angiogenesis in hemangioblastomas by the von Hippel-Lindau tumor suppressor gene. *J. Neuropathol. Exp. Neurol.* **56:** 1242.

Straub J.A., Lipscomb E.A., Yoshida E.S., and Freeman R.S. 2003. Induction of SM-20 in PC12 cells leads to increased cytochrome c levels, accumulation of cytochrome c in the cytosol, and caspase-dependent cell death. *J. Neurochem.* **85:** 318.

Tanimoto K., Makino Y., Pereira T., and Poellinger L. 2000. Mechanism of regulation of the hypoxia-inducible factor-1alpha by the von Hippel-Lindau tumor suppressor protein. *EMBO J.* **19:** 4298.

Vogel K.S., Brannan C.I., Jenkins N.A., Copeland N.G., and Parada L.F. 1995. Loss of neurofibromin results in neurotrophin-independent survival of embryonic sensory and sympathetic neurons. *Cell* **82:** 733.

Vortmeyer A., Gnarra J., Emmert-Buck M., Katz D., Linehan W., Oldfield E., and Zhuang Z. 1997. von Hippel-Lindau gene deletion detected in the stromal cell component of a cerebellar hemangioblastoma associated with von Hippel-Lindau disease. *Hum. Pathol.* **28:** 540.

Wizigmann-Voos S., Breier G., Risau W., and Plate K. 1995. Up-regulation of vascular endothelial growth factor and its receptors in von Hippel-Lindau disease-associated and sporadic hemangioblastomas. *Cancer Res.* **55:** 1358.

Wykoff C., Pugh C., Maxwell P., Harris A., and Ratcliffe P. 2000. Identification of novel hypoxia dependent and independent target genes of the von Hippel-Lindau (VHL) tumour suppressor by mRNA differential expression profiling. *Oncogene* **19:** 6297.

Ye Y., Vasavada S., Kuzmin I., Stackhouse T., Zbar B., and Williams B. 1998. Subcellular localization of the von Hippel-Lindau disease gene product is cell cycle-dependent. *Int. J. Cancer* **78:** 62.

Yu F., White S., Zhao Q., and Lee F. 2001. HIF-1α binding to VHL is regulated by stimulus-sensitive proline hydroxylation. *Proc. Natl. Acad. Sci.* **98:** 9630.

Zatyka M., da Silva N.F., Clifford S.C., Morris M.R., Wiesener M.S., Eckardt K.U., Houlston R.S., Richards F.M., Latif F., and Maher E.R. 2002. Identification of cyclin D1 and other novel targets for the von Hippel-Lindau tumor suppressor gene by expression array analysis and investigation of cyclin D1 genotype as a modifier in von Hippel-Lindau disease. *Cancer Res.* **62:** 3803.

Zhuang Z., Bertheau P., Emmert-Buck M., Liotta L., Gnarra J., Linehan W., and Lubensky I. 1995. A microscopic dissection technique for archival DNA analysis of specific cell populations in lesions <1mm in size. *Am. J. Pathol.* **146:** 620.

Zimmer M., Doucette D., Siddiqui N., and Iliopoulos O. 2004. Inhibition of hypoxia-inducible factor is sufficient for growth suppression of VHL-/- tumors. *Mol. Cancer Res.* **2:** 89.

The Src Substrate Tks5, Podosomes (Invadopodia), and Cancer Cell Invasion

S.A. Courtneidge,[*][†] E.F. Azucena Jr.,[*][†] I. Pass,[*][†] D.F. Seals,[*] and L. Tesfay[*]

[*]The Van Andel Research Institute, Grand Rapids, Michigan 49505; [†]The Burnham Institute, La Jolla, California 92037

Some years ago, we employed a screen of phage cDNA expression libraries to identify novel substrates of the protein tyrosine kinase Src. One of these, Tks5 (previously known as Fish), is a large scaffolding protein with an amino-terminal PX domain and five SH3 domains. In normal fibroblasts, Tks5 is cytoplasmic, but the protein is found in podosomes when the cells are transformed with Src. Using short interfering RNA technology, we have shown that Tks5 is required for podosome formation. Furthermore, cells with reduced Tks5 expression are poorly invasive through Matrigel. Tks5 is expressed and localized to podosomes in invasive human cancer cell lines and in tumor tissue, particularly breast cancers and melanomas. In these cells too, Tks5 is required for invasion. Our future work will focus on the identification of the binding partners of Tks5 that are responsible for podosome formation and invasion, and on determining the role of Tks5 in animal models of metastasis.

The study of tumor viruses has contributed much to our understanding of the mechanisms by which cancer cells arise, resist signals that restrain the growth of normal cells, and metastasize. The study of the oncogene *src* has been particularly informative. Src-transformed cells are morphologically transformed and highly invasive both in vitro and in vivo. The *src* gene product is a membrane-associated protein tyrosine kinase. Since the intrinsic catalytic activity of Src is absolutely required for transformation, identifying and studying its substrates has proved invaluable in understanding many aspects of the cancer phenotype, including factor-independent growth, motility, and escape from apoptosis (Martin 2001; Frame 2002).

Several years ago, we developed a screen to rapidly isolate Src substrates, regardless of their abundance or ability to associate with Src (Lock et al. 1998). This involved using an enriched preparation of Src to phosphorylate proteins produced from phage expressing mammalian cDNA libraries. Positive clones were identified by immunoblotting with anti-phosphotyrosine antibodies. Our screen was validated by the cloning of many established Src substrates. We also implicated several known proteins as Src substrates, and we cloned several novel cDNAs (Courtneidge 2003). Further analysis of each of these novel clones in mammalian cells confirmed that they were indeed Src substrates. One of these substrates, Tks5, is the subject of our current research and is described here.

Tks5: A Src SUBSTRATE AND SCAFFOLD PROTEIN

The partial cDNAs we isolated from the Src substrate screen were designated Tks, for tyrosine kinase substrate. Conceptual translation of one such clone, Tks5, showed that it contained several possible Src phosphorylation sites and part of an SH3 domain (Lock et al. 1998). A full-length clone of Tks5 was then isolated and sequenced.

Two distinct Tks5 transcripts were identified in a mouse embryonic cDNA library. Each transcript encodes a protein with an amino-terminal phox homology (PX) domain, five SH3 domains, and multiple proline-rich motifs. The larger transcript differs from the smaller by the presence of two alternative splices, positioned each side of SH3#1 (Fig. 1). We have yet to explore fully the utilization of these transcripts, although our preliminary data suggest that fibroblasts in culture predominantly express a form of Tks5 containing only the second alternatively spliced exon. No catalytic domain was found in the protein, and it is therefore designated as a scaffolding or adapter protein, whose function is to interact with other proteins and lipids (see below).

We initially named the protein encoded by this locus Fish (for *five SH3* domains). However, because of the potential for confusion, and the difficulty this name creates when searching databases, we have now reverted to the designation Tks5. Note also that in many databases, the gene encoding Tks5 has been given the name SH3MD1.

At the time that we originally cloned Tks5, which is located on human chromosome 10, we found no closely related sequences, although p47[phox], a cytoplasmic component of the NADPH oxidase system of neutrophils, did show some similarity in the arrangement of its PX domain and two SH3 domains. However, in 2004, a sequence (derived from a mouse dendritic cell cDNA library) that more closely resembled Tks5, with an amino-terminal PX domain followed by three SH3 domains, was deposited in databases. Some months ago, genomic databases were used to map this gene to human chromosome 5, and to update and extend it, such that it is now predicted to contain four SH3 domains. Although this gene product remains at this point hypothetical, the fact that similar sequences are conserved in genomes from fish to man suggests that it is a genuine gene. We propose to name the protein Tks4. It is of note that Tks4 shares none of the putative Src phosphorylation sites found in Tks5, although it does have a

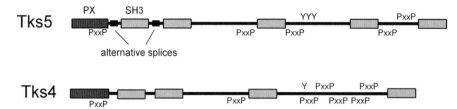

Figure 1. Domain map of Tks5 and the related protein Tks4. Black boxes represent phox homology (PX) domains, and gray boxes denote Src homology 3 (SH3) domains. Proline-rich motifs matching the consensus for SH3 domain binding are denoted PxxP, and each potential Src phosphorylation site is marked with a Y.

distinct canonical Src phosphorylation and SH2 domain binding site (YEEI) in the long linker sequence between the third and fourth SH3 domains. We are currently deriving a cDNA clone of Tks4 in order to study it further.

We observed that the Tks5 mRNA was generally expressed, although it was low in spleen and absent in testis (Lock et al. 1998). We have subsequently found, however, that some cell lines in culture fail to express the Tks5 protein, even when they contain the mRNA. Still others lack mRNA expression (Seals et al. 2005). This suggests that Tks5 expression is likely to be regulated at several levels, both transcriptionally and posttranscriptionally. We are currently exploring this in more depth. Tks5 is phosphorylated by Src in Src-transformed fibroblasts, and in normal cells in response to various stimuli, including growth factors and disruptors of the actin cytoskeleton (Abram et al. 2003). Cytoskeletal disruption in fibroblasts lacking Src, Fyn, and Yes did not result in Tks5 phosphorylation (C. Abram and S.A. Courtneidge, unpubl.). Thus, to date we have no evidence that Tks5 is a substrate of tyrosine kinases other than those of the Src family.

Tks5 LOCALIZES TO PODOSOMES IN NORMAL AND CANCER CELLS

In mouse fibroblasts, Tks5 has a predominantly cytoplasmic localization. However, we noticed a striking relocalization of Tks5 to the ventral membrane when these fibroblasts were transformed by Src (Fig. 2). Tks5 colocalized with F-actin in structures known as rosettes of po-

dosomes (Abram et al. 2003). Podosomes, also known as invadopodia, have been implicated in both tumor cell invasion and the control of proteolysis (David-Pfeuty and Singer 1980; Tarone et al. 1985; Chen 1989; Linder and Aepfelbacher 2003). They are fine ventral protrusions of the plasma membrane, with an actin core, and rich in actin regulatory proteins. Indeed, several studies have shown that the formation of podosomes requires actin turnover. Podosomes also contain several proteases and have been implicated in degradation of the extracellular matrix (ECM). Podosomes are found in many cancer cells, including Src-transformed fibroblasts, as well as in invasive human carcinomas, including breast cancers and melanomas (Kelly et al. 1994; Chen 1996).

Podosomes have also been described in many normal cell types whose physiological roles require motility and ECM degradation, including osteoclasts, macrophages, endothelial cells, and vascular smooth muscle cells (Linder and Aepfelbacher 2003; Buccione et al. 2004). We have yet to examine each of these cell types for Tks5 expression and localization, but, together with Drs. Elson and Geiger (Weizmann Institute), we have detected Tsk5 in the podosomes of mature osteoclasts (Fig. 2). Our current studies have focused on a role for Tks5 in the invasive nature of cancer cells, but it will be interesting in the future to dissect its role in cells such as osteoclasts.

Tks5 IS NEEDED FOR PODOSOME FORMATION AND INVASION IN CANCER CELLS

Malignant tumors are distinguished from their benign counterparts by their ability to metastasize. The process of metastasis involves many steps, including escape from the tissue in which the tumor first arises, passage into the vasculature, exit from the vasculature and movement into a distant tissue, followed by growth at this site. There are two properties in particular that propel this metastatic phenotype: motility and the promotion of proteolysis (Ridley 2000; Chang and Werb 2001). Proteases are not just involved in the degradation of the specialized ECM called basement membrane that surrounds organs, but are also responsible for the turnover and remodeling of ECM that occurs during tumor growth. Several proteases have been implicated in the process of metastasis, including both metalloproteases (particularly of the matrix type) and serine proteases (particularly urokinase plasminogen activator; uPA) (Blasi 1997; McCawley and Matrisian

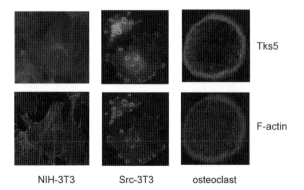

Figure 2. The subcellular localization of Tks5. Cultured NIH-3T3 cells (*left*), T3 cells transformed with an activated form of Src (*middle*), and mature osteoclasts (*right*), were fixed and stained for Tks5 (*top*) or actin (using phalloidin, *bottom*).

2000). Although tumor cells often themselves secrete the required proteases, it is also clear that tumor cells can orchestrate the production and activation of proteases by host cells in the tumor microenvironment, such as macrophages and osteoclasts (van Kempen et al. 2003). Intriguingly, each of these cell types can form podosomes (Linder and Aepfelbacher 2003).

We tested whether Tks5 was required for the formation of podosomes, and for the invasive phenotype (Seals et al. 2005). We generated clones of Src-transformed NIH-3T3 cells expressing a short hairpin RNA vector targeting Tks5, which on average showed a fourfold reduction in Tks5 expression. Cell growth was not affected in the knockdown cells. We fixed and stained these cells with fluorescent phalloidin, to visualize F-actin. Whereas the parental cells and control clones (transfected with an empty vector) contained many rosettes of podosomes, these structures were only rarely observed in the knockdown cells. Rather, the cells appeared to regain some actin stress fibers and focal adhesions. Furthermore, the knockdown cells failed to elicit robust ECM degradation and were poorly invasive through Matrigel, although chemotaxis was unaffected (Fig. 3 and data not shown). Taken together, these data suggest that Tks5 is required both for podosome formation and for the invasive properties of the cells.

We next addressed whether Tks5 was expressed in human cancer cell lines and tissues (Seals et al. 2005). We found measurable expression of Tks5 in three invasive breast cancer cells. In contrast, only barely detectable levels were evident in two breast cancer cell lines that are considered poorly invasive. A similar correlation between Tks5 expression and invasiveness was seen in three prostate cancer cell lines (D. Seals et al., unpubl.). All melanoma cell lines tested expressed Tks5. Furthermore, we detected Tks5 expression in several samples of paraffin-embedded cancers, including breast, prostate, and melanoma (in collaboration with Dr. James Resau,

Van Andel Research Institute). We used short interfering RNAs to probe a possible role for Tks5 in the invasive ability of human cancer cells, particularly breast cancers and melanomas. In each case, we found that inhibition of Tks5 expression reduced the invasiveness of the cells through Matrigel, to the same extent as protease inhibitors. Although the sample sizes were small in these analyses, they do suggest that further study of the relationship between Tks5 expression, invasiveness, and cancer type and stage is warranted.

In other experiments, we have shown that the introduction of Tks5 into cells that do not normally express it (for example, T47D breast cancer cells), along with activated Src, results in the formation of podosomes (Seals et al. 2005). Together, our data suggest that Tks5 is critical for the formation of podosomes. Furthermore, our experiments provide further support for the conclusion that proteolytic degradation of the ECM, and invasive behavior, require podosomes.

THE SCAFFOLDING FUNCTIONS OF TKS5

Given that Tks5 lacks catalytic activity, it must derive its ability to drive the formation of podosomes from its interaction with other molecules. We have begun to characterize these molecules. We first analyzed the PX domain (Abram et al. 2003). Since other PX domains bind to phosphorylated inositol lipids (Sato et al. 2001; Wishart et al. 2001; Xu et al. 2001; Ellson et al. 2002), we tested the ability of the PX domain of Tks5 to bind lipids. We found that, in vitro, the PX domain shows strong binding to both PI3P and $PI3,4P_2$. When expressed in normal fibroblasts, the isolated PX domain of Tks5 shows a punctate intracellular distribution, consistent with the predominantly endosomal localization of PI3P. In Src-transformed cells, however, the PX domain is targeted to podosomes, suggesting that perhaps in this case it is associating with $PI3,4P_2$. Although these data might

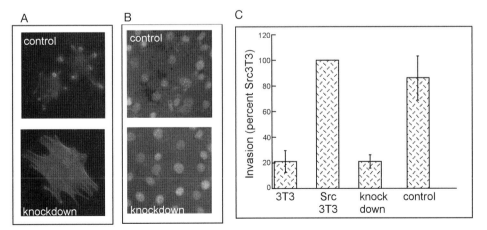

Figure 3. Tks5 is required for podosome formation, ECM degradation, and invasion. (*A*) Src-3T3 cells stably transfected with control vector (*control*), or a vector containing shRNA targeting Tks5 (*knockdown*), were fixed and stained with phalloidin to visualize the actin cytoskeleton. (*B*) Control and knockdown cells were plated onto coverslips coated with FITC-gelatin. After 24 hr, degradation of the gelatin was evaluated by fluorescence microscopy. Cells were also stained with DAPI to visualize the nuclei. (*C*) Parental 3T3 and Src-3T3 cells, as well as control and knockdown cells, were assayed for their ability to invade through Matrigel, using a Boyden chamber assay.

suggest that Tks5 is targeted to podosomes via a PX domain:lipid interaction, we note that its PX domain also contains a polyproline motif that might allow it to associate with SH3 domain-containing proteins. We are currently generating the appropriate mutants that will allow us to test the relative roles of lipid and protein binding in targeting Tks5 to podosomes.

We have also begun to characterize the proteins that bind to the SH3 domains of Tks5. The first technique we used was phage display, using phage carrying inserts from a mammalian cDNA library (Abram et al. 2003). The top hit in this analysis was a carboxy-terminal fragment of ADAM19, which is a member of the ADAMs family of metalloproteases. Subsequent biochemical analyses in mammalian cells confirmed this association and also revealed an association between Tks5 and ADAMs 12 and 15. The ADAMs family is a group of transmembrane proteins, already known to associate with several signaling molecules via their proline-rich tails, and with functions as diverse as shedding of growth factors and cytokines, motility, and cell fate determination (Seals and Courtneidge 2003). We determined the effect of Tks5 association on ADAM12 localization. Whereas ADAM12 showed a predominantly intracellular localization in normal cells (presumably because of its association with the endoplasmic reticulum), in a breast cancer cell line (and in Src-tranformed fibroblasts), some ADAM12 was localized to podosomes (Fig. 4). This relocalization has the effect of orienting the protease domain and the integrin binding domains of ADAM12 to face the extracellular milieu. It will be of great interest in the future to determine whether ADAM12, or the other ADAMs that associate with Tks5, play any role in podosome formation and/or function, and in cancer cell invasion.

We have just begun to isolate binding partners for the other SH3 domains of Tks5. One method we are currently using entails incubating cell extracts with each SH3 domain expressed as a GST fusion protein, resolving the associated proteins by gel electrophoresis, and sequencing

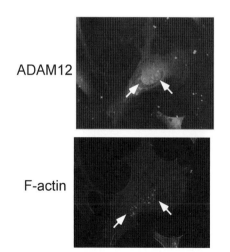

Figure 4. ADAM12 is localized to podosomes in breast cancer cells. Hs578T breast cancer cells were stained with antibodies against ADAM12, or with phalloidin. The arrows indicate the positions of clusters of podosomes.

the proteins by mass spectrometry (in collaboration with Greg Cavey at the Van Andel Research Institute). We are also using co-immunoprecipitation analyses to probe the association of Tks5 with proteins known to be present in podosomes. Although our data are preliminary, and as yet unpublished, they are intriguing. For example, we have detected associations with dynamin, N-WASp, and focal adhesion kinase, all proteins shown by other investigators to be required for podosome formation.

CONCLUSIONS

In the last few years, we have begun the characterization of an intriguing scaffold protein and Src substrate, Tks5. In normal fibroblasts, Tks5 is predominantly cytoplasmic. We have found that it becomes tyrosine phosphorylated by Src family kinases following mitogen stimulation, and upon disruption of the actin cytoskeleton. However, the consequences of this phosphorylation, as well as any potential role for Tks5 in the response to mitogens, have yet to be explored.

In Src-transformed cells, Tks5 is constitutively phosphorylated on tyrosine residues, and associated with podosomes. We know that the PX domain of Tks5 is both necessary and sufficient for podosome localization. Yet in normal cells, in the context of the full-length protein, the PX domain is not available to bind lipid. This is possibly due to intramolecular interactions between the PX domain and one of the SH3 domains, as has been reported for p47[phox] (Hiroaki et al. 2001). Our current working hypothesis is that upon Src transformation, this intramolecular association is weakened, freeing the PX domain for intermolecular interactions. We are currently testing the possible role of the tyrosine phosphorylation of Tks5 in this process.

Our studies show that in vitro, Tks5 is required for invasive behavior and for podosome formation. What about in vivo? We have preliminary evidence that reduction in Tks5 expression affects the subcutaneous growth of Src-transformed fibroblasts in immunocompromised mice (D. Seals and S.A. Courtneidge, unpubl.). We are currently generating a Tks5–GFP fusion protein, so that we may visualize its localization, and the morphology of podosomes, in 3-dimensional culture systems and in tumor explants. However, a full understanding of Tks5 function in cancer progression will require appropriate animal models. To this end, we are in the process of creating mice expressing a conditional allele of Tks5 so that we may ablate Tks5 expression in either tumor cells or host cells such as macrophages or endothelial cells, and test the effect in several mouse models of tumorigenesis. Such mice will also facilitate our analysis of Tks5 during embryogenesis.

ACKNOWLEDGMENTS

We thank former and current lab members Clare Abram, Laila Al-Duwaisan, Rebecca Gordon, Peter Lock, Lisa Maurer, Therese Roth, and Dan Salinsky; and our collaborators Greg Cavey, Ari Elson, Benjamin Geiger, and James Resau, for their contributions to this research.

REFERENCES

Abram C.L., Seals D.F., Pass I., Salinsky D., Maurer L., Roth T.M., and Courtneidge S.A. 2003. The adaptor protein Fish associates with members of the ADAMs family and localizes to podosomes of Src-transformed cells. *J. Biol. Chem.* **278:** 16844.

Blasi F. 1997. uPA, uPAR, PAI-1: Key intersection of proteolytic, adhesive and chemotactic highways? *Immunol. Today* **18:** 415.

Buccione R., Orth J.D., and McNiven M.A. 2004. Foot and mouth: Podosomes, invadopodia and circular dorsal ruffles. *Nat. Rev. Mol. Cell Biol.* **5:** 647.

Chang C. and Werb Z. 2001. The many faces of metalloproteases: Cell growth, invasion, angiogenesis and metastasis. *Trends Cell Biol.* **11:** S37.

Chen W.T. 1989. Proteolytic activity of specialized surface protrusions formed at rosette contact sites of transformed cells. *J. Exp. Zool.* **251:** 167.

———. 1996. Proteases associated with invadopodia, and their role in degradation of extracellular matrix. *Enzyme Protein* **49:** 59.

Courtneidge S.A. 2003. Isolation of novel Src substrates. *Biochem. Soc. Trans.* **31:** 25.

David-Pfeuty T. and Singer S.J. 1980. Altered distributions of the cytoskeletal proteins vinculin and alpha-actinin in cultured fibroblasts transformed by Rous sarcoma virus. *Proc. Natl. Acad. Sci.* **77:** 6687.

Ellson C.D., Andrews S., Stephens L.R., and Hawkins P.T. 2002. The PX domain: A new phosphoinositide-binding module. *J. Cell Sci.* **115:** 1099.

Frame M.C. 2002. Src in cancer: Deregulation and consequences for cell behaviour. *Biochim. Biophys. Acta* **1602:** 114.

Hiroaki H., Ago T., Ito T., Sumimoto H., and Kohda D. 2001. Solution structure of the PX domain, a target of the SH3 domain. *Nat. Struct. Biol.* **8:** 526.

Kelly T., Mueller S.C., Yeh Y., and Chen W.T. 1994. Invadopodia promote proteolysis of a wide variety of extracellular matrix proteins. *J. Cell. Physiol.* **158:** 299.

Linder S. and Aepfelbacher M. 2003. Podosomes: Adhesion hotspots of invasive cells. *Trends Cell Biol.* **13:** 376.

Lock P., Abram C.L., Gibson T., and Courtneidge S.A. 1998. A new method for isolating tyrosine kinase substrates used to identify Fish, an SH3 and PX domain-containing protein, and Src substrate. *EMBO J.* **17:** 4346.

Martin G.S. 2001. The hunting of the Src. *Nat. Rev. Mol. Cell Biol.* **2:** 467.

McCawley L.J. and Matrisian L.M. 2000. Matrix metalloproteinases: Multifunctional contributors to tumor progression. *Mol. Med. Today* **6:** 149.

Ridley A. 2000. Molecular switches in metastasis. *Nature* **406:** 466.

Sato T.K., Overduin M., and Emr S.D. 2001. Location, location, location: Membrane targeting directed by PX domains. *Science* **294:** 1881.

Seals D.F. and Courtneidge S.A. 2003. The ADAMs family of metalloproteases: Multidomain proteins with multiple functions. *Genes Dev.* **17:** 7.

Seals D.F., Azucena, Jr. E.F., Pass I., Tesfay L., Gordon R., Woodrow M., Resau J.H., and Courtneidge S.A. 2005. The adaptor protein Tks5/Fish is required for podosome formation and function, and for the protease-driven invasion of cancer cells. *Cancer Cell* **7:** 155.

Tarone G., Cirillo D., Giancotti F.G., Comoglio P.M., and Marchisio P.C. 1985. Rous sarcoma virus-transformed fibroblasts adhere primarily at discrete protrusions of the ventral membrane called podosomes. *Exp. Cell Res.* **159:** 141.

van Kempen L.C., Ruiter D.J., van Muijen G.N., and Coussens L.M. 2003. The tumor microenvironment: A critical determinant of neoplastic evolution. *Eur. J. Cell Biol.* **82:** 539.

Wishart M.J., Taylor G.S., and Dixon J.E. 2001. Phoxy lipids: Revealing PX domains as phosphoinositide binding modules. *Cell* **105:** 817.

Xu Y., Seet L.F., Hanson B., and Hong W. 2001. The Phox homology (PX) domain, a new player in phosphoinositide signalling. *Biochem. J.* **360:** 513.

Modeling Neurofibromatosis Type 1 Tumors in the Mouse for Therapeutic Intervention

L.F. PARADA, C.-H. KWON, AND Y. ZHU

Center for Developmental Biology, University of Texas Southwestern Medical Center,
Dallas, Texas 75390-9133

Von Recklinghausen's neurofibromatosis is a dominantly inherited cancer syndrome. Its gene encodes neurofibromin, a protein with ras GTPase-activating function (rasGAP) and, therefore, all NF1-associated pathology is thought to originate from selective deregulation of the ras pathway. We have constructed a variety of mouse models for NF1 that permit recapitulation of the most common tumors seen in patients. In addition, these mouse models offer insights into tumor origin and into paracrine interactions. Given the molecular and pathological fidelity of the mouse tumors to the human counterparts, it is hoped that these mouse strains will serve as effective tools for therapeutic discovery.

Von Recklinghausen's neurofibromatosis type 1 (NF1) is a common genetic disease that affects 1 in 3000 individuals worldwide. Individuals born with a germ-line mutation in the NF1 gene are susceptible to many pathological conditions, including intellectual deficits, abnormal bone development, and hypertension (Cichowski and Jacks 2001; Zhu and Parada 2001). However, these abnormalities are of variable penetrance. In contrast, tumor development is a frequent hallmark of NF1. Virtually all NF1 patients develop benign tumors of the peripheral nerves called neurofibromas. Individuals with plexiform neurofibromas, involving large segments of peripheral nerve, are at high risk to develop malignant peripheral nerve sheath tumors (MPNSTs), an incurable form of cancer. NF1 patients also have increased susceptibility to develop astrocytomas. Although estimates vary, as many as 25% of NF1 patients have optic nerve astrocytomas (pilocytic astrocytomas), and the incidence of glioblastoma among NF1 patients is greater than fivefold that of the population at large (Zhu et al. 2005). Thus, NF1 is a classic tumor suppressor locus (Zhu and Parada 2002).

The gene encoding NF1 was cloned independently by two groups in 1990 (Ballester et al. 1990; Xu et al. 1990b). The sequence revealed a large protein of 2900+ amino acids that contains a domain highly homologous to yeast *Ira* sequences which have rasGTPase-enhancing activity (Viskochil 1999). Subsequent studies from many groups have demonstrated that the NF1 protein, neurofibromin, is indeed a functional rasGAP protein (Xu et al. 1990a; Bollag and McCormick 1991). A close NF1 homolog in *Drosophila* has been reported to have predominant activity in cAMP-dependent pathway activation, although these results remain controversial (Guo et al. 1997; The et al. 1997). In summary, the majority of current information supports the idea that NF1 pathology can be attributed to deregulation of the ras pathway in a variety of cellular contexts (Klesse and Parada 1998; Zhu et al. 2002; Le et al. 2004).

In the course of the past decade, we have sought to model NF1 disease in the mouse. Initial studies employed classic gene knockout technology, and resultant NF1 null mice were developed. Several important insights were obtained using these mice, despite the fact that they perish embryonically at about E13.0 of development (Brannan et al. 1994; Jacks et al. 1994; Zhu et al. 2001).

The observation that NF1 heterozygous mice did not develop the frequent tumor types seen in patients was initially confounding. Aged NF1 heterozygotes did show susceptibility to pheochromocytomas, a rare tumor in NF1 but nonetheless more frequent than non-NF1-associated tumors (Jacks et al. 1994). Whereas in NF1 patients MPNSTs only arise in the context of neurofibromas, studies of these malignant tumors have demonstrated the existence of additional mutations, particularly in the p53 and Arf tumor suppressors. To test whether addition of such mutations would enhance tumor susceptibility, we, and T. Jacks independently, generated mice that were doubly heterozygous for both NF1 and p53 in the germ line. These mutations were carried in *cis*, since the tumor suppressors are linked both in mouse and in humans. The outcome was one of fully penetrant development of MPNSTs (Cichowski et al. 1999; Vogel et al. 1999). Histopathological and molecular analysis demonstrated remarkable similarity to human MPNST samples from NF1 patients. These data provide a proof of principle that NF1 could be modeled in mice. The appearance of MPNSTs directly in these mice was always associated with loss of the functional copies of both the NF1 and p53 genes.

We reasoned that one possibility to explain the absence of neurofibromas in NF1 heterozygous mice was essentially a reduced window of opportunity. In humans, loss of heterozygosity (LOH) of the NF1 locus presumably occurs stochastically, in the tumor target population during embryonic development. In mice, the considerably reduced time of gestation and relatively smaller number of neural-crest-derived precursors could simply undermine the likelihood of an effective LOH event in the appropriate cell to induce tumor formation. To develop more precise mouse models for NF1-associated tumorigenicity, we turned to Cre/loxP technology that permits more selective spatial and temporal ablation of NF1 function. LoxP sites were introduced into the NF1 locus to flank exons 32–34, thereby mimicking the original null mutation. The flox allele of NF1 is equivalent to the wild-type allele as determined by crossing to a null allele to create a flox/– genetic configuration. In addition, exposure of the floxed allele to cre recombinase, either via adenovirus exposure of primary cultures or through matings with tissue-specific promoter-driven cre transgenic mouse lines, demonstrated the recombinogenic capacity of the locus (Zhu et al. 2001).

Table 1. Unique Affinity between Null Schwann Cells and Heterozygous Mast Cells

Genotype	Schwann cells	Mast cells	Infiltration	Tumors
NF1$^{flox/-}$ or NF1$^{+/-}$	+/–	+/–	–	–
NF1$^{flox/flox}$;K^{cre+}	–/–	+/+	–	–/+[1]
$NF1^{flox/-}$; K^{cre+}	–/–	+/–	+++	+++

[1]Microscopic Schwann cell hyperplasia.

NF1 AND NEUROFIBROMAS

A predominant feature of NF1 pathology is the appearance of neurofibromas. These tumors are otherwise rare and are always associated with peripheral nerves and contain abnormal Schwann cells, fibroblasts, perineural sheath cells, and mast cells (Zhu and Parada 2001; Zhu et al. 2002). Several studies provided evidence that the target cell of tumor initiation in neurofibromas belongs to the Schwann cell lineage (Rutkowski et al. 2000; Muir et al. 2001; Perry et al. 2001). Using our conditional NF1 knockout mouse strain, we demonstrated that in mice, Schwann cell lineage-specific ablation of NF1 is necessary but not sufficient for generation of tumors resembling plexiform neurofibromas (Zhu et al. 2002). The genetic data demonstrated that tumors only arose when all somatic cells were heterozygous at the NF1 locus (NF1$^{+/-}$). In the case in which mice were configured to be nullizygous for NF1 in the Schwann cell lineage but wild type (NF1$^{flox/flox}$) throughout all other somatic tissues, they showed evidence of microscopic hyperplasia in sensory ganglia but no tumor development. In the course of these studies, we noted the remarkable infiltration of mast cells into sensory ganglia months prior to tumor formation. Thus, the NF1$^{fox/-}$; Krox20-cre mice (containing NF1$^{-/-}$ Schwann cells and NF1$^{+/-}$ mast cells) had mast cell infiltration and developed tumors, whereas the NF1$^{fox/flox}$; Krox20-cre mice (containing NF1$^{-/-}$ Schwann cells and NF1$^{+/+}$ mast cells) did not exhibit mast cell infiltration into sensory nerves and did not develop tumors. In culture studies, Clapp and colleagues have added considerable strength to this model with their elegant experiments showing that haploinsufficiency at *NF1* increased mast cell proliferation, survival, and colony formation in response to Kit Ligand (KitL) (Ingram et al. 2000). Additional recent work from these investigators demonstrated that NF1$^{-/-}$ Schwann cells secreted KitL which stimulates mast cell migration, and NF1$^{+/-}$ mast cells are hypermotile in response to KitL (Yang et al. 2003). Thus, the current working hypothesis is that $NF1^{+/-}$ mast cells contribute in a fundamental way to the formation of neurofibromas in vivo (Table 1). The interactions between *NF1* null Schwann cells and *NF1* heterozygous mast cells are very likely to play important roles during tumorigenesis.

To directly test this hypothesis, adoptive transfer of NF1 heterozygous bone marrow into irradiated $NF1^{fox/flox}$; Krox20-cre mice (containing $NF1^{-/-}$

Schwann cells and $NF1^{+/+}$ mast cells) should allow reconstitution of the capacity to form peripheral nerve tumors. Additionally, pharmacological block of mast cell migration or mast cell function should inhibit early mast cell infiltration of peripheral nerves by heterozygous mast cells and thus block subsequent tumor formation. Further study and identification of gene products that participate in this process in both Schwann cells and mast cells will help us further understand the molecular mechanisms mediating tumor formation and possibly develop new therapies to prevent or delay the onset of tumorigenesis in NF1 individuals. Obvious candidates for preclinical trials are drugs that block Kit receptor function, given the hypersensitivity of mast cells to cytokines and the up-regulation of KitL in nullizygous Schwann cells.

NF1 AND ASTROCYTOMAS

Astrocytic tumors or astrocytomas account for a vast majority of primary central nervous system (CNS) tumors (Kleihues and Cavenee 2000; Holland 2001). Grade II–IV astrocytomas are malignant neoplasms that diffusely infiltrate surrounding brain structures. Grade I pilocytic astrocytomas are benign and are generally not infiltrative (Kleihues and Cavenee 2000; Holland 2001; Maher et al. 2001).

As described above, individuals with NF1 germ-line mutations are predisposed to the development of astrocytomas (Listernick and Gutmann 1999; Listernick et al. 1999). NF1-associated pilocytic astrocytomas are benign, but because of frequent localization to the optic nerve, can cause vision impairment and other neurological symptoms.

Functional activation of the *ras* pathway through up-regulation of receptor tyrosine kinases such as PDGF and EGF receptors has been well documented in human astrocytoma (Kleihues and Cavenee 2000; Holland 2001; Maher et al. 2001; Zhu et al. 2002). In fact, because of the absence of effective conventional chemotherapeutic or radiotherapeutic treatments for astrocytoma, surgical intervention has been a common palliative therapy. Surgical specimens have yielded considerable molecular information concerning oncogenes, tumor suppressors, and cell cycle genes that are aberrant in these tumors. Among low-grade tumors, p53 mutations and amplification of the PDGF receptors is a common feature. Anaplastic (Grade III) tumors exhibit up-regulation of cell cycle genes and loss of the Rb pathway. Finally, Grade IV tumors (GBM) exhibit loss of the Pten tumor suppressor and activation of angiogenic factors such as VEGF. Inspection of such data has led to the hypothesis that inactivation of *p53* and activation of the *ras* pathway might be sufficient to engender astrocytoma in mouse models. Efforts to test this hypothesis by using ablation of NF1 as a surrogate of ras activation, together with p53 inactivation, have yielded evidence that this pathway is sufficient to cause tumor formation (Reilly et al. 2000, 2004; Zhu et al. 2005).

Recent developments in the tumor initiation field of research point to the existence of "cancer stem cells" within tumors that likely represent the self-renewing capacity of the tumor (Singh et al. 2004). The characterization of cancer stem cells has drawn many parallels with typical organ stem cells. A critical question now becomes whether the stem cell niche is the source of the tumor initiation cell. The availability of transgenic mouse lines that reproducibly develop glioblastoma within a predictable time frame permits inspection of mice prior to tumor formation (Zhu et al. 2005).

PERSPECTIVES

The ability to use genetically altered mice to model specific human cancers with molecular fidelity is apparently at hand. Sporadic cancer in humans is a complex process that requires a series of initiating and tumor progression events to occur in successive steps. Our studies using a genetic disease in which the NF1 tumor suppressor is by definition a critical tumor initiation gene greatly simplifies our task. Promising results in the modeling of neurofibromas, MPNSTs, and astrocytomas permit us to probe the tumor genome for critical progression events, be they genetic or epigenetic. In addition, these models that exhibit high penetrance will serve as ideal substrates for experimental therapeutics. It is reasonable to speculate that the lessons learned from studying NF1 mouse tumor models may have general applicability to sporadic cancer. As a negative regulator of the *ras* pathway, loss of NF1 is equivalent to limited ras activation. Ras activation is a common feature of human cancer. Finally, as attention focuses on the role of the microenvironment and inflammation in cancer, the unique interaction of loss of NF1 in the Schwann cell and the heterozygous mast cell should provide insight into the non-cell-autonomous mechanisms of cancer progression.

ACKNOWLEDGMENTS

L.F.P. is an American Cancer Society Professor and is funded by the National Institute of Neurological Disorders and Stroke and the Department of Defense. The authors thank the members of the Parada lab for helpful discussions.

REFERENCES

Ballester R., Marchuk D., Boguski M., Saulino A., Letcher R., Wigler M., and Collins F. 1990. The NF1 locus encodes a protein functionally related to mammalian GAP and yeast IRA proteins. *Cell* **63:** 851.

Bollag G. and McCormick F. 1991. Differential regulation of rasGAP and neurofibromatosis gene product activities. *Nature* **351:** 576.

Brannan C.I., Perkins A.S., Vogel K.S., Ratner N., Nordlund M.L., Reid S.W., Buchberg A.M., Jenkins N.A., Parada L.F., and Copeland N.G. 1994. Targeted disruption of the neurofibromatosis type-1 gene leads to developmental abnormalities in heart and various neural crest-derived tissues (erratum in *Genes Dev.* [1994] **8:** 2792). *Genes Dev.* **8:** 1019.

Cichowski K. and Jacks T. 2001. NF1 tumor suppressor gene function: Narrowing the GAP. *Cell* **104:** 593.

Cichowski K., Shih T.S., Schmitt E., Santiago S., Reilly K., McLaughlin M.E., Bronson R.T., and Jacks T. 1999. Mouse models of tumor development in neurofibromatosis type 1. *Science* **286:** 2172.

Guo H.F., The I., Hannan F., Bernards A., and Y. Zhong Y. 1997. Requirement of *Drosophila* NF1 for activation of adenylyl cyclase by PACAP38-like neuropeptides. *Science* **276:** 795.

Holland E.C. 2001. Gliomagenesis: Genetic alterations and mouse models. *Nat. Rev. Genet.* **2:** 120.

Ingram D.A., Yang F.C., Travers J.B., Wenning M.J., Hiatt K., New S., Hood A., Shannon K., Williams D.A., and Clapp D.W. 2000. Genetic and biochemical evidence that haploinsufficiency of the Nf1 tumor suppressor gene modulates melanocyte and mast cell fates in vivo. *J. Exp. Med.* **191:** 181.

Jacks T., Shih T.S., Schmitt E.M., Bronson R.T., Bernards A., and Weinberg R.A. 1994. Tumour predisposition in mice heterozygous for a targeted mutation in Nf1. *Nat. Genet.* **7:** 353.

Kleihues P. and Cavenee W.K. 2000. *Pathology and genetics of tumours of the nervous system.* IARC Press, Lyon, France.

Klesse L.J. and Parada L.F. 1998. p21 ras and phosphatidylinositol-3 kinase are required for survival of wild-type and NF1 mutant sensory neurons. *J. Neurosci.* **18:** 10420.

Le D.T., Kong N., Zhu Y., Lauchle J.O., Aiyigari A., Braun B.S., Wang E., Kogan S.C., Le Beau M.M., Parada L.F., and Shannon K.M. 2004. Somatic inactivation of Nf1 in hematopoietic cells results in a progressive myeloproliferative disorder. *Blood* **103:** 4243.

Listernick R. and Gutmann D.H. 1999. Tumors of the optic pathway. In *Neurofibromatosis: Phenotype, natural history, and pathogenesis* (ed. J.M. Friedman et al.), pp. 75–89. Johns Hopkins University Press, Baltimore, Maryland.

Listernick R., Charrow J., and Gutmann D.H. 1999. Intracranial gliomas in neurofibromatosis type 1. *Am. J. Med. Genet.* **89:** 38.

Maher E.A., Furnari F.B., Bachoo R.M., Rowitch D.H., Louis D.N., Cavenee W.K., and DePinho R.A. 2001. Malignant glioma: Genetics and biology of a grave matter. *Genes Dev.* **15:** 1311.

Muir D., Neubauer D., Lim I.T., Yachnis A.T., and Wallace M.R. 2001. Tumorigenic properties of neurofibromin-deficient neurofibroma Schwann cells. *Am. J. Pathol.* **158:** 501.

Perry A., Roth K.A., Banerjee R., Fuller C.E., and Gutmann D.H. 2001. NF1 deletions in S-100 protein-positive and negative cells of sporadic and neurofibromatosis 1 (NF1)-associated plexiform neurofibromas and malignant peripheral nerve sheath tumors. *Am. J. Pathol.* **159:** 57.

Reilly K.M., Loisel D.A., Bronson R.T., McLaughlin M.E., and Jacks T. 2000. Nf1;Trp53 mutant mice develop glioblastoma with evidence of strain-specific effects. *Nat. Genet.* **26:** 109.

Reilly K.M., Tuskan R.G., Christy E., Loisel D.A., Ledger J., Bronson R.T., Smith C.D., Tsang S., Munroe D.J., and Jacks T. 2004. Susceptibility to astrocytoma in mice mutant for Nf1 and Trp53 is linked to chromosome 11 and subject to epigenetic effects. *Proc. Natl. Acad. Sci.* **101:** 13008.

Rutkowski J.L., Wu K., Gutmann D.H., Boyer P.J., and Legius E. 2000. Genetic and cellular defects contributing to benign tumor formation in neurofibromatosis type 1. *Hum. Mol. Genet.* **9:** 1059.

Singh S.K., Hawkins C., Clarke I.D., Squire J.A., Bayani J., Hide T., Henkelman R.M., Cusimano M.D., and Dirks P.B. 2004. Identification of human brain tumour initiating cells. *Nature* **432:** 396.

The I., Hannigan G.E., Cowley G.S., Reginald S., Zhong Y., Gusella J.F., Hariharan I.K., and Bernards A. 1997. Rescue of a *Drosophila* NF1 mutant phenotype by protein kinase A. *Science* **276:** 791.

Viskochil D.H. 1999. The structure and function of the NF1 gene: Molecular pathology. In *Neurofibromatosis: Phenotype, natural history, and pathogenesis* (ed. J.M. Friedman et al.), p. 119. Johns Hopkins University Press, Baltimore, Maryland.

Vogel K.S., Klesse L.J., Velasco-Miguel S., Meyers K., Rushing E.J., and Parada L.F. 1999. Mouse tumor model for neurofibromatosis type 1. *Science* **286:** 2176.

Xu G.F., Lin B., Tanaka K., Dunn D., Wood D., Gesteland R., White R., Weiss R., and Tamanoi F. 1990a. The catalytic domain of the neurofibromatosis type 1 gene product stimulates ras GTPase and complements ira mutants of *S. cerevisiae*. *Cell* **63:** 835.

Xu G.F., O'Connell P., Viskochil D., Cawthon R., Robertson M., Culver M., Dunn D., Stevens J., Gesteland R., and White R., et al. 1990b. The neurofibromatosis type 1 gene encodes a protein related to GAP. *Cell* **62:** 599.

Yang F.C., Ingram D.A., Chen S., Hingtgen C.M., Ratner N., Monk K.R., Clegg T., White H., Mead L., Wenning M.J., Williams D.A., Kapur R., Atkinson S.J., and Clapp D.W. 2003. Neurofibromin-deficient Schwann cells secrete a potent migratory stimulus for Nf1+/– mast cells. *J. Clin. Invest.* **112:** 1851.

Zhu Y. and Parada L.F. 2001. Neurofibromin, a tumor suppressor in the nervous system. *Exp. Cell Res.* **264:** 19.

———. 2002. The molecular and genetic basis of neurological tumours. *Nat. Rev. Cancer* **2:** 616.

Zhu Y., Ghosh P., Charnay P., Burns D.K., and Parada L.F. 2002. Neurofibromas in NF1: Schwann cell origin and role of tumor environment. *Science* **296:** 920.

Zhu Y., Guignard F., Zhao D., Liu L., Burns D.K., Mason R.P., Messing A., and Parada L.F. 2005. Early inactivation of p53 tumor suppressor gene cooperating with NF1 loss induces malignant astrocytoma. *Cancer Cell* **8:** 119.

Zhu Y., Romero M.I., Ghosh P., Ye Z., Charnay P., Rushing E.J., Marth J.D., and Parada L.F. 2001. Ablation of NF1 function in neurons induces abnormal development of cerebral cortex and reactive gliosis in the brain. *Genes Dev.* **15:** 859.

Stem Cell Self-Renewal and Cancer Cell Proliferation Are Regulated by Common Networks That Balance the Activation of Proto-oncogenes and Tumor Suppressors

R. PARDAL,* A.V. MOLOFSKY, S. HE, AND S.J. MORRISON

Howard Hughes Medical Institute and Departments of Internal Medicine and Cell and Developmental Biology, University of Michigan, Ann Arbor, Michigan 48109-0934

Networks of proto-oncogenes and tumor suppressors that control cancer cell proliferation also regulate stem cell self-renewal and possibly stem cell aging. Proto-oncogenes promote regenerative capacity by promoting stem cell function but must be balanced with tumor suppressor activity to avoid neoplastic proliferation. Conversely, tumor suppressors inhibit regenerative capacity by promoting cell death or senescence in stem cells. For example, the polycomb family proto-oncogene, *Bmi-1*, is consistently required for the self-renewal of diverse adult stem cells, as well as for the proliferation of cancer cells in the same tissues. Bmi-1 promotes stem cell self-renewal partly by repressing the expression of *Ink4a* and *Arf*, tumor suppressor genes that are commonly deleted in cancer. Despite ongoing Bmi-1 expression, *Ink4a* expression increases with age, potentially reducing stem cell frequency and function. Increased tumor suppressor activity during aging therefore may partly account for age-related declines in stem cell function. Thus, networks of proto-oncogenes and tumor suppressors have evolved to coordinately regulate stem cell function throughout life. Imbalances within such networks cause cancer or premature declines in stem cell activity that resemble accelerated aging.

Mammals depend on stem cells in diverse tissues to replace cells throughout adult life and to repair tissues after injury or disease. For example, hematopoietic stem cells in the bone marrow produce millions of new blood cells daily, and stem cells in intestinal crypts constantly replace diverse types of gut epithelial cells. The depletion of stem cells from critical adult tissues, such as the hematopoietic system or gut epithelium, quickly leads to a loss of tissue integrity and death (for review, see Joseph and Morrison 2005). The persistence of stem cells throughout life in diverse tissues is therefore essential. The mechanism by which stem cells persist throughout life involves self-renewal, the process by which stem cells divide to form more stem cells (Morrison et al. 1997; Molofsky et al. 2004).

The persistence and continued mitotic activity of stem cells throughout life makes these cells a potential reservoir for the accumulation of oncogenic mutations (Reya et al. 2001). The self-renewal mechanisms that allow stem cells to persist consistently involve proto-oncogenic pathways such as Wnt, Shh, and Notch (Reya et al. 2001; Taipale and Beachy 2001). The activation of these pathways in stem cells throughout life may predispose these cells to neoplastic transformation, as it may take fewer mutations to constitutively activate such pathways in stem cells as compared to postmitotic cells in which pathway components are no longer expressed. There is evidence that some cancers arise from mutations that transform stem cells; however, the target cells for most cancers have not been rigorously identified, and many cancers may be capable of arising either from mutated

stem cells or from restricted progenitors/differentiated cells that acquire self-renewal capacity as a result of mutations (Sell and Pierce 1994; Reya et al. 2001; Pardal et al. 2003). In either case, the danger of neoplastic transformation from mutations that constitutively activate self-renewal pathways makes it critical to incorporate tumor suppressor mechanisms into this process.

Tumor suppressors come in two varieties: "caretakers," such as ATM (ataxia telangiectasia mutated), that prevent mutations by detecting and promoting the repair of DNA damage, and "gatekeepers," such as Rb and p53, that promote senescence or cell death when cells become mutated or stressed (Kinzler and Vogelstein 1997; Campisi 2005). Cellular senescence is a specialized form of terminal differentiation that is induced at the end of the replicative life of a cell, making the cell irreversibly postmitotic. These tumor suppressor functions take on added importance in stem cells as any mutations that occur in highly proliferative stem cells could be propagated throughout large numbers of progeny, increasing the probability of accumulating the additional mutations required for neoplastic transformation. Caretaker tumor suppressors would be expected to sustain normal stem cell activity by reducing the rate of mutagenesis. In contrast, gatekeeper tumor suppressors would be expected to reduce stem cell function by promoting cell death or senescence. Caretaking and gatekeeping tumor suppressors would thus be expected to have opposing effects on stem cell maintenance.

Tumor suppressors are also likely to influence stem cell aging. Tumor suppressors can induce cellular senescence in response to a variety of stimuli, including telomere shortening, oxidative stress, and oncogene activation—each of which activates tumor suppressors (Lowe and Sherr 2003; Itahana et al. 2004; Campisi 2005). Although the relationship between cellular senescence (which is typ-

*Present address: Laboratorio de Investigaciones Biomédicas, Departamento de Fisiología and Hospital Universitario Virgen del Rocío, Universidad de Sevilla, E-41013, Seville, Spain.

PARDAL ET AL.

ically studied in vitro) and aging is not clear, it is thought that cellular senescence reflects some of the changes that occur during aging (Chang et al. 2004; Campisi 2005). Senescent cells have been reported to accumulate in aging human skin (Dimri et al. 1995), primate retina (Mishima et al. 1999), and human liver (Paradis et al. 2001). Senescent cells have also been detected at sites of age-related pathology (Vasile et al. 2001), and genes that overcome senescence can enhance the regenerative capacity of tissues exposed to chronic injury (Rudolph et al. 2000). These observations suggest that the senescence of progenitors in aging or damaged tissues may contribute to the age-related decline in the regenerative capacity of tissues.

The foregoing suggests that we have struck an evolutionary balance between proto-oncogenes that promote regeneration but also contribute to neoplastic proliferation, and tumor suppressors that inhibit carcinogenesis but also limit regenerative capacity. This raises the question of whether these pathways are coordinately regulated in stem cells, which are required for the regeneration of adult tissues, and which are thought to frequently be the targets of transforming mutations. Furthermore, aging is associated with decreased capacity for repair, increased incidence of degenerative disease, and increased incidence of cancer in many tissues that contain stem cells. This raises the additional question of whether the effects of proto-oncogenes and tumor suppressors on stem cells at least partially explain the changes observed in mammalian tissues with age. Recent evidence suggests that networks of proto-oncogenes and tumor suppressors coordinately regulate self-renewal and age-related changes in stem cells, as well as the generation and proliferation of cancer cells in the same tissues. This indicates that common networks of genes regulate stem cell self-renewal, cancer cell proliferation, and stem cell aging.

Bmi-1 PROMOTES STEM CELL SELF-RENEWAL AND CANCER CELL PROLIFERATION

Bmi-1 was first identified in 1991 as a proto-oncogene that cooperates with c-myc in oncogenesis (Haupt et al. 1991; van Lohuizen et al. 1991) and that causes leukemia when overexpressed in mice (Haupt et al. 1993). It is a member of the Polycomb group of proteins, transcriptional repressors that modify chromatin structure in a heritable way to maintain gene expression patterns established during prenatal development (Valk-Lingbeek et al. 2004). It has since been found to be overexpressed in multiple human cancers, including mantle cell lymphomas (Bea et al. 2001), non-small-cell lung cancer (Vonlanthen et al. 2001), and medulloblastomas (Leung et al. 2004).

Bmi-1-deficient mice are born in normal numbers and appear normal except for a relatively mild skeletal patterning abnormality (van der Lugt et al. 1994) that is presumably caused by the dysregulation of *Hox* gene expression upon loss of *Bmi-1* (Alkema et al. 1995). In contrast to their nearly normal prenatal development, *Bmi-1*$^{-/-}$ mice exhibit progressive growth retardation postnatally and typically die by early adulthood with

hematopoietic failure, and neurological abnormalities including ataxia and seizures (van der Lugt et al. 1994).

The onset of growth retardation, hematopoietic failure, and neurological abnormalities correlates with the depletion of stem cells from every adult tissue yet examined in *Bmi-1*-deficient mice. Stem cells in the hematopoietic system and in the central and peripheral nervous systems form in normal numbers in the absence of *Bmi-1*, and appear to differentiate normally during fetal development, but exhibit a postnatal self-renewal defect that leads to their depletion by early adulthood (Fig. 1) (Lessard and Sauvageau 2003; Molofsky et al. 2003; Park et al. 2003). Overexpression of Bmi-1 is also sufficient to promote the self-renewal of hematopoietic stem cells (Iwama et al. 2004). Interestingly, some restricted neural progenitors from the forebrain and gut proliferate normally in the absence of *Bmi-1*, indicating that *Bmi-1* is not generically required for the proliferation of all cells (Molofsky et al. 2003). These results indicate that *Bmi-1* is preferentially and consistently required for the postnatal maintenance of stem cells.

In addition to being essential for the maintenance of adult stem cells, *Bmi-1* is similarly required for the maintenance of cancer stem cells (Reya et al. 2001; Pardal et al. 2003). It is required for the maintenance of leukemic stem cells in a manner very similar to its requirement for the maintenance of normal hematopoietic stem cells (Lessard and Sauvageau 2003), and it is likely to be required for the proliferation of medulloblastoma cells as well (Leung et al. 2004). Bmi-1 overexpression also promotes the generation/maintenance of cancer cells, as Bmi-1 overexpression in lymphocytes leads to lymphoma (Haupt et al. 1993) and, in mammary epithelial cells, leads to their immortalization (Dimri et al. 2002). These data support the idea that cancer cells generally, and cancer stem cells in particular, depend on similar pathways as normal stem cells for their proliferation/self-renewal.

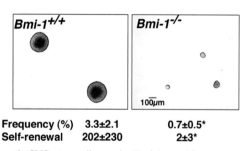

| Frequency (%) | 3.3±2.1 | 0.7±0.5* |
| Self-renewal | 202±230 | 2±3* |

Figure 1. CNS stem cells require Bmi-1 to self-renew postnatally. The photos depict typical neurospheres (neural stem cell colonies that arise from single cells in nonadherent cultures) that formed after 10 days in culture from CNS subventricular zone cells. By postnatal day 30, the frequency of CNS subventricular zone cells that formed multipotent neurospheres in culture was significantly lower in the absence of Bmi-1, and the self-renewal of these cells in culture was also significantly reduced (*, $p <$ 0.05). Self-renewal is expressed as the number of secondary neurospheres generated per primary neurosphere upon subcloning. Similar results were obtained for multipotent neural crest stem cells from the peripheral nervous system (data not shown). (Photos reprinted, with permission, from Molofsky et al. 2003 [©Nature Publishing Group].)

OTHER PROTO-ONCOGENES ALSO PROMOTE STEM CELL SELF-RENEWAL

Bmi-1 is not unusual among proto-oncogenes in promoting the self-renewal of normal stem cells and the proliferation of cancer cells from the same tissues (Reya et al. 2001). The Wnt/β-catenin signaling pathway promotes the self-renewal of intestinal epithelial stem cells, and mutations that increase signaling through this pathway promote the generation and proliferation of colorectal cancer cells (Kinzler and Vogelstein 1996; Batlle et al. 2002; van de Wetering et al. 2002). This pathway also promotes normal stem cell self-renewal and tumorigenesis in other tissues, including the skin and the hematopoietic system (for review, see Kleber and Sommer 2004; Reya and Clevers 2005). Similarly, Sonic Hedgehog signaling is necessary for the maintenance of neural stem cells in the central nervous system (Lai et al. 2003; Machold et al. 2003), and overactivation of this pathway is involved in the generation of diverse types of brain tumors (Ruiz i Altaba et al. 2002). These are only a few of many examples of pathways that promote normal stem cell self-renewal and which lead to tumorigenesis upon overactivation. These results are consistent with the idea that mutations frequently cause cancer by inappropriately activating self-renewal mechanisms in stem cells or other cells.

THE TUMOR SUPPRESSORS *Ink4a* AND *Arf* INHIBIT CANCER CELL PROLIFERATION AND STEM CELL SELF-RENEWAL

To avoid neoplastic proliferation, the activities of proto-oncogenes are balanced against tumor suppressors. Tumor suppressor activity can be induced by inappropriate mitogenic stimuli and can inhibit proliferation by promoting cellular senescence or cell death. The *Ink4a-Arf* locus encodes two gatekeeper tumor suppressors that activate critical senescence pathways (Sherr 2001; Campisi 2005). *Ink4a* encodes p16[Ink4a], a cyclin-dependent kinase inhibitor that promotes Rb activation by disrupting cyclin D–cdk4/6 complexes. *Arf* encodes p19[Arf], which promotes p53 activation by inactivating Mdm2. Induction of p16[Ink4a] and/or p19[Arf] expression in cultured primary cells leads to cellular senescence via the activation of these Rb and p53 pathways (for review, see Campisi 2005). Bmi-1 overexpression, in contrast, can bypass senescence and extend the replicative life span of primary cells by reducing p16[Ink4a] and p19[Arf] expression (Jacobs et al. 1999a; Dimri et al. 2002; Itahana et al. 2003).

Inactivation of these senescence pathways contributes strongly to carcinogenesis. *Ink4a* deletion in mice and humans is associated with lymphoma, lung adenoma, brain tumors, melanoma, and other cancers (Krimpenfort et al. 2001; Sharpless et al. 2001; Sherr and McCormick 2002). *Arf* deletion in mice leads to an increased incidence of sarcomas, lymphomas, and gliomas, as well as other types of cancers (Kamijo et al. 1999). Combined loss of *Ink4a* and *Arf* is often observed in human tumors (for review, see Ruas and Peters 1998; Sherr 1998). These data indicate that p16[Ink4a] and p19[Arf] are critical tumor suppressors in diverse tissues.

p16[Ink4a] and p19[Arf] also inhibit the self-renewal of at least some types of stem cells. Two of the major mechanisms by which Bmi-1 promotes neural stem cell self-renewal are inhibiting *Ink4a* and *Arf* expression (Molofsky et al. 2003, 2005; Bruggeman et al. 2005). Bmi-1 directly or indirectly represses transcription at the *Ink4a-Arf* locus (Jacobs et al. 1999a,b; Itahana et al. 2003). Deletion of *Ink4a-Arf* rescues the ability of *Bmi-1*[−/−] mouse embryonic fibroblasts to proliferate in culture and partially rescues cerebellum development in *Bmi-1*[−/−] mice (Jacobs et al. 1999a). Although p16[Ink4a] and p19[Arf] are not generally expressed by normal cells in young mice in vivo (Zindy et al. 1997), these proteins become strongly expressed in stem cells and other progenitors in the absence of *Bmi-1* (Molofsky et al. 2003, 2005; Park et al. 2003). Deletion of either *Ink4a* or *Arf* from *Bmi-1*-deficient mice substantially, although only partially, rescues neural stem cell self-renewal, neural stem cell frequency, and various aspects of

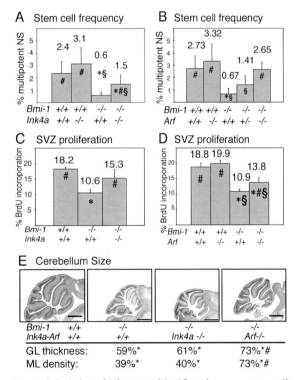

Figure 2. Deletion of *Ink4a* or *Arf* significantly rescues stem cell frequency and proliferation in the forebrain subventricular zone (SVZ) of *Bmi-1*[−/−] mice but exhibits differential effects on cerebellum rescue. *Ink4a* deficiency (*A*) or *Arf* deficiency (*B*) partially rescues the percentage of SVZ cells from *Bmi-1*[−/−] mice that form multipotent stem cell colonies in culture. The rate of proliferation (percentage of cells that incorporate a pulse of BrdU) in the forebrain SVZ of *Bmi-1*[−/−] mice is also significantly increased by *Ink4a* deficiency (*C*) or by *Arf* deficiency (*D*). (*E*) Hematoxylin and eosin-stained sagittal sections of adult cerebellum show that deletion of *Arf*, but not *Ink4a*, partially rescues the overall cerebellum size in *Bmi-1*[−/−] mice. Thickness of the cerebellum granule cell layer (GL) and cell density in the molecular layer (ML) for each genotype is quantified as a percentage of wild-type. * indicates significantly different (*p* < 0.05 by *t*-test) from wild-type, # indicates significantly different from *Bmi-1*[−/−]*Ink4a*[+/+] or *Bmi-1*[−/−]*Arf*[+/+], and § indicates significantly different from *Bmi-1*[+/+]*Ink4a*[−/−] or *Bmi-1*[+/+]*Arf*[−/−].

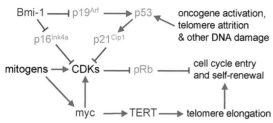

Figure 3. Networks of proto-oncogenes (*purple*) and tumor suppressors (*orange*) control stem cell self-renewal. The ability of adult stem cells to self-renew depends on a network of proto-oncogenes that activate cell cycle entry, and tumor suppressors that block cell cycle progression. External stimuli like mitogen activation promote cell cycle entry, whereas oncogene activation, telomere attrition, or DNA damage can promote senescence or cell death via p53 activation.

neural development (Fig. 2) (Molofsky et al. 2003, 2005; Bruggeman et al. 2005). These results indicate that the *Ink4a* and *Arf* senescence pathways must be repressed in order to maintain neural stem cells throughout adult life. Adult stem cell self-renewal thus reflects a balance in which proto-oncogene activity promotes self-renewal and tumor suppressor activity inhibits self-renewal (Fig. 3). Mutational overactivation of proto-oncogenes can cause cancer, whereas substantial increases in tumor suppressor activity can cause premature senescence of stem cells, potentially impairing tissue growth and regeneration (Fig. 4).

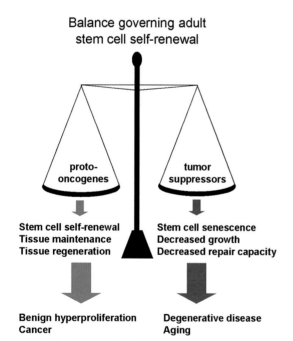

Figure 4. Adult stem cell self-renewal represents a balance between proto-oncogenes that promote stem cell self-renewal but which can cause cancer when overactivated, and gatekeeper tumor suppressors that keep self-renewal in check but which can lead to premature depletion of stem cells when overactivated. Tissue regeneration is likely favored by the activation of proto-oncogene pathways whereas the activation of gatekeeper tumor suppressors may contribute to reduced regenerative capacity, increased degenerative disease, and perhaps aging.

THE *Ink4a* TUMOR SUPPRESSOR MAY ALSO PROMOTE STEM CELL AGING

A central feature of aging in mammals is the reduced capacity for regeneration in tissues that contain stem cells. Stem cell function declines with age in diverse tissues, including the hematopoietic system (Morrison et al. 1996b; Chen et al. 2000), muscle (Conboy et al. 2003, 2005), and brain (Kuhn et al. 1996; Maslov et al. 2004). Indeed, differences among mouse strains in the frequency and proliferation of hematopoietic stem cells during aging correlate with differences in life span, suggesting that stem cell aging is regulated by mechanisms that also determine life span (de Haan et al. 1997). These observations raise the possibility that certain aspects of mammalian aging are caused by age-related reductions in stem cell function.

The expression of p16^{Ink4a} and p19^{Arf} increases substantially with age in multiple mouse tissues (Zindy et al. 1997; Krishnamurthy et al. 2004). This raises the question of whether these increases in p16^{Ink4a} and p19^{Arf} expression cause age-related declines in tissue function (Sharpless 2004). Although moderately increased expression of p16^{Ink4a} and p19^{Arf} in transgenic mice did not detectably accelerate aging or change life span (Matheu et al. 2004), the increase in p16^{Ink4a} and p19^{Arf} expression in these mice was small relative to the increase observed in old mice. The levels of p16^{Ink4a} and p19^{Arf} that are required to promote aging may be qualitatively higher than the levels that are required to inhibit cancer. To assess the physiological role of these proteins in normal aging, it will therefore be necessary to examine mice that are deficient for *Ink4a* and/or *Arf* (Fig. 5).

Although *Ink4a* may regulate stem cell aging, the relationship between stem cell aging and overall organismal aging or life span remains unclear. The age-related decline in stem cell function may be a major cause of the decline in regenerative capacity and the increase in degenerative disease that are observed in many aging tissues. On the other hand, increases in the death or dysfunction of mature cells in many aging tissues must also contribute to age-related morbidity. It is similarly unknown whether physiological differences in the rate at which stem cell activity declines with age have a detectable impact on longevity. It is likely that there will be important differences between tissues, and perhaps between stem cells and differentiated cells, in terms of the genes that regulate

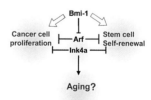

Figure 5. Stem cell self-renewal, stem cell aging, and cancer cell proliferation may be coordinately regulated by pathways that balance the activation of proto-oncogenes like *Bmi-1* and tumor suppressors like *Ink4a* and *Arf*.

the aging process. Although many of these big picture questions remain unanswered, it may be possible to gain important new insights into the aging process at a cellular level by studying individual cell types that have known physiological functions in vivo, such as hematopoietic or neural stem cells.

OTHER TUMOR SUPPRESSORS MAY ALSO REGULATE AGING

Other tumor suppressors also regulate aging in mice, although few studies have specifically examined their ability to promote age-related changes in stem cells. p53 is a powerful gatekeeping tumor suppressor that responds to a variety of cellular stresses, including DNA damage, hypoxia, and oncogene activation, to induce cell death or cell cycle arrest (Levine 1997; Serrano et al. 1997; Giaccia and Kastan 1998). p53 is also one of the most commonly deleted genes in human cancer (Lozano and Elledge 2000; Sherr and McCormick 2002). Recent reports about genetically engineered mice with altered longevity phenotypes implicate p53 as a mediator of aging (Migliaccio et al. 1999; Vogel et al. 1999; Lim et al. 2000). Mice expressing a mutant form of p53 that augments wild-type p53 activity exhibit enhanced resistance to spontaneous tumors and display an early onset of phenotypes associated with aging (Tyner et al. 2002). The short isoform of p53, p44, promotes IGF-1 signaling (Maier et al. 2004), a pathway that controls both aging and cancer cell proliferation in mammals (Holzenberger et al. 2003; Pollak et al. 2004). Mice overexpressing p44 exhibit phenotypes consistent with accelerated aging (Maier et al. 2004). Moderate overexpression of p53 in BAC transgenic mice increased cancer resistance but did not accelerate aging (Garcia-Cao et al. 2002), suggesting that aging requires higher levels of p53 activity than tumor suppression. This raises the question of whether physiological levels of p53 expression regulate aging; the levels of p53 activation that are required to accelerate aging may never be achieved under physiological circumstances. Nonetheless, p53 is likely to regulate the self-renewal of stem cells because p53 activation promotes p21^{Cip1} expression, and p21^{Cip1} regulates stem cell self-renewal in diverse tissues (Cheng et al. 2000; Kippin et al. 2005).

Telomere length is another crucial checkpoint that regulates neoplastic proliferation, as well as stem cell function and aging (Sharpless and DePinho 2004). Telomeres are repetitive DNA sequences at the ends of eukaryotic chromosomes that prevent the fusion of chromosomes (McEachern et al. 2000). In most somatic tissues, telomeric DNA undergoes progressive shortening with each round of cell division, resulting from incomplete replication by DNA polymerases (McEachern et al. 2000). Telomere shortening to a critical length can activate DNA damage pathways that trigger cell cycle arrest or apoptosis (Chiu and Harley 1997). Thus, telomere attrition limits the number of times that progenitors can divide in the absence of mechanisms like telomerase expression that maintain or lengthen telomeres.

Stem cells express telomerase and depend on it to maintain their tremendous self-renewal potential (Morrison et al. 1996a; Lee et al. 1998; Allsopp et al. 2003a); however, telomere length in stem cells still declines with age and can limit stem cell proliferation after repeated injury (Chiu et al. 1996; Rudolph et al. 2000; Allsopp et al. 2003b). Inbred laboratory mice have hyper-long telomeres (Starling et al. 1990) and therefore take three generations to critically deplete telomeres in the absence of telomerase; however, upon reaching this point, telomerase-deficient mice exhibit proliferation defects in a variety of tissues and show signs of premature aging (Blasco et al. 1997; Lee et al. 1998). These phenotypes are rescued to a considerable extent by p53 deficiency, indicating that telomere attrition causes senescence via p53 activation (Chin et al. 1999). By regulating the number of times a cell can divide before triggering senescence, telomeres and telomerase can inhibit neoplastic proliferation and determine the replicative life span of normal stem cells. Since humans have a much longer life span and much shorter telomeres than inbred mice, these observations raise the possibility that the proliferation of some human cells could be limited by telomere erosion during normal aging in vivo.

Although gatekeeper tumor suppressors promote aging phenotypes, other tumor suppressors can slow the aging process while linking stem cell self-renewal and cancer cell proliferation. ATM is a caretaker tumor suppressor that is activated in response to oxidative stress, DNA damage, or telomere instability, and which can promote DNA damage repair as well as cellular senescence (Shiloh 2003). Mutational inactivation of *Atm* causes ataxia telangiectasia, a recessive disorder characterized by neuronal degeneration, premature aging, and high cancer incidence (Shiloh 2003). Loss of both *Atm* and telomerase function in mice leads to premature aging with multiple stem cell populations apparently affected (Wong et al. 2003). ATM also regulates the maintenance of hematopoietic stem cells (Ito et al. 2004). In the absence of *Atm*, an increase in reactive oxygen species leads to activation of p16^{ink4a} and to the depletion of hematopoietic stem cells, which could be rescued by treatment with antioxidants or by overexpression of Bmi-1. ATM therefore slows the aging process and avoids carcinogenesis by reducing DNA damage and other oxidative damage in diverse cells, including stem cells.

The tumor suppressor PTEN negatively regulates signaling through the PI3 kinase pathway, which promotes cell growth, proliferation, and survival (Stiles et al. 2004). PTEN negatively regulates the self-renewal of fetal CNS stem cells (Backman et al. 2001; Groszer et al. 2001) as well as the proliferation of CNS and other cancer cells (Suzuki et al. 1998; Di Cristofano and Pandolfi 2000; Wechsler-Reya and Scott 2001). PTEN negatively regulates signaling through the insulin/insulin-like growth factor pathway, which promotes aging in an evolutionarily conserved manner (Tatar et al. 2003), and the *Caenorhabditis elegans* homolog of Pten, Daf-18, promotes life span extension in nematodes (Mihaylova et al. 1999; Solari et al. 2005). Human *Pten* complements the Daf-18 mutation in worms (Solari et al. 2005), raising the question of whether PTEN promotes life span extension, or at least maintenance of adult stem cell activity, in mammals as well.

CONCLUSIONS: AN EVOLVED BALANCE BETWEEN PROTO-ONCOGENES AND TUMOR SUPPRESSORS

Stem cells must self-renew throughout life to promote tissue maintenance and repair. This makes these cells particularly susceptible to the accumulation of potentially transforming mutations. To promote tissue regeneration while avoiding malignant transformation, a tightly regulated balance between the expression of proto-oncogenes and tumor suppressors has evolved. Proto-oncogenes promote stem cell self-renewal and tissue regeneration, but mutations that activate these pathways can lead to cancer. Gatekeeping tumor suppressors are activated by mutations and prevent neoplastic proliferation by promoting cellular senescence. This reduces cancer incidence but also contributes to aging by reducing the regenerative capacity of tissues. Hence, aging is in some ways a by-product of mechanisms that evolved to prevent the neoplastic transformation of stem cells and other progenitors.

The balance of proto-oncogene and tumor suppressor activity in stem cells changes throughout life (Fig. 6). Fetal development is a time of rapid tissue growth before cells have an opportunity to accumulate mutations. As a result, proto-oncogene activity dominates tumor suppressor activity in stem cells during fetal development to promote rapid proliferation. In contrast, most adult stem cells are quiescent most of the time (Morshead et al. 1994; Cheshier et al. 1999). Whereas this quiescence is likely critical for stem cell maintenance and probably reflects the increased influence of tumor suppressors during adult life (Cheng et al. 2000), the regulation of stem cell quies-

cence remains poorly understood. In concert with these developmental changes in stem cell function, adult mammals also exhibit an increased incidence of cancer in all proliferative tissues that contain stem cells. Whether because of accumulating damage/dysfunction or because of a developmentally programmed senescence process, tumor suppressors such as p16[Ink4a] appear to exhibit increasing activity in aging stem cells. This could contribute to age-related morbidity by reducing the regenerative capacity of aging tissues, perhaps increasing the incidence of degenerative disease.

These observations raise the question of whether polymorphisms that cause partial increases or decreases in the activity of proto-oncogenes and tumor suppressors cause physiological variations in tissue regenerative capacity or aging just as such polymorphisms are already known to affect cancer predisposition. A human polymorphism that reduces p53 activity increases cancer risk but may also be associated with significantly increased survival into old age, despite the increased cancer risk (van Heemst et al. 2005). More studies confirming findings of this type could greatly increase our understanding of how relatively small functional changes in tumor suppressor function could lead to natural variations in human longevity and regenerative capacity (Donehower 2005). A key question is whether by better understanding these networks of proto-oncogenes and tumor suppressors it will be possible to pharmacologically enhance tissue regeneration or delay changes associated with aging without increasing the risk of cancer and vice versa.

ACKNOWLEDGMENTS

This work was supported by the National Institutes of Health (R01 NS40750), the James S. McDonnell Foundation, and the Howard Hughes Medical Institute. R.P. was supported by a postdoctoral fellowship from the Spanish Ministry of Science and Technology but is now a Ramon y Cajal Fellow at the University of Seville. A.V.M. was supported by a National Research Service Award from the National Institutes of Health (F30 NS048642). S.H. was supported by a fellowship from the University of Michigan Cellular and Molecular Biology program. Thanks to Maarten van Lohuizen for providing *Bmi-1*[+/−] mice, to Charles Sherr for providing *Arf*[+/−] mice, and to Ronald DePinho for providing *Ink4a*[+/−] and *Ink4a-Arf*[+/−] mice.

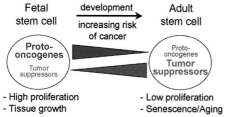

Figure 6. Developmental changes in the balance between proto-oncogenes and tumor suppressors. Stem cells proliferate rapidly during fetal development to accomplish the necessary tissue growth. This suggests that pathways which favor proliferation are strongly activated during fetal development and may not be subject to some of the gatekeeping tumor suppressor mechanisms that limit the proliferation of adult cells. Evolutionarily it may be possible to promote rapid fetal growth by removing tumor suppressor mechanisms because there is little opportunity to accumulate carcinogenic mutations during fetal development. In contrast, adult stem cells are quiescent most of the time, and appear to be subject to many more constraints upon their rate and extent of proliferation. This suggests that more tumor suppressor mechanisms are expressed in adult cells, which are at risk of accumulating transforming mutations.

REFERENCES

Alkema M.J., van der Lugt N.M.T., Bobeldijk R.C., Berns A., and van Lohuizen M. 1995. Transformation of axial skeleton due to overexpression of bmi-1 in transgenic mice. *Nature* **374:** 724.

Allsopp R.C., Morin G.B., DePinho R., Harley C.B., and Weissman I.L. 2003a. Telomerase is required to slow telomere shortening and extend replicative lifespan of HSCs during serial transplantation. *Blood* **102:** 517.

Allsopp R.C., Morin G.B., Horner J.W., DePinho R., Harley C.B., and Weissman I.L. 2003b. Effect of TERT over-expression on the long-term transplantation capacity of hematopoietic stem cells. *Nat. Med.* **9:** 369.

Backman S.A., Stambolic V., Suzuki A., Haight J., Elia A., Pretorius J., Tsao M.-S., Shannon P., Bolon B., Ivy G.O., and

Mak T.W. 2001. Deletion of Pten in mouse brain causes seizures, ataxia, and defects in soma size resembling Lhermitte-Duclos disease. *Nat. Genet.* **29:** 396.

Batlle E., Henderson J.T., Beghtel H., van den Born M.M., Sancho E., Huls G., Meeldijk J., Robertson J., van de Wetering M., Pawson T., and Clevers H. 2002. Beta-catenin and TCF mediate cell positioning in the intestinal epithelium by controlling the expression of EphB/ephrinB. *Cell* **111:** 251.

Bea S., Tort F., Pinyol M., Puig X., Hernandez L., Hernandez S., Fernandez P.L., van Lohuizen M., Colomer D., and Campo E. 2001. BMI-1 gene amplification and overexpression in hematological malignancies occur mainly in mantle cell lymphomas. *Cancer Res.* **61:** 2409.

Blasco M.A., Lee H.-W., Hande M.P., Samper E., Lansdorp P.M., DePinho R.A., and Greider C.W. 1997. Telomere shortening and tumor formation by mouse cells lacking telomerase RNA. *Cell* **91:** 25.

Bruggeman S.W.M., Valk-Lingbeek M.E., van der Stoop P.P.M., Jacobs J.J.L., Kieboom K., Tangier E., Hulsman D., Leung C., Arsenijevic Y., Marino S., and van Lohuizen M. 2005. Ink4a and Arf differentially affect cell proliferation and neural stem cell self-renewal in Bmi-1-deficient mice. *Genes Dev.* **19:** 1438.

Campisi J. 2005. Senescent cells, tumor suppression, and organismal aging: Good citizens, bad neighbors. *Cell* **120:** 513.

Chang S., Multani A.S., Cabrera N.G., Naylor M.L., Laud P., Lombard D., Pathak S., Guarente L., and DePinho R.A. 2004. Essential role of limiting telomeres in the pathogenesis of Werner syndrome. *Nat. Genet.* **36:** 877.

Chen J., Astle C.M., and Harrison D.E. 2000. Genetic regulation of primitive hematopoietic stem cell senescence. *Exp. Hematol.* **28:** 442.

Cheng T., Rodrigues N., Shen H., Yang Y.-G., Dombkowski D., Sykes M., and Scadden D.T. 2000. Hematopoietic stem cell quiescence maintained by p21cip1/waf1. *Science* **287:** 1804.

Cheshier S., Morrison S.J., Liao X., and Weissman I.L. 1999. In vivo proliferation and cell cycle kinetics of long-term self-renewing hematopoietic stem cells. *Proc. Natl. Acad. Sci.* **96:** 3120.

Chin L., Artandi S.E., Shen Q., Tam A., Lee S.L., Gottlieb G.J., Greider C.W., and DePinho R.A. 1999. p53 deficiency rescues the adverse effects of telomere loss and cooperates with telomere dysfunction to accelerate carcinogenesis. *Cell* **97:** 527.

Chiu C.P. and Harley C.B. 1997. Replicative senescence and cell immortality: The role of telomeres and telomerase. *Proc. Soc. Exp. Biol. Med.* **214:** 99.

Chiu C.-P., Dragowska W., Kim N.W., Vaziri H., Yui J., and Lansdorp P. 1996. Differential expression of telomerase activity in hematopoietic progenitors from adult human bone marrow. *Stem Cells* **14:** 239.

Conboy I.M., Conboy M.J., Smythe G.M., and Rando T.A. 2003. Notch-mediated restoration of regenerative potential to aged muscle. *Science* **302:** 1575.

Conboy I.M., Conboy M.J., Wagers A.J., Girma E.R., Weissman I.L., and Rando T.A. 2005. Rejuvenation of aged progenitor cells by exposure to a young systemic environment. *Nature* **433:** 760.

de Haan G., Nijhof W., and Van Zant G. 1997. Mouse strain-dependent changes in frequency and proliferation of hematopoietic stem cells during aging: Correlation between lifespan and cycling activity. *Blood* **89:** 1543.

Di Cristofano A. and Pandolfi P.P. 2000. The multiple roles of PTEN in tumor suppression. *Cell* **100:** 387.

Dimri G.P., Martinez J.L., Jacobs J.J., Keblusek P., Itahana K., van Lohuizen M., Campisi J., Wazer D.E., and Band V. 2002. The Bmi-1 oncogene induces telomerase activity and immortalizes human mammary epithelial cells. *Cancer Res.* **62:** 4736.

Dimri G.P., Lee X., Basile G., Acosta M., Scott G., Roskelley C., Medrano E.E., Linskens M., Rubelj I., and Pereira-Smith O., et al. 1995. A biomarker that identifies senescent human cells in culture and in aging skin in vivo. *Proc. Natl. Acad. Sci.* **92:** 9363.

Donehower L.A. 2005. p53: Guardian AND suppressor of longevity? *Exp. Gerontol.* **40:** 7.

Garcia-Cao I., Garcia-Cao M., Martin-Caballero J., Criado L.M., Klatt P., Flores J.M., Weill J.C., Blasco M.A., and Serrano M. 2002. "Super p53" mice exhibit enhanced DNA damage response, are tumor resistant and age normally. *EMBO J.* **21:** 6225.

Giaccia A.J. and Kastan M.B. 1998. The complexity of p53 modulation: Emerging patterns from divergent signals. *Genes Dev.* **12:** 2973.

Groszer M., Erickson R., Scripture-Adams D.D., Lesche R., Trumpp A., Zack J.A., Kornblum H.I., Liu X., and Wu H. 2001. Negative regulation of neural stem/progenitor cell proliferation by the Pten tumor suppressor gene in vivo. *Science* **294:** 2186.

Haupt Y., Bath M.L., Harris A.W., and Adams J.M. 1993. BMI-1 transgene induces lymphomas and collaborates with Myc in tumorigenesis. *Oncogene* **8:** 3161.

Haupt Y., Alexander W.S., Barri G., Klinken S.P., and Adams J.M. 1991. Novel zinc finger gene implicated as myc collaborator by retrovirally accelerated lymphomagenesis in E mu-myc transgenic mice. *Cell* **65:** 753.

Holzenberger M., Dupont J., Ducos B., Leneuve P., Geloen A., Even P.C., Cervera P., and Le Bouc Y. 2003. IGF-1 receptor regulates lifespan and resistance to oxidative stress in mice. *Nature* **421:** 182.

Itahana K., Campisi J., and Dimri G.P. 2004. Mechanisms of cellular senescence in human and mouse cells. *Biogerontology* **5:** 1.

Itahana K., Zou Y., Itahana Y., Martinez J.L., Beausejour C., Jacobs J.J., Van Lohuizen M., Band V., Campisi J., and Dimri G.P. 2003. Control of the replicative life span of human fibroblasts by p16 and the polycomb protein Bmi-1. *Mol. Cell. Biol.* **23:** 389.

Ito K., Hirao A., Arai F., Matsuoka S., Takubo K., Hamaguchi I., Nomiyama K., Hosokawa K., Sakurada K., Nakagata N., Ikeda Y., Mak T.W., and Suda T. 2004. Regulation of oxidative stress by ATM is required for self-renewal of haematopoietic stem cells. *Nature* **431:** 997.

Iwama A., Oguro H., Negishi M., Kato Y., Morita Y., Tsukui H., Ema H., Kamijo T., Katoh-Fukui Y., Koseki H., van Lohuizen M., and Nakauchi H. 2004. Enhanced self-renewal of hematopoietic stem cells mediated by the polycomb gene product Bmi-1. *Immunity* **21:** 843.

Jacobs J.J., Kieboom K., Marino S., DePinho R.A., and van Lohuizen M. 1999a. The oncogene and Polycomb-group gene bmi-1 regulates cell proliferation and senescence through the ink4a locus. *Nature* **397:** 164.

Jacobs J.J., Scheijen B., Voncken J.W., Kieboom K., Berns A., and van Lohuizen M. 1999b. Bmi-1 collaborates with c-Myc in tumorigenesis by inhibiting c-Myc-induced apoptosis via INK4a/ARF. *Genes Dev.* **13:** 2678.

Joseph N.M. and Morrison S.J. 2005. Toward an understanding of the physiological function of stem cells. *Dev. Cell* **9:** 173.

Kamijo T., Bodner S., van de Kamp E., Randle D.H., and Sherr C.J. 1999. Tumor spectrum in ARF-deficient mice. *Cancer Res.* **59:** 2217.

Kinzler K.W. and Vogelstein B. 1996. Lessons from hereditary colorectal cancer. *Cell* **87:** 159.

———. 1997. Cancer-susceptibility genes. Gatekeepers and caretakers. *Nature* **386:** 761.

Kippin T.E., Martens D.J., and van der Kooy D. 2005. p21 loss compromises the relative quiescence of forebrain stem cell proliferation leading to exhaustion of their proliferation capacity. *Genes Dev.* **19:** 756.

Kleber M. and Sommer L. 2004. Wnt signaling and the regulation of stem cell function. *Curr. Opin. Cell Biol.* **16:** 681.

Krimpenfort P., Quon K.C., Mooi W.J., Loonstra A., and Berns A. 2001. Loss of p16Ink4a confers susceptibility to metastatic melanoma in mice. *Nature* **413:** 83.

Krishnamurthy J., Torrice C., Ramsey M.R., Kovalev G.I., Al-Regaiey K., Su L., and Sharpless N.E. 2004. Ink4a/Arf expression is a biomarker of aging. *J. Clin. Invest.* **114:** 1299.

Kuhn H.G., Dickinson-Anson H., and Gage F.H. 1996. Neurogenesis in the dentate gyrus of the adult rat: Age-related decrease of neuronal progenitor proliferation. *J. Neurosci.* **16:** 2027.

Lai K., Kaspar B.K., Gage F.H., and Schaffer D.V. 2003. Sonic hedgehog regulates adult neural progenitor proliferation in vitro and in vivo. *Nat. Neurosci.* **6:** 21.

Lee H.-W., Blasco M.A., Gottlieb G.J., Horner J.W., Greider C.W., and DePinho R.A. 1998. Essential role of mouse telomerase in highly proliferative organs. *Nature* **392:** 569.

Lessard J. and Sauvageau G. 2003. Bmi-1 determines the proliferative capacity of normal and leukemic stem cells. *Nature* **423:** 255.

Leung C., Lingbeek M., Shakhova O., Liu J., Tanger E., Saremaslani P., van Lohuizen M., and Marino S. 2004. Bmi1 is essential for cerebellar development and is overexpressed in human medulloblastomas. *Nature* **428:** 337.

Levine A.J. 1997. p53, the cellular gatekeeper for growth and division. *Cell* **88:** 323.

Lim D.S., Vogel H., Willerford D.M., Sands A.T., Platt K.A., and Hasty P. 2000. Analysis of ku80-mutant mice and cells with deficient levels of p53. *Mol. Cell. Biol.* **20:** 3772.

Lowe S.W. and Sherr C.J. 2003. Tumor suppression by Ink4a-Arf: Progress and puzzles. *Curr. Opin. Genet. Dev.* **13:** 77.

Lozano G. and Elledge S.J. 2000. p53 sends nucleotides to repair DNA. *Nature* **404:** 24.

Machold R., Hayashi S., Rutlin M., Muzumdar M.D., Nery S., Corbin J.G., Gritli-Linde A., Dellovade T., Porter J.A., Rubin L.L., Dudek H., McMahon A.P., and Fishell G. 2003. Sonic hedgehog is required for progenitor cell maintenance in telencephalic stem cell niches. *Neuron* **39:** 937.

Maier B., Gluba W., Bernier B., Turner T., Mohammad K., Guise T., Sutherland A., Thorner M., and Scrable H. 2004. Modulation of mammalian life span by the short isoform of p53. *Genes Dev.* **18:** 306.

Maslov A.Y., Barone T.A., Plunkett R.J., and Pruitt S.C. 2004. Neural stem cell detection, characterization, and age-related changes in the subventricular zone of mice. *J. Neurosci.* **24:** 1726.

Matheu A., Pantoja C., Efeyan A., Criado L.M., Martin-Caballero J., Flores J.M., Klatt P., and Serrano M. 2004. Increased gene dosage of Ink4a/Arf results in cancer resistance and normal aging. *Genes Dev.* **18:** 2736.

McEachern M.J., Krauskopf A., and Blackburn E.H. 2000. Telomeres and their control. *Annu. Rev. Genet.* **34:** 331.

Migliaccio E., Giorgio M., Mele S., Pelicci G., Reboldi P., Pandolfi P.P., Lanfrancone L., and Pelicci P.G. 1999. The p66shc adaptor protein controls oxidative stress response and life span in mammals. *Nature* **402:** 309.

Mihaylova V.T., Borland C.Z., Manjarrez L., Stern M.J., and Sun H. 1999. The PTEN tumor suppressor homolog in *Caenorhabditis elegans* regulates longevity and dauer formation in an insulin receptor-like signaling pathway. *Proc. Natl. Acad. Sci.* **96:** 7427.

Mishima K., Handa J.T., Aotaki-Keen A., Lutty G.A., Morse L.S., and Hjelmeland L.M. 1999. Senescence-associated beta-galactosidase histochemistry for the primate eye. *Invest. Ophthalmol. Vis. Sci.* **40:** 1590.

Molofsky A.V., Pardal R., and Morrison S.J. 2004. Diverse mechanisms regulate stem cell self-renewal. *Curr. Opin. Cell Biol.* **16:** 700.

Molofsky A.V., He S., Bydon M., Morrison S.J., and Pardal R. 2005. Bmi-1 promotes neural stem cell self-renewal and neural development but not mouse growth and survival by repressing the p16Ink4a and p19Arf senescence pathways. *Genes Dev.* **19:** 1432.

Molofsky A.V., Pardal R., Iwashita T., Park I.K., Clarke M.F., and Morrison S.J. 2003. Bmi-1 dependence distinguishes neural stem cell self-renewal from progenitor proliferation. *Nature* **425:** 962.

Morrison S.J., Shah N.M., and Anderson D.J. 1997. Regulatory mechanisms in stem cell biology. *Cell* **88:** 287.

Morrison S.J., Prowse K.R., Ho P., and Weissman I.L. 1996a. Telomerase activity in hematopoietic cells is associated with self-renewal potential. *Immunity* **5:** 207.

Morrison S.J., Wandycz A.M., Akashi K., Globerson A., and Weissman I.L. 1996b. The aging of hematopoietic stem cells. *Nat. Med.* **2:** 1011.

Morshead C.M., Reynolds B.A., Craig C.G., McBurney M.W., Staines W.A., Morassutti D., Weiss S., and van der Kooy D. 1994. Neural stem cells in the adult mammalian forebrain: A relatively quiescent subpopulation of subependymal cells. *Neuron* **13:** 1071.

Paradis V., Youssef N., Dargere D., Ba N., Bonvoust F., Deschatrette J., and Bedossa P. 2001. Replicative senescence in normal liver, chronic hepatitis C, and hepatocellular carcinomas. *Hum. Pathol.* **32:** 327.

Pardal R., Clarke M.F., and Morrison S.J. 2003. Applying the principles of stem-cell biology to cancer. *Nat. Rev. Cancer* **3:** 895.

Park I.-K., Qian D., Kiel M., Becker M., Pihalja M., Weissman I.L., Morrison S.J., and Clarke M. 2003. Bmi-1 is required for the maintenance of adult self-renewing hematopoietic stem cells. *Nature* **423:** 302.

Pollak M.N., Schernhammer E.S., and Hankinson S.E. 2004. Insulin-like growth factors and neoplasia. *Nat. Rev. Cancer* **4:** 505.

Reya T. and Clevers H. 2005. Wnt signalling in stem cells and cancer. *Nature* **434:** 843.

Reya T., Morrison S.J., Clarke M.F., and Weissman I.L. 2001. Stem cells, cancer, and cancer stem cells. *Nature* **414:** 105.

Ruas M. and Peters G. 1998. The p16INK4a/CDKN2A tumor suppressor and its relatives. *Biochim. Biophys. Acta* **1378:** F115.

Rudolph K.L., Chang S., Millard M., Schreiber-Agus N., and DePinho R.A. 2000. Inhibition of experimental liver cirrhosis in mice by telomerase gene delivery. *Science* **287:** 1253.

Ruiz i Altaba A., Sanchez P., and Dahmane N. 2002. Gli and hedgehog in cancer: Tumours, embryos and stem cells. *Nat. Rev. Cancer* **2:** 361.

Sell S. and Pierce G.B. 1994. Maturation arrest of stem cell differentiation is a common pathway for the cellular origin of teratocarcinomas and epithelial cancers. *Lab. Invest.* **70:** 6.

Serrano M., Lin A.W., McCurrach M.E., Beach D., and Lowe S.W. 1997. Oncogenic ras provokes premature cell senescence associated with accumulation of p53 and p16INK4a. *Cell* **88:** 593.

Sharpless N.E. 2004. Ink4a/Arf links senescence and aging. *Exp. Gerontol.* **39:** 1751.

Sharpless N.E. and DePinho R.A. 2004. Telomeres, stem cells, senescence, and cancer. *J. Clin. Invest.* **113:** 160.

Sharpless N.E., Bardeesy N., Lee K.H., Carrasco D., Castrillon D.H., Aguirre A.J., Wu E.A., Horner J.W., and DePinho R.A. 2001. Loss of p16Ink4a with retention of p19Arf predisposes mice to tumorigenesis. *Nature* **413:** 86.

Sherr C.J. 1998. Tumor surveillance via the ARF-p53 pathway. *Genes Dev.* **12:** 2984.

———. 2001. The INK4a/ARF network in tumour suppression. *Nat. Rev. Mol. Cell Biol.* **2:** 731.

Sherr C.J. and McCormick F. 2002. The RB and p53 pathways in cancer. *Cancer Cell* **2:** 103.

Shiloh Y. 2003. ATM and related protein kinases: Safeguarding genome integrity. *Nat. Rev. Cancer* **3:** 155.

Solari F., Bourbon-Piffaut A., Masse I., Payrastre B., Chan A.M., and Billaud M. 2005. The human tumour suppressor PTEN regulates longevity and dauer formation in *Caenorhabditis elegans*. *Oncogene* **24:** 20.

Starling J.A., Maule J., Hastie N.D., and Allshire R.C. 1990. Extensive telomere repeat arrays in mouse are hypervariable. *Nucleic Acids Res.* **18:** 6881.

Stiles B., Groszer M., Wang S., Jiao J., and Wu H. 2004. PTEN-less means more. *Dev. Biol.* **273:** 175.

Suzuki A., de la Pompa J.L., Stambolic V., Elia E.J., Sasaki T., del Barco Barrantes I., Ho A., Wakeham A., Itie A., Khoo W., Fukumoto M., and Mak T.W. 1998. High cancer susceptibility and embryonic lethality associated with mutation of the PTEN tumor suppressor gene in mice. *Curr. Biol.* **8:** 1169.

Taipale J. and Beachy P.A. 2001. The hedgehog and Wnt signaling pathways in cancer. *Nature* **411:** 349.

Tatar M., Bartke A., and Antebi A. 2003. The endocrine regulation of aging by insulin-like signals. *Science* **299:** 1346.

Tyner S.D., Venkatachalam S., Choi J., Jones S., Ghebranious

N., Igelmann H., Lu X., Soron G., Cooper B., Brayton C., Hee Park S., Thompson T., Karsenty G., Bradley A., and Done- hower L.A. 2002. p53 mutant mice that display early ageing- associated phenotypes. *Nature* **415:** 45.

Valk-Lingbeek M.E., Bruggeman S.W., and van Lohuizen M. 2004. Stem cells and cancer; the polycomb connection. *Cell* **118:** 409.

van der Lugt N.M.T., Domen J., Linders K., van Roon M., Robanus-Maandag E., te Riele H., van der Valk M., De- schamps J., Sofroniew M., van Lohuizen M., and Berns A. 1994. Posterior transformation, neurological abnormalities, and severe hematopoietic defects in mice with a targeted dele- tion of the bmi-1 proto-oncogene. *Genes Dev.* **8:** 757.

van de Wetering M., Sancho E., Verweij C., de Lau W., Oving I., Hurlstone A., van der Horn K., Batlle E., Coudreuse D., Haramis A.P., Tjon-Pon-Fong M., Moerer P., van den Born M., Soete G., Pals S., Eilers M., Medema R., and Clevers H. 2002. The beta-catenin/TCF-4 complex imposes a crypt pro- genitor phenotype on colorectal cancer cells. *Cell* **111:** 241.

van Heemst D., Mooijaart S.P., Beekman M., Schreuder J., de Craen A.J., Brandt B.W., Slagboom P.E., and Westendorp R.G. 2005. Variation in the human TP53 gene affects old age survival and cancer mortality. *Exp. Gerontol.* **40:** 11.

van Lohuizen M., Verbeek S., Scheijen B., Wientjens E., van der Gulden H., and Berns A. 1991. Identification of cooperating

oncogenes in E mu-myc transgenic mice by provirus tagging. *Cell* **65:** 737.

Vasile E., Tomita Y., Brown L.F., Kocher O., and Dvorak H.F. 2001. Differential expression of thymosin beta-10 by early passage and senescent vascular endothelium is modulated by VPF/VEGF: Evidence for senescent endothelial cells in vivo at sites of atherosclerosis. *FASEB J.* **15:** 458.

Vogel H., Lim D.S., Karsenty G., Finegold M., and Hasty P. 1999. Deletion of Ku86 causes early onset of senescence in mice. *Proc. Natl. Acad. Sci.* **96:** 10770.

Vonlanthen S., Heighway J., Altermatt H.J., Gugger M., Kap- peler A., Borner M.M., van Lohuizen M., and Betticher D.C. 2001. The bmi-1 oncoprotein is differentially expressed in non-small cell lung cancer and correlates with INK4A-ARF locus expression. *Br. J. Cancer* **84:** 1372.

Wechsler-Reya R. and Scott M.P. 2001. The developmental bi- ology of brain tumors. *Annu. Rev. Neurosci.* **24:** 385.

Wong K.K., Maser R.S., Bachoo R.M., Menon J., Carrasco D.R., Gu Y., Alt F.W., and DePinho R.A. 2003. Telomere dysfunction and Atm deficiency compromises organ home- ostasis and accelerates ageing. *Nature* **421:** 643.

Zindy F., Quelle D.E., Roussel M.F., and Sherr C.J. 1997. Ex- pression of the p16(INK4a) tumor suppressor versus other INK4 family members during mouse development and aging. *Oncogene* **15:** 203.

Prostate Stem Cells and Prostate Cancer

D.A. Lawson,* L. Xin,* R. Lukacs,* Q. Xu,* D. Cheng,† and O.N. Witte*†‡

*Department of Microbiology, Immunology and Molecular Genetics, ‡Department of Molecular and
Medical Pharmacology, David Geffen School of Medicine, †Howard Hughes Medical Institute,
University of California, Los Angeles, California 90095-1662

Understanding prostate stem cells (PSCs) may provide insight for the design of therapeutics for prostate cancer. We have developed a quantitative in vivo colony-forming assay and have demonstrated that the Sca-1 antigen is present on the surface of a prostate cell subpopulation that possesses multiple stem cell properties. Immunofluorescent analysis demonstrates that Sca-1 is expressed by both basal and luminal cells in the proximal region of the adult prostate, but is not expressed by either lineage in more distal regions. The proximal region has been suggested as the PSC niche based on BrdU label-retention studies and the presence of distinct smooth-muscle cells that produce high levels of TGF-β. Sca-1 is also expressed by nearly all cells within fetal prostate epithelial chords, suggesting Sca-1 may be conserved on PSCs throughout development. Malignant epithelial cells from TRAMP mice, as well as normal prostate cells with lentiviral-mediated alteration of the PTEN/AKT signaling pathway, give rise to PIN lesions and prostate cancer in vivo. Alteration of PTEN/AKT signaling in Sca-1-enriched PSCs also results in PIN lesions, suggesting that PSCs can serve as one target for prostate carcinogenesis.

Stem cells are defined by their capacity for self-renewal, multilineage differentiation, and replication quiescence. Pluripotent embryonic stem cells possess the most plasticity and can give rise to all tissues of an organism. Demonstration of stem cells in adult tissues was first realized in experiments in which lethally irradiated mice were rescued by transfer of bone marrow from donor mice. The existence of hematopoietic stem cells (HSCs) was later confirmed in limit-dilution experiments demonstrating that small numbers of bone marrow cells could give rise to clonal colonies in the spleens of lethally irradiated hosts (for review, see Shizuru et al. 2005). Adult stem cells have since been identified in tissue systems from all three embryonic germ layers, including the lung, intestine, brain, breast, skin, and prostate. Debate still ensues over the existence of adult stem cells in some organs such as the pancreas, in which mature insulin-producing islet β-cells rather than stem cells may divide to replenish the islet β-cell compartment (Dor et al. 2004).

Mutation of somatic stem cells may contribute to many types of human pathology such as cancer. Stem cells may be particularly vulnerable to malignant transformation because of their unique capacity for long-term self-renewal and multilineage differentiation. Many tumor types have been shown to be hierarchical with respect to differentiation status, where only a discrete subpopulation of "cancer stem cells" within the tumor are capable of initiating and sustaining tumor growth (for review, see Huntly and Gilliland 2005).

Investigation of the potential role of prostatic stem cells in tumorigenesis may provide valuable insight for the development of more efficacious therapeutics against prostate cancer. In this paper, we focus on current approaches for the isolation of prostate stem cells, their dependence on a niche for survival and function, and current knowledge about the role of stem cells in prostate cancer initiation and progression.

EXPERIMENTAL PROCEDURES

In vivo prostate regeneration. For development of the in vivo prostate colony-forming (CFU) assay, dissociated prostate cells were prepared from 6- to 10-week-old C57BL/6 and β-actin GFP transgenic mice as described previously and mixed in the ratios listed (Xin et al. 2003). β-Actin GFP transgenic mice were purchased from the Jackson Laboratory (C57BL/6-TgN[ACTbEGFP]1Osb). Each sample was resuspended in collagen, incubated overnight, and implanted under the kidney capsule of SCID mice as described previously (Xin et al. 2003).

For evaluation of the regenerative activity of Sca-1+ and Sca-1− prostate cells, cells were dissociated from β-actin GFP mice and were sorted into Sca-1+ and Sca-1− fractions using magnetic bead sorting, as described previously (Xin et al. 2005). 5×10^4 cells from each fraction were then mixed with 1×10^5 cells from C57BL/6 mice and placed in the regeneration system for 8 weeks. Fluorescent signal in resulting grafts was observed by fluorescent microscopy and measured by the IVIS optical imaging system (Xenogen) as described previously (Xin et al. 2005).

For development of the in vivo prostate tumorigenesis assay, dissociated prostate cells were prepared from 6- to 10-week-old β-actin GFP and TRAMP mice. 1×10^5 cells from each source were mixed and implanted under the kidney capsule. Tumorigenic activity was measured by fluorescence microscopy and histological analysis.

Immunohistochemistry and Immunofluorescence.
Frozen sections were prepared from adult and fetal (embryonic day [E]16–17) tissue and stained with rat monoclonal anti-Sca-1 (1:250, Pharmingen), mouse monoclonal anti-CK8 (1:1000, Covance), or rabbit monoclonal anti-CK5 (1:1000, Covance). Sca-1 stained sections were subsequently incubated with a biotin-conjugated rabbit anti-rat antibody (1:200, DakoCytomation), and incubated with FITC-conjugated streptavidin (1:200, Jackson

ImmunoResearch). CK5 and CK8 sections were stained with Alexa594-conjugated anti-rabbit (1:1000, Molecular Probes) and FITC-conjugated anti-mouse (1:250, Jackson ImmunoResearch) antibodies, respectively. Sections were counterstained with PI in mounting medium and analyzed by fluorescent microscopy.

IDENTIFICATION OF PROSTATE STEM CELLS

The concept of an adult prostatic stem cell (PSC) first emerged to explain the profound capacity of the organ for tissue regeneration. Androgen cycling experiments demonstrating that the rodent prostate can undergo more than 30 cycles of involution and regeneration revealed the presence of cells possessing self-renewal and multipotentiality (Isaacs 1987). Hoechst staining and FACS analysis of dissociated human prostate cells has further shown that stem-like cells more efficient at dye efflux, called side population cells, are present in the prostate (Bhatt et al. 2003). Extension of this operational definition of PSCs is essential to gain an in-depth understanding of PSC function. Recent efforts have therefore focused on the development of in vivo stem cell assays for isolating PSCs for functional analysis.

Some of the best assays for comparing stem cell enrichment strategies have been developed for the hematopoietic and central nervous systems. The spleen colony-forming assay (CFU-S) developed by Till and McCulloch in 1961 was used to first identify the antigenic profile (Thy-1^{lo}Lin$^-$Sca-1$^+$) of murine HSCs (Spangrude et al. 1988). In this assay, nodules appear within the spleen representing the clonal outgrowth of single myeloerythroid progenitor cells following the intravenous transfer of bone marrow cells into lethally irradiated mice. The number of nodules can be counted in limit-dilution experiments to quantify the number of progenitor cells transferred (Wu et al. 1967). In the competitive repopulation (CRU) assay, HSC number is measured by coinjecting a decreasing number of fractionated cells with differentially marked unfractionated "helper" cells in order to count the number of recipients with donor-derived repopulation by the fractionated population (Harrison 1980). Neural stem cell (NSC) number can be assessed using an in vitro colony assay in which NSCs give rise to clonal clusters of floating cells called neurospheres (Reynolds et al. 1992). This assay was used by Uchida et al. (2000) to demonstrate that the CD133$^+$ CD24$^{-/lo}$ population of cells is enriched for neural stem cells.

The prostate tissue fragment recombination procedure developed by Cunha and Lung (1978) is an excellent system for the study of prostate development and epithelial–mesenchymal interactions. This system uses tissue fragments dissected from rat or mouse urogenital sinus mesenchyme (UGSM) in combination with adult epithelial tissue to regenerate prostate-like tissues when implanted under the kidney capsule of immunodeficient mice. To define PSCs using the cell-fractionation approaches utilized for HSC and NSC enrichment, we modified this system to utilize dissociated cell populations of adult mouse epithelial cells in combination with E16 UGSM cells (Fig. 1) (Xin et al. 2003). Tissue regenerated using this method possesses a normal prostate marker profile and most closely resembles the anterior and ventral lobes of the murine prostate.

Previously, we modified the prostate regeneration system for use as a CFU assay to identify murine PSC markers. Analogous to the CFU-S and CRU assays used in studies of HSC enrichment, serial dilution experiments were performed using decreasing numbers of GFP$^+$ prostate cells from β-actin GFP mice in combination with a constant number of cells from wild-type C57BL/6 mice. The lack of chimeric tubules containing both GFP$^+$ and GFP$^-$ cells in prostate tissue regenerated from these mixed populations suggests that each tubule is clonal and derived from the outgrowth of a single cell (Fig. 2). Because each tubule appears to be clonal, GFP$^+$ tubules can be counted as in the CFU-S assay to quantify the number of cells contributing to graft formation. This analysis suggests that, on average, about 1 in 2500 prostate cells dissociated from 8-week-old murine prostate tissue possesses stem cell activity, which is significantly lower than previous in vitro reports of 1–4% for both human and rodent prostate cells (Hudson et al. 2000; Sawicki and Rothman 2002). This may be because in vitro and in vivo techniques measure different cell entities. For example, both stem cells and progenitors may grow in vitro, whereas whole tubule structures may only be regenerated from true stem cells in vivo. Alternatively, the seeding efficiency of PSCs may be lower in vivo than in vitro. Perhaps more stringent niche requirements are necessary for tubule growth in vivo than for colony growth in vitro.

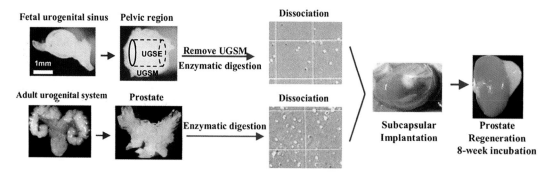

Figure 1. Schematic representation of dissociated cell prostate regeneration system. Cells dissociated from adult murine prostate tissue are mixed with dissociated UGSM cells from E16 fetuses and implanted under the kidney capsule of immunedeficient mice for the regeneration of prostatic tissues.

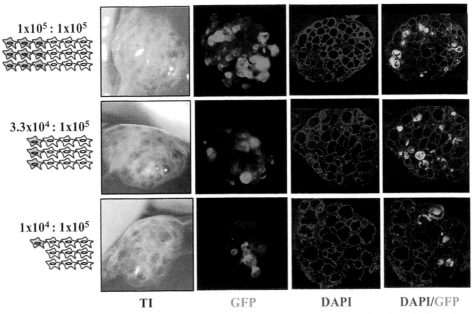

Figure 2. Development of in vivo CFU assay. Decreasing numbers of dissociated prostate cells from β-actin GFP mice are combined with a constant number (1×10^5) of wild-type prostate cells and implanted under the kidney capsule for 8 weeks. Transillumination (TI) and fluorescent (GFP) images of regenerated tissues and tissue sections.

Short-term in vitro cell culture assays have been used to monitor PSCs and progenitor cells in multiple studies. Collins and colleagues (2001) demonstrated that CD44$^+$ human prostate basal cells can be fractionated into integrin $\alpha_2\beta_1$ high- and low-expressing populations based on differential adherence to type I collagen in vitro. Rapidly adherent cells possess 3.8-fold greater colony-forming efficiency (CFE) in vitro and can develop into phenotypically normal glands when grafted onto the flanks of athymic mice. Later studies by the same group found that subdivision of the $\alpha_2\beta_1$^{hi} basal cell compartment using CD133, an NSC and HSC marker, results in an 11-fold increase in CFE in vitro (Richardson et al. 2004). CD133$^+$ $\alpha_2\beta_1$^{hi} cells can also give rise to glandular tissue in vivo, but the efficiency of tubule regeneration following this enrichment is unclear.

Stem cell antigen 1 (Sca-1), a glycosylphosphatidyl inositol (GPI)-linked cell surface protein, has been used as a marker for the enrichment of hematopoietic, mammary, and lung stem cells (Spangrude et al. 1988; Welm et al. 2002; Kim et al. 2005). We previously used the dissociated prostate CFU assay to show that Sca-1 can also be used to enrich for murine prostate stem cells (Fig. 3) (Xin et al. 2005). Because each regenerated tubule is thought to be clonal in origin, the presence of both basal and luminal cells in each tubule suggests that Sca-1$^+$ cells are at least bipotential. Using similar techniques, another group further demonstrated that the Sca-1^{hi} population contains more regenerative activity in vivo than either the Sca-1^{lo} or Sca-1$^-$ population (Burger et al. 2005). Castration, which results in an enrichment for PSCs and progenitor cells, causes a concomitant increase in the percentage of Sca-1$^+$ cells, and Sca-1$^+$ cell fractions have been shown to contain increased percentages of replication-quiescent cells that localize to the proximal region of the murine prostate nearest to the urethra (Burger et al.

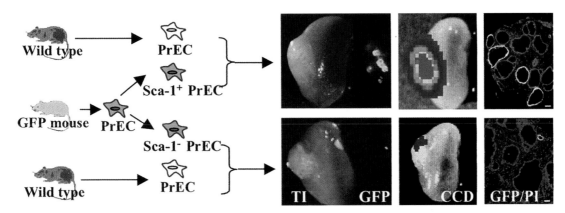

Figure 3. Cells dissociated from β-actin GFP mouse prostate tissue were separated into Sca-1$^+$ and Sca-1$^-$ fractions using magnetic beads. 1×10^5 cells from each fraction were combined with wild-type prostate cells and incubated under the kidney capsule. Transillumination (TI) and fluorescent (GFP) images of grafts and tissue sections are shown. Fluorescent signal was quantified by CCD camera (CCD). (Reprinted, with permission, from Xin et al. 2005 [©National Academy of Sciences].)

2005; Xin et al. 2005). The Sca-1 antigen, however, is present on a much larger population (10–15%) of prostate cells than could be true stem cells and, therefore, most likely enriches for both PSCs and more differentiated progenitors. The key characteristic of self-renewal activity must also be evaluated in Sca-1-enriched prostate cell subpopulations.

THE PROSTATE STEM CELL NICHE

The careful balance of quiescence, self-renewal, and differentiation of somatic stem cells is maintained by specific interactions with supportive cells and extracellular materials that comprise their specialized microenvironment, or niche (Fuchs et al. 2004). Intra- and intercellular signaling of stem cells with neighboring cells in the niche is thought to occur through three main pathways: Wnt, Sonic hedgehog (Shh), and Notch. For example, inhibition of Wnt receptors by the transgenic expression of Dickkopf-1, a secreted antagonist of Wnt signaling, results in a complete loss of intestinal epithelial stem cell niches called crypts (Kuhnert et al. 2004). Ablation of Notch-1 in transgenic mice abrogates PSC function, resulting in the inhibition of cell growth, differentiation, and branching morphogenesis of the prostate in vitro as well as in vivo following androgen replacement after castration (Wang et al. 2004). Shh signaling is also an important component of fetal prostate development. Shh expression at epithelial evaginations of the urogenital sinus epithelium activates the transcription factor Gli-1 in the mesenchyme to promote early ductal morphogenesis. Shh expression then becomes strongest in advancing distal regions of budding tubules until expression stabilizes in the adult organ (Lamm et al. 2002; Freestone et al. 2003).

PSCs are traditionally thought to reside in the basal cell layer of the prostate, where they divide to give rise to highly proliferative transit-amplifying cells (TACs) that in turn differentiate to produce neuroendocrine cells and terminal, secretory luminal cells (Bonkhoff and Remberger 1996). Several lines of evidence support this theory. The preferential survival of basal cells and loss of terminal, androgen-dependent cells following androgen deprivation suggests that the self-renewal and proliferative activities that confer tissue regeneration following androgen replacement are most likely possessed by basal cells (English et al. 1987). Cell kinetic studies demonstrating that 70% of proliferating human epithelial cells localize to the basal compartment suggest this compartment may house both the stem and transit-amplifying elements (Bonkhoff et al. 1994). Human basal cells also uniformly express bcl-2, a protein frequently found up-regulated in many types of stem cells, which is known to protect cells from apoptosis (Verhagen et al. 1992). The discovery of subsets of human cells with basal/luminal and basal/neuroendocrine intermediate phenotypes suggests that basal cells are precursors to both luminal and neuroendocrine lineages (Verhagen et al. 1992). The most striking evidence, however, supporting the concept that PSCs reside in the basal cell compartment is the discovery that mice with a homozygous knockout of p63, a prostate basal cell marker, are born without limbs or epithelial organs such as the mam-

mary and prostate glands (Mills et al. 1999; Yang et al. 1999; Signoretti et al. 2000).

An intriguing modification of this model was recently proposed by Tsujimura et al. (2002). Using BrdU labeling to identify slow-cycling cells, this group found that approximately 25% of both basal and luminal cells in the proximal region of the murine prostate nearest to the urethra retain the label following repeated rounds of androgen cycling. However, the majority of label-retaining cells in the intermediate and distal regions of the prostatic ducts were of the basal phenotype (Tsujimura et al. 2002). These data suggest that although slow-cycling stem-like cells are not confined to the basal cell lineage in the proximal region, only basal cells function like stem cells in the distal regions of prostatic tubules. This group also found that rapidly cycling TACs were predominantly localized in the distal and intermediate ductal regions where the fastest cycling cells displayed a luminal phenotype. This is consistent with prior findings that actively proliferating cells are located at the tips of prostatic ducts (Sugimura et al. 1986).

Murine prostate stem cell populations identified by functional analysis in in vivo regeneration assays also appear to localize to the proximal region of the murine prostate. Both groups identifying Sca-1 as a murine PSC marker demonstrated that the proximal region contains at least a 3- to 4-fold higher percentage of Sca-1[+] cells than more distal regions of the prostate (Burger et al. 2005; Xin et al. 2005). In an attempt to resolve some of the debate regarding the location of PSCs, we investigated the relationship of basal, luminal, and Sca-1[+] cells in the proximal region. Immunofluorescent analysis of serial sections of murine prostate tissue demonstrates that Sca-1[+] cells colocalize with both basal (CK5) and luminal (CK8) cell markers in the proximal region of prostatic ducts (Fig. 4). The basement membrane and/or some of the stromal cells in the region may also stain positive for Sca-1. However, neither basal, luminal, nor stromal cells in the distal tips of prostatic tubules express the Sca-1 antigen.

Sca-1 has been used to enrich for both fetal and adult murine HSCs and therefore may be conserved on HSCs during development (Jordan et al. 1995). To determine whether Sca-1 is also present on both fetal and adult PSCs, we harvested urogenital sinus tissue from E16 fetuses. At E16–17, solid epithelial chords begin to bud into the fetal mesenchyme where they later canalize in a proximal to distal manner (Hayward et al. 1996). Immunofluorescent analysis indicates that Sca-1 is expressed by nearly all cells within developing epithelial chords (Fig. 5). Sca-1 expression also appears to overlap with CK5 and CK8 expression at this developmental stage. These data suggest that Sca-1 expression may be conserved on the surface of fetal and adult prostate stem and progenitor cells throughout prostate development.

Many hypotheses can be proposed to explain the fact that subsets of Sca-1[+] cells possess basal and/or luminal markers. It is possible that true PSCs are not confined to the basal cell lineage. This would explain the label retention and Sca-1 expression of both basal and luminal cells in the proximal region of the prostate. Recent work by Kurita et al. (2004) supports this model. Using tissue recombinant strategies, this group demonstrated that lu-

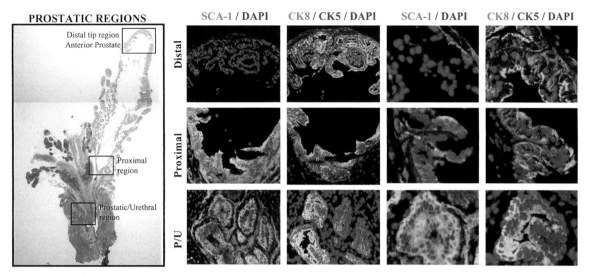

Figure 4. Analysis of cytokeratin expression profile of Sca-1⁺ prostate cells. Longitudinal sections were prepared from 8-week-old wild-type prostate tissue. Immunofluorescent analysis for Sca-1 (*green*, columns 1 and 3), CK5 (*red*, columns 2 and 4), and CK8 (*green*, columns 2 and 4) was performed and sections were counterstained with DAPI (*blue*) for visualization of cell nuclei. Fluorescent images were taken at three anatomical locations: the distal tips of tubules of the anterior lobe (Distal), the proximal region of anterior lobe tubules near the urethra (Proximal), and the prostatic/urethral epithelium (P/U).

minal and neuroendocrine cells, but not basal cells, can develop from urogenital sinus tissue of p63⁻/⁻ fetuses. Although the ductal morphology in regenerated tissue was not completely normal, this indicates that luminal cells may arise by pathways other than basal cell differentiation.

An alternative hypothesis is that PSCs may lie specifically in the basal cell layer of the proximal murine prostate. On the basis of their work, Tsujimura et al. (2002) proposed a model in which prostate stem cells in the proximal region give rise to early TACs that migrate distally where they contribute to the periodic replenishment of mature secretory cells along the tubule axis. In this model, perhaps Sca-1⁺ basal stem cells in the proximal region differentiate to give rise to early TACs possessing a more luminal-like morphology that retain the Sca-1 marker (Tsujimura et al. 2002). This would explain findings that the Sca-1⁺ prostate cell subset contains both quiescent and actively dividing cells, and the fact that Sca-1 is expressed on a larger population (15%) of prostate cells than could be true stem cells (Xin et al. 2005). Furthermore, the small numbers of Sca-1⁺ cells in more distal regions previously identified by fluorescence-activated cell sorting (FACS) analysis may constitute the

micro-niches of slow-cycling stem-like cells and early TACs identified by Tsujimura et al. (2002). Differentiation of the progeny of TACs into terminal luminal cells may then accompany loss of the Sca-1 marker.

The proximal region of the murine prostate near the urethral/prostatic boundary is an excellent candidate for the stem niche. The tubules in this region appear to form concave pocket structures highly analogous to the structures of other niches such as the intestinal crypt. Additionally, the proximal region contains a thick band of smooth muscle cells that produce high levels of the mitogen transforming growth factor-β (TGF-β), whereas stromal cells in more proliferative distal regions resemble fibroblasts and produce lower levels of the mitogen (Nemeth and Lee 1996; Nemeth et al. 1997). TGF-β has been implicated in maintaining the quiescence of HSCs (Cashman et al. 1990; Tumbar et al. 2004). Absence of TGF-β or its receptor has been shown to induce prostate epithelial cell proliferation and to diminish normal levels of apoptosis in the proximal region of transgenic mice (Kundu et al. 2000). Furthermore, recent studies by Salm et al. (2005) have demonstrated that the proximal–distal gradient of active TGF-β signaling is reversed following androgen ablation, resulting in apoptosis of distal tip cells

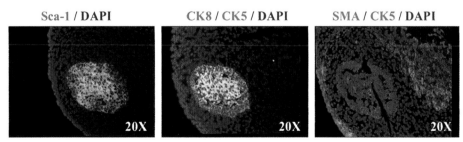

Figure 5. Sca-1 expression during fetal prostate branching morphogenesis. Immunofluorescent staining for Sca-1 in E16 epithelial chord is shown in left panel. CK5 (*red*) and CK8 (*green*) staining in the same region is shown in middle panel. Left panel shows immunostaining for CK5 (*red*) and SMA (*green*). Nuclei were counterstained with DAPI (*blue*).

and a sensitization of proximal cells to growth stimulation by cytokines that induce prostate regeneration following androgen replacement. This group suggests a model in which high levels of active TGF-β signaling in the proximal region maintain stem cell quiescence in intact animals, whereas low levels of signaling in more distal regions allow the proliferation and differentiation of TACs (Salm et al. 2005).

PROSTATE STEM CELLS IN PROSTATE CANCER

Most human cancers are considered clonal diseases in which one cell that has accumulated sufficient transforming mutations initiates unrestrained cancerous growth. De Marzo et al. (1998) have suggested that most human prostate cancers are derived from the accumulation of oncogenic events in non-terminally differentiated secretory luminal cells that still maintain some proliferative activity. In this model, mutational events disrupting cell cycle control may result in the production of secretory cells that do not undergo terminal differentiation, thereby causing the development of high-grade prostatic intraepithelial neoplasia (HGPIN). This is supported by findings that basal cells are not readily identifiable in most human prostate cancers, and that the bulk of cancer cells express luminal-cell-specific markers such as cytokeratin 8 (CK8), cytokeratin 18 (CK18), and prostate-specific antigen (PSA) (Okada et al. 1992).

This model is difficult to reconcile, however, with the identification of prostate cancer cells coexpressing both basal and luminal cell markers that may represent less-differentiated cells preceding secretory cell development in the traditional lineage hierarchy. Verhagen et al. (1992) suggested that the presence of intermediate cells indicates that prostate cancers are more likely to arise from intermediate, transit-amplifying basal cells that normally express both basal and luminal cell markers. Finding that PSCA, a putative marker of normal late-intermediate prostate cells, is also up-regulated in most stages of prostate cancer further supports this model (Reiter et al. 1998; Tran et al. 2002).

One prevailing theory for tumor initiation in many tissues implicates somatic stem cells as the predominant targets for transformation. Since stem cells persist in organisms for longer than differentiated cells, they theoretically have more opportunity to accumulate the mutations necessary for transformation (Reya et al. 2001). More mutational events would also be required to confer stem cell properties such as self-renewal in more differentiated cells. Additionally, tumorigenesis and normal organogenesis are similar. The cells comprising most tumors are heterogeneous with respect to cellular morphology, differentiation status, and function, indicating that cancer-initiating clones must have some degree of multipotentiality that is characteristic of somatic stem cells (Reya et al. 2001). Similarly, most prostate tumors contain cells resembling three of the four known cell types, such as CK8+CK18+ luminal cells, intermediate cells expressing CK5 and CK8, and scattered neuroendocrine cells expressing markers such as serotonin (Okada et al. 1992;

Verhagen et al. 1992; Aprikian et al. 1993).

The overexpression of genes typically associated with stem cells in prostate cancers further suggests that PSCs may be targets for prostate tumor initiation. The anti-apoptotic protein bcl-2 frequently present in stem cells and prostate basal cells is up-regulated in hormone-refractory prostate cancer (HRPC) (McDonnell et al. 1992; Colombel et al. 1993). Telomerase, a reverse transcriptase that promotes cell immortality by preventing telomere shortening, is another typical stem cell gene commonly expressed in prostate cancers (Sommerfeld et al. 1996). Furthermore, both telomerase and bcl-2 are present in HGPIN, which is a generally accepted precursor lesion of prostate cancer.

Another phenomenon supporting the stem cell model of tumorigenesis is the frequent dysregulation in cancer cells of pathways typically involved in the self-renewal and homeostasis of normal stem cells. Loss of the adenomatous polyposis coli (APC) gene, a scaffolding protein that binds β-catenin in the Wnt signaling pathway, is found in at least 60% of sporadic colorectal cancers and is the principal cause of familial adenomatous polyposis (Powell et al. 1992; Kinzler and Vogelstein 1996). Mutation and loss of heterozygosity of the APC gene in human prostate tumor samples have been reported by several groups (Brewster et al. 1994; Phillips et al. 1994; Watanabe et al. 1996). Disruptions in Wnt signaling may also contribute to the progression of prostate cancer to androgen independence. A higher percentage of hormone-refractory (38%) than hormone-sensitive (23%) prostate cancers present abnormal β-catenin staining (de la Taille et al. 2003). This may be explained by recent observations that nuclear β-catenin can act as an activator of the androgen receptor (AR). Overexpression of β-catenin in prostate cancer cell lines results in enhanced androgen-stimulated transcription by the AR and reduces the antagonistic capacity of bicalutamide against AR signaling (Truica et al. 2000; Chesire et al. 2002). Wnt signaling changes may therefore represent a cause of oncogenic alteration of AR signaling that is commonly found in the progression to HRPC.

The Notch and Shh pathways critical in PSC function during development also play key roles in prostate tumorigenesis. Immunohistochemical analysis has shown that expression of the Notch1 ligand Jagged1 is higher in metastases than in benign prostate tissue or localized prostate cancer (Santagata et al. 2004). Karhadkar et al. (2004) demonstrated that Shh expression is 200- to 400-fold increased in prostate cancer cell lines such as PC3, DU145, and LnCAP relative to normal epithelial cells. This group further found that stable expression of the transcription factor Gli in normal prostate epithelial cells results in the formation of aggressive tumors in vivo (Karhadkar et al. 2004). Prostate tumors are also dependent on sustained Shh signaling for vitality (Stecca et al. 2005). Significant inhibition of prostate cancer growth has been achieved by the administration of anti-hedgehog antibodies, small inhibitory RNAs (siRNAs) against GLI, and cyclopamine that antagonizes smoothened, a receptor for hedgehog proteins (Karhadkar et al. 2004; Sanchez et al. 2004).

Dysregulation of signaling in neighboring cells in the stem cell niche, rather than PSC themselves, may also contribute to cancer initiation. For example, conditional inactivation of the TGF-β type II receptor in the fibroblasts of transgenic mice results in an increase in fibroblast number as well as epithelial proliferation and the formation of PIN lesions (Bhowmick et al. 2004). Since the production of TGF-β by stromal cells in the putative PSC niche is thought to function in maintaining the quiescent state of PSCs, disruption of this signaling in stromal cells by inactivation of the TGF-β receptor may cause sufficient oncogenic insult to induce transformation of PSCs and initiate tumorigenesis.

In most types of tumors, only small subpopulations of cancer cells possess the stem-like capacity to initiate and sustain tumor growth. These cells, called "cancer stem cells," may represent the cancerous progeny of the initial transformed stem cell clone of origin of the tumor and therefore support the stem cell theory of tumor initiation. Cancer stem cells were identified in human acute myeloid leukemia (AML) by Bonnet and Dick (1997), who demonstrated that the CD34$^+$CD38$^-$ cell fraction representing only 0.1–1% of the AML cell population contained all of the tumor-initiating capacity when transplanted into NOD/SCID mice. The discovery of cancer stem cells in solid tumors such as the brain and mammary gland suggest cancer stem cells may also exist in prostate tumors (Al-Hajj et al. 2003; Singh et al. 2004). Since normal PSCs are androgen-independent, the presence of prostate cancer stem cells in primary tumors may explain the rise of androgen-independent cancer following androgen ablation therapies. Small numbers of preexisting androgen-independent cancer stem cells residing within primary tumors may become selected during androgen withdrawal and expand to produce new tumors composed entirely of androgen-independent cells. This model also explains the overexpression of stem and basal cell genes

such as bcl-2 in HRPC, and provides a mechanism for which luminal, transit-amplifying neuroendocrine cells are all produced within clonally derived tumors.

It is equally possible that differentiated cells initiate prostate tumorigenesis and then evolve to display the PSC property of androgen independence when placed under selective pressure during androgen ablation. It is also possible that initial oncogenic events take place in PSCs that do not themselves become transformed, but require additional mutations in their progeny to lead to tumor initiation. Recent efforts to investigate tumor initiation have therefore taken a reductionist approach to directly assess the tumorigenic potential of different somatic cell populations. For example, Passegue et al. (2004) inactivated *junB*, a transcriptional regulator of myelopoiesis, in HSCs and later progenitor cells to demonstrate that only HSCs could give rise to myeloproliferative disorders similar to human chronic myelogenous leukemia (CML) in transgenic mice.

Direct comparison of different prostate cell populations has so far been hindered mostly by the absence of cell surface markers for cell separation, and lack of in vivo tumorigenesis assays to assess tumor initiation and progression. To develop an in vivo tumorigenesis assay, we tested whether cells with known oncogenic potential could initiate tumorigenesis in the dissociated cell prostate regeneration system. Dissociated prostate cells from TRAMP mice expressing the viral SV40 small t and large T antigens (Greenberg et al. 1995) were mixed with prostate cells from β-actin GFP mice and UGSM and implanted in the subcapsular renal space (Fig. 6A). Eight weeks later, grafts were harvested, and sectioned tissue was examined for cancerous lesions. Figure 6B shows the presence of GFP$^-$ PIN lesions and GFP$^+$ normal tissue (panel 3). PIN lesions also stained positive for the SV40 antigen as expected (panel 2), indicating that PIN lesions were derived from TRAMP cells.

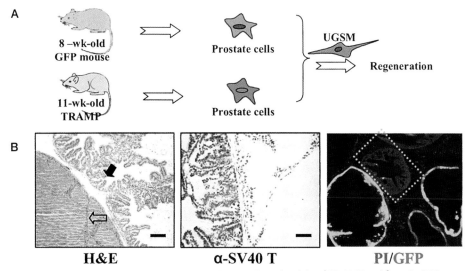

Figure 6. Development of in vivo tumorigenesis assay. (*A*) Cells were dissociated from TRAMP and β-actin GFP mouse prostate tissue, mixed, and implanted in the renal subcapsular space. (*B*) Left panel shows hematoxylin and eosin (H&E) staining of regenerated tissue. Solid arrow indicates PIN lesion, and open arrow indicates normal tissue. Middle panel shows immunohistochemical staining for the SV40 T antigen. An immunofluorescent image regenerated tissue counterstained with the nuclear stain propidium iodide (pI) is shown in right panel. Box indicates PIN lesion.

This regeneration assay can also be used to assess the impact of introducing oncogenic stimuli in normal murine prostatic epithelial cells. Infection of adult murine prostate cells with a lentivirus producing a constitutively active form of AKT, a serine/threonine kinase in the PTEN/AKT signaling pathway that is often dysregulated in human prostate cancer, results in the growth of low- and high-grade PIN, as well as some areas of carcinoma in older grafts. Infection of normal prostate cells by lentivirus containing siRNA to knock down PTEN expression also results in the formation of PIN lesions and prostate cancer in vivo (Xin et al. 2005).

Since Sca-1 has been identified as a putative murine prostate stem/progenitor cell marker, some insight about the tumor-initiating capacity of primitive prostate cells can be gained by investigating the oncogenic potential of these cells. We have demonstrated that murine prostate Sca-1$^+$ stem/progenitor cells expressing activated AKT can give rise to PIN lesions following an 8-week incubation in vivo (Xin et al. 2005). Interestingly, tumor tissue derived from normal prostate cells infected with lentivirus containing AKT contains high (75%) percentages of Sca-1$^+$ cells. This phenomenon is also observed in tumors from transgenic mice expressing the c-*myc* oncogene and mice with a conditional knockout of PTEN (H. Wu, pers. comm.). This assay will be useful in future studies to quantitatively compare the tumorigenic activity of highly enriched stem cell populations and more differentiated prostate cells, as well as for the potential identification of murine and human prostate cancer stem cells.

CONCLUSION

Although cancer stem cells have been identified as the true malignant cells within tumors, most current therapeutic strategies actually target more differentiated tumor cells. Gleevec, a targeted anticancer therapy, is a Bcr-Abl kinase inhibitor that induces remission in over 90% of newly diagnosed patients with CML (Kantarjian et al. 2002). However, the majority of cells eliminated by Gleevec are differentiated leukemic cells. Multiple studies have identified residual CML stem/progenitor cells in patients following Gleevec exposure, indicating that these cells may be preferentially resistant to the drug (Graham et al. 2002; Bhatia et al. 2003; Chu et al. 2005; Michor et al. 2005).

A similar problem may exist in current treatments for metastatic prostate cancer. Although surgical resection is an effective treatment for clinically localized prostate cancer, androgen ablation therapies to eradicate androgen-dependent metastatic prostate cancer cells are only effective for a short period of time before HRPCs appear in the absence of androgen (Klein et al. 1997). Since primitive PSCs and TACs survive but do not proliferate in the absence of androgen, it is plausible that small numbers of androgen-independent prostate cancer stem cells survive androgen ablation therapy. Theoretically, such prostate cancer stem cells should remain quiescent, or give rise to androgen-dependent progeny that die rapidly due to their androgen dependency. However, mutations conferring an-

drogen independence may arise in prostate cancer stem cells or their progeny, enabling more differentiated prostate cancer cells to survive in androgen-depleted environments. Revival of androgen receptor signaling via amplification, mutation, and/or cross-talk with other signaling pathways has been documented in patients with HRPC and in prostate cancer cell lines (Visakorpi et al. 1995; Tilley et al. 1996; Hobisch et al. 1998).

The existence of many cell types and complex intercellular interactions within most tumors make them a challenging target for therapeutic design. The increasing evidence for the role of adult stem cells in tumor initiation suggests that most cancers are developmental disorders in which pathological stem cell function results in aberrant tissue development. Therapies aimed at treating epithelial cancer as a chronic developmental disorder may therefore prove to be as efficacious as those aimed at proliferative events.

ACKNOWLEDGMENTS

We thank Hong Wu and Charles Sawyers for helpful suggestions and for permission to cite unpublished data. This work was supported by funds from the Prostate Cancer Foundation, UCLA Specialized Program of Research Excellence in Prostate Cancer (Jean Dekernion, Principal Investigator), and the Department of Urology at UCLA. O.N.W. is an Investigator of the Howard Hughes Medical Institute. D.A.L. is supported by National Institutes of Health Tumor Cell Biology Training Grant PHS T32 CA09056.

REFERENCES

Al-Hajj M., Wicha M.S., Benito-Hernandez A., Morrison S.J., and Clarke M.F. 2003. Prospective identification of tumorigenic breast cancer cells. *Proc. Natl. Acad. Sci.* **100:** 3983.

Aprikian A.G., Cordon-Cardo C., Fair W.R., and Reuter V.E. 1993. Characterization of neuroendocrine differentiation in human benign prostate and prostatic adenocarcinoma. *Cancer* **71:** 3952.

Bhatia R., Holtz M., Niu N., Gray R., Snyder D.S., Sawyers C.L., Arber D.A., Slovak M.L., and Forman S.J. 2003. Persistence of malignant hematopoietic progenitors in chronic myelogenous leukemia patients in complete cytogenetic remission following imatinib mesylate treatment. *Blood* **101:** 4701.

Bhatt R.I., Brown M.D., Hart C.A., Gilmore P., Ramani V.A., George N.J., and Clarke N.W. 2003. Novel method for the isolation and characterisation of the putative prostatic stem cell. *Cytometry A* **54:** 89.

Bhowmick N.A., Chytil A., Plieth D., Gorska A.E., Dumont N., Shappell S., Washington M.K., Neilson E.G., and Moses H.L. 2004. TGF-beta signaling in fibroblasts modulates the oncogenic potential of adjacent epithelia. *Science* **303:** 848.

Bonkhoff H. and Remberger K. 1996. Differentiation pathways and histogenetic aspects of normal and abnormal prostatic growth: A stem cell model. *Prostate* **28:** 98.

Bonkhoff H., Stein U., and Remberger K. 1994. The proliferative function of basal cells in the normal and hyperplastic human prostate. *Prostate* **24:** 114.

Bonnet D. and Dick J.E. 1997. Human acute myeloid leukemia is organized as a hierarchy that originates from a primitive hematopoietic cell. *Nat. Med.* **3:** 730.

Brewster S.F., Browne S., and Brown K.W. 1994. Somatic allelic loss at the DCC, APC, nm23-H1 and p53 tumor suppressor gene loci in human prostatic carcinoma. *J. Urol.* **151:** 1073.

Burger P.E., Xiong X., Coetzee S., Salm S.N., Moscatelli D., Goto K., and Wilson E.L. 2005. Sca-1 expression identifies stem cells in the proximal region of prostatic ducts with high capacity to reconstitute prostatic tissue. *Proc. Natl. Acad. Sci.* **102:** 7180.

Cashman J.D., Eaves A.C., Raines E.W., Ross R., and Eaves C.J. 1990. Mechanisms that regulate the cell cycle status of very primitive hematopoietic cells in long-term human marrow cultures. I. Stimulatory role of a variety of mesenchymal cell activators and inhibitory role of TGF-beta. *Blood* **75:** 96.

Chesire D.R., Ewing C.M., Gage W.R., and Isaacs W.B. 2002. In vitro evidence for complex modes of nuclear beta-catenin signaling during prostate growth and tumorigenesis. *Oncogene* **21:** 2679.

Chu S., Xu H., Shah N.P., Snyder D.S., Forman S.J., Sawyers C.L., and Bhatia R. 2005. Detection of BCR-ABL kinase mutations in CD34+ cells from chronic myelogenous leukemia patients in complete cytogenetic remission on imatinib mesylate treatment. *Blood* **105:** 2093.

Collins A.T., Habib F.K., Maitland N.J., and Neal D.E. 2001. Identification and isolation of human prostate epithelial stem cells based on alpha(2)beta(1)-integrin expression. *J. Cell Sci.* **114:** 3865.

Colombel M., Symmans F., Gil S., O'Toole K.M., Chopin D., Benson M., Olsson C.A., Korsmeyer S., and Buttyan R. 1993. Detection of the apoptosis-suppressing oncoprotein bc1-2 in hormone-refractory human prostate cancers. *Am. J. Pathol.* **143:** 390.

Cunha G.R. and Lung B. 1978. The possible influence of temporal factors in androgenic responsiveness of urogenital tissue recombinants from wild-type and androgen-insensitive (Tfm) mice. *J. Exp. Zool.* **205:** 181.

de la Taille A., Rubin M.A., Chen M.W., Vacherot F., de Medina S.G., Burchardt M., Buttyan R., and Chopin D. 2003. Beta-catenin-related anomalies in apoptosis-resistant and hormone-refractory prostate cancer cells. *Clin. Cancer Res.* **9:** 1801.

De Marzo A.M., Nelson W.G., Meeker A.K., and Coffey D.S. 1998. Stem cell features of benign and malignant prostate epithelial cells. *J. Urol.* **160:** 2381.

Dor Y., Brown J., Martinez O.I., and Melton D.A. 2004. Adult pancreatic beta-cells are formed by self-duplication rather than stem-cell differentiation. *Nature* **429:** 41.

English H.F., Santen R.J., and Isaacs J.T. 1987. Response of glandular versus basal rat ventral prostatic epithelial cells to androgen withdrawal and replacement. *Prostate* **11:** 229.

Freestone S.H., Marker P., Grace O.C., Tomlinson D.C., Cunha G.R., Harnden P., and Thomson A.A. 2003. Sonic hedgehog regulates prostatic growth and epithelial differentiation. *Dev. Biol.* **264:** 352.

Fuchs E., Tumbar T., and Guasch G. 2004. Socializing with the neighbors: Stem cells and their niche. *Cell* **116:** 769.

Graham S.M., Jorgensen H.G., Allan E., Pearson C., Alcorn M.J., Richmond L., and Holyoake T.L. 2002. Primitive, quiescent, Philadelphia-positive stem cells from patients with chronic myeloid leukemia are insensitive to STI571 in vitro. *Blood* **99:** 319.

Greenberg N.M., DeMayo F., Finegold M.J., Medina D., Tilley W.D., Aspinall J.O., Cunha G.R., Donjacour A.A., Matusik R.J., and Rosen J.M. 1995. Prostate cancer in a transgenic mouse. *Proc. Natl. Acad. Sci.* **92:** 3439.

Harrison D.E. 1980. Competitive repopulation: A new assay for long-term stem cell functional capacity. *Blood* **55:** 77.

Hayward S.W., Baskin L.S., Haughney P.C., Cunha A.R., Foster B.A., Dahiya R., Prins G.S., and Cunha G.R. 1996. Epithelial development in the rat ventral prostate, anterior prostate and seminal vesicle. *Acta Anat.* **155:** 81.

Hobisch A., Eder I.E., Putz T., Horninger W., Bartsch G., Klocker H., and Culig Z. 1998. Interleukin-6 regulates prostate-specific protein expression in prostate carcinoma cells by activation of the androgen receptor. *Cancer Res.* **58:** 4640.

Hudson D.L., O'Hare M., Watt F.M., and Masters J.R. 2000.

Proliferative heterogeneity in the human prostate: Evidence for epithelial stem cells. *Lab. Invest.* **80:** 1243.

Huntly B.J. and Gilliland D.G. 2005. Leukaemia stem cells and the evolution of cancer-stem-cell research. *Nat. Rev. Cancer* **5:** 311.

Isaacs J., Ed. 1987. *Control of cell proliferation and cell death in the normal and neoplastic prostate: A stem cell model.* Department of Health and Human Services, National Institutes of Health, Bethesda, Maryland.

Jordan C.T., Astle C.M., Zawadzki J., Mackarehtschian K., Lemischka I.R., and Harrison D.E. 1995. Long-term repopulating abilities of enriched fetal liver stem cells measured by competitive repopulation. *Exp. Hematol..* **23:** 1011.

Kantarjian H., Sawyers C., Hochhaus A., Guilhot F., Schiffer C., Gambacorti-Passerini C., Niederwieser D., Resta D., Capdeville R., Zoellner U., Talpaz M., Druker B., Goldman J., O'Brien S.G., Russell N., Fischer T., Ottmann O., Cony-Makhoul P., Facon T., Stone R., Miller C., Tallman M., Brown R., Schuster M., Loughran T., Gratwohl A., Mandelli F., Saglio G., Lazzarino M., Russo D., Baccarani M., Morra E., and the International STI571 CML Study Group. 2002. Hematologic and cytogenetic responses to imatinib mesylate in chronic myelogenous leukemia. *N. Engl. J. Med.* **346:** 645.

Karhadkar S.S., Bova G.S., Abdallah N., Dhara S., Gardner D., Maitra A., Isaacs J.T., Berman D.M., and Beachy P.A. 2004. Hedgehog signalling in prostate regeneration, neoplasia and metastasis. *Nature* **431:** 707.

Kim C.F., Jackson E.L., Woolfenden A.E., Lawrence S., Babar I., Vogel S., Crowley D., Bronson R.T., and Jacks T. 2005. Identification of bronchioalveolar stem cells in normal lung and lung cancer. *Cell* **121:** 823.

Kinzler K.W. and Vogelstein B. 1996. Lessons from hereditary colorectal cancer. *Cell* **87:** 159.

Klein K.A., Reiter R.E., Redula J., Moradi H., Zhu X.L., Brothman A.R., Lamb D.J., Marcelli M., Belldegrun A., Witte O., and Sawyers C.L. 1997. Progression of metastatic human prostate cancer to androgen independence in immunodeficient SCID mice. *Nat. Med.* **3:** 402.

Kuhnert F., Davis C.R., Wang H.T., Chu P., Lee M., Yuan J., Nusse R., and Kuo C.J. 2004. Essential requirement for Wnt signaling in proliferation of adult small intestine and colon revealed by adenoviral expression of Dickkopf-1. *Proc. Natl. Acad. Sci.* **101:** 266.

Kundu S.D., Kim I.Y., Yang T., Doglio L., Lang S., Zhang X., Buttyan R., Kim S.J., Chang J., Cai X., Wang Z., and Lee C. 2000. Absence of proximal duct apoptosis in the ventral prostate of transgenic mice carrying the C3(1)-TGF-beta type II dominant negative receptor. *Prostate* **43:** 118.

Kurita T., Medina R.T., Mills A.A., and Cunha G.R. 2004. Role of p53 and basal cells in the prostate. *Development* **131:** 4955.

Lamm M.L., Catbagan W.S., Laciak R.J., Barnett D.H., Hebner C.M., Gaffield W., Walterhouse D., Iannaccone P., and Bushman W. 2002. Sonic hedgehog activates mesenchymal Gli1 expression during prostate ductal bud formation. *Dev. Biol.* **249:** 349.

McDonnell T.J., Troncoso P., Brisbay S.M., Logothetis C., Chung L.W., Hsieh J.T., Tu S.M., and Campbell M.L. 1992. Expression of the protooncogene bcl-2 in the prostate and its association with emergence of androgen-independent prostate cancer. *Cancer Res.* **52:** 6940.

Michor F., Hughes T.P., Iwasa Y., Branford S., Shah N.P., Sawyers C.L., and Nowak M.A. 2005. Dynamics of chronic myeloid leukaemia. *Nature* **435:** 1267.

Mills A.A., Zheng B., Wang X.J., Vogel H., Roop D.R., and Bradley A. 1999. p63 is a p53 homologue required for limb and epidermal morphogenesis. *Nature* **398:** 708.

Nemeth J.A. and Lee C. 1996. Prostatic ductal system in rats: Regional variation in stromal organization. *Prostate* **28:** 124.

Nemeth J.A., Sensibar J.A., White R.R., Zelner D.J., Kim I.Y., and Lee C. 1997. Prostatic ductal system in rats: Tissue-specific expression and regional variation in stromal distribution of transforming growth factor-beta 1. *Prostate* **33:** 64.

Okada H., Tsubura A., Okamura A., Senzaki H., Naka Y., Komatz Y., and Morii S. 1992. Keratin profiles in normal/hyperplastic prostates and prostate carcinoma. *Virchows Arch. A Pathol. Anat. Histopathol.* **421:** 157.

Passegue E., Wagner E.F., and Weissman I.L. 2004. JunB deficiency leads to a myeloproliferative disorder arising from hematopoietic stem cells. *Cell* **119:** 431.

Phillips S.M., Morton D.G., Lee S.J., Wallace D.M., and Neoptolemos J.P. 1994. Loss of heterozygosity of the retinoblastoma and adenomatous polyposis susceptibility gene loci and in chromosomes 10p, 10q and 16q in human prostate cancer. *Br. J. Urol.* **73:** 390.

Powell S.M., Zilz N., Beazer-Barclay Y., Bryan T.M., Hamilton S.R., Thibodeau S.N., Vogelstein B., and Kinzler K.W. 1992. APC mutations occur early during colorectal tumorigenesis. *Nature* **359:** 235.

Reiter R.E., Gu Z., Watabe T., Thomas G., Szigeti K., Davis E., Wahl M., Nisitani S., Yamashiro J., LeBeau M.M., Loda M., and Witte O.N. 1998. Prostate stem cell antigen: A cell surface marker overexpressed in prostate cancer. *Proc. Natl. Acad. Sci.* **95:** 1735.

Reya T., Morrison S.J., Clarke M.F., and Weissman I.L. 2001. Stem cells, cancer, and cancer stem cells. *Nature* **414:** 105.

Reynolds B.A., Tetzlaff W., and Weiss S. 1992. A multipotent EGF-responsive striatal embryonic progenitor cell produces neurons and astrocytes. *J. Neurosci.* **12:** 4565.

Richardson G.D., Robson C.N., Lang S.H., Neal D.E., Maitland N.J., and Collins A.T. 2004. CD133, a novel marker for human prostatic epithelial stem cells. *J. Cell Sci.* **117:** 3539.

Salm S.N., Burger P.E., Coetzee S., Goto K., Moscatelli D., and Wilson E.L. 2005. TGF-β maintains dormancy of prostatic stem cells in the proximal region of ducts. *J. Cell Biol.* **170:** 81.

Sanchez P., Hernandez A.M., Stecca B., Kahler A.J., DeGueme A.M., Barrett A., Beyna M., Datta M.W., Datta S., and Ruiz i Altaba A. 2004. Inhibition of prostate cancer proliferation by interference with SONIC HEDGEHOG-GLI1 signaling. *Proc. Natl. Acad. Sci.* **101:** 12561.

Santagata S., Demichelis F., Riva A., Varambally S., Hofer M.D., Kutok J.L., Kim R., Tang J., Montie J.E., Chinnaiyan A.M., Rubin M.A., and Aster J.C. 2004. JAGGED1 expression is associated with prostate cancer metastasis and recurrence. *Cancer Res.* **64:** 6854.

Sawicki J.A. and Rothman C.J. 2002. Evidence for stem cells in cultures of mouse prostate epithelial cells. *Prostate* **50:** 46.

Shizuru J.A., Negrin R.S., and Weissman I.L. 2005. Hematopoietic stem and progenitor cells: Clinical and preclinical regeneration of the hematolymphoid system. *Annu. Rev. Med.* **56:** 509.

Signoretti S., Waltregny D., Dilks J., Isaac B., Lin D., Garraway L., Yang A., Montironi R., McKeon F., and Loda M. 2000. p63 is a prostate basal cell marker and is required for prostate development. *Am. J. Pathol.* **157:** 1769.

Singh S.K., Hawkins C., Clarke I.D., Squire J.A., Bayani J., Hide T., Henkelman R.M., Cusimano M.D., and Dirks P.B. 2004. Identification of human brain tumour initiating cells. *Nature* **432:** 396.

Sommerfeld H.J., Meeker A.K., Piatyszek M.A., Bova G.S., Shay J.W., and Coffey D.S. 1996. Telomerase activity: A prevalent marker of malignant human prostate tissue. *Cancer Res.* **56:** 218.

Spangrude G.J., Heimfeld S., and Weissman I.L. 1988. Purification and characterization of mouse hematopoietic stem cells. *Science* **241:** 58.

Stecca B., Mas C., and Altaba A.R. 2005. Interference with HH-GLI signaling inhibits prostate cancer. *Trends Mol. Med.* **11:** 199.

Sugimura Y., Cunha G.R., and Donjacour A.A. 1986. Morphogenesis of ductal networks in the mouse prostate. *Biol. Reprod.* **34:** 961.

Tilley W.D., Buchanan G., Hickey T.E., and Bentel J.M. 1996. Mutations in the androgen receptor gene are associated with progression of human prostate cancer to androgen independence. *Clin. Cancer Res.* **2:** 277.

Tran C.P., Lin C., Yamashiro J., and Reiter R.E. 2002. Prostate stem cell antigen as a marker of late intermediate prostate epithelial cells. *Mol. Cancer Res.* **1:** 113.

Truica C.I., Byers S., and Gelmann E.P. 2000. Beta-catenin affects androgen receptor transcriptional activity and ligand specificity. *Cancer Res.* **60:** 4709.

Tsujimura A., Koikawa Y., Salm S., Takao T., Coetzee S., Moscatelli D., Shapiro E., Lepor H., Sun T.T., and Wilson E.L. 2002. Proximal location of mouse prostate epithelial stem cells: A model of prostatic homeostasis. *J. Cell Biol.* **157:** 1257.

Tumbar T., Guasch G., Greco V., Blanpain C., Lowry W.E., Rendl M., and Fuchs E. 2004. Defining the epithelial stem cell niche in skin. *Science* **303:** 359.

Uchida N., Buck D.W., He D., Reitsma M.J., Masek M., Phan T.V., Tsukamoto A.S., Gage F.H., and Weissman I.L. 2000. Direct isolation of human central nervous system stem cells. *Proc. Natl. Acad. Sci.* **97:** 14720.

Verhagen A.P., Ramaekers F.C., Aalders T.W., Schaafsma H.E., Debruyne F.M., and Schalken J.A. 1992. Colocalization of basal and luminal cell-type cytokeratins in human prostate cancer. *Cancer Res.* **52:** 6182.

Visakorpi T., Hyytinen E., Koivisto P., Tanner M., Keinanen R., Palmberg C., Palotie A., Tammela T., Isola J., and Kallioniemi O.P. 1995. In vivo amplification of the androgen receptor gene and progression of human prostate cancer. *Nat. Genet.* **9:** 401.

Wang X.D., Shou J., Wong P., French D.M., and Gao W.Q. 2004. Notch1-expressing cells are indispensable for prostatic branching morphogenesis during development and re-growth following castration and androgen replacement. *J. Biol. Chem.* **279:** 24733.

Watanabe M., Kakiuchi H., Kato H., Shiraishi T., Yatani R., Sugimura T., and Nagao M. 1996. APC gene mutations in human prostate cancer. *Jpn. J. Clin. Oncol.* **26:** 77.

Welm B.E., Tepera S.B., Venezia T., Graubert T.A., Rosen J.M., and Goodell M.A. 2002. Sca-1(pos) cells in the mouse mammary gland represent an enriched progenitor cell population. *Dev. Biol.* **245:** 42.

Wu A.M., Till J.E., Siminovitch L., and McCulloch E.A. 1967. A cytological study of the capacity for differentiation of normal hemopoietic colony-forming cells. *J. Cell. Physiol.* **69:** 177.

Xin L., Lawson D.A., and Witte O.N. 2005. The Sca-1 cell surface marker enriches for a prostate-regenerating cell subpopulation that can initiate prostate tumorigenesis. *Proc. Natl. Acad. Sci.* **102:** 6942.

Xin L., Ide H., Kim Y., Dubey P., and Witte O.N. 2003. In vivo regeneration of murine prostate from dissociated cell populations of postnatal epithelia and urogenital sinus mesenchyme. *Proc. Natl. Acad. Sci.* (suppl. 1) **100:** 11896.

Yang A., Schweitzer R., Sun D., Kaghad M., Walker N., Bronson R.T., Tabin C., Sharpe A., Caput D., Crum C., and McKeon F. 1999. p63 is essential for regenerative proliferation in limb, craniofacial and epithelial development. *Nature* **398:** 714.

Telomere-related Genome Instability in Cancer

T. DE LANGE

The Rockefeller University, New York, New York 10021

Genome instability is a hallmark of most human cancers. Although a mutator phenotype is not required for tumorigenesis, it can foster mutations that promote tumor progression. Indeed, several inherited cancer-prone syndromes are due to mutations in DNA repair pathways. However, sporadic tumors are usually proficient in DNA repair, making it unlikely that unrepaired lesions are a major source of genome instability in sporadic cancers. A decade ago, I argued in another CSHL Press publication that a "collapse in telomere function can explain a significant portion of the genetic instability in tumors" (de Lange 1995). Since that time, the structure of mammalian telomeres has been analyzed, the consequences of telomere dysfunction have been determined, a mouse model for cancer-relevant aspects of telomere biology has been developed, and the nature and magnitude of cancer genome rearrangements have been revealed. In light of these developments, this is an opportune time to revisit the conjecture that telomere dysfunction contributes to genome instability in human cancer.

The genomes of human carcinomas and several other tumor types are in an astonishing state of disarray. The extent of genome scrambling was only appreciated after development of high-resolution techniques. Spectral karyotyping (M-FISH, SKY) has painted a picture of extensive reshuffling of chromosome segments. Techniques that display the differences between normal and cancer genomes, combined with DNA microarrays (array-CGH, Pinkel et al. 1998; ROMA, Lucito et al. 2003), have revealed countless copy number changes. What is the origin of this genome instability? Recent findings make a compelling case for the view that genome instability in human cancer is largely rooted in telomere dysfunction. Dysfunctional telomeres can explain most genome alterations observed in human cancer (Fig. 1). Moreover, the telomere-

shortening process that gives rise to dysfunctional telomeres takes place in the majority of human somatic cells, potentially explaining genome instability in many different human tumor types. Finally, a brief period of telomere dysfunction early in tumorigenesis can explain the transient nature of cancer genome instability. New data relating to these issues are discussed below.

TELOMERES AND THEIR FUNCTIONAL COLLAPSE

The molecular features of human telomeres are now understood in sufficient depth to permit formulation of a working model for how these elements protect chromosome ends (Fig. 2). In human cells, chromosomes termi-

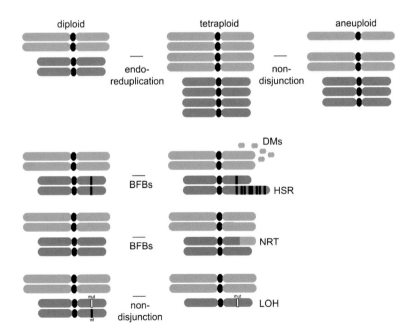

Figure 1. Telomere-related genome instability. Schematic of various types of karyotypic alterations that can be the result of telomere dysfunction.

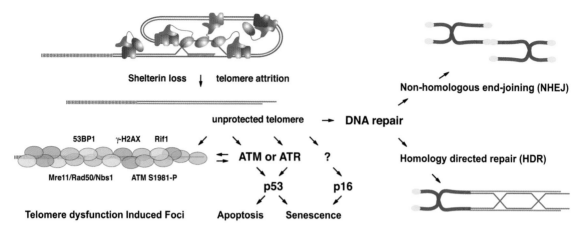

Figure 2. Telomere function and dysfunction. Schematic of the mammalian telomeric complex in the t-loop configuration associated with shelterin. The consequences of shelterin inhibition (through TRF2 deletion) and telomere attrition are depicted below.

nate in a long array of direct repeats that originate from telomerase, a telomere-specific reverse transcriptase with an RNA component that contains the template for the telomeric TTAGGG sequence (Chen and Greider 2005; Cristofari and Lingner 2005). Although DNA replication leads to progressive loss of telomeric DNA, most human and mouse cells have an adequate telomere reserve for extensive proliferation without telomerase. Ultimately, however, telomere attrition limits the proliferative life span of human cells so that activation of telomerase or an alternative pathway for telomere lengthening (ALT) is required for cellular immortalization (Neumann and Reddel 2005; Shay and Wright 2005). The ability of telomerase to counteract telomere attrition explains its virtual omnipresence in human cancer.

At the end of the telomeric repeat array, single-stranded TTAGGG repeats form a 50–300-nucleotide 3′ overhang. This tail is thought to be important for telomere function. EM analysis showed that the single-stranded TTAGGG repeats pair with CCCTAA repeats within the duplex telomeric repeat array, generating a large double-stranded loop, the t-loop (de Lange 2005a). Because the t-loop conceals the physical end of the chromosome, it might explain how cells distinguish natural chromosome ends from double-strand breaks (DSBs), but other aspects of the telomeric complex are likely to contribute to the protective function of telomeres as well.

The telomeric DNA is associated with a telomere-specific protein complex, called shelterin (de Lange 2005b). Shelterin contains three telomeric DNA-binding proteins (TRF1, TRF2, and POT1) that together confer exquisite specificity for the sequence and structure of telomeric DNA. The complex is sufficiently abundant at chromosome ends to coat the whole duplex telomeric repeat array. Shelterin is at telomeres throughout the cell cycle and present in all human cells regardless of their proliferative state. Unlike telomerase, deletion of most shelterin components results in embryonic lethality in the mouse.

Shelterin has three main functions at telomeres. It protects telomeres from DNA repair enzymes and helps conceal chromosome ends from the DNA damage response signaling pathways. The third function of shelterin is to

govern telomere length. Shelterin can control telomerase through a *cis*-acting negative feedback loop that maintains telomeres within a set size range (Smogorzewska and de Lange 2004). The challenge is to understand how shelterin and its associated factors execute these functions. In part, the answer may be found in the DNA remodeling activities of TRF1 and TRF2. Both proteins alter telomeric DNA into looped structures, suggesting that they promote t-loop formation in vivo. The t-loop structure has been invoked as an architectural mechanism to conceal chromosome ends from the repair enzymes that threaten telomere integrity and could explain why the DNA damage response does not get activated by natural chromosome ends.

Telomere function collapses when shelterin is inhibited or when the telomeric DNA has been shortened beyond a critical (but as yet undefined) minimal length. These two sources of telomere dysfunction have similar outcomes, suggesting that shortened telomeres fail to function because of insufficient loading of shelterin. Studies of the consequences of telomere attrition and shelterin inhibition have illuminated the types of genome damage resulting from telomere dysfunction.

TELOMERE-RELATED GENOME INSTABILITY

The Root Cause: Repair of Dysfunctional Telomeres

Telomere-related genome instability is caused by inappropriate DNA repair taking place at dysfunctional telomeres (Fig. 2). Damaged telomeres are processed by the two pathways that repair most DSBs: nonhomologous end-joining (NHEJ) and homology-directed repair (HDR). Both have potentially detrimental outcomes.

When the shelterin component TRF2 is inhibited or when telomeres become too short, chromosome end fusions are formed. Genetic dissection of the fusions generated by TRF2 loss indicates that they are dependent on DNA ligase IV, implicating the NHEJ pathway (Smogorzewska et al. 2002; Celli and de Lange 2005). The importance of the NHEJ pathway in this context is that it generates covalently joined chromosomes that are not readily resolved during mitosis. The resulting problems in anaphase are one of the sources of telomere-related genome instability. A challenge in telomere biology is to understand the mechanism by which shelterin and other telomere-associated factors impede NHEJ and thereby prevent telomere-related genome instability. The most likely explanation is that the t-loop structure itself provides a major hurdle for NHEJ. NHEJ involves the loading of Ku70/80 on a DNA end, which is not available in the t-loop configuration.

HDR at telomeres can also threaten genome integrity. Inappropriate recombination between two telomeres can elongate one telomere at the expense of another. Furthermore, HDR between a telomere and a chromosome-internal stretch of telomere-related sequences can result in translocations, inversions, and deletions (see Fig. 4 below).

Telomere-initiated BFB Cycles Generating Loss of Heterozygosity, Amplification, and Non-reciprocal Translocations

A main source of telomere-related chromosomal aberrations are the dicentric chromosomes formed when damaged telomeres are processed by NHEJ. Dicentrics are unstable, except when the two centromeres are so close that they function in concert. End-to-end fusions in human cells usually produce fused chromosomes with two independently functioning centromeres. Such dicentrics enter the so-called breakage-fusion-bridge (BFB) cycles

originally described by Barbara McClintock (1941). Upon breakage of the dicentric, the newly formed broken ends can initiate a second round of fusion, resulting in another dicentric chromosome and further BFB cycles. Unless the broken ends are healed with a functional telomere, the cells will have ongoing genome instability.

The BFB cycles initiated by a dicentric chromosome can have three outcomes pertinent to cancer genetics: gene losses (LOH), gene amplification, and non-reciprocal translocations (NRTs) (Fig. 3). LOH at cancer-relevant loci can occur upon breakage of a dicentric and concomitant asymmetric segregation of chromosome segments. Gene amplification is also a predicted outcome of BFB cycles, but requires the particularity that the fusion take place after DNA replication and involves sister chromatids (Fig. 3). BFB-driven gene amplification generates amplicons organized in inverted repeats, a structure frequently encountered in cancer. The integrity of the genome can further deteriorate when a broken dicentric recombines with another chromosome, giving rise to NRTs.

Inversions, Translocations, and Deletions

HDR of telomeres can induce a different set of aberrations (Fig. 4). Dysfunctional telomeres can recombine with each other, potentially giving rise to uncontrolled changes in telomere length. Since sequences with substantial homology to telomeric DNA occur at interstitial sites, a dysfunctional telomere could recombine with such an internal stretch of telomeric DNA on the same or

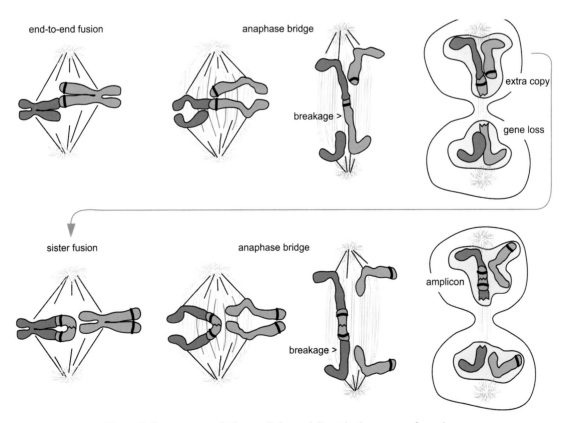

Figure 3. Consequences of telomere fusion and dicentric chromosome formation.

another chromosome. These events can generate inversions, deletions, and NRTs (Fig. 4). Indirect evidence for the participation of telomeres in HDR events with chromosome internal telomeric DNA has been obtained from ERCC1$^{-/-}$ deficient cells (Zhu et al. 2003). These cells form extrachromosomal fragments containing telomeric DNA, called telomeric DNA-containing double-minute chromosomes, TDMs, which are the predicted product of homologous recombination between interstitial telomeric DNA and a dysfunctional telomere (see Fig. 4C).

Telomere-related Tetraploidy and Aneuploidy

Telomere dysfunction is also a potential source of aneuploidy because damaged telomeres can induce endoreduplication (Fig. 5). The tetraploid cells formed by endoreduplication are the likely precursor to aneuploid genomes (Fig. 1). How cells manage to enter S phase without completing mitosis is not known. It appears that reentry into S phase occurs before anaphase. This follows from analysis of primary human cells which have become tetraploid in response to TRF2 inhibition (Smogorzewska and de Lange 2002). The metaphase spreads of such cells often show the presence of diplochromosomes, made up of four chromatids that are closely apposed or connected at the centromere. This indicates that the centromeric cohesin was still present at the time that the cell entered the second round of DNA replication. Since the centromeric cohesin is degraded at anaphase, the presence of diplochromosomes indicates that endoreduplication took place in a cell that had passed through S phase but had not yet entered anaphase. Tetraploid cells with multiple centrosomes are also observed in primary cells undergoing replicative senescence and appear to be a general outcome of telomere dysfunction. However, the frequency of these events is generally low, affecting at most 15% of the population.

Once a cell has become tetraploid, chromosome missegregation can generate aneuploid daughter cells (Fig.

1). A tetraploid cell is better able to survive genome damage, since loss of essential functions is less likely. Thus, tetraploidy and its associated aneuploidy form an ideal setting for the accumulation of oncogenic lesions.

Repression of Telomere-related Genome Instability by DNA Damage Checkpoints

Telomere-related genome instability can be prevented by the activation of the DNA damage response resulting in the culling of cells with dysfunctional telomeres. This telomere damage response has also been invoked as a pathway that limits the proliferative potential of incipient tumor cells once their telomere reserve has been depleted. It is therefore important to understand how cells detect dysfunctional telomeres. Recent data have shown that damaged telomeres activate the canonical DNA damage response (Fig. 2). The ATM kinase is activated, resulting in phosphorylation of Chk2, up-regulation of p53, and induction of p21. The DNA damage response can be detected at the dysfunctional telomeres themselves in the form of the so-called *T*elomere dysfunction *I*nduced *F*oci (TIFs), which contain DNA damage response markers such as the Mre11 complex, 53BP1, and γ-H2AX (d'Adda di Fagagna et al. 2003; Takai et al. 2003). Activation of the ATM pathway by damaged telomeres can block entry into S phase through p21-mediated inhibition of Cdk2-cycE, and p53 can induce apoptosis or senescence if the telomere damage persists.

Although the ATM kinase is a prominent transducer of the telomere damage signal, the ATR kinase, and possibly other PIKKs, can respond to dysfunctional telomeres as well (Herbig et al. 2004). For example, A-T cells retain the ability to arrest in response to dysfunctional telo-meres, and global inhibition of PIKKs with caffeine and wortmannin is required to extinguish the TIFs (Takai et al. 2003). Redundancy in the telomere damage signal is also present at the level of the effectors. Most data suggest that

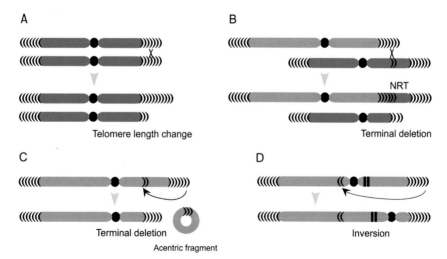

Figure 4. Potential consequences of homology-directed repair at dysfunctional telomeres. (*A*) Telomere sister chromatid exchanges can elongate one telomere at the expense of another. (*B*) HDR involving a telomere and interstitial telomeric DNA on another chromosome can give rise to terminal deletions and NRTs. (*C,D*) Recombination between a telomere and interstitial telomeric DNA on the same chromosome can give rise to a terminal deletion and an acentric fragment or an inversion, depending on the orientation of the interstitial telomeric tract.

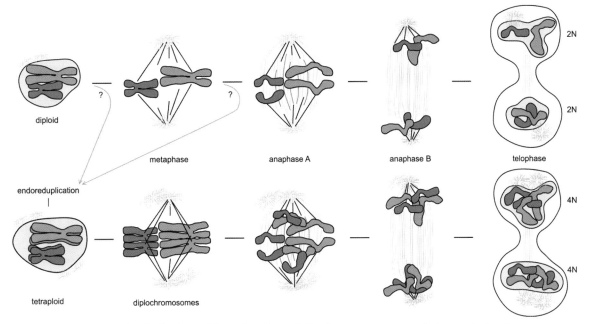

Figure 5. Endoreduplication and formation of tetraploid cells as a consequence of telomere dysfunction.

the p53 pathway is the dominant effector of telomere damage as it is for general DNA damage. However, p53-deficient fibroblasts, although dampened in their response to dysfunctional telomeres, still have the ability to undergo senescence. This secondary pathway is dependent on p16^{INK4a}. Ablation of both p53 and p16 is required to allow fibroblasts with telomere damage to enter S phase unimpeded (Jacobs and de Lange 2004; for a contrasting view, see Herbig et al. 2004). The telomere damage response is also abrogated in cells lacking p21, consistent with the proposal that p21 is the ultimate arbiter of G_1/S regulation in response to DNA damage (Brown et al. 1997).

Synthesis and Scenario

What is known about telomere dynamics, telomere function, checkpoint status, and telomerase activity can be synthesized into a scenario that plays out early in tumorigenesis before invasive characteristics have been attained. This scenario describes three distinct stages of telomere dysfunction, each with different consequences for tumorigenesis.

1. Telomere attrition and p53-dependent tumor suppression. Telomere shortening in the early stages of tumorigenesis will eventually induce a DNA damage response, and the accompanying apoptosis or senescence can block tumorigenic potential. In the epithelial compartment and in lymphoid cells, apoptosis is the predominant outcome of telomere dysfunction, whereas senescence is observed in fibroblasts. Although mouse models (see below) suggest a tumor-suppressive effect of shortening telomeres, it is not yet clear whether telomere-driven apoptosis and senescence contribute to tumor suppression in humans. Because both pathways rely heavily on p53 activation, loss of p53 (or

other components of this pathway) would curb the immediate tumor-suppressive effect of telomere shortening. In this regard, the order of events is crucial. Is p53 still functional when the telomeres become too short? The answer depends on the replicative history of the cells and the other challenges faced by the transformed cells. For instance, selection for loss of p53 function can occur when hyperplastic and neoplastic growths experience hypoxia (Graeber et al. 1996) or when cells experience a DNA damage response due to inappropriate entry into S phase (Bartkova et al. 2005; Gorgoulis et al. 2005). In p53-deficient fibroblasts, p16 can impede proliferation in response to telomere dysfunction, but it is not yet clear whether this second effector can block other cell types from proliferating beyond the telomere barrier (Jacobs and de Lange 2005). Thus, this first stage in the telomere–cancer scenario is still speculative in human cancer.

2. Crisis due to lethal levels of telomere-related genome instability. Several types of selective pressure, including telomere dysfunction, can explain the emergence of p53-deficient cells in the early stages of tumorigenesis. Such cells are expected to proliferate even if some of their telomeres are defective. If the cell has become tetraploid due to the initial telomere damage response, it may tolerate a considerable level of telomere-related genome instability. Chromosome non-disjunction and ongoing BFB cycles would not necessarily generate daughter cells with lethal genetic deficiencies.

Upon further proliferation, the genome will become increasingly unstable. As more telomeres shorten beyond the minimal functional length, more chromosome end fusions and BFB cycles will follow. The accumulating stress on the genome eventually will curb the proliferative potential of these cells, precipitating a growth crisis. There are no clear genetic determinants of the way in which a cell population perishes at this point, suggesting nonspecific cell death events due to different genetic deficiencies in the daughter cells. At this stage, cells can only survive if telomerase heals the dysfunctional telomeres and adds telomeres to the DSBs that have resulted from telomere-related chromosome breakage.

3. Telomerase keeps telomeres on the verge. Telomerase up-regulation, the final step in this scenario, often occurs early in tumor development. For instance, in breast cancer, telomerase activity becomes robust at the DCIS stage, before an invasive phenotype is acquired (Herbert et al. 2001; Meeker and Argani 2004). At this stage, telomere attrition has already removed much of the telomere reserve, providing a selective pressure for a telomere maintenance system. A similar scenario seems to apply to other epithelial cancers (Meeker et al. 2004). Once telomerase is activated, the level of telomere-related genome instability will diminish and BFB cycles can be abrogated by de novo telomere addition. The abrogation of BFB cycles will provide telomerase-positive cells with a considerable proliferative advantage.

Even though telomerase is expressed, tumor telomeres tend to be short (de Lange et al. 1990; Hastie et al. 1990). Work on telomere length maintenance has revealed how cells can attain short but stable telomeres. The length of telomeres is determined by at least three parameters: the activity telomerase, the rate of telomere shortening, and a telomere length homeostasis pathway governed by shelterin. Shelterin is part of a negative feedback loop which inhibits telomerase at a telomere that has become too long (Smogorzewska and de Lange 2004). As more shelterin is loaded onto a telomere, telomerase's ability to act on its end is diminished. The primary role of this homeostasis pathway is thought to control telomere length in the germ line and during early development so that the appropriate telomere length is transferred to all offspring. However, telomere length homeostasis is also operational in human tumor cell lines and presumably also affects telomere length in tumors in vivo. Thus, high levels of shelterin can keep tumor telomeres at a short length setting, even though telomerase is highly active.

The short telomere length of most human tumors suggests that their telomeres never regain full function, and many human tumor cell lines show evidence of partial telomere dysfunction (e.g., telomere fusions). The mild genome instability associated with such partially functional telomeres could confer a selective advantage during tumor progression while not curbing the proliferation rate of the cells.

Inherent in the Scenario: A Transient Burst of Telomere-related Genome Instability

One of the most compelling arguments in favor of telomere dysfunction as a source of genome instability in cancer is based on its transient occurrence. A mutator phenotype is favored when extrinsic or intrinsic forces require generation of variants. Through hitchhiking with selected mutations, a mutator phenotype can become fixed in the population. Such persistence of a mutator allele comes at a cost, since most mutations are deleterious. A brief episode of high mutation rate followed by return to a more stable genome would avoid a potential mutational load that might hamper proliferation. In this regard, telomere dysfunction is different from other sources of genome instability, since it is reversible through the up-regulation of telomerase. Upon acquisition of sufficient telomerase levels, this period of telomere-related scrambling will end, resulting in more stable, yet altered, genomes. The notion that tumors develop through a brief period of telomere dysfunction that generates extensive genetic diversity is borne out by data on genomic alterations during the development of breast cancer (Chin et al. 2004).

Alternative Scenarios: Tumors Lacking Telomere-related Genome Instability

If telomerase is active before malignant transformation, telomere-related genome instability is less likely to occur. Examples are the lymphomas and leukemias, probably arising in telomerase-competent cell types. The genomes of these types of cancer, while carrying telltale balanced translocations, often lack the complex karyotypes seen in carcinomas (Hilgenfeld et al. 1999; Roschke et al. 2003). Another scenario is represented by the solid tumors of early childhood, which may have ample telomere reserve and emerge as clinically detectable malignancies in a relatively short time period, thus limiting the impact of replicative telomere attrition. For example, retinoblastomas have simple karyotypes and often lack telomerase (Gupta et al. 1996). Neuroblastoma can also arise without telomerase activation and, in this tumor type, absence of telomerase is correlated with better outcome (Hiyama et al. 1995, 1997; Streutker et al. 2001).

Modeling in the Mouse

In order to mimic the telomere biology of human cells, telomerase-deficient mice have to be propagated over several generations so that their telomeres become sufficiently short. When such mice are challenged with DMBA/TPA to promote skin tumors, short telomeres have a tumor-suppressive effect (Gonzalez-Suarez et al. 2000). Similar results were obtained in the INK4a(delta 2/3) mouse model (Greenberg et al. 1999), several models for hepatocellular carcinoma (Farazi et al. 2003), and ApcMin-induced intestinal carcinoma (Rudolph et al. 2001). In these settings, telomere shortening has little or no effect on the incidence of early-stage lesions; rather, the telomere tumor suppressor pathway appears to limit tumor progression.

Although telomere attrition can limit tumor outgrowth in several mouse models, dysfunctional telomeres promote tumorigenesis in mice with a deficient p53 pathway.

This difference is likely to be due to the role of p53 in enforcing cell cycle arrest after telomere damage. Mouse cells that lack p53 continue to proliferate despite telomere dysfunction, so that the tumor-suppressive aspect of telomere dysfunction is abrogated. In that setting, the ability of telomere dysfunction to promote tumorigenesis emerges (Chin et al. 1999). A seminal experiment showed that dysfunctional telomeres specifically promote malignant transformation of epithelial cells (Artandi et al. 2000). The telomere attrition generated in the mTERC$^{-/-}$ mouse induced a remarkable shift in the tumor spectrum associated with heterozygosity for p53. Whereas p53$^{+/-}$ mice which usually develop lymphomas and sarcomas, when combined with telomere dysfunction, p53$^{+/-}$ status leads to a predominance of carcinomas. As expected, these tumors have lost the wild-type p53 allele. Karyotypic analysis indicates a higher burden of genome rearrangements in the tumors, including both clonal and nonclonal NRTs. Furthermore, these tumors show amplification and LOH, as predicted based on the known outcomes of telomere dysfunction.

Although the telomerase knockout mouse model has been extremely informative, there are two aspects of human tumorigenesis it does not reflect. In this model, tumorigenesis takes place in the context of persistent telomere dysfunction. Telomerase is absent and cannot be activated. As argued above, human tumorigenesis is more likely to progress through a transient burst of telomere-related genome instability, followed by telomerase-mediated (partial) stabilization of the genome. A second potential difference is found in the telomere damage signaling pathway in murine and human cells. Human fibroblasts can respond to telomere damage through the up-regulation of either p53 or p16, whereas mouse fibroblasts lack the p16 response. Therefore, loss of p53 is sufficient to abrogate the cell cycle arrest upon telomere damage in the mouse system. The challenge will be to create mouse models that address these issues and more accurately reflect telomere biology in human cells.

ACKNOWLEDGMENTS

The research in my laboratory is supported by grants from the National Institutes of Health (CA76027, AG16642, and GM49046) and by a grant from the Breast Cancer Research Foundation.

REFERENCES

Artandi S.E., Chang S., Lee S.L., Alson S., Gottlieb G.J., Chin L., and DePinho R.A. 2000. Telomere dysfunction promotes non-reciprocal translocations and epithelial cancers in mice. *Nature* **406:** 641.

Bartkova J., Horejsi Z., Koed K., Kramer A., Tort F., Zieger K., Guldberg P., Sehested M., Nesland J.M., Lukas C., Orntoft T., Lukas J., and Bartek J. 2005. DNA damage response as a candidate anti-cancer barrier in early human tumorigenesis. *Nature* **434:** 864.

Brown J.P., Wei W., and Sedivy J.M. 1997. Bypass of senescence after disruption of p21CIP1/WAF1 gene in normal diploid human fibroblasts. *Science* **277:** 831.

Celli G. and de Lange T. 2005. DNA processing not required for

ATM-mediated telomere damage response after TRF2 deletion. *Nat. Cell Biol.* **7:** 712.

Chen J.-L. and Greider C.W. 2005. Telomerase biochemistry and biogenesis. In *Telomeres*, 2nd edition (ed. T. de Lange et al.), p. 49. Cold Spring Harbor Laboratory Press, Cold Spring Harbor, New York.

Chin K., De Solorzano C.O., Knowles D., Jones A., Chou W., Rodriguez E.G., Kuo W.L., Ljung B.M., Chew K., Myambo K., Miranda M., Krig S., Garbe J., Stampfer M., Yaswen P., Gray J.W., and Lockett S.J. 2004. In situ analyses of genome instability in breast cancer. *Nat. Genet.* **36:** 984.

Chin L., Artandi S.E., Shen Q., Tam A., Lee S.L., Gottlieb G.J., Greider C.W., and DePinho R.A. 1999. p53 deficiency rescues the adverse effects of telomere loss and cooperates with telomere dysfunction to accelerate carcinogenesis. *Cell* **97:** 527.

Cristofari G. and Lingner J. 2005. The telomerase ribonucleoprotein particle. In *Telomeres*, 2nd edition (ed. T. de Lange et al.), p. 21. Cold Spring Harbor Laboratory Press, Cold Spring Harbor, New York.

d'Adda di Fagagna F., Reaper P.M., Clay-Farrace L., Fiegler H., Carr P., Von Zglinicki T., Saretzki G., Carter N.P., and Jackson S.P. 2003. A DNA damage checkpoint response in telomere-initiated senescence. *Nature* **426:** 194.

de Lange T. 1995. Telomere dynamics and genome instability in human cancer. In *Telomeres* (ed. E.H. Blackburn and C.W. Greider), p. 265. Cold Spring Harbor Laboratory Press, Cold Spring Harbor, New York.

―――. 2005a. Mammalian telomeres. In *Telomeres*, 2nd edition (ed. T. de Lange et al.), p. 387. Cold Spring Harbor Laboratory Press, Cold Spring Harbor, New York.

―――. 2005b. Shelterin: The protein complex that shapes and safeguards human telomeres. *Genes Dev.* **19:** 2100.

de Lange T., Shiue L., Myers R.M., Cox D.R., Naylor S.L., Killery A.M., and Varmus H.E. 1990. Structure and variability of human chromosome ends. *Mol. Cell. Biol.* **10:** 518.

Farazi P.A., Glickman J., Jiang S., Yu A., Rudolph K.L., and DePinho R.A. 2003. Differential impact of telomere dysfunction on initiation and progression of hepatocellular carcinoma. *Cancer Res.* **63:** 5021.

Gonzalez-Suarez E., Samper E., Flores J.M., and Blasco M.A. 2000. Telomerase-deficient mice with short telomeres are resistant to skin tumorigenesis. *Nat. Genet.* **26:** 114.

Gorgoulis V.G., Vassiliou L.V., Karakaidos P., Zacharatos P., Kotsinas A., Liloglou T., Venere M., Ditullio R.A.J., Kastrinakis N.G., Levy B., Kletsas D., Yoneta A., Herlyn M., Kittas C., and Halazonetis T.D. 2005. Activation of the DNA damage checkpoint and genomic instability in human precancerous lesions. *Nature* **434:** 907.

Graeber T.G., Osmanian C., Jacks T., Housman D.E., Koch C.J., Lowe S.W., and Giaccia A.J. 1996. Hypoxia-mediated selection of cells with diminished apoptotic potential in solid tumours. *Nature* **379:** 88.

Greenberg R.A., Chin L., Femino A., Lee K.H., Gottlieb G.J., Singer R.H., Greider C.W., and DePinho R.A. 1999. Short dysfunctional telomeres impair tumorigenesis in the INK4a(delta2/3) cancer-prone mouse. *Cell* **97:** 515.

Gupta J., Han L.P., Wang P., Gallie B.L., and Bacchetti S. 1996. Development of retinoblastoma in the absence of telomerase activity. *J. Natl. Cancer Inst.* **88:** 1152.

Hastie N.D., Dempster M., Dunlop M.G., Thompson A.M., Green D.K., and Allshire R.C. 1990. Telomere reduction in human colorectal carcinoma and with ageing. *Nature* **346:** 866.

Herbert B.S., Wright W.E., and Shay J.W. 2001. Telomerase and breast cancer. *Breast Cancer Res.* **3:** 146.

Herbig U., Jobling W.A., Chen B.P., Chen D.J., and Sedivy J.M. 2004. Telomere shortening triggers senescence of human cells through a pathway involving ATM, p53, and p21(CIP1), but not p16(INK4a). *Mol. Cell* **14:** 501.

Hilgenfeld E., Padilla-Nash H., Schrock E., and Ried T. 1999. Analysis of B-cell neoplasias by spectral karyotyping (SKY). *Curr. Top. Microbiol. Immunol.* **246:** 169.

Hiyama E., Hiyama K., Yokoyama T., Matsuura Y., Piatyszek M.A., and Shay J.W. 1995. Correlating telomerase activity levels with human neuroblastoma outcomes. *Nat. Med.* **1:** 249.

Hiyama E., Hiyama K., Ohtsu K., Yamaoka H., Ichikawa T., Shay J.W., and Yokoyama T. 1997. Telomerase activity in neuroblastoma: Is it a prognostic indicator of clinical behaviour? *Eur. J. Cancer* **33:** 1932.

Jacobs J.J. and de Lange T. 2004. Significant role for p16(INK4a) in p53-independent telomere-directed senescence. *Curr. Biol.* **14:** 2302.

———. 2005. p16INK4a as a second effector of the telomere damage pathway. *Cell Cycle* **4:** 1360.

Lucito R., Healy J., Alexander J., Reiner A., Esposito D., Chi M., Rodgers L., Brady A., Sebat J., Troge J., West J.A., Rostan S., Nguyen K.C., Powers S., Ye K.Q., Olshen A., Venkatraman E., Norton L., and Wigler M. 2003. Representational oligonucleotide microarray analysis: A high-resolution method to detect genome copy number variation. *Genome Res.* **13:** 2291.

McClintock B. 1941. The stability of broken ends of chromosomes in *Zea mays*. *Genetics* **26:** 234.

Meeker A.K. and Argani P. 2004. Telomere shortening occurs early during breast tumorigenesis: A cause of chromosome destabilization underlying malignant transformation? *J. Mammary Gland Biol. Neoplasia* **9:** 285.

Meeker A.K., Hicks J.L., Iacobuzio-Donahue C.A., Montgomery E.A., Westra W.H., Chan T.Y., Ronnett B.M., and De Marzo A.M. 2004. Telomere length abnormalities occur early in the initiation of epithelial carcinogenesis. *Clin. Cancer Res.* **10:** 3317.

Neumann A.A. and Reddel R.R. 2005. Telomerase-independent maintenance of mammalian telomeres. In *Telomeres* (ed. T. de Lange et al.), p. 163. Cold Spring Harbor Laboratory Press, Cold Spring Harbor, New York.

Pinkel D., Segraves R., Sudar D., Clark S., Poole I., Kowbel D., Collins C., Kuo W.L., Chen C., Zhai Y., Dairkee S.H., Ljung B.M., Gray J.W., and Albertson D.G. 1998. High resolution analysis of DNA copy number variation using comparative genomic hybridization to microarrays. *Nat. Genet.* **20:** 207.

Roschke A.V., Tonon G., Gehlhaus K.S., McTyre N., Bussey K.J., Lababidi S., Scudiero D.A., Weinstein J.N., and Kirsch I.R. 2003. Karyotypic complexity of the NCI-60 drug-screening panel. *Cancer Res.* **63:** 8634.

Rudolph K.L., Millard M., Bosenberg M.W., and DePinho R.A. 2001. Telomere dysfunction and evolution of intestinal carcinoma in mice and humans. *Nat. Genet.* **28:** 155.

Shay J.W. and Wright W.E. 2005. Telomerase and human cancer. In *Telomeres*, 2nd edition (ed. T. de Lange et al.), p. 81. Cold Spring Harbor Laboratory Press, Cold Spring Harbor, New York.

Smogorzewska A. and de Lange T. 2002. Different telomere damage signaling pathways in human and mouse cells. *EMBO J.* **21:** 4338.

———. 2004. Regulation of telomerase by telomeric proteins. *Annu. Rev. Biochem.* **73:** 177.

Smogorzewska A., Karlseder J., Holtgreve-Grez H., Jauch A., and de Lange T. 2002. DNA ligase IV-dependent NHEJ of deprotected mammalian telomeres in G1 and G2. *Curr. Biol.* **12:** 1635.

Streutker C.J., Thorner P., Fabricius N., Weitzman S., and Zielenska M. 2001. Telomerase activity as a prognostic factor in neuroblastomas. *Pediatr. Dev. Pathol.* **4:** 62.

Takai H., Smogorzewska A., and de Lange T. 2003. DNA damage foci at dysfunctional telomeres. *Curr. Biol.* **13:** 1549.

Zhu X.D., Niedernhofer L., Kuster B., Mann M., Hoeijmakers J.H., and de Lange T. 2003. ERCC1/XPF removes the 3′ overhang from uncapped telomeres and represses formation of telomeric DNA-containing double minute chromosomes. *Mol. Cell.* **12:** 1489.

Telomerase and Cancer Stem Cells

M. ARMANIOS* AND C.W. GREIDER*†

*Departments of *Oncology and †Molecular Biology and Genetics, Johns Hopkins University
School of Medicine, Baltimore, Maryland 21205*

Telomerase is critical for the integrity of stem cell compartments. Mutations in telomerase components lead to telomere shortening and hematopoietic stem cell failure in autosomal dominant dyskeratosis congenita and aplastic anemia. Telomerase activity is readily detected in most cancers but not in adult somatic cells. The telomere hypothesis for cancer states that telomerase is reactivated in late stages of carcinogenesis. However, recent evidence has suggested a stem cell origin for certain cancers, implying that the genetic alterations that lead to cancer accumulate in tissue-specific stem cells and not in adult somatic cells. In these cancers, stem cells would already have telomerase and it would not need to be reactivated. Here, we reconsider the telomere hypothesis in view of this evidence and propose that, rather than telomerase reactivation, enzyme activity may increase in later stages of carcinogenesis due to increased expression or efficient assembly of telomerase components. Understanding these mechanisms will refine approaches to telomerase inhibition in cancer.

Telomeres protect chromosome ends and distinguish them from DNA breaks. In humans, the telomeric complex consists of 5–10 kb of TTAGGG repeats bound to specialized telomere-binding proteins. Telomerase synthesizes telomeric repeats onto chromosomes to maintain telomere length (Greider and Blackburn 1985). Telomerase contains a catalytic protein component hTERT and an intrinsic RNA component hTR (Greider and Blackburn 1987; Feng et al. 1995; Nakamura et al. 1997). The RNA contains a small region that serves as a template for telomere repeat addition (Greider and Blackburn 1989). In the absence of telomerase, telomeres shorten because of the end replication problem (reviewed in Greider 1996). Critically short telomeres activate a DNA-damage response that can lead to cell cycle arrest or apoptosis (Lee et al. 1998; Hemann et al. 2001a,b; d'Adda di Fagagna et al. 2003; Hao et al. 2004). Cancers appear to have an unlimited replicative capacity and must develop mechanisms of maintaining telomere function. The telomere hypothesis for cancer proposes that normal somatic cells lack telomerase; however, in cancer cells, telomerase is reactivated and can compensate for telomere loss as cancer cells proliferate (Harley et al. 1990). Here, we reexamine the telomere hypothesis in view of accumulating evidence that the genetic events which lead to some cancers take place, not in somatic cells, but in primitive cells that have the capacity to self-renew and differentiate (Reya et al. 2001; Taipale and Beachy 2001). The fact that telomerase is already present in stem cells and need not be reactivated has implications for the ongoing pursuit of anti-telomerase therapies in cancer.

THE TELOMERE HYPOTHESIS

The telomere hypothesis was first articulated in the 1990s and was based on the fact that telomerase is active in germ cells, not readily detectable in somatic cells, and must be reactivated in cancer. This idea was based on multiple observations in human cells. First, in primary human fibroblasts, which appear to lack telomerase activity, telomeres shorten in vitro and in vivo with aging (Harley et al. 1990). Telomere shortening eventually leads to senescence, which can be bypassed by expressing hTERT, the protein component of telomerase (Bodnar et al. 1998). Second, transformation of primary cells with SV40 bypasses senescence and leads to further telomere shortening (Counter et al. 1992). The immortal cells that then arise after crisis have activated telomerase and can maintain telomere length. Unlike in primary fibroblasts, telomerase activity is readily detectable in germ cells and hematopoietic stem cells (Kim et al. 1994). The majority of cancers also have telomerase activity (Kim et al. 1994). On the basis of this evidence, it was hypothesized that cancers, presumably arising as clonal populations from somatic cells, activate telomerase, and those clones where it is active have a selective advantage in that they can divide indefinitely. In this model, telomere shortening occurs initially in the absence of telomerase and provides an environment of genomic instability, which then leads to the activation of oncogenes, silencing of tumor suppressors, and reactivation of telomerase (Hackett and Greider 2002; Feldser et al. 2003).

STEM CELLS AND CANCER

In recent years, interest in cancer as a disorder of stem cells has emerged. The stem cell theory of cancer holds that the initial events which lead to cancer occur in primitive or stem cells. By definition, these cells divide over long periods of time and are more likely to accumulate genetic defects that can lead to neoplasia. In addition, similar to cancer, stem cells possess the capacity to both self-renew and differentiate (Reya et al. 2001; Taipale and Beachy 2001). The idea gained support when it became apparent that in acute myelogenous leukemia, only rare cells occurring at a frequency of 1–100 in 10^{-6}, and not blasts, are capable of inducing leukemia in immune-deficient mice (Lapidot et al. 1994; Guenechea et al.

2001). In solid tumors, similar findings have established the likely presence of a cancer stem cell in breast cancer and glioblastoma multiforme (Al-Hajj et al. 2003; Singh et al. 2004). These cancers consist of heterogeneous populations of cells with only a minority capable of sustaining tumor growth. These subpopulations of cells may represent expansions of tissue-specific progenitors (Pardal et al. 2003). Additionally, many cancers show constitutive activation of pathways that determine stem cell identity and number. For example, up-regulated hedgehog pathway activity has been documented in upper gastrointestinal cancers, small cell lung cancer, and prostate cancer (Berman et al. 2003; Watkins et al. 2003; Karhadkar et al. 2004). In colorectal cancers, mutations in either *APC* or β-*catenin* lead to aberrant Wnt pathway activity (Morin et al. 1997). Current research is aimed at isolating and identifying the genetic determinants of cancer stem cells with the hope of designing targeted therapies that can lead to durable clinical responses.

The cancer stem cell theory is intrinsically at odds with a model of telomerase activation in cancer. Indeed, stem cells normally express telomerase, and tumors that arise from stem cells would already have telomerase and it need not be reactivated. If this is so, how then do we reconcile the fact that telomere shortening occurs in most tumors? Short telomeres appear to be present in early preneoplastic lesions (Meeker et al. 2004). For example, in prostatic intraepithelial neoplastic lesions, telomeres are short compared with neighboring benign prostatic epithelium in the same patient (van Heek et al. 2002). This is surprising, since these lesions are relatively static and do not have high mitotic rates. Advanced prostate cancers also have short telomeres, implying that there may be little change in telomere length between early and late lesions despite the higher mitotic rates in advanced carcinomas (van Heek et al. 2002). If neoplastic lesions represent genetic alterations in stem cells that are telomerase-positive, why are the telomeres short? New insights come from the rare inherited syndrome, autosomal dominant dyskeratosis congenita, where telomere shortening occurs despite the presence of telomerase and leads to stem cell failure.

STEM CELL FAILURE IN SYNDROMES OF TELOMERE SHORTENING

Dyskeratosis congenita is a rare hereditary syndrome initially described on the basis of a triad of mucocutaneous features: skin hyperpigmentation, oral leukoplakia, and nail dystrophy (Dokal and Vulliamy 2003). The main cause of morbidity is aplastic anemia, a failure of hematopoiesis due to the loss of bone marrow stem cells. In recent years, germ-line mutations in both *hTR* and *hTERT* have been identified in subsets of patients with apparently sporadic aplastic anemia (Vulliamy et al. 2002; Yamaguchi et al. 2005). Mutations in both components of telomerase are also present in families with autosomal dominant dyskeratosis congenita (Vulliamy et al. 2001; Armanios et al. 2005). Affected individuals develop idiopathic pulmonary fibrosis, liver fibrosis, hy-

pogonadism, and premature graying, which characterize this disease complex. Families with autosomal dominant dyskeratosis congenita display genetic anticipation, an earlier and more severe onset of phenotypes with successive generations. This anticipation correlates with telomere shortening, as was initially noted in the telomerase knockout mouse (Blasco et al. 1997; Vulliamy et al. 2004). The presence of heterozygous mutations in autosomal dominant dyskeratosis congenita and aplastic anemia patients suggests that haploinsufficiency of telomerase underlies the loss of stem cells.

DYSKERATOSIS CONGENITA IS A CANCER-PREDISPOSING SYNDROME

Both aplastic anemia and dyskeratosis congenita patients have an increased predisposition to malignancies, which occur in 10% of cases (Dokal 2000). The cancers that arise are generally limited to tissues of high turnover where stem cell failure is also present. For example, aplastic anemia patients are predisposed to developing acute myelogenous leukemia and myelodysplasia. In dyskeratosis congenita, there is an increased incidence of squamous cell carcinomas of the skin and upper aerodigestive tract, which arise where hyperpigmentation and oral leukoplakia also appear. Taken together, these observations imply that in humans, telomere shortening preferentially leads to stem cell loss, which is most prominent in tissues of high turnover: the skin and bone marrow. Despite the limited number of remaining stem cells, genomic instability may occur and can lead to tumor initiation.

We recently described a mouse model of autosomal dominant dyskeratosis congenita on a wild-derived Castaneus (CAST/EiJ) genetic background that has telomere lengths similar to those of humans (Hao et al. 2005). The CAST/EiJ mTR$^{-/-}$ mice developed bone marrow failure, villous atrophy, and germ cell loss similar to the phenotypes seen in dyskeratosis congenita patients. In the lower gastrointestinal tract, the mice also developed dysplastic microadenomas interspersed between atrophic lesions. The concurrent presence of both atrophy and dysplasia in the gastrointestinal tract of these CAST/EiJ mice highlights the paradoxical effect of telomere shortening on stem cell function and resembles both the degenerative and cancer-predisposition phenotypes in dyskeratosis congenita.

TELOMERE SHORTENING IN THE PRESENCE OF TELOMERASE

Since autosomal dominant dyskeratosis congenita patients are heterozygous for telomerase, we examined successive generations of CAST/EiJ mTR$^{+/-}$ mice. These mice developed progressive telo-mere shortening in later generations, which correlated with worsening cytopenias and germ cell loss (Hao et al. 2005). The evidence for haploinsufficiency of telomerase in the CAST/EiJ mTR$^{+/-}$ mouse, along with evidence of hTR and hTERT haploinsufficiency in patients with autosomal dominant dyskeratosis congenita and aplastic anemia, implies that telomere maintenance in stem cells is exquisitely sensitive to the level of telomerase (Armanios et al. 2005; Hao et al. 2005; Ly et al. 2005; Yamaguchi et al. 2005). Despite the presence of half the dose of telomerase, telomeres shorten, and defects in tissue renewal arise because of stem cell depletion. The fact that telomere shortening can be seen in cells that express telomerase supports the concept that cancers which arise from stem cells may show extensive telomere shortening even though telomerase is present.

TELOMERASE ACTIVATION OR TELOMERASE DETECTION?

The telomere hypothesis for cancer suggests that most tumors have short telomeres because they arise from telomerase-negative cells, and that telomerase is activated during tumorigenesis. Here, we suggest that tumors may arise from telomerase-positive stem cells. If telomerase is present in stem cells that give rise to a tumor, rather than being activated later, how then do we account for the absence of telomerase activity in the majority of precursor lesions (Blasco et al. 1996)?

There are at least two explanations for this. First, telomerase activity may be present in a few cells within the bulk of a premalignant lesion but may escape detection by conventional methods. As the number of cells that are telomerase-positive within a tumor expands, the level of telomerase activity detected will increase but may only reflect differences in sampling within a tumor, rather than an "off-to-on" phenomenon. Second, the level of telomerase per cell may increase as tumors progress from premalignant to malignant states. Telomerase activity is usually measured by the telomere repeat amplification protocol assay, which is not ideal for precise measurement. The lack of reliable in situ assays for telomerase activity does not allow quantitation of activity at the cellular level. One study using an in situ assay for TERT expression showed low mRNA levels in premalignant lesions, and there was an increase in both the amount of hTERT per cell and the total number of cells expressing the transcript during tumor progression (Kolquist et al. 1998). This supports the idea that both an increase in level and an increase in the number of cells expressing telomerase may occur during tumorigenesis. As methods to identify cancer stem cells improve, along with better cell-based assays of enzyme activity, these hypotheses can be further tested.

TELOMERASE LEVELS IN CANCER STEM CELLS

As we reconsider the telomere hypothesis in light of the presence of cancer stem cells, we propose that altered telomerase levels may be integral to events of tumorigenesis. The stem cells from which tumors are derived have telomerase, but telomere shortening still occurs, giving rise to premalignant lesions that have short telomeres. As cells accumulate mutations that activate oncogenes or in-

activate tumor suppressors, expression of hTERT, which is generally tightly controlled, can be deregulated and can lead to an increase in telomerase activity (Lin and Elledge 2003). Increased telomerase will then allow maintenance or even lengthening of telomeres in tumors. There is also evidence that localization of telomerase components within the nucleus is altered in cancer cells and may lead to more efficient assembly of telomerase components and, thus, increased enzyme activity (Zhu et al. 2004). Further support for the idea that increased levels of telomerase can prevent telomere shortening comes from transgenic models where TERT overexpression stabilizes telomere length in hematopoietic stem cells (Allsopp et al. 2003). Thus, an up-regulation of telomerase activity to levels at which telomeres can be maintained in cancer stem cells may be an essential step in tumorigenesis.

SUMMARY

In summary, telomerase is critical for the integrity of stem cell compartments. In autosomal dominant dyskeratosis congenita, where half the dose of telomerase is limiting, stem cell failure predominates. However, despite the presence of telomerase, telomeres shorten and likely contribute to genomic instability that leads to tumor initiation. The evidence that many cancers originate in tissue-specific stem cells contradicts the original telomere hypothesis which assumes a somatic cell origin for cancer. Here, we propose that in cancer stem cells, telomerase rather than being reactivated, is more efficient at telomere maintenance. A better understanding of these molecular events will help refine approaches to targeting telomerase in cancer stem cells.

ACKNOWLEDGMENTS

We thank Drs. John Lee and Phillip Beachy for helpful discussions. Work from our lab described here was supported by the Richard S. Ross Clinician Scientist Award to M.A., by National Institutes of Health grant P01 CA16519 to C.W.G., and by a pilot grant from the Johns Hopkins Institute for Cell Engineering to C.W.G.

REFERENCES

Al-Hajj M., Wicha M.S., Benito-Hernandez A., Morrison S.J., and Clarke M.F. 2003. Prospective identification of tumorigenic breast cancer cells. *Proc. Natl. Acad. Sci.* **100:** 3983.

Allsopp R.C., Morin G.B., Horner J.W., DePinho R., Harley C.B., and Weissman I.L. 2003. Effect of TERT over-expression on the long-term transplantation capacity of hematopoietic stem cells. *Nat. Med.* **9:** 369.

Armanios M., Chen J.L., Chang Y.P., Brodsky R.A., Hawkins A., Griffin C.A., Eshleman J.R., Cohen A.R., Chakravarti A., Hamosh A., and Greider C.W. 2005. Haploinsufficiency of telomerase reverse transcriptase leads to anticipation in autosomal dominant dyskeratosis congenita. *Proc. Natl. Acad. Sci.* **102:** 15960.

Berman D.M., Karhadkar S.S., Maitra A., Montes De Oca R., Gerstenblith M.R., Briggs K., Parker A.R., Shimada Y., Eshleman J.R., Watkins D.N., and Beachy P.A. 2003. Widespread requirement for Hedgehog ligand stimulation in growth of digestive tract tumours. *Nature* **425:** 846.

Blasco M.A., Rizen M., Greider C.W., and Hanahan D. 1996.

Differential regulation of telomerase activity and telomerase RNA during multi-stage tumorigenesis. *Nat. Genet.* **12:** 200.

Blasco M.A., Lee H.W., Hande M.P., Samper E., Lansdorp P.M., DePinho R.A., and Greider C.W. 1997. Telomere shortening and tumor formation by mouse cells lacking telomerase RNA. *Cell* **91:** 25.

Bodnar A.G., Ouellette M., Frolkis M., Holt S.E., Chiu C.P., Morin G.B., Harley C.B., Shay J.W., Lichtsteiner S., and Wright W.E. 1998. Extension of life-span by introduction of telomerase into normal human cells. *Science* **279:** 349.

Counter C.M., Avilion A.A., LeFeuvre C.E., Stewart N.G., Greider C.W., Harley C.B., and Bacchetti S. 1992. Telomere shortening associated with chromosome instability is arrested in immortal cells which express telomerase activity. *EMBO J.* **11:** 1921.

d'Adda di Fagagna F., Reaper P.M., Clay-Farrace L., Fiegler H., Carr P., Von Zglinicki T., Saretzki G., Carter N.P., and Jackson S.P. 2003. A DNA damage checkpoint response in telomere-initiated senescence. *Nature* **426:** 194.

Dokal I. 2000. Dyskeratosis congenita in all its forms. *Br. J. Haematol.* **110:** 768.

Dokal I. and Vulliamy T. 2003. Dyskeratosis congenita: Its link to telomerase and aplastic anaemia. *Blood Rev.* **17:** 217.

Feldser D.M., Hackett J.A., and Greider C.W. 2003. Telomere dysfunction and the initiation of genome instability. *Nat. Rev. Cancer* **3:** 623.

Feng J., Funk W.D., Wang S.S., Weinrich S.L., Avilion A.A., Chiu C.P., Adams R.R., Chang E., Allsopp R.C., and Yu J., et al. 1995. The RNA component of human telomerase. *Science* **269:** 1236.

Greider C.W. 1996. Telomere length regulation. *Annu. Rev. Biochem.* **65:** 337.

Greider C.W. and Blackburn E.H. 1985. Identification of a specific telomere terminal transferase activity in *Tetrahymena* extracts. *Cell* **43:** 405.

——. 1987. The telomere terminal transferase of *Tetrahymena* is a ribonucleoprotein enzyme with two kinds of primer specificity. *Cell* **51:** 887.

——. 1989. A telomeric sequence in the RNA of *Tetrahymena* telomerase required for telomere repeat synthesis. *Nature* **337:** 331.

Guenechea G., Gan O.I., Dorrell C., and Dick J.E. 2001. Distinct classes of human stem cells that differ in proliferative and self-renewal potential. *Nat. Immunol.* **2:** 75.

Hackett J.A. and Greider C.W. 2002. Balancing instability: Dual roles for telomerase and telomere dysfunction in tumorigenesis. *Oncogene* **21:** 619.

Hao L.Y., Strong M.A., and Greider C.W. 2004. Phosphorylation of H2AX at short telomeres in T cells and fibroblasts. *J. Biol. Chem.* **279:** 45148.

Hao L.-Y., Armanios M., Strong M.A., Karim B., Feldser D.M., Huso D., and Greider C.W. 2005. Short telomeres, even in the presence of telomerase, limit tissue renewal capacity. *Cell* **123:** 1121.

Harley C.B., Futcher A.B., and Greider C.W. 1990. Telomeres shorten during ageing of human fibroblasts. *Nature* **345:** 458.

Hemann M.T., Strong M.A., Hao L.Y., and Greider C.W. 2001a. The shortest telomere, not average telomere length, is critical for cell viability and chromosome stability. *Cell* **107:** 67.

Hemann M.T., Rudolph K.L., Strong M.A., DePinho R.A., Chin L., and Greider C.W. 2001b. Telomere dysfunction triggers developmentally regulated germ cell apoptosis. *Mol. Biol. Cell* **12:** 2023.

Karhadkar S.S., Bova G.S., Abdallah N., Dhara S., Gardner D., Maitra A., Isaacs J.T., Berman D.M., and Beachy P.A. 2004. Hedgehog signalling in prostate regeneration, neoplasia and metastasis. *Nature* **431:** 707.

Kim N.W., Piatyszek M.A., Prowse K.R., Harley C.B., West M.D., Ho P.L., Coviello G.M., Wright W.E., Weinrich S.L., and Shay J.W. 1994. Specific association of human telomerase activity with immortal cells and cancer. *Science* **266:** 2011.

Kolquist K.A., Ellisen L.W., Counter C.M., Meyerson M., Tan L.K., Weinberg R.A., Haber D.A., and Gerald W.L. 1998. Expression of TERT in early premalignant lesions and a subset of cells in normal tissues. *Nat. Genet.* **19:** 182.

Lapidot T., Sirard C., Vormoor J., Murdoch B., Hoang T., Caceres-Cortes J., Minden M., Paterson B., Caligiuri M.A., and Dick J.E. 1994. A cell initiating human acute myeloid leukaemia after transplantation into SCID mice. *Nature* **367:** 645.

Lee H.W., Blasco M.A., Gottlieb G.J., Horner J.W., II, Greider C.W., and DePinho R.A. 1998. Essential role of mouse telomerase in highly proliferative organs. *Nature* **392:** 569.

Lin S.Y. and Elledge S.J. 2003. Multiple tumor suppressor pathways negatively regulate telomerase. *Cell* **113:** 881.

Ly H., Calado R.T., Allard P., Baerlocher G.M., Lansdorp P.M., Young N.S., and Parslow T.G. 2005. Functional characterization of telomerase RNA variants found in patients with hematologic disorders. *Blood* **105:** 2332.

Meeker A.K., Hicks J.L., Iacobuzio-Donahue C.A., Montgomery E.A., Westra W.H., Chan T.Y., Ronnett B.M., and De Marzo A.M. 2004. Telomere length abnormalities occur early in the initiation of epithelial carcinogenesis. *Clin. Cancer Res.* **10:** 3317.

Morin P.J., Sparks A.B., Korinek V., Barker N., Clevers H., Vogelstein B., and Kinzler K.W. 1997. Activation of beta-catenin-Tcf signaling in colon cancer by mutations in beta-catenin or APC. *Science* **275:** 1787.

Nakamura T.M., Morin G.B., Chapman K.B., Weinrich S.L., Andrews W.H., Lingner J., Harley C.B., and Cech T.R. 1997. Telomerase catalytic subunit homologs from fission yeast and human. *Science* **277:** 955.

Pardal R., Clarke M.F., and Morrison S.J. 2003. Applying the principles of stem-cell biology to cancer. *Nat. Rev. Cancer* **3:** 895.

Reya T., Morrison S.J., Clarke M.F., and Weissman I.L. 2001. Stem cells, cancer, and cancer stem cells. *Nature* **414:** 105.

Singh S.K., Hawkins C., Clarke I.D., Squire J.A., Bayani J., Hide T., Henkelman R.M., Cusimano M.D., and Dirks P.B. 2004. Identification of human brain tumour initiating cells. *Nature* **432:** 396.

Taipale J. and Beachy P.A. 2001. The Hedgehog and Wnt signalling pathways in cancer. *Nature* **411:** 349.

van Heek N.T., Meeker A.K., Kern S.E., Yeo C.J., Lillemoe K.D., Cameron J.L., Offerhaus G.J., Hicks J.L., Wilentz R.E., Goggins M.G., De Marzo A.M., Hruban R.H., and Maitra A. 2002. Telomere shortening is nearly universal in pancreatic intraepithelial neoplasia. *Am. J. Pathol.* **161:** 1541.

Vulliamy T., Marrone A., Dokal I., and Mason P.J. 2002. Association between aplastic anaemia and mutations in telomerase RNA. *Lancet* **359:** 2168.

Vulliamy T., Marrone A., Szydlo R., Walne A., Mason P.J., and Dokal I. 2004. Disease anticipation is associated with progressive telomere shortening in families with dyskeratosis congenita due to mutations in TERC. *Nat. Genet.* **36:** 447.

Vulliamy T., Marrone A., Goldman F., Dearlove A., Bessler M., Mason P.J., and Dokal I. 2001. The RNA component of telomerase is mutated in autosomal dominant dyskeratosis congenita. *Nature* **413:** 432.

Watkins D.N., Berman D.M., Burkholder S.G., Wang B., Beachy P.A., and Baylin S.B. 2003. Hedgehog signalling within airway epithelial progenitors and in small-cell lung cancer. *Nature* **422:** 313.

Yamaguchi H., Calado R.T., Ly H., Kajigaya S., Baerlocher G.M., Chanock S.J., Lansdorp P.M., and Young N.S. 2005. Mutations in TERT, the gene for telomerase reverse transcriptase, in aplastic anemia. *N. Engl. J. Med.* **352:** 1413.

Zhu Y., Tomlinson R.L., Lukowiak A.A., Terns R.M., and Terns M.P. 2004. Telomerase RNA accumulates in Cajal bodies in human cancer cells. *Mol. Biol. Cell* **15:** 81.

Regulation of Telomerase by Human Papillomaviruses

D.A. Galloway,* L.C. Gewin,*[†] H. Myers,*[‡] W. Luo,*[¶] C. Grandori,*
R.A. Katzenellenbogen,*[§] and J.K. McDougall*[††]

*Program in Cancer Biology, Divisions of Human Biology and Public Health Sciences,
Fred Hutchinson Cancer Research Center, Seattle, Washington 98109-1024; §Department of Pediatrics,
University of Washington, Seattle, Washington 98195

The E6 oncoprotein of human papillomaviruses (HPVs) induces telomerase activity in primary human epithelial cells. This activity is dependent on association of E6 with E6AP, a cellular ubiquitin ligase. E6 activates the transcription of *hTERT*, the catalytic subunit of telomerase. E boxes near the start of *hTERT* transcription are required for E6; however, acetylated histones are only present in the E6 cells. We identified two isoforms of NFX1, a new binding partner of E6/E6AP. The NFX1-91 isoform binds to an X-box motif located adjacent to the proximal E box, binds Sin3A and HDACs, repressing *hTERT* transcription. It preferentially binds E6/E6AP and is targeted for ubiquitin-mediated degradation. The NFX1-123 isoform has the opposite activity, increasing *hTERT* transcription or translation. This is the first example of viral oncoproteins disrupting regulation of telomerase, a critical event in tumorigenesis.

Nearly 20% of cancers worldwide have a component of their etiology that is due to infectious agents. In some cases, infection has an indirect effect, such as the immunosuppression caused by HIV or the inflammation caused by *Helicobacter pylori*, but in other cases, such as human papillomaviruses (HPVs), viral gene products persist in the cancer and directly promote neoplasia. Understanding the mechanisms by which the viral genes disrupt the checkpoints that normally protect cells from cancer will likely provide insights into cancers in which the underlying critical abnormalities are more difficult to discern.

Both epidemiologic observations and molecular data firmly support a causal role for a group of HPVs in the etiology of virtually 100% of cervical carcinomas, as well as the majority of other anogenital cancers and a subset of head and neck cancers (Cogliano et al. 2005). Of these HPV types, HPV-16 DNA is found in more than 50% of tumors (Walboomers et al. 1999). Two viral genes, E6 and E7, are invariably retained and expressed in cervical cancers, and together E6 and E7 efficiently immortalize human epithelial cells. The E7 protein associates with the retinoblastoma (Rb) family of proteins through a LXCXE motif and promotes the ubiquitin-mediated degradation of Rb, p107, and p130 (Munger et al. 2001). Degradation of Rb is necessary but not sufficient for E7's role in cellular immortalization, which also requires sequences in the carboxy-terminal zinc-like finger (Helt and Galloway 2001). HPV-16 E6 associates with a cellular protein, E6AP, and together the complex functions as a ubiquitin ligase (Huibregtse et al. 1993). The p53 tumor suppressor is the best-studied target of E6/E6AP, and its degradation eliminates several checkpoints that normally maintain genetic stability (Kessis et al. 1993; Demers et al. 1994).

Disruption of the Rb and p53 pathways is critical for transformation of many human cell types, but it is also essential to prevent telomere shortening (Hahn et al. 1999). In some strains of human fibroblasts, the introduction of hTERT, the catalytic subunit of telomerase, is sufficient for immortalization (Bodnar et al. 1998; Kiyono et al. 1998; Vaziri and Benchimol 1998; Wang et al. 1998). Telomerase may play additional roles in tumorigenic transformation, because hTERT was necessary for transformation of cells that maintained long telomeres by the ALT pathway (Stewart et al. 2002). Nearly all tumors and cells transformed in culture express hTERT at levels that provide sufficient telomerase activity to keep telomeres above a critically short level (Kim et al. 1994). Multiple mechanisms are likely responsible for regulation of telomerase activity, including changes in transcription factors (Xu et al. 2001), loss of transcriptional repressors (Horikawa et al. 1998; Ducrest et al. 2001; Lin and Elledge 2003), changes in chromatin structure (Takakura et al. 2001; Hou et al. 2002), and altered levels of telomere-binding proteins (van Steensel et al. 1998). Additionally, cancers may arise in stem cells in which telomerase is constitutively active.

Immortalization of cells by oncogenes such as SV40 T antigen is accompanied by a stage known as crisis, or M2, in which there is both proliferation and apoptosis, and massive chromosomal instability resulting from cycles of fusion and breakage (Shay et al. 1991). A small population of cells emerge from crisis that have activated telomerase by unknown mechanisms. In contrast, immortalization of human epithelial cells by HPV E6 and E7 shows very little, if any, evidence of crisis (McDougall 1994). Although cells expressing E6/E7 show some telomere shortening, a significant proportion of cells in the culture express sufficient telomerase activity to proliferate indefinitely (Klingelhutz et al. 1994). This suggested that, unlike T antigen, the HPV oncoproteins might directly activate telomerase.

††This work is dedicated to J.K.M., who died September 13, 2003, in recognition of his seminal contributions to the papillomavirus field.
Present addresses: †Salk Institute, La Jolla, California; ‡University of California at San Francisco Medical School, San Francisco, California; ¶Vanderbilt University, Nashville, Tennessee.

Indeed, expression of HPV-16 E6, but not E7, was shown to induce telomerase activity (Klingelhutz et al. 1996). The effects of E6 were observed in two epithelial cell types, keratinocytes, and mammary epithelial cells, but not in fibroblasts (Klingelhutz et al. 1996; Wang et al. 1998). Using mutated E6 proteins, we showed that the induction of telomerase was distinct from the degradation of p53. Further studies indicated that E6 was able to activate transcription of *hTERT* (Gewin and Galloway 2001; Oh et al. 2001; Veldman et al. 2001). However, clones of E6-expressing cells had variable levels of telomerase activity, suggesting epigenetic influences on *hTERT* transcription. In this paper, we discuss what is known about the mechanism by which HPV-16 E6 activates *hTERT* transcription, and we speculate on a role for telomerase induction in the life cycle of HPVs.

E6, c-Myc, AND hTERT TRANSCRIPTION

The *hTERT* promoter contains many known transcription-factor-binding sites, including several E boxes and Sp1 sites (Horikawa and Barrett 2003). Although c-Myc is able to bind the E boxes in the *hTERT* promoter and can induce *hTERT* expression in many cell types (Wang et al. 1998; Greenberg et al. 1999; Wu et al. 1999), we and other investigators have found no correlation between the level of c-Myc expression and the ability of E6 to induce *hTERT* (Gewin and Galloway 2001; Oh et al. 2001; Veldman et al. 2001). We have, however, determined that the promoter region including the proximal E box is important for E6-mediated *hTERT* induction (Gewin and Galloway 2001; Veldman et al. 2001). Mutations in the E boxes that disrupt c-Myc binding severely diminish the ability of either c-Myc or E6 to *trans*-activate the *hTERT* promoter.

To determine whether c-Myc binding to the *hTERT* promoter was influenced by E6, chromatin immunoprecitption assays (ChIP) were performed on human foreskin keratinocytes (HFKs) expressing HPV-16 E6 or a control vector (LXSN) (Fig. 1). c-Myc occupied the *hTERT* promoter in E6 expressing HFKs in which hTERT was expressed, as well as in the LXSN-HFKs that had little or no hTERT expression. Although the overall levels of c-Myc were equivalent in the two cell types, the E6-HFKs reproducibly showed more c-Myc at the *hTERT* promoter than did the LXSN-HFKs, but never even a twofold difference, which was not enough to explain the apparent on–off switch of *hTERT* expression. Interestingly, when the *hTERT* promoter was interrogated for markers of transcriptionally active chromatin, such as acetylated histone H3 and H4, only the E6-HFKs showed these markers at the *hTERT* promoter (Fig. 1B). This indicated that although c-Myc was able to bind to the *hTERT* promoter, it was unable to recruit the necessary machinery, including histone acetyltransferases to activate *hTERT* transcription. The minimal *hTERT* promoter contains two c-Myc-binding sites, one that is 40 bp downstream of the transcription start site and another that is 220 bp upstream of the start. We have not been able to determine whether c-Myc occupies one or both of these sites, or whether E6 changes the occupation. Although c-Myc steady-state levels do not change upon E6 expression, it is possible that this is a result of balanced c-Myc induction (Kinoshita et al. 1997) and increased degradation (Gross-Mesilaty et al. 1998). E6/E6AP has been demonstrated to ubiquitinate c-Myc in vitro and in vivo (Gross-Mesilaty et al. 1998). In fact, E6 has been found at the *hTERT* promoter, and E6 can immunoprecipitate c-Myc from cell lysates (Veldman et al. 2003). Although we have been unable to demonstrate an interaction be-

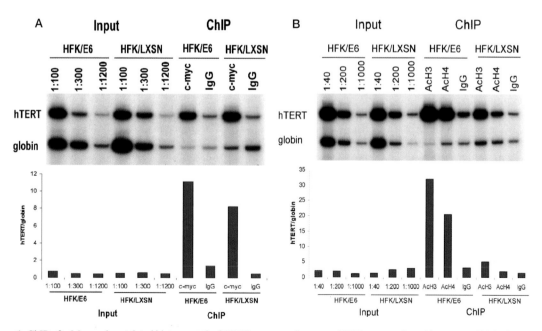

Figure 1. ChIP of c-Myc and acetylated histones at the *hTERT* promoter. Lysates of HFKs expressing either vector (LXSN) or E6 were crosslinked and immunoprecipitated with antibodies to c-Myc (*A*), acetylated histone H3 (*B*), or acetylated histone H4. After reversal of the crosslink, PCR was performed with primers spanning the two c-Myc-binding sites in the *hTERT* promoter, and to a region of human β-globin. A nonspecific IgG antibody was used as a control and the hTERT signal was normalized to a β-globin control.

tween c-Myc and E6, it remains possible that these proteins do interact in a complex at the *hTERT* promoter.

Many of the activities of the high-risk E6 proteins require their association with E6AP and degradation of target proteins. When we used mutated E6 proteins to identify domains of E6 that were necessary for activation of *hTERT*, we noted that binding of E6AP was correlated with hTERT activation but was independent of binding to p53 (Kiyono et al. 1998; Gewin and Galloway 2001). To test for the requirement for E6AP activation of *hTERT* transcription, we knocked down the expression of E6AP using shRNAs (Fig. 2). Of three shRNAs to E6AP, Esh1 expression most efficiently restored the levels of p53 in E6-expressing cells (Fig. 2B). Similarly, Esh1 strongly reduced telomerase activity as measured in a telomerase repeat amplification protocol (TRAP) assay, and it reduced the level of *hTERT* RNA. Furthermore, knockdown of E6AP in E6-expressing cells reduced the levels of acetylated histones H3 and H4. These data indicate that E6AP is required for the ability of E6 to activate *hTERT* transcription. We have not been able to show that the ubiquitin ligase activity of E6AP is required for *hTERT* transcription by expressing a catalytically dead form of E6AP (E6AP-C833A) (L. Gewin, unpubl.); however, the endogenous E6AP may be recruited to E6/E6AP-C833A complexes.

NFX1-91 IS A NOVEL REPRESSOR OF hTERT TRANSCRIPTION

Finding that E6AP was required for E6 activation of *hTERT* transcription prompted us to look for novel targets of E6/E6AP that might repress *hTERT* transcription. A survey of previously identified cellular targets of E6/E6AP did not reveal any logical contenders for *hTERT* transcriptional regulators; therefore, we began to search for new targets of E6/E6AP by a yeast two-hybrid screen. The bait construct consisted of E6AP-C833A fused to the Gal4 DNA-binding domain. To ensure equal dosage of both E6 and E6AP, the plasmid also encoded the E6 oncoprotein. In a screen of both fetal brain and HeLa cell cDNA libraries, several known E6/E6AP interactors were identified. In addition, a new E6/E6AP target protein identified in the screen was NFX1 (nuclear *f*actor binds to the *X1* box), a transcriptional repressor of MHC class II genes (Song et al. 1994). NFX1 was originally described and cloned in a screen for proteins that bound to the X-box region of MHC class II genes and is thought to be involved in a feedback loop to limit the immune response following infection.

Recent advances in the annotation of the human genome revealed that *NFX1* has two splice variants encoding isoforms with identical amino termini and variant carboxyl termini (Fig. 3, Unigene Hs. 413074). We will specify the longer 1120-amino acid isoform here as NFX1-123, because it is approximately 123 kD, and the shorter 833-amino acid isoform as NFX1-91 (~91 kD). We demonstrated that both isoforms of NFX1 are expressed in HFKs. Both isoforms have a RING finger/ PHD finger domain; found in many E3 ubiquitin ligases, this domain has been shown to confer autoubiquitination activity to NFX1 in in vitro assays (Lorick et al. 1999). The RING finger domain is followed by several cys-

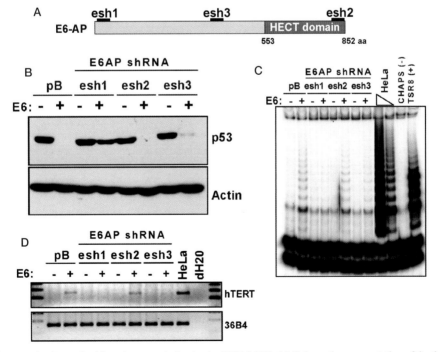

Figure 2. *E6AP* expression is required for telomerase induction by HPV-16 E6. (*A*) Schematic representation of the three shRNA constructs targeting *E6AP* (esh1,2,3). (*B*) HFKs expressing the *E6AP* shRNA constructs were subsequently transduced with LXSN empty vector (–) or LXSN-16E6 (+). p53 levels were examined by western blot. Actin is a loading control. (*C*) TRAP assay. Extracts from the same cells shown in *B* were assayed for telomerase activity. HeLa cells are a positive control lysate. CHAPS is a lysis buffer negative control. TSR8 is a synthetic template of eight telomeric repeats used as a PCR-positive control. (*D*) RT-PCR. Expression of *hTERT* RNA was examined by RT-PCR of RNA extracts. *36B4* is a loading control.

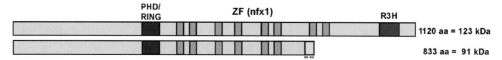

Figure 3. Schematic representation of the two NFX1 isoforms. The blue box represents a PHD/RING finger domain. Multiple green boxes indicate NFX1-type zinc-finger domains. The red box represents an R3H domain present only in NFX1-123. The yellow box indicates the unique lysine-rich carboxy-terminal domain of NFX1-91.

teine/histidine-rich sequences identified as NFX1-type zinc fingers by the Pfam database (www.sanger.ac.uk//cgi-bin/Pfam/getacc?PF01422). Identified as the DNA-binding domain of NFX1 (Song et al. 1994), these zinc fingers (C-X[1-6]-H-X-C-X3-C-[H/C]-X[3-4]-[H/C]-X[1-10]-C) are highly homologous to one another but do not exhibit the typical spacing of traditional zinc fingers. NFX1-91 contains the first six zinc fingers followed by a unique lysine-rich stretch of 25 amino acids, whereas NFX1-123 contains eight zinc fingers as well as a region known as an R3H domain believed to be involved in single-stranded nucleic acid binding (Fig. 3). The *NFX1* gene is highly conserved among eukaryotic species, although little is known about the functions of its homologs.

In reporter assays using *hTERT* promoter constructs that encoded either 219 bp or 710 bp upstream of the transcription start site, NFX1-91 repressed basal transcription or transcription that had been activated by either E6, c-Myc, or both (Gewin et al. 2004). Because NFX1 was originally identified in a screen for proteins that bind the X box of MHC class II genes, the presence of similar sequences in the *hTERT* promoter was investigated. The MHC class II X-box sequence is <u>CCTAGC</u>A<u>ACAGA</u>TG (highly conserved residues are underlined) (Song et al. 1994). Sequence scanning of the promoter found two possible X-box-like sequences within the *hTERT* proximal promoter. One of these X-box-like sequences (<u>CGTGGGAAG</u>CCCTG) overlapped with the proximal E box while the other (<u>CCTGGGAACAGGTG</u>) lay in the reverse orientation approximately 400 bp upstream of the transcription start site. To address whether NFX1-91 directly binds the proximal putative X box within the *hTERT* promoter, recombinant His-tagged NFX1 protein spanning the zinc fingers and novel carboxy-terminal tail was generated and purified for use in electrophoretic mobility shift assays (EMSA). Using titrations of recombinant protein, we found that His-NFX1-91 bound and shifted a 48-bp region surrounding the proximal E box and overlapping putative X box, and binding was slightly diminished upon mutation of five residues within the X box (Gewin et al. 2004).

Although E6 interacted with NFX1-123 in the yeast two-hybrid screen and in in vitro binding assays (L. Gewin, unpubl.), E6 preferentially bound to NFX1-91 and not to NFX1-123 in co-immunoprecipitations from 293Ts transiently transfected with AU1-tagged E6 (Gewin et al. 2004). This is particularly striking because the steady-state level of NFX1-123 is much greater than that of NFX1-123. Furthermore, the association of E6/E6AP with NFX1-91 resulted in a proteosome-dependent degradation of NFX1-91, which was not seen in HFKs expressing mutated E6 proteins that failed to bind E6AP (Gewin et al. 2004). Preliminary data indicated that degradation of

NFX1-91 was dependent on the four lysine residues in the unique carboxy-terminal tail, because mutation of these residues to alanine resulted in a much more stable protein (L. Gewin and R. Katzenellenbogen, unpubl.). Ubiquitinated NFX1-91 was much more prevalent in HFK/E6 cells than in HFK/LXSN cells, and NFX1-123 did not appear to be ubiquitinated. Longer exposures indicated that there is some ubiquitinated NFX1-91 in HFK/LXSN cells, and ubiquitination of NFX1-91 was readily observed in 293T cells (Gewin et al. 2994). These observations are similar to what is seen with p53; i.e., that p53 stability is regulated by E6/E6AP in E6 cells and by a different ubiquitin ligase, MDM2, in non-E6-expressing cells.

To address directly whether NFX1-91 functions as a transcriptional repressor at the endogenous *hTERT* promoter, NFX1-91 expression was reduced using stable shRNA expression in HFKs. We constructed an shRNA construct targeted to the unique 3′ untranslated region (3′UTR) of NFX1-91. The NFX1-91 shRNA (n91sh) reduced NFX1-91 protein levels in HFKs accompanied by derepression of the *hTERT* promoter even in cells lacking E6 expression (Gewin et al. 2004). E6 cells with reduced NFX1-91 expression had a greater than twofold increased expression of hTERT as demonstrated by RT-PCR and TRAP assay. Furthermore, in HFK/LXSN cells with reduced NFX1-91 levels, acetylated H3 and H4 were increased at the *hTERT* promoter in ChIP assays.

Transcriptional repressors often function by recruiting histone deacetylases (HDACs) to the promoter through scaffold proteins such as Sin3A. In vitro co-immunoprecipitation experiments showed that endogenous NFX1-91 directly bound to in vitro translated, ^{35}S-labeled mSin3A, and in vivo co-immunoprecipitation assays also showed that FLAG-tagged NFX1-91 could bind to myc-tagged mSin3A in 293T cells (W. Luo et al., unpubl.). FLAG-tagged-NFX1-91 immunoprecipitates showed high HDAC activity, whereas FLAG-NFX1-123 immunoprecipitates showed relatively lower HDAC activity. Surprisingly, the amino-terminal region of NFX1-91 (upstream of the PHD/RING finger) bound to Sin3A, a region that is in common with NFX1-123. It is unclear why NFX1-91, but not the 123-kD isoform, binds Sin3A; we speculate that the unique carboxy-terminal tails of the two isoforms influence binding to DNA and to other proteins.

Taken together, our data suggest a model (Fig. 4) in which NFX1-91 functions to repress *hTERT* transcription in HFKs by binding to an X-box motif that is located adjacent to the proximal E box in the *hTERT* promoter. NFX1-91 binds to Sin3A and recruits HDACs to the promoter. It is unclear whether binding of NFX1-91 occludes binding of c-Myc to the proximal E-box. Although we know that c-Myc occupies the *hTERT* promoter in HFKs, the resolution of the ChIP assay does not allow us to determine whether

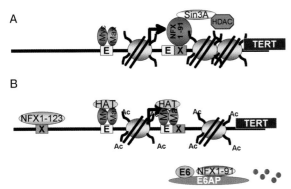

Figure 4. Model for the regulation of the *hTERT* promoter by HPV-16 E6. (*A*) In normal HFKs, NFX1-91 binds to an X box that partially overlaps an E box, perhaps occluding binding of c-Myc to the E-box. NFX1-91 binds Sin3A and recruits HDACs to repress transcription. c-Myc is present at the promoter, although unable to activate transcription. (*B*) In E6-HFKs, NFX1-91 is targeted for ubiquitin-mediated degradation. This may allow occupancy of the proximal E box by c-Myc and recruitment of HATs. NFX1-123 may bind a distal X-box motif contributing to activation.

c-Myc binds one or both E boxes in the minimal promoter. What is clear is that NFX1-91 binding prevents the recruitment or activity of histone acetyltransferases (HATs) at the *hTERT* promoter. In E6-expressing HFKs, NFX1-91 binds to the E6/E6AP complex, and it is ubiquitinated and targeted for proteosomal degradation. It is possible that simply removing NFX1-91 from the promoter is sufficient to allow c-Myc to activate transcription of hTERT; alternatively, this may be only one step in the process of robustly inducing *hTERT* expression by E6. Given that E6/E6AP and the NFX1 RING finger possess E3 ubiquitin ligase activity, it is possible that other proteins at the promoter, such as histone H2B, c-Myc, or other transcriptional regulators, may be ubiquitinated by bringing E6/E6AP to the promoter. An attractive synthesis of this model with our data is that E6/E6AP may function at multiple levels to induce *hTERT*. First, the E6/E6AP complex may target NFX1-91 for increased turnover to derepress the promoter; then, an E3 ligase may ubiquitinate and activate the c-Myc bound at the *hTERT* promoter. This theory and the possible role of the E3 ligase activity of the NFX1 isoforms or the E6/E6AP complex to ubiquitinate either histone H2B or c-Myc remain to be tested.

NFX1-123 AND ITS ROLE IN hTERT TRANSCRIPTION

Reporter assays indicated that NFX1-123 could co-activate the *hTERT* promoter when present with c-Myc, E6, or both. We considered a simple model in which degradation of NFX1-91 by E6/E6AP would lead to replacement

with NFX1-123 at the proximal E box and recruitment of histone acetyltransferases, but that model seems incorrect for several reasons. First, NFX1-123 did not activate transcription in promoter assays when only the 219-bp promoter was used, nor did it bind to the proximal X box in gel-shift assays. Second, NFX1-123 is much more abundant and stable than NFX1-91; thus, one might anticipate that if NX1 could occupy the proximal X box, it would displace NFX1-91. A second X box is located about 400 bp upstream of the proximal X box, and we will examine binding of NFX1-123 to that site.

As another approach to investigate how NFX1-123 might regulate transcription of hTERT, we used tagged forms of NFX1-123 and identified co-immunoprecipitating proteins by mass spectrometry (R.A. Katzenellenbogen et al., unpubl.). Of interest, several poly(A)-binding proteins were identified. Cytoplasmic poly(A)-binding proteins (PABPCs) contain four RNA recognition motifs (RRM) in their amino termini, which define the fidelity with which they bind poly(A) or poly(AU) RNA (Kuhn and Wahle 2004). At their carboxyl termini, PABPCs have a poly(A)-binding protein carboxy-terminal domain, similarly named PABC, and with this domain they interact with other proteins that have a poly(A)-binding interacting motif, named PAM2. Cytoplasmic poly(A)-binding proteins bind to the 3′ poly(A) tail of mRNA and directly interact with 5′ cap proteins, forming a closed loop of RNA. This loop helps recruit the 40S ribosome subunit to the mRNA and may in fact keep ribosomes on the same mRNA, thereby allowing reinitiation of translation. These proteins also stabilize mRNA transcripts by blocking premature decapping of the mRNA and by preventing deadenylation of mRNA. Thus, PABPs work downstream of transcriptional activation; they lengthen the half-life of mRNA and increase protein expression through improved translation. We found that NFX1-123 has a putative PAM2 motif in its amino terminus. In preliminary experiments, we found that NFX1-123 can interact with poly(A)-binding proteins and that mutation of the PAM2 site significantly reduces that interaction. Importantly, mutation of that site reduced expression of luciferase in the hTERT reporter assays. Thus, we are exploring a model (Fig. 5) in which NFX1-123 may augment hTERT expression by a posttranscriptional mechanism. This mechanism may act in concert with direct activation of the *hTERT* promoter through binding of NFX1-123 to the distal X box in the *hTERT* promoter.

ACTIVATION OF TELOMERASE AND THE PAPILLOMAVIRUS LIFE CYCLE

Viruses, particularly those with small genomes, likely only retain gene products that in some way benefit their life cycle. HPVs infect basal cells in cutaneous or mucosal

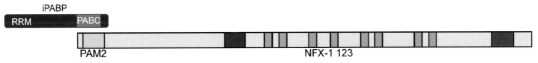

Figure 5. Schematic of interactions between poly(A)-binding proteins with NFX1-123. A PABPC motif in the carboxyl terminus of the inducible poly(A)-binding protein (iPABP) interacts with the PAM2 domain in the amino terminus of NFX1-123.

epithelium and complete their life cycle entirely within the epithelium. HPVs induce cellular replication of otherwise quiescent cells, expanding the proliferative compartment of the epithelial layer, yet epithelial differentiation proceeds and is required for the expression of the capsid proteins (Howley and Schlegel 1988). Overall, the number of population doublings that an HPV-infected epithelial cell will undergo are likely to be too few to critically shorten telomeres. Therefore, we have wondered how induction of telomerase benefits human papillomaviruses and have considered three possible explanations.

First, HPV likely remains latent or persistent in epithelial cells, and the induction of telomerase might confer long-lasting replicative potential. Although this is possible, there is no evidence that cells which harbor HPV undergo extensive replication. Additionally, HPV may remain latent in stem cells in which telomerase is constitutively active.

A second possibility is that NFX1-91 likely represses many genes in addition to *hTERT*, and derepression of some of these other genes by E6/E6AP may be important for the virus life cycle. We are currently identifying other targets of NFX1.

A third possibility is that telomerase has activities other than elongation of telomeres which may be beneficial to HPVs. Several lines of evidence lend support to this hypothesis. hTERT has been shown to be required for tumorigenic transformation of cells that are able to maintain their telomeres by the ALT mechanism (Stewart et al. 2002). Expression of hTERT in two different cell types resulted in increased expression of genes in the EGFR signaling pathway (Lindvall et al. 2003; Smith et al. 2003), implying that hTERT might stimulate growth. Induction of TERT expression in mouse skin lacking the RNA component of telomerase resulted in the proliferation of normally quiescent stem cells in hair follicles (Sarin et al. 2005). Additionally, we reported that expression of hTERT in young fibroblasts with long telomeres increased the density at which the cells could grow and strongly cooperated with activated Ha-Ras to increase saturation density (Benanti and Galloway 2004). Thus, we speculate that the induction of telomerase by human papillomaviruses might provide a growth advantage to HPV-infected cells that is independent of telomere lengthening.

CONCLUSIONS

Induction of telomerase appears to be a common and requisite event in the immortalization and transformation of many cell types, and in the development of human cancers. In our studies to determine how HPV-16 E6 induces telomerase in epithelial cells, we have identified NFX1-91 as a cellular repressor of the human *hTERT* promoter both in vivo and in vitro that is destabilized by the E6/E6AP complex. A related splice variant, NFX1-123, can co-activate the *hTERT* promoter, although its role in telomerase regulation remains to be defined.

A recent study found three different tumor suppressor/oncogene pathways involved in hTERT repression (Lin and Elledge 2003). It is striking that these repressors do not seem redundant; oncogenic stimulation that abrogates any one of them is sufficient to relieve repression. Therefore, it is not implausible that, despite the identification of several *hTERT* repressor proteins, E6/E6AP specifically targets only one transcriptional repressor, NFX1-91, to induce *hTERT* expression. It is likely that future investigations will reveal different cell-type specificities for *hTERT* repressors and variability in the responsiveness of different cell types to perturbations of these repressors. How, or whether, induction of hTERT benefits HPV-infected cells is speculative but may involve telomere-independent activities of hTERT.

ACKNOWLEDGMENTS

We thank members of the Galloway and McDougall labs, past and present, for their many contributions to this work, particularly Al Klingelhutz, Scott Foster, Tohru Kiyono, Jenn Koop, and Jenny Benanti. This work was supported by grants from the National Cancer Institute (CA42792 and CA64795) to D.A.G. and J.K.M. L.C.G. was supported in part by the Viral Oncology Training grant (T32 CA 09229-23), and R.A.K. and L.C.G. were supported in part by a STD/AIDS Research Training grant (T32 AI07140).

REFERENCES

Benanti J.A. and Galloway D.A. 2004. Normal human fibroblasts are resistant to RAS-induced senescence. *Mol. Cell. Biol.* 24: 2842.

Bodnar A.G., Ouellette M., Frolkis M., Holt S.E., Chiu C.P., Morin G.B., Harley C.B., Shay J.W., Lichtsteiner S., and Wright W.E. 1998. Extension of life-span by introduction of telomerase into normal human cells (comment). *Science* 279: 349.

Cogliano V., Baan R., Straif K., Grosse Y., Secretan B., El Ghissassi F., and the W.H.O. International Agency for Research on Cancer. 2005. Carcinogenicity of human papillomaviruses. *Lancet Oncol.* 6: 204.

Demers G.W., Foster S.A., Halbert C.L., and Galloway D.A. 1994. Growth arrest by induction of p53 in DNA damaged keratinocytes is bypassed by human papillomavirus 16 E7. *Proc. Natl. Acad. Sci.* 91: 4382.

Ducrest A.L., Amacker M., Mathieu Y.D., Cuthbert A.P., Trott D.A., Newbold R.F., Nabholz M., and Lingner J. 2001. Regulation of human telomerase activity: Repression by normal chromosome 3 abolishes nuclear telomerase reverse transcriptase transcripts but does not affect c-Myc activity. *Cancer Res.* 61: 7594.

Gewin L. and Galloway D.A. 2001. E box-dependent activation of telomerase by human papillomavirus type 16 E6 does not require induction of c-myc. *J. Virol.* 75: 7198.

Gewin L., Myers H., Kiyono T., and Galloway D.A. 2004. Identification of a novel telomerase repressor that interacts with the human papillomavirus type-16 E6/E6-AP complex. *Genes Dev.* 18: 2269.

Greenberg R.A., O'Hagan R.C., Deng H., Xiao Q., Hann S.R., Adams R.R., Lichtsteiner S., Chin L., Morin G.B., and DePinho R.A. 1999. Telomerase reverse transcriptase gene is a direct target of c-Myc but is not functionally equivalent in cellular transformation. *Oncogene* 18: 1219.

Gross-Mesilaty S., Reinstein E., Bercovich B., Tobias K.E., Schwartz A.L., Kahana C., and Ciechanover A. 1998. Basal and human papillomavirus E6 oncoprotein-induced degradation of Myc proteins by the ubiquitin pathway. *Proc. Natl. Acad. Sci.* 5: 8058.

Hahn W.C., Counter C.M., Lundberg A.S., Beijersbergen R.L., Brooks M.W., and Weinberg R.A. 1999. Creation of human tumour cells with defined genetic elements (comment). *Nature* **400:** 464.

Helt A.M. and Galloway D.A. 2001. Destabilization of the retinoblastoma tumor suppressor by human papillomavirus type 16 E7 is not sufficient to overcome cell cycle arrest in human keratinocytes. *J. Virol.* **75:** 6737.

Horikawa I. and Barrett J.C. 2003. Transcriptional regulation of the telomerase hTERT gene as a target for cellular and viral oncogenic mechanisms. *Carcinogenesis* **24:** 1167.

Horikawa I., Oshimura M., and Barrett J.C. 1998. Repression of the telomerase catalytic subunit by a gene on human chromosome 3 that induces cellular senescence. *Mol. Carcinog.* **22:** 65.

Hou M., Wang X., Popov N., Zhang A., Zhao X., Zhou R., Zetterberg A., Bjorkholm M., Henriksson M., Gruber A., and Xu D. 2002. The histone deacetylase inhibitor trichostatin A derepresses the telomerase reverse transcriptase (hTERT) gene in human cells. *Exp. Cell Res.* **274:** 25.

Howley P.M. and Schlegel R. 1988. The human papillomaviruses: An overview. *Am. J. Med.* **85:** 155.

Huibregtse J.M., Scheffner M., and Howley P.M. 1993. Localization of the E6-AP regions that direct human papillomavirus E6 binding, association with p53, and ubiquitination of associated proteins. *Mol. Cell. Biol.* **13:** 4918.

Kessis T.D., Slebos R.J., Nelson W.G., Kastan M.B., Plunkett B.S., Han S.M., Lorincz A.T., Hedrick L., and Cho K.R. 1993. Human papillomavirus 16 E6 expression disrupts the p53-mediated cellular response to DNA damage. *Proc. Natl. Acad. Sci.* **90:** 3988.

Kim N.W., Piatyszek M.A., Prowse K.R., Harley C.B., West M.D., Ho P.L.C., Coviello G.M., Wright W.E., Weinrich S.L., and Shay J.W. 1994. Specific association of human telomerase activity with immortal cells and cancer. *Science* **266:** 2011.

Kinoshita T., Shirasawa H., Shino Y., Moriya H., Desbarats L., Eilers M., and Simizu B. 1997. Transactivation of prothymosin α and c-myc promoters by human papillomavirus type 16 E6 protein. *Virology* **232:** 53.

Kiyono T., Foster S.A., Koop J.I., McDougall J.K., Galloway D.A., and Klingelhutz A.J. 1998. Both Rb/p16INK4a inactivation and telomerase activity are required to immortalize human epithelial cells (comment). *Nature* **396:** 84.

Klingelhutz A.J., Foster S.A., and McDougall J.K. 1996. Telomerase activation by the E6 gene product of human papillomavirus type 16. *Nature* **380:** 79.

Klingelhutz A.J., Barber S.A., Smith P.P., Dyer K., and McDougall J.K. 1994. Restoration of telomeres in human papillomavirus-immortalized human anogenital epithelial cells. *Mol. Cell. Biol.* **14:** 961.

Kuhn U. and Wahle E. 2004. Structure and function of poly(A) binding proteins. *Biochim. Biophys. Acta* **1678:** 67.

Lin S.Y. and Elledge S.J. 2003. Multiple tumor suppressor pathways negatively regulate telomerase. *Cell* **113:** 881.

Lindvall C., Hou M., Komurasaki T., Zheng C., Henriksson M., Sedivy J.M., Bjorkholm M., Teh B.T., Nordenskjold M., and Xu D. 2003. Molecular characterization of human telomerase reverse transcriptase-immortalized human fibroblasts by gene expression profiling: Activation of the epiregulin gene. *Cancer Res.* **63:** 1743.

Lorick K.L., Jensen J.P., Fang S., Ong A.M., Hatakeyama S., and Weissman A.M. 1999. RING fingers mediate ubiquitin-conjugating enzyme (E2)-dependent ubiquitination. *Proc. Natl. Acad. Sci.* **96:** 11364.

McDougall J.K. 1994. Immortalization and transformation of human cells by human papillomavirus. *Curr. Top. Microbiol. Immunol.* **186:** 101.

Munger K., Basile J.R., Duensing S., Eichten A., Gonzalez S.L., Grace M., and Zacny V.L. 2001. Biological activities and molecular targets of the human papillomavirus E7 oncoprotein. *Oncogene* **20:** 7888.

Oh S.T., Kyo S., and Laimins L.A. 2001. Telomerase activation by human papillomavirus type 16 E6 protein: Induction of human telomerase reverse transcriptase expression through Myc and GC-rich Sp1 binding sites. *J. Virol.* **75:** 5559.

Sarin K.Y., Cheung P., Gilison D., Lee E., Tennen R.I., Wang E., Artandi M.K., Oro A.E., and Artandi S.E. 2005. Conditional telomerase induction causes proliferation of hair follicle stem cells (comment). *Nature* **436:** 1048.

Shay J.W., Wright W.E., and Werbin H. 1991. Defining the molecular mechanisms of human cell immortalization. *Biochim. Biophys. Acta* **1072:** 1.

Smith L.L., Coller H.A., and Roberts J.M. 2003. Telomerase modulates expression of growth-controlling genes and enhances cell proliferation. *Nat. Cell Biol.* **5:** 474.

Song Z., Krishna S., Thanos D., Strominger J.L., and Ono S.J. 1994. A novel cysteine-rich sequence-specific DNA-binding protein interacts with the conserved X-box motif of the human major histocompatibility complex class II genes via a repeated Cys-His domain and functions as a transcriptional repressor. *J. Exp. Med.* **180:** 1763.

Stewart S.A., Hahn W.C., O'Connor B.F., Banner E.N., Lundberg A.S., Modha P., Mizuno H., Brooks M.W., Fleming M., Zimonjic D.B., Popescu N.C., and Weinberg R.A. 2002. Telomerase contributes to tumorigenesis by a telomere length-independent mechanism (comment). *Proc. Natl. Acad. Sci.* **99:** 12606.

Takakura M., Kyo S., Sowa Y., Wang Z., Yatabe N., Maida Y., Tanaka M., and Inoue M. 2001. Telomerase activation by histone deacetylase inhibitor in normal cells. *Nucleic Acids Res.* **29:** 3006.

van Steensel B., Smogorzewska A., and deLange T. 1998. TRF2 protects human telomeres from end-to-end fusions. *Cell* **92:** 401.

Vaziri H. and Benchimol S. 1998. Reconstitution of telomerase activity in normal human cells leads to elongation of telomeres and extended replicative life span. *Curr. Biol.* **8:** 279.

Veldman T., Horikawa I., Barrett J.C., and Schlegel R. 2001. Transcriptional activation of the telomerase hTERT gene by human papillomavirus type 16 E6 oncoprotein. *J. Virol.* **75:** 4467.

Veldman T., Liu X., Yuan H., and Schlegel R. 2003. Human papillomavirus E6 and Myc proteins associate in vivo and bind to and cooperatively activate the telomerase reverse transcriptase promoter. *Proc. Natl. Acad. Sci.* **100:** 8211.

Walboomers J.M., Jacobs M.V., Manos M.M., Bosch F.X., Kummer J.A., Shah K.V., Snijders P.J., Peto J., Meijer C.J., and Munoz N. 1999. Human papillomavirus is a necessary cause of invasive cervical cancer worldwide (comment). *J. Pathol.* **189:** 12.

Wang J., Xie L.Y., Allan S., Beach D., and Hannon G.J. 1998. Myc activates telomerase. *Genes Dev.* **12:** 1769.

Wu K.-J., Grandori C., Amacker M., Simon-Vermot N., Polack A., Lingner J., and Dalla-Favera R. 1999. Direct activation of TERT transcription by c-MYC. *Nat. Genet.* **21:** 220.

Xu D., Popov N., Hou M., Wang Q., Bjorkholm M., Gruber A., Menkel A.R., and Henriksson M. 2001. Switch from Myc/Max to Mad1/Max binding and decrease in histone acetylation at the telomerase reverse transcriptase promoter during differentiation of HL60 cells. *Proc. Natl. Acad. Sci.* **98:** 3826.

Genomic Progression in Mouse Models for Liver Tumors

A.D. Tward,* K.D. Jones,† S. Yant,‡ M.A. Kay,‡ R. Wang,¶ and J.M. Bishop*

*G.W. Hooper Foundation, †Department of Pathology, ¶Departments of Surgery and Anatomy and Pacific Vascular Research Lab, University of California at San Francisco, San Francisco, California 94143; ‡Departments of Pediatrics and Genetics, Stanford University, Stanford, California 94305

The principal cause of human liver cancer is infection with hepatitis viruses B and C, but tumor progression is fueled by ensuing perturbations that confer gain of function on proto-oncogenes or loss of function on tumor suppressor genes. Frequent among these perturbations is overexpression of the proto-oncogene *MET*. We have modeled the pathogenesis of liver tumors by expressing conditional transgenes of *MET* in the hepatocytes of inbred mice. The response to the *MET* transgene varied with both the magnitude and timing of its expression but included hyperplasia of hepatic progenitor cells, as well as benign and malignant tumors that display both phenotypic and genotypic resemblances to human counterparts. The results reveal *MET* to be a crucial switch in the development of the liver; dramatize how different cellular compartments within a developmental lineage can give rise to distinctive tumor stem cells; delineate rules of tumor progression; provide evidence that the experimental tumors in mice are authentic models for human tumors; and support a role for MET in the genesis of human liver tumors. The models should be useful in elucidating the mechanisms of tumorigenesis and in the preclinical testing of new therapeutics.

Neoplastic tumors arise from a stepwise sequence of events known as tumor progression (Nowell 1976; Kinzler and Vogelstein 1996). Each step in the sequence is thought to represent a discrete genetic or epigenetic aberration, typically affecting the structure or expression of either a proto-oncogene or tumor suppressor gene.

This scheme engenders a number of questions. What causes each of the steps in tumor progression? How does each step contribute to tumorigenesis? Are there discrete and specific genotypic pathways to each form of neoplasm? Must the steps in these pathways occur in a particular chronological sequence? How constrained is the tumorigenic pathway, once an initiating event has occurred? Which of the steps in any given pathway might be suitable targets for therapeutic intervention?

We cannot answer these questions solely by the study of human tumors. Instead, we need to reconstruct the events of tumorigenesis in a prospective manner. The most desirable means to this end would be the development of animal models that replicate tumorigenesis as it occurs in humans. For a host of reasons, the animal of choice is the laboratory mouse.

There is a venerable tradition of denigrating mouse models for cancer, and with good cause, but now the tide has turned. Recent years have seen the development of mouse models that are based on the faithful reconstruction of genetic lesions found in human cancer. The result has been models that offer both biological and molecular authenticity. Here we illustrate this advance by describing the development and use of mouse models for benign and malignant tumors of the liver, the genesis of which resembles that of hepatic tumors in humans.

Cancer of the liver is among the most common and grievous of human malignancies (Parkin et al. 2005). Although relatively infrequent in developed nations, at least 600,000 new cases occur worldwide every year. The av-

erage survival time is 6 months. The only therapeutic recourse of note is surgical resection and liver transplantation.

The principal cause of human liver cancer is infection with either hepatitis B virus or hepatitis C virus, although dietary toxins and chronic alcoholism have also been implicated (Llovet et al. 2003). Downstream of these causes, however, lie perturbations that confer gain of function on proto-oncogenes or loss of function on tumor suppressor genes (Thorgeirsson and Grisham 2002). Frequent among these perturbations is overexpression of the proto-oncogene *MET* (Tavian et al. 2000), which encodes a receptor protein-tyrosine kinase (Met), activated by a ligand known as either hepatocyte growth factor or scatter factor (Trusolino and Comoglio 2002).

We have modeled the pathogenesis of liver tumors by expressing conditional transgenes of *MET* in the liver cells of inbred mice. The response to the *MET* transgene varied with both the magnitude and timing of its expression, but included arrested development of the liver, as well as benign and malignant liver tumors that display both phenotypic and genotypic resemblances to human counterparts. Our results provide insight into the genotypic underpinnings of tumor progression. The models should be useful in studying the mechanisms of tumorigenesis and the preclinical testing of new therapeutics.

PATHOGENIC EFFECTS OF *MET* VARY WITH THE MAGNITUDE AND DEVELOPMENTAL TIMING OF GENE EXPRESSION

To replicate the overexpression of *MET* found frequently in human liver tumors, we targeted the expression of a transgene representing human *MET* to liver cells by using the transcriptional control element for the liver-enriched activator protein gene (Wang et al. 2001). Four in-

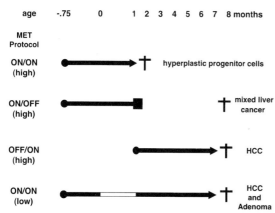

Figure 1. Protocols for the induction of liver tumors with transgenic *MET*. The strains of transgenic mice used here have been described previously (Wang et al. 2001). Expression of the *MET* transgene could be repressed by administration of doxycycline (OFF) or permitted by withholding doxycycline (ON). Two strains of mice expressed the transgene at relatively high levels (Lines 1 and 2 in Wang et al. 2001), two others expressed it at relatively low levels (Lines 3 and 4 in Wang et al. 2001). The first three protocols diagrammed in the figure employed Line 2, the fourth protocol employed Line 3. Doxycycline was administered (*circles*) or withheld (*square*) at the indicated time points. Solid black indicates activity of Met kinase, solid white indicates absence of such activity despite the presence of Met protein.

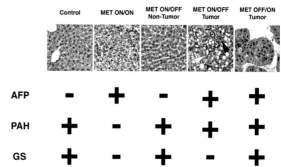

Figure 2. Hepatic phenotypes elicited by overexpression of *MET*. Doxycycline was administered according to the first three protocols outlined in Fig. 1, with the indicated outcomes. Livers were harvested at the following times: (Control) 1 month postpartum; (MET ON/ON) 1 month; (MET ON/OFF, Non-Tumor) 2 months; (MET ON/OFF, Tumor) 16 months; and (MET OFF/ON) 12 months. Specimens were analyzed by microscopy after staining with hematoxylin and eosin (H+E), and by western blotting for the presence of α-fetoprotein (AFP), phenylalanine hydroxylase (PAH), and glutamine synthetase (GS). AFP is a marker for hepatic precursor cells, PAH and GS are markers for mature hepatocytes. (+) Strong expression; (–) little if any expression. The white arrowhead denotes biliary cells, the black arrowhead denotes hepatocytic cells.

dependent strains of transgenic mice were developed, in each of which expression of the *MET* transgene could be inactivated by administration of doxycycline (Wang et al. 2001). Two strains expressed the transgene at relatively high levels (previously designated lines 1 and 2), whereas two expressed it at lower levels (previously designated lines 3 and 4) (for details, see Wang et al. 2001). The phenotypic response was dependent on both the magnitude and timing of expression (Fig. 1).

Physiological expression of *MET* in the normal mouse liver occurs throughout embryogenesis and into adult life (Ishikawa et al. 2001 and data not shown). However, the kinase activity of the gene product subsides soon after birth, apparently in response to controls that act directly on the protein without reducing its abundance (Ishikawa et al. 2001 and data not shown). In contrast, hepatic expression of a *MET* transgene at a high level in utero and continuing after birth produced sustained activity of the kinase (data not shown), and this in turn led to death within 3–8 postnatal weeks (Fig. 1, first protocol). Prior to death, the animals had greatly enlarged, hyperplastic livers composed of immature precursor cells (Fig. 2 and data not shown). Death was apparently caused by the absence of mature liver function.

If instead, the same transgene was inactivated 1 month after birth (Fig. 1, second protocol), the hyperplastic livers were remodeled into mature tissue, and survival of the animals was prolonged (Fig. 2 and data not shown). Within several months, however, the mice developed fatal hepatic carcinomas composed of both biliary and hepatic lineages (Fig. 2). The mixed nature of the tumors suggests that tumorigenesis was initiated from a relatively primitive, bipotential cell. The tumors displayed a marker

of precursor cells (α-fetoprotein, AFP) and a marker of mature hepatocytes (phenylalanine hydroxylase, PAH). A second marker of mature cells, glutamine synthetase (GS), was absent. The extensive proliferation of progenitor cells that occurred during the time that the *MET* transgene was active would have provided an opportunity for the occurrence and fixation of an initiating mutation.

In a third protocol with the same strain of mice, the *MET* transgene was held inactive until 3 weeks after birth, then activated by the withdrawal of doxycycline (Fig. 1, third protocol). Over the ensuing months, the livers first became morphologically dysplastic (data not shown), then developed neoplastic tumors resembling the hepatocellular carcinomas of humans (HCC) without evidence of biliary elements (Fig. 2). The tumor cells displayed molecular markers of both hepatic progenitor cells and mature hepatocytes (Fig. 2). Thus, the tumors may have originated either by transformation of partially differentiated progenitor cells or by partial dedifferentiation of mature hepatocytes—we cannot presently distinguish between these two possibilities.

Expression of a *MET* transgene at a lower level in utero and throughout postnatal life elicited a progression of events that evolved from focal hyperplasia of mature hepatocytes (frequently surrounding central veins) to dysplastic foci and, eventually, to multiple nodules of HCC (Fig. 1, fourth protocol; Fig. 3) (see Wang et al. 2001). The histopathology of the murine tumors closely resembled that of human HCC (Fig. 3) (Wang et al. 2001). No biliary elements were apparent. The tumor cells displayed molecular markers of both immature and mature hepatocytes—AFP for the former, PAH and GS for the latter (data not shown). Similar tumors arose, albeit more slowly, even if activation of the *MET* transgene was delayed until after weaning of the mice (data not shown).

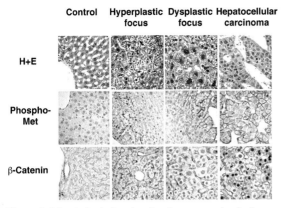

Control   Hyperplastic   Dysplastic   Hepatocellular
           focus   focus   carcinoma

H+E

Phospho-
Met

β-Catenin

Figure 3. Morphological and molecular progression in the genesis of hepatocellular carcinoma elicited by *MET*. Doxycycline was withheld throughout life from a strain of mouse that expresses a *MET* transgene at a relatively low level (fourth protocol in Fig. 1). Stages in tumor progression were evaluated by microscopy (H+E, as in Fig. 2), and by immunohistochemistry for both Met kinase activity, using phosphorylation of Met as a surrogate for enzymatic activity (Phospho-Met), and activation of β-catenin, using nuclear location as an indicator of activity in transcription. Livers were harvested according to the following schedule: (Control) 2 months of age; (Hyperplastic focus) 1 month; (Dysplastic focus) 2 months; and (Hepatocellular carcinoma) 4 months.

Some of these animals also developed benign adenomas interspersed with nodules of HCC (Figs. 1 and 4 and data not shown), but in fewer numbers and over a longer course of time. In contrast to the HCC described above, the adenomas contained no detectable AFP, PAH, or GS. Appearance of the adenomas required relatively extended survival of the animals and may have been limited by death from concurrent HCC. The nature of the stem cell from which the adenomas arose is not clear. Tumorigenesis could conceivably have originated with the same type of cell that engendered HCC, with a diversion of tumor progression occurring in response to a distinctive genotypic change (see below, Conclusions).

GENOTYPIC PROGRESSION IN THE GENESIS OF LIVER TUMORS

The morphological progression to HCC elicited by relatively low expression of transgenic *MET* had biochemical and genomic counterparts. Phosphorylation of the Met protein was used as a surrogate marker for activation of the protein-tyrosine kinase. Despite abundant expression of the transgenic protein (data not shown), no kinase activity could be detected in normal liver of the adult mice (Fig. 3), so it appears that the transgenic protein was susceptible to posttranslational control of its enzymatic activity, reminiscent of that observed for endogenous Met in normal mice (see above). Met kinase activity became apparent in cells of hyperplastic foci, intensified in dysplastic cells, and was abundant in end-stage malignancies (Fig. 3).

It seemed likely that additional genetic events contributed to tumorigenesis in the model. For hints of what these might be, we turned to the example of human HCC. Among the more frequent genetic anomalies in such tumors is the mutational activation of β-catenin, a multifunctional protein that mediates signaling to the transcriptional apparatus through the Wnt pathway (Giles et al. 2003). In the absence of Wnt signaling, β-catenin is located in the cytoplasm and at the plasma membrane. Cytoplasmic β-catenin is situated in a protein complex that facilitates phosphorylation and consequent destruction of the protein. When activated by signaling from Wnt, however, degradation of β-catenin is inhibited and much of the protein moves to the nucleus, where it then serves as a transcription factor. Thus, nuclear localization can be used as a surrogate marker for activation of β-catenin in the Wnt pathway.

Figure 4. Morphological and molecular phenotypes. Hepatic tissue and tumors were obtained from transgenic mice either subjected to the fourth protocol in Fig. 1 or that had received various genes by hydrodynamic transfection at 8 weeks of age. Transfection was performed as described by Yant et al. (2000). The genes introduced by transfection included cDNA representations of a normal allele of human *MET*, a mutant allele of β-catenin that constitutively activates the transcriptional function of the protein (Barth et al. 1997) (ΔNβ-catenin), and a dominant negative allele of HNF-1α (dnHNF-1α)(Vaxillaire et al. 1999). Specimens from liver were analyzed by microscopy (H+E); and for the presence of α-fetoprotein (AFP), phenylalanine hydroxylase (PAH), and glutamine synthetase, as in Fig. 2. The white arrowheads indicate foci of dysplastic cells that appear following transfection of *MET*, the black arrowhead denotes cells that are deficient in PAH following transfection of dnHNF-1α. Fields of normal tissue are designated nt, fields of adenoma, ad.

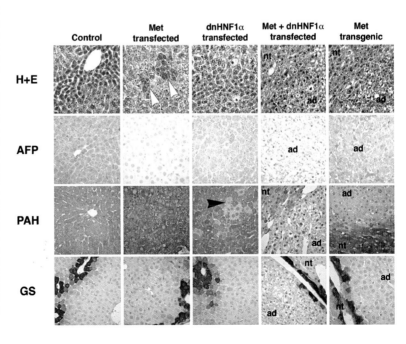

Control | Met transfected | dnHNF1α transfected | Met + dnHNF1α transfected | Met transgenic

H+E

AFP

PAH

GS

Immunostaining for β-catenin revealed intense concentration of the protein at the periphery of normal liver cells, and the cells of both hyperplastic and dysplastic foci (Fig. 3). In contrast, the protein was abundant in the nuclei of most cells in the full-blown HCC (Fig. 3). The activation of β-catenin in malignant cells was attributable to mutations found in the β-catenin gene (Fig, 5). The mutations were analogous to those found in human HCC and included both point mutations and small deletions. These changes preclude the phosphorylations that elicit the degradation of β-catenin (Giles et al. 2003) and thus serve to constitutively activate the protein.

Multiple nodules of HCC developed in most affected livers. Individual nodules always contained a single mutant allele of the β-catenin gene (*CTNNB1*), indicating that the nodule was probably clonal in origin (data not shown). However, the mutations varied from one nodule to another, signaling independent origins of each nodule. The consistency with which the mutations were found in tumors suggests that they confer some selective advantage during clonal evolution of the emerging tumor cells and provides strong circumstantial evidence for a role in tumorigenesis.

The adenomas in transgenic animals displayed activation of the Met kinase, but not of β-catenin (data not shown). Sequencing of the β-catenin gene in adenomas also failed to uncover any mutant alleles (data not shown). In search for other possible genetic lesions, we turned again to the example of human tumors. Hepatic adenomas of humans occur in both congenital and sporadic forms (Zucman-Rossi 2004). In the congenital form, tumor susceptibility is apparently transmitted by a heterozygous deficiency in the HNF-1α gene (*TCF1*) (Bacq et al. 2003), and homozygous deficiencies of HNF-1α are frequent in sporadic adenomas (Bluteau et al. 2002). We have failed to find any genomic damage to HNF-1α in the adenomas of the mouse model (data not

shown), but the signaling pathway to which HNF-1α contributes appears to be deficient, as manifested by an absence of PAH (Fig. 4), production of which is dependent on signaling from HNF-1α (Pontoglio et al. 1997).

RECONSTRUCTION OF TUMORIGENESIS BY HYDRODYNAMIC TRANSFECTION

Knowing that abnormalities of both Met and β-catenin apparently contributed to the genesis of HCC in the transgenic mice, we sought to explore their individual roles in tumor progression. To this end, we used hydrodynamic transfection to introduce and express ectopic genes in the livers of adult mice (Liu et al. 1999; Zhang et al. 1999; Yant et al. 2000). We used a wild-type allele of *MET*, as in the transgenic model, and a mutant allele of the β-catenin gene that encodes a constitutively active protein (Barth et al. 1997). The results are summarized in Figure 6. Introduction of *MET* alone gave rise to microscopic foci of slightly dysplastic cells (Fig. 4), whereas transfection of the β-catenin gene had no apparent effect (data not shown). When the two genes were introduced and expressed together, the recipient animals developed HCC within a month or so (Figs. 4 and 6). Moreover, sequential introduction of the two genes at an interval of one month produced tumors, and the sequence of introduction had no effect on the outcome (data not shown). Thus, cooperation between *MET* and the β-catenin gene in the genesis of HCC appears not to be strictly dependent on the chronological sequence with which the two genes go awry.

We were also able to reconstruct the genesis of hepatic adenomas by hydrodynamic transfection. To do this, we created a dominant negative allele of HNF-1α found in human hepatic adenomas (Vaxillaire et al. 1999), which can mimic the effect of a genetic deficiency in the endogenous gene. Transfection of the inhibitory allele of HNF-1α produced numerous individual cells that were

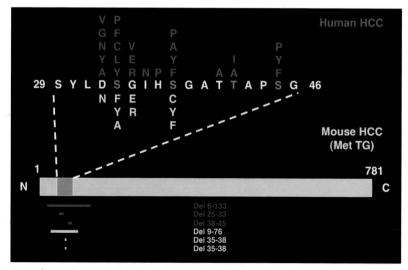

Figure 5. Mutations in the β-catenin gene of human and mouse hepatocellular carcinomas. HCC was elicited by the protocol described for Fig. 3. The β-catenin gene was sequenced in 21 HCCs obtained from 15 mice. An activating mutation was found in all but one HCC. Representative results are shown in yellow. Representative data reported by others for human tumors are given in red. Serine and threonine residues whose phosphorylations elicit degradation of β-catenin are shown in green. The data for human tumors were derived from Buendia (2000).

Gene(s) transfected	Tumor
Met	–
ΔNβ-Catenin	–
dnHNF1α	–
Met + ΔNβ-Catenin	HCC
Met + dnHNF1α	Adenoma
Myc	HBL

Figure 6. Tumorigenesis following hydrodynamic transfection. Hydrodynamic transfection was used to achieve expression of ectopic genes in the livers of 8-week-old mice, as described for Fig. 4. Transfection was also performed with a normal allele of *MYC*. The resulting tumors included HCC, benign adenomas, and a primitive tumor known as hepatoblastoma (HBL), previously elicited with a transgene of *MYC* (Shachaf et al. 2004).

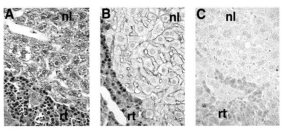

Figure 7. Reconstitution of the normal liver after regression of HCC in mice. HCC was elicited with the protocol described for Fig. 3. When the tumors reached an advanced state, doxycycline was administered to elicit regression, as described previously (Wang et al. 2001). Liver was harvested for examination 6 months following the initiation of doxycycline administration, then examined by microscopy (*A*), and by immunohistochemistry for β-catenin (*B*) and Met kinase (*C*). Fields of normal cells are designated by nl, fields of residual tumor cells by rt.

deficient in PAH (Fig. 4), but no tumors (Fig. 6). When *MET* and the dominant negative HNF-1α were introduced and expressed together, however, they rapidly gave rise to adenomas (Figs. 4 and 6). The tumors displayed histological morphology and differentiation markers identical to those of the adenomas found in transgenic mice (Fig. 4).

Previous work demonstrated that the targeted expression of transgenic normal *MYC* in liver cells gave rise to a primitive tumor known as hepatoblastoma (Shachaf et al. 2004). The same tumor occurred when hydrodynamic transfection was used to express a normal allele of human *MYC* in the liver of adult mice (Fig. 6). The tumors arose rapidly, without any readily apparent intermediate stage, and contained neither detectable Met kinase activity nor mutations in the β-catenin gene (data not shown).

REGRESSION OF HCC AFTER INACTIVATION OF THE INITIATING TRANSGENE

The prevailing scheme of tumor progression raises the question of which steps in that progression remain essential for maintenance of the eventual malignancy and, thus, might be suitable targets for therapeutic intervention. Recent efforts to address this question with mouse models have shown that many forms of malignancy initiated by transgenes will regress when the responsible transgene is inactivated, even if the tumor has reached an advanced stage (Felsher 2004). We previously reported that this is true for HCC elicited by *MET* (Wang et al. 2001). The regression was mediated by both a cessation of tumor cell proliferation and widespread apoptosis, accompanied by regeneration of normal liver tissue.

The regenerated liver contained microscopic foci of residual tumor surrounded by normal liver tissue (Fig. 7A). As anticipated, there was no detectable Met protein or kinase activity in either the residual tumor cells or the normal tissue (Fig. 7C and data not shown). Nuclear β-catenin was apparent in the residual tumor cells, but not in the normal tissue (Fig. 7B). Thus, the liver had apparently been reconstituted from normal stem cells or hepatocytes, rather than by differentiation of malignant cells in the manner reported for the hepatoblastomas elicited by a MYC transgene (Shachaf et al. 2004).

When held for 6 months or more with the *MET* transgene inactivated, the animals often suffered a clinical relapse, again developing fatal HCC (data not shown). The tumor cells still contained activated β-catenin, but there was no indication that the *MET* transgene had been reactivated (data not shown). We conclude that the relapses were driven by a new and different genetic event that bypassed the requirement for Met kinase and presumably cooperated with the activity of β-catenin in tumorigenesis.

CONCLUSIONS

We have developed mouse models for both benign and malignant liver tumors. The results support a role for *MET* in the genesis of liver tumors by complementing previous circumstantial evidence from studies of human tumors; provide insight into the rules of tumor progression; dramatize how different cellular compartments within a developmental lineage can give rise to distinctive tumors in response to the same tumorigenic influence, presumably by generating distinctive tumor stem cells; and provide evidence that the experimental tumors in mice are authentic models for human tumors.

We initiated tumorigenesis by overexpression of a normal allele of the *MET* proto-oncogene. Although this anomaly is common in human HCC, it apparently lies downstream of an external cause, such as chronic infection with either hepatitis B or C virus. It is not presently clear how viral infection might lead to the genetic abnormalities required for tumorigenesis. One hypothesis holds that ongoing death and regeneration of liver tissue in response to chronic infection sets the stage for the occurrence and fixation of genetic damage (Thorgeirsson and Grisham 2002). This view is consistent with the lengthy time that separates the onset of infection from the appearance of malignant tumors. In contrast, tumorigenesis in the mouse models is relatively quick, with tumors arising after a few months at the most. At least three factors may contribute to this difference.

First, by introducing the overexpression of *MET* into numerous, if not all, liver cells, we have both bypassed earlier events that would otherwise be necessary for tumorigenesis and increased the likelihood of subsequent events by creating a vast number of potential tumor stem cells. It is also possible that sustained activity of *MET* might destabilize the genome, much as described for *MYC* (Mai et al. 1996; Felsher and Bishop 1999). Second, the rapidity of tumorigenesis in the models is in accord with the natural history of cancer in mice, which develop spontaneous malignancies much more quickly than do humans (Campisi 2003). This difference may reflect inferior defenses against permanent genetic damage in rodents (Ames et al. 1993). Third, cells in the dysplastic foci induced by *MET* were proliferating (data not shown), providing a permissive environment for the occurrence and fixation of mutations.

Although overexpression of *MET* and mutational activation of β-catenin are common in human HCC, neither is universal. In contrast, the mouse HCC described here contained both abundant Met kinase and activating mutations of β-catenin, almost without exception. The former was by experimental design; the latter must have arisen from spontaneous mutagenesis followed by selection during the course of tumor progression. We suggest that in constructing the mouse model, we have imposed one of several possible genetic pathways to HCC.

In pursuit of this idea, we have surveyed more than 50 human HCCs for the presence of enzymatically active Met and activating mutations of β-catenin. The results indicate that the two were frequently congruent, and in particular, robust Met kinase activity was virtually never present in the absence of a β-catenin mutation (A.D. Tward et al., unpubl.). These correlations have not previously been appreciated. Thus, the findings in the mouse model have led us to a subset of human tumors in which the course of tumorigenesis was apparently akin to that in the model. The remainder of human HCC would arise from at least one additional pathway that has not been replicated by our mouse model. A further inference would be that activation of Met kinase constrains the subsequent pathway of tumorigenesis.

We have not detected Met kinase activity in the normal cells of adult transgenic livers (Fig. 3 and data not shown). Activity became apparent only with the appearance of hyperplastic foci and then persisted throughout the course of tumorigenesis. We presume that only occasional liver cells express the *MET* transgene above the threshold required to initiate tumorigenesis, and that such cells give rise to the hyperplastic foci.

The tumors in our mouse models all arose from overexpression of the *MET* proto-oncogene, but the specific outcome of tumorigenesis was determined by which genetic anomalies occur subsequently. We dramatized this conclusion by using hydrodynamic transfection to introduce various genetic anomalies into the mouse liver in vivo. The results demonstrated that *MET* and β-catenin cooperate to produce HCC, whereas *MET* and a deficiency of HNF-1α cooperate to produce benign adenomas. We have found no evidence that the abnormalities of β-catenin and HNF-1α ever coincide in tumors, and we cannot presently say whether either of these preempts the other, should they occur coincidentally in the same cell, but the issue is amenable to study by hydrodynamic transfection.

The determining nature of genetic lesions in tumorigenesis is further illustrated by the fact that targeted expression of *MYC* in liver cells, using the same control element as in the present work, gave rise to hepatoblastomas, rather than either HCC or adenomas (Shachaf et al. 2004 and data not shown). We were able to recapitulate that finding by using hydrodynamic transfection to express a normal allele of human *MYC* in the liver of adult mice. The transfected mice developed hepatoblastoma.

The reconstruction of tumorigenesis in the transgenic mouse models places overexpression of Met upstream of the other genetic events required for the genesis of either HCC or adenomas. We have not conducted an exhaustive search for such cooperating events, focusing instead on known candidates deduced from data obtained with human tumors. However, the rapidity with which mouse tumors arise after simultaneous transfection of *MET* and mutants of either β-catenin or HNF-1α suggests that, in the mouse at least, relatively few additional spontaneous events may be required. Our results with hydrodynamic transfection also raise the possibility that HCC will arise irrespective of the order in which overexpression of Met and mutation of β-catenin occur, but more extensive experimentation will be required to address this issue in a definitive manner.

A major objective of modeling tumorigenesis in the mouse is to identify individual steps in tumor progression that are suitable targets for therapeutic intervention. Our work with the mouse model for HCC illustrates this prospect. Inactivation of *MET*, even in the most advanced tumors, led to prompt and universal tumor regression. Thus, *MET* not only initiated tumorigenesis, but also served as a tumor maintenance function. The efficiency and relative durability of regression were presumably due to the permanent removal of Met kinase from the tumor cells. The mouse tumors do recur, but only after extended periods of time, and only after the advent of some event that can bypass the need for *MET* and, perhaps, exploit the presence of residual cells with mutant β-catenin. These results highlight Met as a possible target in the treatment of HCC. They also dramatize how occurrence of mutations that bypass any requirement for the target could give rise to drug resistance during the course of therapy.

In aggregate, this and many other reports of similar results with mouse models further justify the pursuit of therapeutics that are targeted at single genetic lesions in human tumors—therapies of the sort represented by the landmark pharmaceutical, Gleevec (Sawyers 2004). Mouse models with the authenticity exemplified by the present work should be useful in evaluating both the suitability of individual targets and the potential efficacy of additional targeted therapies, once they are in hand.

It is now apparent that *MET* is a crucial switch in the development of the liver (Fig. 8). The function of the gene is required to sustain proliferation of hepatic progenitor cells, but it must be inactivated in order to permit differentiation of those cells (A.D. Tward et al., in prep.). Unphysiological activity of the Met kinase can disturb the differentiation of hepatocytes and engender tumorigenesis from both

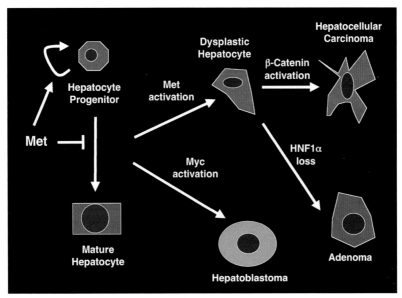

Figure 8. Pathways of tumor progression. The diagram is based on results for tumor progression reported in the present paper and elsewhere (Wang et al. 2001; Shachaf et al. 2004) and on results describing the role of Met in hepatic development, which demonstrate that the physiological activity of Met both drives proliferation and blocks differentiation of hepatic precursor cells (Suzuki et al. 2003, and in prep.).

bipotential and unipotential cells within the hepatocyte lineage, as dramatized by the work presented here.

We cannot discern whether the effects of Met on progenitor proliferation and differentiation are independent of one another. Alternatively, one of the effects might follow the other. For example, the mere withdrawal of progenitor cells from the cell cycle after depletion of Met kinase activity might itself trigger differentiation. Whatever its genesis, the massive hyperplasia of progenitor cells in response to the in utero and postnatal overexpression of *MET* could provide an abundant source of such cells for the experimental study of hepatic differentiation, tumorigenesis, and tissue engineering.

ACKNOWLEDGMENTS

We thank Linda Prentice for assistance with histology, and Luda Urisman for assistance with animal husbandry. The work was supported by funds from the National Cancer Institute (CA009043), the George W. Hooper Research Foundation, and the National Institutes of Health (DK49022 to M.A.K.). ADT was supported by the UCSF Medical Scientist Training Program NIH NIGMS (5T32GMO7618).

REFERENCES

Ames B.N., Shigenaga M.K., and Hagen T.M. 1993. Oxidants, antioxidants, and the degenerative disease of aging. *Proc. Natl. Acad. Sci.* **90:** 7915.

Bacq Y., Jacquemin E., Balabaud C., Jeannot E., Scotto B., Branchereau S., Laurent C., Bourlier P., Pariente D., de Muret A., Fabre M., Bioulac-Sage P., and Zucman-Rossi J. 2003. Familial liver adenomatosis associated with hepatocyte nuclear factor 1 alpha incactivation. *Gastroenterology* **125:** 1470.

Barth A.I., Pollack A.L., Altschuler Y., Mostov K.E., and Nel-son W.J. 1997. NH2-terminal deletion of beta-catenin results in stable colocalization of mutant beta-catenin with adenomatous polyposis coli protein and altered MDCK cell adhesion. *J. Cell Biol.* **136:** 693.

Bluteau O., Jeannot E., Bioulac-Sage P., Marques J.M., Blanc J.F., Bui H., Beaudoin J.C., Franco D., Balabaud C., Laurent-Puig P., and Zucman-Rossi J. 2002. Bi-allelic inactivation of TCF1 in hepatic adenomas. *Nat. Genet.* **32:** 312.

Buendia M.A. 2000. Genetics of hepatocellular carcinoma. *Semin. Cancer Biol.* **10:** 185.

Campisi J. 2003. Cancer and ageing: Rival demons? *Nat. Rev. Cancer* **3:** 339.

Felsher D.W. 2004. Reversibility of oncogene-induced cancer. *Curr. Opin. Genet. Dev.* **14:** 37.

Felsher D.W. and Bishop J.M. 1999. Transient excess of MYC activity can elicit genomic instability and tumorigenesis. *Proc. Natl. Acad. Sci.* **96:** 3940.

Giles R.H., vas Es J.H., and Clevers H. 2003. Caught up in a Wnt storm: Wnt signalling in cancer. *Biochim Biophys Acta.* **1653:** 1.

Ishikawa K.S., Masui T., Ishikawa K., and Shiojiri N. 2001. Immunolocalization of hepatocyte growth factor and its receptor (c-Met) during mouse liver development. *Histochem. Cell Biol.* **116:** 453.

Kinzler K.W. and Vogelstein B. 1996. Lessons from hereditary colon cancer. *Cell* **87:** 159.

Liu F., Song Y., and Liu D. 1999. Hydrodynamics-based transfection in animals by systemic administration of plasmid DNA. *Gene Ther.* **6:** 1258.

Llovet J.M., Burroughs A., and Bruix J. 2003. Hepatocellular carcinoma. *Lancet* **362:** 1907.

Mai S., Fluri M., Siwarski D., and Huppi K. 1996. Genomic instability in MycER-activated Rat1A-MycER cells. *Chromosome Res.* **4:** 365.

Nowell P.C. 1976. The clonal evolution of tumor cell populations. *Science* **194:** 23.

Parkin D.M., Bray F., Ferlay J., and Pisani P. 2005. Global cancer statistics, 2002. *CA Cancer J. Clin.* **55:** 74.

Pontoglio M., Faust D.M., Doyen A., Yaniv M., and Weiss M.C. 1997. Hepatocyte nuclear factor 1alpha gene inactivation impairs chromatic remodeling and demethylation of the phenylalanine hydroxylase gene. *Mol. Cell. Biol.* **17:** 4948.

Sawyers C. 2004. Targeted cancer therapy. *Nature* **432:** 294.

Shachaf C.M., Kopelman A.M., Arvanitis C., Karlsson A., Beer S., Mandl S., Bachmann M.H., Borowsky A.D., Ruebner B., Cardiff R.D., Yang Q., Bishop J.M., Contag C.H., and Felsher D.W. 2004. MYC inactivation uncovers pluripotent differentiation and tumour dormancy in hepatocellular cancer. *Nature* **431:** 1112.

Suzuki A., Iwama A., Miyashita H., Nakauchi H., and Taniguchi H. 2003. Role of growth factors and extracellular matrix in controlling differentiation of prospectively isolated hepatic stem cells. *Development.* **130:** 2513.

Tavian D., De Petro G., Benetti A., Portolani N., Giulini S.M., and Barlati S. 2000. u-PA and c-MET mRNA expression is co-ordinately enhanced while hepatocyte growth factor mRNA is down-regulated in human hepatocellular carcinoma. *Int. J. Cancer* **87:** 644.

Thorgeirsson S.S. and Grisham J.W. 2002. Molecular pathogenesis of human hepatocellular carcinoma. *Nature Genetics* **31:** 339.

Trusolino L. and Comoglio P.M. 2002. Scatter-factor and semaphorin receptors: Cell signalling for invasive growth. *Nat. Rev. Cancer* **2:** 289.

Vaxillaire M., Abderrahmani A., Boutin P., Bailleul B., Froguel P., Yaniv M., and Pontoglio M. 1999. Anatomy of a homeoprotein revealed by the analysis of human MODY3 mutations. *J. Biol. Chem.* **274:** 35646.

Wang R., Ferrell L.D., Faouzi S., Maher J.J., and Bishop J.M. 2001. Activation of the Met receptor by cell attachment induces and sustains hepatocellular carcinomas in transgenic mice. *J. Cell Biol.* **153:** 1023.

Yant S.R., Meuse L., Chiu W., Ivics Z., Izsvak Z., and Kay M.A. 2000. Somatic integration and long-term transgene expression in normal and haemophilic mice using a DNA transposon system. *Nat. Genet.* **25:** 35.

Zucman-Rossi J. 2004. Genetic alterations in hepatocellular adenomas: Recent findings and new challenges. *J. Hepatol.* **40:** 1036.

Zhang G., Budker V., and Wolff J.A. 1999. High levels of foreign gene expression in hepatocytes after tail vein injections of naked plasmid DNA. *Hum. Gene Ther.* **10:** 1735.

Genotype–Phenotype Relationships in a Mouse Model for Human Small-Cell Lung Cancer

J. Calbó, R. Meuwissen, E. van Montfort, O. van Tellingen, and A. Berns

Division of Molecular Genetics and Centre of Biomedical Genetics, The Netherlands Cancer Institute,
1066 CX, Amsterdam, The Netherlands

Lung tumors are usually classified into small-cell lung cancer (SCLC) or non-SCLC (NSCLC) depending on their pathological and histological characteristics. SCLC is defined not only by its characteristic neuroendocrine differentiation, aggressiveness, and metastatic potential, but also by a specific set of genetic aberrations, including the loss of the tumor suppressor genes p53 and Rb1 and the amplification of any member of the Myc family of oncogenes. We have previously described a mouse model of SCLC by somatic conditional disruption of *Trp53* and *Rb1* genes that closely resembles the human condition. Based on the possibility to study early tumor lesions and to culture and subclone progressed tumors and metastases, we discuss here a strategy to define genotype–phenotype relationships that can explain the underlying biology of lung neuroendocrine tumors. We have found that tumors may be constituted by genetically variant cell populations, which might represent different progression stages. Interestingly, we observed L-myc amplification and Ascl-1 expression in those populations showing neuroendocrine differentiation. Non-neuroendocrine cell populations from the same tumors did not show L-myc amplification nor Ascl-1 expression. We propose that this genetic divergence can play a relevant role in the definition of some phenotypic characteristics like metastasis potential or chemoresistance.

Since the description of cancer as a genetic disease, an overwhelming number of data have been generated which show the contribution of numerous oncogenes and tumor suppressor genes to the tumorigenic process. More recently, cancer has been defined as a differentiation disease, due to loss of proliferation constraint (differentiation) rather than acquisition of proliferative capability (Harris 2004), underscoring the relevance of undifferentiated progenitor cells carrying specific mutations that drive tumorigenesis. Conforming to this concept, "cancer stem cells" (CSC) have been observed in tumors of different origins. These cells have the ability to self-renew and to give rise to more differentiated cells that constitute most of the tumor mass, thus dictating the phenotype, metastatic properties, and response to therapy. However, the link between CSC and normal tissue stem cells is still undefined. It is unknown whether CSCs are relatively quiescent as normal stem cells, and whether tumors harbor also a "transit-amplifying" cell pool responsible for most of the proliferation. If so, classic DNA-damaging agents used in chemotherapy would only target dividing cells but would leave unaffected resting CSCs as the seeds for relapse of the tumor (Dean et al. 2005).

The current description of CSC implies that these cells have acquired and sustain a complete set of mutations responsible for the tumorigenic properties. In other words, epigenetic control rather than additional genetic changes distinguishes CSC from differentiated tumor cells, as also happens in normal tissues. In this concept, the tumor mass is an end point in which additional genetic and epigenetic changes occurring beyond the CSC or transit-amplifying compartment do not contribute to tumorigenesis but rather represent background noise. Moreover, the consideration of CSCs as the tumor seeds runs the risk of underestimating the role of less progressed cells in the biology of the tumor.

Tumorigenesis is a selective process in which the initial growth-promoting mutations can largely determine the tumor characteristics. Mitogen-independent proliferation, escape from apoptosis, survival in hypoxic conditions, or increased detoxification efficiency are likely selected for in the primary tumor mass. However, it is less clear how this selective process occurring in the primary tumor would yield genetic changes needed for metastasis. One might argue that alterations facilitating distant spread and growth occur early in tumor progression because of other selective advantages relevant for primary tumor growth. In this case, metastasis-predisposing genes would belong to the classically defined oncogenes and tumor suppressor genes (Bernards and Weinberg 2002). This is in agreement with the detection of poor-prognosis expression signatures in primary tumors that predict a high risk of metastatic spread (van de Vijver et al. 2002; van 't Veer et al. 2002; Ramaswamy et al. 2003). Another possibility is that rare cell populations, sporadically acquiring new genetic aberrations, have an increased ability to metastasize. That would explain why cells derived from metastases have repeatedly been shown to be more metastatic than the bulk population of cells from primary tumors. This is supported by observations that different subpopulations of cells with distinct metastatic potential and target organ preference can be identified in a human breast cancer cell line both by in vivo selection and by in vitro subcloning (Kang et al. 2003; Minn et al. 2005).

Interestingly, those highly predisposed variants also share the "poor prognosis" signature but show in addition a specific set of expressed genes determining organ preference and/or metastatic potential. Therefore, both models appear to be true: There is a general predisposition but also the need for additional changes that may affect more or less rare cell populations of the primary tumor (Hynes 2003).

From the observation that most sporadic tumors are phenotypically heterogeneous, we hypothesize that some phenotypic characteristics might be due to the presence in tumors of genetically variant cell populations representing different evolutionary (progression) steps. Such genetic heterogeneity would give the tumor the opportunity to adapt to new situations (plasticity), required for invasion, metastases, and resistance to chemotherapy or radiotherapy.

One good example illustrating this possibility is the case of relapsed SCLC. Primary and metastatic SCLC are known to be very sensitive to chemotherapy, but drug-resistant relapses occur almost invariably. In addition, some relapsed tumors show clear transdifferentiation, resulting in NSCLC features (Brambilla et al. 1991; Kraus et al. 2002). SCLC tumors are also highly metastatic, producing distant nodules in liver, adrenal glands, brain, and bone. It is worth noting that little is known about the premalignant lesions from which SCLC originates, as patients mostly present with advanced, metastatic disease. Focusing on a unique animal model for SCLC and taking into consideration the likely heterogeneity of tumors, we present here a strategy to establish relevant genotype–phenotype correlations, which can help in understanding the salient features of the underlying tumor biology.

SCLC

Lung cancer is currently the leading cause of cancer deaths worldwide, with a higher morbidity than breast, pancreatic, prostate, and colorectal cancers combined (Landis et al. 1999). SCLC is a histopathologically defined subset of lung cancers formed by small cells with scarce cytoplasm and molded nuclei, showing neuroendocrine (NE) differentiation, and accounts for almost 18% of all lung tumors. Due to the high proliferative and metastatic potential, but especially to the almost certain recurrence after chemotherapy, the 5-year survival rate for SCLC is around 5% (Worden and Kalemkerian 2000). In contrast, 80% of lung tumors show markers of non-neuroendocrine epithelial differentiation, including adenocarcinomas, squamous cell, bronchioalveolar, and large-cell carcinomas, classified altogether as NSCLC. SCLC and NSCLC show major differences in histopathological characteristics that can be explained by the distinct patterns of genetic lesions found in both tumor classes (Zochbauer-Muller et al. 2002). As an important example, oncogenic mutations in Ras proteins are exclusively found in NSCLC tumors, whereas amplification of L-myc (MYCL1) and N-myc (MYCN) genes is exclusively observed in SCLC (Table 1) (Meuwissen and Berns 2005). C-myc gene (MYC) amplification has been observed in both NSCLC and SCLC, but the overall MYC-family amplification is significantly more frequent in SCLC (20–35%) than in NSCLC (5–20%) (Richardson and Johnson 1993). Also intriguing is the tumor-type specificity observed in mutations affecting the p16[INK4a]/

Table 1. Major Genetic Aberrations in Lung Cancer

		SCLC %	NSCLC %
MYC family	amplification	20[a]–35[b]	5[a]–20[b]
MYCL1 or *MYCN*[c]	amplification	20[a]–20[b]	<3[a]–0[b]
RAS	mutations	<1	15–20
EGFR	mutation	—	20
RB1	LOH mutations	70	30
		90	15–30
TP53	LOH mutations	75–100	60
		75	50
INK4a	LOH mutations	50	70
p16[INK4a]		20–50	<5
3p chromosomal region	LOH	90–100	70–80

Data from Meuwissen and Berns (2005).
[a]Tumors.
[b]Cell lines.
[c]Concurrent amplification of multiple members of the *MYC* family is never found in a single tumor.

CycD1/CDK4/RB1 pathway. Inactivation of this pathway is found in virtually all tumor types; despite the mutual exclusiveness of the mutations in these genes, alterations in *p16INK4a, CycD1*, or *CDK4* are most commonly seen in NSCLC, whereas *RB* gene inactivation is a typical feature for SCLC (Zochbauer-Muller et al. 2002; Fong et al. 2003). More than 90% of SCLCs harbor abnormalities in the RB protein (Reissmann et al. 1993; Dosaka-Akita et al. 1997) and rarely show allelic loss, mutation, or promoter hypermethylation of *P16INK4a* (Fong et al. 2003). On the other hand, *TP53* missense mutations are found in 75% of SCLC and 50% of NSCLC (Toyooka et al. 2003). In SCLC, p53 loss is frequently accompanied by elevated Bcl-2 and reduced Bax protein levels (Brambilla et al. 1996). Loss of other tumor suppressor genes might be relevant in the early progression steps, as recurrent chromosome losses do occur. Especially frequent in SCLC is loss of heterozygosity (LOH) of the 3p chromosome region, containing putative tumor suppressor genes like *FHIT, RASSF1, SEMA3B, FUS1*, and *RAR*β.

Deregulation of the external, environmental signals that stimulate or constrain the proliferation of cells is another typical feature of cancer cells. By up-regulating growth factor receptors and their ligands, cancer cells can provide themselves with autocrine or paracrine loops facilitating tumor growth (Maulik et al. 2003). In SCLC, frequent hyperactivation is observed of the autocrine loop composed by gastrin-releasing or other bombesin-like peptides (GRP/BN) and their coupled receptors (GPCR) (Fathi et al. 1996; Rozengurt 1998). However, the mechanism of activation is not known, as no mutations or amplifications have been detected for *GRP* or its receptor (Forgacs et al. 2001). On the other hand, autocrine signaling involving receptors for tyrosine kinase appear to be more relevant in NSCLC. For instance, the neuregulin receptor ERBB-2 is aberrantly expressed in 30% of NSCLC, and the epidermal growth factor receptor (EGFR, ERBB-1) is mutated or overexpressed together with its ligands in a substantial fraction of NSCLC, serving as an appealing target for therapeutic intervention (Paez et al. 2004).

In summary, from the point of view of genetic alterations, SCLC and NSCLC are two markedly different entities, as also reflected by their histological and pathological differences. It is still an unsolved question whether this set of specific genetic changes determines the tumor phenotype or whether the transformation of different target cells drives development of distinct lung tumors. Mouse models can serve as an important tool to answer this question as well as to help to assess the contribution of different aberrations to the tumorigenic process.

STRATEGY TO DEFINE GENOTYPE–PHENOTYPE CORRELATIONS

Mouse models for human cancer have proven to be of great value in the understanding of the underlying tumor biology. Especially, transgenic models facilitate the study of the contribution of oncogene activation or tumor suppressor gene loss to the tumorigenic process. The idea is simple: Introduction of genetic lesions found in specific subsets of human cancer in the mouse may result in the development of tumors with a similar phenotype. Given that most genetic alterations driving human tumorigenesis are sporadic and somatic, the more we can reproduce this loco-temporal tumorigenic process, the closer the mouse model will likely resemble its human counterpart. Conditional transgenesis, and regulatable and lineage-specific directed expression are indispensable tools for building accurate cancer mouse models (Jonkers and Berns 2002).

Our approach to study the molecular determinants of lung tumorigenesis consists of an integrated survey of genotypic changes and phenotypic consequences (Fig. 1). The starting point is the selection of gene mutations relevant for the human disease. In the case of SCLC, we selected *Trp53* and *Rb1* loss, whereas in the case of

NSCLC, we and other investigators have introduced oncogenic *K-Ras* mutants to model lung adenocarcinoma in mice (Fig. 2) (Jackson et al. 2001; Johnson et al. 2001; Meuwissen et al. 2001). By using adenovirus-mediated somatic gene transfer of Cre recombinase, conditional *Trp53* and *Rb1* alleles can be inactivated in the lung epithelium. In this way, we mimicked the site, the time, and the sporadic fashion in which mutations occur in human SCLC. Tumors do arise with high penetrance, showing histopathological features very similar to those of the human disease (more details about this model are described below). Interestingly, targeting the same range of cells with the same Adeno-Cre vector in conditional *K-RasV12* mice resulted in exclusive induction of adenocarcinoma (Meuwissen et al. 2001).

It is currently accepted that tissue stem cells are the most likely target cells, given their ability to self-renew, thereby allowing the accumulation of mutations. Substantial efforts are being made to identify these self-renewing stem cells from different tissues. In lung, different progenitor/stem cell niches have been defined, including the CK14+ cells in the epithelium of proximal airways (Hong et al. 2004), the variant Clara cells associated with NE bodies (Hong et al. 2001), and another type of variant Clara cells found in the bronchioalveolar duct junction in the distal airways (Giangreco et al. 2002). Very recently, Kim et al. have shown the presence in adult mice of a stem cell population able to repopulate damaged epithelium. These stem cells likely give rise to adenocarcinomas upon acquiring an oncogenic K-Ras mutation (Kim et al. 2005). However, much less is known about the progenitors of NE cells in the lung. It is possible, although experimental data supporting this are lacking, that the same stem cells can differentiate into both the epithelial and NE lineage. In that case, the target cell for NSCLC and SCLC would be the same. Which tumor

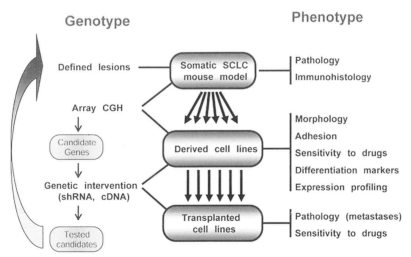

Figure 1. Strategy to establish genotype–phenotype relationships in a mouse model for SCLC. Genetic alterations observed in the human disease are mimicked in mice to initiate tumorigenesis. Tumors are studied both phenotypically (histopathology) and genotypically (array CGH). Derived cloned cell lines facilitate a more extensive study of phenotypic features, which can be matched to genetic data. Observed additional genetic alterations correlating with a specific phenotype can be further studied by genetic manipulation of cell lines. The contribution of these candidate genetic changes to the in vivo phenotype can be initially tested in an orthotopic transplantation model and finally in a spontaneous compound mouse model.

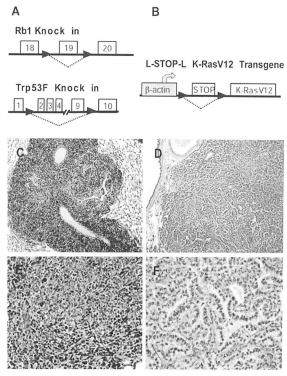

A
Rb1 Knock in

Trp53F Knock in

B
L-STOP-L K-RasV12 Transgene

β-actin STOP K-RasV12

Figure 2. Induced genetic alteration determines tumor phenotype. (*A*) Schematic representation of *Rb1* and *Trp53* conditional alleles. LoxP sites (*red triangles*) were inserted around exon 19 of *Rb1* and exons 2–9 of *Trp53*. After Cre-mediated recombination, the region between LoxP sites is removed (*dotted line*), resulting in loss of function. (*B*) Schematic representation of conditional oncogenic mutant *K-Ras* allele. In this transgene, LoxP sites (*red triangles*) were surrounding a transcriptional STOP cassette. After Cre-mediated recombination, the region between LoxP sites is removed (*dotted line*), resulting in β-actin promoter-directed expression of K-RasV12 oncogenic protein. (*C–F*) Representative hematoxylin & eosin staining on mSCLC tumors (*C* and *E*) or mNSCLC tumors (*D* and *F*).

wide expression of K-RasV12 predominantly results in an early induction of adenocarcinoma in the lung, while other tissues are largely unaffected (Guerra et al. 2003). These mouse models have clearly established a functional relationship between the initiating genetic lesions and the final phenotype of the tumors, offering unique opportunities to study these early lesions.

However, in most, if not all, cases, additional mutations are required both in man and in mouse. Cells carrying initiating mutations will acquire additional genetic alterations followed by clonal expansion, and selective outgrowth will result in the final genotype and phenotype of the tumor. Unfortunately, insight into this evolution history is still poor, mostly due to the complexity of the process and the difficulty to study precursor lesions. This is even more critical in tumors like SCLC, for which no clear premalignant stages have been defined. We can now, using well-defined animal models, look at precursor lesions and at different stages of tumor progression. The other way to learn about this evolutionary process takes advantage of the persistence of clones representative for different progression steps in the tumor. Genetic aberrations observed in these stages can be compared, and the sequence of events can be determined, indicating the order, relevance, and phenotypic consequence of frequently occurring genetic alterations.

Ideally, one would like to know the genotype and potential phenotype of each cell, or at least each distinct cell population, forming a tumor. By using linear amplification of genomic DNA, it is in principle possible to search for genomic aberrations in a single cell by array comparative genomic hybridizaton (CGH), and to establish a hierarchical clustering containing genealogical information. Using this approach, it has been recently described that breast cancer tumor cells might disseminate while harboring far fewer genomic aberrations than observed in primary tumors or in overt metastases (Schmidt-Kittler et al. 2003). This result points to the importance of less progressed tumor cell populations in establishing metastases. Derivation of several cloned cell lines from a single tumor lesion will allow us to study these genealogical relationships, but will also permit us to obtain better insight into the phenotype of each variant (Fig. 1). Expression profiles, in vitro growth characteristics, cell adhesion and migration characteristics, drug sensitivity, resistance to anoikis, in vivo tumor growth, and metastatic potential are examples of phenotypic features that one would like to match with distinct genetic aberrations. For each cell line, one can link genotype and phenotype, and then make a comparison between cells from the same tumor that share a number of genetic alterations but differ with respect to others. In this way, one can obtain information about the relevant genetic events that are responsible for a specific feature. Moreover, observed gene expression patterns can be easily reproduced and monitored in vitro by overexpressing or down-regulating genes. This will provide insight into the role of these genes in determining the phenotypic characteristics of the tumor. However, this approach is only possible when the in vivo–in vitro transition does not cause a major change in cell behavior

arises then would depend on the genetic lesions acquired. In contrast, different progenitor cell populations could generate Clara cells and alveolar type I and II cells on the one hand and NE cells on the other hand. A NE progenitor cell has been found in bronchial epithelia that survived ablation of all cells carrying a Clara-cell-specific marker. However, it is unclear whether this cell represents a genuine stem cell or a transit-amplifying cell. The ablation of all Clara cells in mouse lung does allow only short-term survival of the mice, so the reconstituting potential of the NE progenitors could not be rigorously tested. The presence of NE stem cells in lung is supported by a study showing a similar pattern of sonic hedgehog (SHH) signaling in embryonic NE precursor cells and in a subset of SCLCs (Watkins et al. 2003). Nevertheless, the potential NE precursors in the adult lung are not well defined.

If the precursor cell for SCLC and NSCLC is not the same, this implies that particular progenitor cells can only be transformed by specific mutations, thereby contributing to the tumor-type specificity of distinct mutations. Experimental evidence using a conditional oncogenic K-RasIRESlacZ allele indirectly supports the latter, since or results in a strong selection for specific cell variants. One can consider an orthotopic transplantation experiment resulting in a tumor that is very similar to the primary tumor as an indication for limited culture artifacts. In addition, such study might be further complicated when tumors show a high genomic instability.

Importantly, we can reproduce in compound mutant mice some of the observed genetic aberrations and confirm their contribution to the tumor phenotype. Thus, the role of particular combinations of genetic aberrations found in variant cell populations can be studied. This will help to understand whether some of these variant populations, although relatively small, might in fact determine the prognostic features of the tumor.

Next, we describe the use of this strategy in a mouse model for SCLC developed in our laboratory, and we present initial findings illustrating both the resemblance of the mouse model to the human disease and the suitability of this approach.

SPORADIC MOUSE SCLC MODEL

We have described previously the generation of a murine model for SCLC (mSCLC) (Meuwissen et al. 2003). Somatic application of the Cre-loxP system was used to obtain lung-epithelium-specific deletion of *Rb1* and *Trp53* genes. Somatic inactivation of both *Rb1* and *Trp53* alleles in a broad range of proliferating lung epithelial and alveolar type II cells leads to the development of multiple tumors with a histological morphology and immunophenotype closely resembling human SCLC (Fig. 3). Within a relatively short time period after inoculation of mice with Adeno-Cre virus (6–8 weeks), we observed small foci of NE cell proliferation in the airways, which could represent the precursor lesions for dysplasias

and histologically malignant lung tumors. However, NE proliferative foci were still detected in mice that already had substantial tumor load and even metastases. This might indicate that loss of Rb1 and p53 function leads to the expansion of a population of cells highly prone to SCLC development, but that additional genetic lesions are required for progression. Overt tumors, which could be observed 25–40 weeks after infection, were highly proliferative, invasive, and had a marked capacity to metastasize to liver, brain, adrenal gland, bone, and ovaries. Expression of markers for NE differentiation were observed in both primary tumors and metastases, including synaptophysin, neural-cell adhesion molecule 1 (Ncam1), Calcitonin-gene-related peptide (Cgrp), in association with high Ascl1 expression (Fig. 3). The mammalian achaete scute homolog 1 (*ASCL1, HASH-1*) is a basic helix-loop-helix transcription factor that determines the onset and maintenance of NE differentiation in normal pulmonary epithelial cells and also in lung tumors with NE features (Ball et al. 1993; Borges et al. 1997), and is considered a key marker for human SCLC.

To expand the study of genotype–phenotype relationships to distinct cell populations in these tumors, a number of independent cell lines were derived and characterized. All showed expression of NE markers. All these cell lines have been subcloned, and several of the obtained clonal cell lines are now further characterized by immunophenotyping, expression profiling, and array CGH. In vitro growth properties are also being studied. The initial results indicate that different subclones derived from a single tumor may have distinct phenotypes, even when genetic markers (CGH) point to a clonal origin (data not shown), and both *Trp53* and *Rb1* genes are biallelically inactivated in each case. The vast majority of the subclones tested show strong NE differentiation, which correlates with

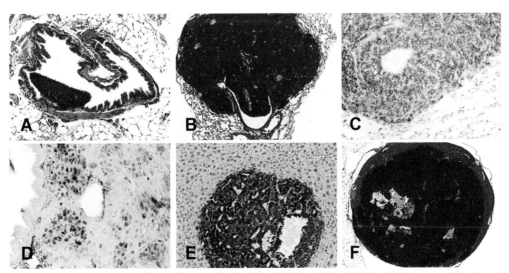

Figure 3. Histopathology of NE tumors from mice carrying *Trp53* and *Rb1* conditional alleles. (*A*) Representative photomicrograph of NE proliferative foci lying in the lumen of bronchioles, visible after 8 weeks of tumor induction. (*B*) Extensive mSCLC tumor, surrounding blood vessels and infiltrating into lung parenchyma. (*C*) NCAM-1 immunodetection of a mSCLC tumor, showing membrane staining. (*D*) Mash-1 (Ascl1) immunodetection of a mSCLC tumor, showing nuclear staining. (*E*) Synaptophysin immunodetection of a liver metastasis from mSCLC. Note cytoplasmic staining in tumor cells but not in liver parenchyma. (*F*) mSCLC metastases into the ovary. (Reprinted, with permission, from Meuwissen et al. 2003 [©Elsevier].)

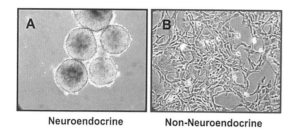

Neuroendocrine   Non-Neuroendocrine

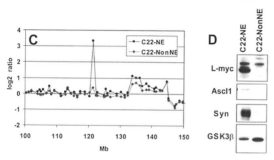

Figure 4. Comparison of distinct cloned cell lines derived from the same original tumor (#22). (*A,B*) Photomicrographs showing the morphology of (*A*) NE-differentiated cells, growing in floating aggregates, and (*B*) non-NE cells, attaching to the plate and featuring spindle-like shape. (*C*) Array CGH profile from a small region on chromosome 4 (100–150 Mb). NE-differentiated cells (*blue line*), but not non-NE cells (*red line*), show a high-level amplification of a BAC-clone-containing *Lmyc1* locus. (*D*) Immunoblotting of L-Myc, Mash-1, synaptophysin, and GSK3β (loading control), showing the correlation between L-myc overexpression and NE-marker expression.

high expression levels of L-myc, N-myc, and Ascl1. These subclones grow as aggregates in suspension resembling "neurospheres." However, other subclones from the same tumors grow attached to substrate and show an expression profile clearly divergent from the NE-differentiated cells. The expression of some stem cell markers in these cells might point to the presence, in mSCLC tumors, of a population of undifferentiated cells, which could be responsible for the metastatic potential of those tumors and especially for the relapse after chemotherapy. In Figure 4, an example of the in vitro morphology of two cloned cell lines is shown. Note that both NE cells, growing in floating aggregates, and non-NE, spindle-like cells were established from the same mSCLC tumor. Some of these cloned cell lines have been orthotopically transplanted into Balb/c nude mice. Only orthotopically transplanted NE cells closely reproduce the tumor growth

properties and marker expression of the original tumors. Variant, non-NE cells that lack some genetic aberrations characteristic of SCLC also do not reproduce the SCLC tumor phenotype upon orthotopic grafting, and might represent a minor subpopulation in the original tumors.

INSIGHT INTO THE MOLECULAR EVENTS

To gain better insight into the separate role of p53 and Rb1 loss in SCLC induction, mice homozygous for both the *Trp53* and *Rb1* conditional alleles were compared to mice carrying either a wild-type (wt) *Trp53* allele (*Trp53F/wt;Rb1F/F*) or a wt *Rb1* allele (*Trp53F/F; Rb1F/wt*) (Meuwissen et al. 2003). Our data show unambiguously that loss of *Rb1* and *Trp53* tumor suppressors acts synergistically in mouse NE tumor formation and that loss of both *Rb1* and *Trp53* is therefore a prerequisite for NE lung tumor formation (Table 2). First, Cre-mediated biallelic deletion of *Trp53* and *Rb1* is found in all NE lung tumors from *Trp53F/F;Rb1F/F* mice. Second, NE lung tumors from *Trp53F/wt;Rb1F/F* mice showed LOH of the remaining wild-type *Trp53* allele, and third, *Trp53F/F;Rb1F/wt* mice only developed mSCLC upon loss of the *wt Rb1* allele; when the *wt Rb1* allele was retained, only adenocarcinomas ensued, similar to those found in *Trp53F/F* mice or in *Trp53⁻/⁻* mice. In summary, complete loss of *Trp53* was observed in all tumors, being an essential event for both adenocarcinoma and SCLC. In contrast, *Rb1* loss per se was unable to initiate lung tumorigenesis but was required together with loss of *Trp53* for the development of NE tumors. This suggests that *Rb1* loss permits the proliferation of cells expressing the NE differentiation program, whereas *Rb1* loss is insufficient to allow proliferation of other cell types, possibly as a result of redundancy of other pocket protein family members. Recent evidence obtained in studies in which targeted disruption was performed of either *Rb1* alone or the three retinoblastoma-protein family members (i.e., *Rb1, p130, p107*) in embryonic lung epithelium further demonstrates a specific role of *Rb1* in the determination of NE cell fate (Wikenheiser-Brokamp 2004). These results also show marked functional redundancy of the pocket proteins in epithelial cell lineages, which could explain, at least in part, the prevalence of p16[INK4a] loss over Rb1 loss in NSCLC.

In addition, loss of *Rb1* appears particularly predominant in tumors originated from neural or NE cells, in line

Table 2. Tumor Phenotypes in Conditional Transgenic Mice

Genotype	Number of mice	No lesions (%)	Only SCLC (%)	Only NSCLC (%)	SCLC and NSCLC (%)	Other lesions (%)	Latency (days)
RbF/F;Trp53F/F	33	—	91	—	6	3	196–350
RbF/wt;Trp53F/F[a]	13	46.1[c]	38.5	7.6	7.6	—	331–584
RbF/F;Trp53F/wt[b]	13	38.5[c]	—	7.6	38.5	15.4	308–588
RbF/F	8	100	—	—	—	—	
Trp53F/F	6	—	—	100	—	—	350–530
LSL-K-RasV12	12	—	—	100	—	—	63–91

[a]LOH in Rb1 was observed in all SCLC tumors tested from heterozygous mice, whereas the wt Rb1 allele was retained in NSCLC lesions.

[b]LOH in Trp53 was observed in all lesions tested, regardless of the tumor phenotype.

[c]These mice were sacrificed at early time points either for examination or due to non-tumor-related sickness.

with the continued expression of neuronal markers including Ascl1 in the majority of these tumors. Whether or not Ascl1 is a direct or indirect downstream effector of Rb1's NE-fate restrictive function, it is clearly necessary to sustain the NE differentiation in human SCLC cell lines (Borges et al. 1997). In fact, Ascl1 immunoreactivity was observed in most mSCLC, and expression levels at the protein and RNA levels correlate very well with the NE differentiation of mSCLC-derived cell lines (Fig. 4).

Also intriguing are our observations regarding L-myc gene (*Lmyc1*) copy number and expression. Array CGH-BAC of primary mSCLC tumor material invariably showed amplification of a narrow genomic stretch containing the *Lung carcinoma derived myc* gene (*Lmyc1*). Even more interestingly, most, if not all, cell clones showing NE phenotype also have a gain in the *Lmyc1* gene copy number, whereas this amplicon is not observed in non-NE-related cell clones (Fig. 4). Expression array data are completely consistent with this finding, as a high level of L-myc expression is observed in mSCLC primary tumors and NE cell clones, but not in non-NE cells. Whether or not *Lmyc1* amplification is functionally responsible for aspects of the NE differentiation, e.g., directly or indirectly regulating *Ascl1* expression, is a question that needs to be addressed in future experiments.

In any case, this confirms that different cell populations in the tumor can harbor distinct genetic alterations, determining or at least correlating with phenotypic divergence. Of note, analysis of whole tumor preparations may neglect the existence of small populations of variant cells that represent a minor component within the tumor. The contribution of these cells to the properties of the tumor (invasion, metastasis, drug resistance) might be easily underestimated, and deserves further study.

CONCLUSIONS

The sporadic mouse SCLC model generated by conditional deletion of *Trp53* and *Rb1* tumor suppressor genes in the mouse lung epithelium has proven to be an invaluable tool for the understanding of neuroendocrine tumor biology because (1) it mimics the histological and pathological characteristics of human SCLC; (2) it presents with a high penetrance, specificity, and relatively short latency; (3) it reproduces some of the additional genetic aberrations and expression changes observed in the human counterpart (i.e., *MYCL1* amplification, *ASCL1* up-regulation); (4) potential target cells and early lesions can be studied; (5) cell lines can be derived and subcloned without being perturbed by major culture artifacts; and (6) derived cell clones may reflect different steps in the tumorigenic process and enable us to establish detailed genotype–phenotype correlations.

Applying the approach described, we can gain a detailed insight into the events that determine tumor phenotype and prognosis. First, we want to define which additional genetic aberrations are necessary for tumor formation and maintenance, as well as when and why these lesions are selected. What is the reason for specific amplification of *Lmyc1* among other *Myc* family members? Second, we want to dissect the signaling pathways that sustain tumor growth, with special interest in the paracrine loops that establish cross-talk relations between cells in a tumor. Finally, we want to assess why distinct populations of cells with different genotypes do persist in the tumor mass. For instance, non-NE cells seem to have little advantage compared to NE cells within the SCLC tumor, but they might contribute to tumor growth by providing growth factors, cytokines, or extracellular matrix components. In addition, this minor cell population can serve as a source of plasticity giving the tumor better chances to adapt to new conditions, like hypoxia, nutrient depletion, or chemotherapy. To test these possibilities further in vivo, we are currently testing the advantage of mixed populations versus pure cloned populations in orthotopically grafted mice.

However, the final goal of any animal model for human pathology is to translate the acquired knowledge into prevention, diagnostic, or treatment strategies, as well as to enable preclinical testing of such strategies. The mSCLC model also offers good opportunities for translational studies. The search for serological markers in mice in early stages of the disease can provide a tool for early detection of lung neuroendocrine lesions. On the other hand, intervention studies using the in vitro and in vivo systems described here can yield new preventive or therapeutic regimens. For example, RNA interference technology applied to cloned cell lines either in vitro or in tumor cell grafts will enable us to test candidate targets even before having target-specific drugs. In addition, cloned cell lines can be labeled with reporter genes (e.g., luciferase, lacZ) to facilitate the longitudinal screening of tumor growth and metastatic spread.

These studies, together with observations made in other mouse tumor models, will undoubtedly increase our understanding not only of cancer as a disease, but also of the selective processes leading to tumor progression. In addition to the mSCLC model, we have generated a number of different well-defined mouse tumor models, like lung adenocarcinoma (Meuwissen et al. 2001), mesothelioma (J. Jongsma et al., in prep.), or melanoma (I. Huijbers et al., in prep.) also showing an important degree of specificity. The goal is now to uncover the Achilles' heel of these tumorigenic processes so that we can intervene in a way that leaves little chance for tumor progression or relapse.

ACKNOWLEDGMENTS

The authors thank Suzanne Jonkheer and John Zevenhoven for technical assistance, and the personnel of the mouse facility for animal care. J.C. was supported by the Centre of Biomedical Genetics. Part of the work was supported by The Dutch Cancer Society (E.vM.).

REFERENCES

Ball D.W., Azzoli C.G., Baylin S.B., Chi D., Dou S., Donis-Keller H., Cumaraswamy A., Borges M., and Nelkin B.D. 1993. Identification of a human achaete-scute homolog highly expressed in neuroendocrine tumors. *Proc. Natl. Acad. Sci.* **90:** 5648.

Bernards R. and Weinberg R.A. 2002. A progression puzzle. *Nature* **418**: 823.

Borges M., Linnoila R.I., van de Velde H.J., Chen H., Nelkin B.D., Mabry M., Baylin S.B., and Ball D.W. 1997. An achaete-scute homologue essential for neuroendocrine differentiation in the lung. *Nature* **386**: 852.

Brambilla E., Negoescu A., Gazzeri S., Lantuejoul S., Moro D., Brambilla C., and Coll J.L. 1996. Apoptosis-related factors p53, Bcl2, and Bax in neuroendocrine lung tumors. *Am. J. Pathol.* **149**: 1941.

Brambilla E., Moro D., Gazzeri S., Brichon P.Y., Nagy-Mignotte H., Morel F., Jacrot M., and Brambilla C. 1991. Cytotoxic chemotherapy induces cell differentiation in small-cell lung carcinoma. *J. Clin. Oncol.* **9**: 50.

Dean M., Fojo T., and Bates S. 2005. Tumour stem cells and drug resistance. *Nat. Rev. Cancer* **5**: 275.

Dosaka-Akita H., Hu S.X., Fujino M., Harada M., Kinoshita I., Xu H.J., Kuzumaki N., Kawakami Y., and Benedict W.F. 1997. Altered retinoblastoma protein expression in nonsmall cell lung cancer: Its synergistic effects with altered ras and p53 protein status on prognosis. *Cancer* **79**: 1329.

Fathi Z., Way J.W., Corjay M.H., Viallet J., Sausville E.A., and Battey J.F. 1996. Bombesin receptor structure and expression in human lung carcinoma cell lines. *J. Cell. Biochem. Suppl.* **24**: 237.

Fong K.M., Sekido Y., Gazdar A.F., and Minna J.D. 2003. Lung cancer. 9: Molecular biology of lung cancer: Clinical implications. *Thorax* **58**: 892.

Forgacs E., Zochbauer-Muller S., Olah E., and Minna J.D. 2001. Molecular genetic abnormalities in the pathogenesis of human lung cancer. *Pathol. Oncol. Res.* **7**: 6.

Giangreco A., Reynolds S.D., and Stripp B.R. 2002. Terminal bronchioles harbor a unique airway stem cell population that localizes to the bronchoalveolar duct junction. *Am. J. Pathol.* **161**: 173.

Guerra C., Mijimolle N., Dhawahir A., Dubus P., Barradas M., Serrano M., Campuzano V., and Barbacid M. 2003. Tumor induction by an endogenous K-ras oncogene is highly dependent on cellular context. *Cancer Cell* **4**: 111.

Harris H. 2004. Tumour suppression: Putting on the brakes. *Nature* **427**: 201.

Hong K.U., Reynolds S.D., Giangreco A., Hurley C.M., and Stripp B.R. 2001. Clara cell secretory protein-expressing cells of the airway neuroepithelial body microenvironment include a label-retaining subset and are critical for epithelial renewal after progenitor cell depletion. *Am. J. Respir. Cell Mol. Biol.* **24**: 671.

Hong K.U., Reynolds S.D., Watkins S., Fuchs E., and Stripp B.R. 2004. Basal cells are a multipotent progenitor capable of renewing the bronchial epithelium. *Am. J. Pathol.* **164**: 577.

Hynes R.O. 2003. Metastatic potential: Generic predisposition of the primary tumor or rare, metastatic variants-or both? *Cell* **113**: 821.

Jackson E.L., Willis N., Mercer K., Bronson R.T., Crowley D., Montoya R., Jacks T., and Tuveson D.A. 2001. Analysis of lung tumor initiation and progression using conditional expression of oncogenic K-ras. *Genes Dev.* **15**: 3243.

Johnson L., Mercer K., Greenbaum D., Bronson R.T., Crowley D., Tuveson D.A., and Jacks T. 2001. Somatic activation of the K-ras oncogene causes early onset lung cancer in mice. *Nature* **410**: 1111.

Jonkers J. and Berns A. 2002. Conditional mouse models of sporadic cancer. *Nat. Rev. Cancer* **2**: 251.

Kang Y., Siegel P.M., Shu W., Drobnjak M., Kakonen S.M., Cordon-Cardo C., Guise T.A., and Massague J. 2003. A multigenic program mediating breast cancer metastasis to bone. *Cancer Cell* **3**: 537.

Kim C.F., Jackson E.L., Woolfenden A.E., Lawrence S., Babar I., Vogel S., Crowley D., Bronson R.T., and Jacks T. 2005. Identification of bronchioalveolar stem cells in normal lung and lung cancer. *Cell* **121**: 823.

Kraus A.C., Ferber I., Bachmann S.O., Specht H., Wimmel A., Gross M.W., Schlegel J., Suske G., and Schuermann M. 2002.

In vitro chemo- and radio-resistance in small cell lung cancer correlates with cell adhesion and constitutive activation of AKT and MAP kinase pathways. *Oncogene* **21**: 8683.

Landis S.H., Murray T., Bolden S., and Wingo P.A. 1999. Cancer statistics, 1999. *CA Cancer J. Clin.* **49**: 8.

Maulik G., Kijima T., and Salgia R. 2003. Role of receptor tyrosine kinases in lung cancer. *Methods Mol. Med.* **74**: 113.

Meuwissen R. and Berns A. 2005. Mouse models for human lung cancer. *Genes Dev.* **19**: 643.

Meuwissen R., Linn S.C., van der Valk M., Mooi W.J., and Berns A. 2001. Mouse model for lung tumorigenesis through Cre/lox controlled sporadic activation of the K-Ras oncogene. *Oncogene* **20**: 6551.

Meuwissen R., Linn S.C., Linnoila R.I., Zevenhoven J., Mooi W.J., and Berns A. 2003. Induction of small cell lung cancer by somatic inactivation of both Trp53 and Rb1 in a conditional mouse model. *Cancer Cell* **4**: 181.

Minn A.J., Kang Y., Serganova I., Gupta G.P., Giri D.D., Doubrovin M., Ponomarev V., Gerald W.L., Blasberg R., and Massague J. 2005. Distinct organ-specific metastatic potential of individual breast cancer cells and primary tumors. *J. Clin. Invest.* **115**: 44.

Paez J.G., Janne P.A., Lee J.C., Tracy S., Greulich H., Gabriel S., Herman P., Kaye F.J., Lindeman N., Boggon T.J., Naoki K., Sasaki H., Fujii Y., Eck M.J., Sellers W.R., Johnson B.E., and Meyerson M. 2004. EGFR mutations in lung cancer: Correlation with clinical response to gefitinib therapy. *Science* **304**: 1497.

Ramaswamy S., Ross K.N., Lander E.S., and Golub T.R. 2003. A molecular signature of metastasis in primary solid tumors. *Nat. Genet.* **33**: 49.

Reissmann P.T., Koga H., Takahashi R., Figlin R.A., Holmes E.C., Piantadosi S., Cordon-Cardo C., and Slamon D.J. 1993. Inactivation of the retinoblastoma susceptibility gene in non-small-cell lung cancer. The Lung Cancer Study Group. *Oncogene* **8**: 1913.

Richardson G.E. and Johnson B.E. 1993. The biology of lung cancer. *Semin. Oncol.* **20**: 105.

Rozengurt E. 1998. V. Gastrointestinal peptide signaling through tyrosine phosphorylation of focal adhesion proteins. *Am. J. Physiol.* **275**: G177.

Schmidt-Kittler O., Ragg T., Daskalakis A., Granzow M., Ahr A., Blankenstein T.J., Kaufmann M., Diebold J., Arnholdt H., Muller P., Bischoff J., Harich D., Schlimok G., Riethmuller G., Eils R., and Klein C.A. 2003. From latent disseminated cells to overt metastasis: Genetic analysis of systemic breast cancer progression. *Proc. Natl. Acad. Sci.* **100**: 7737.

Toyooka S., Tsuda T., and Gazdar A.F. 2003. The TP53 gene, tobacco exposure, and lung cancer. *Hum. Mutat.* **21**: 229.

van de Vijver M.J., He Y.D., van't Veer L.J., Dai H., Hart A.A., Voskuil D.W., Schreiber G.J., Peterse J.L., Roberts C., Marton M.J., Parrish M., Atsma D., Witteveen A., Glas A., Delahaye L., van der Velde T., Bartelink H., Rodenhuis S., Rutgers E.T., Friend S.H., and Bernards R. 2002. A gene-expression signature as a predictor of survival in breast cancer. *N. Engl. J. Med.* **347**: 1999.

van 't Veer L.J., Dai H., van de Vijver M.J., He Y.D., Hart A.A., Mao M., Peterse H.L., van der Kooy K., Marton M.J., Witteveen A.T., Schreiber G.J., Kerkhoven R.M., Roberts C., Linsley P.S., Bernards R., and Friend S.H. 2002. Gene expression profiling predicts clinical outcome of breast cancer. *Nature* **415**: 530.

Watkins D.N., Berman D.M., Burkholder S.G., Wang B., Beachy P.A., and Baylin S.B. 2003. Hedgehog signalling within airway epithelial progenitors and in small-cell lung cancer. *Nature* **422**: 313.

Wikenheiser-Brokamp K.A. 2004. Rb family proteins differentially regulate distinct cell lineages during epithelial development. *Development* **131**: 4299.

Worden F.P. and Kalemkerian G.P. 2000. Therapeutic advances in small cell lung cancer. *Expert Opin. Investig. Drugs* **9**: 565.

Zochbauer-Muller S., Gazdar A.F., and Minna J.D. 2002. Molecular pathogenesis of lung cancer. *Annu. Rev. Physiol.* **64**: 681.

Cell Cycle and Cancer: Genetic Analysis of the Role of Cyclin-dependent Kinases

M. Barbacid, S. Ortega, R. Sotillo, J. Odajima, A. Martín, D. Santamaría, P. Dubus,* and M. Malumbres

*Molecular Oncology Program, Centro Nacional de Investigaciones Oncológicas (CNIO), Melchor Fernández Almagro 3, 28029 Madrid, Spain; *EA2406 University of Bordeaux 2, F-33076 Bordeaux, France*

Most human tumors harbor mutations that misregulate the early phases of the cell cycle. Here, we summarize genetic evidence, mostly obtained in our laboratory using strains of gene-targeted mice, that provides direct experimental support for a role of Cdk4 in tumor development. Moreover, these genetic studies challenge some well-established concepts regarding the role of Cdks during the early phases of the cell cycle. For instance, they have illustrated that Cdk4 and Cdk6 are not essential for cell division during embryonic development except in the hematopoietic system. More surprisingly, mice lacking Cdk2 survive for over 2 years without detectable abnormalities except in their germ cells, indicating that Cdk2 is essential for meiosis but dispensable for the normal mitotic cell cycle. Cdk2 is also dispensable for cell cycle inhibition and tumor suppression by the Cip/Kip inhibitors, p21^{Cip1} and p27^{Kip1}. These observations have important implications not only to understand cell cycle regulation, but also to validate Cdks as potential targets for the development of therapeutic strategies to block proliferation of tumor cells.

To ensure proper progression through the cell cycle, cells have developed a series of checkpoints that prevent them from entering into a new phase of the cycle until they have successfully completed the previous one. Recently divided or quiescent cells also must pass certain checkpoints before they enter a new cycle. For instance, these cells must determine whether they have all the necessary nutrients to carry out cell division. They also need to sense that they have reached proper homeostatic cell size, otherwise they will decrease (or increase) in size with each round of division. Metazoans must also control the number of cells in every organ, a parameter that, coupled with cell size, ultimately determines the size of every individual. In addition, cells must control the amount of mitogenic information required to enter the cycle (for review, see Malumbres and Barbacid 2001). Too stringent requirements would prevent cell proliferation at critical times such as during wound healing or to fight an infection. On the other hand, overly relaxed controls would lead to unscheduled proliferation and possibly neoplastic growth.

The mammalian cell cycle (see Fig. 1) is thought to be driven by heterodimeric kinases composed of a catalytic subunit known as cyclin-dependent kinase (Cdk) and a regulatory subunit, designated as cyclin. Two of these Cdks, Cdk4 and Cdk6, bind to and are activated by the D-type family of cyclins, D1, D2, and D3 (for review, see Sherr and Roberts 1999). The D-type cyclins are critical integrators of mitogenic signaling since their synthesis is one of the main endpoints of the Ras/Raf/MAPK signaling pathway. Interestingly, mouse embryonic fibroblasts that lack the three D-type cyclins can proliferate, indicating that these molecules are not strictly necessary for progression through G$_1$ (Kozar et al. 2004; see below). Whether this activity is mediated by other cyclins, or by alternative mechanisms, remains to be resolved.

The primary role of the D-type cyclin/Cdk4 or Cdk6

complexes is to phosphorylate members of the retinoblastoma (Rb) protein family, pRb, p107, and p130. The Rb proteins are tumor suppressors that in their active, nonphosphorylated state prevent expression of genes necessary for DNA replication (S phase of the cell cycle) and mitosis (M phase). Phosphorylation of pRb by D-type cyclin/Cdk4 or Cdk6 complexes results in its partial inactivation, which, in turn, allows expression of a limited number of transcriptional targets needed to drive cells through the G$_1$ phase of the cell cycle (for review, see Co-

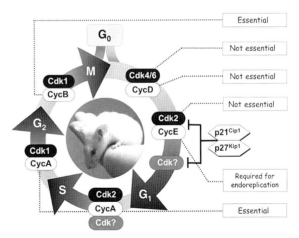

Figure 1. Schematic representation of the mammalian cycle. The distinct phases of the mammalian cell cycle, including quiescence (G$_0$), Gap 1 (G$_1$), DNA synthesis (S), Gap2 (G$_2$), and mitosis (M) are indicated. Those Cdk/cyclin complexes thought to drive each of these phases are also indicated. **Cdk?** represents a putative Cdk responsible for mediating the inhibitory activity of the Cip/Kip proteins in G$_1$ and/or driving DNA synthesis in the absence of Cdk2. Boxes on the right side indicate whether each of these molecules is essential for cell cycle progression based on genetic studies using gene-targeted mice. For more details see Table 1.

Table 1. Genetic Analysis of Mammalian Cell Cycle Cdks

Cdk	Alteration	Viability	Phenotype in vivo	Phenotype in vitro	References
Cdk4	R42C mutant insensitive to INK4 inhibitors	viable	epithelial and mesenchymal tumors with complete penetrance after 14–18 months	faster cell cycles and no "culture crisis"; increased susceptibility to transformation by Ras oncogenes	Sotillo et al. (2001a,b)
Cdk4	null mutation	viable	lack of proliferation of post-natal pancreatic β-cells and pituitary lactotrophs; small size	decreased susceptibility to immortalization or trans-formation by oncogenes	Rane et al. (1999); Tsutsui et al. (1999); Moons et al. (2002); Martín et al. (2003)
Cdk6	null mutation	viable	defective erythroid lineage development	no phenotype in MEFs but delayed proliferation of lymphoid cells	Malumbres et al. (2004)
Cdk4 and Cdk6	double null mutant	late-embryonic lethality	limited proliferation of committed hematopoietic precursors, especially those of erythroid origin	delayed cell cycles and decreased pRb phosphory-lation; cells respond to mitogenic stimuli and become immortal upon passage	Malumbres et al. (2004)
Cdk2	null mutation	viable	male and female sterility due to meiotic defects; no defects in mitotic cells	Early senescence in MEFs in culture; no major cell cycle defects	Ortega et al. (2003)
Cdk2	conditional null mutation	viable	no phenotype observed	no defects in cell proliferation after ablation	our unpublished observations
Cdk2 and Cdk6	double null mutant	viable	phenotype identical to Cdk2 and Cdk6 single mutants	phenotype identical to Cdk2 and Cdk6 single mutants; no synergism	Malumbres et al. (2004)
Cdk3	premature stop codon	viable	normal; most laboratory strains carry this mutation	normal; mutation present in "wild type" MEFs	Ye et al. (2001)

For related information on mice defective in the corresponding cyclins, see Ciemerych and Sicinski (2005).

brinik 2005). Some of these targets include the E-type cyclins (E1 and E2), whose primary role is to activate Cdk2. Active E-type cyclin/Cdk2 complexes further phosphorylate pRb, leading to a wave of transcriptional activity essential to proceed through the G_1/S transition.

Cdk activity can be negatively regulated by Cdk inhibitors (CKI). CKIs come in two flavors. The four-member INK4 family (p16^{INK4a}, p15^{INK4b}, p18^{INK4c}, and p19^{INK4d}) exerts its inhibitory activity by binding to the Cdk4 and Cdk6 kinases and preventing their association with D-type cyclins (Sherr and Roberts 1999). Although INK4 proteins are biochemically indistinguishable from each other in vitro, they are expressed at different times during embryonic and postnatal development. Moreover, generation of gene-targeted mice deficient for each of these proteins has revealed significant functional differences (for review, see Ortega et al. 2002). The three members of the Cip/Kip family, p21^{Cip1}, p27^{Kip1}, and p57^{Kip2}, form heterotrimeric complexes with all the G_1/S Cdks and their cognate cyclins (Sherr and Roberts 1999). However, in stoichiometric amounts, they preferentially inhibit the kinase activity of Cdk2/cyclin E complexes (see below).

CELL CYCLE AND CANCER

Molecular analysis of human tumors has revealed frequent mutations and epigenetic changes within cell cycle regulators (Malumbres and Barbacid 2001). Most of these molecular alterations occur in G_1 regulators, thus underscoring the importance of maintaining proper control of cell cycle commitment to prevent human cancer. They include overexpression of cyclins (mainly cyclins D1 and E1) and Cdks (mainly Cdk4 and Cdk6) as well as loss of CKI expression (mainly p16^{INK4a}, p15^{INK4b}, and p27^{Kip1}) and of pRb. Moreover, Cdk4 has been found mutated in familial melanoma. Although most of these tumor-associated alterations result from DNA mutations, it is becoming increasingly evident that epigenetic silencing of certain promoters (e.g., p16^{INK4a}, p15^{INK4b}, or pRb) also plays a significant role in tumor development (for review, see Esteller 2005).

Direct genetic or epigenetic alteration of Cdk2 has been rarely described. Yet, expression of some of its most direct regulators, p27^{Kip1} and cyclin E1, is frequently altered in human tumors, changes that often correlate with poor prognosis (for review, see Yamasaki and Pagano 2004). Within the Rb protein family, loss or inactivation of pRb is a rather frequent event in human tumors. However, p130 is less frequently lost, and p107 inactivation has not been reported (for review, see Paggi and Giordano 2001). These observations suggest that p107 and p130 may play a primary role in promoting differentiation rather than proliferation, a concept supported by results obtained with gene-targeted mice (for review, see Classon and Harlow 2002). Finally, mutations in the E2F family of transcription factors have not been observed in human tumors.

WIDESPREAD TUMOR INDUCTION IN MICE EXPRESSING A MISREGULATED Cdk4 KINASE

Most human tumors have genetic and/or epigenetic alterations in the cyclin D-INK4-Cdk4/6-pRb pathway. As indicated above, a miscoding mutation (replacement of Arg-24 by Cys) that renders Cdk4 resistant to INK4 inhibitors is associated with the development of human melanoma. To study the effects of such mutation in the regulation of the cell cycle in particular and in tumorigenesis in general, we have engineered knockin mice that carried this mutation within the endogenous mouse $Cdk4$ locus (Rane et al. 1999). $Cdk4^{R24C/R24C}$ mice are born at the expected Mendelian ratio, are fertile, and develop normally. However, these mice developed detectable tumors after 8 months and most of them died by 16 months of age (Sotillo et al. 2001a). Necropsy of more than 100 $Cdk4^{R24C/R24C}$ mice showed a wide spectrum of tumors, including malignancies of mesenchymatous origin (67% incidence); epithelial endocrine (55%); epithelial non-endocrine (24%), and, to a lesser extent, hematopoietic malignancies (3%). Many mice exhibit multiple tumors of independent origin, with an average of almost two tumors per animal. A cohort of 50 mice sacrificed at 14–16 months of age without external signs of disease revealed a similar tumor distribution pattern, except for reduced incidence of sarcomas and pituitary tumors, suggesting that these malignancies are a major cause of death in $Cdk4^{R24C/R24C}$ mice. $Cdk4^{+/R24C}$ mice also succumbed to the same types of malignancies, although with increased latency (Sotillo et al. 2001a).

Cdk4 misregulation synergizes with mutations in other cancer genes such as p53. Double mutant $Cdk4^{R24C/R24C};p53^{-/-}$ mice die before reaching 4 months of age, significantly earlier than their $Cdk4^{+/+};p53^{-/-}$ littermates (Sotillo et al. 2001a). These mice display an increased number of sarcomas, mainly hemangiosarcomas and leiomyosarcomas. Moreover, a significant fraction of these double mutant mice (10%) develop immature teratomas, a tumor not found in any of their single mutant siblings, although a low incidence of teratomas (<2%) has been described previously in $p53^{-/-}$ mice. These results suggest that these key regulators exert growth control at different threshold levels in different cell types.

A MUTANT Cdk4R24C KINASE INDUCES INVASIVE MELANOMAS IN MICE

Interestingly, $Cdk4^{R24C/R24C}$ mice do not develop melanomas, the type of tumor induced by this very same mutation in humans. To determine whether these observations were a consequence of intrinsic mechanistic differences between human and rodents or of phenotypic differences, we submitted the skin of these mutant mice to carcinogenic insults. Specifically, $Cdk4^{R24C/R24C}$ mice were treated with 7,12-dimethylbenz[a]anthracene (DMBA) followed by repeated exposure to 12-O-tetradecanoylphorbol-13-acetate (TPA), a treatment known to induce the rapid development of skin papillomas. Unlike wild-type mice, $Cdk4^{R24C/R24C}$ animals develop a high number of nevi that rapidly grow in size, leading to the formation of tumors of up to 20 mm in diameter by 20 weeks (Sotillo et al. 2001b). Alternative treatments with DMBA plus UVB light also result in the development of similar tumors, albeit with reduced efficiency. No melanocytic tumors are observed after single treatments with either DMBA or UVB light alone.

Histological examination of these lesions confirmed the presence of melanomas in 70% of carcinogen-treated $Cdk4^{R24C/R24C}$ mice (Sotillo et al. 2001b). Unlike other models of melanoma, these tumors are highly melanotic, a property that makes them more reminiscent of those observed in humans. Moreover, as observed in human melanomas, the percentage of melanotic cells decreases in advanced malignancies, since active proliferation and melanocyte dedifferentiation often result in decreased production of melanin. In the more advanced melanomas, $Cdk4^{R24C/R24C}$ tumors are highly cellular, mainly composed of proliferating atypical melanocytes, frequently spindle-shaped with low or no load of melanin. Mitotic figures and areas of necrosis can be easily found. In these cases, melanocyte proliferation is usually invasive to neighbor tissues with infiltrating margins. The neuroectodermal origin of the melanomas is confirmed by positive immunological staining for the S100 antigen. Molecular analysis of $Cdk4^{R24C/R24C}$ melanomas did not reveal either deletion, rearrangement or promoter methylation in $p16^{INK4a}$, $p15^{INK4b}$, or $p19^{ARF}$ loci (Sotillo et al. 2001b). Although these results are expected for those genes encoding upstream INK4 regulators, the absence of $p19^{ARF}$ inactivation suggests that alterations in the p53 pathway are not needed for induction and/or progression of these melanomas.

GENETIC ANALYSIS OF THE ROLE OF Cdks IN VIVO

Targeting the cell cycle is an attractive strategy to block neoplastic growth, since most human tumors carry molecular alterations in genes that regulate cell cycle commitment. Unfortunately, most cell cycle regulators altered in human cancer, such as loss of $p27^{Kip1}$, $p16^{Ink4a}$, or pRb expression, overexpression of cyclin D and cyclin E, etc., are not amenable to classic pharmacological approaches. On the other hand, the Cdks, regardless of whether they are mutated or not, are suitable targets for therapeutic intervention. Indeed, kinase inhibition has already been successfully used for therapeutic purposes in many diseases, including cancer (e.g., Gleevec). Yet, our current knowledge of the cell cycle is not sufficient to ensure the development of optimal strategies. For instance, we do not know which Cdk inhibitors will provide the best therapeutic benefit or whether it would be more efficacious to block two or several Cdks at the same time.

To gain further knowledge about the role of individual Cdks in the proliferation of normal and tumor cells, we have embarked on the systematic analysis of each of the four cell cycle Cdks: Cdk1, Cdk2, Cdk4, and Cdk6, at the genetic level using gene-targeted strategies in embryonic stem cells. A fifth Cdk also implicated in the cell cycle

(Ren and Rollins 2004), Cdk3, is mutated in most strains of laboratory mice (Ye et al. 2001) and will no longer be considered here. Below is a summary of the main results derived from characterizing strains of mice lacking Cdk4, Cdk6, or Cdk2, as well as of double mutant strains lacking Cdk4 and Cdk6 ($Cdk4^{-/-};Cdk6^{-/-}$), Cdk2 and Cdk6 $Cdk2^{-/-};Cdk6^{-/-}$), and Cdk2 and its inhibitors p27^{Kip1} ($Cdk2^{-/-};p27^{Kip1-/-}$) and p21^{Cip1} ($Cdk2^{-/-};p21^{Cip1-/-}$).

Cdk4 null MICE

Ablation of *Cdk4* does not have significant consequences for cell proliferation, at least in mouse embryonic fibroblasts (MEFs). Quiescent *Cdk4 null* ($Cdk4^{n/n}$) MEFs enter S phase with slightly delayed kinetics but proliferate normally (Rane et al. 1999; Tsutsui et al. 1999). In vivo, $Cdk4^{n/n}$ mice are viable, indicating that Cdk4 is not essential for proliferation of most cell types (Rane et al. 1999; Tsutsui et al. 1999). Yet, these mice have limited populations of certain endocrine cell types. For instance, adult $Cdk4^{n/n}$ mice become diabetic due to reduced numbers of insulin-producing pancreatic β-cells (Rane et al. 1999; Tsutsui et al. 1999). Subsequent studies have indicated that Cdk4 is essential for postnatal proliferation of pancreatic β-cells but not for their neogenesis from ductal epithelial cells (Martín et al. 2003). Interestingly, Cdk6 expression is basically undetectable in postnatal pancreatic β-cells, thus providing a possible explanation for their strict dependence on Cdk4 expression.

Cdk4 null mice also have decreased male fertility due to defective spermatogenesis and reduced numbers of Leydig cells (Rane et al. 1999; Tsutsui et al. 1999). Female $Cdk4^{n/n}$ mice are completely sterile due to limited prolactin production, a consequence of their reduced numbers of pituitary lactotrophs (Moons et al. 2002; Jirawatnotai et al. 2004). As in the case of pancreatic β-cells, Cdk4 is essential for postnatal proliferation of the anterior pituitary, but it is not required for embryonal development of the pituitary gland (Moons et al. 2002). Interestingly, siRNA-mediated knockdown of *Cdk4*, but not of *Cdk6*, inhibits GHRH-induced proliferation of GH3 somato/lactotroph cells with restored expression of GHRH receptors, thus suggesting distinct functional roles for these highly related kinases within the same cellular context (Jirawatnotai et al. 2004).

Finally, $Cdk4^{n/n}$ mice are considerably smaller than their wild-type littermates (Rane et al. 1999; Tsutsui et al. 1999). This phenotype is not a consequence of the hormonal defects of *Cdk4 null* animals. $Cdk4^{n/n}$;Rip-*Cre* mice, in which an active Cdk4 kinase is re-expressed in pancreatic β-cells and in pituitary lactotrophs, are normoglycemic and fully fertile, yet they retain their small-size phenotype (Martín et al. 2003). Since the size of *Cdk4 null* cells appears to be similar to that of wild-type cells, it is possible that Cdk4 plays a role in controlling homeotic cell numbers, at least in mice.

Cdk6 null MICE

Mice lacking Cdk6 develop normally and are viable, although hematopoiesis is slightly impaired (Malumbres et al. 2004). This is a somewhat expected result, since Cdk6 is most abundantly expressed in lymphoid organs. In Cdk6-deficient mice, the thymus is reduced in size due to lower cellularity, and its cortical area is atrophic in about one-third of the mutant animals. Their spleens are also reduced in size due to decreased cell density in the red pulp. Whereas in wild-type mice, 70–75% of all spleen cells belong to the erythroid lineage, these figures decrease to 35–40% in $Cdk6^{-/-}$ littermates. Similarly, the number of megakaryocytes is severely reduced to less than one-third of those present in wild-type spleens (Malumbres et al. 2004). *Cdk6 null* mice also exhibit lower numbers of red cells (about 15%) in peripheral blood. Interestingly, $Cdk6^{-/-}$ mice do not display obvious deficiencies in the bone marrow. In vitro, Cdk6 *null* lymphocytes, but not $Cdk6^{-/-}$ MEFs, show delayed entry in the cell cycle upon mitogenic stimulation (Malumbres et al. 2004).

LATE EMBRYONIC LETHALITY OF *Cdk4;Cdk6* DOUBLE MUTANT MICE

Mice lacking both cyclin D-dependent kinases, Cdk4 and Cdk6, are not viable. Yet, $Cdk4^{n/n};Cdk6^{-/-}$ double mutant embryos develop to midgestation with the expected Mendelian frequency, suggesting that they do not have intrinsic cell cycle defects (Malumbres et al. 2004). The percentage of dead embryos increases during late embryonic development. Although some $Cdk4^{n/n};Cdk6^{-/-}$ pups can make it to term, all of them have been found to be dead at birth. These double *null* embryos/pups and their corresponding placentas are well formed and do not present significant abnormalities. Moreover, all tissues, except for those of hematopoietic origin, display normal levels of proliferating and apoptotic cells. E14.5 to E18.5 $Cdk4^{n/n};Cdk6^{-/-}$ embryos have structurally aberrant livers with decreased levels of erythroid precursors. Peripheral blood also reveals a dramatic decrease in the number of red blood cells that display a megaloblastic feature typical of anemia. These findings suggest that $Cdk4^{n/n};Cdk6^{-/-}$ embryos die during the late stages of embryonic development due to limited proliferation of erythroid progenitors.

The relative numbers of $Cdk4^{n/n};Cdk6^{-/-}$ hematopoietic stem cells (HSCs) appear to be normal, although their absolute numbers are decreased due to the lower cellularity of the mutant livers (around 15%). However, the levels of other *Cdk4/Cdk6 null* lineage-committed progenitors are reduced beyond those levels expected from the decreased cellularity (Malumbres et al. 2004). Accordingly, the numbers of more mature hematopoietic cells, such as monocytes, macrophages, or lymphocytes, are also reduced. Interestingly, the phenotype of $Cdk4^{n/n};Cdk6^{-/-}$ double knockout mice is very similar to that observed in mice lacking the three D-type cyclins (Kozar et al. 2004). Yet, D-type cyclin-depleted embryos exhibit a more dramatic reduction of hematopoietic cells. Whether the formation of Cdk2/cyclin D complexes (see below) contributes to alleviate the requirement for Cdk4 and Cdk6 in hematopoietic cells remains to be determined.

Cdk4 AND Cdk6 DEFECTIVE MEFs

Early passage $Cdk4^{n/n}$;$Cdk6^{-/-}$ MEFs proliferate well, albeit at a slower rate than control cells (Malumbres et al. 2004). Moreover, all Cdk4$^{n/n}$;Cdk6$^{-/-}$ double mutant MEFs can immortalize upon continuous passage in culture. These MEFs also proliferate in low serum conditions and respond to mitogenic stimuli induced by addition of EGF and IGF-1. Moreover, they enter S phase upon mitogenic stimulation with normal kinetics, albeit less efficiently than wild-type cells. These observations, taken together, indicate that the D-type cyclin-dependent kinases are not essential either for cell proliferation or for re-entry in the cell cycle, at least in MEFs.

Ablation of Cdk4 and Cdk6 does not affect expression of D-type cyclins. These cyclins, in the absence of their cognate partners, form functional complexes with Cdk2 (Malumbres et al. 2004). Indeed, these Cdk2/cyclin D kinases phosphorylate pRb, at least in vitro. Moreover, $Cdk2$ shRNA significantly decreases the rate of BrdU incorporation in $Cdk4^{n/n}$;$Cdk6^{-/-}$ MEFs. These observations suggest that in the absence of Cdk4 and Cdk6, Cdk2, in association with D-type cyclins, may help to drive cells through the early phases of the cell cycle. Yet, confirmation of this hypothesis must await genetic scrutiny; for instance, by generating Cdk4/Cdk6/Cdk2 triple mutant mice.

ABLATION OF THE *Cdk2* LOCUS REVEALS Cdk2 AS AN ESSENTIAL MEIOTIC KINASE

$Cdk2^{-/-}$ mice are born at the expected Mendelian ratio, indicating that Cdk2 is not essential for cell proliferation in most, if not all, tissues (Berthet et al. 2003; Ortega et al. 2003). Moreover, these mutant mice do not display gross anatomical or behavioral abnormalities for up to 2 years of life except for severe atrophy in their gonads that results in complete sterility. Spermatogenesis defects in $Cdk2^{-/-}$ male mice become visible at P20, a time when germ cells have completed meiosis I. P20 $Cdk2^{-/-}$ animals do not have round spermatids in the seminiferous tubules, and there is massive apoptosis of spermatocytes (Ortega et al. 2003). Analysis of spermatocytes from adult mice by immunoconfocal microscopy shows leptotene, zygotene, and pachytene stages, but no diplotene or later meiotic stages. Studies using immunohistochemical markers firmly established that the absence of Cdk2 triggers the pachytene checkpoint responsible for the massive apoptosis observed in $Cdk2^{-/-}$ spermatocytes (Ortega et al. 2003).

$Cdk2^{-/-}$ oocytes develop normally through the leptotene, zygotene, and pachytene stages (E14.5–E18.5). However, when oocytes reach the dictyate stage (P1–P2), $Cdk2$ mutant oocytes display multiple defects (desynapsed fibers, randomly distributed centromeres, etc.) which indicate that $Cdk2^{-/-}$ oocytes also have a defect in prophase I, albeit at a later developmental stage (Ortega et al. 2003). These observations establish that Cdk2 is essential for completion of the first meiotic division in both male and female germ cells.

Interestingly, mice deficient for both E-type cyclins are not viable, most likely due to a defect in the endoreplication of placental trophoblast giant cells (Geng et al. 2003; Parisi et al. 2003). These observations provide genetic evidence for a differential role of Cdk2 and E-type cyclins, at least during endoreplication. This suggests that E-type cyclins must have a partner(s) other than Cdk2. Whether such partners are Cdks, and whether they are functional in cells other than trophoblasts, remain to be determined.

Cdk2 IS DISPENSABLE FOR THE MITOTIC CELL CYCLE

Primary $Cdk2^{-/-}$ MEFs grow well in culture and proliferate with kinetics similar to those of wild-type cells (Berthet et al. 2003; Ortega et al. 2003). Serum-starved $Cdk2^{-/-}$ MEFs enter S phase with the same kinetics as their wild-type counterparts upon serum stimulation. $Cdk2^{-/-}$ MEFs also become immortalized upon continuous passage in culture. Indeed, we have only observed subtle differences in the timing at which these cells enter culture crisis. Moreover, removal of Cdk2 from $Cdk2^{lox/-}$ MEFs does not have significant consequences in their proliferative properties, indicating that Cdk2 is dispensable for cell proliferation in conditions in which plasticity is unlikely to play a role (Ortega et al. 2003). E-type cyclin-deficient MEFs also proliferate well in culture. However, these cells have a defect in cell cycle re-entry, presumably due to a failure in loading MCM proteins onto DNA replication origins (Geng et al. 2003). These observations provide additional genetic evidence for the existence of E-type cyclin partners other than Cdk2. Whether the putative cyclin E partners responsible for this cell cycle defect are the same as those required for endoreplication remains to be determined.

ABSENCE OF SYNERGISM BETWEEN Cdk6 AND Cdk2 DEFICIENCIES

Crosses between $Cdk6^{+/-}$;$Cdk2^{+/-}$ heterozygous mice yield $Cdk6^{-/-}$;$Cdk2^{-/-}$ double *null* animals with expected Mendelian ratios. Mice defective for Cdk6 and Cdk2 display those phenotypical abnormalities previously observed in Cdk6 and Cdk2 single mutant strains (Ortega et al. 2003; Malumbres et al. 2004). Briefly, $Cdk6^{-/-}$;$Cdk2^{-/-}$ animals are sterile and show marked defects in spermatogenesis and oogenesis, basically indistinguishable from those reported for Cdk2-deficient mice (Ortega et al. 2003). They also have limited defects in hematopoietic cells similar to those described above for $Cdk6$ null mice. Finally, $Cdk6^{-/-}$;$Cdk2^{-/-}$ animals survive for up to 1.5 years without developing obvious additional abnormalities (Malumbres et al. 2004).

Cdk2 IS ALSO DISPENSABLE FOR CELL CYCLE REGULATION MEDIATED BY Cip/Kip INHIBITORS

The above results challenge the central roles attributed to Cdk2 in cell cycle progression. One such role involves mediating the inhibitory properties and tumor-suppressing activities of p21^{Cip1} and p27^{Kip1}, the best character-ized members of the Cip/Kip family of cell cycle in-hibitors (Sherr and Roberts 1999). Infection of primary MEFs with retroviruses expressing p21^{Cip1} or p27^{Kip1} proteins halts their proliferation regardless of the pres-ence or absence of Cdk2 (Martín et al. 2005). About half of the $Cdk2^{-/-}$ MEFs are halted in G_2/M, a result likely due to inhibition of Cdk1. However, most $Cdk2^{-/-}$ cells (60%) are arrested in G_1. Genetic evidence argues against a compensatory role of Cdk4 and Cdk6, since p27^{Kip1} and p21^{Cip1} effectively block cell proliferation in MEFs lack-ing either Cdk4 and Cdk6, or the three D-type cyclins (Kozar et al. 2004; Malumbres et al. 2004). Generation of double Cdk2/Cdk4 mutant cells or cells lacking the three G_1/S Cdks: Cdk2, Cdk4, and Cdk6, should help to deci-pher the functional target(s) of the Cip/Kip inhibitors.

Primary $p27^{Kip1-/-};Cdk2^{-/-}$ and $p21^{Cip1-/-};Cdk2^{-/-}$ MEFs display increased proliferation rates similar to those of $p27^{Kip1}$ null or $p21^{Cip1}$ null cells (Martín et al. 2005). These observations indicate that loss of Cdk2 does not abrogate the proliferative advantage conferred by the absence of p27^{Kip1} or p21^{Cip1} tumor suppressors. More-over, quiescent $p27^{Kip1-/-};Cdk2^{-/-}$ and $p21^{Cip1-/-};Cdk2^{-/-}$ MEFs enter S phase 4–6 hours earlier than wild-type cells upon serum stimulation (Martín et al. 2005), indicating that the shortening in S phase entry cannot be mediated by constitutive activation of Cdk2.

Cdk2 IS NOT ESSENTIAL FOR p21^{Cip1}-MEDIATED CELL CYCLE ARREST AFTER DNA DAMAGE

p21^{Cip1} is one of the major effectors of cell cycle arrest induced following DNA damage. Double mutant $p21^{Cip1-/-};Cdk2^{-/-}$ cells display the same levels of BrdU incorporation as $p21^{Cip1-/-}$ MEFs upon exposure to gamma radiation or to etoposide treatment. Moreover, these double mutant cells also fail to arrest in G_1 after these treatments (Martín et al. 2005). These observations provide genetic evidence against the concept that p21^{Cip1} mediates cell cycle arrest at the DNA damage checkpoint by blocking Cdk2 activity.

THE TUMOR SUPPRESSOR ACTIVITY OF p27^{Kip1} DOES NOT REQUIRE Cdk2

Mice defective for p27^{Kip1} are bigger in size, display organomegaly and retinal defects, and develop frequent pituitary tumors (Fero et al. 1996; Kiyokawa et al. 1996; Nakayama et al. 1996). $p27^{Kip1-/-};Cdk2^{-/-}$ double mutant mice weigh, on average, 50–60% more than wild type and display widespread organomegaly similar to $p27^{Kip1-/-}$ null animals, except in testis and ovaries which were as hypotrophic as in $Cdk2^{-/-}$ mice (Martín et al. 2005). $p27^{Kip1-/-};Cdk2^{-/-}$ mutant animals display the same retinal defects observed in $p27^{Kip1}$ null mice and with similar penetrance (about 10%) (Kiyokawa et al. 1996; Nakayama et al. 1996). More importantly, these double mutant mice develop pituitary tumors with the same high penetrance and latency as p27^{Kip1} single mu-tant animals (Martín et al. 2005). The pituitary tumors of $p27^{Kip1-/-};Cdk2^{-/-}$ mice display the same elevated prolif-erative indexes and volume sizes as those observed in $p27^{Kip1-/-}$ null mice. These results illustrate that Cdk2 is not required to mediate the in vivo tumor suppressor ac-tivity of p27^{Kip1}.

CONCLUSIONS

Cell Cycle Mutations and Cancer

Cancer is frequently considered as a cell cycle disease. Although many cell cycle regulatory mechanisms have been studied at length in vitro, it is still unclear how they are coordinately regulated in vivo and how their misreg-ulation leads to human cancer. Evidence accumulated over the last decade has clearly illustrated that mutation of the same cell cycle regulators known to be mutated or epigenetically altered in human cancer also leads to tu-mor development in mice (Ortega et al. 2002). For in-stance, $pRb^{+/-}$ (Jacks et al. 1992; Lee et al. 1992), $Cdk4^{R24C/R24C}$ (Rane et al. 1999; Sotillo et al. 2001a), and $Ink4a/Arf^{-/-}$ (Serrano et al. 1996) mice develop tumors with complete penetrance. Other mutations, such as those ablating the INK4 inhibitors p16^{Ink4a} and p15^{Ink4b}, have not led to overt tumor development (Latres et al. 2000; Krimpenfort et al. 2001; Sharpless et al. 2001) but seem to predispose to cancer. Whether these mutations in hu-mans only contribute to carcinogenesis in the presence of other mutations remains to be determined. Finally, am-plification of cyclin D1 or cyclin E in mice also leads to abnormal growth, albeit not to overt tumor growth, sug-gesting that they are contributors, but not "primary drivers" of carcinogenesis.

Cdks and the Regulation of the Cell Cycle

Genetic analysis of the role of Cdks has provided a se-ries of observations that are not compatible with widely accepted models for the mammalian cell cycle. Mainly, neither the D-type cyclins nor their cognate cyclin D-de-pendent kinases, Cdk4 and Cdk6, are essential for cell proliferation or exit from quiescence in most cell types. Only cells of hematopoietic origin appear to require at least one of these D-type cyclins or their kinase partners for proper proliferation. Several issues need to be ad-dressed before we can fully evaluate the requirements for the D-type cyclin-dependent kinases in mammalian cells. For instance, we need to determine whether they are re-quired in adult tissues, since it could be argued that dur-ing embryonic development most cells do not exit the cy-cle. Alternatively, it is possible that exit from quiescence during embryogenesis might be regulated by mechanisms distinct from those that regulate cell cycle re-entry in adult cells.

It is also possible that in the absence of Cdk4 and Cdk6, cellular plasticity allows Cdk2 to interact with the D-type cyclins and to compensate for their absence. Likewise, it could be argued that the Cdk2/cyclin E kinases may func-tionally compensate for the lack of D-cyclin-dependent kinase activity (Geng et al. 1999). Generation of triple Cdk4/Cdk6/Cdk2 *null* mice should help to resolve some of these issues.

Regardless of potential compensatory effects by other Cdks, or even by other less related kinases, the absolute dispensability of Cdk2 in mitotic cells in vivo is an unexpected finding. Despite extensive bibliography linking Cdk2 to many critical cellular processes such as DNA replication and centrosome duplication (Sherr and Roberts 1999), available genetic evidence to date has failed to demonstrate a role for Cdk2 in these processes. Equally surprising have been recent genetic observations indicating that Cdk2 is not essential for mediating the cell cycle inhibitory properties of the Cip/Kip inhibitors p21^{Cip1} and p27^{Kip1} (Aleem et al. 2005; Martín et al. 2005). Likewise, the presence or absence of Cdk2 has no effect on the incidence or latency of pituitary tumors caused by loss of p27^{Kip1}. These observations have direct implications in the design of therapeutic strategies to fight tumors in which there is loss of p27^{Kip1} expression, or even loss of P53, since this tumor suppressor controls the synthesis of p21^{Cip1}. Although the essential targets for p21^{Cip1} and p27^{Kip1} tumor suppressors remain to be identified, it is likely that they block cell cycle progression, at least partially, by inhibiting Cdk1. Whether inhibition of Cdk1 will have a selective effect on tumor cells is a key issue that should be addressed by genetic means before selective inhibitors are developed.

In summary, our results illustrate the need to continue interrogating the cell cycle by genetic means. An integrated view from biochemical studies, experimental animal models, and the analysis of cancer mutations will undoubtedly help to exploit this knowledge to develop rational therapeutic approaches with which to target those tumors exhibiting a deregulated cell cycle.

REFERENCES

Aleem E., Kiyokawa H., and Kaldis P. 2005. Cdc2-cyclin E complexes regulate the G1/S phase transition. *Nat. Cell Biol.* **7**: 831.

Berthet C., Aleem E., Coppola V., Tessarollo L., and Kaldis P. 2003. Cdk2 knockout mice are viable. *Curr. Biol.* **13**: 1775.

Ciemerych M.A. and Sicinski P. 2005. Cell cycle in mouse development. *Oncogene* **24**: 2877.

Classon M. and Harlow E. 2002. The retinoblastoma tumour suppressor in development and cancer. *Nat. Rev. Cancer* **2**: 910.

Cobrinik D. 2005. Pocket proteins and cell cycle control. *Oncogene* **24**: 2796.

Esteller M. 2005. Aberrant DNA methylation as a cancer-inducing mechanism. *Annu. Rev. Pharmacol. Toxicol.* **45**: 629.

Fero M.L., Rivkin M., Tasch M., Porter P., Carow C.E., Firpo E., Polyak K., Tsai L.H., Broudy V., Perlmutter R.M., Kaushansky K., and Roberts J.M. 1996. A syndrome of multiorgan hyperplasia with features of gigantism, tumorigenesis, and female sterility in p27(^{Kip1})-deficient mice. *Cell* **85**: 733.

Geng Y., Whorískey W., Park M.Y., Bronson R.T., Medema R.H., Li T., Weinberg R.A., and Sicinski P. 1999. Rescue of cyclin D1 deficiency by knockin cyclin E. *Cell* **97**: 767.

Geng Y., Yu Q., Sicinska E., Das M., Schneider J.E., Bhattacharya S., Rideout W.M., Bronson R.T., Gardner H., and Sicinski P. 2003. Cyclin E ablation in the mouse. *Cell* **114**: 431.

Jacks T., Fazeli A., Schmitt E.M., Bronson R.T., Goodell M.A., and Weinberg R.A. 1992. Effects of an Rb mutation in the mouse. *Nature* **359**: 295.

Jirawatnotai S., Aziyu A., Osmundson E.C., Moons D.S., Zou X., Kineman R.D., and Kiyokawa H. 2004. Cdk4 is indispensable for postnatal proliferation of the anterior pituitary. *J. Biol. Chem.* **279**: 51100.

Kiyokawa H., Kineman R.D., Manova-Todorova K.O., Soares V.C., Hoffman E.S., Ono M., Khanam D., Hayday A.C., Frohman L.A., and Koff A. 1996. Enhanced growth of mice lacking the cyclin-dependent kinase inhibitor function of p27(Kip1). *Cell* **85**: 721.

Kozar K., Ciemerych M.A., Rebel V.I., Shigematsu H., Zagozdzon A., Sicinska E., Geng Y., Yu Q., Bhattacharya S., Bronson R.T., Akashi K., and Sicinski P. 2004. Mouse development and cell proliferation in the absence of D-cyclins. *Cell* **118**: 477.

Krimpenfort P., Quon K.C., Mooi W.J., Loonstra A., and Berns A. 2001. Loss of p16Ink4a confers susceptibility to metastatic melanoma in mice. *Nature* **413**: 83.

Latres E., Malumbres M., Sotillo R., Martín J., Ortega S., Martín-Caballero J., Flores J.M., Cordon-Cardo C., and Barbacid M. 2000. Limited overlapping roles of P15(INK4b) and P18(INK4c) cell cycle inhibitors in proliferation and tumorigenesis. *EMBO J.* **19**: 3496.

Lee E.Y., Chang C.Y., Hu N., Wang Y.C., Lai C.C., Herrup K., Lee W.H., and Bradley A. 1992. Mice deficient for Rb are nonviable and show defects in neurogenesis and haematopoiesis. *Nature* **359**: 288.

Malumbres M. and Barbacid M. 2001. To cycle or not to cycle: A critical decision in cancer. *Nat. Rev. Cancer* **1**: 222.

Malumbres M., Sotillo R., Santamaria D., Galan J., Cerezo A., Ortega S., Dubus P., and Barbacid M. 2004. Mammalian cells cycle without the D-type cyclin-dependent kinases Cdk4 and Cdk6. *Cell* **118**: 493.

Martín J., Hunt S.L., Dubus P., Sotillo R., Nehme-Pelluard F., Magnuson M.A., Parlow A.F., Malumbres M., Ortega S., and Barbacid M. 2003. Genetic rescue of Cdk4 null mice restores pancreatic beta-cell proliferation but not homeostatic cell number. *Oncogene* **22**: 5261.

Martín A., Odajima J., Hunt S.L., Dubus P., Ortega S., Malumbres M., and Barbacid M. 2005. Cdk2 is dispensable for cell cycle inhibition and tumor suppression mediated by p27^{Kip1} and p21^{Cip1}. *Cancer Cell* **7**: 591.

Moons D.S., Jirawatnotai S., Tsutsui T., Franks R., Parlow A.F., Hales D.B., Gibori G., Fazleabas A.T., and Kiyokawa H. 2002. Intact follicular maturation and defective luteal function in mice deficient for cyclin-dependent kinase-4. *Endocrinology* **143**: 647.

Nakayama K., Ishida N., Shirane M., Inomata A., Inoue T., Shishido N., Horii I., Loh D.Y., and Nakayama K. 1996. Mice lacking p27(^{Kip1}) display increased body size, multiple organ hyperplasia, retinal dysplasia, and pituitary tumors. *Cell* **85**: 707.

Ortega S., Malumbres M., and Barbacid M. 2002. Cyclin D-dependent kinases, INK4 inhibitors and cancer. *Biochim. Biophys. Acta* **1602**: 73.

Ortega S., Prieto I., Odajima J., Martín A., Dubus P., Sotillo R., Barbero J.L., Malumbres M., and Barbacid M. 2003. Cyclin-dependent kinase 2 is essential for meiosis but not for mitotic cell division in mice. *Nat. Genet.* **35**: 25.

Paggi M.G. and Giordano A. 2001. Who is the boss in the retinoblastoma family? The point of view of Rb2/p130, the little brother. *Cancer Res.* **61**: 4651.

Parisi T., Beck A.R., Rougier N., McNeil T., Lucian L., Werb Z., and Amati B. 2003. Cyclins E1 and E2 are required for endoreplication in placental trophoblast giant cells. *EMBO J.* **22**: 4794.

Rane S.G., Dubus P., Mettus R.V., Galbreath E.J., Boden G., Reddy E.P., and Barbacid M. 1999. Loss of Cdk4 expression

Due to space limitations we could not include all the appropriate references. The reader is referred to the reviewed articles for specific references.

causes insulin-deficient diabetes and Cdk4 activation results in β-cell hyperplasia. *Nat. Genet.* **22:** 44.

Ren S. and Rollins B.J. 2004. Cyclin C/cdk3 promotes Rb-dependent G0 exit. *Cell* **117:** 239.

Serrano M., Lee H., Chin L., Cordon-Cardo C., Beach D., and DePinho R.A. 1996. Role of the INK4a locus in tumor suppression and cell mortality. *Cell* **85:** 27.

Sharpless N.E., Bardeesy N., Lee K.H., Carrasco D., Castrillon D.H., Aguirre A.J., Wu E.A., Horner J.W., and DePinho R.A. 2001. Loss of p16Ink4a with retention of p19Arf predisposes mice to tumorigenesis. *Nature* **413:** 86.

Sherr C.J. and Roberts J.M. 1999. CDK inhibitors: Positive and negative regulators of G1-phase progression. *Genes Dev.* **13:** 1501.

Sotillo S., Dubus P., Martín J., de la Cueva E., Ortega S., Malumbres M., and Barbacid M. 2001a. Wide spectrum of tumors in knock in mice carrying a Cdk4 protein insensitive to INK4 inhibitors. *EMBO J.* **20:** 6637.

Sotillo R., García J.F., Ortega S., Martín J., Dubus P., Barbacid M., and Malumbres M. 2001b. Invasive melanoma in Cdk4 targeted mice. *Proc. Natl. Acad. Sci.* **98:** 13312.

Tsutsui T., Hesabi B., Moons D.S., Pandolfi P.P., Hansel K.S., Koff A., and Kiyokawa H. 1999. Targeted disruption of Cdk4 delays cell cycle entry with enhanced p27Kip1 activity. *Mol. Cell. Biol.* **19:** 7011.

Yamasaki L. and Pagano M. 2004. Cell cycle, proteolysis and cancer. *Curr. Opin. Cell. Biol.* **16:** 623.

Ye X., Zhu C., and Harper J.W. 2001. A premature-termination mutation in the *Mus musculus* cyclin-dependent kinase 3 gene. *Proc. Natl. Acad. Sci.* **98:** 1682.

Mouse Models of Human Non-Small-Cell Lung Cancer: Raising the Bar

C.F.B. Kim,* E.L. Jackson,[†] D.G. Kirsch,*[‡] J. Grimm,[¶] A.T. Shaw,*[§] K. Lane,* J. Kissil,**
K.P. Olive,[††] A. Sweet-Cordero,[‡‡] R. Weissleder,[¶] and T. Jacks*[¶¶]

*Center for Cancer Research and Department of Biology, Massachusetts Institute of Technology,
Cambridge, Massachusetts 02139; [‡]Department of Radiation Oncology, [¶]Center for Molecular Imaging Research,
and [§]Cancer Center, Massachusetts General Hospital and Harvard Medical School, Boston, Massachusetts;
[¶¶]Howard Hughes Medical Institute, Center for Cancer Research, Cambridge, Massachusetts 02139

Lung cancer is a devastating disease that presents a challenge to basic research to provide new steps toward therapeutic advances. The cell-type-specific responses to oncogenic mutations that initiate and regulate lung cancer remain poorly defined. A better understanding of the relevant signaling pathways and mechanisms that control therapeutic outcome could also provide new insight. Improved conditional mouse models are now available as tools to improve the understanding of the cellular and molecular origins of adenocarcinoma. These models have already proven their utility in proof-of-principle experiments with new technologies including genomics and imaging. Integrated thinking to apply technological advances while using the appropriate mouse model is likely to facilitate discoveries that will significantly improve lung cancer detection and intervention.

Lung cancer is the leading cause of death from cancer worldwide (Parkin et al. 2005). Despite the extensive characterization of genetic changes associated with this disease, as well as the development of genetic and chemically induced mouse models, lung cancer remains very difficult to cure.

Little is known about the cellular origins of lung tumors or the process of tumor initiation because of the inability to detect early-stage tumors. The 5-year survival rate for lung cancer patients with distant metastasis is only 2%. However, the survival rate for patients with early-stage, localized lung cancer is 50%. Unfortunately, the majority of lung cancers are detected at an advanced stage of disease (National Cancer Institute 2005). Therefore, studies to facilitate early detection are predicted to significantly affect mortality of lung cancer patients. With this goal in mind, it is imperative to understand the earliest cellular and molecular changes in lung tumorigenesis.

In parallel with an understanding of early events in lung tumorigenesis, the high mortality rate for lung cancer patients compared to other tumor sites highlights the great need for more effective treatment of lung cancer (National Cancer Institute 2005). Advances will likely require better insight into the cellular and molecular factors regulating tumor progression, invasion, and metastasis. Improved techniques for predicting and monitoring therapeutic response are also needed. Even for current therapies that provide benefit for some patients, the mechanisms behind tumor response are poorly understood, hindering the ability to build upon current therapies with more rational drug design and treatment. A combination of accurate mouse models of lung cancer and new technologies currently in hand now make it possible to investigate questions that cannot be addressed with patient samples.

MURINE K-ras CONDITIONAL LUNG CANCER MODELS

Human lung cancer is divided into subtypes based on histological appearance: Two major types are small-cell lung carcinoma (SCLC), which resembles neuroendocrine cells, and non-small-cell lung carcinoma (NSCLC). Classification into these subtypes often determines the course of treatment (Rosai and Sobin 1995). Most chemically induced and genetically manipulated mouse models of lung cancer resemble the most common subtype of NSCLC, adenocarcinoma (Rosai and Sobin 1995; Jackson et al. 2004).

Several genetic mouse models of lung cancer have relied on initiation by oncogenic K-ras. K-ras mutations are found in 15–50% of human lung adenocarcinomas (Rodenhuis et al. 1988; Kobayashi et al. 1990; Mills et al. 1995). Codons 12, 13, and 61 of K-ras are mutated to an oncogenic form thought to limit its GTPase activity (Campbell et al. 1998). Since these mutations occur spontaneously in humans, many groups have sought to create "conditional" mouse models, in which the oncogene is expressed under temporal and spatial constraints. This situation more closely resembles the human condition than do mouse models in which all cells express a mutant protein from development through adulthood.

A first-generation K-ras-conditional model of lung cancer provided an unbiased means to analyze the consequences of physiological levels of oncogenic Ras expression in vivo (Johnson et al. 2001). This $K-ras^{LA}$ model allowed expression of an oncogenic mutation, G12D, of K-ras only after spontaneous recombination of the endogenous allele in somatic cells to resolve an intra-chromosomal exon-1 duplication. Surprisingly, the lung was

Present addresses: [†] University of California, San Francisco, California; **Wistar Institute, Philadelphia, Pennsylvania; [††]University of Pennsylvania, Philadelphia, Pennsylvania; [‡‡]Stanford University Medical Center, Stanford, California.

particularly susceptible to this process, and K-ras^{LA} mice rapidly developed multiple lung adenocarcinomas (Johnson et al. 2001). Other tumors and hyperplasia did develop in K-ras^{LA} mice, including thymic lymphomas and intestinal hyperplasia, but death due to lung tumor burden limited analysis of the tumor spectrum resulting from expression of K-ras^{G12D}. In this system, it remains to be determined whether differential rates of recombination between tissues can account for these observations or whether physiological, oncogenic Ras only affects certain tissues.

Several second-generation models have been created to allow more precise spatial and temporal regulation of oncogenic K-ras expression (Fisher et al. 2001; Jackson et al. 2001; Meuwissen et al. 2001). In K-ras^{LSL} mice, the same oncogenic G12D mutation is encoded in exon 1, but the transcription of the mutant allele is prevented by the presence of a stop cassette flanked by loxP sites (LSL). Upon exposure to Cre recombinase, the stop cassette is removed, allowing active transcription and expression of oncogenic Ras. Intranasal infection with adenovirus containing the Cre recombinase (AdCre) allows the expression of oncogenic Ras in multiple types of lung epithelia. It is also conceivable to use cell- or developmental-stage-specific Cre mice (e.g., Cre driven by a lung-cell-specific promoter) to further restrict tumorigenesis. In addition to its utility in studying lung cancer, the K-ras^{LSL} strain has provided a strategy for modeling hematopoietic, pancreatic, and ovarian malignancies (Aguirre et al. 2003; Hingorani et al. 2003; Braun et al. 2004; Chan et al. 2004; Dinulescu et al. 2005). Meuweissen et al. (2001) have employed a similar strategy to model adenocarcinoma using a transgenic K-ras$^{G12V-IRES-PLAP-pA}$ cDNA construct regulated by the β-actin promoter and a LSL cassette. Distinct from the K-ras^{LSL} and K-ras$^{G12V-IRES-PLAP-pA}$ strains, Fisher et al. used bitransgenic mice, CCSP-rtTA; TetO7- K-ras4b^{G12D} mice, in which a doxycycline-inducible Clara cell secretory protein (CCSP, aka CCA, CC10) promoter (CCSP-rtTA) drives murine K-ras4b^{G12D} expression in alveolar type II cells. One advantage of this model is the ability to switch Ras expression on or off, which allowed the demonstration that K-ras^{G12D} was needed for both tumor initiation and maintenance (Fisher et al. 2001).

Using the K-ras^{LSL}, K-ras4b^{G12D}, and K-ras$^{G12V-IRES-PLAP-pA}$ strains, the precise timing of tumor initiation is defined, making it possible to examine the first effects of oncogenic Ras expression in the lung. In K-ras^{LSL} mice, atypical adenomatous hyperplasias (AAH), or hyperproliferation of alveolar type II (AT2) cells, was observed as soon as 5 days after exposure to Cre. By 6 weeks after Cre, adenomas appeared, and fewer AAH were seen. By 16 weeks after Cre, Kras^{LSL} mice have adenomas and overt adenocarcinomas. Intratracheal instillation of AdCre in K-ras$^{G12V-IRES-PLAP-pA}$ mice and doxycycline treatment of CCSP-rtTA; TetO7- K-ras4b^{G12D} mice resulted in lung tumors comparable to those observed in AdCre; K-ras^{LSL} mice (Fisher et al. 2001; Meuwissen et al. 2001). The timing of lesion development suggests that AAH, which have been proposed to be the precursor to adenocarcinomas in humans (Mori et al. 1993, 2001), progress into

adenomas that in turn progress into adenocarcinomas. It is unclear whether all AAH and adenomas have equal ability to give rise to adenocarcinomas, or furthermore, whether some AAH can skip the intermediate stage and rapidly take on carcinoma features. These issues can be addressed through clonal analyses and imaging of individual tumors.

Another conditional allele of K-ras has provided some evidence for tissue-specific susceptibility to oncogenic Ras. Guerra et al. inserted an IRES-B-geo cassette within the 3′ untranslated region of a K-ras allele encoding oncogenic K-ras^{G12V} under the regulation of a LSL cassette. In K-ras$^{G12V-IRES-BGeo}$ mice crossed with an inducible Cre strain that can be activated by exposure to 4-hydroxytamoxifen (4-OTH), only the lung appeared to be hyperproliferative or to develop carcinomas. Endogenous expression of K-ras^{G12V} had no apparent effect on most tissues, such as the colon and pancreas, despite efficient activation of the BGeo reporter (Guerra et al. 2003). In contrast to the results of Guerra et al., expression of oncogenic Ras in K-ras^{LSL} mice had proliferative effects on salivary gland, skin, hematopoietic, ovarian, lung, and gastrointestinal cells and was not compatible with viability in combination with Protamine-Cre, a transgene that yields efficient recombination in the male germ line. Differences in the properties of K-ras^{G12V} and K-ras^{G12D}, mouse genetic background, or the presence of the 3′BGeo reporter may account for differences in these observations (Tuveson et al. 2004). Despite different conclusions about the effect of Ras on various tissues, the different K-ras conditional alleles present valuable tools to further dissect lung tumorigenesis.

NEW DIRECTIONS FOR MURINE MODELS: EGFR

In addition to mutations in K-RAS, many other genetic lesions have been characterized in human lung tumors, including those in RB, p53, MYC, and INK4a/ARF (Minna et al. 2002). The mechanisms by which these lesions lead to tumor initiation and progression, as well as how they may affect therapeutic outcomes, are yet to be determined. Particularly relevant to understanding response to therapy and rational drug design, it has recently been determined that lung cancer patients who responded favorably to treatment with inhibitors of the EGF receptor, Iressa and Tarceva, harbor mutations in the EGFR gene (Lynch et al. 2004; Paez et al. 2004; Pao et al. 2004). Interestingly, many of these patients share several characteristics, including their tumor subtype (NSCLC, adenocarcinoma), heritage (Asian descent), gender (female), and smoking history (many are never-smokers). EGFR mutations and K-RAS mutations appear to be mutually exclusive (Pao et al. 2005), and there is some evidence that patients with K-RAS mutations have a worse prognosis after Iressa treatment (Eberhard et al. 2005). Furthermore, a subset of patients that initially responded to Iressa but later developed resistant disease harbor secondary mutations in EGFR (Kobayashi et al. 2005; Pao et al. 2005). The discovery of EGFR mutations provides perhaps a first opportunity to develop tools with which to understand therapeutic response. These studies also raise many questions: Are EGFR mutations sufficient for tumor initiation? How does mutant EGFR affect the Ras downstream effectors? Which effectors are important for the observed clinical response and drug resistance?

In an effort to begin to address these issues, several laboratories are now working to create mouse models of lung cancer using the identified EGFR mutations. Varmus and colleagues (this volume) have shown that transgenic mice carrying the L858R mutation under the direction of a doxycycline-dependent, lung-specific promoter indeed develop lung lesions. In an attempt to more closely mimic the situation in human tumors, a knockin strategy to create germ-line constitutive and conditional alleles of the most frequently occurring Iressa-sensitive mutations: the point mutation L858R and the deletion L746-E749, A750P, is also under way in our laboratory. Similar to the K-ras^{LSL} strain, the conditional $EGFR$ mice will not express the oncogenic form until exposure to Cre recombinase. Experiments are ongoing to determine the outcome in conditional $EGFR^{L858R}$ mice after intranasal infection with AdCre (K. Lane and T. Jacks, unpubl.). These conditional mice will be an important resource with which to understand the role of these mutant $EGFR$ alleles in the initiation and maintenance of NSCLC, the dependency of late-stage chemorefractory tumors on signaling through the EGFR, and the biology behind the exclusive nature of $EGFR$ and K-RAS mutations. They will also provide a means to examine resistance to Iressa, both primary, as in the case of tumors harboring K-RAS mutations, and secondary resistance; i.e., tumors with $EGFR$ mutations that initially respond to Iressa but then relapse.

The spatial context in which a mutation occurs may influence its oncogenic potential. Little is known about whether the timing of oncogene activation may also modulate the kinetics of tumor development. The idea that a germ-line and a somatic mutation are not equivalent is supported by (1) a recent report demonstrating that mice with germ-line activation of an oncogenic $ErbB2$ allele have complete resistance to tumor development, whereas conditional activation of the same allele in the mammary gland resulted in the development of mammary tumors, with greater than 90% of mice being affected by 2 years of age (Andrechek et al. 2004), and (2) the existence of a tumor-free mouse strain that harbors an ENU-induced germ-line $Egfr$ mutation equivalent to one found in human tumors responsive to Iressa (Fitch et al. 2003; Lynch et al. 2004). The generation of strains of mice harboring mutant $Egfr$ alleles will provide a means to ask whether temporal regulation of oncogene activation can influence lung tumor formation.

IMPROVING MURINE MODELS: COOPERATIVE EFFECTS OF K-ras AND p53 MUTATION

Whereas the EGFR models in development will provide insight for newly discovered mutations and mechanisms of tumorigenesis related to observed clinical re-

sponse, improvement of the current mouse models of NSCLC is also needed. In contrast to human adenocarcinomas, both genetically and chemically induced murine lung tumors typically do not exhibit invasion, stromal desmoplasia, or metastasis and thus appear more similar to early-stage human lesions. Mouse lung tumors may even be regarded to more closely resemble bronchioalveolar carcinoma (BAC) than adenocarcinoma. Over 50% of human lung cancers are diagnosed at an advanced stage of disease with distant metastases (National Cancer Institute 2005). Therefore, mouse studies with therapeutic implications for patients would likely be more insightful if murine tumors more closely resembled invasive, metastatic human adenocarcinoma.

Analysis of compound mutations in K-ras^{LSL}:$p53$ conditional mice has led to a more "humanized" version of the K-ras^{LSL} NSCLC model, indicating that there is a clear cooperation between loss of p53 function and activation of K-ras (Jackson et al. 2005). Indeed, alterations in the p53 tumor suppressor gene occur in ~50% of human NSCLC cases (Chiba et al. 1990). Direct comparison of the effects of p53 mutations on lung tumor growth and progression was performed by generating compound conditional K-ras^{LSL} mice with one of three $p53$ conditional knockin alleles: a contact mutant ($p53^{R270H}$), a structural mutant ($p53^{R172H}$) (Olive et al. 2004), or a null allele ($p53^{flox/flox}$) (Jonkers et al. 2001). p53 loss or mutation strongly promoted the progression of K-ras^{G12D}-induced lung adenocarcinomas, yielding tumors that more accurately recapitulate several aspects of human lung adenocarcinoma (Fig. 1A–F). In particular, K-ras^{LSL}:$p53$ tumors exhibited a large stromal component in which nests of tumor cells could be found growing within a field of desmoplastic stroma, production of collagen was abundant, and expression of smooth muscle actin was observed (Fig. 1E–G). Double mutant tumors were highly invasive, growing into the hilus, heart, and overlying pleura and along the luminal surfaces of blood and lymphatic vessels, demonstrating extravasation (Fig. 1H). Lymph node metastases were present in over 50% of K-ras^{LSL}:$p53$ mice, and distant metastases were also observed (Jackson et al. 2005). With its similarities to advanced-stage human NSCLC, the K-ras^{LSL}:$p53$ model of lung cancer represents a better tool for studying the human disease.

IMAGING TOOLS FOR MURINE LUNG CANCER MODELING

Related to improvements to "humanize" mouse models of NSCLC, it is equally important to develop new technologies with which to observe tumor development and monitor progression in vivo in order to make any strides in lung cancer therapy. Progression of lung cancer can be easily followed in mice by harvesting tissue at various time points and analyzing histological sections. However, because patients typically have one tumor rather than the multiple tumors present in mouse models, a more powerful approach for better understanding and prediction of patient responses would be to follow individual tumors within individual mice. Aside from the scientific advan-

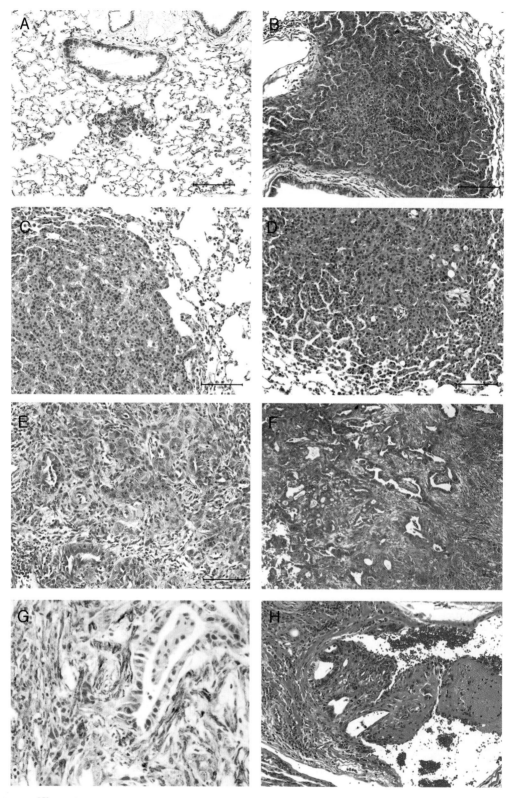

Figure 1. *K-ras^{LSL}; p53* lung tumors display characteristics of advanced adenocarcinomas. (*A,B*) H&E images show atypical adeno-matous hyperplasia (*A*) and adenocarcinoma (*B*) present 6 weeks after AdCre infection in *K-ras^{LSL}; p53^{flox/+}* and *K-ras^{LSL}; p53^{flox/flox}* mice, respectively. (*C,D*) Low-grade adenocarcinomas from *K-ras^{LSL}; p53^{+/+}* mice 10 months after AdCre infection. (*E,F*) Typical high-grade adenocarcinomas from *K-ras^{LSL}; p53^{270/flox}* and *K-ras^{LSL}; p53^{flox/flox}* mice 3 months after AdCre infection, respectively. (*G*) Smooth muscle actin staining (*brown*) of a *K-ras^{LSL}; p53^{flox/flox}* tumor to demonstrate stromal desmoplasia. (*H*) A *K-ras^{LSL}; p53^{flox/flox}* tumor invading a blood vessel. All images: 200x magnification; bars, 100 μm.

tage of analyzing single lesions, this approach also takes into account an important practical point that is crucial for drug trials in mice: Imaging makes it possible to reduce the number of mice used in a study, reducing costs for generation, maintenance, and treatment of animals and thus making it possible to carry out more variations than when each step requires euthanasia.

Imaging of murine lung tumors using the same techniques and equipment as that used for patients, and innovative tools for mouse tumor imaging, have already been used to demonstrate initial phenotype and regression of oncogenic K-ras-induced lung tumors. MRI scans of K-$ras4b^{G12D}$ mice revealed multiple tumor masses 3 months after exposure to doxycycline, and reduced tumor volume was detected 8 days after doxycycline withdrawal (Fisher et al. 2001). A Cre-activated luciferase reporter allele has also proven useful for measuring murine lung tumors in individual mice over time after AdCre infection (Lyons et al. 2003).

The progress of imaging has been accelerated by the development of dedicated small-animal imaging equipment for micro-computed tomography (CT). Using a micro-CT with a voxel resolution of 72 microns, K-ras^{LSL} lung tumors can be detected with sub-millimeter resolution (Grimm et al. 2005). Images collected after AdCre infection have led to several interesting observations. First, new tumors that were not detected in the first scan developed over time. Second, serial imaging of the same mice during a period of 6 months after AdCre administration demonstrates that some tumors grew larger rapidly, whereas the size of other tumors increased slowly (D.G. Kirsch et al., unpubl.). Similarly, micro-CT imaging of K-ras^{LA} lung tumors revealed both tumor growth and shrinkage within individual mice (Cody et al. 2005). These data make it clear that some lung tumors grow quickly, whereas others appear to progress with slower kinetics. It remains to be determined whether the heterogeneity in lung tumor behavior is attributable to different mutational events, cellular context, microenvironments, or a combination of such factors. Despite these unanswered questions, imaging techniques will clearly be important for determining response to therapy in mouse-based drug trials. Proof-of-principle experiments using CT imaging in mice will be important for drawing parallels between results from detection or therapeutic trials in mice and predicted response in patients.

ANALYSIS OF Ras EFFECTOR PATHWAYS IN TUMORIGENESIS

Improved therapy for NSCLC may follow from a detailed understanding of the relevant effector pathways operative downstream of oncogenic Ras. It is conceivable that differential tumor behavior between patients may be related to variation in use of effector pathways. Studies in primary fibroblasts have linked high levels of Raf-MAPK-ERK activity to Ras-induced premature senescence, suggesting that this arm of Ras effectors may be an important therapeutic target (Lin et al. 1998; Zhu et al.

1998). In contrast, studies in MEFs expressing oncogenic K-ras at physiological levels have failed to demonstrate an overt up-regulation of this pathway. However, the use of pharmacological inhibitors of the MAPK and PI3K pathways, U0216 and LY294002, respectively, indicated that these pathways do contribute to morphological changes seen in Lox-K-ras^{G12D} MEFs (Tuveson et al. 2004). Remarkably, early-stage tumors in K-ras^{LSL} mice also do not have appreciable activation of the pathway, and only 13% of late-stage tumors contained large foci of positive cells following staining with anti-phospho-p42/44MAPK antisera (Tuveson et al. 2004; E. Jackson and T. Jacks, unpubl.). Collectively, the data suggest that the Raf-MAPK-ERK pathway may not be driving K-ras-mediated lung tumorigenesis, but do not rule out a role for this pathway in some aspects of disease phenotype.

Numerous lines of evidence have implicated the Rac pathway as a downstream effector of Ras signaling in tumorigenesis, making it a relevant pathway for investigation of lung cancer therapy. K-ras is an effective activator of the Rac1 GTPase, and Rac1 is required for Ras-induced focus formation (Khosravi-Far et al. 1995; Qiu et al. 1995; Walsh and Bar-Sagi 2001). Furthermore, the Rac-GEF Tiam1 is required for Ras-induced skin tumors (Malliri et al. 2002). To further explore the role of Rac1 during lung tumorigenesis after expression of oncogenic Ras in vivo, a proof-of-principle genetics experiment has been performed. Compound mutant K-ras^{LSL};$Rac1^{flox/flox}$ mice (Walmsley et al. 2003) were infected intranasally with AdCre to analyze the effects on tumorigenesis. Rac1 deficiency resulted in a dramatic inhibition of tumor formation in the K-ras^{LSL} background. Whereas there was not a complete elimination of tumors, all tumors that arose in double mutant mice failed to recombine both Rac1 alleles (J. Kissil and T. Jacks, unpubl.). These data suggest that Rac1 function is necessary for oncogenic K-ras-induced tumorigenesis, turning attention to the JNK and/or NF-κB arms of the Ras effector pathway as potentially important therapeutic targets.

GENOMICS APPROACHES TO ANALYZING LUNG CANCER

Aside from analyzing individual candidate pathways, genomics approaches are proving useful for gaining a better understanding of mechanisms of tumorigenesis in mouse models and for comparing these models to the human disease. For example, the gene expression profile of K-ras-induced murine lung tumors has been compared to normal lung tissue using microarray analysis. These data revealed that K-ras^{G12D} lung tumors resemble human tumors, and particularly human lung adenocarcinomas, at the molecular level, further validating this model (Sweet-Cordero et al. 2005).

Data from gene expression analyses have gone beyond model validation to show that mouse models can provide instruction for potential druggable targets and insight into molecular mechanisms important for human disease. Whereas the difference in gene expression pattern in K-ras

mutant versus wild-type tumors in mice was clear, it was not possible to separate the genes differentially expressed in human tumors with K-*RAS* mutations versus those without K-*RAS* mutations with data from human tumors alone. However, using cross-species gene expression studies between murine and human lung adenocarcinomas, a pattern of gene expression indicative of mutant K-*RAS* was identified from the human data (Sweet-Cordero et al. 2005).

In addition to gene expression analyses of tumors, other genomic approaches of importance include comprehensive analyses of the chromosomal changes that occur during lung tumor formation and progression. Both whole- and sub-chromosomal changes in *K-ras*^{LSL} lung tumors are currently being examined using BAC arrays and representational oligonucleotide microarray analysis (ROMA) (Lucito et al. 2003). Similar work in human lung tumors (Tonon et al. 2005) has demonstrated that novel alterations in tumors can be detected with these methods. Finally, comparison of RNA and DNA changes will likely provide even further molecular insight.

Aside from identifying pathways for analysis of mechanism and treatment, genomic approaches can also be useful for finding biomarkers of lung cancer. A biomarker allows tumorigenic tissue or the presence of a tumor to be distinguished from the non-tumorigenic situation; there is no requirement that a biomarker be biologically important. Proteomics platforms, in particular, are likely to contribute significantly to the search for lung cancer biomarkers (Shaw et al. 2005). Proteomics simply refers to the systematic study of protein expression patterns, protein interactions, and protein pathways in complex biological systems, such as cells, tissues, and organs. Recent work has focused on analysis of the serum or plasma proteome for cancer biomarker discovery, given that blood should (in theory) contain any altered or overexpressed proteins shed into the circulation during tumorigenesis (Petricoin et al. 2002). Serum proteomic analysis of patient specimens has proven to be a formidable challenge, due in part to genetic and environmental variables (Check 2004). Many of these variables can be readily controlled using the appropriate animal models. Consequently, several groups are now applying proteomic technologies to validated mouse models, including the *K-ras*^{LSL} conditional mouse model of lung cancer described above. Preliminary analysis of pooled mouse plasma samples has identified over 50 candidate biomarkers of early lung cancer. These candidates await verification in individual mouse samples followed by validation in patient plasma samples (A. Shaw and T. Jacks, unpubl.).

Another method to discover and validate potential biomarkers is to combine genomics data and imaging technology. Molecular imaging characterizes and measures molecular events in living animals with high sensitivity and spatial resolution (Weissleder 1999). Imaging molecular events is achieved by utilizing novel imaging agents including "smart sensor probes" that can be activated upon interaction with their biological targets (Tung et al. 2000). Fluorescence molecular tomography (FMT) is capable of resolving molecular functions in deep tissues by reconstructing the in vivo distribution of an intravenously injected fluorescent probe (Ntziachristos et al. 2005).

Using gene expression profiling, cathepsin cysteine proteases were identified as highly up-regulated genes in K-ras-induced murine tumors. Overexpression of cathepsin proteases was confirmed by immunohistochemistry and western blotting. Therefore, an optical probe activated by cathepsin proteases was selected to detect murine lung tumors in vivo. Three-dimensional maps of the fluorescence signal fused with anatomical CT images showed a close correlation between fluorescence signal and tumor burden (Fig. 2) (Grimm et al. 2005). Cathepsin proteases are also overexpressed in some patients with lung cancer, and their expression has been associated with tumor invasion and poor prognosis (Schweiger et al. 2000; Joyce et al. 2004). It remains to be determined whether these molecules will be useful in imaging human tumors, but this work highlights the feasibility of using gene expression profiling to identify molecular targets for imaging lung cancer.

DETERMINING THE CELL OF ORIGIN OF LUNG CANCER

Development of imaging technologies brings to mind further questions: Will it be possible to image early lesions in patients at risk for lung cancer? Will detection of one or a few tumorigenic cells within a normal respiratory system be feasible? Furthermore, what is the identity of these first tumorigenic cells? A better understanding of the earliest cellular contexts in lung cancer could make

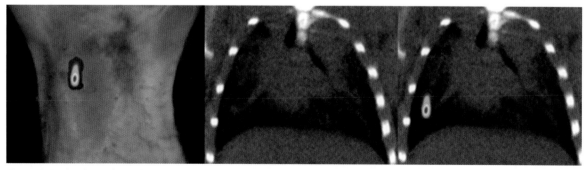

Figure 2. Molecular tools combined for lung tumor imaging. (*Left*) FMT superimposed on white light image; (*middle*) CT; (*right*) FMT-CT fusion images. The fluorescence signals (*color*) from cathepsin probe-based-FMT detect tumors.

significant improvements in early tumor detection and chemoprevention.

It has been proposed that tumors originate from adult stem cells, the self-renewing cells that maintain multiple types of specialized cells within a tissue, in contrast to the view that differentiated cells of a given tissue are the cells of origin of cancer (Reya et al. 2001). The best evidence for a stem cell origin of cancer comes from analyses of the hematopoietic system (Bonnet and Dick 1997; Passegue et al. 2004), yet this issue remains to be explored in epithelial tissues. The pulmonary system is composed of over 40 specialized cell types, and methods to isolate stem cells from the lung are largely unknown. Lack of knowledge of pulmonary stem cells and their relationship to differentiated lung cells precludes understanding their role in cancer and lung disease.

A variety of epithelial cell types in the lung each reside in distinct anatomical locations, or niches. Interestingly, many of the subtypes of NSCLC share characteristics with cells found in each of the distinct pulmonary cell niches in which the tumors most frequently arise. For example, squamous cell carcinomas exhibit keratinization, as do cells of the trachea and proximal airways, and these tumors generally arise in bronchi. In contrast, most adenocarcinomas and BACs display features of Clara cells, the non-ciliated bronchiolar epithelial cells, or AT2 cells, the surfactant-producing alveolar epithelia, and the location of these tumors is generally peripheral or endobronchial (Rosai and Sobin 1995). It is reasonable to hypothesize that each of these subtypes of lung cancer originates from a cell population that resides in its related niche, but little evidence presently exists to support this hypothesis. The observation that K-ras^{LSL} adenocarcinomas stained positively for the AT2 cell-specific marker pro-surfactant apoprotein-C (SP-C) corroborated previous studies that implicated AT2 cells as the target cells in rodent and human lung adenocarcinomas. However, evidence in other murine models and human specimens points to Clara cells as the cell of origin of adenocarcinoma (Dermer 1982; Gunning et al. 1991; Thaete and Malkinson 1991; Wikenheiser et al. 1992; Mori et al. 1993, 2001; Mason et al. 2000).

Cells expressing both SP-C and the Clara-cell-specific marker CCA (also known as CC10 or CCSP) were found in K-ras^{LSL} adenomas and adenocarcinomas, representing a very small proportion of the total tumor cell population that largely consisted of SP-C-positive cells (Fig. 3) (Jackson et al. 2001). Interestingly, Guerra et al. and Wootton et al. also reported the existence of rare CC10-positive cells among SP-C-positive cells in murine lung tumors induced by Ras or the Jaagsiekte sheep retrovirus (Guerra et al. 2003; Wootton et al. 2005). It was possible that SP-C-positive, CCA-positive cells might have originated from expansion of a rare stem cell population in the adult lung, which is reminiscent of embryonic lung epithelial precursors (Wuenschell et al. 1996). Alternatively, as a consequence of oncogenic K-ras, abnormal AT2 cells may have reacquired the ability to express markers of bronchiolar cells.

Careful examination of normal lung cell biology to ad-

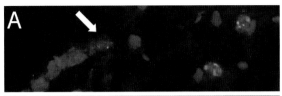

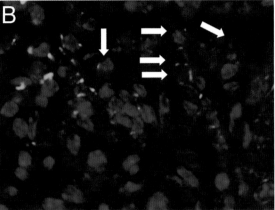

Figure 3. BASCs in normal and tumorigenic lung. Dual color immunofluorescence to detect BASCs (*arrows*) is shown. (*A*) In normal murine lung, an individual BASC (*arrow*) is observed at the bronchioalveolar duct junction, the branch point between a terminal bronchiole lined with Clara cells positive for CCA (*red*) and the alveolar space lined with alveolar epithelium including AT2 cells positive for SP-C (*green*). (*Blue*) DAPI. BASCs are positive for both CCA and SP-C. (*B*) Clusters of BASCs are identified within a K-ras^{LSL} lung tumor largely composed of SP-C-positive cells.

dress these possibilities led to the identification of a stem cell population in the distal lung epithelium, termed bronchioalveolar stem cells (BASCs) (Kim et al. 2005). BASCs expressing both CCA and SP-C were found in normal lung in the bronchioalveolar duct junction (Fig. 3A), a proposed bronchiolar stem cell niche (Giangreco et al. 2002). Important for their definition as stem cells, BASCs were shown to proliferate in response to bronchiolar damage in vivo (Kim et al. 2005). A FACS-based method to isolate BASCs was developed based on the presence of staining for the surface markers Sca-1 and CD34 with exclusion of hematopoietic and endothelial cells. BASCs purified by FACS can be manipulated in culture to remain undifferentiated and self-renew, or to differentiate into bronchiolar and alveolar lung cell lineages even after multiple passages in culture, demonstrating the key features of stem cells. These data support the hypothesis that BASCs are a regional lung stem cell population that maintains the bronchiolar cells and alveolar cells of the distal lung during homeostasis.

Several lines of evidence suggest that although adenocarcinomas are traditionally thought to arise from Clara or AT2 cells, transformed BASCs may be the cells of origin for this subtype of lung cancer (Kim et al. 2005). In K-ras^{LSL} mice, BASC expansion was coexistent with the earliest tumorigenic lesions. Further suggesting that BASC expansion is a key early event in tumorigenesis, K-ras^{G12D} activation increased the proliferation of cells in

BASC cultures, whereas AT2 cell cultures did not have a proliferative response to oncogenic Ras. Finally, stimulation of BASC proliferation by airway damage prior to tumor initiation resulted in an increase in tumor number and size, further implicating BASCs in tumorigenesis.

Further characterization of lung stem cells is needed for insight into lung tumor biology. Whereas the lineage from long-term hematopoietic stem cells to specialized blood cells has been well defined, it remains to be determined whether a classic hierarchy of stem, progenitor, and differentiated cells exists for pulmonary epithelia. Knowing the connections between adult lung cell lineages and how they are regulated at the molecular level will be a crucial foundation for studying the mechanisms of lung disease and tumorigenesis. Gene expression analyses to identify specific markers for BASCs, bronchiolar cells, and alveolar cells, and for comparison of expression patterns in normal and tumorigenic cells, will be important to identify factors regulating putative cells of origin of lung cancer, as well as to find genes that are specifically activated in response to oncogenic Ras. By generating mouse strains to spatially and temporally restrict expression of oncogenic *K-ras* to lung stem cells or more differentiated lung epithelia, the tools will be available to determine which cells are sufficient for lung tumor initiation. Further understanding of NSCLC subtypes other than adenocarcinoma as well as SCLC will likely require knowledge of the identity of stem, progenitor, and differentiated cell populations in niches distinct from the bronchioalveolar region. Finally, it will be important to determine whether murine lung stem cell populations have counterparts in normal human lung and human lung tumors.

EXAMINING LUNG CANCER STEM CELLS

In parallel to studies of lung cancer cells of origin, it is also important to examine the relationship between these cells and the cells of established tumors that are required for tumor maintenance. It has been demonstrated that some types of tumors (e.g., breast, brain, and lymphoid tumors) harbor a "cancer stem cell" population (often the minority of the tumor cells) that is required to maintain malignancy (Bonnet and Dick 1997; Al-Hajj et al. 2003; Singh et al. 2003, 2004). Importantly, it is hypothesized that cancer stem cells might be more resistant to chemotherapy than other cancer cells (Reya et al. 2001). Therefore, in order to cure cancer, it may be crucial to develop rational treatments that specifically target cancer stem cells. There is currently no experimental system to determine whether a stem cell population exists within lung cancers. BASCs were observed in established tumors in *K-ras^{LSL}* mice (Fig. 3B) (Jackson et al. 2001; Kim et al. 2005), suggesting that they may play a role in later stages of tumorigenesis in addition to a role in tumor initiation. Transplantation of specific cell subsets, including AT2 cells or BASCs, from primary tumors into secondary hosts is currently being performed for comparison of their capacity for tumorigenesis (C. Kim and T. Jacks, unpubl.). It will be important to determine whether human lung tumors have a similar cancer stem cell population.

CONCLUSIONS

This is an opportune time to further dissect lung tumorigenesis using mouse modeling. Clearly, it will be important to precisely define the cells, microenvironmental influence, and the specific gene products that should be targeted for novel therapeutics and early disease detection. Tools now in hand, including improved mouse models of lung cancer, genomics, proteomics, and imaging technologies, and enhanced understanding of lung cell biology and pathways involved in development, apoptosis, proliferation, and differentiation, make it possible to address these issues.

Key to success in elucidating targets for lung cancer therapy will be the ability to incorporate multiple concepts and technologies in combination for experimental design and interpretations. For example, the cell of origin of lung adenocarcinoma should be considered when choosing the cells to use in experiments to determine the relevant downstream Ras effector pathways operative in adenocarcinoma. If distinct lung cell populations utilize different effectors, the unique use of effectors in less abundant cell types that control tumorigenesis may be missed using total tumor or total lung protein extracts or RNA. Integrated thinking and "systems biology" approaches should become a part of the daily research plan.

Mouse models that accurately recapitulate human lung cancer at the genetic, histological, and molecular levels, such as the *K-ras^{LSL};p53* models, should be better suited for therapeutic and translational studies than xenograft models or studies using established cell lines. The successful treatment of xenografts is often a key step in the development of anticancer drugs, but these have too often led to disappointment in the clinic (Sridhar and Shepherd 2003). Models such as the *K-ras^{LSL};p53* adenocarcinomas provide an in vivo tool that takes into account the genetic changes that occur as tumors form and progress, as well as the relevant microenvironment that cannot be accurately represented with xenografts. The challenge facing researchers today is thus not to create a mouse model of lung cancer that can be cured, but rather to start with advanced, invasive, and metastatic murine lung tumors that present the same therapeutic challenges as is presented by advanced lung cancer in humans. If we can successfully control, and one day cure, such diseases in the mouse, we will be significantly closer to doing the same for lung cancer patients.

ACKNOWLEDGMENTS

We apologize to those whose work we could not cite because of space constraints. The authors thank Amber Woolfenden and Jacks lab members for experimental and collaborative contributions to the work described. C.F.B.K. is a Merck Fellow of The Jane Coffin Childs Memorial Fund for Medical Research. T.J. is a Howard Hughes Medical Institute Investigator.

REFERENCES

Aguirre A.J., Bardeesy N., Sinha M., Lopez L., Tuveson D.A., Horner J., Redston M.S., and DePinho R.A. 2003. Activated

Kras and Ink4a/Arf deficiency cooperate to produce metastatic pancreatic ductal adenocarcinoma. *Genes Dev.* **17:** 3112.

Al-Hajj M., Wicha M.S., Benito-Hernandez A., Morrison S.J., and Clarke M.F. 2003. Prospective identification of tumorigenic breast cancer cells. *Proc. Natl. Acad. Sci.* **100:** 3983.

Andrechek E.R., Hardy W.R., Laing M.A., and Muller W.J. 2004. Germ-line expression of an oncogenic erbB2 allele confers resistance to erbB2-induced mammary tumorigenesis. *Proc. Natl. Acad. Sci.* **101:** 4984.

Bonnet D. and Dick J.E. 1997. Human acute myeloid leukemia is organized as a hierarchy that originates from a primitive hematopoietic cell. *Nat. Med.* **3:** 730.

Braun B.S., Tuveson D.A., Kong N., Le D.T., Kogan S.C., Rozmus J., Le Beau M.M., Jacks T.E., and Shannon K.M. 2004. Somatic activation of oncogenic Kras in hematopoietic cells initiates a rapidly fatal myeloproliferative disorder. *Proc. Natl. Acad. Sci.* **101:** 597.

Campbell S.L., Khosravi-Far R., Rossman K.L., Clark G.J., and Der C.J. 1998. Increasing complexity of Ras signaling. *Oncogene* **17:** 1395.

Chan I.T., Kutok J.L., Williams I.R., Cohen S., Kelly L., Shigematsu H., Johnson L., Akashi K., Tuveson D.A., Jacks T., and Gilliland D.G. 2004. Conditional expression of oncogenic K-ras from its endogenous promoter induces a myeloproliferative disease. *J. Clin. Invest.* **113:** 528.

Check E. 2004. Proteomics and cancer: Running before we can walk? *Nature* **429:** 496.

Chiba I., Takahashi T., Nau M.M., D'Amico D., Curiel D.T., Mitsudomi T., Buchhagen D.L., Carbone D., Piantadosi S., and Koga H., et al. 1990. Mutations in the p53 gene are frequent in primary, resected non-small cell lung cancer. Lung Cancer Study Group. *Oncogene* **5:** 1603.

Cody D.D., Nelson C.L., Bradley W.M., Wislez M., Juroske D., Price R.E., Zhou X., Bekele B.N., and Kurie J.M. 2005. Murine lung tumor measurement using respiratory-gated micro-computed tomography. *Invest. Radiol.* **40:** 263.

Dermer G.B. 1982. Origin of bronchioloalveolar carcinoma and peripheral bronchial adenocarcinoma. *Cancer* **49:** 881.

Dinulescu D.M., Ince T.A., Quade B.J., Shafer S.A., Crowley D., and Jacks T. 2005. Role of K-ras and Pten in the development of mouse models of endometriosis and endometrioid ovarian cancer. *Nat. Med.* **11:** 63.

Eberhard D.A., Johnson B.E., Amler L.C., Goddard A.D., Heldens S.L., Herbst R.S., Ince W.L., Janne P.A., Januario T., Johnson D.H., Klein P., Miller V.A., Ostland M.A., Ramies D.A., Sebisanovic D., Stinson J.A., Zhang Y.R., Seshagiri S., and Hillan K. J. 2005. Mutations in the epidermal growth factor receptor and in KRAS are predictive and prognostic indicators in patients with non-small-cell lung cancer treated with chemotherapy alone and in combination with erlotinib. *J. Clin. Oncol.* **23:** 5900.

Fisher G.H., Wellen S.L., Klimstra D., Lenczowski J.M., Tichelaar J.W., Lizak M.J., Whitsett J.A., Koretsky A., and Varmus H.E. 2001. Induction and apoptotic regression of lung adenocarcinomas by regulation of a K-Ras transgene in the presence and absence of tumor suppressor genes. *Genes Dev.* **15:** 3249.

Fitch K.R., McGowan K.A., van Raamsdonk C.D., Fuchs H., Lee D., Puech A., Herault Y., Threadgill D.W., Hrabe de Angelis M., and Barsh G.S. 2003. Genetics of dark skin in mice. *Genes Dev.* **17:** 214.

Giangreco A., Reynolds S.D., and Stripp B.R. 2002. Terminal bronchioles harbor a unique airway stem cell population that localizes to the bronchoalveolar duct junction. *Am. J. Pathol.* **161:** 173.

Grimm J., Kirsch D.G., Windsor S.D., Kim C.F.B., Santiago P.M., Ntziachristos V., Jacks T., and Weissleder R. 2005. Use of gene expression profiling to direct in vivo molecular imaging of lung cancer. *Proc. Natl. Acad. Sci.* **102:** 14404.

Guerra C., Mijimolle N., Dhawahir A., Dubus P., Barradas M., Serrano M., Campuzano V., and Barbacid M. 2003. Tumor induction by an endogenous K-ras oncogene is highly dependent on cellular context. *Cancer Cell* **4:** 111.

Gunning W.T., Stoner G.D., and Goldblatt P.J. 1991. Glyceraldehyde-3-phosphate dehydrogenase and other enzymatic activity in normal mouse lung and in lung tumors. *Exp. Lung Res.* **17:** 255.

Hingorani S.R., Petricoin E.F., Maitra A., Rajapakse V., King C., Jacobetz M.A., Ross S., Conrads T.P., Veenstra T.D., Hitt B.A., Kawaguchi Y., Johann D., Liotta L.A., Crawford H.C., Putt M.E., Jacks T., Wright C.V., Hruban R.H., Lowy A.M., and Tuveson D.A. 2003. Preinvasive and invasive ductal pancreatic cancer and its early detection in the mouse. *Cancer Cell* **4:** 437.

Jackson E.L., Kim C.F.B., and Jacks T. 2004. Lung Cancer Models, National Cancer Institute, Mouse Models of Human Cancers Consortium. (http://emice.nci.nih.gov/mouse_models/organ_models/lung_models).

Jackson E.L., Olive K.P., Tuveson D.A., Bronson R.T., Crowley D., Brown M., and Jacks T. 2005. The differential effects of mutant p53 alleles on advanced murine lung cancer. *Cancer Res.* **65:** 10280.

Jackson E.L., Willis N., Mercer K., Bronson R.T., Crowley D., Montoya R., Jacks T., and Tuveson D.A. 2001. Analysis of lung tumor initiation and progression using conditional expression of oncogenic K-ras. *Genes Dev.* **15:** 3243.

Johnson L., Mercer K., Greenbaum D., Bronson R.T., Crowley D., Tuveson D.A., and Jacks T. 2001. Somatic activation of the K-ras oncogene causes early onset lung cancer in mice. *Nature* **410:** 1111.

Jonkers J., Meuwissen R., van der Gulden H., Peterse H., van der Valk M., and Berns A. 2001. Synergistic tumor suppressor activity of BRCA2 and p53 in a conditional mouse model for breast cancer. *Nat. Genet.* **29:** 418.

Joyce J.A., Baruch A., Chehade K., Meyer-Morse N., Giraudo E., Tsai F.Y., Greenbaum D.C., Hager J.H., Bogyo M., and Hanahan D. 2004. Cathepsin cysteine proteases are effectors of invasive growth and angiogenesis during multistage tumorigenesis. *Cancer Cell* **5:** 443.

Khosravi-Far R., Solski P.A., Clark G.J., Kinch M.S., and Der C.J. 1995. Activation of Rac1, RhoA, and mitogen-activated protein kinases is required for Ras transformation. *Mol. Cell. Biol.* **15:** 6443.

Kim C.F., Jackson E.L., Woolfenden A.E., Lawrence S., Babar I., Vogel S., Crowley D., Bronson R.T., and Jacks T. 2005. Identification of bronchioalveolar stem cells in normal lung and lung cancer. *Cell* **121:** 823.

Kobayashi S., Boggon T.J., Dayaram T., Janne P.A., Kocher O., Meyerson M., Johnson B.E., Eck M.J., Tenen D.G., and Halmos B. 2005. EGFR mutation and resistance of non-small-cell lung cancer to gefitinib. *N. Engl. J. Med.* **352:** 786.

Kobayashi T., Tsuda H., Noguchi M., Hirohashi S., Shimosato Y., Goya T., and Hayata Y. 1990. Association of point mutation in c-Ki-ras oncogene in lung adenocarcinoma with particular reference to cytologic subtypes. *Cancer* **66:** 289.

Lin A.W., Barradas M., Stone J.C., van Aelst L., Serrano M., and Lowe S.W. 1998. Premature senescence involving p53 and p16 is activated in response to constitutive MEK/MAPK mitogenic signaling. *Genes Dev.* **12:** 3008.

Lucito R., Healy J., Alexander J., Reiner A., Esposito D., Chi M., Rodgers L., Brady A., Sebat J., Troge J., West J.A., Rostan S., Nguyen K.C., Powers S., Ye K.Q., Olshen A., Venkatraman E., Norton L., and Wigler M. 2003. Representational oligonucleotide microarray analysis: A high-resolution method to detect genome copy number variation. *Genome Res.* **13:** 2291.

Lynch T.J., Bell D.W., Sordella R., Gurubhagavatula S., Okimoto R.A., Brannigan B.W., Harris P.L., Haserlat S.M., Supko J.G., Haluska F.G., Louis D.N., Christiani D.C., Settleman J., and Haber D.A. 2004. Activating mutations in the epidermal growth factor receptor underlying responsiveness of non-small-cell lung cancer to gefitinib. *N. Engl. J. Med.* **350:** 2129.

Lyons S.K., Meuwissen R., Krimpenfort P., and Berns A. 2003. The generation of a conditional reporter that enables bioluminescence imaging of Cre/loxP-dependent tumorigenesis in mice. *Cancer Res* **63:** 7042.

Malliri A., van der Kammen R.A., Clark K., van der Valk M.,

Michiels F., and Collard J.G. 2002. Mice deficient in the Rac activator Tiam1 are resistant to Ras-induced skin tumours. *Nature* 417: 867.

Mason R.J., Kalina M., Nielsen L.D., Malkinson A.M., and Shannon J.M. 2000. Surfactant protein C expression in urethane-induced murine pulmonary tumors. *Am. J. Pathol.* 156: 175.

Meuwissen R., Linn S.C., van der Valk M., Mooi W.J., and Berns A. 2001. Mouse model for lung tumorigenesis through Cre/lox controlled sporadic activation of the K-Ras oncogene. *Oncogene* 20: 6551.

Mills N.E., Fishman C.L., Rom W.N., Dubin N., and Jacobson D.R. 1995. Increased prevalence of K-ras oncogene mutations in lung adenocarcinoma. *Cancer Res.* 55: 1444.

Minna J.D., Roth J.A., and Gazdar A.F. 2002. Focus on lung cancer. *Cancer Cell* 1: 49.

Mori M., Chiba R., and Takahashi T. 1993. Atypical adenomatous hyperplasia of the lung and its differentiation from adenocarcinoma. Characterization of atypical cells by morphometry and multivariate cluster analysis. *Cancer* 72: 2331.

Mori M., Rao S.K., Popper H.H., Cagle P.T., and Fraire A.E. 2001. Atypical adenomatous hyperplasia of the lung: A probable forerunner in the development of adenocarcinoma of the lung. *Mod. Pathol.* 14: 72.

National Cancer Institute. 2005. SEER Cancer Statistics Review 1975-2002, National Cancer Institute. (http://seer.cancer.gov/csr/1975_2002/).

Ntziachristos V., Ripoll J., Wang L.V., and Weissleder R. 2005. Looking and listening to light: The evolution of whole-body photonic imaging. *Nat. Biotechnol.* 23: 313.

Olive K.P., Tuveson D.A., Ruhe Z.C., Yin B., Willis N.A., Bronson R.T., Crowley D., and Jacks T. 2004. Mutant p53 gain of function in two mouse models of Li-Fraumeni syndrome. *Cell* 119: 847.

Paez J.G., Janne P.A., Lee J.C., Tracy S., Greulich H., Gabriel S., Herman P., Kaye F.J., Lindeman N., Boggon T.J., Naoki K., Sasaki H., Fujii Y., Eck M.J., Sellers W.R., Johnson B.E., and Meyerson M. 2004. EGFR mutations in lung cancer: Correlation with clinical response to gefitinib therapy. *Science* 304: 1497.

Pao W., Miller V.A., Politi K.A., Riely G.J., Somwar R., Zakowski M.F., Kris M.G., and Varmus H. 2005. Acquired resistance of lung adenocarcinomas to gefitinib or erlotinib is associated with a second mutation in the EGFR kinase domain. *PLoS Med.* 2: e73.

Pao W., Miller V., Zakowski M., Doherty J., Politi K., Sarkaria I., Singh B., Heelan R., Rusch V., Fulton L., Mardis E., Kupfer D., Wilson R., Kris M., and Varmus H. 2004. EGF receptor gene mutations are common in lung cancers from "never smokers" and are associated with sensitivity of tumors to gefitinib and erlotinib. *Proc. Natl. Acad. Sci.* 101: 13306.

Parkin D.M., Bray F., Ferlay J., and Pisani P. 2005. Global cancer statistics, 2002. *CA Cancer J. Clin.* 55: 74.

Passegue E., Wagner E.F., and Weissman I.L. 2004. JunB deficiency leads to a myeloproliferative disorder arising from hematopoietic stem cells. *Cell* 119: 431.

Petricoin E.F., Zoon K.C., Kohn E.C., Barrett J.C., and Liotta L.A. 2002. Clinical proteomics: Translating benchside promise into bedside reality. *Nat. Rev. Drug Discov.* 1: 683.

Qiu R.G., Chen J., Kirn D., McCormick F., and Symons M. 1995. An essential role for Rac in Ras transformation. *Nature* 374: 457.

Reya T., Morrison S.J., Clarke M.F., and Weissman I.L. 2001. Stem cells, cancer, and cancer stem cells. *Nature* 414: 105.

Rodenhuis S., Slebos R.J., Boot A.J., Evers S.G., Mooi W.J., Wagenaar S.S., van Bodegom P.C., and Bos J.L. 1988. Incidence and possible clinical significance of K-ras oncogene activation in adenocarcinoma of the human lung. *Cancer Res.* 48: 5738.

Rosai J. and Sobin L.H., Eds. 1995. *Atlas of tumor pathology: Tumors of the lower respiratory tract*. Armed Forces Institute of Pathology, Washington, D.C.

Schweiger A., Staib A., Werle B., Krasovec M., Lah T.T., Ebert W., Turk V., and Kos J. 2000. Cysteine proteinase cathepsin H in tumours and sera of lung cancer patients: Relation to prognosis and cigarette smoking. *Br. J. Cancer* 82: 782.

Shaw A.T., Kirsch D.G., and Jacks T. 2005. Future of early detection of lung cancer: The role of mouse models. *Clin. Cancer Res.* 11: 4999s.

Singh S.K., Clarke I.D., Terasaki M., Bonn V.E., Hawkins C., Squire J., and Dirks P.B. 2003. Identification of a cancer stem cell in human brain tumors. *Cancer Res.* 63: 5821.

Singh S.K., Hawkins C., Clarke I.D., Squire J.A., Bayani J., Hide T., Henkelman R.M., Cusimano M.D., and Dirks P.B. 2004. Identification of human brain tumour initiating cells. *Nature* 432: 396.

Sridhar S.S. and Shepherd F.A. 2003. Targeting angiogenesis: A review of angiogenesis inhibitors in the treatment of lung cancer. *Lung Cancer* (suppl. 1) 42: S81.

Sweet-Cordero A., Mukherjee S., Subramanian A., You H., Roix J.J., Ladd-Acosta C., Mesirov J., Golub T.R., and Jacks T. 2005. An oncogenic KRAS2 expression signature identified by cross-species gene-expression analysis. *Nat. Genet.* 37: 48.

Thaete L.G. and Malkinson A.M. 1991. Cells of origin of primary pulmonary neoplasms in mice: Morphologic and histochemical studies. *Exp. Lung Res.* 17: 219.

Tonon G., Wong K.K., Maulik G., Brennan C., Feng B., Zhang Y., Khatry D.B., Protopopov A., You M.J., Aguirre A.J., Martin E.S., Yang Z., Ji H., Chin L., and Depinho R.A. 2005. High-resolution genomic profiles of human lung cancer. *Proc. Natl. Acad. Sci.* 102: 9625.

Tung C.H., Mahmood U., Bredow S., and Weissleder R. 2000. In vivo imaging of proteolytic enzyme activity using a novel molecular reporter. *Cancer Res.* 60: 4953.

Tuveson D.A., Shaw A.T., Willis N.A., Silver D.P., Jackson E.L., Chang S., Mercer K.L., Grochow R., Hock H., Crowley D., Hingorani S.R., Zaks T., King C., Jacobetz M.A., Wang L., Bronson R.T., Orkin S.H., DePinho R.A., and Jacks T. 2004. Endogenous oncogenic K-ras(G12D) stimulates proliferation and widespread neoplastic and developmental defects. *Cancer Cell* 5: 375.

Walmsley M.J., Ooi S.K., Reynolds L.F., Smith S.H., Ruf S., Mathiot A., Vanes L., Williams D.A., Cancro M.P., and Tybulewicz V.L. 2003. Critical roles for Rac1 and Rac2 GTPases in B cell development and signaling. *Science* 302: 459.

Walsh A.B. and Bar-Sagi D. 2001. Differential activation of the Rac pathway by Ha-Ras and K-Ras. *J. Biol. Chem.* 276: 15609.

Weissleder R. 1999. Molecular imaging: Exploring the next frontier. *Radiology* 212: 609.

Wikenheiser K.A., Clark J.C., Linnoila R.I., Stahlman M.T., and Whitsett J.A. 1992. Simian virus 40 large T antigen directed by transcriptional elements of the human surfactant protein C gene produces pulmonary adenocarcinomas in transgenic mice. *Cancer Res.* 52: 5342.

Wootton S.K., Halbert C.L., and Miller A.D. 2005. Sheep retrovirus structural protein induces lung tumours. *Nature* 434: 904.

Wuenschell C.W., Sunday M.E., Singh G., Minoo P., Slavkin H.C., and Warburton D. 1996. Embryonic mouse lung epithelial progenitor cells co-express immunohistochemical markers of diverse mature cell lineages. *J. Histochem. Cytochem.* 44: 113.

Zhu J., Woods D., McMahon M., and Bishop J.M. 1998. Senescence of human fibroblasts induced by oncogenic Raf. *Genes Dev.* 12: 2997.

Generation and Analysis of Genetically Defined Liver Carcinomas Derived from Bipotential Liver Progenitors

L. ZENDER,* W. XUE,* C. CORDÓN-CARDO,† G.J. HANNON,* R. LUCITO,* S. POWERS,*
P. FLEMMING,‡ M.S. SPECTOR,* AND S.W. LOWE*¶

*Cold Spring Harbor Laboratory, Cold Spring Harbor, New York 11724;
†Division of Molecular Pathology, Memorial Sloan-Kettering Cancer Center, New York, New York 10021;
‡Department of Pathology, Medical School Hannover, Hannover, Germany;
¶Howard Hughes Medical Institute, Cold Spring Harbor, New York, New York 11724

Hepatocellular carcinoma is a chemoresistant cancer and a leading cause of cancer mortality; however, the molecular mechanisms responsible for the aggressive nature of this disease are poorly understood. In this study, we developed a new liver cancer mouse model that is based on the ex vivo genetic manipulation of embryonic liver progenitor cells (hepatoblasts). After retroviral gene transfer of oncogenes or short hairpin RNAs targeting tumor suppressor genes, genetically altered liver progenitor cells are seeded into the liver of otherwise normal recipient mice. We show that histopathology of the engineered liver carcinomas reveals features of the human disease. Furthermore, representational oligonucleotide microarray analysis (ROMA) of murine liver tumors initiated by two defined genetic hits revealed spontaneously acquired genetic alterations that are characteristic for human hepatocellular carcinoma. This model provides a powerful platform for applications like cancer gene discovery or high-throughput preclinical drug testing.

Hepatocellular carcinoma (HCC) represents the fifth most frequent neoplasm worldwide. However, due to the lack of treatment options, it constitutes the third leading cause of cancer death (>500,000 deaths per year) (Parkin et al. 2001). The only curative treatment options for HCC are surgical resection or liver transplantation. Unfortunately, at the time of diagnosis the majority of patients present with advanced tumor growth and are therefore not candidates for surgical therapy. Local ablative therapies like transarterial chemoembolization (TACE) or percutaneous ethanol injection (PEI) are being used as treatment options but are only feasible in selected patients and are not curative (Bruix et al. 2004). Systemic chemotherapeutic treatment is ineffective against HCC. For example, whereas doxorubicin or cisplatinum has marginal activity, these agents have no impact on long-term patient survival (Llovet et al. 2003).

More than 80% of all HCCs in humans are due to infection with hepatitis B virus (HBV) or hepatitis C virus (HCV) or aflatoxin B1 (AFB1) intake. The precise mechanisms by which HBV and HCV predispose to liver cancer are not fully elucidated. However, it is certain that chronic infection with HBV or HCV leads to a chronic turnover of hepatocytes, and this provides a suitable context for oncogenic genetic alterations. Furthermore, recent studies have shown that the HBx antigen of HBV can bind and functionally inactivate the tumor suppressor p53 (Wang et al. 1994; Ueda et al. 1995; Huo et al. 2001). In fact, mice transgenic for the HBx antigen develop hepatic adenomas and HCC (Ueda et al. 1995). Similar studies have been performed for proteins of HCV. It has been reported that the HCV core protein transcriptionally represses the p53 promoter in different cell types (Ray et al. 1997). In non-virus-induced liver cancers, p53 mutations may also play a role. For exam-

ple, liver cancers arising from aflatoxin exposure frequently have mutations in p53 at codon 249.

A number of other genetic alterations have been linked to the development of HCC. For example, Rb and/or the insulin growth factor receptor 1 (IGFR1) are frequently mutated or deleted (Murakami et al. 1991; Kim et al. 1996), whereas c-myc and cyclin D1 are often amplified (Peng et al. 1993; Nishida et al. 1994; Kusano et al. 1999; Wong et al. 1999; Niketeghad et al. 2001). Alterations in the Wnt-signaling pathway may also be important during hepatocarcinogenesis. Thus, mutations that activate β-catenin, or inactivate its negative regulator axin, occur in 30–40% of human HCCs, and nuclear overexpression of β-catenin occurs in 10–90% of these tumors (Nhieu et al. 1999; Buendia 2000; Wong et al. 2001). Deregulation of β-catenin leads to transcriptional activation of Wnt-pathway target genes like cyclin D1, c-myc, or PPARγ, which in turn promote tumor progression by enhancing proliferation.

Despite its impact on human health, liver cancer is understudied compared to other major lethal cancers. In addition, the field has a limited arsenal of model systems in which to study the development of this disease and to test potential intervention strategies. For the most part, the traditional study of human cancers only provides a snapshot of the final result, rather than a detailed roadmap of the route taken by the tumor cell to reach its destination. The ability to model intermediate stages of tumor formation is essential for a complete understanding of the disease—not only in terms of our understanding of disease biology, but also in terms of effectively using biological information for the development of new treatments and therapies.

The use of genetically engineered mouse models to study cancer enables an assessment of how specific genetic alterations occurring in the human disease affect the tumor phenotype. Currently, mouse models of liver cancer are based mainly on classic transgenic approaches, tetracycline-regulated transgene expression or chemically induced carcinogenesis (Sandgren et al. 1989; Jhappan et al. 1990; Murakami et al. 1993; Verna et al. 1996a,b; Deane et al. 2001; Manickan et al. 2001; Wang et al. 2001; Harada et al. 2004; Shachaf et al. 2004). Although these models have produced important insights into the molecular mechanisms of hepatocarcinogenesis, they have several disadvantages. First, the expression of transgenes by tissue-specific promoters may not target all epithelial cells within the organ (stem-cell and non-stem-cell compartment) and thus may alter the cell of origin from that occurring in the human disease. Furthermore, the expression of the oncogene (or deletion of a tumor suppressor gene) in all cells within a tissue creates a field effect such that all cells have altered gene expression, which does not mimic the situation of spontaneous tumorigenesis and may alter a tumor's evolutionary trajectory. Second, it is very cost- and time-intensive to generate germ-line transgenic and knockout animals, and production of compound mutant animals can involve complicated intercrossing strategies that are extremely slow. Third, some lesions also produce developmental abnormalities resulting in embryonic lethality or developmental compensation in the resulting tissue, such that the consequences of the mutation may not reflect the acute activation or loss that occurs in tumorigenesis. Obviously, a mouse model that allows bypass of these limitations would be extremely valuable.

Over the last few years, chimeric mouse models based on the genetic manipulation and retransplantation of hematopoietic stem cells have provided new insights into mechanisms of tumor initiation, progression, and treatment response in hematopoietic malignancies (see, e.g., Pear et al. 1998; Schmitt et al. 2002a,b; Hemann et al. 2005). Such models have the advantage of generating genetically defined tumors at a fraction of the time and cost required to produce comparable germ-line models, allowing more genes and gene combinations to be studied. Because the cancers that arise in these animals are derived from targeting stem and/or progenitor cells, they may more accurately reflect the evolution of corresponding human malignancies. Finally, these models are produced by transplantation of genetically altered cells into recipient mice, thereby yielding genetic mosaics where the developing cancer cell is surrounded by otherwise normal counterparts. For example, using such systems, we have shown that mutant Myc alleles obtained from Burkitt's lymphoma are highly oncogenic because they fail to induce the pro-apoptotic protein Bim (Heman et al. 2005), and that p53 can influence the antitumor activity of certain oncogene-targeted therapeutics (H.G. Wendel et al., in prep.). Nevertheless, these powerful systems have been largely limited to the hematopoietic system.

Combining our previous experience with these novel chimeric mouse model systems, and our desire to easily and accurately model HCCs, we developed and characterized a new mouse model for HCC that is based on the ex vivo manipulation of liver progenitor cells followed by the seeding of these cells into normal recipients. These methods allowed us to rapidly produce in situ liver cancers of defined genetic origin. The generation of the model and its potential applications are the topic of this report.

MATERIALS AND METHODS

Isolation, culture, and retroviral infection of E-Cadherin-positive liver progenitor cells. Liver cell suspensions from fetal livers of ED12.5–15 C57BL/6 mice (Jackson Laboratories, Rochester, New York), were prepared as described previously (Nitou et al. 2002). Purification of E-Cadherin-positive hepatoblasts from liver suspensions was performed using the MACS® magnetic cell-sorting system (Miltenyi, Auburn, California) in the indirect labeling option together with the rat anti-mouse E-Cadherin (ECCD-1) antibody (Calbiochem, San Diego, California). Columns of the "MS" size were used. Purification was performed by a modification of the protocol recommended by the manufacturer. Briefly, goat anti-rat IgG microbeads were first incubated with the ECCD-1 antibody for 45 minutes at room temperature with gentle resuspension by pipetting every 5 minutes. 20 μl of immunomagnetic beads were incubated with 4 μg of ECCD-1 antibody for later incubation with up to 10^7 positive cells. Complexes of primary and secondary antibody were washed using a MS column according to the manufacturer's instructions. Liver cell suspensions were incubated with the antibody complexes in DMEM 10% FBS in plastic tubes for 45 minutes at 4°C. After loading onto MACS MS columns, cells were washed and subsequently eluted in 1 ml of hepatocyte growth medium (Block et al. 1996). The harvest from one embryonic liver was split into two portions and plated in two wells of a 6-well plate that were coated with gelatin (Specialty Media, Phillipsburg, New Jersey) and contained irradiated (30 Gy) NIH-3T3 feeder layers (3×10^3 cells/cm²). Hepatocyte growth medium was supplemented with hepatocyte growth factor (HGF)/SF (40 ng/ml) (Peprotech, Rocky Hill, New Jersey) and epidermal growth factor (EGF) (20 ng/ml) (Peprotech, Rocky Hill, New Jersey).

After 68 hours, cultured hepatoblasts were transduced with various lentiviral or murine stem cell virus (MSCV)-based retroviral vectors as described previously (Schmitt et al. 2002a), each coexpressing a green fluorescent protein (GFP) reporter. Briefly, retrovirus was produced in Phoenix packaging cells and collected in hepatocyte growth medium. High-titer viral supernatant was passed through a 0.45-μm filter and supplemented with polybrene (2 μg/ml), HGF (40 ng/ml), and EGF (20 ng/ml). The infection procedure was repeated three times every 8 hours. 24 hours after the last infection, the fraction of GFP-positive cells was assessed by GFP fluorescence microscopy.

Immunofluorescence, immunohistochemistry, and histopathology. Mouse monoclonal antibodies against cytokeratin AE1 (Biocare Medical, Walnut Creek, California) (1:100), OV-6 (R&D systems, Minneapolis, Minnesota) (1:50), rabbit anti-mouse albumin antiserum (Biogenesis, Poole, United Kingdom) (1:200), rabbit anti-human α-fetoprotein (AFP) antiserum (Dako, Glostrup,

Denmark) (1:200), mouse monoclonal antibodies against cytokeratin 8 (RDI, Concord, Massachusetts) (1:100), or rabbit polyclonal antibodies against GFP (1:200) (Abcam, Cambridge, Massachusetts) were used as primary antibodies. For immunofluorescence of cultured hepatoblasts, cells were either plated on gelatin-coated coverslips/NIH-3T3 feeder layers (CK AE1, OV-6, CK8) or on NIH-3T3 feeder layers grown on gelatin-coated plastic wells (AFP, Alb). Cells were fixed with 4% PFA at room temperature for 15 minutes, permeabilized with 0.2% Triton, 5% goat serum in phosphate-buffered saline (PBS) for 5 minutes and subsequently washed with 0.1% PBS-T, 5% normal goat serum. Incubation with the primary antibody was performed for 1 hour in 0.1% PBS-T, 5% normal goat serum at room temperature. Control samples were incubated with 0.1% PBS-T, 5% normal goat serum. Secondary antibodies used were goat anti-mouse Alexa Fluor 594-labeled antibody (Invitrogen, Carlsbad, California) and goat anti-rabbit Alexa Fluor-labeled antibodies (Invitrogen, Carlsbad, California). Anti-GFP immunofluorescence was performed on paraffin-embedded liver sections. Standard Proteinase K antigen-retrieval was used. Detailed protocols for anti-cytokeratin-8 immunohistochemistry on paraffin-embedded liver tumor sections are available upon request. Histopathological evaluation of murine liver carcinomas was done by an experienced liver pathologist (P.F.) using paraffin-embedded liver tumor sections that were stained with hematoxylin/eosin (H&E) according to standard protocols.

Conditioning of recipient mice and transplantation. Pathogen-free female C57BL/6 mice (Jackson Laboratories, Rochester, New York), 8–12 weeks of age, weighing 20–30 g were used as recipients for genetically modified liver progenitor cells. Retrorsine and CCl_4 stock solutions were prepared as described previously (Guo et al. 2002). Before injection, retrorsine stock solution was diluted 1:5 in sterile PBS. Mice received retrorsine, 70 mg/kg i.p. This dose was repeated after 7 days and the mice were allowed to recover for 10 days prior to hepatoblast transplantation.

For transplantation of genetically modified hepatoblasts, animals were anesthetized with isolflurane, and a small left subcostal laparotomy was performed. The spleen was retracted and the lower spleen pole looped with a 4-0 vicryl ligation. 2×10^6 cells were injected in 0.2 ml of medium in the lower pole of the spleen in an injection time of 2 minutes. The lower spleen pole was ligated and resected. The abdomen was sutured using 4-0 vicryl (Ethicon, Norderstedt, Germany). Transplanted cells were allowed to migrate to the recipient liver and engraft the liver. 5 days after intrasplenic cell transplantation, CCl_4 was administered in a dose of 0.5 ml/kg i.p. CCl_4 treatment was repeated on d10 and d15 after cell transplantation. Animals were subsequently monitored for tumor formation by abdominal palpation of whole-body fluorescence imaging. For external GFP-tumor imaging, mice were anesthetized with isolflurane, abdominal fur was removed with depilating cream, and animals were monitored by whole-body fluorescence imaging for the retrovirally expressed GFP reporter as described previously (Schmitt et al. 2002a). All procedures were per-

formed in accordance with the guidelines of the Institutional Animal Care and Use committee of Cold Spring Harbor Laboratory.

Generation of cell lines and retransplantation. To generate cells from primary HCCs, a tumor nodule of at least 3×3 mm was removed and diced into small pieces. To obtain a single-cell suspension, minced tumor suspensions were incubated in HEPES-buffered DMEM containing 1000 U/ml dispase for 30–60 minutes at 37°C. The suspension was washed twice in DMEM to remove dispase completely. Before plating, the cell suspension was filtered through a sterile metal sieve to remove clumps. To facilitate the initial attachment, isolated tumor cells were plated on gelatin-coated culture plates.

For retransplantation into recipient mice, 2×10^6 cells were injected in 100 µl of medium into the left liver lobe. Briefly, mice were anesthetized as described above. A small ventral midline laparotomy was performed. The left liver lobe was retracted and 2×10^6 cells were injected subcapsularly in 100 µl of medium. The injection site was compressed for at least two minutes to prevent bleeding and peritoneal spreading of tumor cells. The intra-abdominal operation field was rinsed with distilled water to osmotically kill accidentally leaked tumor cells. The abdominal wall was closed using 4-0 vicryl suture material (Ethicon, Norderstedt, Germany).

RESULTS

Isolation and Transduction of Liver Progenitor Cells

There is increasing evidence that bipotential liver stem cells (oval cells in rodents and hepatic progenitor cells in humans) are the cellular targets for transformation in the development of HCC (Braun et al. 1987; Dumble et al. 2002; Alison and Lovell 2005) and eventually also biliary tract cancer (Tsao and Grisham 1987; Steinberg et al. 1997). Oval cells are bipotential liver stem cells, existing in the healthy adult liver in low numbers around the periportal region. During chronic liver damage, oval cells can proliferate extensively (Thorgeirsson 1996; Dabeva and Shafritz 2003), suggesting that they might be good candidates to target with genetic modifications to model liver cancer. Numerous protocols are available to induce the oval-cell compartment in rodents (for review, see Dabeva and Shafritz 2003), and purification procedures for oval cells have been established (Dumble et al. 2002; Dabeva and Shafritz 2003). However, a major disadvantage of these protocols is that they are based on carcinogen treatment, which may introduce undefined genetic mutations that contribute to tumorigenesis.

Bipotential hepatoblasts are the embryonic counterpart to oval cells from the adult liver (Thorgeirsson 1996; Dabeva and Shafritz 2003). These cells also give rise to cells of both the hepatocytic and bile duct lineage (Fig. 1A) and share almost every marker with oval cells. They exist in large quantities in the murine fetal liver, which also contains hematopoietic cells, endothelial cells, connective tissue cells, and precursors of hepatic stellate cells. Recently, it was reported that hepatoblasts can be purified from the ED12.5 mouse liver using antibodies recognizing the extracellular epitopes of E-Cadherin molecules in combination with immunomagnetic beads (Nitou et al. 2002) to a purity of about 98%. These hepatoblasts were capable of spontaneously differentiating into hepatocytes when cocultured with the nonparenchymal fraction of the embryonic liver (Nitou et al. 2002). We therefore reasoned that these embryonic hepatoblasts would serve as an excellent source of liver progenitor cells for further manipulation, and we set out to isolate, culture, and genetically manipulate mouse embryonic hepatoblasts using procedures analogous to our previous efforts in hematopoietic systems.

We isolated E-Cadherin-positive liver progenitor cells using an immunomagnetic-bead-based procedure. After plating, aggregates of hepatoblasts attach in close proximity to the feeder layer cells (Fig. 1B, left). A major limitation to propagating pure hepatoblasts is that the growth and survival of these cells in vitro is limited due to the requirement for hepatoblast–nonparenchymal cell interactions for survival and growth (Nitou et al. 2002). However, we noted that hepatoblasts grown on gelatin-coated culture plates with irradiated NIH-3T3 feeder layers in chemically defined medium (Block et al. 1996) enriched with HGF and EGF are capable of extensive proliferation (Fig. 1B, middle).

Transgenes were introduced into these cells by retrovirus-mediated gene transfer using MSCV-based vectors coexpressing GFP. Using a standard protocol, we typically were able to infect 20–50% of cells, as assessed by monitoring GFP in the target cell population (Fig. 1B, right). To determine whether these cells retained markers of bipotential liver progenitors, we examined their immunophenotype using several well-established markers (AFP, albumin, CK8, CKAE1, and OV-6) that allow (1) the discrimination of parenchymal from non-parenchymal cells and (2) a classification of the parenchymal cells into progenitor cells, cells of the hepatocytic lineage, and cells of the bile duct lineage.

Immunofluorescence against AFP and albumin (Alb) can be performed on hepatoblasts grown on gelatin-coated plastic dishes, thus allowing a quantification of the Alb\AFP-double positive fraction. As expected, the E-Cadherin-positive liver progenitor cells displayed abundant expression of Alb and AFP, with >98% being Alb\AFP-double positive cells. Note that AFP is a marker for bipotential liver progenitor cells that is usually not found in differentiated hepatocytes or bile duct cells. Furthermore, we performed immunofluorescence on the E-Cadherin-positive liver progenitor cells using a monoclonal antibody directed against the acidic (Type 1) family of cytokeratins. This family consists of cytokeratins 10, 14, 15, 16, and 19. Cytokeratins 10, 15, and 16 are mainly found expressed in the skin. Cytokeratins 14 and 19, however, are known to be markers for bipotential liver progenitor cells (for review, see Thorgeirsson 1996). Positive results were also found in immunofluorescence analyses using antibodies directed against the "liver cytokeratin" cytokeratin 8 and the oval-cell antigen OV-6. The expression levels of CK8, CKAE1, and OV-6 were notably lower than those of Alb and AFP. The re-

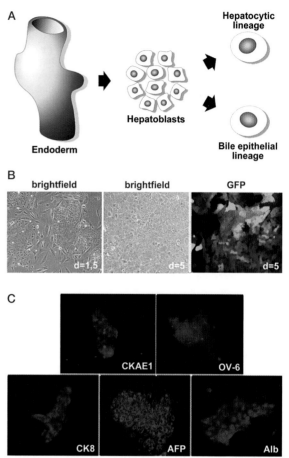

Figure 1. (*A*) Schematic representation showing the embryonic derivation of hepatic cell lineages. (*B*) E-Cadherin-positive fetal liver progenitor cells (LPCs, also known as hepatoblasts) can be purified by immunomagnetic beads. E-Cadherin[+] fetal liver progenitor cells are isolated from ED = 12.5–15 fetal mouse livers using the MACS® system with indirect labeling. Freshly harvested hepatoblasts are grown in gelatin-coated plates on irradiated NIH-3T3 feeder layers. Islands of LPCs are growing in close proximity to 3T3 feeder cells (*left*). E-Cadherin[+] LPCs show an extensive growth potential in vitro when grown on feeder layers in HGF/EGF-enriched hepatocyte growth medium (*middle*). E-Cadherin[+] LPCs can be infected efficiently with standard retroviral vectors as shown by GFP fluorescence (*right*). (*C*) Characterization of the E-Cadherin[+] liver progenitor cells with established hepatoblast/oval cell markers. E-Cadherin[+] LPCs reveal strong positivity for AFP, Alb, and CKAE1; positivity for CK8; and weak positivity for OV-6.

sults of the characterization of the expression pattern of these purified E-Cadherin-positive liver progenitor cells strongly suggest that they are bipotential liver progenitor cells, or hepatoblasts.

Intrahepatic Seeding of Genetically Modified Liver Progenitor Cells

We next sought to explore whether purified hepatoblasts could be genetically modified and incorporated into the liver. It is known that liver cell transplantation into the spleen of healthy recipient mice leads to an inefficient repopulation of the host liver (0.03–0.5% of the total liver mass) (Gupta et al. 1991; Ponder et al. 1991). Different approaches to facilitate the engraftment of transplanted hepatocytes within the recipient liver have been described. All these approaches share the feature that hepatocytes are transplanted into a predamaged liver which provides a regenerative environment for transplanted cells (Shafritz and Dabeva 2002; Dabeva and Shafritz 2003). Recently, Guo et al. (2002) reported an enhanced repopulation of the mouse liver after pretreatment of the animals with retrorsine. Retrorsine is an alkaloid that exerts a strong and persistent block of native hepatocyte proliferation (Laconi et al. 1999). After hepatocyte transplantation, CCl4 was used to induce a regenerative environment in which transplanted cells can proliferate, while proliferation of recipient cells remains blocked. Using this protocol, Guo et al. (2002) demonstrated repopulation rates of up to 20% of the liver mass. We reasoned that such procedures in combination with transplantation of genetically modified hepatocytes which exert a proliferation advantage should allow a highly efficient engraftment of transplanted cells.

A schematic representation of our approach is shown in Figure 2A. E-Cadherin-positive bipotential liver progenitor cells are purified and grown in primary culture. Cells are infected with retroviral constructs, expressing oncogenes or short hairpin RNAs (shRNAs) directed against tumor suppressor genes. After infection, 2×10^6 liver progenitor cells are transplanted into the spleens of recipient mice that were conditioned with retrorsine. One week after intrasplenic injection of the cells, a cycle of three CCl4 treatments is started. The timeline of the retrorsine pretreatment and subsequent CCl4 treatment is shown in Figure 2B. One week after intrasplenic injection of GFP-tagged liver progenitor cells, livers were harvested and processed for immunofluorescence with an antibody directed against GFP. We found that approximately 1% of the whole liver consisted of the "seeded," GFP-positive liver progenitor cells. Interestingly, on H&E sections these transplanted cells are indistinguishable from the surrounding normal hepatocytes (Fig. 2C).

Generation of Liver Cancers In Situ

Our next goal was to generate primary liver carcinomas with defined genetic lesions previously linked to the development of human HCC. For example, mutations in p53, Rb, and IGFR1 are frequently found in HCC (Murakami et al. 1991; Kim et al. 1996), and the oncogenes c-myc and cyclin D1 are frequently found to be overexpressed (Peng et al. 1993; Nishida et al. 1994). To generate primary liver carcinomas of the genetic compound lesion "p53$^{-/-}$;c-myc," we purified hepatoblasts from p53-deficient embryonic mouse livers. These cells were transduced with an MSCV-based retroviral vector coexpressing c-myc with a GFP reporter and transplanted into the spleen of retrorsine-pretreated recipient mice as described above. Animals were continuously monitored for general health and tumor formation by abdominal palpation and external GFP fluorescence imaging.

Figure 2D shows a tumor-bearing mouse with a swollen abdomen due to ascites (digital picture, right panel). The tumor is detectable by whole-body fluorescence imaging (left panel). The asterisks indicate remnants of GFP-positive transplanted hepatocytes in the spleen. GFP imaging of the explanted liver (lower panel, left) shows an advanced liver carcinoma filling a whole liver lobe. It is apparent that the external GFP signal is not proportional to the real tumor size, because about 70% of the GFP signal is absorbed by the ribcage/abdominal wall. Presumably, more sensitive imaging techniques, such as bioluminescence using a luciferase reporter, would enable the detection of small liver tumors and precise assessment of partial responses in treatment studies.

We also generated in situ liver carcinomas by seeding genetically manipulated adult liver cells (no separation of adult hepatocytes from liver progenitor cells) obtained by collagenase perfusion from livers of p53-deficient mice (data not shown). Because the infection efficiency of differentiated hepatocytes with standard retroviral vectors is much lower compared to hepatoblasts (data not shown), we used lentiviral vectors in this setting. Infection of p53-deficient adult liver cells with a lentivirus expressing an HA-tagged form of c-myc (Hemann et al. 2005) and seeding of these cells into the livers of conditioned recipient mice gave rise to in situ liver carcinomas with lower penetrance than the hepatoblast cultures. We also found that tumorigenicity of p53$^{-/-}$ embryonic liver cells isolated from the late-stage mouse embryo (ED16–18) and infected with a c-myc-expressing retrovirus is significantly lower than tumorigenicity of cells of the same genotype that were harvested around ED12.5 (data not shown). Interestingly, embryonic hepatocytes that were harvested from ED18 p53$^{-/-}$ embryonic mouse livers and infected with a retrovirus encoding c-myc are only immortalized but not transformed (0/8 tumors subcutaneously on nude mice, 0/12 tumors in situ).

We next established a protocol for the culture and expansion of hepatoma cells from primary murine HCCs of a defined genetic origin (see Materials and Methods for details). In most instances, this procedure allowed the establishment of a stable population of cultured hepatoma cells. After expansion, the cells could be directly injected into the liver of recipient mice. Figure 2E shows an explanted liver several weeks after direct infiltration of 2×10^6 "p53$^{-/-}$;c-myc" hepatoma cells into the left liver lobe. The tumor is readily visualized by GFP imaging as shown in the left panel of the figure. The ability to generate multiple tumors of exactly the same genetic background should enable side-by-side comparisons of different treatment regimens in tumors of the same genetic background.

Suppression of Gene Expression in Murine HCC Using Stable RNA Interference

Historically, mouse models of human liver cancer have involved the germ-line manipulation of either oncogenes or tumor suppressor genes. In the case of tumor suppressor genes, one either constitutively deletes the tumor suppressor gene or produces a conditional

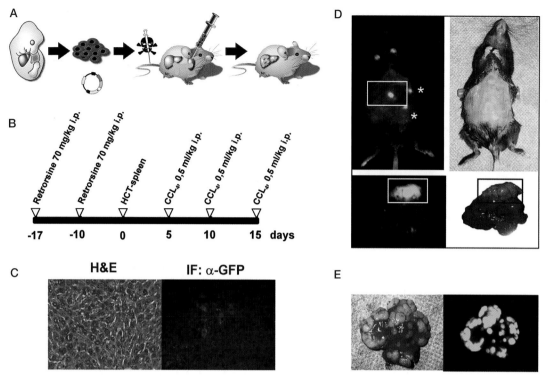

Figure 2. Generation of genetically defined in situ liver cancers. (*A*) Technical outline. E-Cadherin-positive fetal liver progenitor cells (hepatoblasts) are purified and cultured as described above. Using the murine stem cell virus (MSCV) optimized to drive long-term gene expression in vivo, the cells are infected with oncogenes and/or shRNAs directed against tumor suppressor genes. After infection and expansion, the cells are transplanted into the spleens of conditioned recipient mice. Because all retroviral vectors used for infections are GFP-tagged, development of in situ HCCs can be monitored by external GFP imaging. (*B*) Schematic representation of the timeline of the approach. Mice undergo two pretreatments with the liver cell cycle inhibitor retrorsine. After transplantation of the cells into the spleen, the transplanted hepatoblasts are selectively expanded by CCl4 treatment of the mice. (*C*) GFP+ transplanted hepatoblasts can be detected in the recipient liver by anti-GFP immunofluorescence (*right*). H&E staining of an adjacent section of the liver (*left*). (*D*) External GFP imaging of a p53; c-myc tumor-bearing mouse (*left*). The GFP-positive spot in the square represents the intrahepatic tumor mass. The two additional spots (marked by asterisks) represent transplanted cells residing in the spleen after transplantation. Mice with advanced intrahepatic tumor growth present with swollen, ascites-containing abdomen allowing detection of tumor burden by palpation. GFP imaging of the explanted liver (*bottom panel*) reveals an advanced intrahepatic tumor, filling out a whole liver lobe. (*E*) Primary liver tumors can be outgrown in culture and retransplanted in situ into recipient mice. Shown is a tumor that was retransplanted by direct liver injection of 2×10^6 tumor cells. Note the extensive intrahepatic metastasis of the transplanted cells.

"knockout" animal where the gene is flanked by loxP sites such that the tumor suppressor gene can be inactivated in specific settings using cre recombinase. Although extremely powerful, these approaches can be extremely time- and cost-intensive and, in the case of constitutive knockout strains, are subject to developmental compensation that can mask aspects of the null phenotype (Sage et al. 2003). However, over the last several years, RNA interference (RNAi) has emerged as a complementary and effective tool to homologous recombination to study the consequences of gene suppression in cultured mammalian cells and in mice (Hemann et al. 2003; Hannon and Rossi 2004; Dickins et al. 2005). Furthermore, improved reagents for stable RNAi have been reported where the silencing triggers mimic a natural microRNA primary transcript, and each target sequence has been selected on the basis of thermodynamic criteria for optimal shRNA performance (Dickins et al. 2005; Silva et al. 2005). We were therefore interested in evalu-

ating whether stable RNAi technology could be harnessed to create dominantly acting inhibitors of tumor suppressor function in a chimeric (genetic mosaic) model of hepatocarcinogenesis.

To test the feasibility of such an approach, we sought to generate in situ liver carcinomas by genetic manipulation of bipotential liver progenitor cells with synthetic microRNAs directed against p53 in combination with different oncogenes. The predicted folding of the primary microRNA is shown in Figure 3A. The red bars indicate the predicted mature small interfering RNA. Figure 3B shows in situ liver carcinomas derived either from p53-deficient liver progenitor cells (LPCs) overexpressing oncogenic Ras or from wild-type LPCs that were double infected with a microRNA-based sh-construct directed against p53 (MLS.1224), together with a vector expressing oncogenic Ras. The infected cell populations were seeded into the liver or injected subcutaneously into an immunocompromised mouse.

GFP fluorescence revealed that liver carcinomas developed rapidly in the livers of transplanted recipient mice (<3 weeks), irrespective of whether they were derived from p53$^{-/-}$ hepatoblasts or wild-type hepatoblasts expressing sh-p53. Indeed, tumors arising from both configurations displayed a highly aggressive and disseminated growth pattern in the liver (Fig. 3B). Tumors also arose rapidly in the subcutaneous setting, where they could be readily monitored using standard caliper measurements. The growth rates of liver carcinomas derived from "p53$^{-/-}$;H-RasV12" tumors show no significant difference from "shp53;H-RasV12" tumors (Fig. 3C), implying that, in this setting, RNAi was as effective at promoting tumorigenesis as a null allele. Representative GFP images from both groups are shown along with their respective tumor growth curves. To our knowledge, this is the first demonstration of the generation of in situ carcinomas by stable RNAi.

Murine Liver Cancers Resemble Primary Human Liver Cancer

For a mouse model to have maximal utility, it is important to understand the extent to which it recapitulates the histopathology of the corresponding human disease. In humans, the histopathological appearance of HCC is extremely varied, with several distinct growth patterns. These different histopathological patterns have no clinical or prognostic significance in humans with the exception of "fibrolamellar carcinoma" (a rare variant of HCC that can respond to chemoradiation therapy). To validate that the tumors of our mouse model resemble the human pathology, we analyzed a large panel of tumors based on the compound genetic lesion "p53$^{-/-}$;c-myc" for the appearance of different histopathological subtypes. H&E-stained sections from paraffin-embedded tissues were examined by an experienced liver pathologist (P.F.). More than 80% of the examined "c-myc;p53$^{-/-}$ HCCs" were classified as moderately well to poorly differentiated HCCs with a mostly solid, sometimes mixed solid/trabecular growth pattern (Fig. 4). All tumors were additionally stained with cytokeratin 8 to confirm the affiliation with the liver lineage (Thorgeirsson 1996). A much smaller proportion of tumors (<20%) represented histological growth patterns resembling human trabecular HCC or pseudoglandular HCC (Fig. 4). Thus, tumors arising through liver seeding of genetically altered liver progenitor cells show a remarkable similarity to human liver cancers.

DISCUSSION

A New Mouse Model of Liver Cancer

Although HCC is one of the most frequent neoplasms worldwide, there is an insufficient genetic and biological understanding of the disease. Based on our technological foundations from mouse models of blood-related malignancies (Schmitt et al. 2002a,b; Hemann et al. 2005), we sought to develop a chimeric new orthotopic, genetically tractable mouse model for HCC that would allow a more

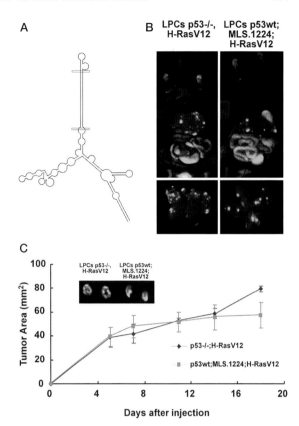

Figure 3. Second-generation, microRNA-based shRNA expression vectors can be used to model hepatocarcinogenesis in vivo. (*A*) Predicted folding for the pri-microRNA. The predicted mature siRNA duplex is labeled with red bars. (*B*) Liver carcinomas were generated either by infecting p53$^{-/-}$ liver progenitor cells (LPCs) with oncogenic Ras or by coinfecting wild-type LPCs with a microRNA-based shRNA construct directed against p53 (MLS.1224) together with oncogenic Ras. (*C*) To facilitate the exact measurement of tumor growth, "p53$^{-/-}$;H-RasV12" and "sh-p53;H-RasV12" liver carcinomas were also grown subcutaneously on NCR nu/nu mice. Shown are representative external GFP imagings of the subcutaneously grown tumors and tumor growth curves for each group. Growth rates of "p53$^{-/-}$;H-RasV12" and "sh-p53;H-RasV12" liver carcinomas were assessed by caliper measurements (*n* = 6 in each group).

effective analysis of this disease. Our approach allows genetic manipulation of bipotential liver progenitor cells ex vivo with subsequent seeding of these cells into the livers of conditioned recipient mice. Following the introduction of appropriate genetic combinations, this procedure results in the development of in situ liver tumors that resemble human HCC.

Our model is based on the targeting of liver progenitor cells with initiating oncogenic lesions. It is an emerging concept that tissue-specific stem or progenitor cells can be the target for transformation in different types of human cancer (Smalley and Ashworth 2003; Al Hajj and Clarke 2004; Baik et al. 2004; Tai et al. 2005). For liver cancer, it remains under debate whether carcinomas are derived from differentiated hepatocytes or from liver progenitor cells. However, there is increasing evidence that bipoten-

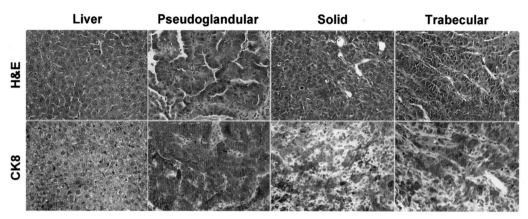

Figure 4. Mouse HCCs derived from E-Cadherin$^+$ liver progenitor cells reveal histopathological subtypes of human HCC. Three common variegations of human HCCs (solid, trabecular, and pseudoglandular growth pattern) are lined up with corresponding mouse HCCs derived from genetically modified hepatoblasts. All shown mouse HCCs are derived from p53$^{-/-}$ hepatoblasts overexpressing c-myc. Mouse HCCs were stained for cytokeratin 8 as a typical liver cytokeratin.

tial liver stem cells, so-called oval cells, are the cellular targets for transformation in the development of HCC (Braun et al. 1987; Dumble et al. 2002; Alison and Lovell 2005). In our model, bipotential liver progenitor cells from the fetal mouse liver are the target for transformation in the development of liver carcinomas. Tumors derived from genetically modified hepatoblasts closely resemble the histopathology of human liver cancer, with respect to both their general pathology and underlying genetics.

Genes were introduced into liver progenitor cells by retroviral transduction, and infected populations were introduced into livers of "conditioned" recipient mice under circumstances that facilitiate engraftment of these cells into the liver. Of note, direct delivery of concentrated lentivirus overexpressing c-myc into the livers of p53-deficient mice gave no liver tumors in an observation period of 1 year (L. Zender and S.W. Lowe, unpubl.). This observation suggests that infiltration of lentivirus into the adult mouse liver predominantly infected differentiated hepatocytes, providing further support for a stem cell theory of hepatocarcinogenesis. Our observations are in accordance with a recent study of Lewis et al. (2005), who demonstrated that c-myc delivered in RCAS vectors into the livers of Alb-TVA p53-deficient mice was not capable of forming liver tumors. The fact that these investigators were able to generate liver carcinomas by delivering the mouse polyomavirus middle-T antigen (PyMT) in RCAS vectors into p53-deficient Alb-TVA may be due to the fact that PyMT-induced transformation is more efficient than c-myc-induced transformation, and a small subfraction of targeted bipotential liver progenitor cells (oval cells) is sufficient to give rise to tumors.

Our approach to generate genetically defined liver carcinomas has several advantages compared to classic transgenic approaches. First, it is a very time- and cost-effective way to produce high numbers of genetically defined HCCs. Second, mosaics are generated, such that genetically modified cells are surrounded by otherwise normal counterparts, allowing the development of tumors that resembles the pathogenesis of human HCC. Third, all

experiments can be conducted in a single genetic background using the same constitutively active promoter, which facilitates the comparison of results between different investigators. Fourth, because the retroviruses used to produce the tumors can have imaging reporters, the resulting tumors can be detected and monitored using inexpensive imaging technologies, such as whole-body fluorescence imaging. Fifth, primary liver carcinomas of defined genetic origin can be grown ex vivo and retransplanted directly into the livers of recipient mice, a property that facilitates the use of this model in preclinical trials to test new treatment regimens against HCC. Finally, tumor-bearing mice can be generated without the use of germ-line methods, thereby circumventing some of the constraints of the "Oncomouse" patent.

Probing HCC Genetics and Biology

Despite the fact that HCC has a huge impact on human health, relatively little is known about the molecular mechanisms of hepatocarcinogenesis. To gain further insights into liver cancer genetics and to define possible therapeutic targets against liver cancer, we applied a high-resolution genome-wide scanning technology to murine liver carcinomas that were initiated by two defined hits. We demonstrate that a mouse liver tumor that was primarily driven by oncogenic ras acquired a focal genomic amplification containing c-myc, a gene highly established as associated with human liver cancer (data not shown).

These results underscore the potential of our approach to identify new candidate genes for hepatocarcinogenesis. Indeed, in a parallel study (L. Zender et al., in prep.), we have taken advantage of our model to identify, validate, and characterize a novel oncogene linked to human HCC. Specifically, we conducted ROMA on a series of murine HCCs arising in the presence of Myc, Akt, or oncogenic Ras, and noted that the Myc-expressing HCCs (and not those expressing Akt or Ras) frequently harbored an amplification on mouse chromosome 9. Interestingly, by analyzing a series of human HCCs, we found a corresponding amplification on chromosome 11, which is syntenic to mouse chromosome 9 and contained the same set of genes. Through further cross-species analysis and expression studies, we narrowed down one gene—the cellular inhibitor of apoptosis gene cIAP1—as the most likely "driver" gene in this amplicon.

One powerful aspect of this system is that genes identified as altered in the tumors can be rapidly examined for oncogenic potential in the mouse using the precise genetic configuration in which the spontaneous lesion arose. Thus, by returning to the mouse, we demonstrated that enforced expression of cIAP1 in the genetic context in which the amplification occurred ($p53^{-/-}$;c-Myc) accelerated tumorigenesis and, conversely, suppression of cIAP1 in cells harboring the amplicon reduced tumor growth. These effects were highly genotype-specific—thus, cIAP1 had no impact on promoting tumors initiated with Akt or Ras, and shRNAs targeting cIAP did not delay the growth of tumors that did not contain the cIAP amplicon. In addition to validating cIAP1 as a bona fide oncogene, these studies define an integrative approach to cancer genetics and biology that may facilitate the annotation of the cancer genome (for more discussion, see L. Zender et al., in prep.).

In addition to identifying new genes involved in HCC using genome-scanning approaches followed by "reverse genetics," our model is amenable to forward genetics approaches using new, low-complexity cDNA or RNAi libraries to identify new oncogenes and tumor suppressor genes, respectively. In principle, one can envision introducing defined "pools" of cDNAs or shRNAs into hepatoblasts from a "sensitized" genetic background followed by transplantation into the livers of recipient mice. In principle, if a given pool harbors an oncogenic cDNA or shRNA, tumors should arise more rapidly than controls. Here, we provide a proof-of-principle experiment that microRNA-based shRNAs can be used to generate in situ liver carcinomas. This HCC mouse model should prove to be a valuable tool to further explore molecular mechanisms of hepatocarcinogenesis and to help define new molecular targets.

A Preclinical Mouse Model for Testing New Therapies

Human liver cancer currently represents the third leading cause of cancer deaths; in part, because no effective chemotherapeutic regimens are currently available. Thus, a major effort of HCC research is to develop the molecular and modeling infrastructure to identify new drug targets and test their potential efficacy. As mentioned above, our chimeric mouse model of HCC has many features that should enable it to provide new insights into the molecular genetics of HCC. In addition, as shown in this study, all of the liver tumors we produce can be monitored by GFP imaging, and most can be propagated in vitro or by transplanting into the livers of syngeneic recipients. Although more sensitive imaging techniques such as bioluminescence should improve monitoring ca-

pabilities, the availability of defined tumors and simple imaging modalities should enable relatively high-throughput preclinical studies using new drugs or drug combinations on HCC. Such approaches, particularly with new molecularly targeted therapies, may identify new treatment regimens that may be effective against liver cancers with a defined set of underlying genetic lesions.

ACKNOWLEDGMENTS

We thank Amy Brady, Christine Rosenthal, Lisa Bianco, and Maria S. Jiao for excellent technical assistance, and Dr. Eva Hernando for assistance with histology. We also acknowledge Michael Wigler, Lakshmi Muthuswamy, and other members of the Wigler group for providing the bioinformatics required for the mouse ROMA chip and ROMA data analysis, and the members of the Lowe lab for constructive criticism and discussions throughout the course of this work. L.Z. was supported by the German Research foundation (Emmy Noether Programme). This work was also supported by a grant from the Alan Seligson foundation, and by grants CA13106, CA87497, and CA105388 from the National Institutes of Health. S.W.L. and G.J.H. are Howard Hughes Medical Institute investigators.

REFERENCES

Al Hajj M. and Clarke M.F. 2004. Self-renewal and solid tumor stem cells. *Oncogene* **23:** 7274.

Alison M.R. and Lovell M.J. 2005. Liver cancer: The role of stem cells. *Cell Prolif.* **38:** 407.

Baik I., Becker P.S., DeVito W.J., Lagiou P., Ballen K., Quesenberry P.J., and Hsieh C.C. 2004. Stem cells and prenatal origin of breast cancer. *Cancer Causes Control* **15:** 517.

Block G.D., Locker J., Bowen W.C., Petersen B.E., Katyal S., Strom S.C., Riley T., Howard T.A., and Michalopoulos G.K. 1996. Population expansion, clonal growth, and specific differentiation patterns in primary cultures of hepatocytes induced by HGF/SF, EGF and TGF alpha in a chemically defined (HGM) medium. *J. Cell Biol.* **132:** 1133.

Braun L., Goyette M., Yaswen P., Thompson N.L., and Fausto N. 1987. Growth in culture and tumorigenicity after transfection with the ras oncogene of liver epithelial cells from carcinogen-treated rats. *Cancer Res.* **47:** 4116.

Bruix J., Boix L., Sala M., and Llovet J.M. 2004. Focus on hepatocellular carcinoma. *Cancer Cell* **5:** 215.

Buendia M.A. 2000. Genetics of hepatocellular carcinoma. *Semin. Cancer Biol.* **10:** 185.

Dabeva M.D. and Shafritz D.A. 2003. Hepatic stem cells and liver repopulation. *Semin. Liver Dis.* **23:** 349.

Deane N.G., Parker M.A., Aramandla R., Diehl L., Lee W.J., Washington M.K., Nanney L.B., Shyr Y., and Beauchamp R.D. 2001. Hepatocellular carcinoma results from chronic cyclin D1 overexpression in transgenic mice. *Cancer Res.* **61:** 5389.

Dickins R.A., Hemann M.T., Zilfou J.T., Simpson D.R., Ibarra I., Hannon G.J., and Lowe S.W. 2005. Probing tumor phenotypes using stable and regulated synthetic microRNA precursors. *Nat. Genet.* **37:** 1289.

Dumble M.L., Croager E.J., Yeoh G.C., and Quail E.A. 2002. Generation and characterization of p53 null transformed hepatic progenitor cells: Oval cells give rise to hepatocellular carcinoma. *Carcinogenesis* **23:** 435.

Guo D., Fu T., Nelson J.A., Superina R.A., and Soriano H.E. 2002. Liver repopulation after cell transplantation in mice treated with retrorsine and carbon tetrachloride. *Transplantation* **73:** 1818.

Gupta S., Aragona E., Vemuru R.P., Bhargava K.K., Burk R.D., and Chowdhury J.R. 1991. Permanent engraftment and function of hepatocytes delivered to the liver: Implications for gene therapy and liver repopulation. *Hepatology* **14:** 144.

Hannon G.J. and Rossi J.J. 2004. Unlocking the potential of the human genome with RNA interference. *Nature* **431:** 371.

Harada N., Oshima H., Katoh M., Tamai Y., Oshima M., and Taketo M.M. 2004. Hepatocarcinogenesis in mice with beta-catenin and Ha-ras gene mutations. *Cancer Res.* **64:** 48.

Hemann M.T., Fridman J.S., Zilfou J.T., Hernando E., Paddison P.J., Cordon-Cardo C., Hannon G.J., and Lowe S.W. 2003. An epi-allelic series of p53 hypomorphs created by stable RNAi produces distinct tumor phenotypes in vivo. *Nat. Genet.* **33:** 396.

Hemann M.T., Bric A., Teruya-Feldstein J., Herbst A., Nilsson J.A., Cordon-Cardo C., Cleveland J.L., Tansey W.P., and Lowe S.W. 2005. Evasion of the p53 tumour surveillance network by tumour-derived MYC mutants. *Nature* **436:** 807.

Huo T.I., Wang X.W., Forgues M., Wu C.G., Spillare E.A., Giannini C., Brechot C., and Harris C.C. 2001. Hepatitis B virus X mutants derived from human hepatocellular carcinoma retain the ability to abrogate p53-induced apoptosis. *Oncogene* **20:** 3620.

Jhappan C., Stahle C., Harkins R.N., Fausto N., Smith G.H., and Merlino G.T. 1990. TGF alpha overexpression in transgenic mice induces liver neoplasia and abnormal development of the mammary gland and pancreas. *Cell* **61:** 1137.

Kim S.O., Park J.G., and Lee Y.I. 1996. Increased expression of the insulin-like growth factor I (IGF-I) receptor gene in hepatocellular carcinoma cell lines: Implications of IGF-I receptor gene activation by hepatitis B virus X gene product. *Cancer Res.* **56:** 3831.

Kusano N., Shiraishi K., Kubo K., Oga A., Okita K., and Sasaki K. 1999. Genetic aberrations detected by comparative genomic hybridization in hepatocellular carcinomas: Their relationship to clinicopathological features. *Hepatology* **29:** 1858.

Laconi S., Curreli F., Diana S., Pasciu D., De Filippo G., Sarma D.S., Pani P., and Laconi E. 1999. Liver regeneration in response to partial hepatectomy in rats treated with retrorsine: A kinetic study. *J. Hepatol.* **31:** 1069.

Lewis B.C., Klimstra D.S., Socci N.D., Xu S., Koutcher J.A., and Varmus H.E. 2005. The absence of p53 promotes metastasis in a novel somatic mouse model for hepatocellular carcinoma. *Mol. Cell. Biol.* **25:** 1228.

Llovet J.M., Burroughs A., and Bruix J. 2003. Hepatocellular carcinoma. *Lancet* **362:** 1907.

Lucito R., Healy J., Alexander J., Reiner A., Esposito D., Chi M., Rodgers L., Brady A., Sebat J., Troge J., West J.A., Rostan S., Nguyen K.C., Powers S., Ye K.Q., Olshen A., Venkatraman E., Norton L., and Wigler M. 2003. Representational oligonucleotide microarray analysis: A high-resolution method to detect genome copy number variation. *Genome Res.* **13:** 2291.

Manickan E., Satoi J., Wang T.C., and Liang T.J. 2001. Conditional liver-specific expression of simian virus 40 T antigen leads to regulatable development of hepatic neoplasm in transgenic mice. *J. Biol. Chem.* **276:** 13989.

Murakami H., Sanderson N.D., Nagy P., Marino P.A., Merlino G., and Thorgeirsson S.S. 1993. Transgenic mouse model for synergistic effects of nuclear oncogenes and growth factors in tumorigenesis: Interaction of c-myc and transforming growth factor alpha in hepatic oncogenesis. *Cancer Res.* **53:** 1719.

Murakami Y., Hayashi K., Hirohashi S., and Sekiya T. 1991. Aberrations of the tumor suppressor p53 and retinoblastoma genes in human hepatocellular carcinomas. *Cancer Res.* **51:** 5520.

Nhieu J.T., Renard C.A., Wei Y., Cherqui D., Zafrani E.S., and Buendia M.A. 1999. Nuclear accumulation of mutated beta-catenin in hepatocellular carcinoma is associated with increased cell proliferation. *Am. J. Pathol.* **155:** 703.

Niketeghad F., Decker H.J., Caselmann W.H., Lund P., Geissler F., Dienes H.P., and Schirmacher P. 2001. Frequent genomic imbalances suggest commonly altered tumour genes in human hepatocarcinogenesis. *Br. J. Cancer* **85:** 697.

Nishida N., Fukuda Y., Komeda T., Kita R., Sando T., Furukawa M., Amenomori M., Shibagaki I., Nakao K., and Ikenaga M., et al. 1994. Amplification and overexpression of the cyclin D1 gene in aggressive human hepatocellular carcinoma. *Cancer Res.* **54:** 3107.

Nitou M., Sugiyama Y., Ishikawa K., and Shiojiri N. 2002. Purification of fetal mouse hepatoblasts by magnetic beads coated with monoclonal anti-e-cadherin antibodies and their in vitro culture. *Exp. Cell Res.* **279:** 330.

Parkin D.M., Bray F., Ferlay J., and Pisani P. 2001. Estimating the world cancer burden: Globocan 2000. *Int. J. Cancer* **94:** 153.

Pear W.S., Miller J.P., Xu L., Pui J.C., Soffer B., Quackenbush R.C., Pendergast A.M., Bronson R., Aster J.C., Scott M.L., and Baltimore D. 1998. Efficient and rapid induction of a chronic myelogenous leukemia-like myeloproliferative disease in mice receiving P210 bcr/abl-transduced bone marrow. *Blood* **92:** 3780.

Peng S.Y., Lai P.L., and Hsu H.C. 1993. Amplification of the c-myc gene in human hepatocellular carcinoma: Biologic significance. *J. Formos. Med. Assoc.* **92:** 866.

Ponder K.P., Gupta S., Leland F., Darlington G., Finegold M., DeMayo J., Ledley F.D., Chowdhury J.R., and Woo S.L. 1991. Mouse hepatocytes migrate to liver parenchyma and function indefinitely after intrasplenic transplantation. *Proc. Natl. Acad. Sci.* **88:** 1217.

Ray R.B., Steele R., Meyer K., and Ray R. 1997. Transcriptional repression of p53 promoter by hepatitis C virus core protein. *J. Biol. Chem.* **272:** 10983.

Sage J., Miller A.L., Perez-Mancera P.A., Wysocki J.M., and Jacks T. 2003. Acute mutation of retinoblastoma gene function is sufficient for cell cycle re-entry. *Nature* **424:** 223.

Sandgren E.P., Quaife C.J., Pinkert C.A., Palmiter R.D., and Brinster R.L. 1989. Oncogene-induced liver neoplasia in transgenic mice. *Oncogene* **4:** 715.

Schmitt C.A., Fridman J.S., Yang M., Baranov E., Hoffman R.M., and Lowe S.W. 2002a. Dissecting p53 tumor suppressor functions in vivo. *Cancer Cell* **1:** 289.

Schmitt C.A., Fridman J.S., Yang M., Lee S., Baranov E., Hoffman R.M., and Lowe S.W. 2002b. A senescence program controlled by p53 and p16INK4a contributes to the outcome of cancer therapy. *Cell* **109:** 335.

Shachaf C.M., Kopelman A.M., Arvanitis C., Karlsson A., Beer S., Mandl S., Bachmann M.H., Borowsky A.D., Ruebner B., Cardiff R.D., Yang Q., Bishop J.M., Contag C.H., and Felsher D.W. 2004. MYC inactivation uncovers pluripotent differentiation and tumour dormancy in hepatocellular cancer. *Nature* **431:** 1112.

Shafritz D.A. and Dabeva M.D. 2002. Liver stem cells and model systems for liver repopulation. *J. Hepatol.* **36:** 552.

Silva J.M., Li M.Z., Chang K., Ge W., Golding M.C., Rickles R.J., Siolas D., Hu G., Paddison P.J., Schlabach M.R., Sheth N., Bradshaw J., Burchard J., Kulkarni A., Cavet G., Sachidanandam R., McCombie W.R., Cleary M.A., Elledge S.J., and Hannon G.J. 2005. Second-generation shRNA libraries covering the mouse and human genomes. *Nat. Genet.* **37:** 1281.

Smalley M. and Ashworth A. 2003. Stem cells and breast cancer: A field in transit. *Nat. Rev. Cancer* **3:** 832.

Steinberg P., Frank H., Odenthal M., Dienes H.P., and Seidel A. 1997. Role of the Ha-ras gene in the malignant transformation of rat liver oval cells. *Int. J. Cancer* **71:** 680.

Tai M.H., Chang C.C., Kiupel M., Webster J.D., Olson L.K., and Trosko J.E. 2005. Oct4 expression in adult human stem cells: Evidence in support of the stem cell theory of carcinogenesis. *Carcinogenesis* **26:** 495.

Thorgeirsson S.S. 1996. Hepatic stem cells in liver regeneration. *FASEB J.* **10:** 1249.

Tsao M.S. and Grisham J.W. 1987. Hepatocarcinomas, cholangiocarcinomas, and hepatoblastomas produced by chemically transformed cultured rat liver epithelial cells. A light- and electron-microscopic analysis. *Am. J. Pathol.* **127:** 168.

Ueda H., Ullrich S.J., Gangemi J.D., Kappel C.A., Ngo L., Feitelson M.A., and Jay G. 1995. Functional inactivation but not structural mutation of p53 causes liver cancer. *Nat. Genet.* **9:** 41.

Verna L., Whysner J., and Williams G.M. 1996a. 2-Acetyl-aminofluorene mechanistic data and risk assessment: DNA reactivity, enhanced cell proliferation and tumor initiation. *Pharmacol. Ther.* **71:** 83.

———. 1996b. N-nitrosodiethylamine mechanistic data and risk assessment: Bioactivation, DNA-adduct formation, mutagenicity, and tumor initiation. *Pharmacol. Ther.* **71:** 57.

Wang R., Ferrell L.D., Faouzi S., Maher J.J., and Bishop J.M. 2001. Activation of the Met receptor by cell attachment induces and sustains hepatocellular carcinomas in transgenic mice. *J. Cell Biol.* **153:** 1023.

Wang X.W., Forrester K., Yeh H., Feitelson M.A., Gu J.R., and Harris C.C. 1994. Hepatitis B virus X protein inhibits p53 sequence-specific DNA binding, transcriptional activity, and association with transcription factor ERCC3. Proc. *Natl. Acad. Sci.* **91:** 2230.

Wong C.M., Fan S.T., and Ng I.O. 2001. β-Catenin mutation and overexpression in hepatocellular carcinoma: Clinicopathologic and prognostic significance. *Cancer* **92:** 136.

Wong N., Lai P., Lee S.W., Fan S., Pang E., Liew C.T., Sheng Z., Lau J.W., and Johnson P.J. 1999. Assessment of genetic changes in hepatocellular carcinoma by comparative genomic hybridization analysis: Relationship to disease stage, tumor size, and cirrhosis. *Am. J. Pathol.* **154:** 37.

Oncogene-dependent Tumor Suppression: Using the Dark Side of the Force for Cancer Therapy

G.I. Evan, M. Christophorou, E.A. Lawlor, I. Ringshausen, J. Prescott, T. Dansen, A. Finch, C. Martins, and D. Murphy

Cancer Research Institute and Department of Cellular and Molecular Pharmacology,
University of California, San Francisco, California 94143-0875

Cancers arise by an evolutionary process that involves the protracted acquisition by somatic cells of suites of interlocking mutations that uncouple proliferation, survival, migration, and damage responses from the mechanisms (selective pressures) that normally restrain or restrict them in time and space. The relative rareness of cancer cells within the soma, in the face of huge numbers of available cell targets, substantial rates of mutation, and an abundance of proto-oncogenes and tumor suppressor gene targets, indicates that the evolutionary space available to incipient tumor cells is highly restricted. The principal way in which this is achieved is through intrinsic tumor suppression pathways—innate growth arrest and apoptotic programs that fulfill an essentially analogous functional role to checkpoints in the cell cycle machinery by antagonizing the tumorigenic potential of oncogenic mutations. Using switchable transgenic and knockin mouse models, it is possible to identify these various tumor suppressor programs and establish where, when, how, and why they act to forestall neoplasia in each tissue type and, consequently, how and why their failure leads to cancer.

Natural selection works on any replicating biological entity in which genetic diversity arises. Consequently, the lifestyle of long-lived, physically large organisms with regenerative potential like vertebrates encompasses a permanent tension between the forces of selection working at the level of the organism to foster reproductive fitness, and the forces of selection at the level of somatic cells, fostering outgrowth of lethal neoplastic clones. Most metazoans sidestep the entire cancer problem by handing the whole business of organismal reproduction over to ephemeral, small body plans in which extensive somatic cell proliferation in the adult is neither necessary nor possible. In contrast, vertebrate genes consign their long-term futures to versatile corpora of potentially traitorous cells. The rarity of cancer in vertebrates, amid the profligacy of normal somatic cell proliferation and tissue remodeling and regeneration, represents a remarkable example of evolutionary footwork.

Clearly, long-lived organisms require the capacity throughout life to maintain self-renewing tissues like superficial epithelia, immune and hematopoietic systems, and to repair damage. Hence, many somatic cell types must be able to engage, with ease, all the machinery necessary for reconstruction of tissues, including the capacity to expand themselves and to remodel adjacent stroma, vasculature, and accessory cells while keeping infection at bay through proactive establishment of the inflammatory and immune responses. On the other hand, too easy an engagement of such powerful regenerative programs would appear to leave them prey to subversion by mutation, with disastrous neoplastic consequences, given the appreciable mutation rate in somatic cells. The rarity of the cancer cell indicates that, somehow, vertebrate cells have squared the regenerative circle by making the programs required for tissue expansion and remodeling both easy to activate, in the right place at the right time, and at

the same time virtually impossible to subvert through mutation. Arguably, this "achievement" is the cornerstone of cancer-free vertebrate longevity (Green and Evan 2002).

In retrospect, the first clue to how vertebrates solve this conundrum came in the early 1980s with the discovery of oncogene cooperation. These seminal observations indicated that individual oncogenic mutations, such as activation of Ras or Myc, or of E1A or E1B, were "insufficient" for phenotypic transformation of normal fibroblastic cells (Land et al. 1983; Van den Elsen et al. 1983). However, the nature of this insufficiency proved elusive. A common interpretation was that no single individual oncogenic lesion was able to engage the full suite of diverse biological programs necessary for oncogenesis. In this scenario, oncogenes cooperate in an additive way by providing elements missing from each other. In the early 1990s, however, the growing appreciation that individual oncogenic mutations can be potent triggers of growth suppression, senescence, and cell death suggested an alternative explanation for oncogene cooperation. According to this idea, the insufficiency of individual oncogenes is because their powerful abilities to orchestrate many, perhaps all, aspects of malignancy are thwarted by their inbuilt tumor suppressor mechanisms. Oncogenes cooperate when they reciprocally gate each other's intrinsic tumor suppressor functions (Fig. 1B)—in effect, individual (proto)oncogenes lie as nodes in networks rather than on linear, cause-and-effect pathways, and specific information is conveyed by the network as a whole rather than parsed through separate modular pathways. From a micro-evolutionary perspective, the great power of the network scenario is that the innate growth-suppressor functions attached to individual nodes in the network effectively mask any immediate selective advantage that might be conferred on a cell from mutating that node—effectively converting it into a potent selective disadvan-

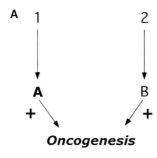

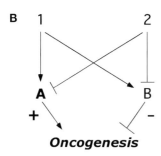

Figure 1. Alternative models describing how signals cooperate to drive malignant transformation. (*A*) Transformation requires the additive cooperation of two signaling modules, each alone insufficient to drive all the necessary programs required for transformation. (*B*) Transformation requires the simultaneous activation of two nodes within a network. Neither node is alone sufficient because each node acts both positively and negatively on the transformed phenotype. Only when both nodes are triggered together do the positive effects of each node gate the negative effects of the other, uncovering the transforming potential inherent in each node.

tage. Subversion of the network through mutation becomes almost impossible because individual mutations obligatorily trigger a shutdown of the very biological response that they also activate. Hence, individual mutations are unstable and cannot accumulate one by one, effectively stalling natural selection at the somatic level and so quelling the risk of neoplasia. On the other hand, when A and B are activated together in a normal cell responding to appropriate trophic and growth factors (signals 1 and 2), the negative impact of A is gated by B and vice versa, unlocking the full potential of the cell's growth, proliferative, angiogenic, and tissue-remodeling programs (Fig. 1B).

Arguably, the most important contra-predictions of the linear versus network models for oncogene interaction pertain to the complexity of tumors and the treatment of cancers. In a linear signaling framework, individual aspects of cell behavior are handled by discrete signaling modules, each of which has to be subverted through the long and protracted accumulation of cognate mutations in each module in order to assemble the wherewithal for the cell to become malignant. Consequently, cancer cells are complex ensembles of mutations, highly polymorphic in nature, and requiring the targeting of multiple pathways to achieve therapeutic efficacy. In contrast, the network idea would suggest that cancer cells are driven and underpinned by a small set of interlocking, interdependent

molecular lesions and that the apparent complexity of the neoplastic phenotype merely reflects the highly pleiotropic nature of these underlying lesions. If this is true, then targeting such pivotal lesions would have a powerful therapeutic impact on established cancers.

Determining which of these two models is correct is complicated in human tumors because of their high level of genomic instability, at least in part arising from processes such as telomere erosion that are secondary to the activation of oncogenes or loss of tumor suppressor genes which presumably initiate and drive early neoplastic clonal expansion. The effect of this is to introduce a large level of mutagenic noise that obscures any underlying causal molecular lesions. For this reason, the laboratory mouse, with its outsized telomeres and its experimental tractability, offers many advantages. By installing defined oncogenic lesions, alone and in combination in specific tissues, it is then possible to evaluate how and why such lesions promote neoplasia. In recent years, a further refinement has been the addition of acutely switchable systems with which to toggle oncogenes between normal and activated or tumor suppressor genes between functional and nonfunctional states. This latter refinement has proven critical for assessing the immediate, often growth-inhibitory impact of acute oncogene activation or tumor suppressor ablation, and how this leads to the eventual onset of malignancy.

MYC—A PARADIGM FOR INTRINSIC TUMOR SUPPRESSION

Against this backdrop, the Myc oncoprotein is a paradigm for the complexities dictating selection for oncogenic traits in cancer. Myc is a basic helix-loop-helix-leucine zipper (bHLH-LZ) transcription factor encoded by the c-*myc* proto-oncogene. It is generally assumed that Myc exerts its protean biological effects through modulation of target genes, some genes being repressed by Myc while others are activated. Most Myc-induced genes have a consensus CACGTG E-box element in their promoters which is recognized by Myc in partnership with its heterodimeric bHLH-LZ partner Max. In Myc-repressed genes, E-box elements are often absent, and the precise recognition element is less well-defined. Upon binding, Myc:Max exhibits contextual interactions with various components of the basal transcriptional machinery. For example, Myc recruitment of TRAAP correlates with transcriptional activation, whereas Myc interaction with the SP-1 and Miz-1 zinc finger proteins mediates its down-regulation of the *p21*^{cip1} and *p15*^{ink4b} promoters. More generally, Myc acts as a network node that orchestrates the wide variety of diverse biological processes required for proliferation of somatic cells. These include both cell-intrinsic processes such as cell growth, biogenesis, metabolism, and proliferation, telomere maintenance, DNA damage and repair; and social processes that coordinate and integrate cell expansion with the somatic environment, such as cell-stromal interactions, angiogenesis, cell migration and invasion. Importantly, many of the biological consequences of Myc activity are indirect and conditional consequences of the transcriptional programs it executes—highly dependent on subtle and ephemeral factors such as cell type, status, and local environment. This pleiotropic and contingent nature of Myc action makes any simplistic distillation of Myc "function" unrealistic. Rather, it seems that Myc serves to establish an eclectic platform of transcriptional changes that empowers the cell with a wide variety of potential biological options.

In normal cells, expression of Myc is tightly dependent on the actions of appropriate mitogens, essentially restricting its pleiotropic activities to cells in receipt of the appropriate extracellular signals for expansion. In contrast, expression of Myc is deregulated in most cancer cells, either through direct mutation or, more commonly, indirectly through the constitutive activation of upstream signaling pathways. This is consistent with the eclectic role played by Myc in promoting cell expansion, which makes Myc a perfect target, at least in principle, for subversion by oncogenic mutation. However, powerful counterselective mechanisms serve to greatly diminish the immediate selective advantage afforded by Myc activation. The first clue that Myc activation, by itself, is insufficient for deregulated cell proliferation came from the early oncogene cooperation studies of Land et al. These studies indicated that Myc is unable to induce in vitro transformation of primary fibroblasts without the aid of auxiliary lesions such as Ras activation (Land et al. 1983). Together with the significant time lag preceding sporadic emergence of clonal tumors in the target tissues of Myc transgenic mice, they reinforced the notion that Myc alone is insufficient to drive tumorigenesis without the cooperation of additional sporadic oncogenic lesions that bestow other aspects of the neoplastic phenotype. The unexpected discovery of Myc-induced apoptosis (Askew et al. 1991; Evan et al. 1992; Harrington et al. 1994a) offered a potential explanation for this obligate need for cooperating oncogenic lesions by indicating that Myc alone is insufficient for tumorigenesis because it harbors an innate lethality that staunches its neoplastic potential (Evan and Littlewood 1998; Evan and Vousden 2001; Lowe et al. 2004).

Two general models have been proposed to explain the conundrum of how Myc can induce apoptosis when activated by oncogenic mutation but not when activated as part of the normal proliferative process. One idea is that cells can innately discriminate between normal and "hyperproliferative" signals, triggering an apoptotic program only in response to the latter. Indeed, recent studies have indicated that cells do possess an intrinsic threshold buffer which insulates some components of their innate ARF/p53 tumor surveillance machinery from levels of Myc activation in normal cells (Zindy et al. 2003). However, it remains unclear to what extent this pathway is involved in determining cell viability/death (see below). An alternative idea is that the choice of whether a Myc-expressing cell should live or die is determined by the dynamic relationship between the cell and its trophic environment. In this "dual pathways" model (Harrington et al. 1994a,b), Myc activation always primes the cellular apoptotic program, but so long as the cell remains in its orthotopic somatic environment, activation of the apoptotic program is suppressed by local trophic signals. Only when an incipient tumor cell expands beyond the capacity of the local environment to quell the apoptotic program does cell death emerge as a biological output of Myc activity.

There is abundant in vitro evidence supporting the "dual pathways" idea that availability of survival factors determines the apoptotic proclivity of Myc (see, e.g., Askew et al. 1993; Harrington et al. 1994b; Kauffmann-Zeh et al. 1997; Rohn et al. 1998). However, we know so little about the abundance and nature of endogenous survival factors for any cell type in vivo that there is no way a priori of deducing whether acute activation of Myc in any particular somatic cell type would lead to cell expansion (abundant survival signals) or involution (insufficient survival signals). Therefore, to assess the relevance of Myc-induced apoptosis in limiting Myc oncogenic activity in vivo, we have established a number of transgenic models in which an acutely activatable form of Myc has been targeted to various cell types. To do this, we made use of the MycER^{TAM} fusion protein in which Myc has been fused to a modified ligand-binding domain of the estrogen receptor. The resulting MycER^{TAM} protein is completely dependent on continuous provision of 4-hydroxytamoxifen (4-OHT) for Myc function: Consequently, MycER^{TAM} transgenic mice have reversibly switchable Myc function in their target tissues that can be regulated by systemic administration or withdrawal of 4-OHT.

TUMOR COMPLEXITY—FACT OR FICTION?

To explore the consequences of Myc activation in a very different type of tissue, we have established a transgenic mouse model in which c-MycER^{TAM} is targeted to pancreatic β cells via the insulin promoter. Although not a common source of human cancers, β cells nonetheless possess several inherent advantages as a model tissue for tumorigenesis. Normal β cells have an intrinsically low proliferative rate, can be easily targeted using the almost completely β-cell-specific insulin promoter, have a well-described ontogeny and lineage relationship with neighboring endocrine and exocrine pancreatic cells, and, most strikingly, reside in 300–400 discrete islet populations dispersed throughout the pancreas. This latter makes possible the simultaneous observation of hundreds of independent foci following acute Myc activation, allowing discrimination between immanent effects of the transgene (which would be expected to arise synchronously in all islets) and those arising from stochastic secondary events (which would appear sporadically in isolated islets). As expected from the potent oncogenic activity of Myc, acute activation of MycER^{TAM} in pancreatic β cells of *pIns-MycER^{TAM}* mice triggers abundant entry of quiescent β cells into S phase, which is synchronous throughout the β-cell populations in each of the 300–400 discrete islets within the pancreas. However, acute Myc activation also triggers profuse apoptosis, which rapidly overwhelms Myc-induced proliferation and leads to the rapid involution of all islets—formal evidence that Myc-induced apoptosis can act as a powerful innate tumor suppressor in cells in vivo (Pelengaris et al. 2002). To test directly the importance of apoptosis in limiting Myc oncogenic activity, the same mice were then crossed into a strain in which the apoptosis inhibitor Bcl-x_L is constitutively expressed in β cells. Activation of MycER^{TAM} in the β cells of these *pIns-MycER^{TAM}* × *RIP7-Bcl-x_L* mice triggered immediate and progressive β-cell expansion, synchronously in all islets (Pelengaris et al. 2002). Moreover, sustained Myc activation in the presence of Bcl-x_L rapidly led to synchronous acquisition of many traits characteristic of advanced neoplastic lesions, including loss of cell–cell contact, profuse angiogenesis, dysplasia, anaplasia, local invasion, and metastasis within only a few days (Pelengaris et al. 2002). The rapidity and synchrony with which such traits emerge in each of the hundreds of discrete pancreatic islets argue strongly against the need for sporadic secondary events and, instead, indicate that all of these diverse aspects of tissue reorganization that accompany tumor evolution are encoded by activated Myc, requiring only suppression of apoptosis to unmask them. This is consistent with the highly diverse nature of genes identified as Myc targets (see below) and strengthens the intriguing possibility outlined earlier that the complexity of the tumor phenotype, rather than being the unhappy confluence of very many disparate mutations, each responsible for governing a specific neoplastic trait, is the consequence of a quite small number of interdependent mutations, each in key pleiotropic regulators of cell and tissue fate. In the case of Myc and Bcl-2/Bcl-x_L, the dramatic oncogenic synergy they exhibit arises because Bcl-2/Bcl-x_L blocks Myc-induced apoptosis while c-Myc overcomes the powerful ability of Bcl-2-Bcl-x_L to suppress cell proliferation (Fig. 2). Thus, neither Myc nor Bcl-2/Bcl-x_L alone can promote cell expansion, whereas coordinate activation of the two together is sufficient to unlock the full potential of β cells

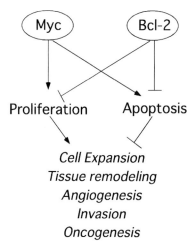

Figure 2. Schematic depiction of the relationship between Myc and Bcl-2 in oncogenesis. Myc drives proliferation, but this is undercut by the dominant role of Myc-induced apoptosis. Bcl-2 suppresses apoptosis, but at the cost of inhibiting cell proliferation. Activation of either alone is an evolutionary cul-de-sac for any cell. However, when Myc is activated together with Bcl-2, Myc overcomes the antiproliferative effect of Bcl-2, and Bcl-2 suppresses the apoptotic action of Myc, allowing activation of cell proliferative programs.

to expand, generate requisite neovasculature, and remodel local tissue architecture to cope with that expansion. This interlocking relationship between Myc and Bcl-2/Bcl-x_L is remarkably similar to that depicted in the interactive network outlined earlier in Figure 1B.

The potent oncogenic synergy between Myc and Bcl-2 raises the issue of whether the only oncogenic lesions that can cooperate with Myc are those that suppress apoptosis. In this context, loss of the ARF or p53 tumor suppressors is especially intriguing. A large number of studies indicate that the ARF/p53 tumor suppressor pathway plays an important role in limiting Myc oncogenic activity and that loss of either ARF or p53 is strongly selected during tumorigenesis (Eischen et al. 1999). Consistent with this, direct ablation of ARF or p53 accelerates tumorigenesis in Myc transgenic mouse models in all tested tissues. Furthermore, Myc activation induces up-regulation of ARF which, in turn, triggers accumulation of p53 (Zindy et al. 1998), and such activation of p53 has been implicated in mediating a component of the Myc-induced apoptotic signal (Hermeking and Eick 1994; Wagner et al. 1994; Zindy et al. 1998). To test directly the roles of ARF and p53 in mediating Myc-induced apoptosis in vivo, *pIns-MycER^{TAM}* mice were crossed into either ARF$^{-/-}$ or p53$^{-/-}$ backgrounds and Myc was activated. In both cases, synchronous eruption of tumors was observed in every islet, essentially phenocopying the tumorigenesis in the *pIns-MycER^{TAM}* × *RIP7-Bcl-x_L* mice (Fig. 3). However, close inspection of the dynamics of tumor growth in each case revealed fundamental differences in the mechanism by which tumors formed in each instance. In the *pIns-MycER^{TAM}* × *RIP7-Bcl-x_L* mice, Myc induced significant proliferation without any measurable apoptosis (Fig. 4). In contrast, activation of Myc in the absence of ARF induced far more pervasive and sustained proliferation, but this was accompanied by significant cell death (Fig. 4): Indeed, the extent of Myc-induced cell death in *pIns-MycER^{TAM}* × ARF$^{-/-}$ islets exceeded that in single transgenic *pIns-MycER^{TAM}* islets at each measured time point. The unexpected conclusion from this analysis is that inactivation of the ARF/p53 pathway promotes Myc oncogenic activity not by forestalling apoptosis but, rather, by enhancing Myc-induced β-cell proliferation to such an extent that it overwhelms apoptosis.

Two important conclusions can be drawn from such analysis. First, it shows that in addition to its well-described ability to prime the apoptotic program, Myc also triggers a second, discrete, innate tumor suppressor pathway that acts to suppress cell proliferation through activation of ARF/p53. As with Myc-induced apoptosis, activation of this antiproliferative program is likely to be extensively modulated by extracellular and social signals. Indeed, there is evidence that ARF expression is, like apoptosis, suppressed by growth and survival factors (Inoue et al. 1999). Nonetheless, elegant experiments by Sherr and colleagues, in which a GFP reporter is inserted into the endogenous *ARF* locus (Zindy et al. 2003), also indicate that induction of ARF is "insulated" from the low levels of Myc induced during normal mitogenesis by some form of innate buffer that, in effect, discriminates between normal and abnormal levels of Myc. The extent

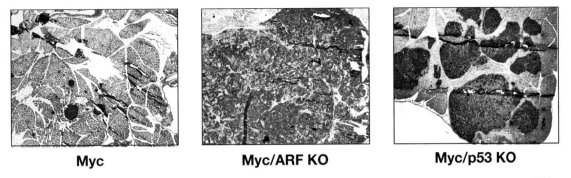

Figure 3. Loss of either ARF or p53 uncovers Myc oncogenic potential in vivo. Myc was activated in β cells of *pIns-MycER^TAM* mice for 21 days (in the absence of ARF, *center panel*) or 15 days (in the absence of p53, *right panel*). In both cases, rapid β-cell expansion and neoplasia were induced.

to which the apoptotic versus antiproliferative programs act to suppress Myc-dependent oncogenesis, or oncogenesis induced by other dominant oncogenic lesions, is unclear, although it seems plausible that the relative contributions each makes will vary between cell types and with circumstance.

Second, tumor formation requires only that net cell gain exceeds net cell loss. It is therefore possible for secondary oncogenic lesions to cooperate with Myc by either of two distinct mechanisms—through suppression of concomitant apoptosis, as in the case of Bcl-x$_L$ expression, or by leaving apoptosis unaffected and enhancing proliferative rate, as in the removal of the intrinsic brake to Myc proliferative potential through inactivation of ARF/p53. This conclusion has one important addi-

tional implication. Either apoptosis suppression or enhanced proliferation is, alone, sufficient to foster lethal outgrowth of a tumor in combination with activated Myc.

DECONSTRUCTING THE ROLE OF MYC IN TUMOR MAINTENANCE

Driving relentless cell proliferation without concomitant compensating apoptosis is sufficient for cell expansion, but is it sufficient to drive and maintain tumorigenesis? Classic models of multistage carcinogenesis posit that tumors are the result of the protracted acquisition of multiple mutations, each adding its own suite of traits to the final malignant mix. A need for multiple mutations

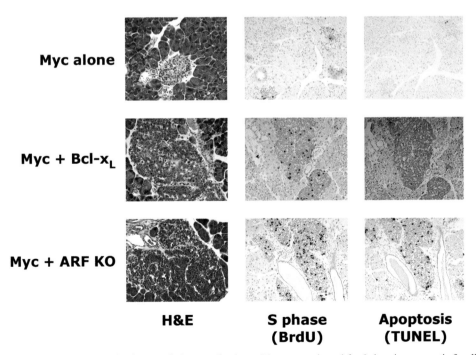

Figure 4. Myc-induced tumors can arise by two distinct mechanisms. Myc was activated for 9 days in pancreatic β cells, inducing substantial islet involution due to the preponderance of Myc-induced apoptosis (*top row*). When apoptosis is suppressed, for example, by overexpression of Bcl-x$_L$ or loss of the obligate apoptotic protein Bax, Myc activation induces progressive β-cell/islet expansion characterized by sustained β-cell proliferation (BrdU) and lack of TUNEL-positive apoptotic β cells (*middle row*). Activation of Myc for 9 days in the absence of ARF also leads to dramatic islet hyperplasia and tumorigenesis. However, this tumorigenesis is characterized by very high levels of proliferation that overwhelm the substantial extent of apoptosis still occurring (*bottom row*).

explains both the remarkable rarity of cancer cells within the soma and the complex phenotypes of established tumors, and is lent credibility by the extensive genomic aberrations seen in many human epithelial tumors. On the other hand, just because tumor cells harbor many genetic lesions need not imply that they are all necessary for maintenance of the established tumor. Tumors arise by an evolutionary process, so some mutations may reflect adaptation to selective pressures early in tumor evolution that are irrelevant at later times. Yet others may be irrelevant bystanders that become co-amplified, co-deleted, or co-mutated during the epochs of genome instability known to occur during tumor evolution due to telomere erosion or inactivation of DNA maintenance/repair genes. Importantly, only those mutations that are continuously required for the maintenance of established tumors will be targets for function-based cancer therapies. Consequently, there is a pressing need to filter out of the extensive mutagenic noise in cancer cells those mutations that are causally responsible for tumor maintenance. Switchable oncogenic models offer a unique way to assess directly, in vivo, how far defined oncogenic lesions (alone and in combinations) can drive normal somatic cells along the pathway to true malignancy and whether, once there, those same lesions are required to maintain an established tumor.

In this context, it is especially intriguing that sustained activation of MycER^{TAM} in β cells under circumstances where Myc-induced apoptosis is overcome by Myc-induced proliferation, whether this is by direct blockade (as in overexpression of Bcl-x$_L$) or overwhelmed (as in loss of ARF or p53), leads seamlessly to synchronous transformation of all islets into large, dysplastic, angiogenic, and invasive β-cell masses. The rapidity (days) and synchrony with which each of the several hundred discrete islets transforms into tumors precludes requirement for any secondary mutations to orchestrate these pleiomorphic traits and, instead, indicates that all these attributes of advanced neoplasia—angiogenesis, dysplasia, anaplasia, local invasion, and metastasis—are orchestrated by Myc, becoming overt only under circumstances where apoptosis is sufficiently overwhelmed to allow progressive cell expansion. The rapid and complete regression of all the tumors upon subsequent deactivation of Myc confirms the notion that all these diverse aspects of the tumor phenotype are directly and continuously dependent on sustained Myc function. Although such findings suggest that Myc may be a critical node in the maintenance of the intertwined network of aberrant signaling pathways that sustain established tumors, it is difficult to extrapolate from artificial, Myc-induced transgenic tumors to spontaneous human tumors where Myc activation may be secondary (in both function and timing) to other oncogenic lesions or to the many tumors where Myc appears not to be mutated itself but acting as a passive conduit for upstream oncogenic flux. Such concerns can only be addressed by construction of wholly new types of switchable mouse models in which the activities of endogenously expressed proto-oncogenes can be ectopically regulated at will.

Nonetheless, the highly pleiotropic nature of Myc suggests that it would make an excellent target for pharma-cological perturbation in cancers. Unfortunately, Myc is a transcription factor, and all evidence indicates that it implements all of its diverse biological functions (tumor promoting and tumor suppressing) through modulation of target genes. Myc interacts with its obligate bHLH-LZ partner Max via an extensive, coiled-coil interactive surface that is difficult to disrupt with small molecules, and with a variegated and redundant ensemble of components within the basal transcription machinery. Currently, such considerations are thought to rule out Myc as a "druggable" target and have, instead, focused attention on defining critical downstream transcriptional targets of Myc, in the hope of finding obligate Myc effectors more amenable to therapeutic intervention. In this context, a "critical" Myc target can be defined as one whose continuous modulation by Myc is required for maintenance of Myc-driven tumors. Unfortunately, the breadth of Myc target genes is huge: Expression microarray or SAGE studies of Myc target genes in lymphocytes or fibroblasts in vitro indicate that hundreds, perhaps over a thousand, genes are directly modulated by Myc (Coller et al. 2000; Guo et al. 2000; Menssen and Hermeking 2002; O'Connell et al. 2003; Zeller et al. 2003). More recent chromatin immunoprecipitation studies have suggested that Myc may be associated with perhaps 5–10% of all genes (Fernandez et al. 2003; Haggerty et al. 2003; Mao et al. 2003). Even a cursory survey of Myc gene targets indicates an enormously broad range of biological activities encompassing virtually all aspects of the cell, including tissue function, cell growth, proliferation, metabolism, biogenesis, cytoskeleton trafficking, intracellular and intercellular signaling, and tissue organization. The highly pleiotropic nature and large number of Myc target genes support the emerging notion that Myc acts as a contextual regulator of global transcription rather than as a driver of specific biological programs (Orian et al., this volume).

Unfortunately, dissecting out from such a large, diffuse and functionally heterogeneous ensemble of gene targets those that are "critical" for specific aspects of the Myc neoplastic phenotype is extremely difficult. Hitherto, the general approach has been to use an unbiased genome-wide approach such as gene expression arrays or chromatin immunoprecipitation to construct a look-up table of Myc target genes and then use human bias, based on preconceived ideas of what genes are important, to filter the candidates down to a "manageable" number that is experimentally testable. Although state-of-the-art, this strategy is an unhappy marriage of objectivity and subjectivity, given the parlous nature of our knowledge of gene functions. In contrast, reversibly switchable transgenic Myc tumor models offer a completely unbiased strategy for deconvoluting the complexity of Myc function, at least with respect to tumorigenesis and tumor maintenance. Following acute Myc activation, it is possible to correlate temporally Myc-induced transcriptional changes in an orthotopic tissue with the cell and tissue changes that accompany tumor progression. Likewise, subsequent deactivation of Myc in established tumors allows temporal correlation of onset of tumor regression with the underlying transcriptional changes that precipitate it. Furthermore, by combining these two analyses, it is possible to define an even more limited cohort of Myc target genes whose expression is inversely regulated upon Myc activation (tumor progression) and subsequent deactivation (tumor regression). Since Myc function is continuously required to maintain tumors in these switchable Myc models, this cohort comprises candidate genes required for tumor maintenance (E.A. Lawlor et al., in prep.).

Figure 5 illustrates such a kinetic progression–regression analysis of Myc-responsive genes. For the tumor progression study, MycER^{TAM} was acutely activated in pancreatic β cells of *pIns-MycER^{TAM}* × *RIP7-Bcl-x$_L$* mice by systemic administration of 4-OHT and, at various times thereafter, islets were isolated by laser capture micro-dissection. RNA was then extracted, amplified, and used to probe an Affymetrix U74Av2 mouse gene array. For the regression study, daily 4-OHT administration to *pIns-MycER^{TAM}* × *RIP7-Bcl-x$_L$* mice was stopped after 21 days, and the β-cell tumors were isolated by laser capture after 0, 1, 2, or 3 days. Gene expression was assayed on the same Affymetrix chips. 4-OHT has a tissue half-life of ~30 hours, so Myc deactivation occurs between 1 and 2 days after 4-OHT surcease.

During both Myc activation and subsequent deactivation, expression of several hundred genes is significantly modulated. Of the genes regulated upon Myc activation,

those whose expression is modulated within 2–4 hours of acute Myc activation are most likely to be direct Myc targets, whereas genes modulated only later (24 hours) are more likely the indirect consequences of programs engaged by those early transcriptional targets. Consistent with this, most (75%) of the genes up-regulated by Myc at either 2 or 4 hours have consensus Myc:Max-binding E-box elements in their promoters, compared with only 30% of those up-regulated at 24 hours. By comparing the Myc activation and deactivation cohorts at all time points, we can identify 257 candidate tumor maintenance probe sets based on the fact that their expression is inversely modulated following Myc activation (tumor induction) versus subsequent Myc deactivation (tumor regression). Importantly, of these 257, only 11 genes qualify as direct Myc targets (the rest are most likely indirect consequences of Myc action)—a number that is small enough to allow direct experimental validation of each candidate, alone and in combination. Clearly, such functional analyses will be needed to validate the role each plays in maintenance of Myc-dependent tumors. Nonetheless, the approach suggests that rapidly switchable and reversible genetic models, by marrying dynamic changes in cell and tissue biology to the molecular changes that cause them, can be used to filter the diffuse abundance of data generated by genome-wide screens in a completely unbiased way into tractable numbers of candidates for further testing.

PARTNERS IN CRIME—THE ROLE OF p53 AS A COOPERATING ONCOGENIC LESION IN TUMOR MAINTENANCE

The dramatic oncogenic synergy between deregulated Myc and inactivation of the ARF/p53 pathway attests to the importance of the p53 pathway in restricting Myc's oncogenic proclivities. Similar tumor-suppressive roles for the p53 pathway have been defined for essentially every type of oncogenic mutation, most notably oncogenic mutations of Ras.

p53 appears to have evolved early in metazoan evolution and, since neoplasia is unlikely to have been a major risk factor for such ephemeral progenitor species, it seems most likely that p53 first evolved as a transcriptional integrator of the DNA damage response to preserve genome integrity in germ-line and somatic cells. This ancestral DNA damage response function has been retained in vertebrates and is thought by many to constitute the critical component of p53's tumor-suppressive mechanism. According to this "Guardian of the Genome" idea (Lane 1992), p53 staunches the capacity of mutated or genomically unstable cells to propagate within the soma by implementing either a suicidal or growth-arrest response to genotoxic injury. In addition to this DNA damage response, however, p53 has also evolved the capacity to respond to a variety of non-genotoxic insults—most pertinently, aberrations in proliferative pathways. Thus, activation of multiple oncogenes such as Myc, Ras, E2F, and Wnt trigger a profound p53 response in the absence of any overt or detectable injury to cellular DNA, an attribute that may reflect an evolutionarily more recent

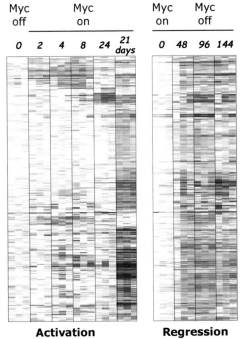

Figure 5. Kinetic analysis of Myc-regulated changes in gene expression in β cells during tumor initiation and subsequent regression. Myc was activated in pancreatic β cells of *pIns-Myc-ER^{TAM}* mice, and at 0, 2, 4, 8, and 24 hr thereafter, RNA was isolated from laser-captured, microdissected islets and analyzed by Affymetrix MG-U74Av2 array. Myc activation was then sustained for 21 days to generate β-cell tumor RNA (21-day time point). After 21 days, daily administration of 4-OHT was stopped and RNA was isolated from regressing tumors after 2, 4, and 6 days (tumor regression cohorts). SAM analysis identified significantly modulated genes, of which those that were reciprocally modulated during Myc activation and deactivation are shown. Red indicates induction of expression; blue, repression.

adaptation to deal with the risk of neoplasia in large, long-lived organisms with self-renewing tissues like mammals. As already outlined above, the principal molecular mediator of this growth-deregulation response pathway is the ARF tumor suppressor that acts to stabilize p53 by blocking p53 degradation by its E3-ubiquitin ligase, Mdm-2. Furthermore, p53 is activated by a wide range of other cell stresses that are not obviously genotoxic in nature, including nutrient privation, virus infection, and hypoxia, many of which are likely to be relevant to tumor cells in vivo.

The relative importance of DNA-damage versus growth-deregulatory or other pathways as triggers of p53 tumor-suppressive function during tumorigenesis and tumor evolution remains unclear, mainly because we have little idea as to which of these p53-activating pathways is triggered, or why and when, during the genesis and progression of any tumor type. Hence, defining the temporal requirements for p53-mediated tumor suppression would shed much needed light on what types of genetic lesions initiate, drive, and maintain cancers in any particular tissue. Importantly, for any therapeutic strategy based around restoring p53 function in cancer cells, it is vital to know whether the signals that activate p53 in tumor cells are transient and episodic or, instead, sustained throughout tumor progression. For example, were p53 to act solely to mediate growth-suppressive responses to hit-and-run mutagenic damage in somatic cell DNA, its tumor-suppressive activity would be confined only to cells harboring acute damage, and any therapeutic effect of restoring p53 function to tumors would be restricted to cancer cells in receipt of ongoing genotoxic injury. In contrast, if p53 is activated by signals that are sustained in tumor cells (for example, deregulated oncogenes, abnormal chromosome content or architecture, nutrient or hypoxic stress), its restoration would presumably exert a therapeutic effect at any time.

Classic gene knockout strategies in mice have, of course, provided important validation of the global significance of p53 in tumor suppression. More recently, conditional knockouts using *cre-lox* recombinase technology have refined such studies by circumventing the ill-defined and often occult developmental compensation that frequently arises in germ-line knockouts and allowing study of the acute consequences of p53 elision. However, even the latter are limited by the fact that gene inactivation is, typically, far from uniform within the target tissue population and, moreover, is irreversible. This means it is not possible to explore what the consequences of p53 functional restoration, transient or permanent, might be during the course of development, tissue maintenance of tumorigenesis. Therefore, to establish a mouse in which p53 functionality can be reversibly toggled between wild-type and knockout states in tissues in vivo, we turned to the ER^{TAM} switch technology we had already established in our switchable MycER^{TAM} transgenic models. In prior in vitro studies, we had already shown the p53ER^{TAM} fusion protein to be reliably and tightly regulated by 4-OHT for all measurable aspects of p53 function (Vater et al. 1996). Importantly, p53ER^{TAM} is not activated by the 4-OHT ligand but, instead, rendered competent to become activated by appropriate p53-activating signals. Hence, a cell expressing p53ER^{TAM} in place of p53 is effectively p53$^{-/-}$ in the absence of 4-OHT ligand and *p53^{wt}* in its presence. By inserting the ER^{TAM} switch in-frame into the carboxy-terminal exon 11 of the endogenous *p53* gene, we generated a mouse expressing p53ER^{TAM} in place of p53. Expression of p53ER^{TAM} in these *p53ER^{TAM} Knockin (KI)* mice is controlled by the same orthotopic transcriptional regulatory sequences that normally regulate *p53* expression in each tissue in vivo. However, since the expressed p53ER^{TAM} protein is functionally competent only in the presence of 4-OHT ligand, the *p53ER^{TAM} KI* mouse provides an unparalleled platform for the specific and temporally controlled perturbation analysis of p53 function, both in mouse tissues in vivo and in explanted primary cells derived from such tissues in vitro (Christophorou et al. 2005).

As expected, *p53ER^{TAM} KI* mice in the absence of 4-OHT resemble classic p53 knockouts in their high incidence of spontaneous tumors—principally lymphoma—whereas their radiosensitive tissues (spleen, thymus, intestinal epithelium) exhibit significant refractoriness to radiation-induced apoptosis (Christophorou et al. 2005). Systemic administration of 4-OHT to *p53ER^{TAM} KI* mice rapidly restores p53 function in all tissues, reestablishing radiosensitivity in thymus, spleen, and intestinal epithelium in vivo, as well as in cells derived from *p53ER^{TAM} KI* mice in vitro (Fig. 5).

Both normal and neoplastic cells in vitro and in vivo exhibit a marked proclivity to undergo genomic catastrophe in the absence of p53 (Harvey et al. 1993; Fukasawa et al. 1996, 1997). Consequently, tissues of non-4-OHT-treated *p53ER^{TAM} KI* mice acquire an appreciable load of cells harboring genetic defects during the course of embryonic development and postnatal life (Fukasawa et al. 1997). The unresolved damage residing in such aberrant somatic cells might be expected to trigger p53 upon its functional restoration in adult mice, inducing diverse tissue pathologies. Surprisingly, however, restoration of p53 function for the first time to adult mice that have hitherto been devoid of p53 activity induces neither any observable pathology nor detectable expression of p53 target genes in any tissue (Christophorou et al. 2005). One possible explanation for this is that, in the absence of a p53-mediated arrest or apoptotic response, DNA damage or chromosomal defects are rapidly resolved, at least at the biochemical level, such that the p53-activating signal rapidly attenuates. Using the *p53ER^{TAM} KI* mouse model, it is possible to test this hypothesis directly by subjecting animals to a single radiation dose in the absence of p53 function, and then restoring p53 function at various times thereafter. Such studies indicate that the p53-activating signal induced by radiation in signal radiosensitive tissues (thymus, spleen, intestinal epithelium) is, indeed, very transient—decaying to baseline within 48–72 hours of the original insult.

Such studies raise some important questions as to what the triggers are in inchoate tumor cells that activate p53 and suppress the emergence of neoplastic cells within the soma. Our experiments reveal that the DNA damage signal activating p53 is fleeting, so unless tumor cells harbor chronic DNA damage, this is unlikely to be other than an episodic trigger of p53, perhaps critical only at the time of exposure to carcinogens or during crisis following telomere erosion. On the other hand, several non-genotoxic triggers can activate p53, and some of these, most notably activated oncogenes, will be persistent features of tumor cells throughout their tortuous evolutionary trajectories.

To investigate directly the role of the DNA damage response in p53-mediated tumor suppression, $p53ER^{TAM}$ KI mice were exposed to a lymphomagenic dose of radiation with $p53ER^{TAM}$ nonfunctional, functional during the time of irradiation but not thereafter, or nonfunctional during irradiation but transiently restored at a later time well after the DNA damage response had attenuated. Mice in which $p53ER^{TAM}$ was nonfunctional throughout showed no ill effects from the radiation but 100% mortality from lymphoma by 24 weeks. Mice in which p53 was functional at the time of irradiation exhibited all the expected radiation-induced pathologies, yet 85% were dead from lymphoma at 24 weeks, indicating only modest tumor suppression. Mice in the third group, in which p53 function was transiently restored at later times, showed no pathology nor measurable activation of p53 target genes in target lymphoid tissues at the time of irradiation, nor at the time of delayed p53 restoration. Nonetheless, 80% of the mice were alive and well at 24 weeks, indicating profound suppression of tumorigenesis. These data indicate that long after their non-tumorigenic siblings have successfully recovered from acute genotoxic injury, the few incipient tumor cells that have acquired oncogenic mutations still harbor persistent signals which can be engaged by p53 to suppress their outgrowth. Exactly what these signals are remains unclear: However, obvious candidates are mutations that deregulate cell proliferative machinery, since these are known to activate p53 and must be persistent features of tumor progression and maintenance.

p53 AS "GUARDIAN OF GENOME"—SHIVA OR SHIBBOLETH?

Much has been made recently of the potential for p53 and other tumor suppressors to exhibit "antagonistic pleiotropy"—in effect, an evolutionary compromise in which provision of effective tumor suppression up to reproductive age comes at the cost of eroding post-reproductive life span (Green and Evan 2002; Campisi 2003; Lowe et al. 2004). Studies such as ours are consistent with such ideas and, moreover, raise the disquieting possibility that the DNA damage response, far from being the linchpin of p53-mediated tumor suppression, is instead an "unfortunate" relic of p53's evolutionary origins. "Unfortunate" because the p53-mediated DNA damage response indiscriminately kills or arrests cells with damaged DNA, even though the vast majority of such cells would never become tumors (as evidenced by the clonality of tumors that arise following such genotoxic insults, even in p53-deficient mice). The result of such indiscriminate culling is a wide range of pathologies, includ-

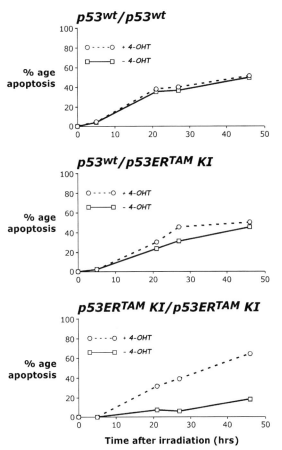

Figure 6. Systemic administration of the ER^{TAM} ligand 4-OHT to $p53ER^{TAM}$ KI mice restores DNA damage sensitivity to thymocytes. Thymocytes of $p53^{wt}$, $p53^{wt}/p53ER^{TAM}$ KI heterozygous, and $p53ER^{TAM}$ homozygous KI mice were irradiated with 3 Gy gamma radiation either in the absence or presence of 4-OHT. In $p53ER^{TAM}$ KI mice, thymocyte apoptosis occurs only when 4-OHT is present and $p53ER^{TAM}$ has been functionally restored.

ing iatrogenic responses to radiation and chemotherapy and, perhaps, through the cumulative attrition of stem cells that encounter damage throughout life, even to organismal aging (Fig. 6).

In contrast to the DNA damage response, however, the response of p53 to growth deregulating mutations is highly specific only for those rare cells that, as a consequence of DNA damage, acquire oncogenic mutations and are therefore likely to evolve into tumors (Fig. 7). Moreover, such oncogenic mutations are likely to be persistent features of tumor cells, throughout their tortuous evolution, and may therefore constitute more efficient triggers of p53 activation than ephemeral DNA damage signals. One radical idea emerging from such considerations is that decoupling p53 from the DNA damage response while retaining the p53 response to growth deregulation might offer the benefits of effective tumor suppression without the demerits of the pathologies associated with acute and chronic DNA damage. Unfortunately, the pathways directly or indirectly linking DNA damage with p53 activation are extremely diverse and re-

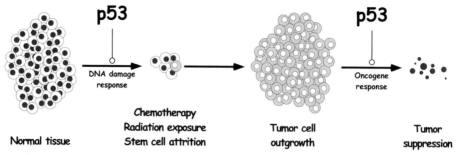

Figure 7. Schematic depiction of the two discrete putative roles of p53 in tumor suppression.

dundant, so it is probably not possible to block them all. An alternative strategy, however, might be to use pharmacological means to limit temporally p53 function throughout life. Our studies using the *p53ER^TAM KI* mice indicate that only a relatively short burst of p53 function may be sufficient to cull incipient tumors, even long after the insult that initiated them. Hence, temporally restricting p53 function to short metronomic periods throughout life might provide sufficient periodic p53 function to staunch incipient tumors while offering substantial protection from DNA damage-induced pathologies in, say, patients receiving radio- or chemotherapy or astronauts sustaining chronic radiological exposure en route to Mars. A predominately "p53-free lifestyle" such as this might even ameliorate the otherwise ineluctable erosion of stem cell compartments and enhance longevity. Such notions are obviously very radical. However, the reversibly switchable *p53ER^TAM KI* mouse model not only allows such ideas to be tested in principle, but also provides a test bed for fine-tuning the metronomic timing of p53 functionality so as to find the optimal balance between tumor suppression and radio resistance.

CONCLUSIONS

The rarity of spontaneous cancers is a strong clue that the evolutionary terrain available to somatic cells is severely constrained, limiting their autonomy and enforcing their obligatorily social nature. However, the mechanism by which such evolution is constrained remains an area of fierce debate. Switchable mouse models indicate that surprisingly small numbers of oncogenic mutation, when combined in highly specific, interdependent sets, carry all the information necessary to generate the full gamut of the neoplastic phenotype—a phenotype driven by the same programs that orchestrate and integrate developmental and regenerative expansion of normal tissues. In the future, such acutely switchable models will also serve as unique, in vivo preclinical test beds with which to establish not only which combinations of oncogenic lesions are required for the evolution and maintenance of cancers, but also what specific properties each type of lesion confers on the tumor phenotype. Knowing this will help direct interventions at the most effective targets for future cancer therapies.

REFERENCES

Askew D.S., Ihle J.N., and Cleveland J.L. 1993. Activation of apoptosis associated with enforced myc expression in myeloid progenitor cells is dominant to the suppression of apoptosis by interleukin-3 or erythropoietin. *Blood* **82:** 2079.

Askew D., Ashmun R., Simmons B., and Cleveland J. 1991. Constitutive c-*myc* expression in IL-3-dependent myeloid cell line suppresses cycle arrest and accelerates apoptosis. *Oncogene* **6:** 1915.

Campisi J. 2003. Cancer and ageing: Rival demons? *Nat. Rev. Cancer* **3:** 339.

Christophorou M.A., Martin-Zanca D., Soucek L., Lawlor E.R., Brown-Swigart L., Verschuren E.W., and Evan G.I. 2005. Temporal dissection of p53 function in vitro and in vivo. *Nat. Genet.* **37:** 718.

Coller H.A., Grandori C., Tamayo P., Colbert T., Lander E.S., Eisenman R.N., and Golub T.R. 2000. Expression analysis with oligonucleotide microarrays reveals that MYC regulates genes involved in growth, cell cycle, signaling, and adhesion. *Proc. Natl. Acad. Sci.* **97:** 3260.

Eischen C.M., Weber J.D., Roussel M.F., Sherr C.J., and Cleveland J.L. 1999. Disruption of the ARF-Mdm2-p53 tumor suppressor pathway in Myc-induced lymphomagenesis. *Genes Dev.* **13:** 2658.

Evan G. and Littlewood T. 1998. A matter of life and cell death. *Science* **281:** 1317.

Evan G.I. and Vousden K.H. 2001. Proliferation, cell cycle and apoptosis in cancer. *Nature* **411:** 342.

Evan G., Wyllie A., Gilbert C., Littlewood T., Land H., Brooks M., Waters C., Penn L., and Hancock D. 1992. Induction of apoptosis in fibroblasts by c-*myc* protein. *Cell* **63:** 119.

Fernandez P.C., Frank S.R., Wang L., Schroeder M., Liu S., Greene J., Cocito A., and Amati B. 2003. Genomic targets of the human c-Myc protein. *Genes Dev.* **17:** 1115.

Fukasawa K., Wiener F., Vande Woude G.F., and Mai S. 1997. Genomic instability and apoptosis are frequent in p53 deficient young mice. *Oncogene* **15:** 1295.

Fukasawa K., Choi T., Kuriyama R., Rulong S., and Vande Woude G.F. 1996. Abnormal centrosome amplification in the absence of p53. *Science* **271:** 1744.

Green D. and Evan G. 2002. A matter of life and death. *Cancer Cell* **1:** 19.

Guo Q.M., Malek R.L., Kim S., Chiao C., He M., Ruffy M., Sanka K., Lee N.H., Dang C.V., and Liu E.T. 2000. Identification of c-myc responsive genes using rat cDNA microarray. *Cancer Res.* **60:** 5922.

Haggerty T.J., Zeller K.I., Osthus R.C., Wonsey D.R., and Dang C.V. 2003. A strategy for identifying transcription factor binding sites reveals two classes of genomic c-Myc target sites. *Proc. Natl. Acad. Sci.* **100:** 5313.

Harrington E.A., Fanidi A., and Evan G.I. 1994a. Oncogenes and cell death. *Curr. Opin. Genet. Dev.* **4:** 120.

Harrington E.A., Bennett M.R., Fanidi A., and Evan G.I. 1994b. c-Myc-induced apoptosis in fibroblasts is inhibited by specific cytokines. *EMBO J.* **13:** 3286.

Harvey M., Sands A.T., Weiss R.S., Hegi M.E., Wiseman R.W., Pantazis P., Giovanella B.C., Tainsky M.A., Bradley A., and Donehower L.A. 1993. In vitro growth characteristics of embryo fibroblasts isolated from p53-deficient mice. *Oncogene* **8:** 2457.

Hermeking H. and Eick D. 1994. Mediation of c-Myc-induced apoptosis by p53. *Science* **265:** 2091.

Inoue R., Asker C., Klangby U., Pisa P., and Wiman K.G. 1999. Induction of the human ARF protein by serum starvation. *Anticancer Res.* **19:** 2939.

Kauffmann-Zeh A., Rodriguez-Viciana P., Ulrich E., Gilbert C., Coffer P., and Evan G. 1997. Suppression of c-Myc-induced apoptosis by Ras signalling through PI 3-kinase and PKB. *Nature* **385:** 544.

Land H., Parada L.F., and Weinberg R.A. 1983. Tumorigenic conversion of primary embryo fibroblasts requires at least two cooperating oncogenes. *Nature* **304:** 596.

Lane D.P. 1992. Cancer. p53, guardian of the genome. *Nature* **358:** 15.

Lowe S.W., Cepero E., and Evan G. 2004. Intrinsic tumour suppression. *Nature* **432:** 307.

Mao D.Y., Watson J.D., Yan P.S., Barsyte-Lovejoy D., Khosravi F., Wong W.W., Farnham P.J., Huang T.H., and Penn L.Z. 2003. Analysis of Myc bound loci identified by CpG island arrays shows that Max is essential for Myc-dependent repression. *Curr. Biol.* **13:** 882.

Menssen A. and Hermeking H. 2002. Characterization of the c-MYC-regulated transcriptome by SAGE: Identification and analysis of c-MYC target genes. *Proc. Natl. Acad. Sci.* **99:** 6274.

O'Connell B.C., Cheung A.F., Simkevich C.P., Tam W., Ren X., Mateyak M.K., and Sedivy J.M. 2003. A large scale genetic analysis of c-Myc-regulated gene expression patterns. *J. Biol. Chem.* **14:** 14.

Pelengaris S., Khan M., and Evan G.I. 2002. Suppression of Myc-induced apoptosis in beta cells exposes multiple oncogenic properties of Myc and triggers carcinogenic progression. *Cell* **109:** 321.

Rohn J.L., Hueber A.O., McCarthy N.J., Lyon D., Navarro P., Burgering B.M., and Evan G.I. 1998. The opposing roles of the Akt and c-Myc signalling pathways in survival from CD95-mediated apoptosis. *Oncogene* **17:** 2811.

Van den Elsen P., Houweling A., and Van der Eb A. 1983. Expression of region E1b of human adenoviruses in the absence of region E1a is not sufficient for complete transformation. *Virology* **128:** 377.

Vater C., Bartle L., Dionne C., Littlewood T., and Goldmacher V. 1996. Induction of apoptosis by tamoxifen-activation of a p53-estrogen receptor fusion protein expressed in E1A and T24 *H-ras* transformed p53$^{-/-}$ mouse embryo fibroblasts. *Oncogene* **13:** 739.

Wagner A.J., Kokontis J.M., and Hay N. 1994. Myc-mediated apoptosis requires wild-type p53 in a manner independent of cell cycle arrest and the ability of p53 to induce p21$^{waf1/cip1}$. *Genes Dev.* **8:** 2817.

Zeller K.I., Jegga A.G., Aronow B.J., O'Donnell K.A., and Dang C.V. 2003. An integrated database of genes responsive to the Myc oncogenic transcription factor: Identification of direct genomic targets. *Genome Biol.* **4:** R69.

Zindy F., Eischen C.M., Randle D.H., Kamijo T., Cleveland J.L., Sherr C.J., and Roussel M.F. 1998. Myc signaling via the ARF tumor suppressor regulates p53-dependent apoptosis and immortalization. *Genes Dev.* **12:** 2424.

Zindy F., Williams R.T., Baudino T.A., Rehg J.E., Skapek S.X., Cleveland J.L., Roussel M.F., and Sherr C.J. 2003. Arf tumor suppressor promoter monitors latent oncogenic signals in vivo. *Proc. Natl. Acad. Sci.* **100:** 15930.

Chromosomal Translocation Engineering to Recapitulate Primary Events of Human Cancer

A. Forster, R. Pannell, L. Drynan, F. Cano, N. Chan, R. Codrington, A. Daser,
N. Lobato, M. Metzler, C.-H. Nam, S. Rodriguez, T. Tanaka, and T. Rabbitts
MRC Laboratory of Molecular Biology, Cambridge CB2 2QH, United Kingdom

Mouse models of human cancers are important for understanding determinants of overt disease and for "preclinical" development of rational therapeutic strategies; for instance, based on macrodrugs. Chromosomal translocations underlie many human leukemias, sarcomas, and epithelial tumors. We have developed three technologies based on homologous recombination in mouse ES cells to mimic human chromosome translocations. The first, called the knockin method, allows creation of fusion genes like those typical of translocations of human leukemias and sarcomas. Two new conditional chromosomal translocation mimics have been developed. The first is a method for generating reciprocal chromosomal translocations de novo using Cre-*loxP* recombination (translocator mice). In some cases, there is incompatible gene orientation and the translocator model cannot be applied. We have developed a different model (invertor mice) for these situations. This method consists of introducing an inverted cDNA cassette into the intron of a target gene and bringing the cassette into the correct transcriptional orientation by Cre-*loxP* recombination. We describe experiments using the translocator model to generate MLL-mediated neoplasias and the invertor method to generate EWS-ERG-mediated cancer. These methods mimic the situation found in human chromosome translocations and provide the framework for design and study of human chromosomal translocations in mice.

The molecular pathology of cancer and possible new therapies have been a major concern of molecular biology since the first gene cloning experiments opened the possibility to clone, sequence, and study mutations in tumor cells. The very early observations of chromosomal changes in tumor cells (Boveri 1914) reflected genomic instability and raised the possibility of mutant proteins on the cancer cell surface to which antibodies might bind and elicit specific cell killing. There are a few examples of this, and most mutant proteins are firmly ensconced inside the cells and not available for antibody-mediated cell killing. Thus, although many mutations have been discovered, few specific therapies have been developed based on the molecular observations. Nevertheless, the cancer-specific mutations remain tantalizing targets for new cancer therapies.

Cancers have somatic mutations ranging from point mutations in genes like those of the *RAS* family (for review, see Hanahan and Weinberg 2000), which create constitutively active signal transduction molecules (Fig. 1), to genes activated after chromosomal translocations, such as the *CMYC* gene in Burkitt's lymphoma, and to fusion genes created uniquely in cancer cells by chromosomal translocations, such as the *BCR-ABL* gene fusion (for review, see Rabbitts 1994). As a range of genes involved in chromosomal translocations was identified, some common features began to emerge, especially in the acute cancers (hematopoietic and mesenchymal tumors) which invariably involve transcription factors whose normal role in cell fate decisions (Cleary 1991; Rabbitts 1991) is subverted (the master gene model; Rabbitts 1991). These transcription factors are often involved in protein–protein interactions. For instance, the T-cell leukemia genes *LMO2* and *TAL1/SCL* are activated by distinct chromosomal translocations, and their encoded proteins interact with each other to form a complex that binds to a bipartite site on DNA (Fig. 1). In addition, the recurrent finding of protein fusions resulting from chromosomal translocations (e.g., MLL or EWS fusions; Fig. 1) has again raised the specter of tumor-specific antigens for targeted therapies. However, the fact that many chromosomal translocation gene products are transcription factors, nuclear in location, and involved in protein–protein interactions moderates enthusiasm for them as therapeutic targets for small-molecule drugs.

New molecular therapeutic entities (macromolecular drugs), such as intracellular antibodies (intrabodies), siRNA molecules, or peptide aptamers (for review, see Rabbitts and Stocks 2003), could be therapeutic reagents based on the properties of, for instance, a chromosomal translocation gene product. However, there are many issues that need to be resolved before any possible use of such molecules (Rabbitts and Stocks 2003). Intrabodies can be effective in blocking protein–protein interactions and could form the basis of highly specific macromolecular drugs (Fig. 1). We have shown that single immunoglobulin variable region domains are most effective as intrabodies (IDAbs; Tanaka et al. 2003) and that the intra-chain disulfide bonds are dispensable for their function (Tanaka and Rabbitts 2003; Tanaka et al. 2003). Aside from the direct therapeutic use of intrabodies, macromolecular drugs of this type may serve as leads to identify small molecules (i.e., conventional drugs) that bind to the same place on the protein targets.

Animal models of spontaneous cancer will allow systematic evaluation of macromolecular drugs as well as leading to an understanding of the mechanism of tumorigenesis. It is not feasible to trial macromolecular drugs in

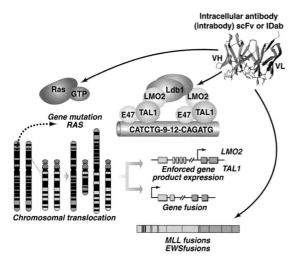

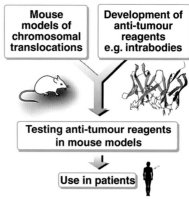

Figure 1. Mutations in cancer cells yield intracellular targets for therapy. Cancer cells have a number of mutations that contribute to the malignant phenotype. These may include point mutations in genes such as the *RAS* family, encoding plasma membrane-associated GTP-binding molecules involved in signal transduction. Commonly, chromosomal translocations are present, especially in hematopoietic and mesenchymal tumors, that either result in oncogene activation or formation of a tumor-specific fusion gene (Rabbitts 1994). Examples of the former are *LMO2* or *TAL1/SCL* activated in T-cell acute leukemia (forming multiprotein complexes involved in transcriptional regulation), and of the latter are *MLL* or *EWS*-fusion genes found, respectively, in hematopoietic or mesenchymal (sarcoma) tumors. The proteins made from these mutant genes are attractive targets for therapeutics, for instance, utilizing novel entities such as intracellular antibody fragments (intrabodies) that can bind with high affinity to their targets in vivo. We have developed a method of Intracellular Antibody Capture (IAC) (Tse et al. 2002) to develop these reagents; and protocols appear at www2.mrc-lmb.cam.ac.uk/PNAC/Rabbitts_T/ group. (scFv) Single-chain Fv comprising a VH and a VL segment joined by a flexible linker region. (IDab) Single immunoglobulin domain VH or VL intrabody.

Figure 2. A strategy for preclinical testing of macrodrugs. Although mutations in cancer cells lead to expression of RNA and protein molecules that could be disrupted by macrodrugs, such as siRNA oligonucleotides or intracellular antibody fragments (intrabodies) (Rabbitts and Stocks 2003), there are major technical problems for their use in vivo. Model systems of tumor development, such as may be offered by mouse models of chromosomal translocations, are possible settings for development of novel methods to investigate use of molecular therapeutic entities (macrodrugs). Having first identified a target gene (e.g., via a chromosomal translocation), generating a mouse model that emulates the human cancer from which it was identified provides a preclinical test-bed for trialing new macrodrugs, prior to use in patients.

cancer patients due to the considerable challenge of developing methods of delivery to tumor sites and to limited numbers of suitable patients, together with concurrent use of conventional treatment. A preclinical strategy is outlined in Figure 2 that defines an initial therapeutic target from a chromosomal translocation, followed by development of a mouse cancer model based on that target. Independently developed anticancer reagents (e.g., intrabodies) can be tested for efficacy in the mouse model and parameters of delivery, toxicity, specificity, and effectiveness experimentally established, prior to any use in clinical settings.

The main options for making transgenic mouse models of human disease are indicated in Figure 3. The transgenic method is the conventional approach to make gain-of-function mice (Fig. 3A), and this can be an inducible system using antibiotic-responsive promoters. Alternatively, retroviral vectors can be used to deliver expression systems to target cells (Fig. 3B), followed by re-introduction into recipient mice. Our approach has been to use gene targeting by homologous recombination in mouse embryonic stem (ES) cells to make specific single genetic changes which form the basis of chromosomal transloca-

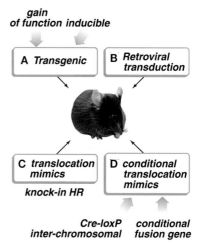

Figure 3. Options of developing mouse models of chromosomal translocations. Chromosomal translocation mimics can be made in various ways in mice. The most commonly used method to make mouse tumor models is transgenesis (*A*). An alternative is retroviral transduction of target cells with a vector expressing the gene of interest (*B*). Using homologous recombination (HR) in ES cells to generate targeted alleles offers an alternative approach to chromosomal translocation mimics. In an initial form, HR was used to knock-in a cDNA element into a target gene to achieve gene fusion (*C*). Conditional forms of chromosomal translocation mimics can both recapitulate the lineage-specific synthesis of the translocation gene and allow conditional, cell-specific activation of chromosomal translocation genes (*D*). We have used two methods: first, to create chromosomal translocations de novo in mice using Cre-*loxP* interchromosomal translocations (Collins et al. 2000; Forster et al. 2003), and second, to create chromosomal translocation mimics involving conditional formation of translocation fusion genes (Codrington et al. 2005; Forster et al. 2005).

tion mimics or actual de novo chromosomal translocations (Fig. 3C,D, respectively). An advantage of using homologous recombination in ES cells is that the genetic changes made, when transmitted through the germ line of mice, are precisely defined by the format of the targeting event. If tumor formation occurs, it is because of the targeting event, together with any secondary mutations that may be necessary for overt disease to appear. Furthermore, targeting offers advantages over xenograft models, which are limited to immunodeficient hosts and generally involve growth of human cells on a mouse background.

We outline in this paper the development of methods for making mouse models of tumors arising from the equivalent of human chromosomal translocations. These models are translocation mimics involving knockin gene fusion, a conditional version or a direct recapitulation of interchromosomal translocations using recombination in mice.

HOMOLOGOUS RECOMBINATION TO CREATE CHROMOSOMAL TRANSLOCATION MIMICS

The most common consequence of reciprocal chromosomal translocations is gene fusion due to breaks within the introns of genes resulting in amalgamation into a chimeric gene, encoding a chimeric protein (for review, see Rabbitts 1994). We developed a simple approach to mimic the effect of gene fusion by knock-in of a cDNA element into the exon of a mouse target gene, equivalent to where a human translocation would occur (Corral et al. 1996; Dobson et al. 1999). We used the *MLL* gene fusion with *AF9* as a model to establish the knockin approach to translocation mimics (Fig. 4). An *AF9* cDNA sequence was introduced into an *Mll* exon 10 gene targeting vector, together with a transcriptional termination polyadenyla-

tion (pA) site and neomycin selectable marker, and the construct was used for homologous recombination in ES cells (Fig. 4A). ES cell lines were isolated with one normal *Mll* allele and one targeted allele in which the *AF9* cDNA sequence was fused in-frame with *Mll* exon 10 (Fig. 4B). Mice were produced by injecting the targeted ES cells into blastocysts, and leukemias arose both in chimeric mice and in mice with germ-line transmission of the *Mll-AF9* fusion gene (Corral et al. 1996; Dobson et al. 1999). This established the knockin procedure for making translocation mimics in mice.

The knockin fusion gene allele in mice is a germ-line mutation and should, in principle, be expressed wherever the promoter of the targeted gene is active. This is undesirable if the experimental protocol is designed for assessing the effects of the translocation mimic in specific tissues or within specific cells of a tissue. Knockin alleles can also have unexpected consequences, due to the gain-of-function effects of expressing the fusion gene in embryos, resulting in embryonic lethality in some cases, such as observed for *Mll-AF4* knockin (N. Lobata et al., unpubl.). These considerations make it desirable to create conditional forms of chromosomal translocation mimics; accordingly, we have developed two independent methods of doing this; namely, the translocator and the invertor mouse models.

THE TRANSLOCATOR MOUSE MODEL OF DE NOVO CHROMOSOMAL TRANSLOCATIONS

The Cre-*loxP* recombination system is very efficient and versatile to allow deletion, inversion, or translocation of DNA sequences (Hoess et al. 1982; Ramirez-Solis et al. 1995; Yu and Bradley 2001). The utility of this recombination system in generating chromosomal translocations in ES cells was shown for two independent selection systems (Smith et al. 1995; van Deursen et al. 1995), suggesting that interchromosomal translocations might be achievable between diverse loci in mice, offering an experimental system of de novo chromosomal translocations, conditional on Cre expression. We have tested the concept in mice using the equivalent of the human *MLL* translocations, and our first studies showed that *Mll-Af9* chromosomal translocations could be detected in peripheral tissues where Cre recombinase was expressed (Collins et al. 2000). We concluded that chromosomal translocations could be made de novo in mouse tissues and at sufficient frequency to be detected in the absence of any selection.

We further demonstrated that interchromosomal translocations could be made in mice resulting in development of hematopoietic tumors (Forster et al. 2003). *LoxP* sites were engineered into the appropriate introns of *Mll*, *Af9*, and *Enl* genes, and mice were made from these targeted cells. Interbreeding of the mice produced lines with both *Mll* and *Af9* loxP alleles (depicted as *Mll-Af9* translocator mice; Fig. 5A) or both *Mll* and *Enl* loxP alleles (depicted as *Mll-Enl* translocator mice; Fig. 5B). The effect of making de novo chromosomal transloca-

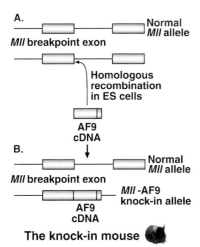

Figure 4. The *Mll-AF9* knockin mouse model. Homologous recombination was used in ES cells to fuse a segment of *AF9* cDNA to an exon of the mouse *Mll* gene (*A*), each corresponding to the gene segments involved in the human chromosomal translocation t(9;11) (Collins et al. 2000). The targeted ES cells are heterozygous for the *Mll-AF9* gene fusion (*B*) and mice made with these ES cells developed acute myeloid-lineage leukemia in 6–12 months.

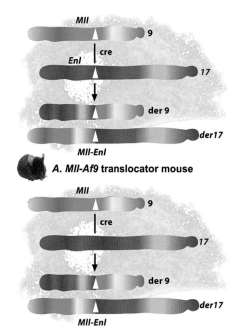

A. Mll-Af9 translocator mouse

B. Mll-Enl translocator mouse

Figure 5. Translocator model of chromosomal translocations. The Cre-*loxP* system was used to create de novo chromosomal translocations in mice. *LoxP* sites were recombined into appropriate introns of *Mll*, *Af9* (*A*) or *Enl* (*B*) genes in ES cells. Mice carrying these alleles were made and interbred with each other and with mice expressing Cre recombinase (McCormack et al. 2003). Interchromosomal translocations occur de novo in cells expressing the *Cre* allele, equivalent to the human translocations t(9;11) (*A*) and t(11;19) (*B*), respectively. This translocator mouse model generates de novo reciprocal translocations and recapitulates the features of de novo human chromosomal translocations. *LoxP* sites are depicted by white triangles.

than in the corresponding *Mll*; *Af9*; *Lmo2-Cre* mice, and showed complete penetrance by 120 days. Considering that neoplasia was dependent on the presence of the *Mll-Enl* translocations, the short time to tumor appearance was remarkable and could mean that only the *Mll-Enl* fusion gene is necessary for overt disease in this model.

In both models, abundance of circulating myeloid lineage cells appeared, showing variable levels of maturity (Fig. 7A is a representative blood film from *Mll*; *Enl*; *Lmo2-Cre* mice). The chromosomes from neoplasias of both *Mll*; *Enl* and *Mll-Af9* translocators include reciprocal chromosomal translocations demonstrated by fluorescence in situ hybridization (Fig. 7B shows painted metaphase chromosomes from a *Mll*; *Enl*; *Lmo2-Cre* mouse tumor). Both of the translocator models shown in Figures 5 and 6 developed neoplasias of the myeloid lineage (Forster et al. 2003) (myeloproliferative disease-like [MPD] myeloid leukemia according to the proposed Bethesda classification [Kogan et al. 2002]).

These studies show that conditional formation of chromosomal translocations in hematopoietic progenitor cells, using an *Lmo2-Cre* knockin allele, can result in myeloid neoplasia (Fig. 7C) and that a similar type of disease occurs in the presence of the fusion gene made by the translocation of *Mll-Enl* or *Mll-Af9*. These models therefore emulate the human disease counterparts that arise from these fusions resulting from t(11;19) and t(9;11), respectively. The translocator approach therefore should allow the study of *MLL* gene fusions in other specific cells and lineages in hematopoiesis by using the appropriate specific expression of Cre recombinase. In addition, the translocator model is a recapitulation of the primary events of human cancers by allowing the formation of reciprocal translocations in single cell precursors of the overt tumor. This should provide an ideal setting for testing drugs and new approaches, such as the intrabody technology mentioned briefly earlier (Fig. 1). As a first step, it will be valuable to ascertain whether the translocator mice with the *Mll* fusions respond to the chemotherapies currently used for treating the equivalent childhood acute leukemia.

tions was studied via interbreeding mice expressing Cre in hematopoietic progenitors from a knockin of *Cre* in the *Lmo2* gene (Fig. 6A). Both sets of compound genotype mice developed hematopoietic neoplasias (Fig. 6B shows the survival curves for the mice). Notably, the rate of tumor occurrence in *Mll*; *Enl*; *Lmo2-Cre* mice was higher

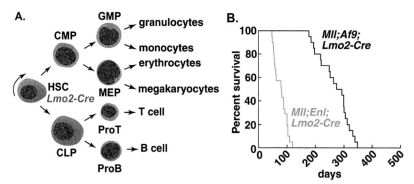

Figure 6. Leukemias occur in *Mll-Af9* and *Mll-Enl* translocator mice. As described in Fig. 5, *loxP* sites were incorporated into *Mll*, *Af9*, and *Enl* mouse genes facilitating the interchromosomal translocation mediated by Cre recombinase. In the experiments described here, Cre was produced from a knockin allele in the *Lmo2* gene, driving Cre expression in hematopoietic progenitor cells (McCormack et al. 2003) (*A* shows a simplified pathway of hematopoiesis indicating pluripotent, self-renewing progenitor cells [HSC] giving rise to myeloid and lymphoid progenitors, respectively CMP and CLP, and in turn to mature, committed cells of myeloid and lymphoid lineage). Leukemias arise in both *Mll-Enl* and *Mll-Af9* translocators (*B* shows Kaplan-Meyer survival curves for the two groups).

Figure 7. Myeloid leukemia in *Mll-Af9* and *Mll-Enl* translocator mice have reciprocal chromosomal translocations. Both *Mll-Enl* and *Mll-Af9* translocator mice develop myeloid leukemias (MPD-like acute myeloid leukemia according to the Bethesda classification), characterized by typical pathology and circulating myeloid cells of varying maturity (*A* shows a blood smear from an *Mll-Enl; Lmo2-Cre* translocator). The tumor cells in these mice show normal ploidy and carry reciprocal chromosomal translocations (*B* shows a metaphase spread from an *Mll-Enl; Lmo2-Cre* tumor with *Mll* and *Enl* chromosomes painted green and red, respectively). Our findings show that the fusion of *Mll* with either *Enl* or *Af9* in hematopoietic progenitors results in tumors of the myeloid lineage (*C*), typical of the types of tumors found in humans with these translocations. The translocator model recapitulates these primary events in human cancer.

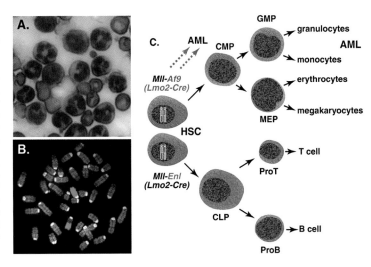

ISSUES CONCERNING THE TRANSLOCATOR MODEL

The translocator model relies on homologous recombination to insert *loxP* recombination sites into introns of interest to potentiate the formation of interchromosomal translocations in a desired cell type using specific *Cre*-expressing alleles. In principle, this should be adaptable to mimic any human reciprocal chromosomal translocation. There are three main caveats to this proposition. First is that the spatial, nuclear organization of mouse chromosomes may preclude certain interactions that could support interchromosomal translocations. Second, the prevailing dogma is that genes should be accessible before a genomic rearrangement can take place, implying that only certain chromosomal regions could interact and be translocated.

A third potential problem is gene orientation. In the cases described here (i.e., *Mll*, *Enl*, and *Af9*), the relative transcriptional orientation on each respective chromosome arm is the same as depicted in Figure 8A. This situation is compatible with the formation of two reciprocal chromosomes from a *loxP*-Cre-mediated translocation. However, if the two genes to be translocated are in the opposite transcriptional orientation (as depicted in Fig. 8B), *loxP*-Cre-mediated recombination would result in two abnormal reciprocal chromosomes, one dicentric and the other lacking a centromere. These chromosomes would be lost at mitosis and the cell would presumably not be viable. In these situations, the mouse translocator model would not be applicable and a different conditional translocation mimic is needed. For this purpose, we developed the invertor model (see below).

THE INVERTOR CHROMOSOMAL TRANSLOCATION MIMIC

To generate a fully conditional fusion gene model, we have made use of the ability of Cre recombinase to invert sequences flanked by appropriately oriented *loxP* sites, and developed the invertor model of chromosomal translocations (Codrington et al. 2005; Forster et al.

2005). In this approach, an inverted cassette, flanked by *loxP* sites, is knocked into the intron of the gene to which a gene fusion is required (e.g., *Ews* as described below). The cassette comprises a short region of intron including an acceptor splice site, a cDNA segment for fusing with the target gene, a pA site for transcription termination, and the MC1-neo-pA fragment for selecting homologous recombinant ES cells. The invertor cassette is knocked in with the opposite transcription orientation to the target gene (Fig. 9A, inactive form). When mice are made from the invertor ES cells and crossed with Cre-expressing strains, the *loxP* sites flanking the invertor cassette are sites for recombinational inversion of the cassette, to make the functional form of the invertor allele (Fig. 9A, active form). In this configuration, transcription of the invertor allele proceeds from the target gene promoter to the pA site in the cassette, forming a pre-mRNA of ex-

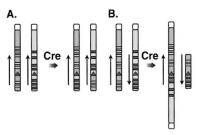

Figure 8. The translocator model is dependent on gene orientation. The translocator model can, in principle, recapitulate any human chromosomal translocation. However, mouse chromosomes are acrocentric (the centromeres are located at one end of each chromosome) and the orientation of the genes to be translocated is crucial to the success of the translocator strategy. In the situation depicted in *A* (such as the case of *Mll-Enl* and *Mll-Af9*), the gene orientation on each chromosome is identical, and therefore Cre-*loxP*-mediated interchromosomal translocation maintains the chromosomal organization of the genes on the derivation chromosomes. Conversely, if the genes are oriented in the opposite transcriptional direction (*B*), Cre-*loxP*-mediated interchromosomal translocation results in two abnormal chromosomes (one dicentric and one lacking a centromere) unable to participate in mitosis. *LoxP* sites are depicted by red triangles and the centromeres by open boxes.

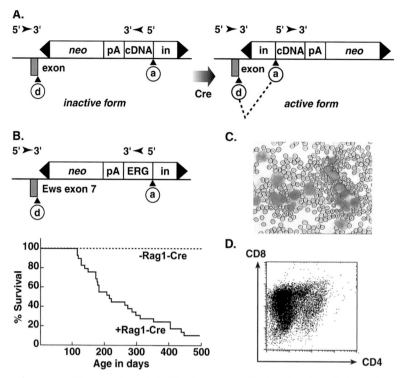

Figure 9. The invertor chromosomal translocation mimic. The invertor knockin translocation mimic involves introducing a cassette into the intron of a relevant gene. The invertor cassette comprises a short intronic sequence with an acceptor splice site, a segment of cDNA sequence for fusion with the targeted gene, and a poly(A) site. It is initially knocked-in in the opposite orientation for transcription (inactive form; *A*) and is flanked by *loxP* sites to allow Cre-mediated inversion in Cre-expressing mice. After inversion, the acceptor site can be spliced to the donor splice site of the adjacent exon of the targeted gene (*A*, active form). The *EWS-ERG* fusion found in human sarcoma was used to test this method. *Ews-ERG* invertor mice (*B*) were bred with *Rag1-Cre* mice. *Ews-ERG*; *Rag1-Cre* mice begin to show hematopoietic neoplasia after about 100 days (*B*), developing T-cell tumors characterized by circulating lymphocytes (*C* shows a blood smear), mostly mature T cells (*D* shows an example of flow cytometry using CD8 and CD4 markers).

ons from the target gene and the cDNA from the invertor cassette.

As a model system to test the invertor method, we constructed a chromosomal translocation mimic of the *EWS-ERG* fusion. *EWS* is a translocation gene found in many human sarcomas and some leukemias, where it is fused to many different partners including *ERG* (Rabbitts 1994). A homologous gene *FUS* is also fused with *ERG* in human acute myeloid leukemias. The invertor model was used to assess whether the *Ews-Erg* fusion could cause neoplasia in mice (Codrington et al. 2005; Forster et al. 2005). The invertor knockin cassette is depicted in Figure 9B. Cohorts of mice were established with the *Ews-ERG* or *Ews-ERG* plus a *Rag1-Cre* knockin allele (Fig. 9B, –Rag-Cre and +Rag-Cre, respectively) (McCormack et al. 2003). Leukemias developed in the *Ews-ERG*; *Rag1-Cre* invertor mice, starting around 110 days; by 500 days, >90% of these mice had succumbed to leukemia (Fig. 9B). The neoplasias were diagnosed as large-cell anaplastic T-cell lymphoma by a number of criteria, including presence of high numbers of circulating lymphocytes (Fig. 9C) and expression of markers, such as CD8, characteristic of mature T cells (Fig. 9D).

These data both validate the invertor model as a Cre-dependent chromosomal translocation mimic (Forster et al. 2005) and show that the Ews-ERG fusion protein can be oncogenic in committed cells (Codrington et al. 2005).

CONCLUSIONS

We have developed three methods to make chromosomal translocation mimics in mice via homologous recombination in ES cells; namely, knockin, translocator, and invertor mice. Our mouse models with these approaches are summarized in Table 1. We have applied the gene knockin approach to one model (viz. *Mll-AF9*). Conditional forms using the invertor approach as a universal translocation mimic have induced lymphoid tumors with this method using *Ews-ERG*, *Bcr-ABL*, and *Mll-AF4* fusions. The most faithful recapitulation of the reciprocal translocations found in human hematopoietic and mesenchymal neoplasias occurs in the translocator model where *loxP* sites on two (non-)homologous chromosomes serve as recombination signals for interchromosomal translocations. We are currently developing second-generation translocator models designed to accelerate the process of creating the translocator lines of mice and introducing elements in the design that will facilitate creating transcriptional options on both reciprocal chromosomes.

An interesting point of similarity exists between our results with mouse *Mll* translocators and the *MLL* fusion genes in man. There are a large number of different translocations to *MLL* on human chromosome 11, and indeed, almost every chromosome arm has been implicated in *MLL*-associated leukemias. Thus, chromosome terri-

Table 1. Gene Targeting Approaches to Chromosomal Translocations Mimics Result in Hematopoietic Tumors in Mice

Targeting strategy	Gene fusion	Cre expressor	Neoplasia (Bethesda classification)
Knock-in			
	Mll-AF9	N.A.	acute myeloid leukemia
Translocator			
	Mll-Af9	Lmo2-Cre	MPD-like acute myeloid leukemia
	Mll-Enl	Lmo2-Cre	MPD-like acute myeloid leukemia
	Mll-Enl	Lck-Cre	small T-cell lymphoma or myeloid leukemia without maturation
Invertor			
	Ews-ERG	Rag1-Cre	large-cell anaplastic T-cell lymphoma
	Mll-AF4	Rag1-Cre	diffuse large B-cell lymphoma
	Mll-AF4	Cd19-Cre	diffuse large B-cell lymphoma
	Mll-AF4	Lck-Cre	diffuse large B-cell lymphoma
	Bcr-Abl	Mx-Cre	B-cell acute leukemia

N.A. indicates not applicable.

tory does not seem to impose much restriction in interchromosomal events in the precursor cell of human leukemias. Our data in the mouse models suggest similar flexibility. We find that chromosomal translocations occur with comparable efficiency between *Mll* and *Enl* or *Af9* genes, all located on separate chromosomes. In human cancer, selection processes presumably engender tumor appearance from rare cells in which a chance, but low probability, chromosomal translocation occurs. This cannot be so in the mouse translocators, since we can observe chromosomal translocations between *Mll* and *Enl* and between *Mll* and *Af9* within days after birth. In all, this suggests fluidity with which chromosomes are able to interact.

Mouse models of human cancer are relevant for the elucidation of factors influencing features of disease but are also important for developing rational therapeutic strategies and testing macromolecular drugs. With the advent of efficient recombination systems in mice, we have developed compound genetic systems to mimic the formation and effects of chromosomal translocations in human cancer. We have described three methods for this objective and hope that the next few years will see the use of these models as preclinical settings for drug development and validation.

ACKNOWLEDGMENTS

We thank the Medical Research Council for funding the work described in this paper. R.C. was a Leukaemia Research Fund Gordon Pillar Student, N.C. was a Croucher Foundation student, and F.C. is a C. Milstein Memorial student of the Darwin Trust, Edinburgh. N.L. was funded by the Kay Kendall Leukaemia Fund and by the Leukaemia Research Fund, M.M. by the German Research Foundation, C.H.N. by the Kay Kendall Leukaemia Fund and by the Lady Tata Memorial Fund, S.R. by the Ministerio de Educación y Ciencia, and T.T. by the National Foundation for Cancer Research. We thank Ms. A. Lenton for the illustration work.

REFERENCES

Boveri T. 1914. *Zur Frage der Entstehung Maligner Tumoren.* Gustav Fischer, Germany.

Cleary M.L. 1991. Oncogenic conversion of transcription factors by chromosomal translocations. *Cell* **66:** 619.

Codrington R., Pannell R., Forster A., Drynan L.F., Daser A., Lobato M.N., Metzler M., and Rabbitts T.H. 2005. The Ews-ERG fusion protein can initiate neoplasia from lineage committed haematopoietic cells. *Publ. Lib. Sci. Biol.* **3:** 242.

Collins E.C., Pannell R., Simpson E.M., Forster A., and Rabbitts T.H. 2000. Inter-chromosomal recombination of *Mll* and *Af9* genes mediated by cre-*loxP* in mouse development. *EMBO Rep.* **1:** 127.

Corral J., Lavenir I., Impey H., Warren A.J., Forster A., Larson T.A., Bell S., McKenzie A.N.J., King G., and Rabbitts T.H. 1996. An *Mll-Af9* fusion gene made by homologous recombination causes acute leukemia in chimeric mice: A method to create fusion oncogenes. *Cell* **85:** 853.

Dobson C.L., Warren A.J., Pannell R., Forster A., Lavenir I., Corral J., Smith A.J.H., and Rabbitts T.H. 1999. The *Mll-AF9* gene fusion in mice controls myeloproliferation and specifies acute myeloid leukaemogenesis. *EMBO J.* **18:** 3564.

Forster A., Pannell R., Drynan L.F., McCormack M., Collins E.C., Daser A., and Rabbitts T.H. 2003. Engineering *de novo* reciprocal chromosomal translocations associated with *Mll* to replicate primary events of human cancer. *Cancer Cell* **3:** 449.

Forster A., Pannell R., Drynan L.F., Codrington R., Daser A., Metzler M., Lobato M.N., and Rabbitts T.H. 2005. The invertor knock-in conditional chromosomal translocation mimic. *Nat. Methods* **2:** 27.

Hanahan D. and Weinberg R.A. 2000. The hallmarks of cancer. *Cell* **100:** 57.

Hoess R.H., Ziese M., and Sternberg N. 1982. P1 site-specific recombination: Nucleotide sequence of the recombining sites. *Proc. Natl. Acad. Sci.* **79:** 3398.

Kogan S.C., Ward J.M., Anver M.R., Berman J.J., Brayton C., Cardiff R.D., Carter J.S., de Coronado S., Downing J.R., Fredrickson T.N., Haines D.C., Harris A.W., Harris N.L., Hiai H., Jaffe E.S., MacLennan I.C., Pandolfi P.P., Pattengale P.K., Perkins A.S., Simpson R.M., Tuttle M.S., Wong J.F., and Morse H.C. 2002. Bethesda proposals for classification of nonlymphoid hematopoietic neoplasms in mice. *Blood* **100:** 238.

McCormack M.P., Forster A., Drynan L.F., Pannell R., and Rabbitts T.H. 2003. The *LMO2* T-cell oncogene is activated via chromosomal translocations or retroviral insertion during gene therapy but has no mandatory role in normal T-cell development. *Mol. Cell. Biol.* **23:** 9003.

Rabbitts T.H. 1991. Translocations, master genes, and differences between the origins of acute and chronic leukemias. *Cell* **67:** 641.

———. 1994. Chromosomal translocations in human cancer. *Nature* **372:** 143.

Rabbitts T.H. and Stocks M.R. 2003. Chromosomal translocation products engender novel intracellular therapeutic technologies. *Nat. Med.* **9:** 383.

Ramirez-Solis R., Liu P., and Bradley A. 1995. Chromosome engineering in mice. *Nature* **378:** 720.

Smith A.J.H., De Sousa M.A., Kwabi-Addo B., Heppell-Parton A., Impey H., and Rabbitts P.H. 1995. A site-directed chromosomal translocation induced in embryonic stem cells by Cre-loxP recombination. *Nat. Genet.* **9:** 376.

Tanaka T. and Rabbitts T.H. 2003. Intrabodies based on intracellular capture frameworks that bind the RAS protein with high affinity and impair oncogenic transformation. *EMBO J.* **22:** 1025.

Tanaka T., Lobato M.N., and Rabbitts T.H. 2003. Single domain intracellular antibodies: A minimal fragment for direct *in vivo* selection of antigen-specific intrabodies. *J. Mol. Biol.* **331:** 1109.

Tse E., Lobato M.N., Forster A., Tanaka T., Chung G.T.Y., and
    Rabbitts T.H. 2002. Intracellular antibody capture technol-
    ogy: Application to selection of single chain Fv recognising
    the BCR-ABL oncogenic protein. *J. Mol. Biol.* **317:** 85.
van Deursen J., Fornerod M., van Rees B., and Grosveld G.

1995. Cre-mediated site-specific translocation between non-
    homologous mouse chromosomes. *Proc. Natl. Acad. Sci.* **92:**
    7376.
Yu Y. and Bradley A. 2001. Engineering chromosomal rear-
    rangements in mice. *Nat. Rev. Genet.* **2:** 780.

Deciphering Cancer Complexities in Genetically Engineered Mice

K. SIMIN,* R. HILL,[†] Y. SONG,* Q. ZHANG,* R. BASH,* R.D. CARDIFF,[‡] C. YIN,* A. XIAO,[¶]
K. MCCARTHY,* AND T. VAN DYKE*

*University of North Carolina School of Medicine, Chapel Hill, North Carolina 27599;
[†]University of California at Los Angeles, Los Angeles, California 90095;
[‡]Department of Pathology, University of California, Davis, California 95616

Because the pRb pathway is disrupted in most solid human cancers, we have generated genetically engineered mouse cancer models by inactivating pRb function in several cell types, including astrocytes and mammary, prostate, ovarian, and brain choroid plexus epithelia. In every case, proliferation and apoptosis are acutely induced, predisposing to malignancy. Cell type dictates the pathways involved in tumor progression. In the astrocytoma model, we developed strategies to induce events in the adult brain, either throughout the tissue or focally. Both K-Ras activation and Pten inactivation play significant roles in progression. In the prostate model, adenocarcinoma progression depends on Pten inactivation. However, nonautonomous induction of p53 in the mesenchyme leads to evolution of both compartments, with p53 loss occurring in the mesenchyme. Thus, studies in these models continue to identify key tumorigenesis mechanisms. Furthermore, we are hopeful that the models will provide useful preclinical systems for diagnostic and therapeutic development.

In an effort to model and understand human cancers, we have generated several genetically engineered mouse (GEM) cancer models based on highly penetrant tumor suppressor gene aberrations observed in human tumors. Because the pRb pathway is disrupted in most solid human cancers, we have inactivated pRb function cell-specifically in the mouse by transgenic expression of T_{121}, a truncated SV40 T antigen that binds and inactivates pRb and related proteins p107 and p130. In numerous cell types, including mammary (Simin et al. 2004), prostate (Hill et al. 2005a,b), ovarian (C. Yin and T. Van Dyke, unpubl.), and brain choroid plexus (Symonds et al. 1994), epithelia and astrocytes (Xiao et al. 2002), inactivation of pRb, p107, and p130 leads to similar induction of aberrant proliferation and concomitant apoptosis (Fig. 1). In addition, these cellular responses have predisposed to malignancy in each case, producing fully penetrant preclinical models for cancer initiation and progression.

In exploring the genetic basis for tumor progression, we have discovered that the specific pathways involved depend on cell type. Whereas mammary and brain epithelia are similar in that p53 mediates most of the apoptotic response and its loss is the predominant mechanism for tumor progression (Symonds et al. 1994; Lu et al. 2001; Simin et al. 2004), astrocytic and prostate epithelial apoptosis depend on Pten (Xiao et al. 2002; Hill et al. 2005a). Brain and mammary epithelia are also divergent in their requirement for E2F1 for proliferation. In choroid plexus epithelium, proliferation is mediated by E2F1 activity (Pan et al. 1998), in contrast to mammary epithelium, where E2F1 activity is dispensable (M. Sardo and T. Van Dyke, unpubl.). These differences have significant impli-

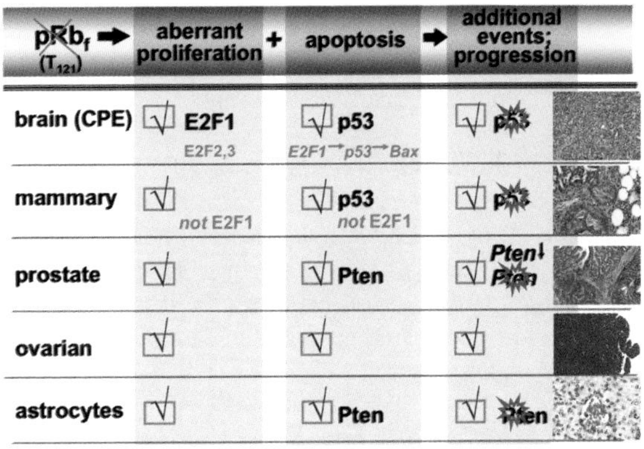

Figure 1. Summary of cancer progression mechanisms. A similar course of events occurs in each system analyzed: T_{121} blocks pRb activity and causes aberrant proliferation and concomitant increased apoptosis; a selective pressure exists for reduced apoptosis among these neoplastic cells, leading to a subsequent loss of apoptosis and acquisition of other tumor-promoting alterations. However, despite the similarity of events, cells differ in the mechanisms they employ for these functions; brain epithelial cells (CPE) and breast cells rely on p53-mediated apoptosis, whereas astrocytes and prostate epithelial cells depend on Pten-mediated apoptosis. Likewise, whereas E2F1 is required for apoptosis and optimal cellular proliferation in CPE, E2F1 is dispensable in mammary epithelial cells. These differences affect the evolution and biology of each tumor type and may ultimately influence the way we diagnose and treat these cancers.

cations for the mechanisms of tumor progression and the biological behaviors of respective tumor types.

In recent studies, we have examined the complex mechanisms of tumor progression in astrocytic and prostate cancers, including the contribution of multiple Pten-regulated pathways to multiple aspects of tumor progression, such as cell survival, invasion, and angiogenesis (Hill et al. 2005a; Xiao et al. 2005), and of stro-

---

[¶]Present address: Rockefeller University, New York, New York 10021.

mal p53 loss to the progression of prostate tumor (Hill et al. 2005b). Thus, the complex dynamics of tumor evolution are being deciphered for these significant human cancers. Our current efforts to understand these mechanisms are discussed.

MATERIALS AND METHODS

Mice. The generation and the characterization of $TgGZT_{121}$, $TgG(\Delta Z)T_{121}$ (Xiao et al. 2002), and $TgAPT_{121}$ (Hill et al. 2005a) mice have been described previously. We generated $TgG(\Delta Z)T_{121}$ by mating $TgGZT_{121}$ mice to $Tg\beta$-*actinCre* mice (Lewandoski and Martin 1997) to generate bi-transgenic mice, selecting for pure $TgG(\Delta Z)T_{121}$ mice in subsequent generations. Screening of the *Pten* nullizygous allele has been described previously (Di Cristofano et al. 1998). Characterization and screening of the *p53* null allele (Jacks et al. 1994), the conditional Pten allele (Trotman et al. 2003; Xiao et al. 2005), and the *LSL-K-ras^{G12D}* allele (Jackson et al. 2001) have been described. *TgGFAP-CreER* mice were constructed and characterized in the McCarthy lab (K. McCarthy et al., unpubl.) and are genotyped using the following parameters: primers are 5′-TGATGAGGTTCGCAAGAACC-3′ and 5′-CCATGAGTGAACGAACCTGG-3′. PCR conditions: 94°C 1.5 min, 35 cycles of 94°C 30 sec, 59°C 1 min, and 72°C 5 min, and finally 72°C 5 min.

Tamoxifen-induced Cre *expression.* *Cre* recombinase was activated in *TgGFAP-CreER* mice by daily i.p. injections of 1 mg of 4-hydroxytamoxifen (4-OHT) over 5 days. Tamoxifen was dissolved in a 1:9 mixture of ethanol and sunflower oil (100 μl), facilitated by 10-minute sonication at mid power. Vehicle-only injections served as a control.

Brain histology and immunohistochemistry. Brain tissue was fixed in formalin (10%) for 20–24 hours and then stored in ethanol (70%). Paraffin-embedded sections (5 μm thick) were processed using standard immunohistochemical methods. The antibodies and their dilution were: anti-p-Erk 42/44 (Cell Signaling, 1:50) and anti-SV40 Tag (1:200, mouse monoclonal, Oncogene). Briefly, samples were deparaffinized with Histo-Clear (National Diagnostics), then hydrated through a graded ethanol series. Boiling-mediated antigen retrieval was performed using citrate buffer (pH 6.0) and microwave heating for 2 minutes at high power followed by 7 minutes at low power. Endogenous peroxidases were quenched with H_2O_2 (3%). Immunohistochemistry was performed using the Vectastain ABC kit with the NovaRED (Vector Laboratories, Burlingame, California) peroxidase substrate as chromogen. Samples were counterstained with Harris hematoxylin (Sigma, St. Louis, Missouri). A subset of samples were stained with ABC-AP substrate kit (Vector Laboratories) and counterstained with Nuclear Fast Red.

Prostate histopathology and in situ assays. Prostate samples were prepared and analyzed as reported previously (Hill et al. 2005a,b).

Laser capture microdissection and LOH analysis. Laser capture microdissection (LCM) of H&E-stained sections was performed using a Leica AS LMD (Leica Microsystems Inc., Bannockburn, Illinois) as described previously (Hill et al. 2005b). Briefly, formalin-fixed paraffin-embedded tissue sections were mounted onto Glass Foiled PEN slides (Vashaw Scientific, Atlanta, Georgia). Cells were collected in 50 μl of lysis buffer (10 mM Tris-HCl, pH 8.0, 1% Tween-20) with addition of 5 μl of proteinase K (100 mg/ml), and incubated at 55°C overnight. Proteinase K was inactivated at 99°C for 10 minutes, and 5–10-μl aliquots were used for PCR analysis. The primers for semi-quantitative PCR and quantitative real-time PCR analysis were as described previously (Hill et al. 2005b). The data were analyzed using SDS 2.1 software (Applied Biosystems, Foster City, California) and standard protocols (http://www.appliedbiosystems.com) as previously described (Hill et al. 2005b).

Statistical analysis. Binomial exact test was performed using SAS 9.1 (Cary, North Carolina) to determine whether loss of the wild-type *p53* allele was statistically significant in tumor stroma of $TgAPT_{121};p53^{+/-}$ and $TgAPT_{121};p53^{+/+}$ mice. The probability of random wild-type *p53* allele loss in the tumor stroma was arbitrarily set at 1%. However, results remain significant ($p < 0.0001$) even if the probability of random loss is as high as 10%.

RESULTS

An Astrocytoma Model and New Systems for Inducing T_{121}

Astrocytoma is the most common primary brain tumor in humans and is rarely amenable to standard therapies. We have engineered mouse models to gain insight to the mechanisms of this poorly understood and often lethal disease, because to fully understand the complexities of such pathologies requires investigation in vivo. The vast majority (70–80%) of high-grade anaplastic astrocytomas (WHO grade III) and glioblastomas (WHO grade IV, GBM) harbor mutations in the pRb pathway (Henson et al. 1994; Ueki et al. 1996) in addition to other genetic alterations such as p53 (~30%) and PTEN loss-of-function (~50%) and EGFR gain-of-function (50%) mutations (Louis and Cavenee 1997; Maher et al. 2001; Reilly and Jacks 2001). Such high frequencies indicate that these defects are often concurrent with pRb pathway loss. Therefore, we designed experiments to investigate the combined effects of these perturbations in the defined experimental setting of GEM.

We used a promoter from the human gene encoding *glial fibrillary acidic protein* (*GFAP*) to direct T_{121} expression within the astrocyte lineage of the central nervous system (CNS) (Fig. 2A) (Xiao et al. 2002). However, expression of T_{121} is dependent on Cre recombinase activity, since a *lacZ* reporter gene flanked by lox P sites lies between the promoter and the T_{121} gene (*TgGZT$_{121}$* mice). In *TgG(ΔZ)T$_{121}$* (generated after crossing to *Tgβ-actinCre* mice; see Materials and Methods) (Lewandoski and Martin 1997), T_{121} is expressed from embryonic day

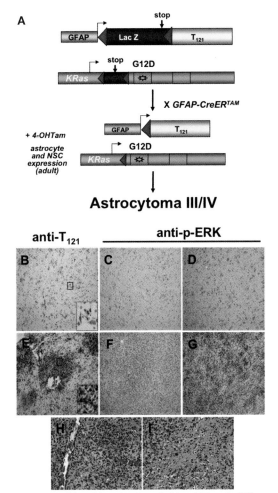

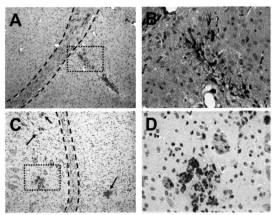

Figure 3. Focal inactivation of pRb function in adult astrocytes by lentiviral *Cre* delivery. As an alternative to germ-line transgenesis using tissue-specific promoter elements, we introduced lentivirus harboring a self-excising-*Cre* construct (unpublished, Tal Kafri, UNC) into the frontal cortex of $TgGZT_{121}$ transgenic mice via stereotaxic injection to initiate localized tumorigenesis. Nineteen days postinjection, T_{121} (*dark brown stain*) can be detected along the needle track (*dashed lines*) in astrocytic cells (*A*). Six months postinjection, clusters of astrocytic cells (*arrows*) can be seen along the injection site (*C*) and as far as 1500 μm away. Magnifications: *A, C,* 100×; *B, D,* 400×. *B* and *D* are higher magnifications of the regions boxed in *A* and *C,* respectively.

Figure 2. Conditional inactivation of pRb, p107, and p130 combined with Ras activation in adult astrocytes causes progression to high-grade astrocytoma. Two *Cre*-conditional alleles, encoding T_{121} ($TgGZT_{121}$) and an activating K-ras point mutant (*LSL-K-ras^{G12D}*), were used to test the consequences of pRb function inactivation and Ras activation, respectively, singly and combined (*A*). Both genes were activated in adult mice at 2–3 months of age using a tamoxifen-inducible Cre recombinase encoded by the *GFAP-CreER* transgene to avoid confounding developmental effects. Two months post-4-OHT, mice with a combination of T_{121} and activated K-ras (*E–G*) show a dramatic expansion of astrocytes that express T_{121} (*E*) as compared to mice expressing T_{121} alone (*B–D*). Ras-dependent activation of the MAPK pathway is indicated in cortical neoplastic cells by phospho-Erk staining (*G*) but not in those of the thalamus (*F*). At 4 months post-4-OHT, both angiogenesis (*H*) and necrosis are apparent (*I*) in mice with both T_{121} and activated K-ras. Samples *B, C, E, F, H,* and *I* are thalamus; *D* and *G* are cortex.

11.5 onward and ultimately results in high-grade astrocytoma in adult mice with 100% penetrance (Xiao et al. 2002). Although we observed diffuse grade III astrocytomas, none had progressed to malignant grade IV astrocytoma (also called glioblastoma multiforme, or GBM). A secondary phenotype we observed in brains of these mice was an expansion of cells in the subventricular zone (SVZ), a cell population of neuronal lineage and not a glial lineage, which we hypothesize was due to the early expression of GFAP promoter in neuronal progenitor cells. To circumvent the possible effects of T_{121} activity during CNS development and to better model the human disease, we crossed $TgGZT_{121}$ mice with $TgGFAP$-*CreER* mice (K. McCarthy, UNC), such that Cre activity can be controlled by treatment with 4-OHT (Fig. 3A). Indeed, T_{121} was inducible in astrocytes of adult mice (2–3 months of age) and yielded diffuse astrocytoma over time as observed in $TgG(\Delta Z)T_{121}$ mice, establishing a valuable inducible model of astrocytoma initiation.

We investigated the possibility that cooperating mutations would synergize with pRb pathway loss to facilitate tumor progression to more severe grades of disease. Although not frequently mutated, Ras is frequently activated in human high-grade astrocytomas (Bos 1989), likely through amplification or mutation of the epidermal growth factor receptor (EGFR; ~40–60% of high-grade tumors) or platelet-derived growth factor (PDGF). Thus, Ras activation generally coexists with aberrations of the pRb pathway. Previous studies showed that overexpression of mutant H-Ras in transgenic astrocytes (Ding et al. 2001), or of activated K-ras in combination with activated Akt (Holland et al. 2000), predisposed GBM-like lesions. We examined the consequences of astrocyte-specific endogenous K-ras activation alone and together with astrocytic T_{121} expression. Through matings, we generated $TgGZT_{121}$;$TgGFAP$-*CreER*, *LSL-K-ras$^{G12D/+}$*; $TgGFAP$-*CreER*, and $TgGZT_{121}$; *LSL-K-ras$^{G12D/+}$*; $TgGFAP$-*CreER* mice (Fig 2A). At 2–3 months of age, Cre activity was induced by treating the mice with 4-OHT (see Materials and Methods) and brains were analyzed at 2 and 4 months postinduction. Activation of Ras alone in astrocytes had no apparent effects up to 4 months post 4-OHT injection (not shown), whereas activation of T_{121} in astrocytes induced an astrocytic expansion within 2 months as described above (Fig. 2B). However, a more dramatic phenotype was observed when both T_{121} and K-ras were activated simultaneously; by 2 months following 4-OHT injections, brains showed features characteristic of human astrocytoma, including peri-neuron and peri-vascular satellitosis (Fig. 2E). Neoplastic astrocytes were positive for T_{121}, and evidence for Ras-specific activation of the MAPK pathway was demonstrated by phospho-Erk IHC. Importantly, phospho-Erk was detectable in the cortex, but not in the thalamus (Fig. 2E, F), suggesting region-specific effects.

Significantly, by 4 months post 4-OHT, angiogenesis (Fig. 2H) and necrosis (Fig. 2I), both properties of GBM, were apparent when both Ras and T_{121} were activated, but not when either was singly activated (data not shown). We conclude from these results that pRb pathway loss is sufficient to predispose astrocytes to tumorigenesis, and that additional events, such as Ras activation, are required for astrocytoma tumor progression to GBM.

Somatic Induction of T_{121} Using *Cre*-expressing Lentivirus Vectors

The recombinase-mediated experiments outlined above provide temporal, but not spatial, control of tumor induction. Since human cancers likely evolve from a single cell, initiating tumorigenesis focally rather than in a large cell population may provide a more authentic model of sporadic cancer, mimicking the scenario in which a transformed cell originates within a microenvironment of wild-type cells. As an alternative to germ-line transgenesis using tissue-specific promoter elements, we are developing retroviral approaches to somatically deliver Cre recombinase in adult cells in more limited regions. In one model, lentivirus harboring a self-excising-*Cre* gene (a kind gift of Tal Kafri, UNC) was introduced into brains of $TgGZT_{121}$ transgenic mice via stereotaxic injection to initiate local tumorigenesis by expressing T_{121} in a limited number of astrocytes. One microliter of lentivirus (10^9 IU/ml) was injected into the cortex of adult $TgGZT_{121}$ mice ($n = 4$). Nineteen days post injection, T_{121} was detected by IHC along the needle track in astrocytic cells ($n = 2$, Fig. 3A,B). To determine whether local T_{121} expression was sufficient to generate astrocytoma, the remaining mice ($n = 2$) were aged for 6 months. Despite T_{121} expression in clusters of astrocytic cells along the injection site (Fig. 3C,D), and as far as 1500 μm away, these conditions were insufficient for astrocytoma development. Although we did not observe tumors in this small cohort, the results of this pilot study show promise for this technique; therefore, we continue to explore the consequences of limited regional pRb pathway inactivation together with additional events such as *K-ras* activation and *Pten* inactivation, and evaluate its effectiveness as a new paradigm for modeling sporadic cancer.

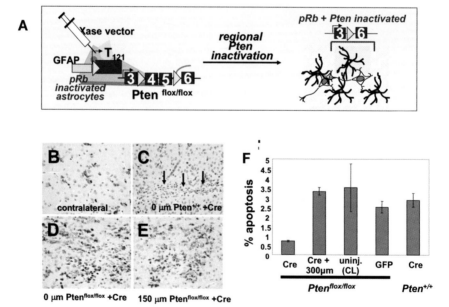

Figure 4. Regional somatic *Pten* inactivation in pRb$_f$-inactivated astrocytes. Somatic delivery of *Cre* (*A*) induces accumulation of neoplastic cells. PCNA immunohistochemical staining of brains 5 weeks after retroviral delivery. Viral-*Cre* delivery to $TgG(\Delta Z)T_{121};Pten^{loxp/loxp}$ brains induced dense neoplastic cell foci at the injection sites (*D*) and in the regions as far as 150 μm away (*E*). The highly dense neoplastic cell foci were not present at the comparable region of the uninjected contralateral hemisphere (*B*). Focal tumor development was not due to retrovirus infection ($TgG(\Delta Z)T_{121};Pten^{loxp/loxp}$ + GFP) or Cre protein ($TgG(\Delta Z) T_{121};Pten^{+/+}$ + Cre; *C*) alone, because no such nodules were found in these controls. The only morphologic difference observed between these brains and those not injected (data not shown) is the needle track (*C, arrows*). In $TgG(\Delta Z)T_{121};Pten^{loxp/loxp}$ brains, the apoptotic level was decreased in tumor cell clusters near injection sites ($0.69 \pm 0.04\%$,), compared with contralateral regions ($3.31 \pm 1.24\%$) and distant adjacent regions (300 μm from the injection site) where injection tracks were not present ($3.51 \pm 0.20\%$). Similar levels of apoptosis were also found at the injected sites of controls ($2.50 \pm 0.53\%$ and $2.86 \pm 0.30\%$). The $TgG(\Delta Z)T_{121};Pten^{loxp/loxp}$ + Cre group is compared with each of the other groups; $p < 0.05$ is considered statistically significant. (Portions of this figure adapted from Xiao et al. 2005.)

In a similar experimental approach, we used somatic viral delivery to measure direct and long-term effects of depleting Pten locally in initiated cells already deficient in pRb pathway function, reminiscent of the clonal changes acquired by human cancers during tumor progression (Xiao et al. 2005). *Pten* mutations are associated with a significant fraction of human high-grade astrocytomas (30–50%). We employed an *MSCV-Cre* viral vector (a kind gift from L. Su, UNC) to assay the effects of Pten loss *within* initiated tumor cells (Fig. 4A). Because normal astrocytes are non-dividing when terminally differentiated, we reasoned that cells expressing T_{121} would be more susceptible to retroviral gene delivery because they are highly proliferative at all ages. Indeed, tumor cells along the injection tracks of $TgG(\Delta Z)T_{121}$; $Pten^{loxp/loxp}$ mice had significantly reduced apoptosis ($p < 0.05$), which is evoked by pRb pathway inactivation, as compared with a distant contralateral region (Fig. 4F). Furthermore, tumor-cell-dense foci were detected at some distance from the injection tracks in $TgG(\Delta Z)T_{121}$; $Pten^{loxp/loxp}$ brains (Fig. 4E), but not $TgG(\Delta Z)T_{121}$; $Pten^{+/+}$ brains (Fig. 4C), indicating *Pten* loss may also facilitate tumor cell invasion.

Using primary astrocytes from $TgG(\Delta Z)T_{121}$; $Pten^{loxp/loxp}$ newborn mice, we showed that *Pten* inactivation by adenovirus-*MSCV-Cre* induced invasion through Matrigel. This primary cell model facilitates analysis of pathways involved in tumorigenic properties and should provide a valuable resource for therapeutic target discovery and validation. In preliminary tests using inhibitors, we showed that invasion induced by *Pten* inactivation was inhibited by both a PI3 kinase inhibitor and a pan protein kinase C (PKC) inhibitor. Furthermore, treatment of cells

with a peptide inhibitor of the atypical PKC-ζ also significantly suppressed Matrigel invasion (Xiao et al. 2005).

These studies indicate that *Pten* loss can potentiate multiple tumorigenic properties in neoplastic astrocytes initiated by inactivation of pRb function and provide both primary cell and animal models for further assessment of the pathways and mechanisms involved. Current studies are exploring the relative contributions of both *K-ras* activation and *Pten* inactivation to astrocytoma progression using each of the above-described strategies.

Complexity of Tumor Progression in a Model of Prostate Cancer

A number of useful transgenic models of prostate cancer have provided the means to investigate one of the most common epithelial cancers afflicting men (Greenberg et al. 1994; Yoshidome et al. 1998). However, because these previous strategies employed wild-type SV40 Large T antigen or the full SV40 early region, these models do not permit assessment of the individual contributions of pRb family loss versus the multiple other concomitant perturbations, some of which have demonstrated roles in tumorigenesis, such as p53 or p300 deficiency, or blocked phosphatase PP2A function. We have shown that inactivation of pRb function mediated by modified rat *probasin* promoter-driven expression of T_{121} ($TgAPT_{121}$) is sufficient for tumor initiation, produces widespread intraepithelial neoplasia (PIN) consisting of high rates of epithelial cell proliferation and apoptosis (Fig. 5B), and ultimately progresses to locally invasive adenocarcinoma

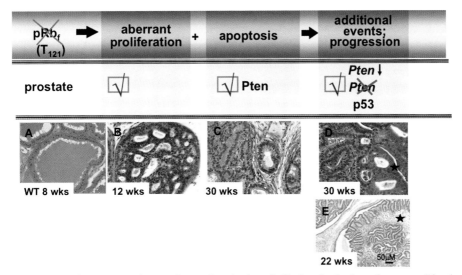

Figure 5. $TgAPT_{121}$ mice develop prostate adenocarcinoma. Inactivation of pRb function leads to aberrant proliferation, and apoptosis is mediated by Pten, not p53. Additional events such as loss of *Pten* and/or *p53* lead to heterogeneous tumor progression. Prostate sections (5 μm) shown are from an 8-week-old nontransgenic littermate (*A*) and $TgAPT_{121}$ mice of different ages (*B,C*). Normal prostate displays a single layer of luminal cells and a thin fibromuscular stromal cell layer (*A*). By 12 weeks (*B*), mouse PIN (mPIN) appears broadly where glands are filled with atypical cells in a cribriform pattern. More advanced lesions are present in prostates of 30-week-old $TgAPT_{121}$ mice, including microinvasive glands with a desmoplastic response and well-differentiated adenocarcinoma (*C*). *Pten* heterozygosity accelerates the onset of mPIN and adenocarcinoma in $TgAPT_{121}$ mice (*D*). In addition, morphologically distinct areas of adenocarcinoma progression also appear (*D*, 30-week-old, *star*). *p53* heterozygosity does not accelerate the onset of mPIN; however, stromal tumors develop as young as 22 weeks of age (*E*) and consist of an abundance of stromal cells (*star*). All sections were stained with hematoxylin and eosin (H&E). (*A–D*, Adapted from Hill et al. 2005a; *E*, adapted from Hill et al. 2005b.)

with no evidence of neuroendocrine tumors (Fig. 5C) (Hill et al. 2005a). Therefore, the $TgAPT_{121}$ mouse line provides a fully penetrant mouse model of prostate cancer initiation with which to dissect the mechanisms of tumor progression.

Roles of *Pten* in Prostate Cancer Suppression

Because apoptosis induced by pRb functional loss is mediated through different mechanisms in different cell types, we examined the pathway(s) used by $TgAPT_{121}$ prostates with a genetic approach. Using the TUNEL assay, we quantified prostate apoptosis levels in 8-week-old mice of the following genotypes: wild type, $TgAPT_{121}$, $TgAPT_{121};Pten^{+/-}$, $TgAPT_{121};p53^{+/-}$, and $TgAPT_{121};$ $p53^{-/-}$. In $TgAPT_{121}$ prostates, hemizygosity or nullizygosity of $p53$ caused no reduction in the apoptotic index, whereas hemizygosity at *Pten* caused a 50% reduction in the apoptotic index accelerating progression to adenocarcinomas with heterogeneous composition (Fig. 6A). Het-

erogeneity is associated with concurrent *Pten* haploinsufficiency and selective focal tumor progression identifiable by concomitant *Pten* loss (Fig. 6C), the appearance of membrane-bound phospho-Akt (p-Akt)(Fig. 6D), a further reduction in apoptosis levels (Fig. 7E), and distinct morphology (Fig. 6B).

Unexpected Roles for p53 in Epithelial/Mesenchymal Interactions

Although p53 is not involved in epithelial apoptosis in $TgAPT_{121}$ mice, we found that it plays a critical role in tumor evolution. T_{121} expression in prostate epithelium resulted in p53 induction in both epithelial and mesenchymal compartments (Hill et al. 2005b). p53 appears to

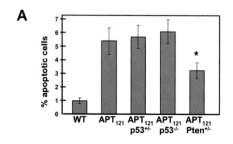

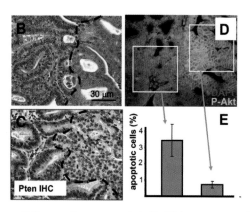

Figure 6. Pten mediates apoptosis in $TgAPT_{121}$ prostate, and its loss contributes to focal tumor progression. (*A*) Prostates from 8-week-old non-transgenic, $TgAPT_{121}$, $TgAPT_{121};p53^{+/-}$, $TgAPT_{121};p53^{-/-}$, and $TgAPT_{121};Pten^{+/-}$ mice were analyzed for apoptosis levels quantified by calculating the number of TUNEL-positive cells (*brown*) as a percentage of the total (*methyl green*). $n = 4$ for each genotype. (*B*) A representative H&E-stained section shows a transition where focal adenocarcinoma develops from neoplastic areas with back-to-back gland structure. (*C*) Immunohistochemistry for Pten (*red/brown*) shows loss of cytoplasmic staining in regions of focal progression. In such regions of Pten loss, cells express membrane-bound p-Akt staining (*D*; *green*). (*E*) Apoptosis assay was performed via TUNEL in those p-Akt expressed and nonexpressed regions (*white boxes*). p-Akt expressed cells, indicating loss of Pten, have further reduction of apoptosis. (Adapted from Hill et al. 2005a.)

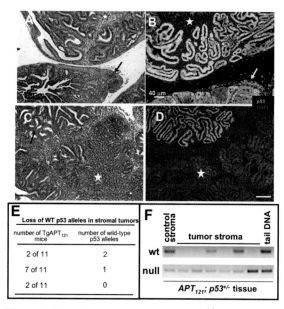

Figure 7. Stromal p53 loss in $TgAPT_{121};p53^{+/-}$ and $TgAPT_{121}$ tumors. Serial sections of an emerging stromal tumor in $TgAPT_{121};p53^{+/-}$ mice with expanding mesenchyme (*star*) and adjacent mPIN (*arrow*) are shown (*A*; H&E) and (*B*; p53 IF). p53 expression is lost in the tumor mesenchyme (*B*, *star*) and retained in the epithelium in addition to the mPIN-associated stroma (*arrow*). A total of 18 $APT_{121};p53^{+/-}$ mice with stromal tumors were examined, and all were found to have lost p53 expression in the stroma. Epithelial p53 loss subsequent to stromal p53 loss compounds heterogeneous tumor progression. In H&E-stained $TgAPT_{121};p53^{+/-}$ tumor sections (*C*), regions of dense epithelial cell growth morphologically distinct from surrounding epithelium (*arrows*) grow in small back-to-back circular glands (*star*). IF for p53 (*yellow*) shows that such regions no longer express p53. Representative tumors from 7-month-old $TgAPT_{121};p53^{+/-}$ mice are shown (*D*). PCR analysis on stromal DNA extracted from laser-captured microdissected (LCM) samples in $TgAPT_{121};p53^{+/-}$ mice showed that stromal loss of wild-type $p53$ allele occurred in four of six tumors (*F*). Similar stromal loss of p53 expression is observed in stromal tumors arising in $TgAPT_{121};p53^{+/+}$ mice ($n = 8$). Real-time quantitative PCR was performed on stromal DNA extracted from LCM samples to determine the status of wild-type $p53$ alleles in stromal tumors or tissues of $TgAPT_{121}$ mice. LCM muscle samples were used as controls. Among 11 stromal tumor samples from 11 distinct animals, 7 showed loss of 1 wild-type allele of $p53$, 2 showed loss of both alleles of $p53$, and 2 retained both wild-type alleles. (Portions of this figure adapted from Hill et al. 2005b.)

suppress fibroblast proliferation in the stroma, since these cells proliferated in a $TgAPT_{121}$ p53-deficient, but not wild-type or heterozygous, background (Hill et al. 2005b). Indeed, all $TgAPT_{121};p53^{-/-}$ and $TgAPT_{121};p53^{+/-}$ (Fig. 5E) male mice developed large tumors composed of extensive stroma, a phenotype that develops most rapidly in the p53 null background. Tumor fibroblasts of the p53 heterozygous background no longer expressed p53 (Fig. 7B), and laser capture microdissection-PCR analysis showed that the wild-type p53 allele was selectively lost in this compartment in most tumors (Fig. 7B,F). Similar stromal loss of p53 expression is observed in stromal tumors arising in $TgAPT_{121};p53^{+/+}$ mice ($n = 8$). Real-time quantitative PCR on stromal DNA extracted from LCM samples showed that among 11 stromal tumor samples from 11 distinct animals, 7 lost 1 wild-type allele of p53, 2 lost both alleles of p53, and 2 retained both wild-type alleles (Fig. 7E) (Hill et al. 2005b). Although the epithelium within these tumors initially retained p53 expression (Fig. 7B), focal regions subsequently lost p53 expression as well (Fig. 7D), suggesting an as yet unknown function of p53 as tumor suppressor in this compartment. These studies demonstrate that non-cell-autonomous responses to epithelial tumorigenic lesions can create a microenvironment in which selective genetic changes occur in non-tumor cells, causing coevolution of multiple cell types within the tumor. Current studies are focused on identifying the p53-inductive signal(s) from initiated epithelium to the mesenchyme and on the mechanisms of p53 tumor suppression in multiple prostate compartments.

CONCLUSIONS

By exploiting T_{121} to inactivate pRb and its related family members, we have explored the requirement of pRb tumor suppression in glial cells and multiple epithelial cell types, including brain (CPE), prostate, and breast. This has been a powerful approach to generate highly penetrant mouse models of cancer that are reflective of human tumors in which the pRb pathway is perturbed and that evolve through the accumulation of additional genetic or epigenetic aberrations. We have dissected some of the genetic pathways contributing to tumor progression both by combining the initiated transgenic models with other engineered germ-line mutations and by analyzing the natural evolution of progressing tumors. Through these experiments, we have identified differences in tumor suppressor mechanisms invoked by varying cell types. More specifically, in each of the systems studied, there is a similar course of events: T_{121} expression causes aberrant proliferation and concomitant increased levels of apoptosis, resulting in a strong selective pressure for reduced apoptosis. Tumors progress when a major tumor suppressor is inactivated, resulting in reduced apoptosis, but also in additional tumor-promoting functions. In response to pRb function loss, CPE and breast cells rely on p53-mediated apoptosis, whereas astrocytes and prostate epithelium depend on Pten activity. These differences significantly affect the dynamics of cancer evolution, and therefore may have wide-ranging implications in the interpretation of diagnostic tumor mutation analysis and in the development of appropriately targeted therapies.

Because T_{121} so effectively evokes illicit cellular proliferation and apoptosis, we have until recently relied on gene regulatory sequences to direct T_{121} expression only in adult cells to avoid secondary developmental defects. We have further refined our strategy by engineering conditional alleles using Cre-LoxP technology to more finely restrict the timing and location of T_{121} expression. Building on this conditional approach, we now also employ retroviral vectors to manipulate more limited cell populations to investigate the consequences of focal events, both in tumor initiation and in events that may contribute to tumor progression. This paradigm more closely mimics natural spontaneous tumor evolution. Combined, these strategies facilitate the analysis of acute consequences to specific genetic lesions, both intrinsic and extrinsic, and the dissection of natural events in the evolution of specific tumors. We are hopeful that the GEM models produced in these studies will also provide useful preclinical systems for diagnostic and therapeutic development.

ACKNOWLEDGMENTS

We thank Jim Pipas (University of Pittsburgh) for generating and characterizing the T_{121} (dl1137) mutant T antigen and for sharing reagents and insightful discussions in the early stages of this work. We thank Hua Wu and Lucy Lu for expert technical assistance in generating transgenic mice, and also Drew Fogarty, Ginger Muse, Daniel Roth, Anne Wolthusen, and Chunyu Yang for colony maintenance and mouse genotyping. We also thank Tal Kafri and Lishan Su (University of North Carolina) for providing Cre-expressing viral vectors, and Tyler Jacks (Massachusetts Institute of Technology) for providing LSL-K-ras^{G12D} mice. This work was supported by grants from the National Cancer Institute (U01-CA84314 and R01-CA046283 to T.V.D. and U01-CA84294 to R.D.C.), the Susan B. Komen Foundation (T.V.D.), the Department of Defense (breast and prostate cancer programs; T.V.D.), the Brain Tumor Society (T.V.D.), and the Goldhirsh Foundation (T.V.D.).

REFERENCES

Bos J.L. 1989. ras oncogenes in human cancer: A review. Cancer Res. **49:** 4682.

Di Cristofano A., Pesce B., Cordon-Cardo C., and Pandolfi P.P. 1998. Pten is essential for embryonic development and tumour suppression. Nat. Genet. **19:** 348.

Ding H., Roncari L., Shannon P., Wu X., Lau N., Karaskova J., Gutmann D.H., Squire J.A., Nagy A., and Guha A. 2001. Astrocyte-specific expression of activated p21-ras results in malignant astrocytoma formation in a transgenic mouse model of human gliomas. Cancer Res. **61:** 3826.

Greenberg N.M., DeMayo F.J., Sheppard P.C., Barrios R., Lebovitz R., Finegold M., Angelopoulou R., Dodd J.G., Duckworth M.L., and Rosen J.M., et al. 1994. The rat probasin gene promoter directs hormonally and developmentally regulated expression of a heterologous gene specifically to the prostate in transgenic mice. Mol. Endocrinol. **8:** 230.

Henson J.W., Schnitker B.L., Correa K.M., von Deimling A.,
    Fassbender F., Xu H.J., Benedict W.F., Yandell D.W., and
    Louis D.N. 1994. The retinoblastoma gene is involved in ma-
    lignant progression of astrocytomas. *Ann. Neurol.* **36:** 714.
Hill R., Song Y., Cardiff R.D., and Van Dyke T. 2005a. Hetero-
    geneous tumor evolution initiated by loss of pRb function in
    a preclinical prostate cancer model. *Cancer Res.* **65:** 10243.
————. 2005b. Selective evolution of stromal mesenchyme with
    p53 loss in response to epithelial tumorigenesis. *Cell* **123:**
    1001.
Holland E.C., Celestino J., Dai C., Schaefer L., Sawaya R.E.,
    and Fuller G.N. 2000. Combined activation of Ras and Akt in
    neural progenitors induces glioblastoma formation in mice.
    Nat. Genet. **25:** 55.
Jacks T., Shih T.S., Schmitt E.M., Bronson R.T., Bernards A.,
    and Weinberg R.A. 1994. Tumour predisposition in mice het-
    erozygous for a targeted mutation in Nf1. *Nat. Genet.* **7:** 353.
Jackson E.L., Willis N., Mercer K., Bronson R.T., Crowley D.,
    Montoya R., Jacks T., and Tuveson D.A. 2001. Analysis of
    lung tumor initiation and progression using conditional ex-
    pression of oncogenic K-ras. *Genes Dev.* **15:** 3243.
Lewandoski M. and Martin G.R. 1997. Cre-mediated chromo-
    some loss in mice. *Nat. Genet.* **17:** 223.
Louis D.N. and Cavenee W.K. 1997. Molecular biology of cen-
    tral nervous system tumors. In *Cancer: Principles and prac-
    tice of oncology* (ed. V.T. DeVita et al.), p. 2013. Lippincott-
    Raven, Philadelphia, Pennsylvania.
Lu X., Magrane G., Yin C., Louis D.N., Gray J., and Van Dyke
    T. 2001. Selective inactivation of p53 facilitates mouse ep-
    ithelial tumor progression without chromosomal instability.
    Mol. Cell. Biol. **21:** 6017.
Maher E.A., Furnari F.B., Bachoo R.M., Rowitch D.H., Louis
    D.N., Cavenee W.K., and DePinho R.A. 2001. Malignant
    glioma: Genetics and biology of a grave matter. *Genes Dev.*
    15: 1311.

Pan H., Yin C., Dyson N., Harlow E., Yamasaki L., and Van
    Dyke T. 1998. A key role for E2F1 in p53-dependent apopto-
    sis and cell division within developing tumors. *Cell* **2:** 283.
Reilly K.M. and Jacks T. 2001. Genetically engineered mouse
    models of astrocytoma: GEMs in the rough (review)? *Semin.
    Cancer Biol.* **11:** 177.
Simin K., Wu H., Lu L., Pinkel D., Albertson D., Cardiff R.D.,
    and Van Dyke T. 2004. pRb inactivation in mammary cells re-
    veals common mechanisms for tumor initiation and progres-
    sion in divergent epithelia. *PLoS Biol.* **2:** E22.
Symonds H., Krall L., Remington L., Saenz-Robles M., Lowe S.,
    Jacks T., and Van Dyke T. 1994. p53-dependent apoptosis sup-
    presses tumor growth and progression in vivo. *Cell* **78:** 703.
Trotman L.C., Niki M., Dotan Z.A., Koutcher J.A., Cristofano
    A.D., Xiao A., Khoo A.S., Roy-Burman P., Greenberg N.M.,
    Dyke T.V., Cordon-Cardo C., and Pandolfi P. 2003. Pten dose
    dictates cancer progression in the prostate. *PLoS Biol.* **1:** E59.
Ueki K., Ono Y., Henson J.W., Efird J.T., von Deimling A., and
    Louis D.N. 1996. CDKN2/p16 or RB alterations occur in the
    majority of glioblastomas and are inversely correlated. *Can-
    cer Res.* **56:** 150.
Xiao A., Wu H., Pandolfi P.P., Louis D.N., and Van Dyke T.
    2002. Astrocyte inactivation of the pRb pathway predisposes
    mice to malignant astrocytoma development that is acceler-
    ated by PTEN mutation. *Cancer Cell* **1:** 157.
Xiao A., Yin C., Yang C., Di Cristofano A., Pandolfi P.P., and
    Van Dyke T. 2005. Somatic induction of Pten loss in a pre-
    clinical astrocytoma model reveals major roles in disease pro-
    gression and avenues for target discovery and validation.
    Cancer Res. **65:** 5172.
Yoshidome K., Shibata M.A., Maroulakou I.G., Liu M.L., Jor-
    cyk C.L., Gold L.G., Welch V.N., and Green J.E. 1998. Ge-
    netic alterations in the development of mammary and prostate
    cancer in the C3(1)/Tag transgenic mouse model. *Int. J. On-
    col.* **12:** 449.

The Evolving Portrait of Cancer Metastasis

P.B. Gupta,[*][†] S. Mani,[†] J. Yang,[†] K. Hartwell,[*][†] and R.A. Weinberg[*][†]

*Department of Biology, Massachusetts Institute of Technology, Cambridge, Massachusetts 02142;
†Whitehead Institute for Biomedical Research, Cambridge, Massachusetts 02142

The phenomenon of cancer metastasis remains poorly understood. We discuss here various conceptual frameworks that attempt to rationalize the mechanisms by which tumors acquire metastatic ability. Portrayal of cancer as a somatic Darwinian process occurring within a tissue fails to fully explain the phenomenon of metastatic competence. The biology of pre-neoplastic cells also complicates this picture, since the phenotypes of normal cellular precursors are clearly relevant to metastatic behavior following transformation. Recent experimental results help to shed light on these and other considerations regarding the molecular mechanisms of malignant progression.

THE DARWINIAN PARADIGM OF TUMOR PROGRESSION

Research over the past three decades has provided a solid foundation for comprehending the genetic basis of tumor formation and progression. As a consequence, we now understand that the requirement for accumulated genetic lesions underlies the progressive development of adult cancers, many of which arise over a span of decades. This multifactorial genetic requirement is reflected in the extensive genomic instability of cancer cells. Indeed, dysregulation of the cellular apparatus that ensures genomic integrity appears to be one common mechanism by which premalignant clones acquire the multiple lesions that are necessary to attain high-grade malignancy (Lengauer et al. 1997; Shih et al. 2001; Goel et al. 2003; Grady 2004; Hiyama et al. 2004).

A second mechanism by which cancer cells acquire multiple genomic lesions depends on repeated cycles of mutation and clonal selection, resulting in the sequential fixation of mutations in the bulk tumor cell population. According to this Darwinian model, tumors evolve toward greater malignancy over time as a result of the expansion of individual cell clones that have sustained novel genetic lesions conferring a selective advantage within the primary tumor microenvironment (Wolman 1983, 1986; Mertens et al. 1991; Chung et al. 1996; Mora et al. 2001). The functional contribution of specific genetic lesions to cancer pathogenesis has been established, in many cases, by associating their presence with particular cancer phenotypes using in vitro and in vivo tumor models. This Darwinian paradigm provides a compelling rationale for the presence of many of the genetic lesions commonly observed in human tumors. Examples of the selective advantage that specific lesions provide include Bcl-2 overexpression (Ehlert and Kubbutat 2001; Kirkin et al. 2004) and p53 function loss (Sidransky et al. 1992; Li et al. 1998; Ehlert and Kubbutat 2001), which confer resistance to apoptosis; pRb loss, which confers resistance to growth-inhibitory signals (Sage et al. 2000); and gain-of-function mutations of Ras proteins (Schleger et al. 2000; Bounacer et al. 2004), which confer the ability to proliferate in the absence of normally required mitogenic signals.

The development of distant metastases is the final step in the progression of many adult malignancies. Given its success in explaining the earlier steps of tumor progression, the Darwinian model has naturally been extended by some to encompass the ultimate phenotypes of cancer cell invasiveness and metastasis. In truth, however, the molecular mechanisms of metastasis remain poorly understood, and the experimental basis for such an extension is essentially nonexistent. Indeed, several conceptual problems and, more recently, experimental observations plague the Darwinian paradigm as it relates to the acquisition of metastatic competence.

THEORETICAL DIFFICULTIES IN EXTENDING THE DARWINIAN MODEL TO CANCER METASTASIS

The abilities to proliferate in the absence of mitogenic signals, to resist apoptotic stimuli, and to induce angiogenesis each confer a clear selective advantage on cancer cells growing within the primary tumor microenvironment. In contrast, it is hardly clear how successive cycles of selective pressure for metastatic ability to secondary organ sites (required under the Darwinian framework) would sensibly operate within the primary tumor microenvironment. Thus, it is hardly clear how the acquisition of metastatic competence by a cancer cell would result per se in its clonal expansion within a tumor. Without such an expansion, rare metastasis-competent cells would not accumulate in large numbers within a primary tumor. Given the low efficiency of the various steps of the "invasion-metastasis cascade," the likelihood of successful metastasis would be extraordinarily small.

The invasion-metastasis cascade (Stracke and Liotta 1992; Lawrence and Steeg 1996; Yoon et al. 2003) encompasses local invasiveness, intravasation into and transport through the circulation, extravasation, formation of a micrometastasis, and finally, formation of a macroscopic metastasis (this last step is sometimes referred to as

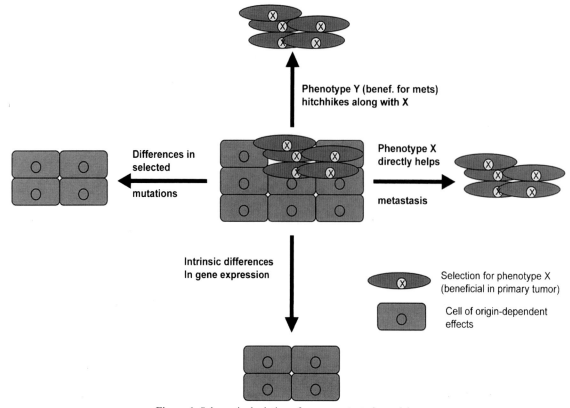

Figure 1. Schematic depiction of cancer metastasis models.

"colonization"). The complexity of this process has caused many to assume that numerous genetic lesions are required within individual cancer cells in order to enable them to complete this cascade. If this were so, the probability of any one of these mutations occurring is small, and, therefore, the likelihood of all requisite lesions occurring together within a single cell is negligibly small.

Alternative scenarios offer resolutions of this conceptual quandary (Fig. 1):

1. Some traits that are advantageous to cancer cells within the primary tumor microenvironment may also contribute to metastatic competence. Resistance to apoptosis, for example, may be dually advantageous for cancer cells—for survival within the primary tumor microenvironment and also for survival in the circulation or at secondary organ sites (prior to colonization), thereby contributing to metastatic competence.

2. Selective pressure within the primary tumor microenvironment for phenotype X may result in the clonal expansion of cancer cells harboring a genetic lesion that also happens to confer a second phenotype Y, the latter contributing to metastatic competence. Thus, cancer cells may acquire a particular phenotype that is advantageous within the primary tumor microenvironment through one of several possible genetic lesions, some of which fortuitously confer additional phenotypes that facilitate cancer cell metastasis.

The possibilities delineated above describe how metastatic phenotypes may hitchhike along with phenotypes that are beneficial within the primary tumor microenvironment, resulting in the clonal expansion of metastasis-competent cells within the primary tumor. These scenarios may help to resolve the *conceptual* difficulties inherent in extending an evolutionary model of tumor progression to include metastasis. However, recent unanticipated observations with tumor specimens obtained from cancer patients call into question the applicability of the Darwinian framework to the acquisition of metastatic competence. In particular, classifiers based on mRNA expression profile arrays have demonstrated that the transcriptional state of relatively early-stage primary tumors is predictive of the ultimate clinical prognosis of patients (van de Vijver et al. 2002; van't Veer et al. 2002; Huang et al. 2003; Ramaswamy et al. 2003; Glinsky et al. 2004a,b; Wang et al. 2005). This surprising finding appears to be fundamentally inconsistent with the stochastic nature of metastasis implied by the Darwinian model. Thus, if it were the case that metastatic competence results from selection operating on a preexisting pool of cancer cell clones that have sustained random genomic alterations, then the ultimate metastatic competence of an early-stage tumor should not be predictable from its cohort of expressed genes. (According to the Darwinian scheme, the ultimate acquisition of metastatic competence is dependent on the nature of lesions that are randomly accumulated by the cells of a tumor late in tumor progression.) The apparent incompatibility of the Darwinian scheme with the existence of a "poor-prognosis" microarray signature remains unresolved by 1 and 2 above.

The ability of early-stage tumor mRNA expression signatures to predict metastatic recurrence has important implications both for our conceptualization of metastasis and for the management of patient treatment. Is it possible to reconcile such observations with the Darwinian mutation/selection model of cancer metastasis? Before returning to these issues, we first turn to a discussion of the role that the cell type of origin can play in influencing tumor biology.

THE INFLUENCE OF CELL TYPE OF ORIGIN ON METASTATIC PROCLIVITY

For more than a century, oncologists have been aware that certain kinds of cancer carry a poorer clinical prognosis than other types of cancer. For instance, melanomas are notorious for rapidly progressing to invasive and metastatic states, whereas basal-cell carcinomas of the skin rarely metastasize. Empirical observations such as these indicate that the cell type from which a particular cancer arises plays a significant role in determining the likelihood that a given tumor will eventually metastasize, independently of genetic variation among individuals. The mechanistic reasons for this are obscure. As tumors become more aggressive, they tend toward greater and greater dedifferentiation. In fact, the most aggressive tumors can be dedifferentiated to a point where it is difficult or impossible to determine their tissue of origin based solely on histological examination (~5% of all cancers are diagnosed as having an unknown primary origin) (Milovic et al. 2002; Dowell 2003; Pavlidis et al. 2003). How is it, then, that malignant cancer cells retain a memory of the cell type from which they originated during later stages of tumor progression, a time at which they are often highly dedifferentiated?

There are two conceptually disparate (but not mutually exclusive) models that could serve to explain the influence of cell type of origin on the natural history and progression of cancer (Fig. 1):

3. The cell type of origin influences metastatic competence by affecting the nature of the genetic lesions that are selected for due to their ability to confer an advantage within the primary tumor microenvironment to a cell that has acquired them. A consequence of this would be that cancers, even at an early stage of development, would have different mutational spectra, depending on their cell type of origin. This model proposes these differences in mutational spectra would be responsible for differences in metastatic propensities (perhaps due to mechanisms 1 or 2 described in the previous subsection).

4. The expression, at various stages of tumor progression, of particular proteins that can influence eventual metastatic competence is in part dependent on the initial differentiation state of a cell prior to neoplastic conversion. Stated differently, the initial differentiation state of a normal founder cell, operating in conjunction with its spectrum of acquired mutations, exerts a strong influence on the eventual expression of metastasis-related proteins in the neoplastic descendants of this founder cell.

Currently available experimental data do not suffice to establish or exclude the importance of either of these mechanisms to human cancer. On the one hand, it is apparent from various genomic profiling studies that certain types of cancers are more prone to possess particular genetic lesions; for example, N-ras mutations or PTEN deletions, providing support for model 3. Experimental evidence in support of model 4 is much harder to come by. Later in this paper, we discuss experiments from our own research group and from other laboratories addressing the plausibility of model 4.

THE RELEVANCE OF CELL TYPE OF ORIGIN TO THE INTERPRETATION OF RECENT TUMOR MICROARRAY DATA

Classifiers based on microarray profiles are readily able to distinguish between different types of cancers and, in some cases, afford a finer distinction between cancer subtypes than is achievable using visual pathological examination alone (Golub et al. 1999; Ramaswamy et al. 2001; Nutt et al. 2003). One can, for example, imagine a situation where the bioinformaticist is supplied with a set of 100 gene expression profiles comprising 50 basal cell carcinomas and 50 melanomas of the skin, all derived from early-stage tumors. One can further envision that the bioinformaticist is given these 100 profiles in a blinded fashion in the absence of any information about the pathological classification of the tumor samples from which they derive, being supplied information only about the clinical outcome of the patient with respect to metastatic recurrence. Having analyzed these data, the bioinformaticist can readily distinguish two subclasses of skin cancer and will be in a position to note that one profile subclass (corresponding to melanomas) affords a significantly poorer prognosis than the other profile subclass (corresponding to basal cell carcinomas). Hence, the bioinformaticist will have constructed classifiers based on gene expression profiles of early-stage tumors that can predict the likelihood of eventual metastatic recurrence and will have done so without knowledge a priori of the intrinsic subclasses into which the tumors segregate.

Similarly, it may be that tumors currently classified as identical on the basis of visual pathological examination alone may be found to harbor subclasses that originate from different cell types and exhibit distinct clinical outcomes, including progression to a metastatic state. If this were indeed the case, then the gene expression analyses would be identifying differences in the cell type of origin, which would in turn underlie differences in both the gene expression profiles and metastatic proclivity. Assuming this scenario, the possibilities 3 and 4 delineated above would have the following respective correlates:

5. Two types of early-stage tumors that appear phenotypically similar may in fact harbor very different sets of genetic lesions. One set of tumors might possess lesions that are permissive of future metastasis-enabling

lesions. A second set of early-stage tumors might possess lesions that, for any number of reasons, are not permissive for additional metastasis-enabling mutations. Gene expression analyses may be able to distinguish between these two types of tumors, which, despite phenotypic similarity, sustain very different genetic alterations and represent different tumor subclasses.

6. Specific proteins that can contribute at some point to metastatic competence may be expressed intensely in some tumors and not in others, depending on the cell type from which the cancer originated. The expression of the aforementioned proteins may not be sufficient to confer metastatic competence, but may collaborate with other proteins to program metastatic ability, perhaps at later stages of tumor progression. Gene expression analyses would be able to distinguish between these two subclasses of tumors.

CAN PREEXISTING CELLULAR STATES INFLUENCE INVASIVE OR METASTATIC BEHAVIOR?

As we have noted in the discussion above, empirical observations suggest that differences in preexisting epigenetic or transcriptional states can provide contributions to cancer cell phenotypes in a manner that is not fully attributable to differences in genetic lesions alone. The question remains as to whether there is experimental evidence to support this notion, particularly with respect to cellular phenotypes that are relevant for metastatic dissemination. Below, we discuss two sets of experimental observations in which epigenetically programmed cellular states provide significant contributions to invasive and metastatic behaviors.

EMTs IN DEVELOPMENT

An important epigenetic program that operates during a variety of morphogenetic processes in early embryogenesis closely resembles the behavior of cancer cells that have progressed to a highly malignant state. This raises the question of whether, during malignant progression, some of these embryonic cell biological programs are resurrected by cancer cells in order to acquire the multiple traits associated with high-grade malignancy, a notion that we explore later. During embryogenesis, subpopulations of cells undergo profound changes in morphology and motility. For example, initiation of gastrulation occurs with the invagination of the ectoderm through the blastopore and subsequent cellular migration along defined tracts within the embryo, resulting in eventual mesoderm specification. As another example, cells of the vertebrate neural crest lineage, which is specified along the dorso-lateral side of the notochord, are characterized by extensive migration throughout the embryo, ultimately giving rise to several adult cell types. In the late 1800s, embryologists observed that these and other developmental migrations were often associated with specific changes in cellular morphology. In particular, they noted that embryonic cells which previously possessed epithelial qualities lost their characteristic polarity, cell–cell junctions, and cytoskeletal components prior to migration. This process was later dubbed an epithelial-to-mesenchymal transition (EMT) (Thiery 2003).

MOLECULAR MEDIATORS OF EMT

What are the physiological stimuli that induce EMTs during development? Embryological tissue engraftment studies have indicated that the initial impetus for a cell to undergo an EMT originates from extracellular cues, e.g,, other nearby cells. Molecular and genetic studies have indicated that TGF-β and Wnt family proteins are important recurrent players in mediating many of the various EMTs that occur during development (Oft et al. 1998; Thiery 2003; Kemler et al. 2004). Also important are HGF and FGF-1, which induce epithelial cell scattering without the concomitant up-regulation of mesenchymal marker (one might call these "partial EMTs") (Thiery and Chopin 1999).

Many of these extracellular signals induce the expression of transcription factors that are prominent regulators of EMT (Martinez-Alvarez et al. 2004; Savagner et al. 2005). These include members of the Snail superfamily of zinc finger proteins (e.g., Snail, Slug, Escargot), as well as bHLH proteins (e.g., Twist, Sip1). In some cases, these factors have been shown to directly repress transcription of the E-cadherin gene, a key epithelial protein. However, little is known about other functional contributions that these transcription factors may provide to EMT, and this remains an important area for future research.

EMT AND CANCER CELL INVASION AND METASTASIS

As a general rule, EMTs are not observed in the adult organism following their transient induction in development. Two notable exceptions include the healing of epithelial injury (where EMT occurs in the cells lining the wound tract) (Tanaka et al. 2004; Savagner et al. 2005) and organs in which there is significant postnatal epithelial development. Accordingly, it is not surprising that the expression of extracellular proteins and transcription factors that can induce EMT is tightly regulated under normal conditions in adult epithelia. However, many factors that induce EMT in development are aberrantly expressed by cancer epithelial cells during tumorigenesis and are implicated in cancer invasion and progression. To name just a few, these include HGF, TGF-β, Rho family proteins, Snail, Slug, and Twist. This observation, together with the association of EMTs with invasive behaviors during development, has naturally led to the proposal that EMTs may play an important role in cancer cell invasion. Experiments in culture have confirmed that the experimental induction of EMT in cancer epithelial cells can enhance their motility and invasiveness using in vitro assays. However, the notion that EMT contributes to cancer cell invasion in vivo has yet to gain widespread acceptance, in large part due to the difficulty in establishing the bona fide occurrence of EMT in human carcinomas.

We note that the current debate over the relevance of the EMT to cancer invasion is reminiscent of a similar debate that raged 5–10 years ago regarding the significance of cellular senescence for tumor suppression (Dimri and Campisi 1994; Wynford-Thomas 1999). At that time, experiments in culture had established that key growth-inhibitory signaling proteins such as p53, pRb, p14ARF, and p16INK4a were clearly relevant to both cellular senescence and tumor formation; however, a convincing demonstration that senescence occurs in vivo was not forthcoming. To a large extent, this difficulty was a direct consequence of the lack of credible and specific functional markers for cellular senescence in vivo (β-galactosidase activity at low pH, although in common use, was of questionable functional relevance). Indeed, the principal criterion for gauging senescence in vitro is morphological and cannot be readily translated to an in vivo setting (Harley 1991; Urquidi et al. 2000). The resolution of this debate proceeded from the recognition that, regardless of whether cellular senescence occurs in vivo, the established overlap between tumor-suppressor pathways and pathways governing the onset of senescence ensured the relevance of this phenomenon to cancer genetics.

Many of these characteristics are shared by the EMT phenomenon: (1) An EMT is most readily observed in pure populations of epithelial cells in culture on the basis of morphologic and motility alterations; (2) an EMT is not readily identifiable in vivo, due to the nature of the criterion just described together with the difficulty in distinguishing epithelial cells that have undergone an EMT from nearby bona fide mesenchymal cells in the tumor stroma; (3) there is a significant overlap between molecular pathways controlling the invasive and migratory behaviors of cancer cells and the pathways governing the induction of EMT. Similar to the situation with cellular senescence, we believe that the overlap between signal transduction pathways mediating EMT and pathways involved in cancer cell invasiveness ensures its relevance to the biology of cancer.

How does all this affect the previous discussion pertaining to experiments indicating that gene expression data can predict invasive behavior? EMT is the prime example of an epigenetically programmed "cellular differentiation state" that (1) does not require genetic alterations for its induction or propagation, (2) is discernible using gene expression profile-based classifiers, and (3) can significantly influence the invasive and migratory properties of normal and carcinomatous epithelial cells. In this respect, the EMT is an example of an experimental phenomenon supporting the plausibility of model 4 described above. In particular, the finding that cancer cells which have undergone an EMT can display increased invasive behaviors demonstrates the plausibility of the notion that cellular differentiation states can affect cancer cell invasiveness in a significant manner independently of genomic lesions.

MELANOMA AND METASTASIS

A second experimental observation supporting model 5 involves the neoplastic transformation of primary human cell types via the introduction in vitro of a defined series of genetic elements. This system utilizes the Simian Virus 40 early region (SV40ER), which encodes the viral large T (LT) and small T (st) oncoproteins, in conjunction with a gene encoding the catalytic subunit of the telomerase holoenzyme (hTERT) to immortalize primary human cells; the resulting immortalized cells are then transformed by introducing a *ras* oncogene. A variety of human cell types transformed in this manner generate localized tumors that have minimal ability to metastasize (Hahn et al. 1999; Elenbaas et al. 2001; Rich et al. 2001; Lundberg et al. 2002). A surprising exception is observed with primary human melanocytes, which exhibit a highly penetrant metastatic phenotype following transformation (Gupta et al. 2005). Because the above-described procedure generates cancer cell lines transformed with an identical set of genes, variations in tumor phenotypes arising from genetic differences between cancer cell lines are effectively minimized. In particular, the uniquely metastatic behavior of transformed melanocytes in this system is most likely a consequence of their differentiation program and is, conversely, not due to differences in genetic lesions.

These observations suggested that intrinsic factors associated with the melanocyte differentiation program can provide a significant contribution to melanoma's metastatic ability. In fact, the neural crest cell factor, Slug, is expressed both in the transformed melanocytes and in human melanocytic nevi in situ (Gupta et al. 2005). This transcription factor, which is known to be required for neural crest cell migration during development (Cheung et al. 2005), provided an important functional contribution to the metastatic ability of the experimentally generated melanoma cells. Since dermal melanocytes are derived from the neural crest, these findings raise the intriguing possibility that factors mediating migratory behaviors in particular embryonic cell types might also contribute to invasiveness following transformation of their differentiated progeny in adults.

CONCLUSION

Recent experimental observations have challenged the conventional conceptual underpinnings of cancer metastasis. Although the genetic heterogeneity–clonal selection model remains indispensable for comprehending malignant progression, it appears likely that other molecular and cellular processes are also relevant to the phenomenon of cancer metastasis. A better understanding of the contribution that the originating cell type of a cancer provides to its metastatic potential may be helpful in interpreting the prognosis-prediction ability of tumor gene expression profiling data. A further examination of the interplay between differentiation state, neoplastic transformation, and metastasis is an important area for future investigation and has broad ramifications for our understanding of metastasis.

ACKNOWLEDGMENTS

This work was supported by U.S. Army Pre-doctoral Breast Cancer Fellowship DAMD17-02-1-0468 (P.B.G.) and by National Institutes of Health/National Cancer Institute grant RO1CA78461-05 (R.A.W.). R.A.W. is an

American Cancer Society Research Professor and a Daniel K. Ludwig Foundation Cancer Research Professor.

REFERENCES

Bounacer A., McGregor A., Skinner J., Bond J., Poghosyan Z., and Wynford-Thomas D. 2004. Mutant ras-induced proliferation of human thyroid epithelial cells requires three effector pathways. *Oncogene* **23:** 7839.

Cheung M., Chaboissier M.C., Mynett A., Hirst E., Schedl A., and Briscoe J. 2005. The transcriptional control of trunk neural crest induction, survival, and delamination. *Dev. Cell* **8:** 179.

Chung G.T., Sundaresan V., Hasleton P., Rudd R., Taylor R., and Rabbitts P.H. 1996. Clonal evolution of lung tumors. *Cancer Res.* **56:** 1609.

Dimri G.P. and Campisi J. 1994. Molecular and cell biology of replicative senescence. *Cold Spring Harbor Symp.Quant. Biol.* **59:** 67.

Dowell J.E. 2003. Cancer from an unknown primary site. *Am. J. Med. Sci.* **326:** 35.

Ehlert J.E. and Kubbutat M.H. 2001. Apoptosis and its relevance in cancer therapy. *Onkologie* **24:** 433.

Elenbaas B., Spirio L., Koerner F., Fleming M.D., Zimonjic D.B., Donaher J.L., Popescu N.C., Hahn W.C., and Weinberg R.A. 2001. Human breast cancer cells generated by oncogenic transformation of primary mammary epithelial cells. *Genes Dev.* **15:** 50.

Glinsky G.V., Higashiyama T., and Glinskii A.B. 2004a. Classification of human breast cancer using gene expression profiling as a component of the survival predictor algorithm. *Clin. Cancer Res.* **10:** 2272.

Glinsky G.V., Glinskii A.B., Stephenson A.J., Hoffman R.M., and Gerald W.L. 2004b. Gene expression profiling predicts clinical outcome of prostate cancer. *J. Clin. Invest.* **113:** 913.

Goel A., Arnold C.N., Niedzwiecki D., Chang D.K., Ricciardiello L., Carethers J.M., Dowell J.M., Wasserman L., Compton C., Mayer R.J., Bertagnolli M.M., and Boland C.R. 2003. Characterization of sporadic colon cancer by patterns of genomic instability. *Cancer Res.* **63:** 1608.

Golub T.R., Slonim D.K., Tamayo P., Huard C., Gaasenbeek M., Mesirov J.P., Coller H., Loh M.L., Downing J.R., Caligiuri M.A., Bloomfield C.D., and Landes E.S. 1999. Molecular classification of cancer: Class discovery and class prediction by gene expression monitoring. *Science* **286:** 531.

Grady W.M. 2004. Genomic instability and colon cancer. *Cancer Metastasis Rev.* **23:** 11.

Gupta P.B., Kuperwasser C., Brunet J.P., Ramaswamy S., Kuo W.L., Gray J.W., Naber S.P., and Weinberg R.A. 2005. The melanocyte differentiation program predisposes to metastasis after neoplastic transformation. *Nat. Genet.* **37:** 1047.

Hahn W.C., Counter C.M., Lundberg A.S., Beijersbergen R.L., Brooks M.W., and Weinberg R.A. 1999. Creation of human tumour cells with defined genetic elements. *Nature* **400:** 464.

Harley C.B. 1991. Telomere loss: Mitotic clock or genetic time bomb? *Mutat. Res.* **256:** 271.

Hiyama T., Tanaka S., Yoshihara M., Sasao S., Kose K., Shima H., Tuncel H., Ueno Y., Ito M., Kitadai Y., Yasui W., Haruma K., and Chayama K. 2004. Chromosomal and microsatellite instability in sporadic gastric cancer. *J. Gastroenterol. Hepatol.* **19:** 756.

Huang E., Cheng S.H., Dressman H., Pittman J., Tsou M.H., Horng C.F., Bild A., Iversen E.S., Liao M., Chen C.M., West M., Nevins J.R., and Huang A.T. 2003. Gene expression predictors of breast cancer outcomes. *Lancet* **361:** 1590.

Kemler R., Hierholzer A., Kanzler B., Kuppig S., Hansen K., Taketo M.M., de Vries W.N., Knowles B.B., and Solter D. 2004. Stabilization of beta-catenin in the mouse zygote leads to premature epithelial-mesenchymal transition in the epiblast. *Development* **131:** 5817.

Kirkin V., Joos S., and Zornig M. 2004. The role of Bcl-2 family members in tumorigenesis. *Biochim. Biophys. Acta* **1644:** 229.

Lawrence J.A. and Steeg P.S. 1996. Mechanisms of tumor invasion and metastasis. *World J. Urol.* **14:** 124.

Lengauer C., Kinzler K.W., and Vogelstein B. 1997. Genetic instability in colorectal cancers. *Nature* **386:** 623.

Li G., Tang L., Zhou X., Tron V., and Ho V. 1998. Chemotherapy-induced apoptosis in melanoma cells is p53 dependent. *Melanoma Res.* **8:** 17.

Lundberg A.S., Randell S.H., Stewart S.A., Elenbaas B., Hartwell K.A., Brooks M.W., Fleming M.D., Olsen J.C., Miller S.W., Weinberg R.A., and Hahn W.C. 2002. Immortalization and transformation of primary human airway epithelial cells by gene transfer. *Oncogene* **21:** 4577.

Martinez-Alvarez C., Blanco M.J., Perez R., Rabadan M.A., Aparicio M., Resel E., Martinez T., and Nieto M.A. 2004. Snail family members and cell survival in physiological and pathological cleft palates. *Dev. Biol.* **265:** 207.

Mertens F., Heim S., Mandahl N., Johansson B., Mertens O., Persson B., Salemark L., Wennerberg J., Jonsson N., and Mitelman F. 1991. Cytogenetic analysis of 33 basal cell carcinomas. *Cancer Res.* **51:** 954.

Milovic M., Popov I., and Jelic S. 2002. Tumor markers in metastatic disease from cancer of unknown primary origin. *Med. Sci. Monit.* **8:** MT25 .

Mora J., Cheung N.K., and Gerald W.L. 2001. Genetic heterogeneity and clonal evolution in neuroblastoma. *Br. J. Cancer* **85:** 182.

Nutt C.L., Mani D.R., Betensky R.A., Tamayo P., Cairncross J.G., Ladd C., Pohl U., Hartmann C., McLaughlin M.E., Batchelor T.T., Black P.M., von Deimling A., Pomeroy S.L., Golub T.R., and Louis D.N. 2003. Gene expression-based classification of malignant gliomas correlates better with survival than histological classification. *Cancer Res.* **63:** 1602.

Oft M., Heider K.H., and Beug H. 1998. TGFbeta signaling is necessary for carcinoma cell invasiveness and metastasis. *Curr. Biol.* **8:** 1243.

Pavlidis N., Briasoulis E., Hainsworth J., and Greco F.A. 2003. Diagnostic and therapeutic management of cancer of an unknown primary. *Eur. J. Cancer* **39:** 1990.

Ramaswamy S., Ross K.N., Lander E.S., and Golub T.R. 2003. A molecular signature of metastasis in primary solid tumors. *Nat. Genet.* **33:** 49.

Ramaswamy S., Tamayo P., Rifkin R., Mukherjee S., Yeang C.H., Angelo M., Ladd C., Reich M., Latulippe E., Mesirov J.P. Poggio T., Gerald W., Loda M., Lander E.S., and Golub T.R. 2001. Multiclass cancer diagnosis using tumor gene expression signatures. *Proc. Natl. Acad. Sci.* **98:** 15149.

Rich J.N., Guo C., McLendon R.E., Bigner D.D., Wang X.F., and Counter C.M. 2001. A genetically tractable model of human glioma formation. *Cancer Res.* **61:** 3556.

Sage J., Mulligan G.J., Attardi L.D., Miller A., Chen S., Williams B., Theodorou E., and Jacks T. 2000. Targeted disruption of the three Rb-related genes leads to loss of G(1) control and immortalization. *Genes Dev.* **14:** 3037.

Savagner P., Kusewitt D.F., Carver E.A., Magnino F., Choi C., Gridley T., and Hudson L.G. 2005. Developmental transcription factor slug is required for effective re-epithelialization by adult keratinocytes. *J. Cell. Physiol.* **202:** 858.

Schleger C., Heck R., and Steinberg P. 2000. The role of wildtype and mutated N-ras in the malignant transformation of liver cells. *Mol. Carcinog.* **28:** 31.

Shih I.M., Zhou W., Goodman S.N., Lengauer C., Kinzler K.W., and Vogelstein B. 2001. Evidence that genetic instability occurs at an early stage of colorectal tumorigenesis. *Cancer Res.* **61:** 818.

Sidransky D., Mikkelsen T., Schwechheimer K., Rosenblum M.L., Cavanee W., and Vogelstein B. 1992. Clonal expansion of p53 mutant cells is associated with brain tumour progression. *Nature* **355:** 846.

Stracke M.L. and Liotta L.A. 1992. Multi-step cascade of tumor cell metastasis. *In Vivo* **6:** 309.

Tanaka T., Saika S., Ohnishi Y., Ooshima A., McAvoy J.W., Liu C.Y., Azhar M., Doetschman T., and Kao W.W. 2004. Fibroblast growth factor 2: Roles of regulation of lens cell proliferation and epithelial-mesenchymal transition in response to injury. *Mol. Vis.* **10:** 462.

Thiery J.P. 2003. Epithelial-mesenchymal transitions in development and pathologies. *Curr. Opin. Cell Biol.* **15:** 740.

Thiery J.P. and Chopin D. 1999. Epithelial cell plasticity in development and tumor progression. *Cancer Metastasis Rev.* **18:** 31.

Urquidi V., Tarin D., and Goodison S. 2000. Role of telomerase in cell senescence and oncogenesis. *Annu. Rev. Med.* **51:** 65.

van de Vijver M.J., He Y.D., van 't Veer L.J., Dai H., Hart A.A., Voskuil D.W., Schreiber G.J., Peterse H.L., Roberts C., Marton M.J., Parrish M., Atsma D., Witteveen A.T., Glas A., Delahaye L., van der Velde T., Bartelink H., Rodenhuis S., Rutgers E.T., Friend S.H., and Bernards R. 2002. A gene-expression signature as a predictor of survival in breast cancer. *N. Engl. J. Med.* **347:** 1999.

van 't Veer L.J., Dai H., van de Vijver M.J., He Y.D., Hart A.A., Mao M., Peterse H.L., van der Kooy K., Marton M.J., Witteveen A.T., Schreiber G.J., Kerkhoven R.M., Roberts C.,

Linsley P.S., Bernards R., and Friend S.H. 2002. Gene expression profiling predicts clinical outcome of breast cancer. *Nature* **415:** 530.

Wang Y., Klijn J.G., Zhang Y., Sieuwerts A.M., Look M.P., Yang F., Talantov D., Timmermans M., Meijer-van Gelder M.E., Yu J., Jatkoe T., Berns E.M., Atkins D., and Foekens J.A. 2005. Gene-expression profiles to predict distant metastasis of lymph-node-negative primary breast cancer. *Lancet* **365:** 671.

Wolman S.R. 1983. Karyotypic progression in human tumors. *Cancer Metastasis Rev.* **2:** 257.

———. 1986. Cytogenetic heterogeneity: Its role in tumor evolution. *Cancer Genet. Cytogenet.* **19:** 129.

Wynford-Thomas D. 1999. Cellular senescence and cancer. *J. Pathol.* **187:** 100.

Yoon S.O., Park S.J., Yun C.H. and Chung A.S. 2003. Roles of matrix metalloproteinases in tumor metastasis and angiogenesis. *J. Biochem. Mol. Biol.* **36:** 128.

Genomic Binding and Transcriptional Regulation by the *Drosophila* Myc and Mnt Transcription Factors

A. ORIAN,* S.S. GREWAL, P.S. KNOEPFLER, B.A. EDGAR, S.M. PARKHURST,
AND R.N. EISENMAN
Division of Basic Sciences, Fred Hutchinson Cancer Research Center, Seattle, Washington 98109-1024

Deregulated expression of members of the *myc* oncogene family has been linked to the genesis of a wide range of cancers, whereas their normal expression is associated with growth, proliferation, differentiation, and apoptosis. Myc proteins are transcription factors that function within a network of transcriptional activators (Myc) and repressors (Mxd/Mad and Mnt), all of which heterodimerize with the bHLHZ protein Mad and bind E-box sequences in DNA. These transcription factors recruit coactivator or corepressor complexes that in turn modify histones. Myc, Mxd/Max, and Mnt proteins have been thought to act on a specific subset of genes. However, expression array studies and, most recently, genomic binding studies suggest that these proteins exhibit widespread binding across the genome. Here we demonstrate by immunostaining of *Drosophila* polytene chromosome that *Drosophila* Myc (dMyc) is associated with multiple euchromatic chromosomal regions. Furthermore, many dMyc-binding regions overlap with regions containing active RNA polymerase II, although dMyc can also be found in regions lacking active polymerase. We also demonstrate that the pattern of dMyc expression in nuclei overlaps with histone markers of active chromatin but not pericentric heterochromatin. dMyc binding is not detected on the X chromosome rDNA cluster (*bobbed* locus). This is consistent with recent evidence that in *Drosophila* cells dMyc regulates rRNA transcription indirectly, in contrast to mammalian cells where direct binding of c-Myc to rDNA has been observed. We further show that the dMyc antagonist dMnt inhibits rRNA transcription in the wing disc. Our results support the view that the Myc/Max/Mad network influences transcription on a global scale.

Several papers in this volume describe a striking association between genomic alterations involving *myc* and different human cancers. Indeed, genetic rearrangements involving the *myc* proto-oncogene have long been linked to an extraordinarily wide spectrum of cancers in humans and other animals (for review, see Henriksson and Luscher 1996; Nesbit et al. 1999; Lutz et al. 2002; Popescu and Zimonjic 2002). The notion that *myc* function is deeply tied to cancer etiology has stimulated a great deal of research on the *myc* gene and its protein product (Myc).

The proteins encoded by the mammalian *myc* gene family (c-, N-, L-Myc) are now understood to function as transcription factors through their heterodimerization with the small basic-helix-loop-helix-zipper (bHLHZ) protein Max. Myc-Max heterodimers recognize the E-box sequence CACGTG with high affinity and activate transcription of synthetic reporter genes and endogenous cellular genes that contain promoter-proximal E-box-binding sites (for recent reviews, see Grandori et al. 2000; Amati et al. 2001; Eisenman 2001; Oster et al. 2002). Myc-Max heterodimers also associate with the BTB-POZ domain protein Miz-1 and inhibit *trans*-activation of Miz-1 target genes (Seoane et al. 2001; Staller et al. 2001; Herold et al. 2002). Other modes of transcriptional repression by Myc have also been reported (Brenner et al.

2005; for review, see Adhikary and Eilers 2005; Kleine-Kohlbrecher et al. 2006).

Myc-Max heterodimers also function within the context of an interesting group of antagonists. These include the Max-binding proteins Mxd1–4 (formerly known as Mad1, Mxi1, Mad3, and Mad4, www.gene.ucl.ac.uk/nomenclature/) and Mnt. These proteins heterodimerize with Max and also recognize the CACGTG E-box sequence. However, the Mxd-Max and Mnt-Max heterodimers repress transcription at these E-box-binding sites and thus act as at least partial antagonists of Myc-Max *trans*-activation function (for review, see Eisenman 2001; Luscher 2001; Zhou and Hurlin 2001; Rottmann and Luscher 2006).

The transcriptional activities of the Myc and Mxd/Mnt proteins are governed by their interactions with higher-order complexes. The highly conserved and functionally essential Myc Box II region of Myc family proteins associates with the TRRAP coactivator, which in turn recruits the Tip60/Tip48/Tip49 and GCN5 histone acetyltransferases (HAT). Other regions of Myc bind the HATs p300 and CBP. Furthermore, components of chromatin-remodeling complexes such as BAF53 and INI1 have also been reported to associate with Myc (for review, see Cole and Nikiforov 2006). The recruitment of putative activating complexes by Myc can be contrasted with the recruitment of repression complexes by the Mxd/Mnt proteins. A small amphipathic helical region (SID) near the amino terminus of all Mxd and Mnt family proteins interacts specifically with a conserved domain within the corepressors mSin3A and mSin3B (Ayer et al. 1995; Schreiber-Agus et al. 1995; Brubaker et al. 2000). This interaction is respon-

---

*Present address: Center for Cancer and Vascular Biology, Rappaport Institute for Medical Research, and the Ruth and Bruce Rappaport Faculty of Medicine, Technion-Israel Institute of Technology, P.O.Box 9649, Bat.Galim Haifa 31096, Israel.

sible for Mxd repression (Cowley et al. 2004). The Sin3 proteins function to recruit class I histone deacetylases (HDACs) and other factors also likely to be involved in transcriptional repression. The associations of Myc and Mxd/Mnt proteins with higher-order coactivator and corepressor complexes suggests that the transcriptional activities of Myc and Mxd/Mnt are due at least in part to histone modifications mediated by the recruited HATs and HDACs. Consistent with this are findings demonstrating that binding of Myc to its target genes results in increased acetylation in the vicinity of the binding site (Frank et al. 2001), whereas Mxd1 (Mad1) binding leads to histone deacetylation (Bouchard et al. 2001; for review, see Amati et al. 2001; Cole and Nikiforov 2006).

ORTHOLOGS OF *Myc*, *Max*, AND *Mnt* GENES IN *DROSOPHILA*

Identification and analysis of *myc*, *max*, and *mxd/mnt* homologs in *Drosophila melanogaster* (denoted *dmyc*, *dmax*, and *dmnt*, respectively) have proven useful in revealing the functions of these genes in both flies and vertebrates (Gallant et al. 1996; Schreiber-Agus et al. 1997; Loo et al. 2005; for recent review, see Gallant 2006). *Drosophila* possesses only one version of each gene, in contrast to the extensive vertebrate *myc* and *mad* gene families, thereby facilitating genetic analysis. Like their vertebrate orthologs, the dMyc and dMnt proteins heterodimerize with dMax, bind CACGTG, and activate (in the case of dMyc-dMax) or repress (in the case of dMnt-dMax) transcription. In addition, *dmyc* has been demonstrated to effectively rescue proliferation in c-*myc* null cells (Trumpp et al. 2001; and our unpublished data) and cotransforms primary rat embryo cells (Schreiber-Agus et al. 1997). *dmyc* is an essential gene involved in cell growth and endoreplication, oogenesis, and apoptosis (Gallant et al. 1996; Schreiber-Agus et al. 1997; Johnston et al. 1999; Maines et al. 2004; Pierce et al. 2004). *dmnt* has recently been shown to be a nonessential gene that functions to limit cell growth (Loo et al. 2005). In addition to conservation of the Max network components themselves, key elements of the machinery that regulates their function are also conserved. For example, mammalian Myc proteins are targeted for ubiquitination and proteasome-dependent degradation by the Fbw7-SCF complex (Welcker et al. 2004a,b; Yada et al. 2004) whereas in *Drosophila* the Fbw7 homolog Archipelago carried out the same function for dMyc (Moberg et al. 2004). Interestingly, although the ubiquitin ligase Skp2 has been suggested to target mammalian Myc for degradation (Kim et al. 2003; von der Lehr et al. 2003), the Skp2 homolog in flies is not involved in turnover of dMyc (Moberg et al. 2004).

WIDESPREAD GENOMIC BINDING BY *DROSOPHILA* Myc/Max/Mnt PROTEINS

A major problem in understanding Myc function in both normal and neoplastic cells has been to delineate the number and nature of the genes that it regulates. Because Myc expression or overexpression causes profound ef-

fects on multiple cellular processes, it is not surprising that expression microarray studies have collectively identified Myc-associated expression changes in a large number (~5%) of cellular genes (see Zeller et al. 2003; for an updated list of Myc target genes, see www.myc-cancer-gene.org/). Modulation of the expression of many of these genes might be considered as only due to an indirect or downstream effect of Myc on the biology of the cell. However, regulation of a large number of these genes by the inducible Myc-ER system was insensitive to cyclo-heximide, suggesting that Myc is directly influencing their expression.

To define genomic binding sites for Myc, we employed the recently described DamID method (van Steensel and Henikoff 2000; van Steensel et al. 2001, 2003; Greil et al. 2003). In this approach, a DNA-binding protein is fused to the bacterial DNA adenine methyltransferase (Dam). Such fusion proteins have been previously shown to methylate adenine in the sequence GATC within 1.5–2 kb of the binding site (van Steensel and Henikoff 2000). The location of the factor-binding sites can be determined by methylation-sensitive restriction enzyme cleavage of the genomic DNA followed by microarray analysis. In our experiments, we expressed low levels of either Dam-dMyc, dMax-Dam, or dMnt-Dam in *Drosophila* Kc cells and isolated 0.1–2 kb DNA fragments produced by digestion with *Dpn*I (which cuts only at G-^{m6}A-T-C, the target sequence for Dam methylation). The Cy5 fluorochrome-labeled DNA fragments from cells expressing the Dam fusion proteins were mixed with Cy3-labeled fragments isolated from cells expressing Dam alone and hybridized to a *Drosophila* cDNA array containing 6255 cDNAs and ESTs. The Cy5:Cy3 fluorescence ratio from multiple experiments was used to establish a statistically significant set of targeted regions. We found that 15.4% of *Drosophila* coding regions (968 of 6255 elements on the array) were associated with one or more of the three dMax-network proteins (Orian et al. 2003). Interestingly, whereas many genomic loci exhibit binding by the three network proteins, a significant number of loci appeared to be targets for a subset of the network factors (see below). dMyc/dMax/dMnt-binding sites are extensively distributed over the four major *Drosophila* chromosomes. However, binding was not random—repetitive elements often associated with pericentric heterochromatin and HP1 binding (the latter also determined using the DamID assay [van Steensel et al. 2001]) were largely devoid of dMyc/dMax/dMnt-binding signal. Furthermore, statistical analysis demonstrated that binding by these factors strongly correlates with the presence of the E-box sequence CACGTG, the previously determined binding site for Myc network proteins (see above). Significant association of dMyc-binding sites with the E-box sequences only occurred in the presence of coexpressed dMax. Other sequence motifs also appear to correlate with binding. These include the binding sites for DREF (DNA replication element factor), the transcription factor Cut, and BEAF32 (a boundary element-associated factor). It remains unclear what role the association of Max network proteins with these sites might play. However, given, for example, the well-established association of mammalian

Myc-Max heterodimers with Miz-1, it is likely that association of dMyc and dMnt with other factors, either as heterodimers with Max or as monomers, could direct the targeting of dMax network proteins to non-E-box sites.

Because a large fraction (48.6%) of the genes found associated with all three dMax network proteins displayed altered expression in response to dMyc in microarray analysis of third-instar larvae (Orian et al. 2003), it seems likely that many of the binding regions are functional. Binding regions that do not correspond to genes displaying altered expression may represent genes whose expression is simply not regulated in the larval stage analyzed, perhaps because cooperating factors, as yet unknown, are absent. Alternatively, binding at a particular site could serve another purpose.

LOCALIZATION OF dMyc BY IMMUNOSTAINING OF *DROSOPHILA* POLYTENE CHROMOSOMES

An important finding of the DamID study is the extensive binding displayed by the dMax network proteins. Nonetheless, our assessment that 15% of *Drosophila* genes are bound by dMax network members is likely to be an underestimate because the array used in our analysis contained cDNAs, thus permitting detection only of binding segments that happen to overlap with an encoded region. Binding of dMax network proteins to intergenic, intronic, or upstream promoter regions would not have been detected in the assay. To obtain another view of dMyc association with genomic DNA, we used an anti-dMyc polyclonal antibody to immunostain *Drosophila* polytene chromosomes (see Bianchi-Frias et al. 2004). Figure 1A shows dMyc (red) and DAPI (blue) staining of a third-instar larval salivary gland chromosome. dMyc appears to be bound to multiple chromosomal segments throughout the length of the chromosome and, in general, appears to be associated with most interband regions. The dense DAPI bands largely represent more condensed chromatin domains. Figure 1B shows staining by antibody against the Hairy transcription factor, another bHLH class protein. Hairy binding is intense in several regions but is considerably less widespread than dMyc, a conclusion supported by the merged images (Fig. 1C) as well as by a DamID study with Hairy (Bianchi-Frias et al. 2004). A more detailed image of a more fully spread anti-dMyc stained chromosome is shown is Figure 1D (green). Co-staining of the chromosome with antibody against phosphorylated Ser-5 within the carboxy-terminal domain (CTD) of RNA polymerase II (red) is shown in Figure 1E, with merged images in Figure 1F. This phosphorylated form of RNA polymerase II (Upstate Biotechnology) is associated with an actively transcribing form of the polymerase. It is evident that both the phospho-CTD staining and the dMyc staining occur extensively throughout the chromosome, again in interband, less condensed, regions and that there is considerable overlap between dMyc and active RNA polymerase II. However, there is also clear evidence of anti-dMyc staining to regions that do not stain with anti-phospho-CTD (Fig. 1F merged image and Fig. 1F', higher magnification merged image). This is consistent with the

comparison between the larval expression array data and the DamID-binding data mentioned above and provides support for the notion that dMyc can interact with regions that are not constitutively transcribed.

dMyc ASSOCIATES WITH REGIONS OF ACTIVE CHROMATIN

The association of dMyc binding with coding regions in the DamID experiments, as well as detection of dMyc and active RNA polymerase II in interband, non-heterochromatic regions of polytene chromosomes, suggests that dMyc is largely present in regions of active chromatin. To further explore this idea, we carried out immunostaining with antibodies against acetylated Lys- 9 in histone H3 (H3-Ac-K9) and dimethyl Lys-9 in histone H3 (H3-diME-K9). These histone modifications correlate with either active chromatin, in the case of H3-Ac-K9, or inactive chromatin, in the case of H3-diME-K9 (Berger 2001; Turner 2002). We first examined nurse cells and follicle cells within the *Drosophila* ovariole. Both of these cell types exhibit distinct staining patterns with antibodies against H3-diME-K9 and against H3-Ac-K9 (Fig. 2A–D). Anti-H3-diME-K9 predominantly stains one discrete region near the periphery of each nurse or follicle cell nucleus (Fig. 2A,C). In contrast, anti-H3-Ac-K9 stains most of the nucleoplasm in both nurse and follicle cells (Fig. 2B,D). Immunostaining with a monoclonal antibody against dMyc shows a distribution similar to the nucleoplasmic staining with anti-H3-Ac-K9 (Fig. 2A'–D'). This is confirmed in the merged images shown in Figure 2A''–D'': dMyc largely overlaps with H3-Ac-K9 but shows diminished overlap or exclusion from areas occupied by H3-diME-K9.

dMyc is known to be expressed during oogenesis in *Drosophila*, and hypomorphic mutations in *dmyc* result in degeneration of the ovaries (Gallant et al. 1996). Figure 2E–E'' shows H3-Ac-K9 and dMyc at several stages of ovary development. As shown previously, dMyc can be detected in the germarium, one of the earliest stages in oogenesis (Fig. 2E', asterisk). H3-Ac-K9 can also be detected at this stage and partly overlaps with dMyc expression (Fig. 2E–E''). At later stages, both dMyc and H3-Ac-K9 levels appear to diminish but then increase at more advanced stages where they are both evident in nurse and follicle cells. dMyc and H3-Ac-K9 can be detected in follicle cells at late stages (note intense overlap in the peripherally staining cells in Fig. 2E''). Although dMyc remains detectable in later-stage nurse cells, H3-Ac-K9 staining is markedly diminished at later stages. However, the oocyte nucleus appears to have high H3-Ac-K9 levels but almost no detectable dMyc. Therefore, although H3-Ac-K9 and dMyc staining are coincident in many situations, they can be uncoupled. These changes are consistent with the predicted periods of high and low transcriptional activity during oogenesis. One possibility is that even transient dMyc expression could act to generate a more stable state of increased acetylation. Our results indicate that dMyc is frequently associated with active chromatin, but the relationship between dMyc and H3-Ac-K9 is dynamic.

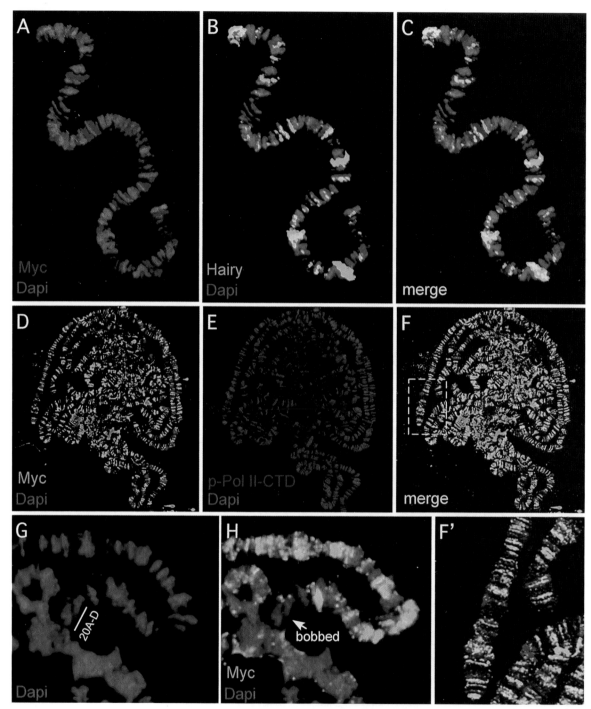

Figure 1. Analysis of the genomic loci bound by dMyc, Hairy, and phospho-RNA polymerase II. (*A–C*) Immunostaining of dMyc (*red*) and Hairy (*green*) on third-instar larval salivary gland polytene chromosome sets counterstained with DAPI (*blue*) to visualize the chromosomes. (*D–F*) Binding of dMyc (*green*) and p-Pol-II CTD (*red*; antibody directed against p-Ser5 CTD PolII). (*F'*) Higher magnification of the rectangle depicted in *F*. (*G–H*) Myc does not bind to the rDNA locus *"bobbed"* (20F). (*G*) Higher magnification of X chromosomal arm regions 17–20 counterstained with DAPI (*blue*) to visualize the chromosomes. (*H*) Myc binding (*green*) and DAPI (*blue*), the rDNA locus *"bobbed"* is indicated by arrow.

dMyc IS NOT ASSOCIATED WITH THE *bobbed* rDNA LOCUS

The DamID study and expression microarray analysis indicate that dMyc binds to multiple sites in the genome in a manner that is associated with transcriptional stimulation of many genes (Orian et al. 2003). In general, most of the genes analyzed in both *Drosophila* and mammalian systems are those transcribed by RNA polymerase II. However, recent work in mammalian cells has provided evidence that among the genes regulated by c-Myc are those that are also transcribed by RNA polymerase I and III. Stimulation of transcription of a subset of small RNAs, many of which are involved in transla-

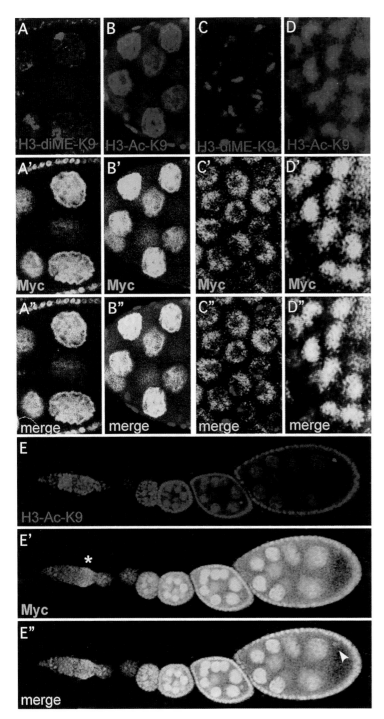

Figure 2. Myc occupies genomic regions that correlate with active chromatin. Immunostaining of *Drosophila* nurse cells (*A-B′′*), follicle cells (*C–D′′*), and during oogenesis (*E–E′′*). (*A–A′′, C–C′′*) dMyc binding is excluded from genomic loci associated with inactive genes. dMyc expression is depicted in green. H3-diME-K9, a marker of inactive chromatin, is shown in red. The lack of overlap in expression is shown in the merged image (lack of yellow staining; A′′, C′′). (*B–B′′, D–D′′*) dMyc binding correlates with genomic regions associated with active chromatin. dMyc expression is depicted in green. H3-Ac-K9, a marker of active chromatin, is shown in red. The overlap in expression is shown in the merged image (extensive yellow staining; B′′, D′′). (*E–E′′*) The pattern of Ac-H3-K9 (*red*; *E*) correlates with dMyc protein expression (*green*; *E′*) during *Drosophila* oogenesis. dMyc expression is observed early in the germarium (*). Regions of overlapping expression are depicted in yellow (merged image; *E′′*). The oocyte nucleus is highly acetylated and is marked by a white arrow (*E′′*).

tion, mediated by RNA polymerase III occurs through association of c-Myc protein with the basal transcription machinery and does not involve direct binding of Myc protein to DNA (Gomez-Roman et al. 2003). In contrast, c-Myc can be detected in nucleoli and binds to multiple E-box sites clustered within the human rDNA regulatory regions and interacts directly with the SL1 subunits of the RNA polymerase I complex, resulting in a marked stimulation of rRNA transcription (Arabi et al. 2005; Grandori et al. 2005). In mammalian cells there is also evidence that c-Myc regulates rRNA abundance indirectly through such targets as UBF (Poortinga et al.

2004), fibrillarin (Coller et al. 2000), and Bop1 (Holzel et al. 2005).

In *Drosophila*, dMyc has been shown to be required for rRNA synthesis and ribosome biogenesis during larval development. However, no direct binding of dMyc to *Drosophila* rDNA genes is detected in DamID analysis or chromatin immunoprecipitation experiments (Grewal et al. 2005; S. Grewal, pers. comm.). Instead, it appears that dMyc indirectly regulates fly rDNA expression entirely through up-regulated transcription of target genes that are involved in ribosome biogenesis. These include the critical RNA-polymerase-I-associated factor dTIF-IA and the second largest subunit of RNA polymerase I, RpI135, as well as multiple genes involved in rRNA processing and ribosomal proteins (Grewal et al. 2005).

Consistent with the above findings, our immunostaining of *Drosophila* polytene chromosomes failed to detect association of dMyc with the rRNA encoding *bobbed* locus in the 20F region of the X chromosome. This lack of dMyc binding is striking, especially considering the extensive association of dMyc with regions adjacent to *bobbed* on the same chromosome (Fig. 1G,H). It is important to note that rDNA is actively transcribed in salivary glands at this stage of larval development (Karpen et al. 1988). These data underscore an interesting divergence of molecular function between the *Drosophila* and mammalian Myc proteins. In both systems, Myc proteins control ribosome biogenesis indirectly by influencing expression of genes involved in rRNA transcription and processing and its assembly into ribosomes. However, in mammalian cells c-Myc has acquired the additional function of stimulating pre-rRNA abundance through direct association with the RNA polymerase I transcriptional apparatus. Because *Drosophila* rDNA genes lack canonical E-boxes (Grewal et al. 2005), whereas mammalian rDNA genes contain multiple E-boxes (Arabi et al. 2005; Grandori et al. 2005), it is possible that mammalian rDNA transcription units have evolved to take advantage of c-Myc transcriptional activity.

dMnt INHIBITS rRNA TRANSCRIPTION

As described above, our DamID analysis demonstrated a striking overlap between binding sites for dMyc and dMnt. dMnt is the single *Drosophila* ortholog of mammalian Mxd/Mnt proteins (Orian et al. 2003). This is consistent with limited chromatin immunoprecipitation data in mammalian cells which demonstrated that c-Myc and Mxd1 (Mad1) have the same binding sites in the cyclin D2 promoter (Bouchard et al. 2001). In addition, T cells overexpressing Mxd1 were found to down-regulate a large number of genes, 80% of whose expression was previously known to be up-regulated by Myc (Iritani et al. 2002). Indeed, there is considerable evidence that mammalian Mxd/Mnt and *Drosophila* dMnt proteins antagonize Myc's biological functions relating to growth, proliferation, transformation, and apoptosis (Lahoz et al. 1994; Cerni et al. 1995; Chen et al. 1995; Koskinen et al. 1995; Roussel et al. 1996; Loo et al. 2005). This antagonism is likely to occur in part through competition for available Max protein and for E-box-binding sites (Walker et al. 2005), as well as through the opposing transcriptional activities of Myc-Max and Mxd-Max heterodimers. The transcriptional repression activity of Mxd and Mnt proteins is mediated by association with mSin3-HDAC corepressor complexes (for review, see Ayer 1999; Knoepfler and Eisenman 1999), and the sole *Drosophila* homolog, dMnt, has been shown to bind dSin3 and to function as a repressor at promoter-proximal E-boxes (Loo et al. 2005).

Because dMyc stimulation of rRNA transcription is a critical function related to cell and organismal growth in

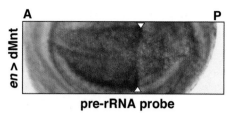

pre-rRNA probe

Figure 3. dMnt inhibits rRNA synthesis. An en-Gal4 driver was used to express a dMnt transgene in the posterior (*P*; *right half*) compartments of wing imaginal discs. Wing discs were analyzed for levels of pre-rRNA by in situ hybridization using a probe to the internal transcribed spacer (ITS1) region of the precursor RNA. The arrowheads represent the A-P posterior border, posterior to the right.

Drosophila, we tested whether dMnt would abrogate rRNA transcription. UAS-dMnt was expressed as a transgene under control of an *engrailed*-Gal4 driver. This driver results in dMnt transgene expression in the posterior compartment (P) of the wing imaginal disc. The amount of rRNA transcription is assessed by in situ hybridization with a probe to the internal transcribed spacer region which only detects the uncleaved precursor rRNA. Because the *engrailed* driver is not expressed in the anterior portion (A) of the disc, this region serves as a control. Figure 3 shows that the levels of pre-rRNA signal are markedly lower throughout the posterior compartment. These findings indicate that expression of dMnt results in down-regulation of pre-rRNA synthesis, consistent with the notion that dMnt antagonizes dMyc's growth-stimulatory effects (Loo et al. 2005). More detailed expression array analysis will be required to determine specifically which dMyc targets are down-regulated by dMnt expression.

CONCLUSIONS

We have presented evidence suggesting that the *Drosophila* dMyc transcription factor exhibits widespread binding to *Drosophila* genomic DNA and that many binding sites are associated with actively transcribed regions of chromatin. This was initially demonstrated in the DamID analysis, which indicated that dMax network proteins associate with approximately 15% of *Drosophila* coding regions on all four major chromosomes (Orian et al. 2003). We surmise that this number is likely to be an underestimate because our approach only detected binding regions located within coding regions and would have excluded intronic and intergenic regions. Our immunostaining of polytene chromosomes shown in Figure 1 provides further support for this idea, since nearly all interband regions appear to be associated with dMyc. Additionally, a majority of regions with actively transcribing RNA polymerase II coincide with the anti-dMyc stained areas, a result consistent with expression array analysis showing that nearly half of dMyc-binding sites correspond to genes whose expression is regulated by dMyc (Orian et al. 2003).

Evidence that dMyc binding and gene regulation are widespread has not been confined to *Drosophila*. Chromatin immunoprecipitation assays in human cells have shown that c-Myc is associated with 8–10% of coding regions and that many of these regions display augmented histone acetylation (Fernandez et al. 2003). Furthermore, array analyses of chromatin immunoprecipitates (ChIP-chip) have confirmed widespread binding by Myc (Cawley et al. 2004; Li et al. 2003), leading to a prediction of 24,000 binding sites in the human genome for c-Myc (Cawley et al. 2004).

The nuclear staining experiments shown in Figure 2 also provide support for the view that dMyc is largely present in active regions of chromatin. dMyc immuno-staining occurs throughout the nucleoplasm, coinciding with H3-Ac-K9, a mark of active chromatin. Importantly, the pericentric heterochromatic regions of the nucleus marked by H3-diMe-K9 are devoid of dMyc staining. Therefore, the DamID studies, and the chromosomal and nuclear immunostaining experiments together, argue that dMyc binding is widespread and correlates with active gene expression. It is important to note, however, that significant amounts of dMyc chromosomal staining do not overlap with anti-phospho-CTD RNA polymerase II immunostained regions (Fig. 1D–F), raising the possibility that dMyc can occupy specific sites which are not undergoing active transcription. Such sites may represent regions that, although transcriptionally inactive, have the potential to be activated or require a component not dependent on the phospho-CTD. Alternatively, they may simply be sites that dMyc occupies without exerting a transcriptional response.

Taken together, the evidence relating to widespread binding and gene activation by both *Drosophila* and mammalian Myc proteins prompts a reassessment of Myc protein function. The view that Myc functions as a standard transcription factor targeting a discrete subset of genes is unlikely to be correct. Instead, Myc can perhaps be considered as a more global DNA-binding protein affecting the transcription or the transcriptional potential of a large number of genes. This view is consistent with the very profound effects on cellular behavior and oncogenesis associated with Myc expression, in that its proximity to such a large number of coding regions implies a direct regulation of many targets, particularly those involved in cell growth. Although less is known about the Mxd/Mnt proteins, our DamID data and the strong effects of dMnt expression on rRNA synthesis make it likely that Mxd/Mnt antagonize Myc activity at many gene targets. To what extent the difference in the ability of vertebrate and invertebrate Myc proteins to directly regulate rRNA transcription accounts for the ability of vertebrate Myc proteins to regulate proliferation and oncogenesis in addition to growth remains an open question. Another important question now under study is whether the widespread binding of Myc occurs as a result of changes in chromatin structure or whether Myc binding itself acts to dictate chromatin structure over large regions of the genome.

ACKNOWLEDGMENTS

We are grateful to Julio Vazquez (Scientific Imagining Facility) and Jeffrey Delrow (Genomics Facility) for discussion, advice, and assistance. This work was supported by grants from the National Institutes of Health to R.N.E. (RO1CA57138), S.M.P. (RO1GM073021), and B.A.E. (RO1 GM51186). A.O. was supported by the Human Frontiers Science Program (CDA 0048/2004C). A.O. and P.S.K. are Special Fellows of the Lymphoma and Leukemia Society. S.S.G. was supported by a research fellowship from the SASS Foundation for Medical Research. R.N.E. is an American Cancer Society Research Professor.

REFERENCES

Adhikary S. and Eilers M. 2005. Transcriptional regulation and transformation by Myc proteins. *Nat. Rev. Mol. Cell Biol.* **6:** 635.

Amati B., Frank S.R., Donjerkovic D., and Taubert S. 2001. Function of the c-Myc oncoprotein in chromatin remodeling and transcription. *Biochim. Biophys. Acta* **1471:** M135.

Arabi A., Wu S., Shiue C., Ridderstrale K., Larsson L.-G., and Wright A.P.H. 2005. c-Myc associates with ribosomal DNA in the nucleolus and activates RNA polymerase I transcription. *Nat. Cell Biol.* **7:** 303.

Ayer D.E. 1999. Histone deacetylases: Transcriptional repression with SINers and NuRDs. *Trends Cell Biol.* **9:** 193.

Ayer D.E., Lawrence Q.A., and Eisenman R.N. 1995. Mad-Max transcriptional repression is mediated by ternary complex formation with mammalian homologs of yeast repressor Sin3. *Cell* **80:** 767.

Berger S.L. 2001. Molecular biology. The histone modification circus. *Science* **292:** 64.

Bianchi-Frias D., Orian A., Delrow J.J., Vazquez J., Rosales-Nieves A.E., and Parkhurst S.M. 2004. Hairy transcriptional repression targets and cofactor recruitment in *Drosophila*. *PLoS Biol.* **2:** E178.

Bouchard C., Dittrich O., Kiermaier A., Dohmann K., Menkel A., Eilers M., and Luscher B. 2001. Regulation of cyclin D2 gene expression by the Myc/Max/Mad network: Myc- dependent TRRAP recruitment and histone acetylation at the cyclin D2 promoter. *Genes Dev.* **15:** 2042.

Brenner C., Deplus R., Didelot C., Loriot A., Vire E., De Smet C., Gutierrez A., Danovi D., Bernard D., Boon T., Pelicci P. G., Amati B., Kouzarides T., de Launoit Y., Di Croce L., and Fuks F. 2005. Myc represses transcription through recruitment of DNA methyltransferase corepressor. *EMBO J.* **24:** 336.

Brubaker K., Cowley S.M., Huang K., Loo L., Yochum G.S., Ayer D.E., Eisenman R.N., and Radhakrishnan I. 2000. Solution structure of the interacting domains of the Mad-Sin3 complex: Implications for recruitment of a chromatin-modifying complex. *Cell* **103:**655.

Cawley S., Bekiranov S., Ng H.H., Kapranov P., Sekinger E.A., Kampa D., Piccolboni A., Sementchenko V., Cheng J., Williams A.J., Wheeler R., Wong B., Drenkow J., Yamanaka M., Patel S., Brubaker S., Tammana H., Helt G., Struhl K., and Gingeras T.R. 2004. Unbiased mapping of transcription factor binding sites along human chromosomes 21 and 22 points to widespread regulation of noncoding RNAs. *Cell* **116:** 499.

Cerni C., Bousset K., Seelos C., Burkhardt H., Henriksson M., and Luscher B. 1995. Differential effects by Mad and Max on transformation by cellular and viral oncoproteins. *Oncogene* **11:** 587.

Chen J., Willingham T., Margraf L.R., Schreiber-Agus N., DePinho R.A., and Nisen P.D. 1995. Effects of the MYC oncogene antagonist, MAD, on proliferation, cell cycling and the malignant phenotype of human brain tumor cells. *Nat. Med.* **1:** 638.

Cole M.D. and Nikiforov M.A. 2006. Transcriptional activation by the Myc oncoprotein. *Curr. Top. Microbiol. Immunol.* **302:** (in press).

Coller H.A., Grandori C., Tamayo P., Colbert T., Lander E.S., Eisenman R.N., and Golub T.R. 2000. Expression analysis with oligonucleotide microarrays reveals MYC regulates genes involved in growth, cell cycle, signaling, and adhesion. *Proc. Natl. Acad. Sci.* **97:** 3260.

Cowley S.M., Kang R.S., Frangioni J.V., Yada J.J., DeGrand A.M., Radhakrishnan I., and Eisenman R.N. 2004. Functional analysis of the Mad1-mSin3A repressor-corepressor interaction reveals determinants of specificity, affinity, and transcriptional response. *Mol. Cell. Biol.* **24:** 2698.

Eisenman R.N. 2001. Deconstructing myc. *Genes Dev.* **15:** 2023.

Fernandez P.C., Frank S.R., Wang L., Schroeder M., Liu S., Greene J., Cocito A., and Amati B. 2003. Genomic targets of the human c-Myc protein. *Genes Dev.* **17:** 1115.

Frank S.R., Schroeder M., Fernandez P., Taubert S., and Amati B. 2001. Binding of c-Myc to chromatin mediates mitogen-induced acetylation of histone H4 and gene activation. *Genes Dev.* **15:** 2069.

Gallant P. 2006. Myc/Max/Mad in invertebrates. The evolution of the Max network. *Curr. Top. Microbiol. Immunol.* **302:** (in press).

Gallant P., Shiio Y., Cheng P.F., Parkhurst S., and Eisenman R.N. 1996. Myc and Max homologs in *Drosophila*. *Science* **274:** 1523.

Gomez-Roman N., Grandori C., Eisenman R.N., and White R.J. 2003. Direct activation of RNA polymerase III transcription by c-Myc. *Nature* **421:** 290.

Grandori C., Cowley S.M., James L.P., and Eisenman R.N. 2000. The MYC/MAX/MAD network and the transcriptional control of cell behavior. *Annu. Rev. Cell Dev. Biol.* **16:** 653.

Grandori C., Gomez-Roman N., Felton-Edkins Z.A., Ngouenet C., Galloway D.A., Eisenman R.N., and White R.J. 2005. c-Myc binds to human ribosomal DNA and stimulates transcription of rRNA genes by RNA polymerase I. *Nat. Cell Biol.* **7:** 311.

Greil F., van der Kraan I., Delrow J., Smothers J.F., de Wit E., Bussemaker H.J., van Driel R., Henikoff S., and van Steensel B. 2003. Distinct HP1 and Su(var)3-9 complexes bind to sets of developmentally coexpressed genes depending on chromosomal location. *Genes Dev.* **17:** 2825.

Grewal S.S., Li L., Orian A., Eisenman R.N., and Edgar B.A. 2005. Myc-dependent regulation of ribosomal RNA synthesis during *Drosophila* development. *Nat. Cell Biol.* **7:** 295.

Henriksson M. and Luscher B. 1996. Proteins of the Myc network: Essential regulators of cell growth and differentiation. *Adv. Cancer Res.* **68:** 109.

Herold S., Wanzel M., Beuger V., Frohme C., Beul D., Hillukkala T., Syvaoja J., Saluz H.P., Haenel F., and Eilers M. 2002. Negative regulation of the mammalian UV response by Myc through association with Miz-1. *Mol. Cell* **10:** 509.

Holzel M., Rohrmoser M., Schlee M., Grimm T., Harasim T., Malamoussi A., Gruber-Eber A., Kremmer E., Hiddemann W., Bornkamm G.W., and Eick D. 2005. Mammalian WDR12 is a novel member of the Pes1-Bop1 complex and is required for ribosome biogenesis and cell proliferation. *J. Cell Biol.* **170:** 367.

Iritani B.M., Delrow J., Grandori C., Gomez I., Klacking M., Carlos L.S., and Eisenman R.N. 2002. Modulation of T-lymphocyte development, growth and cell size by the Myc antagonist and transcriptional repressor Mad1. *EMBO J.* **21:** 4820.

Johnston L.A., Prober D.A., Edgar B.A., Eisenman R.N., and Gallant P. 1999. Drosophila *myc* regulates growth during development. *Cell* **98:** 779.

Karpen G.H., Schaefer J.E., and Laird C.D. 1988. A *Drosophila* rRNA gene located in euchromatin is active in transcription and nucleolus formation. *Genes Dev.* **2:** 1745.

Kim S.Y., Herbst A., Tworkowski K.A., Salghetti S.E., and Tansey W.P. 2003. Skp2 regulates myc protein stability and activity. *Mol. Cell* **11:** 1177.

Kleine-Kohlbrecher D., Adhikary S., and Eilers M. 2006. Mechanisms of transcriptional repression by Myc. *Curr. Top. Microbiol. Immunol.* **302:** (in press).

Knoepfler P.S. and Eisenman R.N. 1999. Sin meets NuRD and other tails of repression. *Cell* **99:** 447.

Koskinen P.J., Ayer D.E., and Eisenman R.N. 1995. Repression of Myc-Ras co-transformation by Mad is mediated by multiple protein-protein interactions. *Cell Growth Differ.* **6:** 623.

Lahoz E.G., Xu L., Schreiber-Agus N., and DePinho R.A. 1994. Suppression of Myc, but not E1a, transformation activity by Max-associated proteins, Mad and Mxi1. *Proc. Natl. Acad. Sci.* **91:** 5503.

Li Z., Van Calcar S., Qu C., Cavenee W.K., Zhang M.Q., and Ren B. 2003. A global transcriptional regulatory role for c-Myc in Burkitt's lymphoma cells. *Proc. Natl. Acad. Sci.* **100:** 8164.

Loo L.W., Secombe J., Little J.T., Carlos L.S., Yost C., Cheng P.F., Flynn E.M., Edgar B.A., and Eisenman R.N. 2005. The transcriptional repressor dMnt is a regulator of growth in *Drosophila melanogaster*. *Mol. Cell. Biol.* **25:** 7078.

Luscher B. 2001. Function and regulation of the transcription factors of the Myc/Max/Mad network. *Gene* **277:** 1.

Lutz W., Leon J., and Eilers M. 2002. Contributions of Myc to tumorigenesis. *Biochim. Biophys. Acta* **1602:** 61.

Maines J.Z., Stevens L.M., Tong X., and Stein D. 2004. *Drosophila* dMyc is required for ovary cell growth and endoreplication. *Development* **131:** 775.

Moberg K.H., Mukherjee A., Veraksa A., Artavanis-Tsakonas S., and Hariharan I.K. 2004. The *Drosophila* F box protein archipelago regulates dMyc protein levels in vivo. *Curr. Biol.* **14:** 965.

Nesbit C.E., Tersak J.M., and Prochownik E.V. 1999. MYC oncogenes and human neoplastic disease. *Oncogene* **18:** 3004.

Orian A., van Steensel B., Delrow J., Bussemaker H.J., Li L., Sawado T., Williams E., Loo L.M., Cowley S.M., Yost C., Pierce S., Edgar B.A., Parkhurst S.M., and Eisenman R.N. 2003. Genomic binding by the *Drosophila* Myc, Max, Mad.Mnt transcription factor network. *Genes Dev.* **17:** 1101.

Oster S.K., Ho C.S., Soucie E.L., and Penn L.Z. 2002. The myc oncogene: MarvelouslY Complex. *Adv. Cancer Res.* **84:** 81.

Pierce S.B., Yost C., Britton J.S., Loo L.W., Flynn E.M., Edgar B.A., and Eisenman R.N. 2004. dMyc is required for larval growth and endoreplication in *Drosophila*. *Development* **131:** 2317.

Poortinga G., Hannan K.M., Snelling H., Walkley C.R., Jenkins A., Sharkey K., Wall M., Brandenburger Y., Palatsides M., Pearson R.B., McArthur G.A., and Hannan R.D. 2004. MAD1 and c-MYC regulate UBF and rDNA transcription during granulocyte differentiation. *EMBO J.* **23:** 3325.

Popescu N.C. and Zimonjic D.B. 2002. Chromosome-mediated alterations of the MYC gene in human cancer. *J. Cell. Mol. Med.* **6:** 151.

Rottmann S. and Luscher B. 2006. The Mad side of the Max network: Antagonising the function of Myc and more. *Curr. Top. Microbiol. Immunol.* **302:** (in press).

Roussel M.F., Ashmun R.A., Sherr C.J., Eisenman R.N., and Ayer D.E. 1996. Inhibition of cell proliferation by the Mad1 transcriptional repressor. *Mol. Cell. Biol.* **16:** 2796.

Schreiber-Agus N., Stein D., Chen K., Goltz J.S., Stevens L., and DePinho R.A. 1997. *Drosophila* Myc is oncogenic in mammalian cells and plays a role in the diminutive phenotype. *Proc. Natl. Acad. Sci.* **94:** 1235.

Schreiber-Agus N., Chin L., Chen K., Torres R., Rao G., Guida P., Skoultchi A.I., and DePinho R.A. 1995. An amino-terminal domain of Mxi1 mediates anti-Myc oncogenic activity and interacts with a homolog of the yeast repressor SIN3. *Cell* **80:** 777.

Seoane J., Pouponnot C., Staller P., Schader M., Eilers M., and Massague J. 2001. TGFβ influences Myc, Miz-1 and Smad to control the CDK inhibitor p15^{INK4b}. *Nat. Cell Biol.* **3:** 400.

Staller P., Peukert K., Kiermaier A., Seoane J., Lukas J., Karsunky H., Möröy T., Bartek J., Massague J., Hänel F., and Eilers M. 2001. Repression of p15^{INK4b} expression by Myc through association with Miz-1. *Nat. Cell Biol.* **3:** 392.

Trumpp A., Refaeli Y., Oskarsson T., Gasser S., Murphy M., Martin G.R., and Bishop J.M. 2001. c-Myc regulates mammalian body size by controlling cell number but not cell size. *Nature* **414:** 768.

Turner B.M. 2002. Cellular memory and the histone code. *Cell*
    111: 285.
van Steensel B. and Henikoff S. 2000. Identification of in vivo
    DNA targets of chromatin proteins using tethered Dam
    methyltransferase. *Nat. Biotechnol.* **18:** 424.
van Steensel B., Delrow J., and Bussemaker H.J. 2003. Genome-
    wide analysis of *Drosophila* GAGA factor target genes re-
    veals context-dependent DNA binding. *Proc. Natl. Acad. Sci.*
    100: 2580.
van Steensel B., Delrow J., and Henikoff S. 2001. Chromatin
    profiling using targeted DNA adenine methyltransferase. *Nat.
    Genet.* **27:** 304.
von der Lehr N., Johansson S., Wu S., Bahram F., Castell A.,
    Cetinkaya C., Hydbring P., Weidung I., Nakayama K.,
    Nakayama K.I., Soderberg O., Kerppola T.K., and Larsson
    L.G. 2003. The F-box protein Skp2 participates in c-Myc pro-
    teosomal degradation and acts as a cofactor for c-Myc-regu-
    lated transcription. *Mol. Cell* **11:** 1189.
Walker W., Zhou Z.Q., Ota S., Wynshaw-Boris A., and Hurlin
    P.J. 2005. Mnt-Max to Myc-Max complex switching regu-

lates cell cycle entry. *J. Cell Biol.* **169:** 405.
Welcker M., Orian A., Grim J.A., Eisenman R.N., and Clurman
    B.E. 2004a. A nucleolar isoform of the Fbw7 ubiquitin ligase
    regulates c-Myc and cell size. *Curr. Biol.* **14:** 1852.
Welcker M., Orian A., Jin J., Grim J.A., Harper J.W., Eisenman
    R.N., and Clurman B.E. 2004b. The Fbw7 tumor suppressor reg-
    ulates glycogen synthase kinase 3 phosphorylation-dependent c-
    Myc protein degradation. *Proc. Natl. Acad. Sci.* **101:** 9085.
Yada M., Hatakeyama S., Kamura T., Nishiyama M., Tsune-
    matsu R., Imaki H., Ishida N., Okumura F., Nakayama K., and
    Nakayama K.I. 2004. Phosphorylation-dependent degrada-
    tion of c-Myc is mediated by the F-box protein Fbw7. *EMBO
    J.* **23:** 2116.
Zeller K.I., Jegga A.G., Aronow B.J., O'Donnell K.A., and Dang
    C.V. 2003. An integrated database of genes responsive to the
    Myc oncogenic transcription factor: Identification of direct
    genomic targets. *Genome Biol.* **4:** R69.
Zhou Z.Q. and Hurlin P.J. 2001. The interplay between Mad and
    Myc in proliferation and differentiation. *Trends Cell Biol.* **11:**
    S10.

Regulation of the *Arf/p53* Tumor Surveillance Network by E2F

P.J. Iaquinta, A. Aslanian,* and J.A. Lees

Center for Cancer Research, Massachusetts Institute of Technology, Cambridge, Massachusetts 02139

Deregulation of the cell cycle machinery plays a critical role in tumorigenesis. In particular, functional inactivation of the retinoblastoma protein (pRB) is a key event. pRB's tumor suppressive activity is at least partially dependent on its ability to regulate the activity of the E2F transcription factors. E2F controls the expression of genes that encode the cellular proliferation machinery. E2F can also trigger apoptosis when it is inappropriately expressed. Here we present evidence that E2F acts to directly regulate the *Arf/p53* tumor surveillance network. In normal cells, a single member of the E2F family, E2F3, participates in the transcriptional silencing of *Arf*. In response to oncogenic stress, the activating E2Fs, E2F1, 2, and E2F3A, all associate with *Arf* and promote its transcription. These findings raise the possibility that E2F acts as a sensor of inappropriate versus normal proliferative signals and determines whether or not the *Arf/p53* tumor surveillance network is engaged.

The retinoblastoma gene (*RB-1*) was the first identified tumor suppressor, and it is mutated in one-third of all human tumors (Sherr 1996). In normal cells, the retinoblastoma protein (pRB) arrests cells in the G_1 phase of the cell cycle. This inhibition is relieved through activation of the cell cycle kinase cyclin D/cdk4 and the sequential phosphorylation of pRB by cyclin D/cdk4 and cyclin E/cdk2. Negative growth signals promote cell cycle arrest by increasing the expression of the cdk inhibitor, p16, a known tumor suppressor. Most, if not all, human tumors carry either inactivating mutations in *Rb* or *p16* or activating mutations that up-regulate cyclin D/cdk4 (Sherr 1996). Thus, functional inactivation of pRB is an essential step in the tumorigenic process.

Molecular studies have identified numerous proteins that bind to the pRB tumor suppressor (Morris and Dyson 2001). The vast majority of these proteins are known components of transcriptional complexes including chromatin regulators (e.g., swi/snf proteins, HDACs, and histone methylases) and transcription factors. Of these interactors, the E2F transcription factors are by far the best characterized (Trimarchi and Lees 2002; Dimova and Dyson 2005). As we outline below, there is overwhelming evidence that pRB's tumor suppressive activity is at least partially dependent on its ability to regulate E2F. In normal cells, E2F controls the expression of genes that encode essential cellular proteins including cell cycle regulators, nucleotide biosynthesis enzymes, histone variants, DNA damage regulators, and DNA repair proteins (Trimarchi and Lees 2002; Cam and Dynlacht 2003). These classic E2F-responsive genes share a highly characteristic pattern of transcription: They are repressed during G_0/G_1, get activated in late G_1, and are switched off again in $S/G_2/M$. This periodic expression is controlled by the concerted action of the E2F proteins and their associated regulatory proteins.

We know that the endogenous E2F activity is generated from the concerted action of multiple E2F complexes (Trimarchi and Lees 2002). Most E2F complexes are heterodimeric, containing one E2F and one DP protein, but recent studies have shown that E2F7 and E2F8 function as homodimers (Trimarchi and Lees 2002; de Bruin et al. 2003; Di Stefano et al. 2003; Christensen et al. 2005; Maiti et al. 2005). The biological properties of individual E2F complexes are determined largely by the E2F subunit. To date, eight *E2f* genes and nine E2F proteins have been identified (Christensen et al. 2005; Dimova and Dyson 2005; Maiti et al. 2005). The discrepancy between these two numbers is explained by the fact that the *E2f3* gene encodes two distinct proteins, called E2F3A and E2F3B, through the use of different promoters and 5′ coding exons (Adams et al. 2000; He et al. 2000; Leone et al. 2000). The E2F proteins can be divided into different subgroups based on significant differences in their roles and upstream regulation (Fig. 1). The most striking distinction is that individual E2Fs appear to be involved predominantly in either the repression or activation of E2F-responsive genes.

As their names imply, E2F6, 7, and 8 were the latest E2F family members to be identified. They share significant sequence homology with the core DNA-binding domain of the other E2F proteins, and the overexpression of E2F6, 7, or 8 is sufficient to enforce the repression of classic E2F-responsive genes (Morkel et al. 1997; Cartwright et al. 1998; Trimarchi et al. 1998; de Bruin et al. 2003; Di Stefano et al. 2003; Christensen et al. 2005; Maiti et al. 2005). We still understand little about the role and regulation of these three E2Fs in vivo. Notably, in contrast to the other E2F family members, E2F6, 7, and 8 are not regulated by their association with pRB or the related pocket proteins, p107 and p130. Without even this circumstantial link, it remains an open question as to whether E2F6, 7, and/or 8 might influence tumorigenesis.

E2F4 and 5 constitute the second E2F subgroup (Trimarchi and Lees 2002; Dimova and Dyson 2005). These E2Fs are thought to play a key role in the transcriptional repression of classic E2F-responsive genes via recruitment of p130 or p107 and their associated histone deacetylases. The nuclear localization of E2F4 and 5 appears to be dependent on their association with the pocket

---

*Present address: Salk Institute, La Jolla, California 92037.

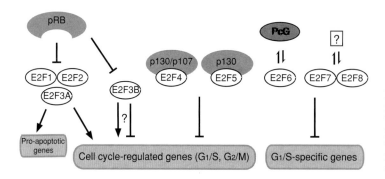

Figure 1. E2F family members are divided into different subgroups, with different functional properties. The different E2F subgroups positively or negatively regulate different subclasses of genes (*shaded boxes*), partially dependent on their upstream regulators and associated proteins (*gray ovals*).

proteins (Verona et al. 1997; Gaubatz et al. 2001). Chromatin immunoprecipitation (ChIP) assays show that E2F4, p107, and p130 bind to classic E2F-responsive promoters in G_0/G_1 when these genes are actively repressed (Ren et al. 2002; Cam et al. 2004). Cells lacking E2F4 and 5 proliferate normally, but they have a defective growth-arrest response due to their inability to appropriately silence E2F-responsive genes (Gaubatz et al. 2000; Landsberg et al. 2003). More recently, E2F3B was cloned and shown to be expressed in quiescent cells in a similar manner to E2F4 and 5 (He et al. 2000; Leone et al. 2000). On the basis of this observation, it was proposed that E2F3B would cooperate with E2F4 and 5 in mediating the transcriptional repression of classic E2F-responsive genes (Leone et al. 2000).

The third E2F subgroup includes E2F1, 2, and 3A (Lees et al. 1993). These E2Fs are potent transcriptional activators, and they are thought to play an important role in the transcriptional activation of classic E2F-responsive genes. E2F1, 2, and 3A are specifically regulated by pRB and not by p107 or p130 in normal cells (Lees et al. 1993). The resulting pRB/E2F1, 2, or 3A complexes are not detected at the promoters of classic E2F-responsive genes in G_0/G_1 cells (Ren et al. 2002; Cam et al. 2004), suggesting that they do not participate in their active repression. However, E2F1, 2, and 3A bind to these promoters in mid to late G_1, coincident with their release from pRB and the activation of these genes (Ren et al. 2002; Cam et al. 2004).

Overexpression studies show that the activating E2Fs can override growth-arrest signals and promote cellular proliferation (Johnson et al. 1994; Qin et al. 1994; Lukas et al. 1996). At the same time, these E2Fs are potent inducers of apoptosis (Qin et al. 1994; Wu and Levine 1994; Hiebert et al. 1995; Hsieh et al. 1997; Phillips et al. 1997, 1999). These opposing forces of proliferation and apoptosis are both classic hallmarks of tumor cells (Hanahan and Weinberg 2000). Mouse models have provided unequivocal proof that the activating E2Fs, *E2f1* and *E2f3*, promote the development of pRB-deficient tumors (Pan et al. 1998; Yamasaki et al. 1998; McCaffrey et al. 1999; Ziebold et al. 2003; Denchi and Helin 2005). Moreover, either directly or indirectly, these E2Fs contribute to both the ectopic proliferation and apoptosis that occur within the developing tumors.

Considerable attention has focused on understanding the mechanism(s) by which the activating E2Fs stimulate

apoptosis. To date, a variety of pro-apoptotic regulators have been identified as candidate E2F-responsive genes. The best-known example is the *Arf* tumor suppressor. The product of the *Arf* gene, called p19^{Arf} (in mouse), is a key component of the *p53* tumor surveillance network. p19^{Arf} exists at low or undetectable levels in most normal cells but is activated by inappropriate proliferative signals (Sherr and Weber 2000). Once it is expressed, p19^{Arf} inhibits mdm2, a ubiquitin ligase, allowing activation of the p53 tumor suppressor and induction of p53-responsive genes. These target genes promote cell cycle arrest or apoptosis and thereby counteract the effect of the abnormal proliferative signals. Essentially, p19^{Arf} acts as a defense against oncogenic signals. This explains why inactivation of the p19^{Arf}-mdm2-p53 network, through either inactivating mutations in *Arf* or *p53* or amplification of *mdm2/hdm2*, is critical for tumor development (Sherr 2001). Importantly, the analysis of a mouse strain that expresses GFP in place of p19^{Arf} provides direct in vivo evidence that *Arf* is not activated by normal proliferation but is reliably induced by the oncogenic signals that trigger tumorigenesis (Zindy et al. 2003).

Understanding the mechanism by which *Arf* responds to inappropriate, but not normal, proliferative signals remains a key goal. A variety of studies suggest a role for E2F in the activation of *Arf* (Phillips and Vousden 2001). The *Arf* promoter contains several consensus E2F-binding sites, and the ectopic expression of the activating E2Fs is sufficient to trigger *Arf* transcription (DeGregori et al. 1997; Phillips et al. 1999). However, it was unclear whether this regulation was direct because the identified E2F sites were dispensable for E2F-dependent *Arf* activation (Parisi et al. 2002; Berkovich et al. 2003) and many oncogenes lead to the activation of *Arf* (Sherr and Weber 2000). Moreover, *Arf* is not expressed in the cell-cycle-dependent manner that is typical of classic E2F-responsive genes. Thus, it was unclear whether *Arf* is a genuine E2F-responsive gene in vivo. As we describe below, our data show that distinct E2F family members contribute to the transcriptional regulation of *Arf* in normal versus tumor cells.

MATERIALS AND METHODS

MEF preparation and culture. *E2f3*$^{+/-}$ mice (Humbert et al. 2000) were intercrossed, and MEFs were prepared from E13.5 embryos as described previously (Humbert et al. 2000). For serum starvation and release experiments, passage-4 MEFs were incubated in low serum (0.1% FCS) for 72 hours, and subsequently fed with media containing 10% FCS. To monitor DNA synthesis, cells were labeled with 5 μCi [³H]thymidine for 1 hour and harvested, and then [³H]thymidine incorporation was measured as described previously (Moberg et al. 1996).

Protein preparation and western blotting. Passage-4 MEFs were plated onto 15-cm dishes at 3×10^6 cells/dish, and cell cycle reentry was performed as described above. For each time point, cells were harvested, and total protein was isolated as described previously (Moberg et al. 1996). Western blotting was performed using 100 μg of whole-cell extract and antibodies specific for cyclin A (Santa Cruz sc-596), p19^Arf (Novus NB200-106), p21^Cip1 (Santa Cruz sc-6246), phospho-p53 (Ser15) (Cell Signaling Technology #9284), or β-Tubulin (TUB2.1, Sigma T4026).

Chromatin immunoprecipitation (ChIP). ChIP was performed essentially as described previously (Takahashi et al. 2000; Aslanian et al. 2004). Sonicated, cross-linked chromatin corresponding to approximately 3×10^6 cells was immunoprecipitated with the following antibodies: normal rabbit IgG (control), sc-2027; E2F1, sc-193; E2F2, sc-633x; E2F3A, sc-879x; E2F3A+B, sc-878x; E2F4, sc-1082x; p130, sc-317x (all from Santa Cruz Biotechnology). 3–4% of the precipitated DNA, or 0.5% of input DNA, was amplified by 30 cycles of PCR using primer sequences for *Arf*, *p107*, or 1 kb upstream of the *E2f1* promoter (Aslanian et al. 2004). PCR products were stained with ethidium bromide after resolution on 8% polyacrylamide gels.

Retroviral infection. Infections were performed exactly as described previously (Serrano et al. 1996). Wild-type MEFs were infected and subsequently selected for 2 days in 2 mg/ml puromycin, grown for an additional 2 days, and then subjected to ChIP analysis as described below. pBabe-Puro and LPC-12S-E1A have been described previously (de Stanchina et al. 1998).

RESULTS

E2f3 Is Required for *Arf* Repression in Unstressed Cells

Our first insight into the role of E2F in the regulation of *Arf* came from the analysis of mouse embryonic fibroblasts (MEFs) derived from an *E2f3* mutant mouse strain. This strain lacks the sequences encoding the E2F DNA-binding domain and consequently is deficient for both the E2F3A and E2F3B proteins (Humbert et al. 2000). The *E2f3*^−/− MEFs have a reduced proliferative capacity and also a dramatic impairment in their ability to reenter the cell cycle in response to growth factor stimulation (Humbert et al. 2000). This cell cycle reentry defect correlates closely with a defect in the cell-cycle-dependent induction of classic E2F-responsive genes (Humbert et al. 2000). We hypothesized that the expression of *Arf* might also be altered in the *E2f3*^−/− MEFs if *Arf* is a genuine E2F-target gene. To test this idea, we used serum deprivation to arrest early-passage wild-type and *E2f3*^−/−

MEFs in G_0/G_1 and harvested cells at various time points after serum re-addition to assess the state of cell cycle reentry (through analysis of incorporated tritiated thymidine) and gene expression (by western blotting). Consistent with our previous studies, the *E2f3*^−/− MEFs showed a dramatic reduction in the level of mitogen-induced DNA replication (Fig. 2A) and the expression of cyclin A, a classic E2F-responsive gene (Fig. 2B). As previously described (Sherr and Weber 2000), p19^Arf was present at very low levels in the arrested wild-type cells, and its expression was not induced during the cell cycle reentry (Fig. 2B). In contrast, p19^Arf was dramatically up-regulated in the *E2f3*^−/− MEFs in both the arrested and the mitogen-treated cells (Fig. 2B). Quantitative RT-PCR shows that this reflects an increase in the level of *Arf* mRNA (data not shown). Thus, *E2f3* inactivation alters the transcription of *Arf* in the opposite manner from its effect on classic E2F-responsive genes.

The predominant function of p19^Arf is to inhibit the ubiquitin ligase mdm2 and consequently trigger the stabilization and activation of p53. Consistent with this scheme, the *E2f3* mutant MEFs displayed the classic hallmarks of p53 activation: There was an increase in the levels of p53 that was phosphorylated on Ser-15 and a dramatic up-regulation in the levels of the cdk inhibitor

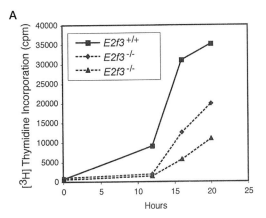

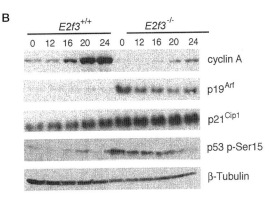

Figure 2. *E2f3*^−/− MEFs are defective in cell cycle reentry, due to activation of p19^Arf and p53. (*A*) Wild-type MEFs (*solid line*) or *E2f3*^−/− MEFs (*dotted lines*) were synchronized by serum starvation, and cell cycle reentry was monitored by [³H]thymidine incorporation into newly synthesized DNA at the indicated times. (*B*) Total protein extracts were prepared at the indicated times after serum stimulation and subjected to western blotting for cyclin A, p19^Arf, p21^Cip1, phospho-p53(Ser15), or β-Tubulin.

p21^{Cip1}, a known transcriptional target of p53 (Fig. 2B). Thus, *E2f3* inactivation leads to the induction of *Arf* and the activation of p53. It is well documented that changes in the levels of p19^{Arf}, p53, and p21^{Cip1} can have a major effect on the properties of MEFs, particularly in their ability to undergo mitogen-induced cell cycle reentry (Sherr and Weber 2000). Consistent with these observations, we found that the loss of either *Arf* or *p53* completely suppressed the cell cycle reentry defects of the *E2f3*$^{-/-}$ MEFs, including the defect in the expression of classic E2F-responsive genes (Aslanian et al. 2004). This genetic rescue could arise in two ways. The loss of *Arf* (or *p53*) could confer a proliferative advantage on the cells that outweighs or overrides the proliferative disadvantage that results from *E2f3* loss. Alternatively, it could reflect the existence of a linear pathway in which E2F3 is required to repress *Arf*, and therefore prevents activation of p53 and p21^{Cip1}.

To determine whether E2F family members are directly involved in the regulation of *Arf* in unstressed wild-type cells, we conducted ChIP assays (Fig. 3). As a positive control, we first examined E2F binding to a classic E2F-responsive promoter, *p107*. In an asynchronous population of MEFs, we were able to detect E2F1, 2, 3, and 4 in association with the *p107* promoter (Fig. 3). This is consistent with the documented role of both repressive (E2F4) and activating (E2F1, 2, and 3A) E2Fs in controlling the cell-cycle-dependent expression of this classic target gene (Trimarchi and Lees 2002). Remarkably, we observed a dramatically different pattern of E2F binding at the *Arf* promoter: It was occupied by E2F3 but not other E2F family members. Notably, this ChIP signal was observed using an antibody that recognizes both E2F3A and E2F3B, but not an antibody that is specific for E2F3A (Fig. 3). This raises the possibility that *Arf* is specifically targeted by the E2F3B isoform.

The transcription of classic E2F-responsive genes is activated in late G$_1$ because of a switch in promoter occupancy from repressive to activating E2F complexes. Given the differential E2F-binding properties of *Arf* versus classic E2F-responsive genes in asynchronous cells, we wanted to establish how *Arf* was regulated at distinct cell cycle stages. To address this issue, we used serum deprivation/restimulation assays to isolate cells at various stages of arrest or cell cycle reentry. As with our previous studies (see Fig. 2, for example), the cells initiate DNA synthesis 16–20 hours after serum stimulation. As expected, we found that the *p107* promoter, a classic E2F target, was bound by the repressive E2F4-p130 complex in arrested cells (0h; Fig. 4). In the enriched S-phase population, the E2F4/p130 signal was reduced and the activating E2Fs, E2F1, and E2F3A, clearly associated with the *p107* promoter (20h; Fig. 4). In striking contrast, E2F3 was the only E2F that was bound to the *Arf* promoter in arrested MEFs. Moreover, this E2F3 binding was maintained during cell cycle reentry and we did not observe recruitment of any other E2Fs to the *Arf* promoter (Fig. 4). This analysis clearly shows that normal proliferative signals encountered during cell cycle entry are insufficient to drive E2F activation of *Arf*. Rather, *Arf* expression is kept low throughout the cell cycle, and this correlates with the binding of E2F3. In the *E2f3*$^{-/-}$ MEFs, the derepression of *Arf* occurs without any detectable binding of the activating E2Fs (data not shown). Thus, we conclude that E2F3 contributes to the transcription repression of *Arf* in unstressed cells.

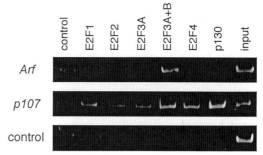

Figure 3. The *Arf* promoter is specifically bound by E2F3. ChIP analysis was performed on asynchronously growing wild-type MEFs, and binding of E2F and pocket protein complexes to the *Arf* and *p107* promoters was monitored. Whereas the classic E2F-responsive promoter, *p107*, is bound by all E2Fs, E2F3 is the only species detected at the *Arf* promoter.

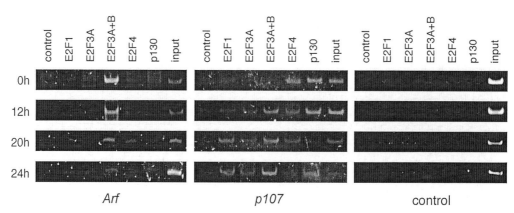

Figure 4. The *Arf* promoter is not activated by E2F during cell cycle reentry. Wild-type MEFs were synchronized by serum withdrawal, stimulated with 10% serum for the indicated times, and then subjected to ChIP analysis. Whereas the activating E2Fs are recruited to the *p107* promoter, the *Arf* promoter is bound only by E2F3 throughout cell cycle reentry.

Activating E2Fs Are Involved in the Oncogenic Activation of *Arf*

The experiments above establish a direct role for E2F3 in repression of *Arf* in unstressed cells. Given these observations, we wanted to determine whether/how the E2F regulation of *Arf* changes when the transcription of this gene is induced by oncogenic challenge. To address this question, we examined the effect of overexpressing the adenoviral oncoprotein, E1A. This is a potent oncogene that promotes both proliferation and apoptosis. E1A acts, at least in part, by sequestering the pocket proteins and relieving the transcriptional inhibition of the endogenous activating E2Fs (Ben-Israel and Kleinberger 2002). We infected early-passage wild-type MEFs with either control or E1A-expressing retroviruses and then used ChIP to assess E2F binding to either the *Arf* or *p107* promoters (Fig. 5). Infection with the control virus did not alter the spectrum of E2F complexes of these cells: *Arf* was still specifically occupied by E2F3 while *p107* was bound by E2F1, 2, 3, and 4. E1A expression had a fairly subtle effect on the spectrum of E2F complexes that were bound to the *p107* promoter. This included a modest reduction in the binding of the repressive E2F, E2F4, and a subtle in-

crease in the binding of the activating E2Fs, E2F1 and 2, that are consistent with E1A's documented ability to promote the expression of classic E2F target genes (Fig. 5). Importantly, E1A had a much more profound effect on *Arf*. There was a dramatic recruitment of the activating E2Fs, E2F1, 2, and 3A, to the *Arf* promoter, and this correlated with a huge increase in the expression of p19^{Arf} (Fig. 5). Given these findings, we conclude that the *endogenous* activating E2Fs participate in the activation of *Arf*, and consequently, the tumor surveillance network engaged by the E1A oncogene.

DISCUSSION

Tumor development is highly dependent on the deregulation of two regulatory networks, the p16^{Ink4a}-cycD/cdk4-pRB-E2F pathway that controls cellular proliferation and the p19^{Arf}-mdm2-p53 axis that mediates the tumor surveillance response (Sherr 2001). Our data reveal a direct connection between these two networks: E2F plays a key role in controlling the transcription of the *Arf* tumor suppressor in both normal and tumor cells.

Through a combination of genetic and biochemical evidence, we have shown that E2F3 contributes directly to the transcriptional repression of *Arf* in unstressed cells. The *E2f3* locus is known to encode two distinct isoforms, E2F3A and E2F3B (He et al. 2000; Leone et al. 2000). E2F3A is expressed in proliferating cells, and it is widely accepted to be an activating E2F (Trimarchi and Lees 2002; Dimova and Dyson 2005). In contrast, E2F3B is expressed in both quiescent and proliferating cells and, based solely on this expression pattern, was proposed to be a transcriptional repressor (Leone et al. 2000). Our ChIP data implicate E2F3B in the transcriptional repression of *Arf*. Specifically, an antibody that is specific for E2F3A yielded a clear ChIP signal at our classic E2F-responsive gene, *p107*, but not at *Arf*, whereas an antibody that recognizes the common carboxyl terminus of both E2F3A and E2F3B detects E2F3 binding to both *Arf* and *p107* promoters. These observations do not rule out the possibility that E2F3A contributes to the transcription repression of *Arf*, but they suggest that E2F3B is the major player. This represents the first functional evidence that the E2F3B protein is a repressor of transcription.

Numerous E2F family members have been classified as repressor E2Fs (Trimarchi and Lees 2002; Dimova and Dyson 2005). Of these, E2F4 and 5 are the best characterized and the most closely related to E2F3B. E2F4 and 5 repress transcription of classic E2F-responsive genes in G_0/G_1 by virtue of their association with the pocket proteins, and their associated histone-modifying enzymes. This repression is relieved as cells enter the cell cycle, when phosphorylation of the pocket protein by CDK activity leads to a disruption of the E2F-pocket protein complex. E2F3B is known to associate specifically with pRB in the G_1 phase (Leone et al. 2000). However, we were not able to detect pRB, or any other pocket protein, binding to the *Arf* promoter (Figs. 3 and 4; data not shown), raising the possibility that E2F3B enforces repression of

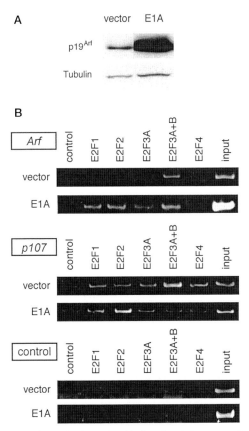

Figure 5. The activating E2Fs bind to the *Arf* promoter in response to oncogenic stress. Wild-type MEFs were infected with retrovirus overexpressing E1A, or an empty virus (vector) and subjected to western (*A*) or ChIP (*B*) analyses with the indicated antisera. MEFs expressing E1A exhibit dramatically increased levels of p19^{Arf}, coincident with recruitment of activating E2Fs (E2F1, E2F2, and E2F3A) to the *Arf* promoter.

Arf in a pRB-independent manner. Notably, the binding of E2F3B to *Arf* persists during cell cycle entry even though CDK activity is high, unlike the E2F4-p130 complex, which is lost from the *p107* promoter during cell cycle entry (Fig. 3). This difference supports the idea that the repressive E2F3B complex is refractory to CDK activity and therefore does not contain pRB. At least two other known repressors of *Arf*, Bmi-1 and CBX7, are members of the Polycomb group of transcriptional repressors (Jacobs et al. 1999; Gil et al. 2004). Since it has been shown previously that another repressive E2F, E2F6, acts in association with Polycomb proteins (Trimarchi et al. 2001; Ogawa et al. 2002; Attwooll et al. 2005), it is feasible that E2F3B may cooperate with Bmi-1 and/or CBX7 to engage repression of *Arf*.

In addition to their well-known role in regulation of cell cycle entry and DNA synthesis, E2F proteins have also been implicated in regulation of genes involved in the apoptotic response. However, there is considerable debate about whether these pro-apoptotic genes are genuine targets in vivo and, more contentiously, which of the E2F family members are capable of inducing apoptosis. A number of studies argue that the induction of apoptosis is a specific property of E2F1 and not other E2F family members (DeGregori et al. 1997; Leone et al. 2001; Denchi and Helin 2005). This specificity could be due, at least in part, to the presence of a domain unique to E2F1 that binds pRB and specifically regulates its apoptotic activity (Dick and Dyson 2003). However, other studies show that the activating E2Fs can all induce apoptosis when they are ectopically expressed (Vigo et al. 1999; Baudino et al. 2003). Clearly, these studies do not rule out the possibility that E2F2 and E2F3A might promote apoptosis indirectly by activating E2F1, a known E2F-responsive gene. Unfortunately, various mouse models give conflicting answers to this issue. For example, it was recently reported that the apoptosis arising in an *E2f3a* transgenic mouse model occurs in an *E2f1*-dependent manner (Denchi and Helin 2005). However, other models clearly show that the absence of *E2f1*, or indeed both *E2f1* and *E2f2*, does not alter the ability of cells to induce *Arf* or undergo apoptosis in response to oncogene activation (Palmero et al. 2002; Baudino et al. 2003). Our data clearly show that E2F1, 2, and 3A all associate with the *Arf* promoter

when this gene is induced by the presence of E1A (Fig. 5). Notably, this validates a role for the endogenous E2Fs, as opposed to overexpressed E2Fs, in the oncogenic response. On the basis of these observations, we conclude that *Arf* is a genuine E2F target and that all three activating E2Fs cooperate in the activation of this pro-apoptotic gene. This redundancy, combined with the need to achieve a certain total level of activating E2Fs, could explain the previous conflicting observations that one or more of the activating E2Fs can be either essential or dispensable for the activation of *Arf* and/or apoptosis in different settings.

Unlike most E2F target genes, *Arf* expression is not induced as cells reenter the cell cycle from a quiescent state (Fig. 2). We show here that this is likely due to the failure of activating E2Fs to bind to the *Arf* promoter during cell cycle entry, as well as the persistence of the repressive E2F3 complex (Fig. 4). However, many questions remain regarding this unique regulation of *Arf*. How is E2F3 specifically targeted to *Arf*? What prevents activation of *Arf* by other E2Fs during cell cycle entry? And how is oncogenic stress sensed, ultimately leading to activating E2F binding to *Arf*? To address this last question: It is possible that the switch from repression to activation requires a modification of either the E2F3-repressive complex or the activating E2F species, which only occurs in conditions of oncogene-induced hyperproliferation. Alternatively, the overall level of E2F activity may be the key determinant. During normal proliferation, perhaps the level of E2F activity is only sufficient to bind and activate the promoters of classic E2F targets. In contrast, the expression of E1A could yield a supra-physiological level of activating E2Fs that allows binding and activation of both classic E2F-responsive genes and additional targets like *Arf*. Importantly, this "supra-activation" model could account for the activity of other cellular oncogenes, including Ras, c-Myc, and Abl. These factors all possess the dual ability to promote cellular proliferation, ultimately by promoting the release of the activating E2Fs, and also activate the *Arf* tumor surveillance network. It is tempting to speculate that some, or all, of these factors would activate *Arf* as an unintended consequence of their need to engage E2F (Fig. 6). At least in the case of *ras*, it is clear that another transcription factor, Dmp1, contributes to

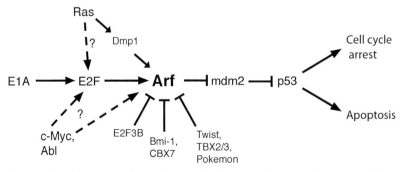

Figure 6. The *Arf*-p53 pathway is subject to complex regulation. *Arf* is known to be regulated, both positively and negatively, by numerous factors (*solid lines*). This study shows that E1A-induced activation of *Arf* occurs via E2F. It remains possible that signaling to *Arf* from other oncogenes (Ras, c-Myc, Abl) may occur through E2F (*dotted lines*).

Arf activation (Fig. 6) (Sreeramaneni et al. 2005). However, the levels of the activating E2Fs could act as a global sensor that would distinguish inappropriate from normal proliferation and mobilize *Arf*.

ACKNOWLEDGMENTS

J.A.L. is a Daniel K. Ludwig Scholar, and P.I. was supported by a Ludwig predoctoral fellowship. This work was supported by a grant from the National Institutes of Health (PO1-CA42063) to J.A.L.

REFERENCES

Adams M.R., Sears R., Nuckolls F., Leone G., and Nevins J.R. 2000. Complex transcriptional regulatory mechanisms control expression of the E2F3 locus. *Mol. Cell. Biol.* **20:** 3633.

Aslanian A., Iaquinta P.J., Verona R., and Lees J.A. 2004. Repression of the Arf tumor suppressor by E2F3 is required for normal cell cycle kinetics. *Genes Dev.* **18:** 1413.

Attwooll C., Oddi S., Cartwright P., Prosperini E., Agger K., Steensgaard P., Wagener C., Sardet C., Moroni M.C., and Helin K. 2005. A novel repressive E2F6 complex containing the polycomb group protein, EPC1, that interacts with EZH2 in a proliferation-specific manner. *J. Biol. Chem.* **280:** 1199.

Baudino T.A., Maclean K.H., Brennan J., Parganas E., Yang C., Aslanian A., Lees J.A., Sherr C.J., Roussel M.F., and Cleveland J.L. 2003. Myc-mediated proliferation and lymphomagenesis, but not apoptosis, are compromised by E2f1 loss. *Mol. Cell* **11:** 905.

Ben-Israel H. and Kleinberger T. 2002. Adenovirus and cell cycle control. *Front. Biosci.* **7:** d1369.

Berkovich E., Lamed Y., and Ginsberg D. 2003. E2F and Ras synergize in transcriptionally activating p14ARF expression. *Cell Cycle* **2:** 127.

Cam H. and Dynlacht B.D. 2003. Emerging roles for E2F: Beyond the G1/S transition and DNA replication. *Cancer Cell* **3:** 311.

Cam H., Balciunaite E., Blais A., Spektor A., Scarpulla R.C., Young R., Kluger Y., and Dynlacht B.D. 2004. A common set of gene regulatory networks links metabolism and growth inhibition. *Mol. Cell* **16:** 399.

Cartwright P., Muller H., Wagener C., Holm K., and Helin K. 1998. E2F-6: A novel member of the E2F family is an inhibitor of E2F-dependent transcription. *Oncogene* **17:** 611.

Christensen J., Cloos P., Toftegaard U., Klinkenberg D., Bracken A.P., Trinh E., Heeran M., Di Stefano L., and Helin K. 2005. Characterization of E2F8, a novel E2F-like cell-cycle regulated repressor of E2F-activated transcription. *Nucleic Acids Res.* **33:** 5458.

de Bruin A., Maiti B., Jakoi L., Timmers C., Buerki R., and Leone G. 2003. Identification and characterization of E2F7, a novel mammalian E2F family member capable of blocking cellular proliferation. *J. Biol. Chem.* **278:** 42041.

DeGregori J., Leone G., Miron A., Jakoi L., and Nevins J.R. 1997. Distinct roles for E2F proteins in cell growth control and apoptosis. *Proc. Natl. Acad. Sci.* **94:** 7245.

Denchi E.L. and Helin K. 2005. E2F1 is crucial for E2F-dependent apoptosis. *EMBO Rep.* **6:** 661.

de Stanchina E., McCurrach M.E., Zindy F., Shieh S.Y., Ferbeyre G., Samuelson A.V., Prives C., Roussel M.F., Sherr C.J., and Lowe S.W. 1998. E1A signaling to p53 involves the p19(ARF) tumor suppressor. *Genes Dev.* **12:** 2434.

Dick F.A. and Dyson N. 2003. pRB contains an E2F1-specific binding domain that allows E2F1-induced apoptosis to be regulated separately from other E2F activities. *Mol. Cell* **12:** 639.

Dimova D.K. and Dyson N.J. 2005. The E2F transcriptional network: Old acquaintances with new faces. *Oncogene* **24:** 2810.

Di Stefano L., Jensen M.R., and Helin K. 2003. E2F7, a novel E2F featuring DP-independent repression of a subset of E2F-regulated genes. *EMBO J.* **22:** 6289.

Gaubatz S., Lees J.A., Lindeman G.J., and Livingston D.M. 2001. E2F4 is exported from the nucleus in a CRM1-dependent manner. *Mol. Cell. Biol.* **21:** 1384.

Gaubatz S., Lindeman G.J., Ishida S., Jakoi L., Nevins J.R., Livingston D.M., and Rempel R.E. 2000. E2F4 and E2F5 play an essential role in pocket protein-mediated G1 control. *Mol. Cell* **6:** 729.

Gil J., Bernard D., Martinez D., and Beach D. 2004. Polycomb CBX7 has a unifying role in cellular lifespan. *Nat. Cell Biol.* **6:** 67.

Hanahan D. and Weinberg R.A. 2000. The hallmarks of cancer. *Cell* **100:** 57.

He Y., Armanious M.K., Thomas M.J., and Cress W.D. 2000. Identification of E2F-3B, an alternative form of E2F-3 lacking a conserved N-terminal region. *Oncogene* **19:** 3422.

Hiebert S.W., Packham G., Strom D.K., Haffner R., Oren M., Zambetti G., and Cleveland J.L. 1995. E2F-1: DP-1 induces p53 and overrides survival factors to trigger apoptosis. *Mol. Cell. Biol.* **15:** 6864.

Hsieh J.K., Fredersdorf S., Kouzarides T., Martin K., and Lu X. 1997. E2F1-induced apoptosis requires DNA binding but not transactivation and is inhibited by the retinoblastoma protein through direct interaction. *Genes Dev.* **11:** 1840.

Humbert P.O., Verona R., Trimarchi J.M., Rogers C., Dandapani S., and Lees J.A. 2000. E2f3 is critical for normal cellular proliferation. *Genes Dev.* **14:** 690.

Jacobs J.J., Kieboom K., Marino S., DePinho R.A., and van Lohuizen M. 1999. The oncogene and Polycomb-group gene bmi-1 regulates cell proliferation and senescence through the ink4a locus. *Nature* **397:** 164.

Johnson D.G., Cress W.D., Jakoi L., and Nevins J.R. 1994. Oncogenic capacity of the E2F1 gene. *Proc. Natl. Acad. Sci.* **91:** 12823.

Landsberg R.L., Sero J.E., Danielian P.S., Yuan T.L., Lee E.Y., and Lees J.A. 2003. The role of E2F4 in adipogenesis is independent of its cell cycle regulatory activity. *Proc. Natl. Acad. Sci.* **100:** 2456.

Lees J.A., Saito M., Vidal M., Valentine M., Look T., Harlow E., Dyson N., and Helin K. 1993. The retinoblastoma protein binds to a family of E2F transcription factors. *Mol. Cell. Biol.* **13:** 7813.

Leone G., Nuckolls F., Ishida S., Adams M., Sears R., Jakoi L., Miron A., and Nevins J.R. 2000. Identification of a novel E2F3 product suggests a mechanism for determining specificity of repression by Rb proteins. *Mol. Cell. Biol.* **20:** 3626.

Leone G., Sears R., Huang E., Rempel R., Nuckolls F., Park C.H., Giangrande P., Wu L., Saavedra H.I., Field S.J., Thompson M.A., Yang H., Fujiwara Y., Greenberg M.E., Orkin S., Smith C., and Nevins J.R. 2001. Myc requires distinct E2F activities to induce S phase and apoptosis. *Mol. Cell* **8:** 105.

Lukas J., Petersen B.O., Holm K., Bartek J., and Helin K. 1996. Deregulated expression of E2F family members induces S-phase entry and overcomes p16INK4A-mediated growth suppression. *Mol. Cell. Biol.* **16:** 1047.

Maiti B., Li J., de Bruin A., Gordon F., Timmers C., Opavsky R., Patil K., Tuttle J., Cleghorn W., and Leone G. 2005. Cloning and characterization of mouse E2F8, a novel mammalian E2F family member capable of blocking cellular proliferation. *J. Biol. Chem.* **280:** 18211.

McCaffrey J., Yamasaki L., Dyson N.J., Harlow E., and Griep A.E. 1999. Disruption of retinoblastoma protein family function by human papillomavirus type 16 E7 oncoprotein inhibits lens development in part through E2F-1. *Mol. Cell. Biol.* **19:** 6458.

Moberg K., Starz M.A., and Lees J.A. 1996. E2F-4 switches from p130 to p107 and pRB in response to cell cycle reentry. *Mol. Cell. Biol.* **16:** 1436.

Morkel M., Wenkel J., Bannister A.J., Kouzarides T., and Hagemeier C. 1997. An E2F-like repressor of transcription. *Nature* **390:** 567.

Morris E.J. and Dyson N.J. 2001. Retinoblastoma protein partners. *Adv. Cancer Res.* **82:** 1.

Ogawa H., Ishiguro K., Gaubatz S., Livingston D.M., and Nakatani Y. 2002. A complex with chromatin modifiers that occupies E2F- and Myc-responsive genes in G0 cells. *Science* **296:** 1132.

Palmero I., Murga M., Zubiaga A., and Serrano M. 2002. Activation of ARF by oncogenic stress in mouse fibroblasts is independent of E2F1 and E2F2. *Oncogene* **21:** 2939.

Pan H., Yin C., Dyson N.J., Harlow E., Yamasaki L., and Van Dyke T. 1998. Key roles for E2F1 in signaling p53-dependent apoptosis and in cell division within developing tumors. *Mol. Cell* **2:** 283.

Parisi T., Pollice A., Di Cristofano A., Calabro V., and La Mantia G. 2002. Transcriptional regulation of the human tumor suppressor p14(ARF) by E2F1, E2F2, E2F3, and Sp1-like factors. *Biochem. Biophys. Res. Commun.* **291:** 1138.

Phillips A.C. and Vousden K.H. 2001. E2F-1 induced apoptosis. *Apoptosis* **6:** 173.

Phillips A.C., Bates S., Ryan K.M., Helin K., and Vousden K.H. 1997. Induction of DNA synthesis and apoptosis are separable functions of E2F-1. *Genes Dev.* **11:** 1853.

Phillips A.C., Ernst M.K., Bates S., Rice N.R., and Vousden K.H. 1999. E2F-1 potentiates cell death by blocking anti-apoptotic signaling pathways. *Mol. Cell* **4:** 771.

Qin X.Q., Livingston D.M., Kaelin W.G., Jr., and Adams P.D. 1994. Deregulated transcription factor E2F-1 expression leads to S-phase entry and p53-mediated apoptosis. *Proc. Natl. Acad. Sci.* **91:** 10918.

Ren B., Cam H., Takahashi Y., Volkert T., Terragni J., Young R.A., and Dynlacht B.D. 2002. E2F integrates cell cycle progression with DNA repair, replication, and G(2)/M checkpoints. *Genes Dev.* **16:** 245.

Serrano M., Lee H., Chin L., Cordon-Cardo C., Beach D., and DePinho R.A. 1996. Role of the INK4a locus in tumor suppression and cell mortality. *Cell* **85:** 27.

Sherr C.J. 1996. Cancer cell cycles. *Science* **274:** 1672.

———. 2001. The INK4a/ARF network in tumour suppression. *Nat. Rev. Mol. Cell Biol.* **2:** 731.

Sherr C.J. and Weber J.D. 2000. The ARF/p53 pathway. *Curr. Opin. Genet. Dev.* **10:** 94.

Sreeramaneni R., Chaudhry A., McMahon M., Sherr C.J., and Inoue K. 2005. Ras-Raf-Arf signaling critically depends on the Dmp1 transcription factor. *Mol. Cell. Biol.* **25:** 220.

Takahashi Y., Rayman J.B., and Dynlacht B.D. 2000. Analysis of promoter binding by the E2F and pRB families in vivo: Distinct E2F proteins mediate activation and repression. *Genes Dev.* **14:** 804.

Trimarchi J.M. and Lees J.A. 2002. Sibling rivalry in the E2F family. *Nat. Rev. Mol. Cell Biol.* **3:** 11.

Trimarchi J.M., Fairchild B., Wen J., and Lees J.A. 2001. The E2F6 transcription factor is a component of the mammalian Bmi1-containing polycomb complex. *Proc. Natl. Acad. Sci.* **98:** 1519.

Trimarchi J.M., Fairchild B., Verona R., Moberg K., Andon N., and Lees J.A. 1998. E2F-6, a member of the E2F family that can behave as a transcriptional repressor. *Proc. Natl. Acad. Sci.* **95:** 2850.

Verona R., Moberg K., Estes S., Starz M., Vernon J.P., and Lees J.A. 1997. E2F activity is regulated by cell cycle-dependent changes in subcellular localization. *Mol. Cell. Biol.* **17:** 7268.

Vigo E., Muller H., Prosperini E., Hateboer G., Cartwright P., Moroni M.C., and Helin K. 1999. CDC25A phosphatase is a target of E2F and is required for efficient E2F-induced S phase. *Mol. Cell. Biol.* **19:** 6379.

Wu X. and Levine A.J. 1994. p53 and E2F-1 cooperate to mediate apoptosis. *Proc. Natl. Acad. Sci.* **91:** 3602.

Yamasaki L., Bronson R., Williams B.O., Dyson N.J., Harlow E., and Jacks T. 1998. Loss of E2F-1 reduces tumorigenesis and extends the lifespan of Rb1(+/-)mice. *Nat. Genet.* **18:** 360.

Ziebold U., Lee E.Y., Bronson R.T., and Lees J.A. 2003. E2F3 loss has opposing effects on different pRB-deficient tumors, resulting in suppression of pituitary tumors but metastasis of medullary thyroid carcinomas. *Mol. Cell. Biol.* **23:** 6542.

Zindy F., Williams R.T., Baudino T.A., Rehg J.E., Skapek S.X., Cleveland J.L., Roussel M.F., and Sherr C.J. 2003. Arf tumor suppressor promoter monitors latent oncogenic signals in vivo. *Proc. Natl. Acad. Sci.* **100:** 15930.

Genetic and Epigenetic Changes in Mammary Epithelial Cells Identify a Subpopulation of Cells Involved in Early Carcinogenesis

H. Berman, J. Zhang, Y.G. Crawford, M.L. Gauthier, C.A. Fordyce, K.M. McDermott, M. Sigaroudinia, K. Kozakiewicz, and T.D. Tlsty

Department of Pathology and UCSF Comprehensive Cancer Center, University of California at San Francisco, San Francisco, California 94143-0511

Morphologically normal foci of epithelial cells exhibiting p16 inactivation have been found in several tissues and may be precursors to cancer. Our previous work demonstrates that cells lacking p16[INK4A] activity exhibit phenotypes associated with malignancy (Romanov et al. 2001). The acquisition of genomic instability occurs through the activation of telomeric and centrosomal dysfunction. Additionally, the activation of stress pathways such as COX-2 provides these cells with the mutagenic potential to survive adverse environments as well as the ability to migrate, evade apoptosis and immune surveillance, and summon sustaining vasculature. Examination of archived tissue from women with DCIS (ductal carcinoma in situ) reveals epithelial cells that overexpress markers of premalignant stress activation pathways and mirror the distinctive expression patterns of these markers observed in vitro. These epithelial cells are found within the premalignant lesion as well as in the field of morphologically normal tissue that surrounds the lesion. Here, we show that p16[INK4A]-silenced vHMEC cells exhibit a gene expression profile which is distinct, reproducible, and extends beyond the changes mediated by p16[INK4A] inactivation. The present work suggests that cells lacking p16[INK4A] activity exhibit critical activities which allow cells to evade differentiation processes that would be expected to terminate proliferation. All of these properties are critical to malignancy. These events may be useful biomarkers to detect the earliest events in breast cancer.

STUDYING CAUSAL EVENTS IN BREAST CANCER

Studies of human mammary epithelial cells (HMEC) from healthy individuals are providing novel insights into how early epigenetic and genetic events affect genomic integrity and fuel carcinogenesis. Key epigenetic changes, such as the hypermethylation of the p16[INK4A] promoter sequences, create a previously unappreciated pre-clonal phase of tumorigenesis in which a subpopulation of mammary epithelial cells is positioned for progression to malignancy (Romanov et al. 2001; Tlsty et al. 2001). These key changes precede the clonal outgrowth of premalignant lesions and occur frequently in healthy, disease-free women. Understanding more about these early events should provide novel molecular candidates for prevention and therapy of breast cancer that target the process, instead of the consequences, of genomic instability. We highlight some of the key alterations that have been studied in HMEC in culture and relate them to events observed in vivo. Heroic efforts over the past three decades have provided culture systems that allow the isolation and propagation of HMEC (Hammond et al. 1984; Band and Sager 1989; Taylor-Papadimitriou et al. 1989; Kao et al. 1995). Understanding the contribution of specific genetic alterations to the transformation of these cells through the expression of viral oncoproteins and selected oncogenes is ongoing in many laboratories (Walen and Stampfer 1989; Foster and Galloway 1996; Kiyono et al. 1998; Hahn et al. 1999) and has increased our knowledge of oncogenesis. Studies in our laboratory have approached this question from a different perspective, analyzing HMEC in the absence of introducing viruses or oncogenes.

Because over 90% of human cancers, including breast cancer, are of epithelial origin, we initiated our studies with the comparison of fibroblasts and epithelial cells from the same tissue, searching for differences in transformation-relevant signal transduction pathways. In contrast to human fibroblasts, HMEC do not exhibit a classic senescent arrest when grown in vitro (Romanov et al. 2001). HMEC obtained from normal human tissues contain a subpopulation of "variant" cells that are resistant to the negative growth signals that initiate a proliferative arrest (selection) in the majority of the HMEC population after several passages in culture (Brenner et al. 1998; Foster et al. 1998; Huschtscha et al. 1998). These variant HMEC (vHMEC), which become visible while the majority of the population is arrested in selection, lack p16INK4a activity, a critical regulator of cell cycle checkpoint control, and proliferate for an extended period of time with eroding telomeric sequences. These cells subsequently exhibit telomeric dysfunction and generate the types of chromosomal abnormalities seen in the earliest lesions of breast cancer (Romanov et al. 2001). Similar subpopulations are not observed in isogenic mammary fibroblasts (Romanov et al. 2001). These differences between epithelial cells and fibroblasts may provide new insights into the mechanistic basis of neoplastic transformation. The existence of this subpopulation of vHMEC cells, their ability to grow past proliferation barriers, and the accompanying acquisition of telomeric and centrosomal dysfunction may be pivotal events in the earliest steps of carcinogenesis, allowing the acquisition of multiple, fundamental genetic changes necessary for oncogenic evolution.

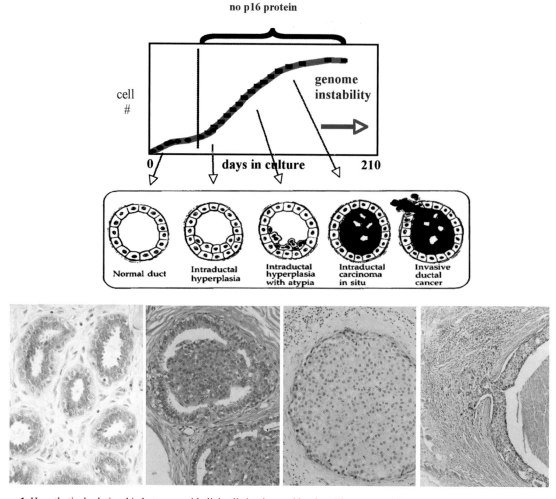

Figure 1. Hypothetical relationship between epithelial cells in vitro and in vivo. The top panel illustrates the growth curve for HMEC isolated from reduction mammoplasties. The (pre-selection) cells increase in number for ~20 population doublings when grown in culture and then enter a proliferation arrest (selection) whose termination is noted by the vertical line. Clonal isolates emerge from the arrested cell lawn and continue proliferation for ~3–5 months in culture until there is no further increase in cell number. These post-selection HMEC (variants) have no detectable p16 protein and contain hypermethylated p16 promoter sequences. 10–20 population doublings prior to an obvious population growth plateau, the cells acquire chromosomal changes (genome instability). We postulate that the growth of vHMEC in vitro may mimic the different premalignant stages of breast cancer (*lower panels*) as illustrated by the arrows.

The long-sought goal of many studies has been to identify the molecular (causal) changes that underlie progression of normal cells to malignancy with hopes that such information will provide selective targets for effective treatment of the disease. In this review, we describe the cellular and molecular evolution of HMEC in vitro and illustrate striking similarities with the evolution of mammary cells as they progress from normal to premalignant to malignant in vivo (Fig. 1).

CHARACTERIZATION OF HMF AND HMEC IN VITRO: IDENTIFICATION OF A SUBPOPULATION OF VARIANT EPITHELIAL CELLS

Fibroblasts have provided the paradigm for cell senescence in culture. It is well known that human fibroblasts

undergo a limited number of cell divisions prior to activating specific cell cycle checkpoints and entering into an irreversible arrest (variously termed the Hayflick limit [Hayflick 1965], irreversible replicative senescence, and mortality stage 1 [M1]). Human mammary fibroblasts (HMF) from healthy individuals were grown as previously described (Hammond et al. 1984) and characterized. Similar to previous studies in human skin fibroblasts (Hammond et al. 1984; Walen and Stampfer 1989; Brenner et al. 1998; Huschtscha et al. 1998; Kiyono et al. 1998), the HMF populations undergo a limited number of population doublings prior to entering a proliferative plateau (Fig. 1) (Romanov et al. 2001). The cells enlarge in size, flatten in shape, vacuolate, and express senescence-associated β-galactosidase (SA-β-gal; Romanov et al. 2001). Low incorporation of bromodeoxyuridine (BrdU) and minimal expression of MCM2 protein indicated a low proliferative index. Additionally, Annexin-V staining indicated a low death index. Further characterization demonstrates that human foreskin fibroblasts and HMF both (1) maintain genomic integrity (Walen and Stampfer 1989; Romanov et al. 2001); (2) maintain intact cell cycle checkpoint control (data not shown); (3) exhibit a 2N to 4N DNA content ratio of ≥ 4 at the growth plateau (Romanov et al. 2001); and (4) have a mean telomere restriction fragment (TRF) length that is similar at senescence (Romanov et al. 2001). By the morphological, behavioral, and molecular criteria described above, HMF could be said to senesce in a manner similar to human skin fibroblasts. If senescence is the result of a signal from shortened telomeres, as has been previously postulated (Bodnar et al. 1998), one would predict that the expression of the catalytic subunit of telomerase, hTERT, would allow cells to bypass "senescence" and continue proliferating. This prediction has been realized in the examination of human fibroblasts expressing hTERT (Bodnar et al. 1998; Jiang et al. 1999); they exhibit an extended life span without acquiring properties of transformed cells (Jiang et al. 1999).

At first glance, it appeared that HMEC do not conform to this paradigm of senescence. In contrast to fibroblasts, HMEC obtained from normal human tissue demonstrate two growth phases (Fig. 1). After an initial phase of active growth (~15–20 population doublings), HMEC exhibit a growth plateau previously termed senescence, selection, or M0 (Hammond et al. 1984; Foster and Galloway 1996; Huschtscha et al. 1998). At this time, the majority of the cell population is arrested in the G_1 phase of the cell cycle. When the flasks containing arrested HMEC are cultured in serum-free media (MCDB 170), colonies of small, proliferative epithelial cells become visible. These cells (post-selection or variant cells) are capable of undergoing an additional 20–50 population doublings before terminating in a population growth plateau that confusingly was also termed senescence or, alternatively, M1 (Foster and Galloway 1996; Huschtscha et al. 1998; Kiyono et al. 1998). On the basis of these observations, it was previously postulated that senescence in HMEC involved two steps, with some cells transitioning past the initial plateau, proliferating, and ultimately entering senescence several months later (Foster and Galloway 1996). We now appreciate that the two growth phases represent the growth of two independent populations of mammary epithelial cells (described below) and that neither population enters replicative senescence as classically defined by experiments in human skin fibroblasts. In keeping with Stampfer's original designation (Hammond et al. 1984), we also term the plateau in which cells containing unmethylated $p16^{INK4a}$ undergo a proliferative arrest, selection. However, because of the recent appreciation for the origin of the (post-selection) HMEC containing hypermethylated $p16^{INK4a}$ promoter sequences, and to avoid a mechanistic implication of their behavior in vivo, we call the $p16^{INK4a}$-deficient cells variant human mammary epithelial cells or vHMEC.

To analyze apparent cell-specific differences, we characterized the two in vitro population-growth plateaus, the first plateau and the second plateau from healthy individuals grown as previously described (Hammond et al. 1984), and compared them to the replicative senescence described in human skin fibroblasts. Similar to previous studies in human skin fibroblasts and HMEC (Hammond et al. 1984; Walen and Stampfer 1989; Brenner et al. 1998; Huschtscha et al. 1998; Kiyono et al. 1998), the epithelial cell populations undergo a limited number of population doublings prior to entering a proliferative plateau (Fig. 1) (Romanov et al. 2001). Just as seen with the fibroblasts described above, the cells enlarge in size, flatten in shape, vacuolate, and express SA-β-gal (Romanov et al. 2001). Low incorporation of BrdU and minimal expression of MCM2 protein indicated a low proliferative index. Additionally, Annexin-V staining indicated a low death index. Further characterization demonstrated that pre-selection HMEC (1) maintain genomic integrity (Walen and Stampfer 1989; Romanov et al. 2001); (2) maintain intact cell cycle checkpoint control (data not shown); (3) exhibit a 2N–4N DNA content ratio of ≥ 4 at the growth plateau (Romanov et al. 2001); and (4) have a mean TRF length that is similar to that of human skin fibroblasts and HMF at replicative senescence (Romanov et al. 2001). Although the morphological, behavioral, and molecular criteria described above suggested that HMEC had entered replicative senescence in a manner similar to human skin fibroblasts, the expression of telomerase did not have a comparable outcome. Experiments (Kiyono et al. 1998; Stampfer et al. 2001) have demonstrated that expression of hTERT in these cells does not prevent their entry into the first growth plateau as described for fibroblasts. This demonstrates that the first growth plateau exhibited by HMEC grown in tissue culture does not correspond to the classic telomere-length-based replicative senescence. As described below, it is only in the epithelial cells which lack $p16^{INK4a}$ expression that telomerase can "immortalize" a population (Kiyono et al. 1998; Stampfer et al. 2001). Intriguingly, recent experiments with fibroblasts also suggest that only fibroblast populations with low $p16^{INK4a}$ activity can be immortalized by expression of telomerase (Benanti and Galloway 2004). If this is so, it raises the question of why fibroblasts do not contain a subpopulation of cells that bypasses the imposed arrest, as is seen in the epithelial population from the same individual.

Strikingly, HMEC and HMF appeared to differ in their ability to spontaneously overcome the observed proliferation barriers by several orders of magnitude. In skin fibroblasts, the terminal growth plateau, senescence, can last for years (>3 years; T.D. Tlsty, unpubl.). Cells remain viable if fed routinely (Romanov et al. 2001), and the frequency of spontaneous emergence is $<10^{-9}$ (data not shown; Romanov et al. 2001). Similarly, HMF fail to produce proliferating cells from senescence even after 5 months in continuous culture ($<6 \times 10^{-7}$, data not shown) (Romanov et al. 2001). In contrast to fibroblasts and consistent with previous reports (Hammond et al. 1984; Huschtscha et al. 1998), epithelial populations maintained at the first plateau sporadically contain clusters of small, refractile cells ($\sim10^{-4}$ to 10^{-5}) that continue to proliferate. Both the epithelial cells growing prior to the selection plateau (pre-selection or HMEC) and the epithelial cells growing after the selection plateau (post-

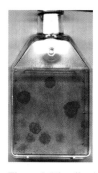

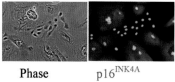

Phase   p16^INK4A

Figure 2. Visualization of vHMEC at selection. HMEC are plated in flasks prior to entering the proliferation barrier. Cells propagate, enter the first plateau, and change morphology, becoming large and flat. After ~2 weeks at the plateau, clonal expansions of small, proliferating cells (vHMEC) are visible (*Phase, middle panel*). ICC shows them to be devoid of p16^INK4a (*red, right panel*). Green fluorescence identifies cell nuclei. The flask (*left panel*) was seeded with 10^5 cells and fed routinely until colonies were visible. The cells were stained with Wright's solution. The number of colonies allows measurement of the clonal events.

selection HMEC or vHMEC) exhibited typical heterogeneous expression of cytokeratins when examined by immunocytochemistry (ICC) (data not shown; Taylor-Papadimitriou et al. 1989). For these and other reasons, the variant cells were believed to be the continued growth of the earlier population. As noted previously by several laboratories, HMEC emerging from the first population-growth plateau lack expression of the *p16^INK4a* protein (Fig. 2) (Brenner et al. 1998; Foster et al. 1998; Huschtscha et al. 1998; Ramirez et al. 2001) due to the hypermethylation of the *p16^INK4a* promoter sequences. This observation provided a viable explanation for the continued growth of the variant cells in culture.

PROMOTER HYPERMETHYLATION OF THE *p16^INK4a* GENE AND CANCER

The lack of *p16^INK4a* activity in the variant HMEC is an intriguing finding (Brenner et al. 1998; Foster et al. 1998; Huschtscha et al. 1998) because it provides an epigenetic marker for the vHMEC population. Although the role of epigenetic *p16^INK4a* silencing in the growth of the vHMEC cells has been relatively uncharacterized, the role of *p16^INK4a* silencing in the carcinogenic process has been extensively studied. The *p16^INK4a* gene product was initially isolated by two-hybrid screening for proteins associated with cyclin-dependent kinase 4 (Serrano et al. 1993) and was found to be a member of a family of proteins that bind and block the activity of cyclin D/cdk4 complexes and induce cell cycle arrest. Forced expression of *p16^INK4a* protein induces a G_1 arrest that is dependent on functional retinoblastoma protein (Rb) (Medema et al. 1995). Homozygous deletion of the chromosomal region containing *p16^INK4a* (and an additional family member, *p15^INK4b*) is the most common genetic event in primary tumors (Cairns et al. 1994). The dissection of the contribution of these two loci in the initiation and progression of different cancers has demonstrated that loss of *p16^INK4a* alone (with retention of p19^Arf) leads to tumor predisposition in mice (Krinferpot et al. 2001). These animals have been shown to be highly susceptible

to spontaneous and carcinogen-induced malignancy (Sharpless et al. 2001). The *p16^INK4a* gene can be inactivated by translocations, by mutations at many sites, and by hypermethylation (Gonzalez-Zulueta et al. 1997). Point mutation in intron 2 (Asp-153) has been identified in tumors that leave cdk4 binding intact while aborting inhibition of cdk activity (Yang et al. 1996). Other temperature-sensitive mutations, Gly-101→Trp and Val-126→Asp, abrogate binding to CDK4/6 and have been demonstrated to increase the fraction of G_1 cells after transfection (Parry and Peters 1996). The hypermethylation of *p16^INK4a* promoter sequences is also seen in over 20% of breast cancers.

The methylation of the *p16^INK4a* gene locus (and the concomitant silencing of *p16^INK4a* activity) is an effective way of modulating gene expression (Gonzalez-Zulueta et al. 1997; Baylin and Herman 2000). In the mammalian genome, methylation can occur at CpG islands that are found in the proximal promoter regions of genes (Baylin and Herman 2000). The change in gene expression is heritable and is tightly linked to the formation of transcriptionally repressed chromatin structure. Cancers often exhibit changes in methylation in gene promoter sequences that are associated with loss of tumor suppressor function (Nguyen et al. 2001), providing an alternative to mutations that disrupt gene function. The importance of CpG island hypermethylation in cancer is obvious, given the frequency of the process and the genes involved. The majority of tumor suppressor genes that cause genetic predisposition to cancer can be silenced by hypermethylation in nonfamilial cancers. The genes that can be methylated include repair genes (MLH1, GST3), cell cycle inhibitors (*p16^INK4a*, p15, p14ARF), tumor suppressor genes (VHL, BRCA1), tissue remodeling enzymes and structures (TIMP3, E-cadherin), and receptors (estrogen receptor), to name a few (Baylin and Herman 2000). Methylation changes often precede the mutagenic events that drive tumor progression.

CHARACTERIZATION OF vHMEC IN VITRO: ACQUISITION OF GENOMIC INSTABILITY VIA TELOMERIC DYSFUNCTION

After they are observed, vHMEC undergo exponential growth that usually extends for several months (Fig. 1, growth past the vertical line), before entering a second population growth plateau (Fig. 1, agonescence). This plateau is critically different from the arrested state that terminates the proliferation of the HMEC population (P1 or first plateau). Although previous studies have referred to this second plateau as senescence or M1, these cells display attributes more similar to cells in crisis, than senescence. vHMEC at this stage are heterogeneous in size and morphology and demonstrate SA-β-gal staining (data not shown). Furthermore, they continue to incorporate BrdU and retain high levels of MCM2 protein (>50% of nuclei strongly staining for MCM2). Upon FACS analysis, the 2N to 4N DNA ratio is approximately 1, similar to a population of cells in crisis (Romanov et al. 2001). This high proliferative index is counterbalanced by an increase in cell death such that the total number of cells remains constant. A significant fraction (~20%) of epithelial cells at the second plateau stain with Annexin-V, an indicator of cell death. In contrast, <1% of isogenic senescent HMF (or HMEC at the first plateau) are Annexin-V-positive. Thus, vHMEC at the second plateau are unlike HMEC at the first plateau or fibroblast cells at senescence (Romanov et al. 2001).

The cytogenetic analysis of vHMEC at selected passages demonstrates that gross chromosomal abnormalities appear in virtually every metaphase spread as the cells approach the second growth plateau (Romanov et al. 2001). In all cases, the abnormalities accumulate rapidly beginning 10–20 population doublings before the final passage of cells (Fig. 3) and coincide with slowing of the proliferation rates. In these cells, both the percentage of abnormal metaphases and the number of abnormalities per metaphase increase. The abnormalities include multiple translocations, deletions, other rearrangements, telomeric associations, polyploidy, and aneuploidy. Substantial polyploidy (~25–35%) is detected by flow cytometric analysis at final passages of vHMEC. Multipolar mitoses are often observed. The accumulation of chromosomal abnormalities is independent of donor age (range, 16–50 years) and total proliferative potential of the epithelial populations (range, 30–60 PD). Characterization of these abnormalities has been described previously (Romanov et al. 2001).

Shortening of telomeres and their associated uncapping has previously been suggested to mediate chromosomal instability through the production of dicentric chromosomes (Van Steensel et al. 1998). Resolution of dicentric chromosomes by chromosome breakage generates translocations, deletions, and duplications. Failure to resolve them can generate anaphase bridges, failed cytokinesis, and polyploid cells. These abnormalities are detected frequently in vHMEC at the second plateau (Romanov et al. 2001). Thus, the subpopulation of vHMEC that emerge from the first proliferation barrier ultimately exhibit telomeric dysfunction. Although vHMEC at the second plateau exhibit many of the cellular characteristics of viral oncoprotein-induced crisis, spontaneous immortalization of variants (an important distinguishing hallmark of crisis) has yet to be detected. In addition, the p53 gene sequence is wild type in these cells and still functional (Romanov et al. 2001). Because of these (and other) differences (Tlsty et al. 2004), we have called these cells "agonescent" to distinguish them from cells in crisis. The Latin root "agon" defines a violent struggle that precedes death or a strong sudden display. The most prominent attributes of the late-passage vHMEC are their dramatic accumulation of chromosomal rearrangements and the dynamic state of proliferation and death.

The vHMEC described in this model system and the existence of an agonescent stage of proliferation provide a compelling argument for acquisition of massive random genomic instability that precedes clonal outgrowth of tumor cells. Indeed, at the point in culture when virtually all of the vHMEC cells exhibit chromosomal abnormalities via karyotypic analysis, analysis by comparative genomic hybridization (CGH) shows the population to be in a diploid non-rearranged state (T.D. Tlsty et al., in prep.). This is because CGH assesses clonal chromosomal changes that are present in a large fraction of the cell population and cannot detect random, non-clonal changes. It is intriguing to speculate that the relatively few chromosomal structural abnormalities observed in hyperplasias and atypical hyperplasias (Burbano et al. 2000), and the transition to the dramatic increase of genomic instability detected in carcinoma in situ (CIS) in vivo using CGH analysis (Berg and Hutter 1995; Pandis 1995), are reflective of a pre-clonal phase of growth followed by clonal expansion in CIS. Therefore, this model system may have uncovered a previously unappreciated pivotal phase in tumorigenesis. In this pre-clonal phase, epithelial cells have the potential to acquire multiple, random chromosomal changes that provide fuel for clonal expansion.

Accumulation of structural chromosomal abnormalities in late passage mammary epithelial cell populations

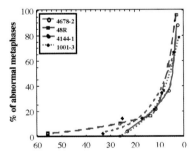

Population doublings before second growth plateau

Figure 3. Chromosomal instability in vHMEC. The kinetics of accumulation of chromosomal abnormalities is diagramed as a function of time. The percentage of metaphase spreads with structural chromosomal abnormalities was plotted as a function of the number of population doublings before the cells entered the population growth plateau (agonescence), designated 0. Each line represents analysis of cells from different women. The women ranged in age from 16 to 50 years old. Karyotypes were performed at each point that comprises the given line.

CHARACTERIZATION OF vHMEC IN VITRO: ACQUISITION OF GENOMIC INSTABILITY VIA CENTROSOMAL DYSFUNCTION

As described previously, many vHMEC exhibit multipolar mitoses as they approach the second plateau, agonescence. To better understand the mechanism responsible for generating cells with more than two centrosomes, we analyzed HMEC obtained from healthy, disease-free women with no predisposition to breast cancer. As these cells are propagated in culture, we observed that vHMEC accumulated centrosome-related (e.g., aneuploidy) genomic abnormalities (Romanov et al. 2001; Tlsty et al. 2001). We demonstrated that, in contrast to HMEC, vHMEC have uncoupled centrosome duplication and DNA replication cycles, and this uncoupling was due to loss of expression of the tumor suppressor protein p16[INK4a]. We also showed that generation of cells with more than two centrosomes was a conditional phenotype, dependent on the inhibition of DNA synthesis. Furthermore, loss of p16^{INK4a} activity and consequent loss of kinase regulation were shown to result in uncoupling of these two cycles in other cell types (i.e., normal diploid human fibroblasts), demonstrating that this is a general role for p16^{INK4a}. Finally, we demonstrated that production of cells with more than two centrosomes gave rise to an aneuploid karyotype.

These results describe a new function of p16^{INK4a} and further demonstrate the importance of p16^{INK4a} in the maintenance of normal cellular properties. In this study, p16^{INK4a} activity was found to be necessary to couple the centrosome duplication and DNA replication cycles. The coupling of these cycles is critical to ensure that the DNA content and the centrosome organelle are duplicated once and only once during the cell cycle. HMEC, with functional p16^{INK4a}, have coupled centrosome and DNA duplication cycles. Suppression of p16^{INK4a} expression was sufficient to relax this control. This conclusion was supported by similar results obtained in multiple cell types (i.e., HMEC, HMF, and HeLa). The uncoupling of the centrosome duplication and DNA replication cycles and subsequent generation of more than two centrosomes was immediately unmasked under conditions that transiently inhibit DNA synthesis and was gradually unmasked during standard growth in culture. This finding offers an explanation for the observed accumulation of centrosome abnormalities in vHMEC during their life span in culture. As vHMEC proliferate in culture, they are increasingly exposed to internal signals (i.e., telomere shortening) and external signals (i.e., oxidative stress) leading to cell cycle checkpoint responses. We hypothesize that these signals result in transient inhibition of DNA synthesis, thereby providing the opportunity for vHMEC to accumulate more than two centrosomes as they mature in culture.

In addition to well-documented effects on genomic integrity, our data suggest that p16^{INK4a} plays a significant role in maintaining cellular integrity via its regulation of centrosome biology. Because the centrosome is directly responsible for instituting proper polarity and microtubule function, abnormal centrosomal function has a direct effect on these properties and, hence, cellular integrity. Loss of proper cell polarity is one of the initial alterations noted in premalignant cells. Although many studies have focused on the role of p16^{INK4a} in initiating a G_1/S DNA replication cell cycle checkpoint, this study is the first to suggest a role for p16^{INK4a} in cellular integrity as well as genomic integrity.

One hallmark of cancer is the accumulation of genomic abnormalities. Aneuploidy is the most frequently observed genomic abnormality and has been shown to occur early in progression, often accompanying premalignant lesions. Aneuploidy is also seen in histologically normal tissue, strongly suggesting that genomic instability is involved in the earliest stages of tumorigenesis (Deng et al. 1996; Larson et al. 1998, 2002; Lakhani et al. 1999; Li et al. 2002). The origin of aneuploidy in these premalignant lesions is unknown. Theodor Boveri hypothesized almost 100 years ago that multipolar mitoses were responsible for genomic abnormalities (Boveri 1914; Boveri et al. 1929). A more modern interpretation of this hypothesis is that events resulting in more than two centrosomes can lead to

multipolar spindles and to improper segregation of the sister chromatids, leading to aneuploidy. The recent discovery of more than two centrosomes in premalignant and malignant lesions of the breast and their correlation with aneuploidy has provided new support for Boveri's hypothesis (Lingle et al. 1998, 2002; Lingle and Salisbury 1999; Salisbury 2001). However, it is still unclear whether centrosome abnormalities drive genomic instability or are merely a marker of cells with genomic abnormalities (Duensing 2005). Our studies are the first to take genomically intact cells with normal numbers of centrosomes, generate more than two centrosomes in these cells, and subsequently demonstrate that they obtain multipolar mitotic spindles and an aneuploid karyotype. These results strongly support the conclusion that centrosome amplification does indeed cause genomic instability.

GENE EXPRESSION PROFILING OF HMEC AND vHMEC IDENTIFIES DIFFERENCES IN EXPRESSION

To further characterize the vHMEC, we compared the expression profiles of isogenic sets of HMEC and vHMEC. Total RNA from pre-selection HMEC was compared to RNA from both mid and late passages of vHMEC using two-color cDNA microarrays (chip content and methods available at http://dir.niehs.nih.gov/microarray). Following this analysis, we identified several genes that were differentially expressed between pre-selection cells and mid- or late-passage vHMEC. One of these genes, prostaglandin-endoperoxide synthase 2 (COX-2), was significantly induced (average, 6.3-fold). We have verified this observation in multiple populations of HMEC using western analysis and immunocytochemistry (Crawford et al. 2004). Subsequent studies demonstrate that this increase in COX-2 expression is causal for phenotypes often associated with malignant cells, such as an increase in angiogenesis, invasion, and proliferation, and a decrease in apoptosis (Crawford et al. 2004).

Strikingly, the gene expression profiles obtained from multiple vHMEC samples each share a significant number of changes (Fig. 4). These changes identify the variant HMEC population as a distinct subset of cells rather than a random outgrowth of mutant cells.

THE ORIGIN OF vHMEC: VARIANT MAMMARY EPITHELIAL CELLS ARE DETECTED IN VIVO

To determine whether cells with characteristics of variant HMEC (inactive *p16^{INK4a}*, overexpression of COX-2, and increased genomic instability) exist in vivo in healthy women, we took several approaches. Using the Luria-Delbrück fluctuation analysis (Luria and Delbrück 1943), we demonstrated that the vHMEC are generated (or exist) prior to the first plateau and do not arise through adaptation (Tlsty et al. 1989; Holst et al. 2003). Since the silencing (most often by methylation; Brenner et al. 1998; Foster et al. 1998; Huschtscha et al. 1998) of the important cell cycle inhibitor *p16^{INK4a}* is a critical distinguishing characteristic of the vHMEC, we also analyzed morphologically normal tissue from reduction mammoplasties us-

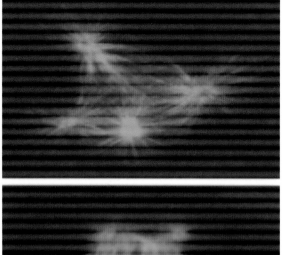

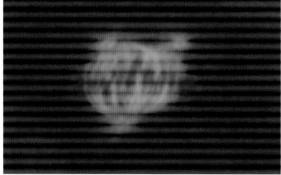

Figure 4. Multipolar mitosis in vHMEC generated via centrosomal dysfunction. Centrosome number was determined by immunocytochemistry with an antibody recognizing the centrosome-associated γ-tubulin protein (centrosome marker, *red*). Note the multipolar mitosis.

ing solution-based methylation-specific PCR to determine whether they contained detectable quantities of cells with $p16^{INK4a}$ promoter methylation. Using techniques that have previously been developed to detect methylated sequences in paraffin-embedded tissues (Herman et al. 1996, 1997), we measured the level of $p16^{INK4a}$ promoter methylation in histological samples in collaboration with Drs. Steve Baylin and James Herman of Johns Hopkins University. Of 15 samples, 4 demonstrated methylated $p16^{INK4a}$ promoter sequences (Holst et al. 2003). Since the removal of tissue from the histological preparations includes both the epithelial cells of the mammary ducts and the stromal cells of the surrounding tissue, we additionally sought a method that would enable us to visualize the HMEC cells embedded in their natural tissue architecture. For this purpose, we collaborated with Dr. Gerard Nuovo, who developed an in situ method for detecting methylated sequences in histological sections from tumors (Nuovo et al. 1999). Ten samples of histological preparations of reduction mammoplasty tissue were examined for cells that contain methylated $p16^{INK4a}$ promoter sequences. Three of the ten samples demonstrated the unequivocal presence of cells (foci) that gave a positive signal, and were mapped using a novel method developed for the purpose of displaying multiple sets of data in the context of whole tissue (Holst et al. 2003). Close examination of the samples revealed that the cells producing a positive signal were luminal epithelial cells. Neither myoepithelial cells nor stromal cells produced

positive signals in any of the samples analyzed. These data demonstrate that epithelial cells with hypermethylation of the $p16^{INK4a}$ promoter sequences exist as foci in morphologically normal tissue of disease-free women (Holst et al. 2003).

Although the in situ methylation-specific PCR assay provided evidence that epithelial cells with a distinguishing characteristic of vHMEC existed in morphologically normal tissue, the assay is too difficult and laborious to apply to large samples. For this purpose, we sought to assess other characteristics of vHMEC in vitro that may also be concomitantly expressed in the foci in vivo. One goal of the expression profile analysis was to identify such distinguishing characteristics of variant cells for the purpose of then examining their expression in vivo. To determine whether the increased expression of COX-2 that is seen in a fraction of the cells containing p16 hypermethylation in vitro is also present in vivo, we analyzed serial histological sections of human mammary tissue for colocalization of these markers (Crawford et al. 2004). Examination of the seven cases that were negative for cells with p16^INK4a hypermethylation did not exhibit intense staining of COX-2. In contrast, examination of the three cases that were positive for cells containing p16^INK4a hypermethylation exhibited areas of intense staining for COX-2 expression in adjacent serial slides. This intense staining colocalized with the areas of p16 promoter hypermethylation and extended to the adjacent areas. Maps were generated to demonstrate the localization of COX-2 in relation to p16^INK4a hypermethylation (Crawford et al. 2004). Further analysis of these regions using an in situ hybridization technique has found them to also have shorter telomeres when compared to other areas of the same slide (C.A. Fordyce et al., in prep.).

The colocalization of intense COX-2 staining in cells with hypermethylated p16 sequences has important implications for the initiation and progression of malignancy in this tissue. COX-2 protein is instrumental in prostaglandin synthesis, and increased expression in tumor cells is accompanied by several phenotypes that are critically relevant to cancer development (Howe et al. 2001). Overexpression of COX-2 leads to stimulation of mammary epithelial cell growth (Bandyopadhyay et al. 1987), increased biosynthesis of estrogens (Harris et al. 1999), and decreased immune surveillance (Huang et al. 1998). Additionally, expression of COX-2 leads to the production of mutagens (Howe et al. 2001), increased invasion, angiogenesis, and the inhibition of apoptosis (Liu et al. 1998; Gately 2000; Howe et al. 2001). The observations described here suggest that the rare foci of cells containing hypermethylated p16 promoters have the ability not only to accumulate genomic instability, but also to induce critical oncogenic phenotypes such as angiogenesis and inhibition of apoptosis. *Thus, these cells represent a potent precursor population for oncogenic progression.*

POTENTIAL RELEVANCE OF vHMEC TO MALIGNANCY

The above data demonstrate that a sizable fraction of women (>30%) have a subpopulation of human mammary ductal and lobular epithelial cells containing hypermethylated p16^{INK4a} promoter sequences and overexpression of COX-2. As noted before, hematoxylin and eosin staining of adjacent serial sections demonstrated that the cells containing the coincident overexpression of COX-2 and methylated p16 promoter sequences retained normal morphology as determined by pathologists. What is the relationship, if any, of these foci to the development of cancer? The first issue to address is that the fraction of women containing any frequency of foci exhibiting the "variant" characteristics is substantially higher than the fraction of women who are diagnosed with breast cancer. In addition, given that these determinations were done on a limited amount of tissue sampled from individual mammary glands, it may be that an even greater fraction of healthy women contain these foci, and/or the reservoir of these cells in healthy women is considerable. At the very least, this could indicate that not all of these foci progress to cancer. Since less than 30% of the population develops breast cancer, it could reasonably be argued that subsequent events are necessary for progression. Of course, alternatively, it could be that these cells do not relate to carcinogenesis at all and may represent some stem cell population or dead-end lineage.

Data exist for the progression of a fraction of less malignant lesions to more malignant ones. In this manner, fewer lesions at each stage would progress to the more advanced state. Using data generated from autopsy series, studies by Nielsen and colleagues (Nielsen et al. 1987) and Alpers and Wellings (1985), among others, shed light on the prevalence of undetected premalignant breast disease. In the Nielsen study of double mastectomy specimens from 110 medicolegal autopsies, whose cause of death was unrelated to breast cancer, nearly one-third of

patients harbored hyperplastic lesions (UDH, 32%), over one-quarter contained atypical ductal hyperplasia (ADH, 27%), almost one-fifth showed ductal carcinoma in situ (DCIS, 18%), and 2% had overt invasive breast cancer. Furthermore, almost half of the women with DCIS had bilateral (41%) and/or multifocal (45%) disease. Alpers and Wellings' study of 185 breast samples from random autopsies confirms this high prevalence of undetected premalignant breast lesions. Several other studies that sampled mastectomy tissue less frequently noted smaller numbers of premalignant lesions (Welch and Black 1997). Additionally, these numbers have been suggested to be high due to the difficulty in accurately diagnosing the various premalignant lesions. In the context of the observations made with the methylation of the p16 promoter in healthy women in vivo, one would hypothesize that the methylation event is an early molecular event and that subsequent events would contribute to the multistep progression of this population of nascent tumor cells through the premalignant stages. If this is so, the characterization of the in vitro vHMEC may provide molecular clues to the subsequent changes required for carcinogenesis.

If cells with variant characteristics do represent precursors to breast cancer, we would predict that some fraction of premalignant lesions would express the relevant characteristics. To test this hypotheis, we examined 65 cases of DCIS for the overexpression of COX-2 (Shim et al. 2003). We found that a large proportion of low- and high-grade DCIS overexpress COX-2 not only in the morphologically distinct DCIS lesion, but also in the adjacent surrounding morphologically normal epithelial cells. Studies are under way to assess the presence of cells with variant characteristics in even earlier premalignant lesions (see Fig. 5).

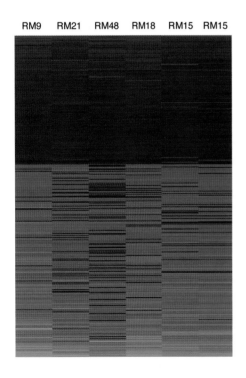

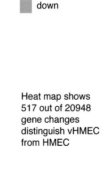

Heat map shows
517 out of 20948
gene changes
distinguish vHMEC
from HMEC

Figure 5. Gene expression profiling identifies a distinct subpopulation of cells in the human mammary gland. Tissues from five different women were processed for the generation of vHMEC populations and subjected to gene expression profiling. A signature of 517 gene changes identified the variant population of cells from the HMEC population. Of these changes, less than half are the result of p16 expression changes.

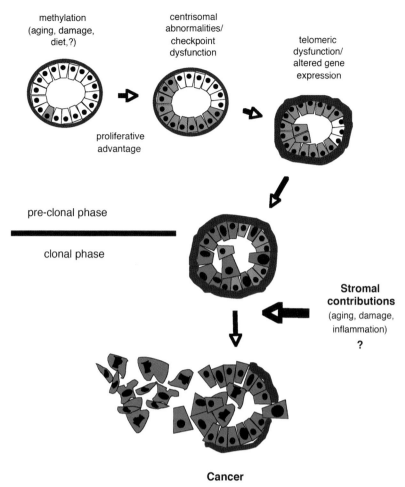

Figure 6. Model for breast cancer evolution.

CONCLUSIONS

We hypothesize that the above-described properties of HMEC in vitro are critically relevant to their transformation processes in vivo and may provide insights into controlling progression to cancer. In the model presented in Figure 6, cells that contain hypermethylated p16 promoter sequences could continue to proliferate under conditions when the p16-expressing cells do not. Since continued proliferation of cells in the absence of p16 expression holds great potential for generating chromosomal abnormalities, this subpopulation of cells is free to accumulate mutations that may facilitate tumorigenesis. When the variant cells proliferate to the point of critically short telomeres, telomeric dysfunction fuels the generation of massive, random pre-clonal genomic instability to allow the emergence of clonal isolates that may progress to tumorigenicity. Selection pressures exerted by the microenvironment would be postulated to generate clonal isolates. The continuing telomeric and centrosomal dysfunction, coupled with the activation of pathways associated with overexpression of COX-2, provides a potent package of events to promote tumorigenesis.

This alternative perception of the tumorigenic process differs from other perceptions in that it recognizes a distinct subpopulation of cells which can be identified in an especially vulnerable stage of carcinogenesis that exists prior to the clonal outgrowth of tumorigenic cells. The majority of therapeutic targets at the present time address the consequences of genomic instability, such as the targeting of Gleevec to the Philadelphia chromosome translocation. Analysis of this model system may provide targets to address the process of genomic instability rather than its consequences.

ACKNOWLEDGMENTS

We gratefully acknowledge Dr. S. Lowe and Dr. G. Hannon for the gift of the shRNA p16[INK4a]. We thank Dr. J. Salisbury for providing antibody for immunocytochemical detection of the centrosome-associated centrin protein (clone 20H5) and for the EGFP-CETN2 plasmid construct. We thank Dr. Alexey Khodjakov for the EGFP-γ-Tubulin plasmid construct. We thank Dr. W. Lingle and V. Negron for technical advice on immunocytochemical techniques. We thank J. Sedivy for the gift of human diploid fibroblasts with inactivated p21, and Karen Chew for help with human tissue acquisition. We thank Dr. W. Hyun for technical assistance with confocal microscopy and flow cytometry. We are also grateful to M. Stampfer for early technical assistance with cell culture. This work was supported by the Avon Foundation, The Cancer League, Inc., grant CA73952 from the National Institutes of Health/National Cancer Institute awarded to T.D.T., and funding from the California Breast Cancer Research Program. K.M.M. and H.B. were supported by funding from the George Williams Hooper Foundation training grant, and K.M.M. by a postdoctoral fellowship to the California Breast Cancer Research Program. C.A.F. was supported by funding from the Department of Defense.

REFERENCES

Alpers C.E. and Wellings S.R. 1985. The prevalence of carcinoma in situ in normal and cancer-associated breasts. *Hum. Pathol.* **16:** 796.

Band V. and Sager R. 1989. Distinctive traits of normal and tumor-derived human mammary epithelial cells expressed in a medium that support long-term growth of both cell types. *Proc. Natl. Acad. Sci.* **86:** 1249.

Bandyopadhyay G.K., Imagawa W., Wallace D., and Nandi S. 1987. Linoleate metabolites enhance the in vitro proliferative response of mouse mammary epithelial cells to epidermal growth factor. *J. Biol. Chem.* **262:** 2750.

Baylin S.B. and Herman J.G. 2000. DNA hypermethylation in tumorigenesis: Epigenetics joins genetics. *Trends Genet.* **4:** 168.

Benanti J.A. and Galloway D.A. 2004. Normal human fibroblasts are resistant to RAS-induced senescence. *Mol. Cell. Biol.* **24:** 2842.

Berg J.W. and Hutter R.V. 1995. Breast cancer. *Cancer* **75:** 257.

Bodnar A.G., Ouellette M., Frolkis M., Holt S.E., Chiu C.P., Morin G.B., Harley C.B., Shay J.W., Lichtsteiner S., and Wright W.E. 1998. Extension of life-span by introduction of telomerase into normal human cells. *Science* **279:** 349.

Boveri T. 1914. *Zur Frage der Entstehung maligner Tumoren,* vol. 4, p. 64. Gustav Fischer, Jena, Germany.

Boveri T. and Boveri M. 1929. *The origin of malignant tumors.* Williams and Wilkins, Baltimore, Maryland.

Brenner A.J., Stampfer M.R., and Aldaz C.M. 1998. Increased p16 expression with first senescence arrest in human mammary epithelial cells and extended growth capacity with p16 inactivation. *Oncogene* **17:** 199.

Burbano R.R., Mederios A., deAmorin M.I., Lima E.M., Mello A., Neto J.B., and Casartelli C. 2000. Cytogenetics of epithelial hyperplasias of the human breast. *Cancer Genet. Cytogenet.* **119:** 62.

Cairns P., Mao L., Merlo A., Lee D.J., Schwab D., Eby Y., Tokino K., Van der Riet P., Blaugrund J.E., and Sidransky D. 1994. Rates of p16 (MTS1) mutations in primary tumors with 9p loss. *Science* **265:** 415.

Crawford Y.G., Gauthier M.L., Joubel A., Mantei K., Kozakiewicz K., Afshari C.A., and Tlsty T.D. 2004. Histologically normal human mammary epithelia with silenced p16(INK4a) overexpress COX-2, promoting a premalignant program. *Cancer Cell* **5:** 263.

Deng G., Lu Y., Zlotnikov G., Thor A.D., and Smith H.S. 1996. Loss of heterozygosity in normal tissue adjacent to breast carcinomas. *Science* **274:** 2057.

Duensing S. 2005. A tentative classification of centrosome abnormalities in cancer. *Cell Biol. Int.* **29:** 352.

Foster S.A. and Galloway D.A. 1996. Human papillomavirus type 16 E7 alleviates a proliferation block in early passage human mammary epithelial cells. *Oncogene* **12:** 1773.

Foster S.A., Wong D.J., Barrett M.T., and Galloway D.A. 1998. Inactivation of p16 in human mammary epithelial cells by CpG island methylation. *Mol. Cell. Biol.* **18:** 1793.

Gately S. 2000. The contributions of cyclooxygenase-2 to tumor angiogenesis. *Cancer Metastasis Rev.* **19:** 19.

Gonzalez-Zulueta M., Bender C.M., Yang A.S., Nguyen T., Beart R.W., Van Tornout J.M., and Jones P.A. 1997. Methylation of the 5′ CpG island of the p16/CDKN2 tumor suppresor gene in normal and transformed human tissue correlates with gene silencing. *Cancer Res.* **55:** 4531.

Hahn W.C., Counter C.M., Lundberg A.S., Beijersbergen R.L., Brooks M.W., and Weinberg R.A. 1999. Creation of human tumor cells with defined genetic elements. *Nature* **400:** 464.

Hammond S.L., Ham R.G., and Stampfer M.R. 1984. Serum-free growth of human mammary epithelial cells: Rapid clonal growth in defined medium and extended passage with pituitary extract. *Proc. Natl. Acad. Sci.* **81:** 5435.

Harris R.E., Robertson F.M., Abou-Issa H.M., Farrar W.B., and Brueggemeier R. 1999. Genetic induction and upregulation of cyclooxygenase (COX) and aromatase (CYP19): An extension of the dietary fat hypothesis of breast cancer. *Med. Hypotheses* **52:** 291.

Hayflick L. 1965. The limited *in vitro* lifetime of human diploid cell strains. *Exp. Cell Res.* **37:** 614.

Herman, J.G., Graff, J.R., Myöhänen S., Nelkin B.D., and Baylin S.B. 1996. Methylation-specific PCR: A novel PCR assay for methylation status of CpG islands. *Proc. Natl. Acad. Sci.* **93:** 9821.

Herman J.G., Civin C.I., Issa J.P., Collector M.I., Sharkis S.J., and Baylin S.B. 1997. Distinct patterns of inactivation of p15INK4B and p16INK4A characterize the major types of hematological malignancies. *Cancer Res.* **57:** 837.

Holst C.R., Nuovo G.J., Esteller M., Chew K., Baylin S.B., Herman J.G., and Tlsty T.D. 2003. Methylation of p16(INK4a) promoters occurs in vivo in histologically normal human mammary epithelia. *Cancer Res.* **63:** 1596.

Howe L.R., Subbaramaiah K., Brown A.M., and Dannenberg A.J. 2001. Cyclooxygenase-2: A target for the prevention and treatment of breast cancer. *Endocr. Relat. Cancer* **8:** 97.

Huang M., Stolina M., Sharma S., Mao J.T., Zhu L., Miller P.W., Wollman J., Herschmann D., and Dubinett S.M. 1998. Non-small cell lung cancer cyclooxygenase-2-dependent regulation of cytokine balance in lymphocytes and macrophages: Up-regulation of interleukin 10 and down-regulation of interleukin 12 production. *Cancer Res.* **58:** 1208.

Huschtscha L.I., Noble J.R., Neumann A.A., Moy E.L., Barry P., Melki J.R., Clark S.J., and Reddel R.R. 1998. Loss of p16INK4 expression by methylation is associated with lifespan extension of human mammary epithelial cells. *Cancer Res.* **58:** 3508.

Jiang X.R., Jimenez G., Chang E., Frolkis M., Kusler B., Sage M., Beeche M., Bodnar A.G., Wahl GM., Tlsty T.D., and Chiu C.P. 1999. Telomerase expression in human somatic cells does not induce changes associated with a transformed phenotype. *Nat. Genet.* **21:** 111.

Kao C.Y., Nomata K., Oakley C.S., Welsh C.W., and Chang C.C. 1995. Two types of normal human breast epithelial cells derived from reduction mammoplasty: Phenotypic characterization and response to SV40 transfection. *Carcinogenesis* **16:** 531.

Kiyono T., Foster S.A., Koop J.I., McDougall J.K., Galloway D.A., and Klingelhutz A.J. 1998. Both Rb/p16INK4a inactivation and telomerase activity are required to immortalize human epithelial cells. *Nature* **396:** 84.

Krinferpot P., Quon K.C., Mooi W.J., Loonstra A., and Berns A. 2001. Loss of p16 Ink4a confers susceptibility to metastatic melanoma in mice. *Nature* **413:** 83.

Lakhani S.R., Chaggar R., Davies S., Jones C., and Collins N. 1999. Genetic alterations in 'normal' luminal and myoepithelial cells of the breast. *J. Pathol.* **189:** 496.

Larson P.S., de las Morenas A., Bennett S.R., Cupples L.A., and Rosenberg C.L. 2002. Loss of heterozygosity or allele imbalance in histologically normal breast epithelium is distinct from loss of heterozygosity or allele imbalance in co-existing carcinomas. *Am. J. Pathol.* **161:** 283.

Larson P.S., de las Morenas A., Cupples L.A., Huang K., and Rosenberg C.L. 1998. Genetically abnormal clones in histologically normal breast tissue. *Am. J. Pathol.* **152:** 1591.

Li Z., Moore D.H., Meng Z.H., Ljung B.M., and Gray J.W.

2002. Increased risk of local recurrence is associated with allelic loss in normal lobules of breast cancer patients. *Cancer Res.* **62:** 1000.

Lingle W.L. and Salisbury J.L. 1999. Altered centrosome structure is associated with abnormal mitosis in human breast tumors. *Am. J. Pathol.* **155:** 1941.

Lingle W.L., Barrett S.L., Negron V.C., D'Assoro A.B., and Boeneman K. 2002. Centrosome and amplification drives chromosomal instability in breast tumor development. *Proc. Natl. Acad. Sci.* **99:** 1978.

Lingle W.L., Lutz W.H., Ingle J.N., Maihle N.J, and Salisbury J.L. 1998. Centrosome hypertrophy in human breast tumors: Implications for genomic stability and cell polarity. *Proc. Natl. Acad. Sci.* **95:** 2950.

Liu X.H., Yao S., Kirschenbaum A., and Levine A.C. 1998. NS398, a selective cyclooxygenase-2 inhibitor, induces apoptosis and down-regulates bcl-2 expression in LNCaP cells. *Cancer Res.* **58:** 4245.

Luria S.E. and Delbrück M. 1943. Mutations of bacteria from virus sensitivity to virus resistance. *Genetics* **28:** 491.

Medema R.H., Herrera R.E., Lam F., and Weinberg R.A. 1995. Growth suppression by p16INK4 requires functional retinoblastoma protein. *Proc. Natl. Acad. Sci.* **92:** 6289.

Nielsen M., Thomsen J.L., Primdahl S., Dyreborg U., and Andersen J.A. 1987. Breast cancer and atypia among young and middle-aged women: A study of 110 medicolegal autopsies. *Br. J. Cancer* **56:** 814.

Nguyen C., Liang G., Nguyen T.T., Tsao-Wei D., Groshen S., Lübbert M., Zhou J.H., Benedict W.F., and Jones P.A. 2001. Susceptibility of nonpromoter CpG islands to de novo methylation in normal and neoplastic cells. *J. Natl. Cancer Inst.* **93:** 1465.

Nuovo G.J., Plaia T.W., Belinsky S.A, Baylin S.B., and Herman J.G. 1999. In situ detection of the hypermethylation-induced inactivation of the p16 gene as an early event in oncogenesis. *Proc. Natl. Acad. Sci.* **96:** 12754.

Pandis N. 1995. Chromosome abnormalities in bilateral breast carcinomas. Cytogenetic evaluation of the clonal origin of multiple primary tumors. *Cancer* **76:** 250.

Parry D. and Peters G. 1996. Temperature-sensitive mutants of p16^{CDKN2} associated with familial melanoma. *Mol. Cell. Biol.* **16:** 3844.

Ramirez R.D., Morales C.P., Herbert B.S., Rohde J.M., Passons C., Shay J.W., and Wright W.E. 2001. Putative telomere-independent mechanisms of replicative aging reflect inadequate growth conditions. *Genes Dev.* **15:** 398.

Romanov S.R., Kozakiewicz B.K., Holst C.R., Stampfer M.R., Haupt L.M., and Tlsty T.D. 2001. Normal human mammary epithelial cells spontaneously escape senescence and acquire genomic changes. *Nature* **409:** 633.

Salisbury J.L. 2001. The contribution of epigenetic changes to

abnormal centrosomes and genomic instability in breast cancer. *J. Mammary Gland Biol. Neoplasia* **6:** 203.

Serrano M., Hannon G.J, and Beach D. 1993. A new regulatory motif in cell-cycle control causing specific inhibition of cyclin D/CDK4. *Nature* **366:** 704.

Sharpless N.E., Bardeesy N., Lee K.H., Carrasco D., Castrillon D.H, Aguirre A.J., Wu E.A., Horner J.W., and DePinho R.A. 2001. Loss of p16Ink4a with retention of p19Arf predisposes mice to tumorigenesis. *Nature* **413:** 86.

Shim V., Gauthier M.L., Sudilovsky D., Mantei K., Chew K.L., Moore D.H., Cha I., Tlsty T.D., and Esserman L.J. 2003. Cyclooxygenase-2 expression is related to nuclear grade in ductal carcinoma in situ and is increased in its normal adjacent epithelium. *Cancer Res.* **63:** 2347.

Stampfer M.R., Garbe J., Levine G., Lichtsteiner S., Vasserot A.P., and Yaswen P. 2001. Expression of the telomerase catalytic subunit, hTERT, induces resistance to transforming growth factor β growth inhibition in p16^{INK4a}(-) human mammary epithelial cells. *Proc. Natl. Acad. Sci.* **98:** 4498.

Taylor-Papadimitriou J., Stampfer M., Bartek J., Lewis A., Boshell M., Lane E.B., and Leigh I.M. 1989. Keratin expression in human mammary epithelial cells cultured from normal and malignant tissue: Relation to *in vivo* phenotypes and influence of medium. *J. Cell Sci.* **94:** 403.

Tlsty T.D., Margolin B.H., and Lum K. 1989. Differences in the rates of gene amplification in nontumorigenic and tumorigenic cell lines as measured by Luria-Delbrück fluctuation analysis. *Proc. Natl. Acad. Sci.* **86:** 9441.

Tlsty T.D., Romanov S.R., Kozakiewicz B.K., Holst C.R., Haupt L.M., and Crawford Y.G. 2001. Loss of chromosomal integrity in human mammary epithelial cells subsequent to escape from senescence. *J. Mammary Gland Biol. Neoplasia* **6:** 235.

Tlsty T.D., Crawford Y.G., Holst C.R., Fordyce C.A., Zhang J., McDermott K., Kozakiewicz K., and Gauthier M.L. 2004. Genetic and epigenetic changes in mammary epithelial cells may mimic early events in carcinogenesis. *J. Mammary Gland Biol. Neoplasia* **9:** 263.

Van Steensel B., Smogorzewska A., and de Lange T. 1998. TRF2 protects human telomeres from end-to-end fusions. *Cell* **92:** 401.

Walen K.H. and Stampfer M.R. 1989. Chromosome analyses of human mammary epithelial cells at stages of chemical-induced transformation progression to immortality. *Cancer Genet. Cytogenet.* **37:** 249.

Welch H.G. and Black W.C. 1997. Using autopsy series to estimate the disease "reservoir" for ductal carcinoma in situ of the breast: How much more breast cancer can we find? *Ann. Intern. Med.* **127:** 1023.

Yang R., Serrano M., Slater J., Leung E., and Koeffler H.P. 1996. Analysis of p16INK4a and its interaction with CDK4. *Biochem. Biophys. Res. Commun.* **218:** 254.

Epigenetic Changes in Cancer and Preneoplasia

J.G. HERMAN

The Sidney Kimmel Comprehensive Cancer Center at Johns Hopkins,
Baltimore, Maryland 21231

Recent studies have identified an increasing number of genes that are inactivated by promoter region methylation in cancer. Some of these genes were initially identified as altered genetically in cancer, but in other tumors they are silenced in association with promoter region CpG island methylation. New approaches for screening the genome add to this list of candidate tumor suppressor genes, and many genes regulated key pathways in cancer, including cell cycle control, DNA repair, and apoptosis. Transcription factors may also be silenced by promoter region methylation, affecting the expression of many downstream target genes and globally altering the cancer phenotype. Determining loss of expression is important in assigning functional importance to promoter region methylation for any gene. Individual cancers have alterations in many different genes, affecting many of these important pathways and contributing to the cancer phenotype. The number of genes targeted for promoter region methylation increases during neoplastic progression. These studies suggest that the epigenetic change of promoter region methylation plays a critical role in neoplastic transformation and progression.

Genetic alterations are a hallmark of human cancer and form the basis of much of what we know about cancer. However, many of the changes that are functionally relevant for the development and progression of cancer occur without changes at the nucleotide level, which is in the absence of mutation. The down-regulation of the expression of many genes has been recently found to be caused by changes in promoter region methylation, which is an epigenetic change. The CpG dinucleotide, which is usually underrepresented in the genome, is clustered in the promoter regions of many genes. These promoter regions have been termed CpG islands (Bird 1986). CpG islands are protected from methylation in normal cells, with the exception of genes on the inactive X chromosome and imprinted genes. This protection is critical, since the methylation of promoter region CpG islands is associated with a loss of expression of these genes through chromatin changes, as discussed below. The following three different alterations in DNA methylation are common in human cancer: (1) global hypomethylation, often seen within the body of genes; (2) dysregulation of DNA methyltransferase I, the enzyme involved in maintaining methylation patterns, and potentially other methyltransferases; and (3) regional hypermethylation in normally unmethylated CpG islands.

EPIGENETIC CHANGES TARGET KEY TUMOR SUPPRESSOR GENES

Extensive work by many investigators over the last several years has demonstrated that promoter hypermethylation commonly silences tumor suppressor genes in human cancer, serving as an alternative mechanism for the loss of tumor suppressor gene function (Baylin et al. 2001; Jones and Baylin 2002; Herman and Baylin 2003). Initial studies commonly focused on classic tumor suppressor genes, which were mutated in some cancers and may have an inherited predisposition associated with

germ-line mutations. For example, the cell-cycle-regulated p16INK4a, a cyclin-dependent kinase inhibitor that regulates another tumor suppressor gene Rb, is commonly deleted in cancers (Kamb et al. 1994). However, if it is not deleted, inactivation can occur in association with promoter region methylation (Merlo et al. 1995) and is associated with loss of gene expression. Although this growth in interest does not displace or diminish the importance of the genetic changes in cancer, in this overview I only discuss the role of epigenetic changes in cancer, specifically, promoter region DNA methylation.

PROMOTER REGION METHYLATION SILENCES THROUGH CHROMATIN CHANGES

DNA hypermethylation in the promoter region of genes is associated with loss of gene expression. By using bisulfite genomic sequencing (including cloning of individual alleles) to obtain a detailed analysis of methylation in acute leukemia, leukemia cell lines, and normal lymphocytes, evidence for the importance of methylation density was shown for p15ink4b/CDKN2B (Cameron et al. 1999a). This gene is frequently methylated in acute lymphocytic and myelogenous leukemia. The entire CpG island region of p15 was largely devoid of methylation in normal lymphocytes, but methylation of varying density was found in primary acute leukemia. Methylation density was generally conserved between the alleles from each sample, but marked heterogeneity for the specific CpG sites methylated was observed. Patterns of methylation were compared and expression was assessed with reverse-transcriptase polymerase chain reaction (RT-PCR). The density of methylation within the CpG island, and not any specific location, correlates best with transcriptional loss (Cameron et al. 1999a). Leukemias with methylation of approximately 40% of the CpG dinucleotides on each allele had complete gene silencing, with variable, but diminished, expression with less dense CpG island methylation.

Promoter region methylation is associated with silencing through changes in chromatin configuration and the histone code. Densely methylated DNA associates with transcriptionally repressive chromatin characterized by the presence of underacetylated histones. Optimal reexpression of silenced genes is accomplished by inhibition of both DNA methyltransferase and histone deacetylases (Cameron et al. 1999b). Using detailed mapping by chromatin immunoprecipitation (ChIP), clearly defined zones of deacetylated histone H3 plus methyl-H3-K9 surround a hypermethylated, silenced promoter, which, when unmethylated and active, is embedded in methyl-H3-K4 and acetylated H3 (Fahrner et al. 2002). Inhibiting DNA methyltransferases, but not histone deacetylases, leads first to promoter demethylation, second to gene reexpression, and finally, to complete histone code reversal (Fahrner et al. 2002). These studies link the changes in DNA methylation to associated changes in the histone code associated with gene silencing and demonstrate the importance of detailed chromatin maps.

HOW FREQUENT ARE PROMOTER REGION METHYLATION CHANGES?

The increasing recognition of epigenetic changes in cancer has been facilitated by technical advances that allow rapid evaluation of promoter region methylation changes, and by screening techniques that can identify novel targets of epigenetic silencing. Evaluation of methylation patterns is largely dependent on the development of bisulfite-based techniques, first used for genomic bisulfite sequencing mentioned above (Frommer et al. 1992). Conversion of cytosine, but not 5′-methyl-cytosine, to uracil allows the epigenetic change of DNA methylation to be converted to a genetic equivalent, thereby permitting the use of genetic analysis. A wide variety of bisulfite-based techniques can be used to determine methylation patterns of genes under study. These include detailed genomic bisulfite sequencing (Clark et al. 1994), methylation-specific PCR (Herman et al. 1996), which has real-time PCR adaptations (Lo et al. 1999; Eads et al. 2000), and restriction analysis following bisulfite treatment (Sadri and Hornsby 1996; Xiong and Laird 1997). Since methylation-associated gene silencing is a regional change associated with gene silencing, as discussed above, analysis is much simpler than the sequencing of the entire coding region of a gene to search for many different mutations. With these techniques, large numbers of samples can be examined at multiple loci.

IDENTIFICATION OF GENES TARGETED FOR PROMOTER REGION METHYLATION

The genes studied for promoter region methylation in cancer are derived from three main sources. First, the group of classic tumor suppressor genes, mutated in some cancers, can be silenced in association with promoter region methylation in many other cancers. For example, *Rb, P16ink4a, MLH1, CDH1, VHL*, and *BRCA1* are all genes with well-defined increased familial risk of cancer associated with germ-line mutations, and for which transcriptional silencing associated with promoter region hypermethylation has been well documented (Herman and Baylin 2003). For these genes, the importance of epigenetic inactivation is supported by the genetic evidence. It is unlikely that many other familial cancer genes of this type will be identified in the future, however, as these low-prevalence genes associated with extremely high cancer risk have largely already been discovered.

However, many other genes have been examined for promoter region methylation in cancer and appear to have important roles, even though little or no genetic evidence for their function in cancer is known. Genes in this second group have in some cases been identified through regions of allelic loss in cancer where mutational inactivation of the second copy is not found. For example, RASSF1a, a gene commonly methylated and silenced in different types of cancer, was identified from a commonly deleted region of the short arm of chromosome 3 in lung cancer (Dammann et al. 2000). In other cases, pathways regulated by the potentially inactivated gene have been so important that an examination of possible inactivation, including those related to epigenetic changes, has been pursued. This group of genes includes *p73*, which shares many important regulatory functions with *p53* (Jost et al. 1997) and is epigenetically, rather than genetically, inactivated in cancers (Corn et al. 1999; Kawano et al. 1999). Finally, epigenetically inactivated genes derived from knowledge of diminished expression in cancer. For example, the loss of expression of the DNA repair protein methyl-guanine methyltransferase (*MGMT*) cannot be explained by genetic losses, but rather is due to promoter region methylation changes (Patel et al. 1997; Esteller et al. 1999).

The recognition of key gene inactivation events playing a role in cancer has led to the development of a number of approaches seeking novel epigenetically silenced genes. Such genome-wide screens either take advantage of methylation-sensitive restriction analysis to find methylated regions in the genome (Liang et al. 1998; Toyota et al. 1999; Costello et al. 2000) or utilize the power of expression analysis using microarrays to find reactivation of silenced genes (Suzuki et al. 2002; Yamashita et al. 2002). Based on the identification of methylation changes through screening approaches, the number of genes methylated in an individual cancer may range in the hundreds (Costello et al. 2000; Suzuki et al. 2002; Yamashita et al. 2002). Given this number, this group of genes represents a challenge for the evaluation of the functional importance of any methylation change, even if clearly associated with loss of gene expression.

FUNCTIONAL SIGNIFICANCE OF PROMOTER METHYLATION

For both genes without mutational inactivation and those identified through screening approaches, however, gene function remains a key component in determining the role that epigenetic changes in the promoter region of a novel gene play in the cancer phenotype. Many of the

- Cell cycle control
  - *Rb, p16, p15, p14, p73, CHFR*
- DNA damage
  - *MLH1, O⁶MGMT, GSTπ, BRCA1, Fanconi-F*
- Apoptosis
  - *DAP-kinase, Caspase-8, ASC/TMS-1*
- Invasion
  - *E-cadherin, VHL, APC, LKB1, TIMP3, THBS1, H-cad*
- Growth factor response
  - *ER, RARβ, AR, SOCS-1, RASSF1a, CRBP, SHP1*
  - *SFRP1, SFRP2, SFRP5*
- Transcription Factors/Repressors
  - *HIC1, PAX5α, PAX5β, AP2, GATA4, GATA5, CDX2*

Figure 1. Promoter region hypermethylation targets critical pathways in human cancer. Promoter region methylation and gene silencing have been demonstrated for these genes in cancer, with resulting alteration in these pathways.

key genes studied extensively for epigenetic silencing in cancer fall into key pathways involved in the malignant phenotype. A select list of such pathway alterations and epigenetically inactivated genes associated with these functions is presented in Figure 1. These involve cell cycle control, DNA repair, apoptosis, and other critical pathways involved in maintaining the normal cell phenotype. The classification of these alterations is in part derived from the well-accepted model of the hallmarks of cancer (Hanahan and Weinberg 2000).

SILENCING OF REGULATORY GENES MAY GLOBALLY AFFECT THE CELL PHENOTYPE

As discussed above, there may be technical advantages in searching for genes methylated in cancer which lead to identification of increased numbers of hypermethylated genes in cancer. However, there may be additional, nontechnical reasons for the large number of reported epigenetic changes in cancer. Although the exact relationship between the number of epigenetic and genetic changes in cancer will not be understood until work in the Cancer Genome Project is complete, providing a comprehensive genetic and hopefully epigenetic map of the cancer genome of specific cancers, it is possible that the number of epigenetic changes in a given cancer exceeds the number of genetic changes. Epigenetic changes are a very powerful modulator of cellular phenotype, as demonstrated by the profound differences in function of differentiated tissues from different organs.

As an example of this normal modulator of the cell phenotype, the wide variety of histological differentiation observed during embryogenesis is mediated through epigenetic mechanisms, not genetic alterations. Tissues of different origins share the same genotype, and the heritable differences in gene expression must be a reflection of epigenetic changes. It is perhaps interesting to speculate that the abnormal gene silencing due to promoter region methylation observed in cancer represents a normal process gone bad; that is, the normal tissue-specific silencing of genes is abnormally utilized by the cancer precursor cell to produce the transformed phenotype. In contrast, the importance of maintenance of the correct DNA sequence

prior to and during DNA replication is reflected by the accuracy of DNA polymerases and the comprehensive and redundant mechanisms for DNA repair pathways that function in human cells (Shcherbakova et al. 2003).

One of the most comprehensive ways to alter a cell phenotype, however, is to alter the expression of genes regulating the expression of other genes. In this case, loss of expression of a transcription factor, for example, would result in altered expression of many downstream target genes. Therefore, it is of interest to note the growing list of recently identified transcription factors that are epigenetically silenced in cancers (Fig. 1). Discussed extensively by Stephen Baylin (Baylin and Chen, this volume) is the HIC-1 gene, a frequently methylated gene in many cancers that can regulate the expression of critical downstream target genes by acting as a transcriptional repressor. Loss of such repressors could lead to increased expression of critical genes, including SIRT1. Also of note are AP2 (Douglas et al. 2004), PAX5 (Palmisano et al. 2003), and GATA4 and GATA5 (Akiyama et al. 2003), all transcription factors potentially modulating the expression of numerous target genes. We have recently determined the methylation-associated silencing of another key transcription factor that modulates the intestinal phenotype. CDX2 is hypermethylated and silenced in certain esophageal cancers, potentially leading to reprogramming of the differentiation of these cells. Loss of CDX2 is associated with loss of the MUC2 gene, normally associated with the adenocarcinoma phenotype.

EPIGENETIC SILENCING AFFECTS MULTIPLE GENES IN INDIVIDUAL TUMORS

Epigenetic silencing can, of course, affect multiple genes within each cancer. Therefore, studies directed at individual loci, although critical for the initial understanding of the role of gene inactivation in these cancers, do not establish this event in the context of the multiple other genetic and epigenetic changes present in a cancer. Indeed, by looking at multiple genes in individual cancers, it can be seen that the majority of cancers contain many aberrantly methylated CpG islands that silence many critical genes (Esteller et al. 2001; Toyota et al. 2001; Chim et al. 2003). These epigenetic profiles differ according to tissue of origin of the cancer and the divergent pathological differentiation followed. In examination of a rarely studied tumor, primary CNS lymphoma, we find frequent methylation of genes involved in cell cycle control, DNA repair, and apoptosis, as well as growth factor response, encompassing each of the fundamental pathways shown in Figure 1. The genes silenced in this malignancy are similar to those found in other non-Hodgkin's lymphomas and Burkitt's lymphoma. Multiple epigenetic changes cooperate to transform a cell from the normal to the transformed state.

EPIGENETIC PROGRESSION OF CANCER

The number of changes observed in these tumors offers another advantage in studying the biology of neoplasia.

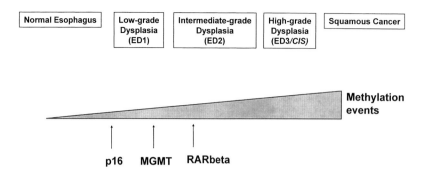

Figure 2. A model for the epigenetic progression of the histological changes found in the development of squamous cell carcinoma. Increases in frequency at individual loci occur as the lesions become more abnormal. In addition, the overall number of genes with aberrant methylation increases as histological atypia increase.

Carcinogenesis is a multistep process that has been described in terms of a tumor progression model, most extensively in the genetic changes found in colon cancer (Vogelstein and Kinzler 1993). We have recently examined the changes in promoter region methylation at multiple loci of invasive tumors, normal tissues, and preinvasive lesions from these same tissues. As an example, the well-defined histology progression of esophageal cancer provides an opportunity to correlate histological progression with molecular progression. The genes targeted for inactivation include those regulating key pathways, as noted in Figure 1. The timing of these events appears to vary, much as has been observed for the genetic models of tumor progression. However, the number of changes present in a lesion increases as the histological changes worsen. We suggest that these observations represent the epigenetic progression that parallels histological progression observed in tumors derived from many organ sites. This is shown in Figure 2.

Because of the frequency and timing of these epigenetic changes, promoter hypermethylation events provide one of the most promising markers for molecular detection of early cancer. DNA-based markers have advantages because of the inherent stability of DNA compared with RNA and some proteins. In addition, the molecular progression observed in many cancers suggests that epigenetic changes might be used to predict progression of preinvasive to invasive cancer, a hypothesis being tested in the preinvasive condition, Barrett's esophagus.

CONCLUSION

In conclusion, extensive work over the last decade by investigators has demonstrated that epigenetic changes, in addition to the previously defined genetic alterations, are a key component in the development and progression of human cancer. Important regulatory pathways are altered by the silencing of genes with tumor suppressor features, and individual cancers normally have promoter region methylation affecting multiple genes. Screening strategies will uncover new targets of epigenetic silencing, for which the evaluation of functional importance will be needed. The development of epigenetic changes parallels the histological progression, suggesting that

many of the phenotypic changes observed histologically are driven by underlying changes in gene expression. The frequency and timing of altered DNA methylation suggest that they may be markers of disease and disease progression.

REFERENCES

Akiyama Y., Watkins N., Suzuki H., Jair K.W., van Engeland M., Esteller M., Sakai H., Ren C.Y., Yuasa Y., Herman J.G., and Baylin S.B. 2003. GATA-4 and GATA-5 transcription factor genes and potential downstream antitumor target genes are epigenetically silenced in colorectal and gastric cancer. *Mol. Cell. Biol.* **23:** 8429.

Baylin S.B., Esteller M., Rountree M.R., Bachman K.E., Schuebel K., and Herman J.G. 2001. Aberrant patterns of DNA methylation, chromatin formation and gene expression in cancer. *Hum. Mol. Genet.* **10:** 687.

Bird A.P. 1986. CpG-rich islands and the function of DNA methylation. *Nature* **321:** 209.

Cameron E.E., Baylin S.B., and Herman J.G. 1999a. p15(INK4B) CpG island methylation in primary acute leukemia is heterogeneous and suggests density as a critical factor for transcriptional silencing. *Blood* **94:** 2445.

Cameron E.E., Bachman K.E., Myohanen S., Herman J.G., and Baylin S.B. 1999b. Synergy of demethylation and histone deacetylase inhibition in the re-expression of genes silenced in cancer. *Nat. Genet.* **21:** 103.

Chim C.S., Wong S.Y., and Kwong Y.L. 2003. Aberrant gene promoter methylation in acute promyelocytic leukaemia: profile and prognostic significance. *Br. J. Haematol.* **122:** 571.

Clark S.J., Harrison J., Paul C.L., and Frommer M. 1994. High sensitivity mapping of methylated cytosines. *Nucleic Acids Res.* **22:** 2990.

Corn P.G., Kuerbitz S.J., van Noesel M.M., Esteller M., Compitello N., Baylin S.B., and Herman J.G. 1999. Transcriptional silencing of the p73 gene in acute lymphoblastic leukemia and Burkitt's lymphoma is associated with 5′ CpG island methylation. *Cancer Res.* **59:** 3352.

Costello J.F., Fruhwald M.C., Smiraglia D.J., Rush L.J., Robertson G.P., Gao X., Wright F.A., Feramisco J.D., Peltomaki P., Lang J.C., Schuller D.E., Yu L., Bloomfield C.D., Caligiuri M.A., Yates A., Nishikawa R., Su Huang H., Petrelli N.J., Zhang X., O'Dorisio M.S., Held W.A., Cavenee W.K., and Plass C. 2000. Aberrant CpG-island methylation has non-random and tumour-type-specific patterns. *Nat. Genet.* **24:** 132.

Dammann R., Li C., Yoon J.H., Chin P.L., Bates S., and Pfeifer G.P. 2000. Epigenetic inactivation of a RAS association domain family protein from the lung tumour suppressor locus 3p21.3. *Nat. Genet.* **25:** 315.

Douglas D.B., Akiyama Y., Carraway H., Belinsky S.A., Esteller M., Gabrielson E., Weitzman S., Williams T., Herman

J.G., and Baylin S.B. 2004. Hypermethylation of a small CpGuanine-rich region correlates with loss of activator protein-2alpha expression during progression of breast cancer. *Cancer Res.* **64:** 1611.

Eads C.A., Danenberg K.D., Kawakami K., Saltz L.B., Blake C., Shibata D., Danenberg P.V., and Laird P.W. 2000. MethyLight: A high-throughput assay to measure DNA methylation. *Nucleic Acids Res.* **28:** e32.

Esteller M., Hamilton S.R., Burger P.C., Baylin S.B., and Herman J.G. 1999. Inactivation of the DNA repair gene O6-methylguanine-DNA methyltransferase by promoter hypermethylation is a common event in primary human neoplasia. *Cancer Res.* **59:** 793.

Esteller M., Fraga M.F., Guo M., Garcia-Foncillas J., Hedenfalk I., Godwin A.K., Trojan J., Vaurs-Barriere C., Bignon Y.J., Ramus S., Benitez J., Caldes T., Akiyama Y., Yuasa Y., Launonen V., Canal M.J., Rodriguez R., Capella G., Peinado M.A., Borg A., Aaltonen L.A., Ponder B.A., Baylin S.B., and Herman J.G. 2001. DNA methylation patterns in hereditary human cancers mimic sporadic tumorigenesis. *Hum. Mol. Genet.* **10:** 3001.

Fahrner J.A., Eguchi S., Herman J.G., and Baylin S.B. 2002. Dependence of histone modifications and gene expression on DNA hypermethylation in cancer. *Cancer Res.* **62:** 7213.

Frommer M., McDonald L.E., Millar D.S., Collis C.M., Watt F., Grigg G.W., Molloy P.L., and Paul C.L. 1992. A genomic sequencing protocol that yields a positive display of 5-methylcytosine residues in individual DNA strands. *Proc. Natl. Acad. Sci.* **89:** 1827.

Hanahan D. and Weinberg R.A. 2000. The hallmarks of cancer. *Cell* **100:** 57.

Herman J.G. and Baylin S.B. 2003. Gene silencing in cancer in association with promoter hypermethylation. *N. Engl. J. Med.* **349:** 2042.

Herman J.G., Graff J.R., Myohanen S., Nelkin B.D., and Baylin S.B. 1996. Methylation-specific PCR: A novel PCR assay for methylation status of CpG islands. *Proc. Natl. Acad. Sci.* **93:** 9821.

Jones P.A. and Baylin S.B. 2002. The fundamental role of epigenetic events in cancer. *Nat. Rev. Genet.* **3:** 415.

Jost C.A., Marin M.C., and Kaelin W.G., Jr. 1997. p73 is a human p53-related protein that can induce apoptosis. *Nature* **389:** 191.

Kamb A., Gruis N.A., Weaver-Feldhaus J., Liu Q., Harshman K., Tavtigian S.V., Stockert E., Day R.S., III, Johnson B.E., and Skolnick M.H. 1994. A cell cycle regulator potentially involved in genesis of many tumor types. *Science* **264:** 436.

Kawano S., Miller C.W., Gombart A.F., Bartram C.R., Matsuo Y., Asou H., Sakashita A., Said J., Tatsumi E., and Koeffler H.P. 1999. Loss of p73 gene expression in leukemias/lymphomas due to hypermethylation. *Blood* **94:** 1113.

Liang G., Salem C.E., Yu M.C., Nguyen H.D., Gonzales F.A., Nguyen T.T., Nichols P.W., and Jones P.A. 1998. DNA methylation differences associated with tumor tissues identified by genome scanning analysis. *Genomics* **53:** 260.

Lo Y.M., Wong I.H., Zhang J., Tein M.S., Ng M.H., and Hjelm N.M. 1999. Quantitative analysis of aberrant p16 methylation using real- time quantitative methylation-specific polymerase chain reaction. *Cancer Res.* **59:** 3899.

Merlo A., Herman J.G., Mao L., Lee D.J., Gabrielson E., Burger P.C., Baylin S.B., and Sidransky D. 1995. 5′ CPG island methylation is associated with transcriptional silencing of the tumour suppressor P16/CDKN2/MTS1 in human cancers. *Nat. Med.* **1:** 686.

Palmisano W.A., Crume K.P., Grimes M.J., Winters S.A., Toyota M., Esteller M., Joste N., Baylin S.B., and Belinsky S.A. 2003. Aberrant promoter methylation of the transcription factor genes PAX5 alpha and beta in human cancers. *Cancer Res.* **63:** 4620.

Patel S.A., Graunke D.M., and Pieper R.O. 1997. Aberrant silencing of the CpG island-containing human O6-methylguanine DNA methyltransferase gene is associated with the loss of nucleosome-like positioning. *Mol. Cell. Biol.* **17:** 5813.

Sadri R. and Hornsby P.J. 1996. Rapid analysis of DNA methylation using new restriction enzyme sites created by bisulfite modification. *Nucleic Acids Res.* **24:** 5058.

Shcherbakova P.V., Bebenek K., and Kunkel T.A. 2003. Functions of eukaryotic DNA polymerases. *Sci. Aging Knowledge Environ.* **2003:** RE3.

Suzuki H., Gabrielson E., Chen W., Anbazhagan R., Van Engeland M., Weijenberg M.P., Herman J.G., and Baylin S.B. 2002. A genomic screen for genes upregulated by demethylation and histone deacetylase inhibition in human colorectal cancer. *Nat. Genet.* **31:** 141.

Toyota M., Kopecky K.J., Toyota M.O., Jair K.W., Willman C.L., and Issa J.P. 2001. Methylation profiling in acute myeloid leukemia. *Blood* **97:** 2823.

Toyota M., Ho C., Ahuja N., Jair K.W., Li Q., Ohe-Toyota M., Baylin S.B., and Issa J.P. 1999. Identification of differentially methylated sequences in colorectal cancer by methylated CpG island amplification. *Cancer Res.* **59:** 2307.

Vogelstein B. and Kinzler K.W. 1993. The multistep nature of cancer. *Trends Genet.* **9:** 138.

Xiong Z. and Laird P.W. 1997. COBRA: A sensitive and quantitative DNA methylation assay. *Nucleic Acids Res.* **25:** 2532.

Yamashita K., Upadhyay S., Osada M., Hoque M.O., Xiao Y., Mori M., Sato F., Meltzer S.J., and Sidransky D. 2002. Pharmacologic unmasking of epigenetically silenced tumor suppressor genes in esophageal squamous cell carcinoma. *Cancer Cell* **2:** 485.

A Genetic Approach to Cancer Epigenetics

A.P. FEINBERG

Departments of Medicine, Molecular Biology & Genetics, and Oncology,
Johns Hopkins University School of Medicine, Baltimore, Maryland 21205

In over 20 years since the discovery of altered methylation in cancer, many epigenetic alterations have been found in human cancer, including global and specific gene hypomethylation, hypermethylation, altered chromatin marks, and loss of genomic imprinting. Cancer epigenetics has been limited by questions of cause and effect, since epigenetic changes can arise secondary to the cancer process and its associated widespread changes in gene expression. Furthermore, mutations in the DNA methylation machinery have not been observed in tumors, whereas they have been for chromatin modification. To address the issue of human cancer etiology, we have taken a genetic approach to cancer epigenetics. One line of investigation has been on the disorder Beckwith-Wiedemann syndrome (BWS). We have found that loss of imprinting (LOI) of the autocrine growth factor gene *IGF2* and of the untranslated antisense RNA *LIT1*, within the K_VLQT1 gene, account for most cases of BWS, and that cancer risk is specifically associated with LOI of *IGF2*. Wilms' tumors, both in BWS and in the general population, involve LOI leading to an expansion of nephrogenic precursor cells. We have also developed an animal model for the role of LOI of *IGF2* in cancer, showing that it cooperates with *Apc* mutations to increase cancer frequency, consistent with human data suggesting a severalfold increased cancer risk for this common epigenetic variant in the adult population. These data suggest that a major component of cancer risk involves epigenetic changes in normal cells that increase the probability of cancer after genetic mutation. They suggest a model of cancer prevention that involves the epigenetic analysis of normal cells for risk stratification and cancer prevention strategies.

Since its inception in 1983 with the discovery of altered DNA methylation of genes in human cancers (Feinberg and Vogelstein 1983), the field of cancer epigenetics has simultaneously become both more and less clear. It has become more clear that epigenetic changes lie at the heart of most tumor processes, and that without a disruption of normal epigenetic programs, tumors would neither arise nor progress (Jones and Baylin 2002; Feinberg and Tycko 2004). The field has become less clear, however, with the discovery of an increasing number of types of epigenetic alteration in tumors, as well as genes that are affected by these changes (Jones and Baylin 2002; Feinberg and Tycko 2004). Perhaps the most dominant genetic feature of any kind in human cancer is a global hypomethylation that appears to occur ubiquitously in tumors, both benign and malignant. That is not to say that every type of tumor shows this change, but neoplasms that have been examined systematically show a marked reduction in the level of DNA methylation (Gama-Sosa et al. 1983; Feinberg and Tycko 2004). This loss of methylation has important consequences. It can lead to increased expression of dominantly acting oncogenes, such as R-ras in gastrointestinal cancer (Nishigaki et al. 2005) and cyclinD2 and maspin in pancreatic cancer (Cho et al. 2000; Akiyama et al. 2003). This hypomethylation-associated gene activation received comparatively less attention than gene silencing until recently, but it is increasingly clear that these changes are as important as those associated with gene silencing. It can also lead to chromosomal instability and loss of heterozygosity (LOH), shown convincingly in mouse models (Gaudet et al. 2003; Yamada et al. 2005). A third epigenetic change is promoter hypermethylation associated with gene silencing. Most tumor suppressor genes that are inactivated by mutation also show epigenetic inactivation, even more

commonly than mutational inactivation with LOH of the wild-type allele (Jones and Baylin 2002). Until recently, it was believed that the methylation was the primary cause of this silencing, but that is not as clear at present. It is now apparent that chromatin changes in the promoters of genes, and possibly within the body of genes as well, may be ultimately responsible for this silencing (Sellers and Loda 2002; Lund and van Lohuizen 2004; Robertson 2005). These chromatin modifications include increased lysine 9 methylation of histones H3 and H4, loss of acetylation at the same residue, and many other specific chromatic modifications. The fact that chromatin changes may precede the methylation changes was indicated by a study in which a cell line engineered to lose DNA methylation by somatic cell knockout of DNA methyltransferases 1 and 3A nevertheless silenced p16 through chromatin modification (Bachman et al. 2003). That is not to understate the importance of hypermethylation, but it may be more important in stabilizing epigenetically silenced genes than their primary inactivation. A recent study showed that global changes in histones may parallel those found in DNA methylation. These global changes include loss of acetylated lysine 16 and trimethylation of lysine 20 of histone H4 (Fraga et al. 2005).

Finally, an intriguing form of epigenetic change in cancer discovered about 10 years ago is loss of genomic imprinting. Imprinting refers to parent-of-origin-specific silencing of one allele of a gene. Many imprinted genes have been discovered, and most appear to be involved, at some level, in growth regulation. The prototype gene involved in LOI in cancer is *IGF2*, which encodes the insulin-like growth factor II protein. *IGF2* is normally expressed exclusively from the paternally inherited allele. LOI of *IGF2*, involving abnormal activation of the normally silent allele, was first found in about half of Wilms' tumors of the kidney, the most common solid tumor of childhood (Ogawa et al. 1993; Rainier et al. 1993). This frequency is about tenfold that of WT1 mutations in Wilms' tumor. In particular, LOI occurs in tumors that have a histopathologic phenotype referred to as perilobar nephrogenic rest-like (Ravenel et al. 2001). Beckwith and colleagues identified this subgroup of tumors as those that arose from nephrogenic stem cells after their commitment to renal development and during fetal life (Beckwith et al. 1990). The overexpression of *IGF2* in these tumors is thought to lead to an increased proliferation of nephrogenic stem cells and their associated perilobar nephrogenic rests (Beckwith et al. 1990; Sharifah et al. 1995). These rests are in fact common in the population at the time of birth, as a study of stillborns showed a prevalence of approximately 1%, but disappear normally over time (Beckwith 1998). Since the discovery of LOI in Wilms' tumor, LOI has been observed in many other human tumors, including common cancers such as colon, lung, hepatocellular, ovarian, and bladder cancer (for review, see Feinberg 1999). Other genes also show LOI in cancer, including *PEG1/MEST* in lung cancer (Nakanishi et al. 2004), $p57^{KIP2}$ in pancreatic cancer (Sato et al. 2005), *ARHI* in breast cancer (Yu et al. 1999), and *p73* in gastric cancer (Kang et al. 2000).

A GENETIC APPROACH TO HUMAN CANCER EPIGENETICS: BECKWITH-WIEDEMANN SYNDROME

Despite these many observations of epigenetic alterations in cancer, it has been difficult for the cancer epigenetics community to persuade the mainstream genetics community that epigenetics changes play a causal role in cancer. The counterarguments have been that epigenetic changes occur secondarily to widespread changes in gene expression in tumors, and/or that they simply reflect the underlying cell type from which tumors arise. Our laboratory has believed that a powerful approach to proving a mechanistic role for epigenetic changes in cancer is through conventional cancer genetics. Thus, we have endeavored to use both human and mouse genetics to build a strong argument for causality. Toward that goal, we borrowed a lesson from Albert Knudson, who pointed out several decades ago that by this study of rare cancer syndromes in the population, one may identify in the germ line genetic alterations that cause cancer which increase the risk of developing tumors many-fold. Knudson further argued that once one identified such changes, they might be present in somatically occurring common tumors, as well (Knudson 1987). We thus endeavored to identify a paradigm genetic syndrome that predisposes to cancer and involves an epigenetic mechanism. That syndrome was Beckwith-Wiedemann syndrome (BWS), a rare disorder that increases the risk of developing Wilms' tumor and other malignancies 850-fold. We thought that BWS might have an epigenetic basis, because it exhibits parent-of-origin-specific transmission, in particular through the mother (Mannens et al. 1994). At the time of our original studies of this disorder, no imprinted human genes had yet been identified, but they were highly suspected, based on studies of the neurological disorders Prader-Willi syndrome and Angelman syndrome, both of which show parental-origin-specific chromosomal alterations. The distinguishing features of BWS are prenatal overgrowth; organomegaly, particularly affecting the liver, kidney, pancreas, and adrenal gland; pancreatic islet cell hyperplasia with hyperinsulinemia and neonatal hypoglycemia; macroglossia (large tongue); midline abdominal wall defects independent of the organomegaly; and dysmorphic features of the face, notably ear pits or creases (DeBaun and Feinberg 2004). These children are at increased risk of developing so-called embryonal tumors that appear to involve an expansion of progenitor cells during prenatal development, such as in the kidney leading to Wilms' tumor, in the liver leading to hepatoblastoma, and in the muscle leading to rhabdomyosarcoma (DeBaun and Feinberg 2004). We initially mapped BWS in two large families to chromosomal band 11p15 by genetic linkage analysis (Ping et al. 1989). At about the same time, Tilghman and others showed that the *H19* gene is imprinted and maps to a syntenic location in the mouse (Bartolomei et al. 1991), and Efstradiatis demonstrated that the *IGF2* gene in mice is imprinted (DeChiara et al. 1991). We and other workers found that *IGF2* and *H19* are imprinted in humans, and that *IGF2* undergoes LOI in Wilms' tumor and in BWS (Zhang and Tycko 1992; Ogawa et al. 1993; Ohlsson et al. 1993; Rainier et al. 1993; Weksberg et al. 1993). Over the next several years, we identified a domain of imprinted genes spread out over approximately one megabase of 11p15, and including a number of growth-related genes, such as $p57^{KIP2}$, a cyclin-dependent kinase inhibitor normally expressed only from the maternal allele (for review, see Feinberg 1999). This gene is also rarely mutated in BWS (Hatada et al. 1996). $p57^{KIP2}$ is part of an imprinted subdomain of genes including *TSSC3*, *TSSC5*, and K_VLQT1, a voltage-gated potassium channel gene (for review, see Feinberg 1999). We found that within the K_VLQT1 gene, which is expressed from the maternal allele, lies a paternally expressed antisense transcript, encoding an untranslated RNA that appears to regulate the expression of other genes within this subdomain (Lee et al. 1999b). We termed this gene *LIT1*, for Long Intronic Transcript 1. *IGF2* and *H19* lie within a separate imprinted subdomain approximately 500 kb telomeric to the group just described (Lee et al. 1999a). *IGF2* and *H19* appear to be independently regulated, and the two subdomains are separated by the non-imprinted genes *TSSC4* and *TSSC6* (Lee et al. 1999a).

The mechanism of BWS turns out to be heterogeneous. 15% of patients demonstrate LOI of *IGF2*, just as in sporadically occurring Wilms' tumors in the general population. Approximately 40% of cases involve LOI of the *LIT1* gene, leading apparently to epigenetic silencing of $p57^{KIP2}$ and possibly other genes within this subdomain. In addition, approximately 5% of patients show mutations of $p57^{KIP2}$. Approximately 1% of patients show balanced or unbalanced chromosomal rearrangements leading to relative duplication of genes on 11p15. Approximately 10% of patients show uniparental disomy with duplication of the paternal alleles throughout both imprinted subdomains of 11p15 (for review, see Beckwith 1998; DeBaun and Feinberg 2004).

To sort out the complexities of the genetics of BWS, we have collaborated over many years with Michael DeBaun and colleagues at Washington University of St. Louis. He has developed a registry of BWS patients that is population-based; i.e., not biased toward malignancy through referrals from oncologists. In a study of 192 BWS patients within the registry, we performed the first epigenotype/phenotype study for any human disorder, asking whether any of the features of BWS were specifically associated with any of the genetic alterations observed in this disorder. The results of that study demonstrated that BWS is a contiguous gene disorder, and that the cancer phenotype is specifically associated with LOI of *IGF2* and associated hypermethylation of *H19* and silencing of *H19* (DeBaun et al. 2002). This represented compelling genetic evidence for a causal role of epigenetic changes in human cancer. Thus, not only is an epigenetic change, namely LOI of *IGF2*, associated with increased cancer risk in this disorder, but it is this particular change rather than alterations of *LIT1*, *p57*[KIP2], or other genes that is associated with that risk. Alterations in these other genes are associated with the midline abdominal wall defects and generalized overgrowth in this disorder (DeBaun et al. 2002).

Considerable progress has also been made in understanding the mechanism of LOI in BWS and Wilms' and other tumors, through basic research in mouse models, as well as human genetic studies. Imprinting of *IGF2* and *H19* are coregulated by a differentially methylated region (DMR) located several kilobases upstream of the *H19* gene and between *IGF2* and *H19* (for review, see Bartolomei and Tilghman 1997; Ohlsson 2004). In mouse, the DMR consists of four binding sites for the insulator protein CTCF, and in humans, the DMR consists of seven binding sites for CTCF. The DMR is normally methylated on the paternal allele and unmethylated on the maternal allele, allowing allele-specific binding of CTCF to the maternal allele. This binding of CTCF insulates the *IGF2* promoter from a shared enhancer downstream of *H19*. Thus, normally, the maternal *H19* allele is active and the paternal *IGF2* allele is active. There is a consequent single dose of *IGF2* protein expression from the paternal allele, as well as a single dose of *H19* expression from the maternal allele (Bartolomei and Tilghman 1997; Ohlsson 2004). The role of *H19* in growth regulation is unclear, as Tycko and colleagues showed that it has a growth-inhibitory effect on tumor cells in vitro (Hao et al. 1993), but Tilghman and colleagues were able to replace the body of the *H19* gene with a luciferase construct, leading to no phenotype within the resulting mice (Jones et al. 1998). In tumors or BWS patients with LOI, the *H19* DMR becomes aberrantly methylated on the maternal allele (Moulton et al. 1994; Steenman et al. 1994). CTCF does not bind to the aberrantly methylated maternal allele, and the enhancer has access to both maternal and paternal *IGF2* alleles, doubling the mRNA and protein levels of *IGF2*, and extinguishing *H19* expression (Ravenel 2001; Ohlsson et al. 2004). Thus, there is a double dose of this growth-promoting factor and loss of a potential growth-inhibitory role of *H19* in these cells.

The study of Wilms' tumor has also provided insight into the mechanism by which LOI increases tumor risk in BWS patients and promotes cancer development in sporadically occurring Wilms' tumors. LOI appears to increase the number of nephrogenic progenitor cells leading to perilobar nephrogenic rests. Abrogation of WT1 expression, in contrast, impairs the development of nephrogenic progenitor cells, leading to an overgrowth of mesonephric blastemal cells, referred to by the pathologist as intralobar nephrogenic rests. This hypothesis is supported by the fact that the perilobar nephrogenic rests themselves show LOI of *IGF2* (Ravenel et al. 2001). Thus, one can hypothesize a model in which epigenetic changes play a role similar to genetic changes in the Knudson hypothesis. The original Knudson model simply states that there are two events that lead to tumors, one occurring rarely and one occurring commonly. Although they may be allelic in the case of tumor suppressor genes, they need not be so. That is because a common and rare event best fit the epidemiology of tumor incidence in familial and sporadic tumors of a given type, without reference to a specific gene. We would therefore argue that LOI represents the common change, albeit an epigenetic one, and that the second event is a more rarely occurring genetic event. In the case of sporadically occurring Wilms' tumors, LOI leads to the presence of perilobar nephrogenic rests (Feinberg and Tycko 2004). Although this is not common, it is far more common than mutational mechanisms in cancer, and may involve as many as 1% of newborn children. In the case of BWS, all of the cells of the kidney would have undergone this epigenetic change, and therefore, the chance of a subsequent genetic mutation affecting a predisposed epigenetically altered precursor cell is much greater than in the general population (Fig. 1) (Feinberg and Tycko 2004).

LOI AND COMMON CANCER RISK

BWS has thus served as a paradigm for understanding both the causal link between epigenetic changes in human cancer and the mechanism for those changes. Nevertheless, it is important to determine whether similar epigenetic changes occur in common human malignancies and contribute significantly to cancer in the general population. Toward that end, about 7 years ago we began to study human colorectal cancer, the original tumor type in which altered DNA methylation was discovered. We found that LOI occurs in approximately one-third of human colon cancers (Cui et al. 1998). What distinguished LOI in colon cancer from other tumor types such as ovarian or bladder cancer was the fact that when LOI was present in the tumor, it was also present in the matched normal colonic mucosa from the same patients. These changes were common even in noncancer patients, occurring in approximately 10% of colon samples (Cui et al. 1998). The fact that LOI was enriched about threefold in cancer patients suggests that either LOI occurs in normal tissue of some individuals and increases the chance of developing cancer, or that it is a normal, perhaps age-dependent, change coincidentally associated with cancer. To distinguish between these possibilities, we performed an epidemiologic study of patients who were undergoing colonoscopic exam in a gastroenterology clinic setting.

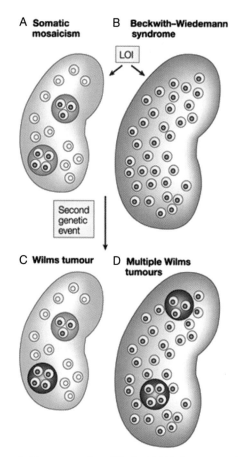

Figure 1. Human genetics of Beckwith-Wiedemann syndrome provides causal support for epigenetics in cancer etiology. (*A*) Loss of imprinting (LOI, dark nuclei) has been shown to arise sporadically as a somatic mosaic epigenetic alteration, because LOI has been found in parenchymal kidney tissue of patients with Wilms' tumor, as well as in premalignant nephrogenic rests (*pink circles*). (*B*) Alternatively, LOI can arise in the germ line or very early in development in BWS, causing nephromegaly (overgrowth of the whole kidney). In both cases, overgrowth is caused by a double dose of *IGF2* expression and possibly silencing of *H19*. (*C*) A second, presumably genetic, event can then lead to Wilms' tumor formation (*red circles*). (*D*) This will be more common in those with BWS, so multiple tumors arise. (Reprinted, with permission, from Feinberg and Tycko 2004 [*Nature Reviews Cancer* © Macmillan Magazines Ltd.; www.nature.com/reviews].)

Over 400 patients were enrolled in the study, of whom 172 were informative for a polymorphism within *IGF2*, allowing us to determine the imprinting status. All of these patients were examined at the level of imprinting in peripheral blood lymphocytes and at multiple locations within the normal colonic mucosa, and they also received a complete assessment of the presence or absence of tumors at the time of examination, as well as a past history of cancer and a history of cancer among first-degree relatives. Surprisingly, the adjusted odds ratio for LOI was 5.15 for those patients who had a positive family history for colorectal cancer among first-degree relatives. Similarly, the adjusted odds ratio for LOI was 4.72 among those patients who had past or present colonic tumors, and this number stratified for the type of tumors with an adjusted odds ratio of 3.26 for adenomas and 21.7 for colorectal cancers

(Cui et al. 2003). It should be noted that among the many genetic mutations that have been identified in the germ line of cancer patients, none occurs commonly. For example, the *BRCA1* mutation occurs in fewer than 1 in 1000 individuals. All of the mutations that increased the risk of developing colorectal cancer, combined, account for only approximately 3% of colorectal cancers in the general population in the United States. Thus, a genetic change that occurs as commonly as in 5–10% of the population, if it increases cancer risk modestly, e.g., two- to threefold, would account for a significant population-attributable risk in the general population. Moreover, the fact that these changes are epigenetic suggests that one might be able to intervene to reverse the abnormality or at least to prevent the consequences of cancer developing late in these patients. Since the original publication of this finding, the results have been confirmed by two other groups. The first examined a series of women with adenomas and found a 5.2 odds ratio for adenomas among patients with LOI. The second study was done on a community-based population that included minority patients (Woodson et al. 2004; M. Cruz-Correa et al., in prep.).

A MOUSE GENETIC MODEL OF HUMAN CANCER EPIGENETICS

More recently, we have developed an animal model to test the hypothesis that LOI of *IGF2* increases the risk of developing intestinal tumors. There have been animal models generated with LOI of *IGF2*, by deleting or mutating the *H19* DMR and/or the associated *H19* gene. Mice that inherit these deletions from their mothers lack the inhibition of maternal *IGF2* expression and show LOI. These mice, although showing biallelic *IGF2* expression, have not exhibited an increased frequency of tumors (Leighton et al. 1995; Ripoche et al. 1997). However, mice with this deletion crossed with a $p57^{KIP2}$ knockout have shown changes consistent with BWS, such as adrenocytomegaly, although the latter mice are perinatal lethals and, therefore, tumors have not been observed (Caspary et al. 1999).

We reasoned that LOI of *IGF2* might not act alone but in conjunction with genetic changes as postulated by the modified epigenetic Knudson model described above. We therefore tested this idea by generating doubly heterozygous mice. The mothers in these matings had a deletion or mutation of the *H19* DMR. The fathers in these matings are the Min mouse with a mutation in the adenomatous polyposis coli gene (APC), which causes intestinal tumors, and involving the same gene that undergoes gatekeeper mutations in virtually all human colon adenomas and carcinomas. The results of this mating led to four possible genotypes. First are mice with mutations in both genes; i.e., showing a predisposition to tumors based on the mutation in APC, as well as LOI of *IGF2* due to the loss of the *H19* gene. A second genotype is the Min mutation without LOI. The third and fourth possibilities are with and without LOI but without the Min mutation. These mice would not be expected to develop tumors but might still show pathological changes of interest. A large number of mice were generated over several years, with a total of 140 mice with the Min mutation, 81 of these with the wild-type *H19* gene, and 59 with the deleted *H19* and consequent LOI. We found that in the normal colon as well as in the tumors themselves, there was a doubling of *IGF2*, similar to what we have seen in other human tumors exhibiting LOI (Sakatani et al. 2005). We confirmed that this doubling of *IGF2* mRNA was associated with a doubling of the *IGF2* protein as well. Thus, although there had been other models of *IGF2* expression that provided compelling evidence for a role of this growth factor in tumor progression (Christofori et al. 1994), a model showing physiological doubling of *IGF2* as one sees with LOI had not previously been generated. The results on tumorigenesis were dramatic. Depending on the method used to score tumors, there was an increase of 1.9- to 2.5-fold in the numbers of tumors in doubly heterozygous mice compared to those with the Min mutation but normal imprinting. This was true in both the intestine and the colon, although the number of colon tumors is much smaller in the Min mouse for reasons that are unknown (Sakatani et al. 2005). These data in and of themselves provide genetic confirmation of our human studies and prove that LOI in normal tissue increases the risk of developing cancer in the intestine.

These mice also provided insight into the mechanism for this increased tumor risk. The ratio of macroadenomas to microadenomas was the same in mice with and without LOI that had the APC mutation. Thus, there was no difference in the rate of progression of tumors once they arose, but there was an increase in tumor initiation in the LOI mice, consistent with the idea that LOI precedes the development of intestinal tumors and in some way increases the risk of developing cancer once an APC mutation has taken place (Sakatani et al. 2005). Histopathologic examination of the intestines of mice with LOI versus mice without LOI revealed that the progenitor cell compartment of the intestine, i.e., the crypts, were enlarged approximately 50%. Furthermore, staining with a variety of histochemical markers for progenitor cells showed a dramatic increase in the number of progenitor cells within the intestinal epithelia of LOI mice, regardless of whether these were mice that also had the APC mutation. Furthermore, this increased presence of progenitor cell markers was also seen in the compartment that should represent relatively differentiated epithelia, namely the villi, and there was a concomitant retreat of differentiated markers within the villi away from the crypt–villus boundary (Sakatani et al. 2005). We also found that within the pancreas, the β-islet cells were hyperplastic in the doubly heterozygous mice. There was also a relative increase in staining in these cells for progenitor cell markers within the double heterozygotes (Sakatani et al. 2005). Taken as a whole, these data support the stem cell hypothesis of cancer, that the source of malignancy in the intestine is an undifferentiated progenitor cell. We would add to this stem cell model the idea that the LOI increases the progenitor cell pool and/or shifts the epigenetic program toward an earlier developmental state. This change in progenitor cells increases the probability of cancer after a genetic mutational insult, in this case, mutation of the APC gene, whether that is in the mouse model or in the development of human colon tumors. This view is also consistent with our earlier studies showing that in BWS there is an overrepresentation of progenitor cells within the renal epithelium. We hypothesize that a primary role of IGF2 in embryogenesis is the careful titration of the progenitor cell pool size. Thus, an overexpression of IGF2 would lead to an increased number of progenitor cells and overall shift toward a less differentiated state, increasing the probability of malignancy, whether in BWS or human colorectal cancer (Fig. 2). These changes might not occur prenatally, but in the case of the colon, might occur postnatally as well, given that this is a highly regenerative tissue source in a state of dynamic equilibrium. An alternative explanation for our data was suggested by George Klein (Klein 2005), who argued that LOI might represent the process of tumor cell promotion first suggested by Berenblum in the 1960s (Berenblum 1962). By this view, LOI could fulfill the dedifferentiation component of tumorigenesis, an appealing idea, since both epigenetic changes and tumor promotion are potentially reversible.

In summary, LOI is a common epigenetic variant in the population, at least in adults. This population variation in epigenetic marks may be due to variable stringency in the maintenance of these marks that may itself be genetically determined. That would explain why we see an association of LOI with cancer in first-degree relatives. In any case, this abnormality appears to represent the first common molecular marker for cancer risk in the general population. Many challenges lie ahead, both in the application of this information to reducing cancer mortality and in cancer epigenetics as a whole. In particular, for an LOI cancer risk test, given that this is epigenetic and also of unclear timing during the human life span, it will be important to study this change serially in individuals who have the abnormality. Furthermore, it will be important to analyze samples that were collected archivally, through nested case/control studies, in order to determine whether LOI is a predictive marker for cancer that occurs eventually in a given individual who was sampled before the tumor arose. Finally, LOI testing is very different from conventional cancer testing. The culture of cancer testing is oriented toward early cancer detection rather than cancer risk assessment. Some type of intervention to ameliorate the risk would be indicated, even though that intervention might be unnecessary in a large number of the patients who were so treated. Still, such an approach has been the most effective one in reducing cardiovascular mortality, and there has been little progress in reducing cancer mortality since the war on cancer was declared in the 1970s. This approach also raises important ethical considerations, because the nature of epigenetic testing is so unfamiliar that it will be difficult to explain to patients in a way that they can understand so as to provide the type of consent that is necessary for long-term prospective studies.

CONCLUSIONS

The field of cancer epigenetics as a whole is now entering its maturity. One of the great challenges will be to identify those changes that occur in cancer prior to the earliest recognizable pathological alterations, even before benign tumors can be detected. It is important to bear this

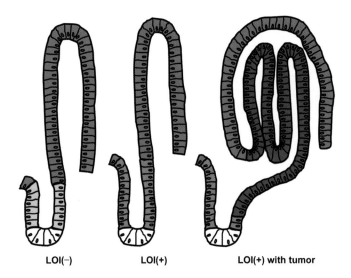

LOI(−)   LOI(+)   LOI(+) with tumor

Figure 2. Mouse genetic model of colorectal cancer provides causal support for epigenetics in cancer etiology. Min mice with a mutation in the *Apc* gene (leading to intestinal tumors) with or without LOI were generated by crossing male Min mice with female mice harboring a deletion in the *H19* gene and differentially methylated region needed for normal *IGF2* silencing. In LOI (−) mice, the progenitor compartment is shown in yellow within the crypts, and the differentiated compartment in the villin in brown, with the Paneth cells in white. In LOI (+) mice, the progenitor compartment is larger and also altered epigenetically (*orange color*). Finally, adenomas (*red*) arise from this altered epithelium but are capable of differentiation given their progenitor cell origin. (Reprinted, with permission, from Feinberg 1999 [© American Association for Cancer Research].)

in mind as experiments are contemplated for a human cancer genome project. As initially conceived, that project called for the comparison of the genetic sequence in pairs of normal tissue and tumor tissue from the same individuals in a relatively large number of tumor types. However, if important epigenetic changes occur in normal tissue even before benign neoplasms arise, then we must compare the epigenetic state in the normal tissue of patients who have developed tumors, to comparable material obtained from control individuals who have not developed tumors. Will this be a technically daunting task, given the large number of potential epigenetic changes that occur throughout the genome? I think not, because the technology for epigenetic analysis genome-wide is advancing very rapidly. For example, it has become possible in other organisms to analyze whole chromosomes for epigenetic alteration using restriction enzymes that cut approximately half of methylated DNA sites, such as McrBC, and then prepare probes from this DNA, compare that to DNA that has not been so digested, and hybridize to arrays of sequence over the genomic region of interest. Although this might not provide a level of resolution at the single-nucleotide level, it might nevertheless provide a very strong indication about epigenetic changes and where they might occur, without our preconceptions interfering with data analysis. I am most hopeful that this new field of epigenomics will be of practical value in identifying patients at risk of cancer and in reducing cancer mortality, while also providing the next wave of mechanistic understanding of the basic biology of cancer.

ACKNOWLEDGMENTS

This work was supported by National Institutes of Health grants CA65145 and CA54358.

REFERENCES

Akiyama Y., Maesawa C., Ogasawara S., Terashima M., and Masuda T. 2003. Cell-type-specific repression of the maspin gene is disrupted frequently by demethylation at the promoter region in gastric intestinal metaplasia and cancer cells. *Am. J. Pathol.* **163:** 1911.

Bachman K.E., Park B.H., Rhee I., Rajagopalan H., Herman J.G., Baylin S.B., Kinzler K.W., and Vogelstein B. 2003. Histone modifications and silencing prior to DNA methylation of a tumor suppressor gene. *Cancer Cell* **3:** 89.

Bartolomei M.S. and Tilghman S.M. 1997. Genomic imprinting in mammals. *Annu. Rev. Genet.* **31:** 493.

Bartolomei M.S., Zemel S., and Tilghman S.M. 1991. Parental imprinting of the mouse *H19* gene. *Nature* **351:** 153.

Beckwith J.B. 1998. Nephrogenic rests and the pathogenesis of Wilms tumor: Developmental and clinical considerations. *Am. J. Med. Genet.* **79:** 268.

Beckwith J.B., Kiviat N.B., and Bonadio J.F. 1990. Nephrogenic rests, nephroblastomatosis, and the pathogenesis of Wilms' tumor. *Pediatr. Pathol.* **10:** 1.

Berenblum I. 1962. The epidemiology of cancer. In *General pathology: Based on lectures delivered at the Sir William Dunn School of Pathology, University of Oxford* (ed. H.B. Florey). W.B. Saunders, Philadelphia.

Caspary T., Cleary M.A., Perlman E.J., Zhang P., Elledge S.J., and Tilghman S.M. 1999. Oppositely imprinted genes p57 (Kip2) and *IGF2* interact in a mouse model for Beckwith-Wiedemann syndrome. *Genes Dev.* **13:** 3115.

Cho M., Grabmaier K., Kitahori Y., Hiasa Y., Nakagawa Y., Uemura H., Hirao Y., Ohnishi T., Yoshikawa K., and Ooesterwijk E. 2000. Activation of the MN/CA9 gene is associated with hypomethylation in human renal cell carcinoma cell lines. *Mol. Carcinog.* **27:** 184.

Christofori G., Naik P., and Hanahan D. 1994. A second signal supplied by insulin-like growth factor II in oncogene-induced tumorigenesis. *Nature* **369:** 414.

Cui H., Horon I.L., Ohlsson R., Hamilton S.R., and Feinberg A.P. 1998. Loss of imprinting in normal tissue of colorectal cancer patients with microsatellite instability. *Nat. Med.* **4:** 1276.

Cui H., Cruz-Correa M., Giardiello F.M., Hutcheon D.F., Kafonek D.R., Brandenburg S., Wu Y., He X., Powe N.R., and Feinberg A.P. 2003. Loss of *IGF2* imprinting: A potential marker of colorectal cancer risk. *Science* **299:** 1753.

DeBaun M.R. and Feinberg A.P. 2004. *IGF2*, *H19*, p57KIP2, and LIT1 and the Beckwith-Wiedemann syndrome. In *Inborn errors of development: The molecular basis of clinical disorders of morphogenesis* (ed. C.J. Epstein et al.). Oxford University Press, New York.

DeBaun M.R., Niemitz E.L., McNeil D.E., Brandenburg S.A., Lee M.P., and Feinberg A.P. 2002. Epigenetic alterations of *H19* and LIT1 distinguish patients with Beckwith-Wiedemann syndrome with cancer and birth defects. *Am. J. Hum. Genet.* **70:** 604.

DeChiara T.M., Robertson E.J., and Efstratiadis A. 1991. Parental imprinting of the mouse insulin-like growth factor II gene. *Cell* **64:** 849.

Feinberg A.P. 1999. Imprinting of a genomic domain of 11p15 and loss of imprinting in cancer: An introduction. *Cancer Res.* **59:** 1743s.

Feinberg A.P. and Tycko B. 2004. The history of cancer epigenetics. *Nat. Rev. Cancer* **4:** 143.

Feinberg A.P. and Vogelstein B. 1983. Hypomethylation distinguishes genes of some human cancers from their normal counterparts. *Nature* **301:** 89.

Fraga M.F., Ballestar E., Villar-Garea A., Boix-Chornet M., Espada J., Schotta G., Bonaldi T., Haydon C., Ropero S., Petrie K., Iyer N.G., Perez-Rosado A., Calvo E., Lopez J.A., Cano A., Calasanz M.J., Colomer D., Piris M.A., Ahn N., Imhof A., Caldas C., Jenuwein T., and Esteller M. 2005. Loss of acetylation at Lys16 and trimethylation at Lys20 of histone H4 is a common hallmark of human cancer. *Nat. Genet.* **37:** 391.

Gama-Sosa M.A., Slagel V.A., Trewyn R.W., Oxenhandler R., Kuo K.C., Gehrke C.W., and Ehrlich M. 1983. The 5-methylcytosine content of DNA from human tumors. *Nucleic Acids Res.* **11:** 6883.

Gaudet F., Hodgson J.G., Eden A., Jackson-Grusby L., Dausman J., Gray J.W., Leonhardt H., and Jaenisch R. 2003. Induction of tumors in mice by genomic hypomethylation. *Science* **300:** 489.

Hao Y., Crenshaw T., Moulton T., Newcomb E., and Tycko B. 1993. Tumour-suppressor activity of *H19* RNA. *Nature* **365:** 764.

Hatada I., Ohashi H., Fukushima Y., Kaneko Y., Inoue M., Komoto Y., Okada A., Ohishi S., Nabetani A., Morisaki H., Nakayama M., Niikawa N., and Mukai T. 1996. An imprinted gene p57KIP2 is mutated in Beckwith-Wiedemann syndrome. *Nat. Genet.* **14:** 171.

Jones B.K., Levorse J.M., and Tilghman S.M. 1998. *IGF2* imprinting does not require its own DNA methylation or *H19* RNA. *Genes Dev.* **12:** 2200.

Jones P.A. and Baylin S.B. 2002. The fundamental role of epigenetic events in cancer. *Nat. Rev. Genet.* **3:** 415.

Kang M.J., Park B.J., Byun D.S., Park J.I., Kim H.J., Park J.H., and Chi S.G. 2000. Loss of imprinting and elevated expression of wild-type p73 in human gastric adenocarcinoma. *Clin. Cancer Res.* **6:** 1767.

Klein G. 2005. Epigenetics: Surveillance team against cancer. *Nature* **434:** 150.

Knudson A.G., Jr. 1987. Prince Takamatsu memorial lecture. Rare cancers: Clues to genetic mechanisms. *Princess Takamatsu Symp.* **18:** 221.

Lee M.P., Brandenburg S., Landes G.M., Adams M., Miller G., and Feinberg A.P. 1999a. Two novel genes in the center of the 11p15 imprinted domain escape genomic imprinting. *Hum. Mol. Genet.* **8:** 683.

Lee M.P., DeBaun M.R., Mitsuya K., Galonek H.L., Brandenburg S., Oshimura M., and Feinberg A.P. 1999b. Loss of imprinting of a paternally expressed transcript, with antisense orientation to KVLQT1, occurs frequently in Beckwith-Wiedemann syndrome and is independent of insulin-like growth factor II imprinting. *Proc. Natl. Acad. Sci.* **96:** 5203.

Leighton P.A., Ingram R.S., Eggenschwiler J., Efstratiadis A., and Tilghman S.M. 1995. Disruption of imprinting caused by deletion of the *H19* gene region in mice. *Nature* **375:** 34.

Lund A.H. and van Lohuizen M. 2004. Epigenetics and cancer. *Genes Dev.* **18:** 2315.

Mannens M., Hoovers J.M., Redeker E., Verjaal M., Feinberg A.P., Little P., Boavida M., Coad N., Steenman M., and Bliek J., et al. 1994. Parental imprinting of human chromosome region 11p15.3-pter involved in the Beckwith-Wiedemann syndrome and various human neoplasia. *Eur. J. Hum. Genet.* **2:** 3.

Moulton T., Crenshaw T., Hao Y., Moosikasuwan J., Lin N., Dembitzer F., Hensle T., Weiss L., McMorrow L., and Loew T., et al. 1994. Epigenetic lesions at the *H19* locus in Wilms' tumour patients. *Nat. Genet.* **7:** 440.

Nakanishi H., Suda T., Katoh M., Watanabe A., Igishi T., Kodani M., Matsumoto S., Nakamoto M., Shigeoka Y., Okabe T., Oshimura M., and Shimizu E. 2004. Loss of imprinting of PEG1/MEST in lung cancer cell lines. *Oncol. Rep.* **12:** 1273.

Nishigaki M., Aoyagi K., Danjoh I., Fukaya M., Yanagihara K., Sakamoto H., Yoshida T., and Sasaki H. 2005. Discovery of aberrant expression of R-RAS by cancer-linked DNA hypomethylation in gastric cancer using microarrays. *Cancer Res.* **65:** 2115.

Ogawa O., Eccles M.R., Szeto J., McNoe L.A., Yun K., Maw M.A., Smith P.J., and Reeve A.E. 1993. Relaxation of insulin-like growth factor II gene imprinting implicated in Wilms' tumour. *Nature* **362:** 749.

Ohlsson R. 2004. Loss of *IGF2* imprinting: Mechanisms and consequences. *Novartis Found. Symp.* **262:** 108.

Ohlsson R., Nystrom A., Pfeifer-Ohlsson S., Tohonen V., Hedborg F., Schofield P., Flam F., and Ekstrom T.J. 1993. *IGF2* is parentally imprinted during human embryogenesis and in the Beckwith-Wiedemann syndrome. *Nat. Genet.* **4:** 94.

Ping A.J., Reeve A.E., Law D.J., Young M.R., Boehnke M., and Feinberg A.P. 1989. Genetic linkage of Beckwith-Wiedemann syndrome to 11p15. *Am. J. Hum. Genet.* **44:** 720.

Rainier S., Johnson L.A., Dobry C.J., Ping A.J., Grundy P.E., and Feinberg A.P. 1993. Relaxation of imprinted genes in human cancer. *Nature* **362:** 747.

Ravenel J.D., Broman K.W., Perlman E.J., Niemitz E.L., Jayawardena T.M., Bell D.W., Haber D.A., Uejima H., and Feinberg A.P. 2001. Loss of imprinting of insulin-like growth factor-II (*IGF2*) gene in distinguishing specific biologic subtypes of Wilms tumor. *J. Natl. Cancer Inst.* **93:** 1698.

Ripoche M.A., Kress C., Poirier F., and Dandolo L. 1997. Deletion of the *H19* transcription unit reveals the existence of a putative imprinting control element. *Genes Dev.* **11:** 1596.

Robertson K.D. 2005. DNA methylation and human disease. *Nat. Rev. Genet.* **6:** 597.

Sakatani T., Kaneda A., Iacobuzio-Donahue C.A., Carter M.G., de Boom Witzel S., Okano H., Ko M.S., Ohlsson R., Longo D.L., and Feinberg A.P. 2005. Loss of imprinting of *IGF2* alters intestinal maturation and tumorigenesis in mice. *Science* **307:** 1976.

Sato N., Matsubayashi H., Abe T., Fukushima N., and Goggins M. 2005. Epigenetic down-regulation of CDKN1C/p57KIP2 in pancreatic ductal neoplasms identified by gene expression profiling. *Clin. Cancer Res.* **11:** 4681.

Sellers W.R. and Loda M. 2002. The EZH2 polycomb transcriptional repressor: A marker or mover of metastatic prostate cancer? *Cancer Cell* **2:** 349.

Sharifah N.A., Yun K., and McLay J. 1995. Insulin-like growth factor II gene expression by congenital mesoblastic nephroma. *Diagn. Mol. Pathol.* **4:** 279.

Steenman M.J., Rainier S., Dobry C.J., Grundy P., Horon I.L., and Feinberg A.P. 1994. Loss of imprinting of *IGF2* is linked to reduced expression and abnormal methylation of *H19* in Wilms' tumour. *Nat. Genet.* **7:** 433.

Waber P.G., Chen J., and Nisen P.D. 1993. Infrequency of ras, p53, WT1, or RB gene alterations in Wilms tumors. *Cancer* **72:** 3732.

Weksberg R., Shen D.R., Fei Y.L., Song Q.L., and Squire J. 1993. Disruption of insulin-like growth factor 2 imprinting in Beckwith-Wiedemann syndrome. *Nat. Genet.* **5:** 143.

Woodson K., Flood A., Green L., Tangrea J.A., Hanson J., Cash B., and Schoenfeld P. 2004. Loss of insulin-like growth factor-II imprinting and the presence of screen-detected colorectal adenomas in women. *J. Natl. Cancer Inst.* **96:** 407.

Yamada Y., Jackson-Grusby L., Linhart H., Meissner A., Eden A., Lin H., and Jaenisch R. 2005. Opposing effects of DNA hypomethylation on intestinal and liver carcinogenesis. *Proc. Natl. Acad. Sci.* **102:** 13580.

Yu Y., Xu F., Peng H., Fang X., Zhao S., Li Y., Cuevas B., Kuo W.L., Gray J.W., Siciliano M., Mills G.B., and Bast R.C., Jr. 1999. NOEY2 (ARHI), an imprinted putative tumor suppressor gene in ovarian and breast carcinomas. *Proc. Natl. Acad. Sci.* **96:** 214.

Zhang Y. and Tycko B. 1992. Monoallelic expression of the human *H19* gene. *Nat. Genet.* **1:** 40.

Microenvironmental Regulators of Tissue Structure and Function Also Regulate Tumor Induction and Progression: The Role of Extracellular Matrix and Its Degrading Enzymes

M.J. Bissell, P.A. Kenny, and D.C. Radisky[*]

*Cancer Biology Department, Life Sciences Division, Lawrence Berkeley National Laboratory,
University of California, Berkeley, California 94720*

It is now widely accepted that elements of the cellular and tissue microenvironment are crucial regulators of cell behavior in culture and homeostasis in vivo, and that many of the same factors influence the course of tumor progression. Less well established is the extent to which extracellular factors actually *cause* cancer, and the circumstances under which this may occur. Using physiologically relevant three-dimensional culture assays and transgenic animals, we have explored how the environmental and architectural context of cells, tissues, and organs controls mammary-specific gene expression, growth regulation, apoptosis, and drug resistance and have found that loss of tissue structure is a prerequisite for cancer progression. Here we summarize this evidence and highlight two of our recent studies. Using mouse mammary epithelial cells, we show that exposure to matrix metalloproteinase-3 (MMP-3) stimulates production of reactive oxygen species (ROS) that destabilize the genome and induce epithelial-mesenchymal transition, causing malignant transformation. Using a human breast cancer progression series, we find that ADAM-dependent growth factor shedding plays a crucial role in acquisition of the malignant phenotype. These findings illustrate how normal tissue structure controls the response to extracellular signals so as to preserve tissue specificity and growth status.

INTRODUCTION AND HISTORICAL BACKGROUND

Key questions in cell and tumor biology include how tissues and organs maintain homeostasis, and how cells within organs lose or overcome these controls in cancer. Developmental pathways may be thought of as a series of extremely rapid short-term events in which each new step depends on the previous state with the final outcome at birth being the organism itself. In mice and humans, these developmental events occur in a mere 21 days or 9 months, respectively, but the stability of the differentiated state and the homeostasis of the organism will last 40–110 times longer. Defining how this extraordinary balance is maintained is key to understanding how the stability is lost in the development of malignancy and aging. The importance of "tissue interaction" to define cellular function was recognized as early as the turn of the previous century (Peebles 1911). However, despite the fact that Alexis Carrel published his landmark articles on maintaining cells and tissues outside the animal around this time (Carrel 1908, 1911), intensive investigations of the factors controlling the stability of the differentiated state did not begin in earnest until the early 1970s, with the recognition that the microenvironment has a profound effect on how cells behave in culture (for a review of the early literature, see Bissell 1981). These early studies concentrated on a few molecules gained or lost in culture—the process we loosely define as differentiation.

The role played by the microenvironment in providing a "congenial soil" for tumor growth was identified at the end of the 19th century (Paget 1889), but the discovery of tumor viruses, oncogenes, and tumor suppressors in the 20th century overshadowed these earlier studies as most workers pursued cell-autonomous mechanisms for cancer cell initiation, progression, and metastasis. However, much important work was done in developmental biology, where it was recognized that the epithelial and stromal tissue components engage in a dynamic cross talk during development and play a crucial role in tissue morphogenesis and differentiation. The groundbreaking transplantation experiments in salamanders of Spemann and Mangold demonstrated the power of certain regions of tissues to interact with, and modulate, the differentiation of adjacent structures (Spemann 1918; Spemann and Mangold 1924). Similarly, mammalian tissue coculture experiments defined some of the reciprocal interactions between epithelial and mesenchymal tissues necessary for the induction of the differentiated state in several organs (Grobstein 1964 and references therein; Sakakura et al. 1976). The identities and roles of many of the key signaling molecules have now been elucidated in several organ systems, including the lung (Cardoso 2001), kidney (Yu et al. 2004), gut (Roberts 2000), and mammary gland (Parmar and Cunha 2004).

With the new molecular and genetic tools available to us at the turn of this new century, we are beginning to understand more fully the complexity of the programs and forces that maintain the unity of form and function in normal organs, and the validity of the instability/plasticity of the differentiated state (Bissell 1981; Blau and Baltimore 1991). These tools and techniques have enabled us to

---

Present address: Mayo Clinic Cancer Center, Griffin Cancer Research Building, 4500 San Pablo Road, Jacksonville, Florida 32224.

show that frank cancer cells can be "reverted" to a phenotypically normal state, and how normal tissues may develop epithelial tumors by alterations in the microenvironment and the stroma.

THE IMPORTANCE OF CELLULAR AND TISSUE CONTEXT

That changes in the stromal component play a role in tumor development has long been obvious to surgeons and pathologists. Resection and analysis of tumors show that they are often tough and fibrotic as a result of deposition of collagens and other extracellular matrix (ECM) molecules by stroma. Dvorak noted extensive parallels between tumor-associated stroma and the stroma induced by wound healing, leading him to suggest that "A tumor is a wound that does not heal" (Dvorak 1986). This is referred to as "reactive" stroma, and the mechanisms by which malignant cells induce these changes in nonmalignant fibroblasts are now beginning to be understood (Ronnov-Jessen et al. 1996). The advent of effective means to separate epithelial and stromal cells and recombine them in culture or in vivo provided a tool to dissect the contributions of these lineages to the malignant state. It is becoming apparent that the tumor stroma is not merely responsive to the developing tumor, but in fact is an active participant in the tumorigenic process. As with normal development, the interaction between epithelium and stroma in tumor initiation and progression is not a monolog but a dialog, or a highly organized group discussion!

Evidence for a cancer-relevant dialog between epithelium and stroma began to accumulate in the 1970s. DeCosse and coworkers showed that a mammary tumor could be induced to differentiate by coculture (across a filter) with embryonic mammary mesenchyme (DeCosse et al. 1973). A comprehensive series of xenograft experiments by Leland Chung demonstrated that co-injection of either nontransformed or transformed fibroblasts greatly enhanced the tumorigenicity in athymic mice of a series of human cancer cell lines from different tissues (Camps et al. 1990). Similarly, Cunha and his collaborators showed that fibroblasts isolated from the reactive tumor stroma had the capacity to transform otherwise nonmalignant immortal prostatic epithelial cells in this assay (Olumi et al. 1999; Cunha et al. 2004). Conversely, prostate cancer cells could be induced to differentiate when co-engrafted with several different types of mesenchyme (Hayashi et al. 1990).

Although these experiments clearly demonstrated that dialog between epithelium and stroma plays a critical role in neoplasia, the language of communication was still a mystery, including the identity of the paracrine signaling molecules and the cell types which produce these signals. Expression analysis of the different cell populations that comprise the normal and malignant breast is now providing insight into the cells that generate and respond to these signals (Allinen et al. 2004), and it is clear that leukocytes, particularly macrophages, play a prominent role (Bingle et al. 2002). Tumor-infiltrating leukocytes

have long been associated with cancer (Virchow 1863) and were long thought to be a hallmark of the immune response to the tumor. It is now appreciated that these tumor-associated macrophages (TAMs) are actually recruited to the tumor as a result of tumor cell expression of chemotactic cytokines. Once recruited, TAMs provide a rich supply of cytokines, proteases, and growth factors that stimulate tumor growth and promote neo-angiogenesis (Pollard 2004). Yet more signaling proteins, such as MSF produced by fibroblasts in the tumor stroma (Schor et al. 2003), exert potent stimulatory effects on malignant cells.

ORGAN ARCHITECTURE AND CONTEXT AS OVERRIDING TUMOR SUPPRESSORS

The maintenance of tissue architecture and organization, as well as tissue polarity and differentiation, is dependent on continued dialog between the cells and their microenvironment. Loss of organization is among the earliest histological hallmarks of malignant progression. Although the role of activated oncogenes and inactivated tumor suppressors in cancer development is clear, studies of large autopsy series reveal that the majority of people who die from causes other than cancer have small neoplastic growths throughout their bodies (Harach et al. 1985; Nielsen et al. 1987; Montie et al. 1989). It is thus also clear that loss of single tumor suppressors, although necessary, is not sufficient to induce tumors, since inherited mutations such as BRCA1, BRCA2, and APC lead to organ-specific tumors, rather than a general increase in all cancers. What is it that constrains these neoplastic growths and keeps the other tissues intact in the absence of the suppressor genes? Early evidence from a number of laboratories, including ours, has indicated that the tissue microenvironment including its "organ-specific form" can exert a potent tumor suppressive effect, even when cells were infected with potent oncogenes.

In a remarkable experiment performed three decades ago, Beatrice Mintz demonstrated that embryonal carcinoma cells (which form malignant tumors upon injection in adult mice), could contribute to cancer-free normal tissues when injected into blastocysts (Mintz and Illmensee 1975). These data are a striking exposition of the power of the tissue context to modify the malignant potential of cancer cells. Similar and complementary experiments were recently reported by Chin and Jaenisch and coworkers (Hochedlinger et al. 2004). In these, nuclei from rastransformed melanoma cells were shown to contribute to adult tissues in chimeric mice, although in this case the mice did develop tumors eventually.

Our laboratory focused on Rous sarcoma virus (RSV). This virus, which encodes the potent transforming oncogene, v-src, causes sarcoma formation in adult birds and mass transformation of cells in culture (for review, see Martin 2004). We found that infection of embryos in ovo with virally encoded Src did not preclude normal embryonic development even though the oncogene was expressed (Dolberg and Bissell 1984), and active (Howlett et al. 1988; Stoker et al. 1990a). Nevertheless, cells isolated from these embryos became transformed en masse when dissociated and placed on tissue culture plastic, demonstrating the importance of context to modify the phenotype of an oncogenically transformed cell. Furthermore, whereas it was widely accepted that viral infection was necessary and sufficient for induction of tumors, we found that RSV-induced tumors would remain local despite circulating virus. We subsequently showed that wounding of infected chickens was in fact necessary and that wounding the chicken at a site different from the original RSV injection was sufficient to induce tumors at the site of wounding. Finally, we showed that TGF-β1 was a key mediator in this process (Sieweke et al. 1990), one of the early demonstrations of the dual role of TGF-β in normal and malignant behavior. These data demonstrated that oncogene expression was compatible with normal nonneoplastic tissue morphogenesis in the embryo, and that the tumorigenic phenotype could be revealed following microenvironmental perturbations such as those induced by cellular cultivation on tissue culture plastic or wounding in the adult chicken.

Several differences exist in wound healing between the embryo and the adult (Ferguson and O'Kane 2004). Embryonic wounds often heal without scar formation, perhaps because at this developmental stage the skin is actively growing and is rich in morphogenetic growth factors. In adults, the skin is more refractory to healing, which results in scar formation. In contrast to adults, embryonic wounds typically have little inflammatory cell infiltration. The isoforms of TGF-β present at the wound site also differ between embryo and adult. TGF-β3 is the predominant isoform in embryonic wounds, whereas TGF-β1 and TGF-β2 are present in adults. Introduction of TGF-β3 into adult wounds promotes scar-free healing (Shah et al. 1995), whereas genetic ablation of TGF-β3 prevents embryonic scar-free healing (Ferguson and O'Kane 2004). These data provide insight into our observations that introduction of RSV by injection in chick embryos did not yield tumors, whereas subsequent wounding of the adult birds, at distant sites, did.

There is much literature (going back to the 19th century) describing the changes that occur in the wounding environment—which included disruption and remodeling of basement membrane (BM), activation of the stroma, immune cell infiltration and degranulation, and, ultimately, scar formation. These events can also provide an oncogenic stimulus to cells with genetic alterations (for a review of the early literature, see Sieweke and Bissell [1994]; for a more recent review see Robinson and Coussens [2005]). But what are the molecular effectors of stability and disruption? One of the problems of trying to define the role of specific components of ECM, BM, or adhesion molecules in development of malignancy is that their very absence is often lethal. Nevertheless, there is increasing evidence that attenuated function of these molecules is indeed instrumental in tumor induction, poor prognosis, and increased progression (Table 1; see the final section of this paper). Dissecting more complex levels of molecular interaction will clearly require robust and more sophisticated models.

THE MAMMARY GLAND AS AN EXPERIMENTAL ORGANISM

To understand the signaling pathways involved in the maintenance of the differentiated state, and to gain insight into the steps that cause and promote malignancy, our laboratory has concentrated for the past 25 years exclusively on one system, that of the mammary gland of mice and humans. We postulated (Bissell et al. 1982), and then demonstrated (for reviews, see Stoker et al. 1990b; Roskelley et al. 1995; Bissell et al. 1999, 2003; Schmeichel and Bissell 2003), that components of the ECM provide critical physical and biochemical cues to epithelial cells, and cooperate with hormones and growth factors to signal to the nucleus and chromatin to maintain mammary-specific gene expression. In parallel, we have been concerned with the loss of tissue organization and polarity, which is among the earliest histological manifestations of an incipient tumor.

The availability of genetic engineering techniques in mice and our ability to culture cells in three-dimensional (3D) gels as a surrogate for normal tissues (Michalopoulos and Pitot 1975; Emerman and Pitelka 1977; Barcellos-Hoff et al. 1989; Petersen et al. 1992) have now made it possible to study the molecular mechanisms involved in how changes in the microenvironment translate into changes in gene expression. One of the first demonstrations that changes in culture substrata and cell shape led to changes in de novo gene expression was performed with murine mammary cells and synthesis and secretion of radiolabeled milk proteins (Lee et al. 1984, 1985). Subsequent studies have demonstrated that expression of tissue-specific genes such as milk proteins are not coordinate but that there is a hierarchy of expression directly related to the nature of the ECM molecules, cell–cell interactions, and complexity of the tissue-specific architecture achieved in culture (Fig. 1A) (for review, see Lin and Bissell 1993). Although not all the transcripts have been interrogated in the case of the mouse mammary cells, it is clear that a number of signaling pathways are shut off and others are turned on; i.e., there is change in the program of tissue-specific gene expression when the cells receive the ECM and cell-shape signals. The postulate that these changes are directly related to cell–ECM interactions was demonstrated by studies that showed β-casein expression is disrupted as a function either of inhibition of specific integrins (Streuli et al. 1991; Muschler et al. 1999) or use of specific inhibitory peptides to chains of laminin-1 (Streuli et al. 1995).

Using β-casein as the prototype, we discovered that there is an ECM-response element in the promoter of the β-casein gene (Fig. 1B, C) that responds to laminin-1 and prolactin. The response was quite dramatic and involved recruitment and activation of transcription factors Stat5 and C/EBPβ, and widespread alterations in chromatin structure (Schmidhauser et al. 1992; Myers et al. 1998; R. Xu et al., in prep.). We later showed that other genes also contain ECM or substrata-response elements, and in some cases, such as that of the TGF-β1 gene, the response to ECM was suppression of expression rather than induction (Streuli et al. 1993).

Table 1. Examples of Inherited Genetic Polymorphisms in Microenvironmental Molecules Which Affect Tumor Incidence, Progression, or Survival

Protein class	Gene	Polymorphism	Type	Molecular phenotype	Tumor phenotype	Tissue	Reference
MMPs	MMP1	2G/1G (-1607)	ins/del	2G: high expression	2G: poor prognosis 2G: poor prognosis 2G: poor prognosis 2G: more advanced tumors	ovarian malignant melanoma colorectal cervical	Kanamori et al. (1999) Ye et al. (2001) Ghilardi et al. (2001) Nishioka et al. (2003)
	MMP3	5A/6A (-1612)	ins/del	5A: high expression	5A: increased incidence	breast	Biondi et al. (2000)
Angiogenesis factors	VEGF	G(-1154)A	SNP	G: low expression	AA: reduces susceptibility AA: thinner tumors	prostate malignant melanoma	McCarron et al. (2002) Howell et al. (2002)
Adhesion proteins	β3-integrin	T(1565)C	SNP		T/T: increases metastasis	breast	Ayala et al. (2003)
	E-cadherin	C(-160)A	SNP	A: low expression	A: more invasive tumors C: more invasive/metastatic	bladder stomach	Ayala et al. (2003) Kuraoka et al. (2003)
Cytokines	TNF-α	G(-308)A	SNP		AA: worse prognosis	breast non-Hodgkin's lymphoma acute lymphoblastic leukemia	Mestiri et al. (2001) Warzocha et al. (1998); Juszczynski et al. (2002) Lauten et al. (2002)
	TNF-β	A(+252)G	intron SNP		AA: better prognosis AA: better prognosis G: worse prognosis	lung stomach non-Hodgkin's lymphoma	Lauten et al. (2002) Shimura et al. (1995) Warzocha et al. (1998)
	IL-6	G(-174)C	SNP	C: low expression	C: better prognosis C: better prognosis	ovarian breast	Hefler et al. (2003) DeMichele et al. (2003)
	IL-10	A(-1080)G, T(-819)C, A(-592)C	SNPs	ACC:intermediate expression	low exp: worse prognosis	cutaneous malignant melanoma	Martinez-Escribano et al. (2002)
				ATA: low expression	low exp: worse prognosis	non-Hodgkin's lymphoma	Cunningham et al. (2003)

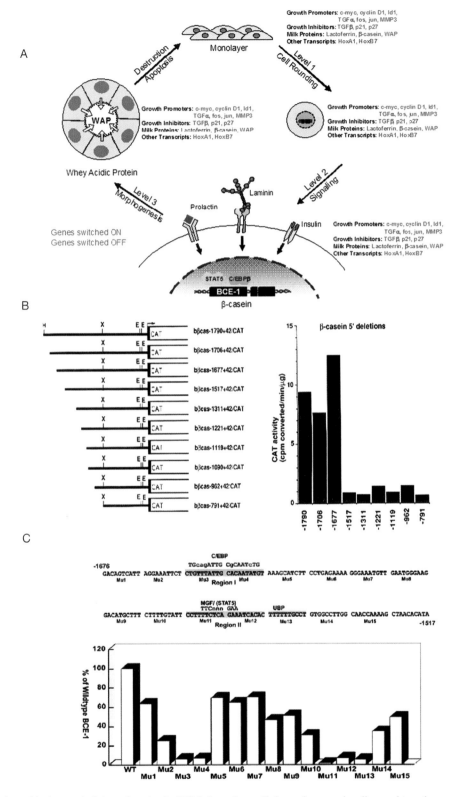

Figure 1. Hierarchical control of tissue function by ECM-dependent cell shape changes, signaling, and morphogenesis. (*A*) Examples of gene products altered by contact with the ECM and by changes in cellular structure. Studies of MECs cultured in the context of a variety of "designer microenvironments" have demonstrated that cells display distinct behaviors in response to changes in cell shape and ECM composition. In these cultures, the inert substratum, polyHEMA, was used to model cell shape change by itself, whereas purified laminin was used as a ligand that stimulates both cell shape change and integrin-dependent signaling. As cells make the transition from 2D to 3D culture, the expression of distinct cassettes of genes is reciprocally modulated. (*B*) Deletion analysis of the β-casein promoter identifies an ECM-response element (BCE-1). (*C*) Systematic mutational analysis of BCE-1 demonstrates that the C/EBPβ and Stat5 binding sites are required for the ECM-dependent transcriptional response. (Modified, with permission, from Schmidhauser et al. 1992; Roskelley et al. 1995; Myers et al. 1998.)

INTERROGATION OF NORMAL AND MALIGNANT HUMAN BREAST CELLS IN 3D REVEALS THAT SIGNALING REGULATION DIFFERS IN 2D AND 3D

Despite differences in the gross anatomy of mouse and human mammary glands, the assays developed for the mouse cells (Barcellos-Hoff et al. 1989) could be used for human cells with an additional bonus: Normal and nonmalignant human breast epithelial cells could be distinguished from premalignant and malignant cells in 3D assays (Petersen et al. 1992). Whereas the normal cells derived from reduction mammoplasty and nonmalignant cell lines became quiescent by day 7 and organized into a replica of human breast acinus with correct tissue polar-ity and proportions, the malignant cells continued to grow, piled up, and formed large, disorganized, tumor-like colonies (Petersen et al. 1992). Using a unique model of human breast cancer progression referred to as HMT3522 (Briand et al. 1987, 1996), we showed that much of the phenotypic difference between the nonma-lignant (S1) and malignant (T4-2) cells was due to changes in the levels and functions of surface receptors for ECM molecules and growth factors leading to aber-rant activation of a number of signaling pathways.

Using a series of signal transduction inhibitors and dominant-negative mutants, we have delineated the path-ways downstream of receptor tyrosine kinases and adhe-sion receptors that contribute to the malignant phenotype of T4-2 cells (Fig. 2). Using blocking antibodies against

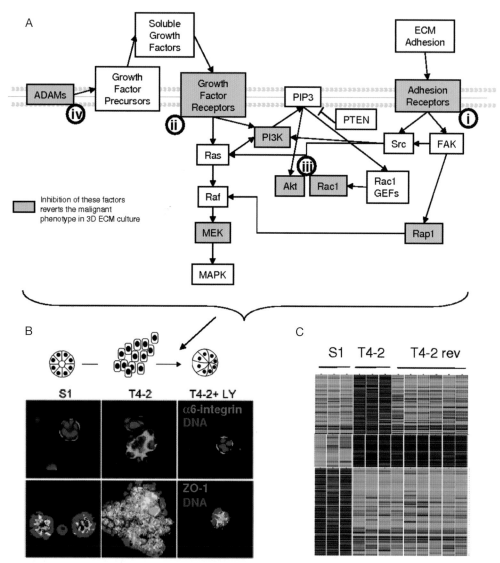

Figure 2. Reversion of the malignant phenotype by modulation of signaling pathways integrated by the ECM. (*A*) Schematic repre-sentation of the signaling pathways downstream of growth factor and adhesion receptors. The activity of some key proteins (*green*) is required for the maintenance of the malignant phenotype. (*B*) The malignant phenotype of T4-2 cells may be reverted in 3D ECM culture using inhibitors of the key signaling receptors and their downstream target proteins described above. A representative exam-ple (PI3K inhibition) is shown. α6-integrin and ZO-1 are markers of basal and apical polarity, respectively. (*C*) Hierarchical cluster-ing of Affymetrix microarray data of S1 and T4-2 cells, and T4-2 cells treated with inhibitors of the regulatory proteins shown in *A*. Reversion of the malignant phenotype using diverse inhibitors elicits a common gene expression pattern (P.A. Kenny and M.J. Bis-sell, unpubl.) (*B*, Modified, with permission, from Liu et al. 2004.).

β1-integrin (Fig. 2Ai), we defined a requirement for increased ECM signaling via this receptor for the maintenance of the malignant phenotype (Weaver et al. 1997). Furthermore, we defined a role for increased signaling by the EGFR pathway, since inhibitors of this receptor and downstream signaling molecules effected a similar reversion of the malignant phenotype (Fig. 2Aii) (Wang et al. 1998). This reversion encompassed a restoration of growth arrest in response to ECM, the restoration of apicobasal acinar polarity, the reorganization of the actin cytoskeleton, and the formation of adherens junctions (Fig. 2B). Inhibition of PI3-kinase (PI3K) resulted in a similar phenotype (Fig. 2Aiii), and we have dissected the different contributions of two critical PI3K effectors, Rac1 and Akt, to malignancy in this model (Liu et al. 2004). Because these malignant breast cells lack mutations in common proto-oncogenes (P.A. Kenny and M.J. Bissell, unpubl.), we have probed the extracellular effectors upstream of EGFR to identify the key endogenous growth factors that drive the malignant phenotype. Using this approach we have identified two EGFR ligands and a protease required for their activity, and demonstrated that the malignant phenotype may also be reverted by targeting this protease (Fig. 2Aiv) (P.A. Kenny and M.J. Bissell, in prep.). Importantly, inhibition of any of these pathways down-modulates the others, as well as the level of the surface receptors β1-integrin, EGFR (Wang et al. 1998), and coxsackievirus and adenovirus receptor, CAR (Anders et al. 2003). This down-modulation does not occur in 2D (Fig. 3) (for review, see Bissell et al. 1999, 2003).

A comparison of cDNA array analysis of nonmalignant and malignant cells indicates that a substantial subset of signaling pathways and programs are altered when cells are placed in 3D (not shown). Furthermore, the array analysis of malignant T4-2 cells treated with these diverse inhibitors indicates that a key subset of genes become "S1-like" in the reverted cells by all the inhibitors tested (Fig. 2C). The contribution of these genes to tissue polarity and growth control is currently under investigation. As such, the reversion model may be used as a screen for how signaling pathways may become integrated as a result of restoration of the tissue architecture. The same approach may be used also for finding new tar-

gets for breast cancer therapy, and a number of laboratories, including ours, are using these assays for such studies at present.

TISSUE POLARITY ALSO REGULATES RESPONSE AND RESISTANCE TO CHEMOTHERAPEUTIC AGENTS

It has long been noted that tumor cells change their response to radiation and chemical treatments when they are aggregated (Kerbel et al. 1996; Durand and Olive 2001). There are well-known pathways by which tumor cells can become resistant to chemotherapy. We reasoned that since tissue structure is so fundamental to phenotypic behavior of tumor cells, one additional mode of resistance could be due to the changes that occur as a result of reestablishment of tissue polarity. That this is indeed the case was shown in a series of experiments we reported in 2002 (Weaver et al. 2002). Briefly, normal and malignant human breast cells become resistant to induction of apoptosis by six different chemotherapeutic agents when they are correctly polarized in 3D (Fig. 4). Both cell types are equally susceptible to cell death when cultivated on tissue culture plastic. That tissue polarity rather than differences in mutation, growth rate, or 3-dimensionality per se is responsible for the observed differences was shown using some of the techniques developed in the laboratory and described above. If normal cells are disorganized in 3D they die. If tumor cells are reverted in laminin-rich ECM, they become resistant; if they are growth-arrested in collagen-I gels where breast tissue polarity is reversed, they still die. These observations were traced to the establishment of the correct tissue polarity through involvement of hemi-desmosomes and α6/β4-integrins (for further details, see Weaver et al. 2002). This is another clear example of the importance of the microenvironment and tissue architecture in function and dysfunction.

	3DlrBM				2D		
	S1	T4-2	T4-2 "treated"		T4-2	T4-2 "treated"	
Inhibitor Added:	–	–	β1-integrin inhibitor	EGFR Inhibitor	–	β1-integrin inhibitor	EGFR Inhibitor
β1-integrin total levels	+	+++	+	+	+++	+++	+++
EGFR total levels	+	++++	+	+	++++	++++	++++
EGFR activated	+	++++	+	+	++++	++++	+

Figure 3. β1-integrin and EGFR protein levels and activities are coordinately modulated in HMT3522 cells in 3D ECM. This reciprocal cross-modulation is not observed in cells cultured on tissue culture plastic. (Reprinted, with permission, from Bissell et al. 1999 [© AACR].)

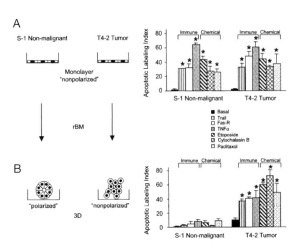

Figure 4. Only nonmalignant cells within mammary acini are resistant to apoptosis. Apoptotic labeling indices calculated for S-1 and T4-2 cells treated with Trail peptide (1 μg/ml), anti-FAS mAb (IgM CH-11, 2 μg/ml), TNF-α (100 nM), etoposide (50 μM), cytochalasin B (1 μM), or paclitaxol (120 nM). Cells were treated (A) as monolayers on a thin coat of collagen I for 24 hr or (B) as 3D structures in rBM for 96 hr. (Reprinted, with permission, from Weaver et al. 2002 [© Elsevier].)

METALLOPROTEINASES AS ONCOGENES; NORMAL STROMA AS A TUMOR SUPPRESSOR

Matrix metalloproteinases (MMPs) regulate a number of pathways relevant to cancer biology, including proliferation, differentiation, apoptosis, migration, and invasion (Egeblad and Werb 2002). Establishment of a causal relationship between MMP overexpression and tumor progression has prompted the development of several MMP inhibitors as anticancer therapeutics, and although clinical trials in which these agents were used to treat late-stage tumors have been disappointing, accumulating evidence suggests that the tumor-promoting activity of MMPs may be most important in the earliest stages of tumor development (Coussens et al. 2002; Egeblad and Werb 2002). We previously observed that transgenic mice expressing an autoactivated form of MMP-3 (stromelysin-1) under control of the whey acidic protein promoter (WAP) to direct expression in mammary epithelial cells in mid-pregnancy (Sympson et al. 1994) develop invasive, genomically unstable mammary tumors (Sternlicht et al. 1999). Development of a culture assay to dissect these effects revealed that treatment with MMP-3 causes mouse mammary epithelial cells to alter cellular morphology, decrease cell–cell interactions, increase motility and invasiveness, down-regulate epithelial cytokeratins, and up-regulate mesenchymal vimentin (Boudreau et al. 1995; Lochter et al. 1997a,b), characteristics of epithelial-to-mesenchymal transition (EMT) that facilitate tumor invasion and metastasis (Thiery 2002). The genomic alterations induced by MMP-3 are strikingly nonrandom, with common patterns of genomic deletions found on chromosome 4 in tumor tissue derived from the WAP-MMP-3 transgenic mice (Fig. 5A) and in cultured mouse mammary epithelial cells exposed to MMP-3 (Fig. 5B) (Sternlicht et al. 1999; Radisky et al. 2005).

A common mechanism underlying both induction of EMT and the development of genomic instability by MMP-3 was suggested by the concomitant appearance of EMT (Fig. 6A) with increased resistance to N-(phosphon-

acetyl)-L-aspartate (PALA) (Fig. 6B) (Johnson et al. 1976), as resistance to PALA is acquired through amplification of the CAD gene (Wahl et al. 1979; Radisky et al. 2005). Our investigations revealed that both the MMP-3-induced phenotypic alterations (e.g., induction of EMT) and genetic changes (e.g., genomic instability) were caused by increases in cellular reactive oxygen species (ROS). Cultured mouse mammary epithelial cells treated with MMP-3 showed significantly increased oxidative DNA damage that was inhibited by treatment with ROS inhibitor N-acetyl cysteine (NAC) and, consistent with the implication that the ROS-mediated DNA damage was related to the induction of genomic instability, we found that NAC inhibited the MMP-3-induced acquisition of PALA resistance, and that elevating cellular redox levels in the absence of MMP-3 by treatment with H_2O_2 was sufficient to stimulate PALA resistance (Radisky et al. 2005). ROS have been implicated as secondary signaling intermediates that control cellular phenotype (Droge 2002; Puri et al. 2002; Finkel 2003), and we found that MMP-3-induced ROS were both necessary and sufficient to induce the EMT phenotypic alterations in target mammary epithelial cells (Radisky et al. 2005).

Previous studies (Kheradmand et al. 1998; Werner and Werb 2002) showed that alterations in cell morphology, a process related to MMP-3-induced EMT, can lead to increased cellular ROS through a Rac1-dependent mechanism. Using pull-down activity assays, we found that MMP-3 treatment stimulated an increase in Rac1 activity and the induction of a higher-molecular-weight form of active Rac1 (Fig. 6C). Rac1b is a highly activated splice isoform of Rac1 that has been found in breast and colorectal tumors (Matos et al. 2003; Fiegen et al. 2004). Quantitative RT-PCR using oligonucleotide primers specific for the Rac1b isoform performed on cells that were treated for up to 4 days with MMP-3 showed a progressively increasing expression of Rac1b for as long as MMP-3 was present, and that Rac1b levels fell off rapidly after MMP-3 withdrawal (Fig. 6D). Consistent with the implication that the MMP-3-induced alterations in Rac1b expression are the trigger for EMT, we observed that expression of Snail and vimentin paralleled the expression of Rac1b (Radisky et al. 2005), and that inhibition of Rac1b expression by RNAi blocked the induction of EMT by MMP-3 (Fig. 6E).

A contrast can be drawn between the phenotypic consequences of MMP-3/Rac1b-induced ROS (i.e., induction of EMT) and the genetic consequences (i.e., DNA damage and genomic instability). Although it seems likely that MMP-3-induced genomic instability is a nonspecific or pathological response, we conjecture that induction of EMT by MMP-3/Rac1b-produced ROS is caused by specific activation of select signaling pathways; indeed, we found that MMP-3-induced ROS were both necessary and sufficient for induction of the Snail transcription factor, implicated previously as a key mediator of EMT (Nieto 2002; Thiery 2002). Although we have shown that MMP-3 can directly cause malignant transformations, it is noteworthy that MMPs are involved in many normal developmental processes, and that genetic deficiency of MMPs

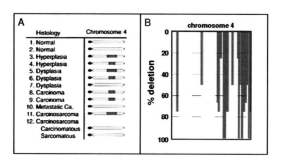

Figure 5. Nonrandom patterns of genomic instability induced by treatment with MMP-3. (*A*) Analysis of normal and tumor tissue from WAP-MMP-3 transgenic mice by cytogenetic comparative genomic hybridization (CGH) reveals common patterns of deletions (*red*) in chromosome 4. (*B*) Cultured SCp2 mouse mammary epithelial cells exposed to MMP-3 become genomically unstable and show deletions in chromosome 4, as revealed by array-based CGH. (*A*, Adapted from Sternlicht et al. 1999; *B*, adapted from Radisky et al. 2005.)

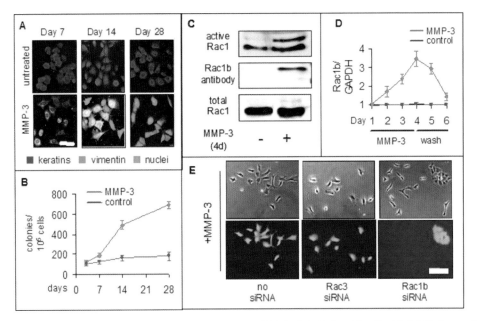

Figure 6. Induction of EMT and genomic instability by treatment with MMP-3: Role of Rac1b. (*A*) MMP-3-treated SCp2 cells, stained for cytokeratins (*red*), vimentin (*green*), and DNA (*blue*); bar, 50 mm. (*B*) Induction of PALA resistance by MMP-3 (*green diamonds*, MMP-3; *red squares*, untreated). (*C*) Treatment with MMP-3 stimulates production of Rac1b, a highly activated splice isoform of Rac1. (*Top*) Active Rac species as assessed by PAK pulldown assay; (*middle*) total cell lysates probed with antibody raised against Rac1b splice insertion; (*bottom*) total cell lysates probed with Rac1 antibody, showing low levels of Rac1b expression relative to Rac1 in lysate from treated cells. (*D*) Time course of Rac1b expression in response to MMP-3 treatment and withdrawal. MMP-3 treatment (days 1–4) and washout (days 5–6) (*green diamonds*, MMP-3-treated; *red squares*, untreated). (*E*) Specific suppression of Rac1b by siRNA blocks MMP3-induced EMT. (Adapted from Radisky et al. 2005.)

can lead to an array of developmental abnormalities (Sternlicht and Werb 2001). In this regard, it is relevant that many other developmental signaling molecules have also been found to facilitate tumor progression, including BMPs, TGF-β (Waite and Eng 2003), Wnts (Moon et al. 2002), Notch (Radtke and Raj 2003), and Hedgehog (Pasca di Magliano and Hebrok 2003). The investigation of the tumor-promoting effects of these factors has been facilitated by an understanding of the cellular signaling mechanisms by which they operate, and our new understanding of the MMP-3-induced signaling pathways provides insight into this parallel process. Since our initial studies on MMP3-induced tumorigenesis, two further extracellular proteases, MT1-MMP and matriptase, have been causally implicated in tumorigenesis using transgenic models (Ha et al. 2001; List et al. 2005).

Demonstrating that these stromal alterations actually facilitate tumor progression is difficult in human studies; however, a number of recently developed animal models address this point and show that genetic lesions in the stroma can make a positive and even causative contribution to epithelial tumorigenesis. Conditional ablation of the Tgfbr2 gene in fibroblasts induced the onset of neoplasia in the prostate and squamous cell carcinoma of the forestomach (Fig. 7) (Bhowmick et al. 2004). It has also been shown that growth of MCF7 xenografts is significantly enhanced in SCID mice null for p53. p53$^{+/-}$ mice exhibit intermediate kinetics of tumor growth and, importantly, loss of the wild-type p53 allele was detected in the tumor stroma arising in six of eight tumors in the heterozygous mice (Kiaris et al. 2005).

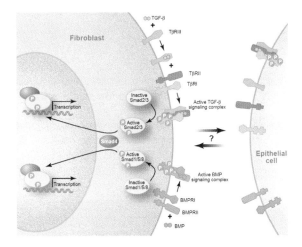

Figure 7. Signaling pathways in stromal cells activated by TGF-β and BMP prevent tumor formation in epithelia. TGF-β signaling can be initiated by association with type III TGF-β receptors prior to formation of an active kinase complex containing receptor types I and II. The active TGF-β signaling complex phosphorylates receptor-regulated R-SMADs such as Smad2 and Smad3, which then bind to common partner co-SMADs such as Smad4. The resulting activated complex can bind to specific DNA sequences and influence the transcription of many tissue-specific genes. Similarly, BMP family members form an active BMP signaling complex, which phosphorylates Smads 1, 5, and 8. These activated R-SMADs then associate with Smad4 to form an active transcriptional complex. Loss of TβRII, Smad4, or BMPRI in stromal cells can stimulate the formation of tumors in adjacent epithelium, although the signals involved in this process have not yet been identified. (Reprinted, with permission, from Radisky and Bissell 2004 [© AAAS].)

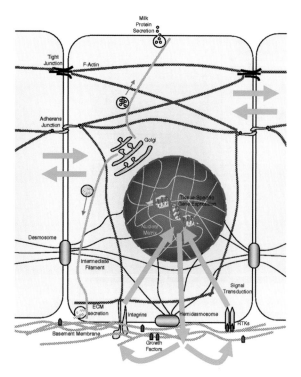

Figure 8. Dynamic reciprocity: The whole is greater than the sum of its parts. Gene expression and function of differentiated tissues is an emergent property arising from the bidirectional flow of biochemical and mechanical signals between the ECM and the nucleus, transduced by transmembrane receptors, signaling molecules, and cytoskeletal elements. In the last analysis, however, the organ itself is the unit of function (Bissell and Hall 1987).

That not only stroma, but the different epithelial cell types, and in fact all cell types that make up the architecture of the organs (Fig. 8), play important roles in the integrity of the function of that organ can be demonstrated further with studies on the role of myoepithelial cells in establishment of tissue polarity in breast acini (Gudjonsson et al. 2002; Adriance et al. 2005).

INHERITED POLYMORPHISMS IN GENES ENCODING MICROENVIRONMENTAL PROTEINS THAT MAY ALTER CANCER SUSCEPTIBILITY AND/OR PROGRESSION KINETICS

Loss of function of tumor suppressor genes such as RB, BRCA1, BRCA2, and CHK2 is a critical component of a large proportion of familial cancers. However, it is clear that other low-penetrance alleles also contribute to this polygenic disease in the wider population. Several case-control studies have examined the effects of germ-line polymorphisms in genes encoding proteins present in the tissue microenvironment to determine whether variation in any of these genes contributes to an increased risk of incidence or progression in several cancers. Such polymorphisms may alter the coding sequence of the protein, with resultant effects on its activity, or they may occur in noncoding regions of the gene, where they may lead to al-

tered levels of gene expression and/or alternative splicing by creating or deleting consensus binding sites for nucleic acid interacting proteins. Although there has been an explosion of interest in this field, it is important to note that many of these studies are relatively small and, despite achieving statistical significance at the threshold set by the investigators, remain to be confirmed in larger studies. We believe that it is important to be fully cognizant of the statistical problems inherent in this methodology, particularly of the propensity of these studies to produce false positives (Risch 2000; Pharoah et al. 2004).

For the purposes of this paper, we confine our discussion to those SNPs which have been demonstrated (or at least imputed) to exert an effect on protein expression or activity. Several of these studies have been reviewed in detail elsewhere (Balasubramanian et al. 2002; Loktionov 2004) and are summarized in Table 1. Polymorphic changes have been reported in genes encoding growth factors, adhesion receptors, proteases, and cytokines—proteins that play crucial roles in the intercellular milieu. Each of these proteins has been implicated in neoplasia. Several of these SNPs are found in the promoter regions of their respective genes and have been associated with alterations in the mRNA expression level for that allele. Although it remains to be seen how many of these findings will be reproduced in larger, independent populations, these data support the hypothesis that dose-dependent alterations in components of the tissue microenvironment may play causative roles in tumorigenesis or may facilitate the neoplastic progression of an incipient tumor cell.

In addition, the importance of epithelial-stromal interactions for cancer progression is underlined by the detection of clones of mutant stromal cells, the expansion of which has been favored by the acquired mutation(s). Several global studies using microdissected samples of tumor epithelium and stroma with subsequent analysis of loss of heterozygosity or allelic imbalance have shown that distinct genetic alterations occur in the epithelial and stromal compartments. Somatically acquired genetic alterations in the stroma have been reported in cancers of the breast (Moinfar et al. 2000; Kurose et al. 2001; Ellsworth et al. 2004; Fukino et al. 2004), colon (Wernert et al. 2001), bladder (Paterson et al. 2003), prostate (McCarthy et al. 2004), and ovary (Tuhkanen et al. 2004). These genomic studies provide a bird's-eye view of the nature and scale of the differing genetic lesions present in the epithelial and stromal compartments. A greater insight into the co-selected mechanisms that drive tumor progression will come from a detailed molecular analysis of these regions, and recent studies have shown that some of the players most familiar from epithelial tumorigenesis are also altered in the stroma. Mutations in p53 and PTEN have been reported in the stroma of breast carcinomas (Kurose et al. 2002), and mutations in EGFR also have been detected in this compartment (Weber et al. 2005). Given the number of mutational and cytogenetic abnormalities detected in stroma to date, it seems likely that epigenetic alterations in stromal cells might also contribute to tumorigenesis. Collectively, these striking data suggest that there is a strong selective pressure in tumors of different epithelial origins for the coevolution of a clonal stromal compartment.

ACKNOWLEDGMENTS

These investigations were supported by grants from the U.S. Department of Energy, Office of Biological and Environmental Research (DE-AC03 SF0098), National Cancer Institute (2 R01 CA064786-09), and an Innovator Award from the Department of Defense Breast Cancer Research Program (BC012005) to M.J.B; and from the National Cancer Institute (CA57621) to M.J.B. and Zena Werb; and by postdoctoral training fellowships (Susan G. Komen Breast Cancer Foundation #2000-223 and DOD BCRP DAMD17-00-1-0224 to P.A.K. and American Cancer Society PF-02-009-01-DDC to D.C.R.).

REFERENCES

Adriance M.C., Inman J.L., Petersen O.W., and Bissell M.J. 2005. Myoepithelial cells: Good fences make good neighbors. *Breast Cancer Res.* **7:** 190.

Allinen M., Beroukhim R., Cai L., Brennan C., Lahti-Domenici J., Huang H., Porter D., Hu M., Chin L., Richardson A., Schnitt S., Sellers W.R., and Polyak K. 2004. Molecular characterization of the tumor microenvironment in breast cancer. *Cancer Cell* **6:** 17.

Anders M., Hansen R., Ding R.X., Rauen K.A., Bissell M.J., and Korn W.M. 2003. Disruption of 3D tissue integrity facilitates adenovirus infection by deregulating the coxsackievirus and adenovirus receptor. *Proc. Natl. Acad. Sci.* **100:** 1943.

Ayala F., Corral J., Gonzalez-Conejero R., Sanchez I., Moraleda J.M., and Vicente V. 2003. Genetic polymorphisms of platelet adhesive molecules: Association with breast cancer risk and clinical presentation. *Breast Cancer Res. Treat.* **80:** 145.

Balasubramanian S.P., Brown N.J., and Reed M.W. 2002. Role of genetic polymorphisms in tumour angiogenesis. *Br. J. Cancer* **87:** 1057.

Barcellos-Hoff M.H., Aggeler J., Ram T.G., and Bissell M.J. 1989. Functional differentiation and alveolar morphogenesis of primary mammary cultures on reconstituted basement membrane. *Development* **105:** 223.

Bhowmick N.A., Chytil A., Plieth D., Gorska A.E., Dumont N., Shappell S., Washington M.K., Neilson E.G., and Moses H.L. 2004. TGF-beta signaling in fibroblasts modulates the oncogenic potential of adjacent epithelia. *Science* **303:** 848.

Bingle L., Brown N.J., and Lewis C.E. 2002. The role of tumour-associated macrophages in tumour progression: Implications for new anticancer therapies. *J. Pathol.* **196:** 254.

Biondi M.L., Turri O., Leviti S., Seminati R., Cecchini F., Bernini M., Ghilardi G., and Guagnellini E. 2000. MMP1 and MMP3 polymorphisms in promoter regions and cancer. *Clin. Chem.* **46:** 2023.

Bissell M.J. 1981. The differentiated state of normal and malignant cells or how to define a "normal" cell in culture. *Int. Rev. Cytol.* **70:** 27.

Bissell M.J. and Hall H.G. 1987. Form and function in the mammary gland: The role of extracellular matrix. In *The mammary gland* (ed. M.C. Neville and C.W. Daniel), p. 97. Plenum Publishing, New York.

Bissell M.J., Hall H.G., and Parry G. 1982. How does the extracellular matrix direct gene expression? *J. Theor. Biol.* **99:** 31.

Bissell M.J., Rizki A., and Mian I.S. 2003. Tissue architecture: The ultimate regulator of breast epithelial function. *Curr. Opin. Cell Biol.* **15:** 753.

Bissell M.J., Weaver V.M., Lelievre S.A., Wang F., Petersen O.W., and Schmeichel K.L. 1999. Tissue structure, nuclear organization, and gene expression in normal and malignant breast. *Cancer Res.* (suppl. 7) **59:** 1757.

Blau H.M. and Baltimore D. 1991. Differentiation requires continuous regulation. *J. Cell Biol.* **112:** 781.

Boudreau N., Sympson C.J., Werb Z., and Bissell M.J. 1995. Suppression of ICE and apoptosis in mammary epithelial cells by extracellular matrix. *Science* **267:** 891.

Briand P., Petersen O.W., and Van Deurs B. 1987. A new diploid nontumorigenic human breast epithelial cell line isolated and propagated in chemically defined medium. *In Vitro Cell. Dev. Biol.* **23:** 181.

Briand P., Nielsen K.V., Madsen M.W., and Petersen O.W. 1996. Trisomy 7p and malignant transformation of human breast epithelial cells following epidermal growth factor withdrawal. *Cancer Res.* **56:** 2039.

Camps J.L., Chang S.M., Hsu T.C., Freeman M.R., Hong S.J., Zhau H.E., von Eschenbach A.C., and Chung L.W. 1990. Fibroblast-mediated acceleration of human epithelial tumor growth in vivo. *Proc. Natl. Acad. Sci.* **87:** 75.

Cardoso W.V. 2001. Molecular regulation of lung development. *Annu. Rev. Physiol.* **63:** 471.

Carrel A. 1908. Results of the transplantation of blood vessels, organs and limbs. *J. Am. Med. Assoc.* **51:** 1662.

———. 1911. Rejuvenation of cultures of tissues. *J. Am. Med. Assoc.* **57:** 1611.

Coussens L.M., Fingleton B., and Matrisian L.M. 2002. Matrix metalloproteinase inhibitors and cancer: Trials and tribulations. *Science* **295:** 2387.

Cunha G.R., Ricke W., Thomson A., Marker P.C., Risbridger G., Hayward S.W., Wang Y.Z., Donjacour A.A., and Kurita T. 2004. Hormonal, cellular, and molecular regulation of normal and neoplastic prostatic development. *J. Steroid Biochem. Mol. Biol.* **92:** 221.

Cunningham L.M., Chapman C., Dunstan R., Bell M.C., and Joske D.J. 2003. Polymorphisms in the interleukin 10 gene promoter are associated with susceptibility to aggressive non-Hodgkin's lymphoma. *Leuk. Lymphoma* **44:** 251.

DeCosse J.J., Gossens C.L., Kuzma J.F., and Unsworth B.R. 1973. Breast cancer: Induction of differentiation by embryonic tissue. *Science* **181:** 1057.

DeMichele A., Martin A.M., Mick R., Gor P., Wray L., Klein-Cabral M., Athanasiadis G., Colligan T., Stadtmauer E., and Weber B. 2003. Interleukin-6 -174G→C polymorphism is associated with improved outcome in high-risk breast cancer. *Cancer Res.* **63:** 8051.

Dolberg D.S. and Bissell M.J. 1984. Inability of Rous sarcoma virus to cause sarcomas in the avian embryo. *Nature* **309:** 552.

Droge W. 2002. Free radicals in the physiological control of cell function. *Physiol. Rev.* **82:** 47.

Durand R.E. and Olive P.L. 2001. Resistance of tumor cells to chemo- and radiotherapy modulated by the three-dimensional architecture of solid tumors and spheroids. *Methods Cell Biol.* **64:** 211.

Dvorak H.F. 1986. Tumors: Wounds that do not heal. Similarities between tumor stroma generation and wound healing. *N. Engl. J. Med.* **315:** 1650.

Egeblad M. and Werb Z. 2002. New functions for the matrix metalloproteinases in cancer progression. *Nat. Rev. Cancer* **2:** 161.

Ellsworth D.L., Ellsworth R.E., Love B., Deyarmin B., Lubert S.M., Mittal V., and Shriver C.D. 2004. Genomic patterns of allelic imbalance in disease free tissue adjacent to primary breast carcinomas. *Breast Cancer Res. Treat.* **88:** 131.

Emerman J.T. and Pitelka D.R. 1977. Maintenance and induction of morphological differentiation in dissociated mammary epithelium on floating collagen membranes. *In Vitro* **13:** 316.

Ferguson M.W. and O'Kane S. 2004. Scar-free healing: From embryonic mechanisms to adult therapeutic intervention. *Philos. Trans. R. Soc. Lond. B Biol. Sci.* **359:** 839.

Fiegen D., Haeusler L.C., Herbrand U., Dvorsky R., Vetter I.R., and Ahmadian M.R. 2004. Alternative splicing of Rac1 generates Rac1b, a self-activating GTPase. *J. Biol. Chem.* **279:** 4743.

Finkel T. 2003. Oxidant signals and oxidative stress. *Curr. Opin. Cell Biol.* **15:** 247.

Fukino K., Shen L., Matsumoto S., Morrison C.D., Mutter G.L., and Eng C. 2004. Combined total genome loss of heterozy-gosity scan of breast cancer stroma and epithelium reveals multiplicity of stromal targets. *Cancer Res.* **64:** 7231.

Ghilardi G., Biondi M.L., Mangoni J., Leviti S., DeMonti M., Guagnellini E., and Scorza R. 2001. Matrix metalloproteinase-1 promoter polymorphism 1G/2G is correlated with colorectal cancer invasiveness. *Clin. Cancer Res.* **7:** 2344.

Grobstein C. 1964. Cytodifferentiation and its controls. *Science* **143:** 643.

Gudjonsson T., Ronnov-Jessen L., Villadsen R., Rank F., Bissell M.J., and Petersen O.W. 2002. Normal and tumor-derived myoepithelial cells differ in their ability to interact with luminal breast epithelial cells for polarity and basement membrane deposition. *J. Cell Sci.* **115:** 39.

Ha H.Y., Moon H.B., Nam M.S., Lee J.W., Ryoo Z.Y., Lee T.H., Lee K.K., So B.J., Sato H., Seiki M., and Yu D.Y. 2001. Overexpression of membrane-type matrix metalloproteinase-1 gene induces mammary gland abnormalities and adenocarcinoma in transgenic mice. *Cancer Res.* **61:** 984.

Harach H.R., Franssila K.O., and Wasenius V.M. 1985. Occult papillary carcinoma of the thyroid. A "normal" finding in Finland. A systematic autopsy study. *Cancer* **56:** 531.

Hayashi N., Cunha G.R., and Wong Y.C. 1990. Influence of male genital tract mesenchymes on differentiation of Dunning prostatic adenocarcinoma. *Cancer Res.* **50:** 4747.

Hefler L.A., Grimm C., Ackermann S., Malur S., Radjabi-Rahat A.R., Leodolter S., Beckmann M.W., Zeillinger R., Koelbl H., and Tempfer C.B. 2003. An interleukin-6 gene promoter polymorphism influences the biological phenotype of ovarian cancer. *Cancer Res.* **63:** 3066.

Hochedlinger K., Blelloch R., Brennan C., Yamada Y., Kim M., Chin L., and Jaenisch R. 2004. Reprogramming of a melanoma genome by nuclear transplantation. *Genes Dev.* **18:** 1875.

Howell W.M., Bateman A.C., Turner S.J., Collins A., and Theaker J.M. 2002. Influence of vascular endothelial growth factor single nucleotide polymorphisms on tumour development in cutaneous malignant melanoma. *Genes Immun.* **3:** 229.

Howlett A.R., Carter V.C., Martin G.S., and Bissell M.J. 1988. pp60v-src tyrosine kinase is expressed and active in sarcoma-free avian embryos microinjected with Rous sarcoma virus. *Proc. Natl. Acad. Sci.* **85:** 7587.

Johnson R.K., Inouye T., Goldin A., and Stark G.R. 1976. Antitumor activity of N-(phosphonacetyl)-L-aspartic acid, a transition-state inhibitor of aspartate transcarbamylase. *Cancer Res.* **36:** 2720.

Juszczynski P., Kalinka E., Bienvenu J., Woszczek G., Borowiec M., Robak T., Kowalski M., Lech-Maranda E., Baseggio L., Coiffier B., Salles G., and Warzocha K. 2002. Human leukocyte antigens class II and tumor necrosis factor genetic polymorphisms are independent predictors of non-Hodgkin lymphoma outcome. *Blood* **100:** 3037.

Kanamori Y., Matsushima M., Minaguchi T., Kobayashi K., Sagae S., Kudo N., Terakawa N., and Nakamura Y. 1999. Correlation between expression of the matrix metalloproteinase-1 gene in ovarian cancers and an insertion/deletion polymorphism in its promoter region. *Cancer Res.* **59:** 4225.

Kerbel R.S., St. Croix B., Florenes V.A., and Rak J. 1996. Induction and reversal of cell adhesion-dependent multicellular drug resistance in solid breast tumors. *Hum. Cell* **9:** 257.

Kheradmand F., Werner E., Tremble P., Symons M., and Werb Z. 1998. Role of Rac1 and oxygen radicals in collagenase-1 expression induced by cell shape change. *Science* **280:** 898.

Kiaris H., Chatzistamou I., Trimis G., Frangou-Plemmenou M., Pafiti-Kondi A., and Kalofoutis A. 2005. Evidence for nonautonomous effect of p53 tumor suppressor in carcinogenesis. *Cancer Res.* **65:** 1627.

Kuraoka K., Oue N., Yokozaki H., Kitadai Y., Ito R., Nakayama H., and Yasui W. 2003. Correlation of a single nucleotide polymorphism in the E-cadherin gene promoter with tumorigenesis and progression of gastric carcinoma in Japan. *Int. J. Oncol.* **23:** 421.

Kurose K., Gilley K., Matsumoto S., Watson P.H., Zhou X.P.,

and Eng C. 2002. Frequent somatic mutations in PTEN and TP53 are mutually exclusive in the stroma of breast carcinomas. *Nat. Genet.* **32:** 355.

Kurose K., Hoshaw-Woodard S., Adeyinka A., Lemeshow S., Watson P.H., and Eng C. 2001. Genetic model of multi-step breast carcinogenesis involving the epithelium and stroma: Clues to tumour-microenvironment interactions. *Hum. Mol. Genet.* **10:** 1907.

Lauten M., Matthias T., Stanulla M., Beger C., Welte K., and Schrappe M. 2002. Association of initial response to prednisone treatment in childhood acute lymphoblastic leukaemia and polymorphisms within the tumour necrosis factor and the interleukin-10 genes. *Leukemia* **16:** 1437.

Lee E.Y., Parry G., and Bissell M.J. 1984. Modulation of secreted proteins of mouse mammary epithelial cells by the collagenous substrata. *J. Cell Biol.* **98:** 146.

Lee E.Y., Lee W.H., Kaetzel C.S., Parry G., and Bissell M.J. 1985. Interaction of mouse mammary epithelial cells with collagen substrata: Regulation of casein gene expression and secretion. *Proc. Natl. Acad. Sci.* **82:** 1419.

Lin C.Q. and Bissell M.J. 1993. Multi-faceted regulation of cell differentiation by extracellular matrix. *FASEB J.* **7:** 737.

List K., Szabo R., Molinolo A., Sriuranpong V., Redeye V., Murdock T., Burke B., Nielsen B.S., Gutkind J.S., and Bugge T.H. 2005. Deregulated matriptase causes ras-independent multistage carcinogenesis and promotes ras-mediated malignant transformation. *Genes Dev.* **19:** 1934.

Liu H., Radisky D.C., Wang F., and Bissell M.J. 2004. Polarity and proliferation are controlled by distinct signaling pathways downstream of PI3-kinase in breast epithelial tumor cells. *J. Cell Biol.* **164:** 603.

Lochter A., Galosy S., Muschler J., Freedman N., Werb Z., and Bissell M.J. 1997a. Matrix metalloproteinase stromelysin-1 triggers a cascade of molecular alterations that leads to stable epithelial-to-mesenchymal conversion and a premalignant phenotype in mammary epithelial cells. *J. Cell Biol.* **139:** 1861.

Lochter A., Srebrow A., Sympson C.J., Terracio N., Werb Z., and Bissell M.J. 1997b. Misregulation of stromelysin-1 expression in mouse mammary tumor cells accompanies acquisition of stromelysin-1-dependent invasive properties. *J. Biol. Chem.* **272:** 5007.

Loktionov A. 2004. Common gene polymorphisms, cancer progression and prognosis. *Cancer Lett.* **208:** 1.

Martin G.S. 2004. The road to Src. *Oncogene* **23:** 7910.

Martinez-Escribano J.A., Moya-Quiles M.R., Muro M., Montes-Ares O., Hernandez-Caselles T., Frias J.F., and Alvarez-Lopez M.R. 2002. Interleukin-10, interleukin-6 and interferon-gamma gene polymorphisms in melanoma patients. *Melanoma Res.* **12:** 465.

Matos P., Collard J.G., and Jordan P. 2003. Tumor-related alternatively spliced Rac1b is not regulated by Rho-GDP dissociation inhibitors and exhibits selective downstream signaling. *J. Biol. Chem.* **278:** 50442.

McCarron S.L., Edwards S., Evans P.R., Gibbs R., Dearnaley D.P., Dowe A., Southgate C., Easton D.F., Eeles R.A., and Howell W.M. 2002. Influence of cytokine gene polymorphisms on the development of prostate cancer. *Cancer Res.* **62:** 3369.

McCarthy R.P., Zhang S., Bostwick D.G., Qian J., Eble J.N., Wang M., Lin H., and Cheng L. 2004. Molecular genetic evidence for different clonal origins of epithelial and stromal components of phyllodes tumor of the prostate. *Am. J. Pathol.* **165:** 1395.

Mestiri S., Bouaouina N., Ahmed S.B., Khedhaier A., Jrad B.B., Remadi S., and Chouchane L. 2001. Genetic variation in the tumor necrosis factor-alpha promoter region and in the stress protein hsp70-2: Susceptibility and prognostic implications in breast carcinoma. *Cancer* **91:** 672.

Michalopoulos G. and Pitot H.C. 1975. Primary culture of parenchymal liver cells on collagen membranes. Morphological and biochemical observations. *Exp. Cell Res.* **94:** 70.

Mintz B. and Illmensee K. 1975. Normal genetically mosaic mice produced from malignant teratocarcinoma cells. *Proc.*

Natl. Acad. Sci. **72:** 3585.

Moinfar F., Man Y.G., Arnould L., Bratthauer G.L., Ratschek M., and Tavassoli F.A. 2000. Concurrent and independent genetic alterations in the stromal and epithelial cells of mammary carcinoma: Implications for tumorigenesis. *Cancer Res.* **60:** 2562.

Montie J.E., Wood D.P., Jr., Pontes J.E., Boyett J.M., and Levin H.S. 1989. Adenocarcinoma of the prostate in cystoprostatectomy specimens removed for bladder cancer. *Cancer* **63:** 381.

Moon R.T., Bowerman B., Boutros M., and Perrimon N. 2002. The promise and perils of Wnt signaling through beta-catenin. *Science* **296:** 1644.

Muschler J., Lochter A., Roskelley C.D., Yurchenco P., and Bissell M.J. 1999. Division of labor among the α6β4 integrin, β1 integrins, and an E3 laminin receptor to signal morphogenesis and beta-casein expression in mammary epithelial cells. *Mol. Biol. Cell* **10:** 2817.

Myers C.A., Schmidhauser C., Mellentin-Michelotti J., Fragoso G., Roskelley C.D., Casperson G., Mossi R., Pujuguet P., Hager G., and Bissell M.J. 1998. Characterization of BCE-1, a transcriptional enhancer regulated by prolactin and extracellular matrix and modulated by the state of histone acetylation. *Mol. Cell. Biol.* **18:** 2184.

Nielsen M., Thomsen J.L., Primdahl S., Dyreborg U., and Andersen J.A. 1987. Breast cancer and atypia among young and middle-aged women: A study of 110 medicolegal autopsies. *Br. J. Cancer* **56:** 814.

Nieto M.A. 2002. The snail superfamily of zinc-finger transcription factors. *Nat. Rev. Mol. Cell Biol.* **3:** 155.

Nishioka Y., Sagae S., Nishikawa A., Ishioka S., and Kudo R. 2003. A relationship between Matrix metalloproteinase-1 (MMP-1) promoter polymorphism and cervical cancer progression. *Cancer Lett.* **200:** 49.

Olumi A.F., Grossfeld G.D., Hayward S.W., Carroll P.R., Tlsty T.D., and Cunha G.R. 1999. Carcinoma-associated fibroblasts direct tumor progression of initiated human prostatic epithelium. *Cancer Res.* **59:** 5002.

Paget S. 1889. The distribution of secondary growths in cancer of the breast. *Lancet* **1:** 571.

Parmar H. and Cunha G.R. 2004. Epithelial-stromal interactions in the mouse and human mammary gland in vivo. *Endocr. Relat. Cancer* **11:** 437.

Pasca di Magliano M. and Hebrok M. 2003. Hedgehog signalling in cancer formation and maintenance. *Nat. Rev. Cancer* **3:** 903.

Paterson R.F., Ulbright T.M., MacLennan G.T., Zhang S., Pan C.X., Sweeney C.J., Moore C.R., Foster R.S., Koch M.O., Eble J.N., and Cheng L. 2003. Molecular genetic alterations in the laser-capture-microdissected stroma adjacent to bladder carcinoma. *Cancer* **98:** 1830.

Peebles F. 1911. On the interchange of limbs of the chick by transplantation. *Biol. Bull.* **20:** 14.

Petersen O.W., Ronnov-Jessen L., Howlett A.R., and Bissell M.J. 1992. Interaction with basement membrane serves to rapidly distinguish growth and differentiation pattern of normal and malignant human breast epithelial cells. *Proc. Natl. Acad. Sci.* **89:** 9064.

Pharoah P.D., Dunning A.M., Ponder B.A., and Easton D.F. 2004. Association studies for finding cancer-susceptibility genetic variants. *Nat. Rev. Cancer* **4:** 850.

Pollard J.W. 2004. Tumour-educated macrophages promote tumour progression and metastasis. *Nat. Rev. Cancer* **4:** 71.

Puri P.L., Bhakta K., Wood L.D., Costanzo A., Zhu J., and Wang J.Y. 2002. A myogenic differentiation checkpoint activated by genotoxic stress. *Nat. Genet.* **32:** 585.

Radisky D.C. and Bissell M.J. 2004. Cancer. Respect thy neighbor! *Science* **303:** 775.

Radisky D.C., Levy D.D., Littlepage L.E., Liu H., Nelson C.M., Fata J.E., Leake D., Godden E.L., Albertson D.G., Nieto M.A., Werb Z., and Bissell M.J. 2005. Rac1b and reactive oxygen species mediate MMP-3-induced EMT and genomic instability. *Nature* **436:** 123.

Radtke F. and Raj K. 2003. The role of Notch in tumorigenesis: Oncogene or tumour suppressor? *Nat. Rev. Cancer* **3:** 756.

Risch N.J. 2000. Searching for genetic determinants in the new millennium. *Nature* **405:** 847.

Roberts D.J. 2000. Molecular mechanisms of development of the gastrointestinal tract. *Dev. Dyn.* **219:** 109.

Robinson S.C. and Coussens L.M. 2005. Soluble mediators of inflammation during tumor development. *Adv. Cancer Res.* **93:** 159.

Ronnov-Jessen L., Petersen O.W., and Bissell M.J. 1996. Cellular changes involved in conversion of normal to malignant breast: Importance of the stromal reaction. *Physiol. Rev.* **76:** 69.

Roskelley C.D., Srebrow A., and Bissell M.J. 1995. A hierarchy of ECM-mediated signalling regulates tissue-specific gene expression. *Curr. Opin. Cell Biol.* **7:** 736.

Sakakura T., Nishizuka Y., and Dawe C.J. 1976. Mesenchyme-dependent morphogenesis and epithelium-specific cytodifferentiation in mouse mammary gland. *Science* **194:** 1439.

Schmeichel K.L. and Bissell M.J. 2003. Modeling tissue-specific signaling and organ function in three dimensions. *J. Cell Sci.* **116:** 2377.

Schmidhauser C., Casperson G.F., Myers C.A., Sanzo K.T., Bolten S., and Bissell M.J. 1992. A novel transcriptional enhancer is involved in the prolactin- and extracellular matrix-dependent regulation of beta-casein gene expression. *Mol. Biol. Cell* **3:** 699.

Schor S.L., Ellis I.R., Jones S.J., Baillie R., Seneviratne K., Clausen J., Motegi K., Vojtesek B., Kankova K., Furrie E., Sales M.J., Schor A.M., and Kay R.A. 2003. Migration-stimulating factor: A genetically truncated onco-fetal fibronectin isoform expressed by carcinoma and tumor-associated stromal cells. *Cancer Res.* **63:** 8827.

Shah M., Foreman D.M., and Ferguson M.W. 1995. Neutralisation of TGF-beta 1 and TGF-beta 2 or exogenous addition of TGF-beta 3 to cutaneous rat wounds reduces scarring. *J. Cell Sci.* **108:** 985.

Shimura T., Hagihara M., Takebe K., Munkhbat B., Ogoshi K., Mitomi T., Nagamachi Y., and Tsuji K. 1995. 10.5-kb homozygote of tumor necrosis factor-beta gene is associated with a better prognosis in gastric cancer patients. *Cancer* (suppl. 6) **75:** 1450.

Sieweke M.H. and Bissell M.J. 1994. The tumor-promoting effect of wounding: A possible role for TGF-beta-induced stromal alterations. *Crit. Rev. Oncog.* **5:** 297.

Sieweke M.H., Thompson N.L., Sporn M.B., and Bissell M.J. 1990. Mediation of wound-related Rous sarcoma virus tumorigenesis by TGF-beta. *Science* **248:** 1656.

Spemann H. 1918. Uber die Determination der ersten Organanlagen des Amphibienembryo. *Wilhelm Roux Arch. Entwicklungsmech. Org.* **43:** 448.

Spemann H. and Mangold H. 1924. Induction of embryonic primordia by implantation of organizers from a different species. In *Foundations of experimental embryology* (ed. B.H. Willier and J.M. Oppenheimer), p. 144. Hafner, New York.

Sternlicht M.D. and Werb Z. 2001. How matrix metalloproteinases regulate cell behavior. *Annu. Rev. Cell Dev. Biol.* **17:** 463.

Sternlicht M.D., Lochter A., Sympson C.J., Huey B., Rougier J.P., Gray J.W., Pinkel D., Bissell M.J., and Werb Z. 1999. The stromal proteinase MMP3/stromelysin-1 promotes mammary carcinogenesis. *Cell* **98:** 137.

Stoker A.W., Hatier C., and Bissell M.J. 1990a. The embryonic environment strongly attenuates v-src oncogenesis in mesenchymal and epithelial tissues, but not in endothelia. *J. Cell Biol.* **111:** 217.

Stoker A.W., Streuli C.H., Martins-Green M., and Bissell M.J. 1990b. Designer microenvironments for the analysis of cell and tissue function. *Curr. Opin. Cell Biol.* **2:** 864.

Streuli C.H., Bailey N., and Bissell M.J. 1991. Control of mammary epithelial differentiation: Basement membrane induces tissue-specific gene expression in the absence of cell-cell interaction and morphological polarity. *J. Cell Biol.* **115:** 1383.

Streuli C.H., Schmidhauser C., Kobrin M., Bissell M.J., and Derynck R. 1993. Extracellular matrix regulates expression of the TGF-beta 1 gene. *J. Cell Biol.* **120:** 253.

Streuli C.H., Schmidhauser C., Bailey N., Yurchenco P., Skubitz A.P., Roskelley C., and Bissell M.J. 1995. Laminin mediates tissue-specific gene expression in mammary epithelia. *J. Cell Biol.* **129:** 591.

Sympson C.J., Talhouk R.S., Alexander C.M., Chin J.R., Clift S.M., Bissell M.J., and Werb Z. 1994. Targeted expression of stromelysin-1 in mammary gland provides evidence for a role of proteinases in branching morphogenesis and the requirement for an intact basement membrane for tissue-specific gene expression. *J. Cell Biol.* **125:** 681.

Thiery J.P. 2002. Epithelial-mesenchymal transitions in tumour progression. *Nat. Rev. Cancer* **2:** 442.

Tuhkanen H., Anttila M., Kosma V.M., Yla-Herttuala S., Heinonen S., Kuronen A., Juhola M., Tammi R., Tammi M., and Mannermaa A. 2004. Genetic alterations in the peritumoral stromal cells of malignant and borderline epithelial ovarian tumors as indicated by allelic imbalance on chromosome 3p. *Int. J. Cancer* **109:** 247.

Virchow R. 1863. Aetologie der neoplastichen Geschwulste/ Pathogenie der neoplastischen Geschwulste. In *Die Krankenhaften Geschwulste*, p. 58. Verlag von August Hirchwald, Berlin, Germany.

Wahl G.M., Padgett R.A., and Stark G.R. 1979. Gene amplification causes overproduction of the first three enzymes of UMP synthesis in N-(phosphonacetyl)-L-aspartate-resistant hamster cells. *J. Biol. Chem.* **254:** 8679.

Waite K.A. and Eng C. 2003. From developmental disorder to heritable cancer: It's all in the BMP/TGF-beta family. *Nat. Rev. Genet.* **4:** 763.

Wang F., Weaver V.M., Petersen O.W., Larabell C.A., Dedhar S., Briand P., Lupu R., and Bissell M.J. 1998. Reciprocal interactions between β1-integrin and epidermal growth factor receptor in three-dimensional basement membrane breast cultures: A different perspective in epithelial biology. *Proc. Natl. Acad. Sci.* **95:** 14821.

Warzocha K., Ribeiro P., Bienvenu J., Roy P., Charlot C., Rigal D., Coiffier B., and Salles G. 1998. Genetic polymorphisms in the tumor necrosis factor locus influence non-Hodgkin's lymphoma outcome. *Blood* **91:** 3574.

Weaver V.M., Petersen O.W., Wang F., Larabell C.A., Briand P., Damsky C., and Bissell M.J. 1997. Reversion of the malignant phenotype of human breast cells in three-dimensional culture and in vivo by integrin blocking antibodies. *J. Cell Biol.* **137:** 231.

Weaver V.M., Lelievre S., Lakins J.N., Chrenek M.A., Jones J.C., Giancotti F., Werb Z., and Bissell M.J. 2002. β4 Integrin-dependent formation of polarized three-dimensional architecture confers resistance to apoptosis in normal and malignant mammary epithelium. *Cancer Cell* **2:** 205.

Weber F., Fukino K., Sawada T., Williams N., Sweet K., Brena R.M., Plass C., Caldes T., Mutter G.L., Villalona-Calero M.A., and Eng C. 2005. Variability in organ-specific EGFR mutational spectra in tumour epithelium and stroma may be the biological basis for differential responses to tyrosine kinase inhibitors. *Br. J. Cancer* **92:** 1922.

Werner E. and Werb Z. 2002. Integrins engage mitochondrial function for signal transduction by a mechanism dependent on Rho GTPases. *J. Cell Biol.* **158:** 357.

Wernert N., Locherbach C., Wellmann A., Behrens P., and Hugel A. 2001. Presence of genetic alterations in microdissected stroma of human colon and breast cancers. *Anticancer Res.* **21:** 2259.

Ye S., Dhillon S., Turner S.J., Bateman A.C., Theaker J.M., Pickering R.M., Day I., and Howell W.M. 2001. Invasiveness of cutaneous malignant melanoma is influenced by matrix metalloproteinase 1 gene polymorphism. *Cancer Res.* **61:** 1296.

Yu J., McMahon A.P., and Valerius M.T. 2004. Recent genetic studies of mouse kidney development. *Curr. Opin. Genet. Dev.* **14:** 550.

How Do Cancer Cells Acquire the Fuel Needed to Support Cell Growth?

C.B. Thompson, D.E. Bauer, J.J. Lum, G. Hatzivassiliou, W.-X. Zong, D. Ditsworth, F. Zhao, M. Buzzai, and T. Lindsten

Abramson Family Cancer Research Institute, Department of Cancer Biology and Department of Medicine, University of Pennsylvania, Philadelphia, Pennsylvania 19104

In this paper we consider whether the dependency of metazoan cells on extracellular signals to maintain cell survival results in an important barrier that must be overcome during carcinogenesis. It is now generally accepted that a major barrier to cancer comes from the inability of cells to enter and progress through the cell cycle in a cell-autonomous fashion. Most of the oncogenes studied over the last two decades contribute to the ability of the cancer cell to enter and progress through the cell cycle in the absence of the instructional signals normally imparted by extracellular growth factors. Over the last two decades, it has begun to be appreciated that there is a second potential barrier to transformation. It appears that all cells in multicellular organisms need extracellular signals not only to initiate proliferation, but also to maintain cell survival. Every cell in our body expresses the proteins necessary to execute its own death by apoptosis. A cell will activate this apoptotic program by default unless it receives signals from the extracellular environment that allow the cell to suppress the apoptotic machinery it expresses. It now appears that the molecular basis of this suppression lies in the signaling pathways that regulate cellular nutrient uptake and direct the metabolic fate of those nutrients.

METAZOAN CELLS LACK THE CELL AUTONOMOUS ABILITY TO TAKE UP NUTRIENTS

Over the last decade, we have been studying the dependency of cells on lineage-specific growth factors. Although this paper focuses on hematopoietic cells, additional data suggest that the findings are equally true of neuronal cells, epithelial cells, and fibroblasts. In all of these cells, the lineage-specific receptors that promote cell survival regulate the ability of the cell to express the transporters needed to take up nutrients from the extracellular environment. Every cell in the human body has an adequate supply of extracellular nutrients to maintain its survival. However, it appears that the cells in multicellular organisms lack the cell-autonomous ability to take up nutrients from the extracellular space. For example, glucose uptake depends on signal transduction that directs the cell to produce glucose transporters, hexokinase, and phosphofructokinase (Vander Heiden et al. 2001). These proteins are required to maintain the supply of glucose utilized by the glycolytic pathway to produce substrates for mitochondrial oxidative phosphorylation. When a cell is deprived of survival signals, the ability of the cell to take up, capture, and metabolize sufficient nutrients to maintain ATP production disappears. In every cell lineage in which this experiment has been done, after 48–96 hours in the absence of the signal transduction that maintains nutrient uptake and metabolism, the cell initiates apoptosis. This apoptotic response depends on the activity of the proapoptotic Bcl-2-related proteins, Bax and Bak (see, e.g., Lindsten et al. 2000).

Bcl-2 PROTEINS REGULATE THE DURATION OF CELL SURVIVAL FOLLOWING GROWTH FACTOR WITHDRAWAL

The first question we have addressed concerns the role of antiapoptotic Bcl-2 proteins in maintaining cell survival following growth factor withdrawal. Surprisingly, we found that Bcl-2 proteins play no role in regulating nutrient uptake. Cells overexpressing antiapoptotic Bcl-2 family members such as Bcl-2 and Bcl-x_L still need survival signal transduction to maintain nutrient transporters. For example, interleukin-3 (IL-3)-dependent cells deprived of IL-3 lose the ability to express both glucose and amino acid transporters. Despite this, antiapoptotic Bcl-2 proteins can keep the cell alive several weeks in the absence of nutrient transporter expression (Rathmell et al. 2000).

Alternative explanations for the decline of nutrient transporters following growth factor withdrawal have been suggested. For example, it could be that the decline in transporters results simply from the cell withdrawing from the cell cycle and no longer requiring a high level of nutrients to support growth. This concept would suggest that changes in nutrient transporter expression are a compensatory response to withdrawal from the cell cycle. In this view, survival receptors regulate cell survival through altering the expression/function of Bcl-2 family members. If Bax and Bak are in excess, apoptosis is initiated by cytochrome c release into the cytosol and activation of caspase 9. If Bcl-2 or other antiapoptotic family members dominate, the cell can survive for a long period of time.

GROWTH FACTOR REGULATION OF CELL SURVIVAL DOES NOT DEPEND ON APOPTOSIS

Cells need a constant supply of energy to maintain themselves even in the absence of growth. Cells need ATP just to "maintain the pumps"—to exclude sodium or to sequester calcium. If a cell cannot take up effective amounts of nutrients from its environment, it will ultimately die a bioenergetic death independent of apoptosis. To test this prediction, we engineered mice that were deficient in Bax and Bak. Bax/Bak-deficient animals have a variety of developmental defects, but a few make it into adulthood, and they have been widely reported (Lindsten et al. 2003). From these mice we have derived cell lines that have allowed us to take our initial experiments one step farther. We have made a variety of cell lines: neural progenitor cell lines, IL-3-dependent hematopoietic cells, and 3T3 fibroblasts (Lindsten et al. 2003; Zong et al. 2004; Lum et al. 2005). All of these cell lines share the property that stress-inducing apoptotic initiators no longer lead to rapid cell death. Thus, Bax and Bak are essential for initiating the apoptotic fate of the cell in response to stress. For example, the apoptotic initiator staurosporine can induce both wild-type cells and p53-deficient cells to die. In contrast, Bax/Bak-deficient cells survive the drug treatment and recover after the drug is removed. If the cells are treated with a chemotherapeutic agent such as etoposide, a topoisomerase inhibitor, a similar result is observed. Normal cells die in a dose- and time-dependent fashion, whereas survival of Bax/Bak-deficient cells is unaffected. Next, we tested the growth factor dependence of these cells: the fibroblasts for serum dependency, the neural progenitor cells for FGF, and the hematopoietic progenitors for IL-3. The IL-3 results have recently been published (Lum et al. 2005). Just as in other

IL-3-dependent cell lines, IL-3 regulates the ability of Bax$^{-/-}$Bak$^{-/-}$ cells to express glucose transporters and catabolize glucose to provide mitochondrial substrates for ATP production. When the cells are deprived of IL-3, the transporters are lost. Thus, cells must catabolize intracellular substrates to maintain ATP production. The IL-3-deprived cells essentially degrade themselves through the process of macroautophagy. As long as a cell can generate metabolites from its intracellular contents to maintain mitochondrial ATP production, the cell survives. Autophagy can keep a cell alive in complete medium for several weeks. After that there is nothing left to catabolize intracellularly, and the cell dies by necrosis. What this suggests is that antiapoptotic Bcl-2 proteins affect the time it takes from the loss of signaling information to the loss of cell viability, but they do not promote cell-autonomous survival. Although activation of proapoptotic family members initiates a more rapid death by apoptosis and the antiapoptotic proteins promote autophagy and longer survival, ultimately, growth-factor-deprived cells still die (Fig. 1).

AUTOPHAGY CAN MAINTAIN TRANSIENT GROWTH FACTOR-INDEPENDENT SURVIVAL

There has recently been a great deal of controversy concerning the role of autophagy in regulating cell survival. Autophagy is a process in which cells sense that they are bioenergetically compromised and initiate the formation of new double membrane vesicles that sequester off regions of the cytosol. These vesicles isolate a region of the cytosol along with its complement of organelles and deliver the contents to the lysosome. Following fusion, the lysosomal degradative enzymes break

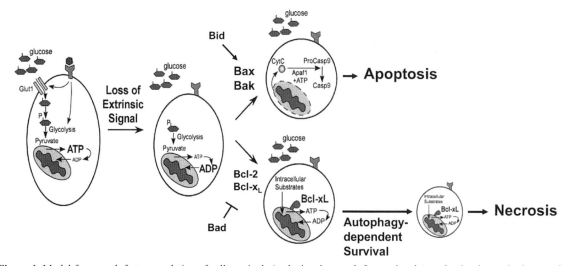

Figure 1. Model for growth factor regulation of cell survival. As depicted, growth factor signal transduction is required to regulate the expression and function of nutrient transporters by which cells take up nutrients needed to maintain ATP production. Loss of growth factor signaling leads inexorably to cell death, unless growth factor-induced nutrient uptake is reestablished. Apoptosis provides a rapid and efficient elimination of unwanted or neglected cells following growth factor deprivation. In the absence of apoptosis, growth-factor-deprived cells persist for several weeks by maintaining their bioenergetics through autophagy. Ultimately, autophagy is a self-limited process and the cells die by necrosis.

the cytosolic and organellar contents into substrates that the mitochondria can utilize to maintain ATP production. Autophagy has been best characterized in yeast and plants, where this process is more easily characterized because there is no apoptosis to complicate the study of the process. The MAP protein, LC3, can be used to identify and study newly forming autophagic vacuoles. Using this marker, we have studied primary IL-3-dependent bone marrow cells out of a Bax/Bak-deficient animal that were subjected to IL-3 withdrawal. In the presence of IL-3, LC3 is diffusely expressed in the cytosol. However, 48 hours after IL-3 depletion, LC3 undergoes redistribution to newly formed autophagic vacuoles. The role of autophagy in maintaining cellular bioenergetics was demonstrated by using either 3-methyladenine or chloroquine to inhibit the degradative process that is initiated by autophagy. In the presence of IL-3, neither of these drugs has any effect on the viability of the bone marrow cells. Viability remains high in IL-3-deprived cells until they are treated with either of the autophagy inhibitors. In the presence of either drug, the IL-3-deprived cells undergo cell death, and only 30% are viable after 24 hours. Over the next 24 hours, the rest of these cells die. The suppression of autophagy kills IL-3-deprived Bax/Bak-deficient cells. This death results from the bioenergetic compromise of the cells, as cell death can be completely reversed by addition of a cell-permeant metabolite, methyl pyruvate, that mitochondria can degrade to produce ATP (Fig. 2).

Autophagy-dependent survival is by its very nature a self-limited survival strategy. Autophagy-dependent cells begin to die several weeks after growth factor deprivation. At the end of this time, the cells appear to be filled with residual autophagolysosomes. These vesicles are filled with degradative debris. Although morphologically the cells look horrible, they retain two properties that suggest they may represent a meaningful biological intermediate in the lineage homeostasis of adult animals. The first is that the cells are capable of moving in response to chemokine signals that normally recruit these progenitor cells to hematopoietic stem cell niches. Even though the cells have undergone profound self-catabolism, they are able to use their remaining energy to move to a chemokine gradient. Hematopoietic progenitors are recruited to hematopoietic niches in the bone marrow by chemokines such as SDF-1. Hematopoietic progenitor cells grown in the presence of IL-3 will respond in a transwell assay to 100 ng/ml of SDF, with essentially all of the cells migrating toward the chemokine gradient. However, the IL-3-deprived cells are even more sensitive and more active to chemokine gradients. It takes one log less chemokine to induce them to migrate. We interpret this to mean that the cells are using their residual energy to find a site with the trophic signals they need to sustain survival.

The one additional signal the cells are capable of responding to is IL-3. IL-3 readdition allows the cells to fully recover glycolysis within 20 hours. Despite the rapid recovery of glycolysis, the cells do not recover the ability to proliferate for a week. In the first 24 hours, the cells recover their ability to take up and metabolize nutrients; they then recover the ability to grow and increase in size over the next 6 days. When the cells reach a size threshold of 700 femtoliters, they are able to resume pro-

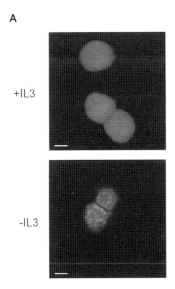

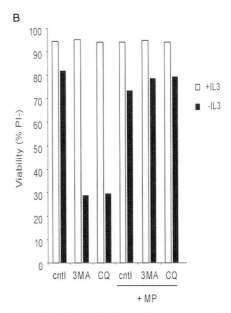

Figure 2. Autophagy maintains the survival of growth-factor-deprived cells. (*A*) Primary bone marrow cells derived from Bax$^{-/-}$Bak$^{-/-}$ mice are placed into culture in the presence of IL-3. Under these conditions, the autophagy marker LC3 exhibits a diffuse cytosolic distribution (*upper panel*). When IL-3 is withdrawn for 48 hours (*lower panel*), LC3 redistributes to newly formed autophagic vesicles. (*B*) Autophagy inhibitors 3-methyladenine (3MA) and chloroquine (CQ) inhibit the survival of growth-factor-deprived Bax$^{-/-}$Bak$^{-/-}$ primary bone marrow cells. Growth-factor-deprived cells, in which autophagy is inhibited by 3MA or CQ, can be rescued from cell death by the addition of a cell-permeant metabolite, methyl pyruvate (MP).

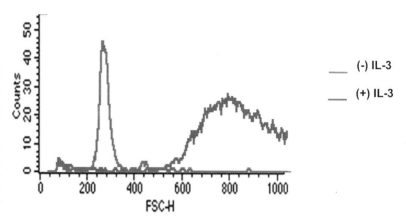

Figure 3. Growth-factor-deprived cells undergo reversible atrophy. Bax$^{-/-}$Bak$^{-/-}$ IL-3-dependent cells were deprived of IL-3. The cells atrophy from 700 femtoliters to ~300 femtoliters in size over the next several weeks. Under these conditions, bioenergetics is maintained by autophagy (–IL-3). Despite this profound autophagy-induced atrophy, cells are able to fully recover following IL-3 readdition. Six days following IL-3 readdition (+IL-3), the cells have recovered their cell volume and reinitiated cell proliferation.

liferation. Upon IL-3 readdition, virtually every cell in the culture increases in size and recovers its ability to engage in exponential growth (Fig. 3).

GROWTH FACTOR SIGNALING PATHWAYS REGULATE NUTRIENT UPTAKE AND METABOLISM

The above results demonstrate that hematopoietic cells lack the ability to maintain sufficient nutrient uptake to maintain cell survival in the absence of instructional signals. This suggests that these cells have two barriers to overcome in order to proliferate in a cell-autonomous fashion. The first is the cell's dependence on growth factor signals to activate the genes needed to enter and progress through the cell cycle. The second is the cell's dependence on survival signals to take up and utilize the nutrients needed to fuel this growth process. A substantial increase in a cell's production of ATP and uptake of

macromolecular precursors is required to support net cell growth.

The major pathway that regulates nutrient uptake in all lineages tested so far is the PI3K/Akt/TOR pathway, which is negatively regulated by the tumor suppressors PTEN, Tsc-1, and Tsc-2 (Bauer et al. 2004). The primary effect of Akt in cellular transformation is to constitutively activate glucose uptake and metabolism. For example, expression of an activated Akt under a doxycyclin promoter in a cell line that lacks constitutive Akt activity leads the cell to increase glycolysis without any significant effect on cell proliferation. The enhanced glycolysis is a specific effect of Akt. There is no generalized increase in metabolism. If anything, the rate of oxidative phosphorylation goes down in response to Akt stimulation of glycolysis. Because Akt transformation does not stimulate increased proliferation, all of the excess carbon taken up as glucose under the direction of activated Akt is secreted into the supernatant as lactate (Fig. 4).

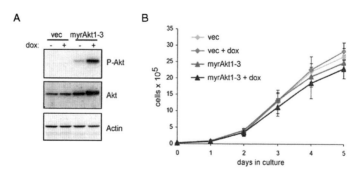

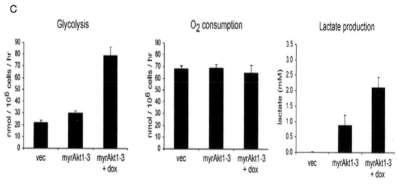

Figure 4. Constitutively active Akt stimulates glycolysis. (*A*) A continuously growing cell line was transfected with a doxycyclin-regulated form of activated Akt (myrAkt1-3). (*B*) Expression of activated Akt does not enhance the growth of the cell line in culture. (*C*) Akt stimulates glycolysis in a dose-dependent fashion, without a commensurate increase in the rate of oxidative phosphorylation. Because Akt stimulation of glycolysis does not result in enhanced cell growth, the excess carbon taken up is secreted into the medium as lactate.

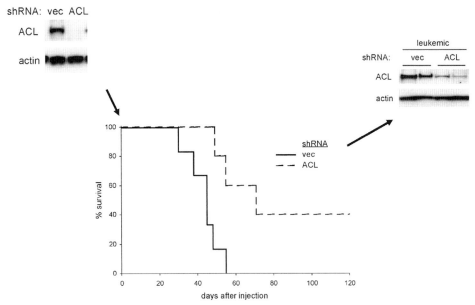

Figure 5. ACL activity is required for cell growth. An Akt-dependent leukemia cell line is stably transfected with an shRNA that suppresses ATP citrate lyase (ACL) (*upper left panel*). Cells exhibiting ACL suppression demonstrated a loss of tumorigenicity when reintroduced in vivo (*middle panel*). Western blot of proteins from the tumors that arise in animals receiving tumors stably transfected with ACL shRNA show recovery of ACL expression (*upper right panel*).

GROWING CELLS RELY ON GLUCOSE-DEPENDENT METABOLISM TO MAINTAIN ATP PRODUCTION AND LIPID BIOSYNTHESIS

Converting to a glucose-dependent form of metabolism is adaptive during cell growth because this conversion allows cells to divert all the amino acids and lipid precursors that they are able to take up into membrane and protein synthesis. The conversion to a glucose-dependent metabolism provides a clear growth advantage in terms of lipid biology. Growing cells do not take up sufficient lipids from their environment to support membrane biosynthesis. Instead they synthesize many of the lipids they need for growth from cytosolic acetyl-CoA. Just as cells use amino acids to produce the new proteins they need, the cells build their own lipids from acetyl-CoA. The ability to engage in net lipid synthesis depends on a novel glucose-dependent metabolic cycle. This mitochondrial-cytosolic cycle turns pyruvate into mitochondrial NADH to maintain electron transport and cytosolic acetyl-CoA that is used for lipid synthesis. During growth, geranylgeranyl and farnesyl groups, membrane phospholipids, and sphingomyelin are all produced in the cytosol from acetyl-CoA. A key Akt-regulated enzyme in this pathway is ATP-citrate lyase (ACL), a direct phosphorylation target of Akt (Bauer et al. 2005). ACL activation appears to play a critical role in Akt-mediated tumorigenesis. We have generated Akt-dependent lymphoma cell lines. When we suppressed ACL in these cell lines by shRNA, the cell lines lost their tumorigenicity (Fig. 5). The few tumors that do arise in the animals no longer display ACL suppression. This suggests that key enzymes associated with metabolic pathways unique to

cell growth may represent potential targets for the treatment of cancer. It is an idea we are just beginning to explore.

ACKNOWLEDGMENTS

The authors thank members of the Thompson laboratory for critical insights and suggestions. We also acknowledge the excellent secretarial assistance of J. Joh and S. Kerns. J.J.L. is supported by a fellowship from the Leukemia and Lymphoma Society. G.H. is supported by a Fellowship Award from the Damon Runyon Foundation. W.X.Z. is supported by a National Cancer Institute Howard Temin Mentored Research Scientist Development Award (KO1). Funding for C.B.T. was provided in part by grants from the NCI and the National Institutes of Health.

REFERENCES

Bauer D.E., Hatzivassiliou G., Zhao F., Andreadis C., and Thompson C.B. 2005. ATP citrate lyase is an important component of cell growth and transformation. *Oncogene* **24:** 6314.

Bauer D.E., Harris M.H., Plas D.R., Lum J.J., Hammerman P.S., Rathmell J.C., Riley J.L., and Thompson C.B. 2004. Cytokine stimulation of aerobic glycolysis in hematopoietic cells exceeds proliferative demand. *FASEB J.* **18:** 1303.

Lindsten T., Golden J.A., Zong W.-X., Minarcik J., Harris M.H., and Thompson C.B. 2003. The proapoptotic activities of Bax and Bak limit the size of the neural stem cell pool. *J. Neurosci.* **23:** 11112.

Lindsten T., Ross A.J., King A., Zong W.-X., Rathmell J.C., Shiels H.A., Ulrich E., Waymire K.G., Mahar P., Frauwirth K., Chen Y., Wei M., Eng V.M., Adelman D.M., Simon M.C., Ma A., Golden J.A., Evan G., Korsmeyer S.J., MacGregor G.R., and Thompson C.B. 2000. The combined functions of proapoptotic Bcl-2 family members Bak and Bax are essential for normal development of multiple tissues. *Mol. Cell* **6:** 1389.

Lum J.J., Bauer D.E., Kong M., Harris M.H., Li C., Lindsten T., and Thompson C.B. 2005. Growth factor regulation of autophagy and cell survival in the absence of apoptosis. *Cell* **120:** 237.

Rathmell J.C., Vander Heiden M.G., Harris M.H., Frauwirth K.A., and Thompson C.B. 2000. In the absence of extrinsic signals, nutrient utilization by lymphocytes is insufficient to maintain either cell size or viability. *Mol. Cell* **6:** 683.

Vander Heiden M.G., Plas D.R., Rathmell J.C., Fox C.J., Harris M.H., and Thompson C.B. 2001. Growth factors can influence cell growth and survival through effects on glucose metabolism. *Mol. Cell. Biol.* **21:** 5899.

Zong W.-X., Ditsworth D., Bauer D.E., Wang Z.-Q., and Thompson C.B. 2004. Alkylating DNA damage stimulates a regulated form of necrotic cell death. *Genes Dev.* **18:** 1272.

Mitochondria and Cancer: Warburg Addressed

D.C. WALLACE

Center for Molecular and Mitochondrial Medicine and Genetics (MAMMAG),
Departments of Biological Chemistry, Ecology and Evolutionary Biology, and Pediatrics,
University of California at Irvine, Irvine, California 92697-3940

Otto Warburg recognized that cancer cells generate excessive lactate in the presence of oxygen (aerobic glycolysis). It now appears that this phenomenon is the product of two factors: a return to the more glycolytic metabolism of the embryo and alterations in oxidative phosphorylation (OXPHOS) to increase mitochondrial reactive oxygen species (ROS) production. Alterations in the *Ras*-PI3K-*Akt* signal transduction pathway can result in induction of hexokinase II and its attachment to mitochondrial porin redirecting mitochondrial ATP to phosphorylate glucose and drive glycolysis. Furthermore, partial inhibition of OXPHOS by mitochondrial gene mutations (germ-line or somatic) can reduce electron flux through the electron transport chain, increasing mitochondrial ROS production. The increased ROS mutagenizes nuclear proto-oncogenes (initiation) and drives nuclear replication (promotion), resulting in cancer. Therefore, hexokinase II and mitochondrial ROS may be useful alternate targets for cancer therapeutics.

More than 70 years ago, Otto Warburg hypothesized that cancer might be caused by defects in the mitochondrion (Warburg 1931). This hypothesis was based on his observation that cancer cells actively metabolize glucose and produce excessive lactate while at the same time consuming oxygen via mitochondrial respiration. This was surprising, since most cells exhibit the "Pasteur Effect," in which glucose consumption is reduced when oxygen is available for the mitochondrial production of ATP by oxidative phosphorylation (OXPHOS) (Gatenby and Gillies 2004). Warburg called this unusual phenomenon "aerobic glycolysis" and suggested that mitochondrial defects might be central to cancer cell biology.

Since Warburg's proposal, many investigators have attempted to determine what defect in mitochondrial OXPHOS could account for tumor cell "aerobic glycolysis" (Pedersen 1978). A variety of differences between cancer mitochondria and normal cell mitochondria have been identified, including a general down-regulation of mitochondrial number and OXPHOS enzymes in cancer cells (Pedersen 1978); the up-regulation of the mRNA levels for individual mitochondrial DNA (mtDNA)-encoded genes including ND5 (LaBiche et al. 1988, 1992) and COII (Glaichenhaus et al. 1986); and the inhibition of mitochondrial ATP hydrolysis after (but not before) the addition of uncoupler (Pedersen 1978).

None of these observations adequately explained aerobic glycolysis, however, nor suggested a mechanism by which mitochondrial dysfunction could cause cancer. Hence, by the end of the 1970s, efforts to identify changes in the mitochondria associated with cancer cells had declined.

In 1988, interest in the role of the mitochondria in disease was rekindled by the discovery that mtDNA mutations can cause age-related diseases (Holt et al. 1988; Wallace et al. 1988a,b; Shoffner et al. 1990). The study of mitochondrial diseases revealed that the role of the mitochondrion in the pathophysiology of diseases was much more complex than previously imagined. It encompasses not only energy production, but also reactive oxygen species (ROS) production, as well as the regulation of programmed cell death (apoptosis) via the mitochondrial permeability transition pore (mtPTP). It was soon discovered that the mtPTP integrated information about the decline of mitochondrial energy metabolism, increased oxidative stress, and Ca^{++} overload to determine whether the mitochondria were sufficiently impaired to justify the destruction of the cell in which they reside. This integration occurred because the mtPTP combined the pro- and anti-apoptotic members of the Bax and Bcl2 gene family; the mitochondrial outer membrane pore protein; porin (voltage-dependent ion channel or VDAC); the mitochondrial inner membrane adenine nucleotide translocator (ANT), which exchanges mitochondrial ATP for cytosolic ADP; cyclophilin D to sense calcium; and the benzodiazepine receptor. VDAC and the ANTs also form a channel for the direct export of the ATP produced in the mitochondrial matrix to the cytosol. Since there are multiple ANT isoforms, the isoform expressed is likely to affect the kinetics of ATP–ADP exchange and/or the modulation of the mtPTP to various pro- and anti-apoptotic effectors (Wallace 2005).

A major advance in understanding aerobic glycolysis came from studies on hepatoma cells relative to normal hepatic cells, specifically that transformation was associated with the increased expression of hexokinase II and the binding of hexokinase II to the mitochondria through VDAC (Bustamante and Pedersen 1977). Hexokinase II is a member of the hexokinase gene family, which consists of four isoforms: hexokinase I, II, III, and IV. Hexokinases I–III are 100-kD proteins and are the result of a duplication of the basic 50-kD enzyme unit seen in hexokinase IV, also known as glucokinase. Even though hexokinases I–III have duplicated components, only in hexokinase II are both of the duplicated segments catalytically active. Moreover, the K_m values for glucose of hexokinases I–III are very low ($K_m = 0.02$–0.03 mM), whereas that of hexokinase IV (glucokinase) is very high

(K_m = 5–8 mM) (Pedersen et al. 2002; Wallace 2005). Hence, expression of hexokinase II in the presence of excess ATP results in the rapid phosphorylation of glucose to glucose-6-phosphate (G6P), the commitment step for glycolysis.

In normal liver cells, glucokinase is actively expressed, whereas hexokinase II is not. However, in hepatomas, hexokinase II is strongly induced and glucokinase expression is reduced. Since hexokinase II has a strong affinity for VDAC, it can occupy the outer membrane pore through which mitochondrial ATP must escape after transport by ANT. Therefore, the hexokinase can trap mitochondrial ATP in its ATP-binding site, priming it to phosphorylate any glucose molecules that become available. The rapid processing of G6P through glycolysis generates excess pyruvate and NADH, which cannot be fully oxidized by the down-regulated cancer cell mitochondria. Consequently, the metabolites build up and are converted to lactate by lactate dehydrogenase. By this mechanism, the cancer cell generates ATP via glycolysis to buffer the effects of hypoxia associated with larger tumor masses.

Concurrent with the induction of hexokinase II, there is a change in the expression of the ANT isoforms, at least in some cell types (Torroni et al. 1990). This may optimize the flow of ATP through VDAC to hexokinase and modulate the sensitivity of the mtPTP. Moreover, since VDAC is part of the mtPTP, the binding of hexokinase II stabilizes the mtPTP and inhibits induction of apoptosis (Pedersen et al. 2002; Gatenby and Gillies 2004).

The induction of hexokinase II in cancer cells is the product of altered transcriptional control. Critical regions of the hexokinase II promoter are methylated in normal hepatocytes, keeping the gene off. However, as these regions become demethylated in hepatomas, gene expression is permitted (Goel et al. 2003). Once activated, the hexokinase II gene's expression can be regulated by glucose, hypoxia, cAMP, phorbol ester, mutated p53, insulin, and glucagon. However, it is most strongly induced by glucose, along with either hypoxia acting through hypoxia-inducible factor-1α (HIF-1α) or through cAMP acting by way of CREB, ATF1, and CREM. This regulation is accomplished through the hexokinase II promoter spanning nucleotides –4000 to +1 and including regulatory elements for Z-DNA, HIF/Ebox, C/EBP, AP1, Oct1, E2F, CCAAT, GRE, multiple GC regions, and a TATA box (Mathupala et al. 1997a,b, 2001; Pedersen et al. 2002; Lee and Pedersen 2003). Hence, the induction of hexokinase II in cancer cells would appear to be the product of derepression by demethylation together with transcriptional induction by glucose, hypoxia, and cAMP.

The binding of hexokinase II to mitochondrial VDAC has recently been shown to be mediated by the action of the *Akt* kinases, also known as protein kinase B (PKB). *Akt* is a serine/threonine kinase and was first described as a retroviral oncogene (Bellacosa et al. 1991). It is now apparent that there are three *Akt*/PKB kinases in mammals (Akt1/PKBα, Akt2/PKBβ, and Akt3/PKBγ). The Akt kinases are activated by the binding of phosphatidylinositol-3,4,5-triphosphate and phosphatidylinositol-3,4-biphosphate to the pleckstrin homology domain at the amino-terminal end of the *Akt* polypeptide. Phosphatidylinositol-3,4,5-triphosphate and phosphatidylinositol-3,4-biphosphate are, in turn, generated by phosphatidylinositol 3-kinase (PI3K) in response to signals from receptor and non-receptor tyrosine kinases via its regulatory subunit, p85. In addition, phosphatidylinositol phosphates are generated through the action of *Ras*, which binds directly to the catalytic p110α subunit of PI3K and activates it. Thus, the *Akt* kinases mediate the signals of a variety of oncogenes, and inhibiting *Akt* inhibits neoplastic transformation (Aoki et al. 1998; Testa and Bellacosa 2001; Brazil et al. 2004; Yanagihara et al. 2005). Activation of the *Akt* kinases promotes the binding of the hexokinases to mitochondrial VDAC. This, in turn, antagonizes the pro-apoptotic action of Bax and Bak (Gottlob et al. 2001; Birnbaum 2004; Majewski et al. 2004a,b). Therefore, during neoplastic transformation, hexokinase II expression restructures the metabolism of the cancer cell mitochondria and inhibits apoptosis.

Although the biology of hexokinase II explains the up-regulation of glycolysis in hypoxic cancer cells, it does not explain why glucose utilization is not down-regulated in cancer cells grown at high oxygen tension. This phenomenon still implies that mitochondrial function is compromised in the cancer cell.

Confirmation that defects in mitochondrial energy metabolism are associated with cancer have come from the discovery that certain chromosomal "oncogenes" are in fact nuclear DNA (nDNA)-encoded proteins involved in mitochondrial energy production. Mutations in the mitochondrial fumarate hydratase gene have been linked to uterine leiomyomas and renal cell carcinomas (Lehtonen et al. 2004), and mutations in three of the four subunits of succinate dehydrogenase (SDH, succinate:ubiquinone oxidoreductase, or OXPHOS complex II) have been linked to paraganglions. The pathophysiological mechanism by which defects in mitochondrial energy metabolism might contribute to cancer is suggested by the function of the various subunits in SDH. SDH (complex II) is assembled from four nDNA-encoded subunits, SDH A, B, C, and D. SDHA collects electrons from succinate in the tricarboxylic acid (TCA) cycle via a flavin adenine dinucleotide (FAD) and passes the electrons through the iron–sulfur components in SDHB to the cytochrome *b* (cytb) and coenzyme Q (CoQ) elements in SDHD and SDHC. This reduces the ubiquinone (CoQ) to ubisemiquinone with a first electron and then ubiquinol with a second. The reduced ubiquinol then transfers the electrons from complex II to complex III for further oxidation. Mutations in SDHB (Astuti et al. 2001; Vanharanta et al. 2004), SDHC (Baysal et al. 2000), and SDHD (Niemann and Muller 2000) all cause paraganglioma. However, mutations in SDHA cause the lethal pediatric neurodegenerative disease Leigh syndrome (Bourgeron et al. 1995), not paraganglioma. In *Caenorhabditis elegans*, inactivation of the cytb subunit of complex II (*mev-1* mutant) markedly increases mitochondrial ROS production in association with a reduction in life span (Ishii et al. 1998; Senoo-Matsuda et al. 2001). The reduced longevity of the *mev-1* mutation can be reversed by treatment with the catalytic antioxidant mimetic EUK134, a salen Mn complex (Melov et al. 2000). Thus, the *C. ele-*

gans studies implicate mitochondrial ROS production in the pathophysiology of paraganglions.

It follows that mutations in the SDHB, C, and D subunits would inhibit electron flow out of complex II, creating an excess of unpaired electrons within the complex which can then be passed directly to O_2 to generate $O_2^{.-}$, the first of the mitochondrially generated ROS. Mutations in SDHA, in contrast, would block the entry of electrons into complex II, keeping the internal electron carriers oxidized and ROS production minimized. However, the absence of electron entry into SDHA would deprive mitochondrial OXPHOS of reducing equivalents to generate ATP, resulting in neurodegenerative disease (Wallace 2005). Thus, mitochondrial ROS production may be the missing mitochondrial link to cancer, not the gross impairment of mitochondrial energy production.

MITOCHONDRIAL BIOENERGETICS

The mitochondria generate ROS as a toxic by-product of the OXPHOS production of cellular energy. Mitochondria generate energy for two main purposes: to synthesize ATP to energize work, and to produce heat that maintains body temperature. In OXPHOS, the calories (reducing equivalents) from the carbohydrates and fats of our diet are oxidized with the oxygen that we breathe via the electron transport chain (ETC). The ETC collects electrons from NADH and H^+ via complex I and from succinate by complex II and transfers each pair of electrons to reduce ubiquinone to ubiquinol. Ubiquinol then transfers the electrons to complex III (the bc_1 complex or ubiquinone:cytocrome *c* oxidoreductase), which in turn donates the electrons to cytochrome *c*, and then finally passes them to complex IV (cytochrome *c* oxidase, COX or reduced cytochrome *c*:oxygen oxidoreductase). Here, the two electrons are passed to an atom of oxygen to generate a molecule of water (or actually, four electrons are transferred to O_2 to give two H_2Os.) The energy that is released by the ETC is used to pump protons out across the mitochondrial inner membrane through complexes I, III, and IV. This creates an electrochemical gradient or capacitance ($\Delta P = \Delta \Psi + \Delta pH$) that is positive and acid on the outside and negative and alkaline on the inside. This capacitance is utilized by complex V (ATP synthase) to generate ATP via the flow of protons back into the matrix through a proton channel in the ATP synthase. The energy that is imparted to the ATP synthase via the proton flux causes the enzyme to condense bound ADP and phosphate (Pi) to generate ATP and to then release the ATP for export to the cytosol through the ANT.

The efficiency with which calories are converted to ATP is known as the coupling efficiency. Coupling efficacy is determined by the efficiency with which the ETC pumps protons out of the mitochondrial matrix and by the efficiency with which the ATP synthase converts this proton capacitance into ATP. The more tightly coupled the mitochondria, the greater the ATP produced per calorie oxidized. The more uncoupled the mitochondria, the less ATP synthesized and the more heat generated.

Mitochondrial OXPHOS produces most of the cellular ROS. This normally occurs because complexes I and III can donate an electron directly to O_2 to generate superoxide ($O_2^{.-}$). These electrons are presumably derived from the half-reduced ubisemiquinone. Superoxide is a potent oxidizing agent. However, the mitochondrial matrix contains a manganese superoxide dismutase (MnSOD) that rapidly dismutates two $O_2^{.-}$s into a hydrogen peroxide (H_2O_2). The H_2O_2 can then be converted to water by glutathione peroxidase (GPx1), but the rate of this reaction is limited by glutathione concentration. Consequently, H_2O_2 persists in the mitochondrial matrix, permitting it to diffuse out into the cytosol and the nucleus.

In the cytosol, H_2O_2 can be removed by the peroxisomal enzyme catalase. However, in the presence of reduced transition metals, H_2O_2 can acquire an additional electron, generating the most reactive oxygen compound, the hydroxyl radical ($^.OH$). The mitochondrial generation of ROS can be substantially enhanced by partially inhibiting electron flux through the ETC either by reducing the efficiency of one of the ETC complexes or by inhibition of the ATP synthase or the ANT, thus increasing ΔP to its maximum potential. Because complexes I, III, and IV cannot pump protons against a maximum ΔP, the ETC stalls. This results in increased electron density in the ETC carriers and increased $O_2^{.-}$. Mitochondrial ROS can then damage mitochondrial enzymes, lipids, and the mtDNA.

Chronically elevated oxidative stress, reduced ΔP, reduced adenine nucleotides, and increased matrix Ca^{++} can all initiate apoptosis by activation of the mtPTP. Within the mtPTP, the ANT serves as a key regulator of permeability transition in response to adenine nucleotide and Ca^{++} concentrations (Kokoszka et al. 2004). Hexokinase modulates the mtPTP's response to Bax and Bak by binding to VDAC (Gottlob et al. 2001; Birnbaum 2004; Majewski et al. 2004a,b). Activation of the mtPTP opens a channel through the mitochondrial inner membrane that short-circuits ΔP. This causes the mitochondria to swell and to release proteins stored in the mitochondrial intermembrane space into the cytosol. The released apoptotic proteins include cytochrome *c* (cytc), procaspase-9, apoptosis initiating factor (AIF), and endonuclease G. Cytocrome *c* binds to cytosolic Apaf-1, which then cleaves and activates procaspase-9. This initiates the digestion of cytosolic proteins by the caspase cascade. AIF and EndoG move to the nucleus and degrade the chromatin. As a consequence of these processes, a cell with the defective mitochondria is removed from the tissue by digestion from within, thus minimizing the inflammatory process (Wallace and Lott 2002).

MITOCHONDRIAL DNA VARIATION IN DISEASE AND CLIMATIC ADAPTATION

The mitochondrial genome consists of 37 mtDNA-encoded genes plus approximately 1500 nDNA-encoded chromosomal genes. The mtDNA genes include a 12S and 16S rRNA, 22 tRNAs, and 13 OXPHOS polypeptide subunits (Wallace and Lott 2002). The 13 mtDNA polypeptides encompass 7 (ND1, 2, 3, 4, 4L, 5, 6) of the 46 subunits of complex I, none of the 4 subunits of complex II, 1 (cytochrome *b*, cytb) of the 11 subunits of complex III, 3 (COI, II, III) of the 13 subunits of complex IV, and 2

(ATP6 and 8) of the 16 subunits of complex V. The mtDNA also contains an approximately 1000-nucleotide (nt) control region which encompasses the promoter for transcribing the G-rich heavy (H) strand (P_H) and the adjacent promoter to transcribe the C-rich light (L) strand (P_L), the intervening mitochondrial transcription factor (mtTFA) binding sites, three conserved sequence boxes (CSB I, II, and III), the origin of H-strand replication, and the termination-associated sequence (TAS). The replication of the mtDNA H-strand has been proposed to start at O_H using a cleaved transcript from P_H as the primer and pausing at TAS to create the 7S DNA, thus forming the triple-stranded displacement (D)-loop. The origin of L-strand replication is located 2/3 around the mtDNA circle.

The nDNA encodes the vast majority of the mitochondrial polypeptides including the mtDNA polymerase γ, the mtRNA polymerase, the mitochondrial ribosomal proteins, the enzymes of mitochondrial metabolism, etc. The genes for these proteins are replicated and transcribed in the nucleus, the mRNAs are translated into protein on cytosolic ribosomes, and the mitochondrial proteins are selectively imported into the mitochondrion using specific import peptide sequences (Wallace and Lott 2002).

Because it is outside the nucleus, the mtDNA has unique genetics. It is inherited exclusively from the mother and is present in thousands of copies per cell which are sequestered within hundreds of mitochondria. It also has a very high mutation rate due to its constant exposure to mitochondrial ROS.

Mutations in both the nDNA and mtDNA genes of the mitochondrial genome have been linked to human degenerative diseases. Pathogenic mtDNA base substitution mutations fall into two broad categories: protein synthesis gene (tRNA and rRNA) mutations and the polypeptide gene mutations (see mitomap.org). When a new mtDNA mutation arises in a cell, this creates a mixed intracellular population of mtDNAs (*heteroplasmy*). As the heteroplasmic cell divides, the mutant and normal molecules segregate randomly, ultimately generating pure mutant or wild-type cell lines (*homoplasmy*). As the percentage of mutant mtDNAs increases, the mitochondrial energetic capacity declines, ROS production increases, and the propensity for apoptosis increases.

The accumulation of ROS damage in the thousands of mtDNAs of the cell progressively inactivates the DNA templates necessary to repair damaged mitochondria. Thus, as mtDNA mutations accumulate, due to oxidative damage, mitochondrial function erodes until the cell dies by apoptosis. As a result, the accumulation of mtDNA mutations acts as the aging clock (Wallace 2005). It is this interaction between the partial defects resulting from inherited mitochondrial defects plus the accumulation of somatic mtDNA mutations that accounts for delayed onset and progressive course of mitochondria-associated diseases. The severity of disease is the product of the extent of the inherited mutation's effect on the mitochondrial function, the percentage of mutant mtDNAs in the tissues at birth, and the additional accumulation of somatic mtDNA mutations with aging (Wallace and Lott 2002; Wallace 2005).

Over tens of thousands of years, the high mtDNA mutation rate has also generated a high degree of mtDNA

single-nucleotide polymorphisms (SNPs) in indigenous populations around the world. The regional specificity of this variation is the result of two factors: (1) the sequential accumulation of mtDNA mutations along radiating female lineages as women moved into new geographical regions and (2) the selective enrichment of functional mutations that were adaptive to the new environments (Mishmar et al. 2003; Ruiz-Pesini et al. 2004; Wallace 2005). These two factors have generated region-specific branches of the mtDNA tree, frequently founded by one or more functional mutations. These regional groups of related mtDNA haplotypes are called haplogroups.

The greatest mtDNA diversity is found in Africa (Johnson et al. 1983; Cann et al. 1987; Merriwether et al. 1991; Mishmar et al. 2003), demonstrating that Africa was the origin of humans about 200,000 years before present (YBP). The most ancient African branches of the mtDNA tree are defined by the nt 3594T polymorphism found in African haplogroups L0, L1, and L2. Many L0–L2 haplotypes also harbor a tRNA^{Asp} variant at nt 7521A. African haplogroup L3, which diverged from L2 and L3 by the T3594C change, subsequently gave rise to haplogroups M and N, the only two lineages that left Africa to colonize all of Eurasia about 65,000 YBP. Macro-haplogroup N was founded by two missense mutations, one in ND3 at nt 10398A causing an A114T amino acid substitution and the other in ATP6 at nt 8701A resulting in an A59T amino acid change. In Europe, macro-haplogroup N gave rise to the European-specific haplogroups H, I, J, Uk, T, U, V, W, and X. These are also founded by distinctive functional polymorphism. For example, haplogroup U was found by the tRNA$^{Leu(CUN)}$ nt 12308G polymorphism, and haplogroup U was later subdivided by the appearance of a 16S rRNA variant at nt 1811G. Similarly, haplogroup J was founded by a reversion of the ND3 10398 back to G (T114A) and the appearance of a ND5 polymorphism at nt 13708A (A458T). Asia was colonized by derivatives of both macro-haplogroups M and N, which gave rise to a plethora of Asian haplogroups, including A, B, F, etc. from N; and C, D, G, etc. from M. Sublineages of Asian haplogroup A and D also acquired the 13708A variant in ND5, demonstrating the frequent convergent evolution that is seen among regional mtDNA variants.

Of all the mtDNA lineages in Central Asia, only three lineages (A, C, and D) became enriched in Northeastern Siberia by 20,000–30,000 years ago, and these were in a position to colonize the Americas when the Bering land bridge became exposed. Hence, the two striking discontinuities in mtDNA diversity occurred as humans migrated from Africa to the Americas, one between the enormous African mtDNA diversity and the colonization of Eurasia by only M and N and the second between the extensive M and N variation in temperate Asia and the colonization of arctic Siberia by only A, C, and D. The best explanation for these geographic discontinuities in mtDNA diversity is that selection has limited the mtDNAs that could move into the higher and colder northern latitudes (Wallace et al. 1999; Mishmar et al. 2003; Ruiz-Pesini et al. 2004; Wallace 2005).

Today, these ancient adaptive mtDNA variants are influencing individual predisposition to disease. For example, mtDNA variation that reduced the coupling efficiency and increased heat production permitted adaptation to cold but also reduced ATP production. The reduced ATP production now increases the individual's susceptibility to ATP deficiency diseases such as clinical depression and Leber's hereditary optic neuropathy (LHON) (Wallace 2005). However, these same uncoupling mutations also keep the ETC more oxidized, reducing ROS production, and thus are protective against age-related degenerative diseases and associated with increased longevity (Wallace 2005).

MITOCHONDRIAL PATHOPHYSIOLOGY OF AGING AND CANCER

The clinical implications of mtDNA variation are not confined to degenerative diseases and aging, but also influence cancer risk, which increases with age. In fact, aging and cancer must be physiologically linked since caloric restriction in rodents both increases life span and reduces cancer risk (Harrison and Archer 1987; Masoro et al. 1992; McCarter and Palmer 1992; Masoro 1993; Sohal et al. 1994). Because calories are the fuel of the mitochondrion, this implicates the mitochondria in both aging and cancer (Fig. 1).

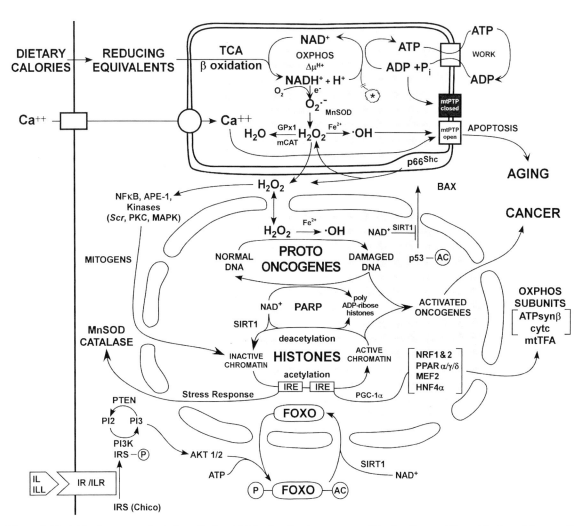

Figure 1. Model for the proposed role for mitochondrial dysfunction in an energy-utilization tissue cell in metabolic and degenerative diseases, aging, and cancer. The mitochondrial pathophysiology of these clinical entities is envisioned to result from the interplay between mitochondrial energy production, ROS generation, and the initiation of apoptosis through activation of the mtPTP. These components of energy metabolism are modulated by environmental constraints such as caloric availability and cold stress through the regulation of the FOXO and PGC-1α transcription factors and the SIRT1 NAD+-dependent deacetylase. The FOXO transcription factors coordinately regulate mitochondrial energy metabolism through PGC-1α as well as the antioxidant and stress response genes necessary to cope with the increased oxidative stress of oxidative metabolism. SIRT1 fine-tunes the interrelationship between energy metabolism and apoptosis through the deacetylation of PGC-1α, p53, and the histone proteins. Caloric overload or inhibition of OXPHOS perturbs the cellular mitochondrial energetic balance, resulting in increased ROS. The increased ROS and decreased mitochondrial energy output sensitize the mtPTP, ultimately driving the cell to apoptotic death. The increased ROS also diffuses into the nucleus as H_2O_2 where it can mutate and activate proto-oncogenes (initiation) and can interact with NF-κB, APE-1, and various kinases to initiate cell division (promotion) leading to neoplastic transformation (cancer). Abbreviations: (PARP) poly ADP-ribose polymerase; (SIRT1) mammalian homolog to Sir2; (FOXO3) the most ubiquitous mammalian forkhead transcription factor; (P) a phosphorylated protein; (Ac) an acetylated protein; (IL) insulin ligand; (ILL) insulin-like ligand; (IR) insulin receptor; (ILR) insulin-like growth factor receptor; (IRE) insulin response element; (PI3K) PI3 kinase; (PI2) membrane-bound phosphatidyl-inositol diphosphate; (PI3) membrane-bound phosphatidyl-inositol triphosphate; (AKT 1/2) the AKT kinases; (ATPsynβ) ATP synthase β subunit; (cytc) cytochrome c (Wallace 2005).

That the accumulation of mtDNA mutations causes aging has been established by introducing a mutator mtDNA polymerase γ into the mouse and showing that these animals age prematurely (Trifunovic et al. 2004; Kujoth et al. 2005). That the natural mtDNA mutagen is mitochondrial ROS has been demonstrated by introducing catalase into the mouse mitochondrial matrix and showing that these animals had an extended life span and reduced mtDNA damage (Schriner et al. 2005). If ROS damage to the mtDNA modulates life span, then it might also influence cancer risk. This possibility is supported by the increased risk of paragangliomas in patients with SDH B, C, or D mutations, by the observations that mice that are heterozygous for a null mutation in the MnSOD gene have greatly increased cancer risk (Van Remmen et al. 2003), that many tumors have reduced MnSOD, that transformation of certain tumors with the MnSOD cDNA reverses the malignant phenotype, and that a cluster of three mutations in the MnSOD gene promoter is found in a number of tumors (Xu et al. 1999; McCord 2000).

If increased mitochondrial ROS production increases cancer risk, then mtDNA mutations that partially inhibit electron transport and increase ROS production might also increase cancer risk. Therefore, both somatic and germline mtDNA mutations should be associated with cancer.

Early indications that cancer cells have alterations in their mtDNAs came from the observations that human leukemia leukocytes had dimeric mtDNAs (Clayton et al. 1970), that sequences of rat liver tumors had partial deletions in the mtDNA tRNA^{Tyr} and tRNA^{Trp} genes (Taira et al. 1983), and that restriction digests of tumor mtDNAs suggested heteroplasmy (Bianchi et al. 1995). However, the first clear evidence that a mtDNA mutation in a cancer cell might be functionally significant came from the report of a renal adenocarcinoma in which 50% of the mtDNAs contained a 294-nt in-frame deletion in the mtDNA ND1 gene which generated a truncated mRNA (Horton et al. 1996). A patient with such a mtDNA mutation would manifest severe mitochondrial disease. Hence, at least some tumor somatic mtDNA mutations must be functionally important.

Subsequently, many publications have reported tumor-specific mtDNA somatic mutations that are absent in the patient's normal tissue but present as somatic mutations in the tumor tissue (Chinnery et al. 2002; Copeland et al. 2002). Analysis of ten colon cancer cell lines revealed that seven (70%) harbored functional tumor-specific mtDNA-coding-region mutations including missense mutations in six lines and a chain termination and a frameshift mutation in the seventh. All of the mutations were homoplasmic except for the missense mutations in two of the cell lines (Alonso et al. 1997; Polyak et al. 1998; Habano et al. 1999). A survey of the mtDNAs of bladder, head and neck, and lung cancers revealed that 64% (9/14) of the bladder, 46% (6/13) of the head and neck, and 43% (6/14) of the lung cancers had tumor-specific mtDNA mutations. Of the 30 apparently functionally important cancer cell somatic mutations identified, 6 altered rRNA or tRNA genes, 4 affected polypeptides, and the remainder altered the control region (Fliss et al. 2000). A survey of mtDNA control region variation in

gastric tumors revealed that 48% (15/31) of the tumors harbored tumor-specific mutations (Wu et al. 2005). Analysis of the mtDNA control region from hepatocellular carcinomas revealed that 39% (24/61) harbored mutations in a Taiwan study (Lee et al. 2004), whereas 68% (13/19) had control region mutations in a Japanese study (Nomoto et al. 2002). Analysis of the mtDNAs in glioblastomas revealed predominately control region variation but also two coding region variants (Kirches et al. 2001), whereas a survey of neurofibromas from neurofibromatosis patients revealed only control region mutations (Kurtz et al. 2004). Analysis of mtDNA variation of thyroid tumors revealed control region somatic mutations in 49% (32/66) of tumors and coding region somatic mutations in 52% (34/66) of tumors in one study (Maximo et al. 2002). Another study found coding region mutants in 23% of 13 papillary thyroid carcinomas (Yeh et al. 2000). However, the thyroid tumors had a relatively low frequency of control region mutants in the hypervariable homopolymeric C region between nt 303 and nt 315 (Tong et al. 2003). Analysis of the complete mtDNA sequence in 10 ovarian tumors revealed both control region and coding region variants in 60% (6/10) of cases (Liu et al. 2001). Control region and coding region mutations were also observed in 61% (11/18) of breast cancer samples (Parrella et al. 2001). Finally, several studies of prostate cancer tumors have revealed somatic control region mutations (Chen et al. 2002, 2003) and control region and coding region mutations (Jeronimo et al. 2001). Three heteroplasmic COI mutations have also been reported in prostate tumors that were clearly functionally important: G5949A-G16X (Stop), T6124C-M74T (interspecific conservation index [CI] = 95%), C6924T-A341S (CI = 100%) (Petros et al. 2005). The importance of the somatic COI mutations is demonstrated by their higher average amino acid CI relative to all prostate cancer COI mutations (CI = 83 ± 25%) and to all COI variants found in the general European population (CI = 71 ± 35%). Moreover, mitochondrial proteomic studies have revealed an increase in the ratio of nDNA to mtDNA-encoded complex IV subunits in prostate cancer patients (Herrmann et al. 2003; Krieg et al. 2004), which could be explained by mtDNA mutations in the COI–III genes.

Collation of the somatic mtDNA mutations reported from these various tumor studies reveals some remarkable associations. One of the most common mtDNA sequence variants seen in the control region of tumor cells is variation in the number of C's in the homopolymer string of C's in the nt region 303–315 (Nomoto et al. 2002; Kurtz et al. 2004; Lee et al. 2004; Wu et al. 2005; Yoneyama et al. 2005). This is also a common variant in normal tissues (Torroni et al. 1994; Trounce et al. 1995). Moreover, the majority of the somatic control region mutations observed in cancer tissues, such as nts 73, 16189, and 16519, have also been reported to be polymorphisms in population studies (Yoneyama et al. 2005). The 16189 T to C variant is particularly intriguing, since it converts at T that disrupts a string of C's {CCCCCT^{16189}CCCC} to a C {CCCCCCCCCC}, thus encouraging slip mispairing and the destabilization of this region on the mtDNA. This same variant has been associated with increased risk for Type 2 diabetes mellitus (Poulton 1998; Poulton et al. 1998), dilated cardiomyopathy (Khogali et al. 2001), and endometrial cancer (Liu et al. 2003). Similarly, in one Taiwanese case of gastric cancer, the patient's tumor was found to be heteroplasmic for a 270-nt insertion between nt 309 and nt 568. This was associated with instability in the number of C's in a homopolymeric string starting at nt 568 (Wu et al. 2005). Interestingly, this same duplication was found to be a characteristic of European haplogroup I (Torroni et al. 1994) and has been implicated in predisposition to mtDNA rearrangements (Brockington et al. 1993). The presence of similar mtDNA control region mutations in tumors and populations raises the possibility that the mitochondria may be exposed to similar selective forces in both populations and tissues.

The concept of selection resulting in convergent mtDNA mutations in human populations and tumors has been further supported by comparing the functional mtDNA variants (rRNA plus tRNA and polypeptide) observed in cancer cells with those in human populations. Focusing on the tumor-specific mtDNA tRNA and rRNA gene mutations, a total of 19 mutations have been reported to be tumor-specific (present in tumors but not in normal tissue) in ovarian (Liu et al. 2001), bladder, head and neck (Fliss et al. 2000), colon (Polyak et al. 1998), thyroid (Yeh et al. 2000), and prostate (Jeronimo et al. 2001) cancer. Most of these somatic mutations are either homoplasmic or approaching homoplasmic in the tumors. Comparison of these "tumor-specific" tRNA and rRNA mutations with our global human mtDNA database of 2453 mtDNA coding region sequences (Brandon et al. 2006) revealed that 53% (10/19) of the somatic tumor mutations have been previously described as population variants (Mishmar et al. 2003; Ruiz-Pesini et al. 2004). For example, in one prostate tumor, a somatic tRNA$^{Leu(CUN)}$ mutation converted nt A12308G (Jeronimo et al. 2001). The 12308G allele defines the European mtDNA haplogroup U and is found in 262 of the 2453 mtDNAs in our collection. Similarly, a 16S rRNA variant found in the head and neck tumors converted nt A1811G (Fliss et al. 2000). The 16S rRNA 1811G allele subdivides haplogroup U and is present in 163/2453 mtDNAs. Finally, in a thyroid tumor, a tRNA^{Asp} mutation changes nt G7521A (Yeh et al. 2000). The 7521A allele is prevalent in African haplogroups L0–L2 and is present in 121/2453 mtDNAs. In contrast, the 7521G allele appears in African haplogroup L3 and is the primary allele in macro-haplogroups M and N (Brandon et al. 2006).

Similarly, multiple tumor mtDNA polypeptide gene variants have also been observed in population samples. Forty-seven functionally relevant somatic mtDNA polypeptide mutations have been reported for ovarian (Liu et al. 2001), glioblastoma (Kirches et al. 2001), bladder, head and neck (Fliss et al. 2000), colon (Polyak et al. 1998), thyroid (Yeh et al. 2000; Maximo et al. 2002), breast (Parrella et al. 2001), and prostate (Jeronimo et al. 2001; Chen et al. 2003) tumors. Five of these are rearrangements and can be excluded from the comparison. The remaining 42 are missense mutations of which 22 (52%) are also population polymorphisms (Brandon et al. 2006).

Some of the cancer somatic mutations are major mtDNA

population markers. For example, one thyroid tumor was reported to have a somatic mutation that changed A10398G (Yeh et al. 2000). Variation at this nucleotide delineates several of the most significant mtDNA lineages. The 10398G allele which determines that the ND3 codon 114 is an alanine (A) is the primary allele for African haplogroups L0–L3 and Asian macro-haplogroup M. However, at the root of macro-haplogroup N, this base changes to 10398A and the ND3 114 amino acid becomes threonine (T). Subsequently, in three sublineages of macro-haplogroup N, specifically European haplogroups J and Uk as well as a sublineage of Asian haplogroup B, the base returns to 10398 G and the ND3 amino acid back to A. Thus, in this thyroid tumor patient, the European A allele of the normal tissue is changed to the African G allele in the tumor tissue. The 10398G allele found in the tumor is present in 1072/2453 mtDNAs. Similarly, two independent thyroid tumor patients were reported to have a somatic A8701G mutation (Maximo et al. 2002). The 8701G allele (ATP6 codon 59A) is prevalent in Africa and in macro-haplogroup M mtDNAs. However, at the base of macro-haplogroup N, the base becomes 8701A and the ATP6 amino acid becomes 59T. Thus, in these thyroid tumor patients, the European 8701A allele in normal tissue is converted to the African 8701G allele in cancerous tissue. The 8701 G allele is found in 762/2453 mtDNAs. Finally, a breast cancer tumor was reported to have acquired a G13708A somatic mutation (Parrella et al. 2001). This variant has arisen several times in human radiation. The founding allele 13708G (ND5 codon 458A) is found in African L0–L3, Asian M, and at the base of Eurasian N mtDNAs. However, at the base of European haplogroup J and in important sublineages of the European X and Asian B haplogroups, the 13708 base changes to A and the associated ND5 amino acid 458 is changed to a T. The 13708A found in the tumor is seen in 209/2453 mtDNAs (Brandon et al. 2006).

One possibility is that these "tumor-specific mtDNA variants" are simply sequencing errors in the patient's tumor or normal mtDNA sample. However, this seems unlikely, since the control region mutations found in tumors also correlate with population variants, different high-frequency population variants have been reported in five independent studies, and the gel for the somatic nt 13708 variant in a breast cancer patient is published and is very convincing. In this breast cancer patient, the nucleotide variant is completely absent in both the peripheral blood sample and the adjacent normal tissue of the patient, but is strongly present in both the tumor tissue and a metastatic node of the same individual (Parrella et al. 2001; Brandon et al. 2006). Hence, we must conclude that at least some tumor mutations are the same as population polymorphisms. As a result, this implies that similar selective forces must be acting on the mtDNAs in both populations and transformed cells. This seems plausible, since in both circumstances the availability of substrates (calories and oxygen) for energy production, the effects of thermal stress, and the function and consequences of ROS production and apoptosis would be equally applicable.

The correlation of population-specific variants and tumor somatic mutations also suggests that individuals who inherit certain population variants might be more prone to cancer. This concept has been supported in two instances. The control region variant at 16189 T to C, which desta-bilizes the mtDNA control region, is associated with in-creased risk for endometrial cancer (Liu et al. 2003), and the 10398 allele has been found to increase the risk for in-vasive breast cancer in both premenopausal and post-menopausal African-American women over women with the 10398G allele. However, the 10398G allele did not in-crease breast cancer risk for Caucasian women (Canter et al. 2005). Interestingly, the 10398G allele is found in sub-Saharan African mtDNAs and in European haplogroup J mtDNAs (Brandon et al. 2006), and an A to G somatic mutation at nt 10398 was found in a patient with papillary thyroid carcinoma (Yeh et al. 2000).

To further investigate the role of germ-line mtDNA variants in cancer risk, we have surveyed the nature and frequency of mtDNA COI gene variants in European-American prostate cancer specimens. We chose to focus on the COI gene because preliminary studies had re-vealed that COI was hypervariable in prostate cancer samples (Petros et al. 2005), proteomic studies had re-ported an increase in the ratio of nDNA/mtDNA-encoded complex IV polypeptides in prostate cancer (Herrmann et al. 2003; Krieg et al. 2004), and haplogroup-specific polymorphisms in COI are rare in Europeans, minimizing background effects (Mishmar et al. 2003; Ruiz-Pesini et al. 2004). The mtDNA COI genes from 260 prostate can-cer specimens from North American patients of predomi-nantly Eurasian descent were sequenced along with blood samples from 54 prostate cancer negative men over age 50 whose PSA was < 1 and in which a prostate nee-dle biopsy was free of cancer cells. This analysis revealed that in European-Americans, COI mutations were found in 11% of the prostate cancer specimens and 0% of the prostate cancer negative controls. Furthermore, four prostate cancer COI mutations were found in multiple in-dependent patient tumors, often on different mtDNA backgrounds. The first mutation, nt T6253C, was found in three independent prostate cancer specimens, all hap-logroup H. This base substitution caused a M117T amino acid substitution (CI of 69%). The second mutation, nt C6340T, was found in six patients on haplogroups J, T, L1, and N and caused an A120T (CI of 97%). The third mutation, nt G6261A, was found in two cases with hap-logroups of H and N, converted amino acid T146I (CI of 79%). The final mutation, nt A6663G, was found in five cases on haplogroups O and L2 and changed amino acid I125V (CI of 95%). Thus, these data prove that germ-line mtDNA COI mutations can cause prostate cancer and thus are oncogenes (Petros et al. 2005).

Surprisingly, a survey of 898 random European mtDNA sequences revealed that 5.5% of the general pop-ulation also harbored COI variants. If COI mutations cause prostate cancer, why would they persist in the pop-ulation? The answer is that only men develop prostate can-cer, whereas only women transmit the mtDNA. Hence, the mutant mtDNAs are insulated against selection.

To demonstrate that mtDNA mutations can indeed be oncogenic, we substituted the mtDNAs of a prostate can-cer cell line, PC-3, with the mtDNAs from a mitochon-drial disease patient who was heteroplasmic for a known

pathogenic mtDNA mutation, T8993G (Holt et al. 1990). By isolating cytoplasmic hybrid (cybrid) cell lines that were homoplasmic for the mutant or wild-type mtDNAs, these cell lines could be used to transfer the two mtDNA genotypes into the presence of a prostate cancer cell nu-cleus, and the effects on tumorigenicity of the mutant and wild-type bases can be assessed. An ATP6 mutant was chosen because we had observed that the prostate tumor which harbored the somatic COI G16X chain termination mutation also harbored a homoplasmic germ-line ATP6 C8932T (P136G) variant with a CI of 64%. Hence, ATP6 mutations may also contribute to the prostate cancer risk of the patient.

The T8993G mutation causes a L156R amino acid change approximately 20 amino acids away from the C8932T mutation. Biochemical analysis of the wild-type T8993T versus the mutant T8993G mtDNA in cybrid lines has revealed that the homoplasmic mutation resulted in an approximately 70% reduction in ATP synthase (complex V) activity (Trounce et al. 1994). An indepen-dent study established that the T8993G mutation also in-creased mitochondrial ROS production (Mattiazzi et al. 2004). To transfer the T8993T and T8993G mtDNAs into the PC-3 cell line, we treated the PC-3 cells with the mi-tochondrial poison, rhodamine 6G (R6G), to destroy their resident mitochondria and mtDNAs. The homoplasmic T8993T or the homoplasmic T8993G cybrids were then enucleated, and cytoplasts were fused to the R6G-treated PC-3 cells (Trounce et al. 1996). The resulting PC-3 (mtDNA T8993T) and PC-3 (mtDNA T8993G) cybrids were then injected into nude mice. Analysis of multiple cybrid clones revealed that the PC-3 cells with the wild-type (T8993T) mtDNA barely grew in the nude mice, whereas the PC-3 cybrids with the mutant (T8993G) mtDNA grew rapidly and required that the animals be eu-thanized due to excessive tumor size. Therefore, we can conclude that mtDNA mutations can contribute substan-tially to tumorigenesis and that a single deleterious base change in the mtDNA can enhance malignant growth (Pet-ros et al. 2005).

To determine whether the increased tumorigenicity of the mutant (T8993G) mtDNA cybrids was due to increased ROS production, we stained the injected cell nodules from the nude mice for ROS production with dihydroethidium. This revealed that the mutant (T8993G) cell line tumors were producing excessive ROS whereas the wild-type T8993T mtDNA nodules were producing very little ROS (Petros et al. 2005). Thus, mitochondrial ROS production is again implicated in the transformation of cells.

A MITOCHONDRIAL PATHOPHYSIOLOGY OF CANCER

These observations suggest that the mitochondrial paradigm of aging and age-related diseases (Fig. 1) (Wal-lace 1992, 2005) can provide a coherent picture of the role of the mitochondria in cancer. Mitochondrial OX-PHOS chronically generates ROS as a toxic by-product. The relative level of ROS production is determined by the coupling efficiency of the individual's mitochondria, which is a consequence of his/her mtDNA and nDNA genotype, the dietary caloric load, and environmental agents that might inhibit mitochondrial energy production. Thus, individuals with cold-adapted, partially uncoupled mitochondria would produce less ROS in the presence of a relatively high caloric load than would individuals with more tightly coupled mitochondria adapted to a warmer climate.

The chronic OXPHOS generation of $O_2^{\cdot-}$ and $\cdot OH$ progressively damages mitochondrial OXPHOS enzymes, membranes, and the mtDNA. The mtDNA template is used to repair the protein damage, but this fails when the mtDNA information becomes corrupted. Excess mitochondrial H_2O_2 diffuses out of the mitochondrion and into the cytosol and the nucleus, where it interacts with mitogenic signal transduction pathways including NF-κB, APE-1, *Fos*, *Jun*, and tyrosine kinases (Src kinase, protein kinase C, MAPK, and receptor tyrosine kinases) and the dual functional apurinic/apyrimidinic endonuclease 1 (APE-1) which redox regulates Fos, Jun, NF-κB, PAX, HIF-1α, and p53 (Evans et al. 2000; Kelley and Parsons 2001), thus driving the cell into mitosis.

Damage to the nDNA also activates the nuclear DNA repair system including poly ADP-ribose polymerase (PARP). PARP converts the nuclear NAD^+ into poly ADP-ribose linked to nuclear proteins, thus depleting nuclear NAD^+. The nuclear NAD^+ level is further depleted by its reduction to NADH as a consequence of the inhibition of the mitochondrial ETC. Depletion of nuclear NAD^+ deprives the protein deacetylase, SIRT2, of its obligatory substrate NAD^+, thus inhibiting deacetylation of histones, the forkhead transcription factors (FOXOs), and p53. The lack of deacetylation of the histones biases them toward the acetylated state, which opens the chromatin, permitting transcription of previously silenced developmental and replication genes, thus permitting expression of the activated oncogenes (Fig. 1).

The activation of the tryrosine kinases and/or *Ras* activates the PI3 kinase, which in turn activates the *Akt*/PKB kinases. The oncogene-induced replication of the pre-transformed cells in solid, unvascularized tissue results in hypoxia and induction of hexokinase II transcription, and the *Akt*/PKB kinases promote the binding of the hexokinase II to mitochondrial VDAC, thus coupling mitochondrial ATP production to driving glycolysis. The activated *Akt*/PKB kinases then phosphorylate the FOXO transcription factors. The phosphorylation of the FOXOs and the lack of SIRT2 deacetylation remove the FOXOs from the nucleus.

When unphosphorylated and unacetylated, the FOXO transcription factors enter the nucleus and bind to the insulin response elements (IREs) in gene promoters. Important IRE-containing genes include antioxidant genes such as the mitochondrial MnSOD gene and the master mitochondrial biogenesis gene regulator, the Peroxisome-Proliferation-Activated Receptor γ (PPARγ)-Coactivator 1α (PGC-1α). Expression of PGC-1α, in turn, activates transcription factors such as NRF-1 and 2 and PPARPγ to up-regulate mitochondrial biogenesis.

Hence, when the FOXOs are rendered inactive by phosphorylation and acetylation, mitochondrial OXPHOS and mitochondrial antioxidant defenses are down-regulated, further increasing mitochondrial ROS production and mtDNA mutagenesis (Fig. 1) (Wallace 2005). This down-regulation of OXPHOS via the *Akt*/PKB and FOXO pathway probably explains the commonly observed reduction of mitochondrial number and OXPHOS enzymes in cancer cells (Pedersen 1978).

The oncogene activation of the *Akt*/PKB kinases also results in the binding of the hexokinase II to the mitochondrial VDAC. This harnesses mitochondrial ATP production to drive glycolysis generating excessive pyruvate and NADH. At the same time, the FOXO-mediated down-regulation of mitochondrial OXPHOS and the inheritance or acquisition of inhibiting mtDNA variants increases mitochondrial ROS production which acts as a mitogen. Moreover, suppression of OXPHOS renders the mitochondria incapable of oxidizing all of the pyruvate and NADH. Consequently, the excess pyruvate and NADH are combined by lactate dehydrogenase to generate lactate in the presence of oxygen "aerobic glycolysis."

The inactivation of p53 further activates the transcription of hexokinase II and inhibits Bax transcription, both inhibiting apoptosis. Moreover, functional p53 is imported into the mitochondrion, where it interacts with the mtDNA polymerase γ and enhances its mtDNA replication function. Hence, the loss of p53 significantly increases mtDNA vulnerability to damage and mtDNA mutation rate (Achanta et al. 2005).

The cumulative ROS damage and loss of p53 fidelity lead to increased mtDNA somatic mutations. Those that partially impede the ETC accentuate ROS production without completely blocking ATP production. The increased ROS drives cellular division, whereas the continued generation of ATP continues to support hexokinase-II-initiated glycolysis.

Increased ROS production can be achieved in multiple ways. Certain mtDNA mutations can impede, but not stop, electron transport. Such mtDNA mutations either can arise de novo in the cancer cells as somatic mutations or can be inherited through the female germ line either as new deleterious germ-line mutations or as ancient adaptive polymorphisms. For individuals harboring mtDNA variants that partially inhibit the ETC, excessive caloric load will increase ROS production, thus increasing cancer risk.

The increased ROS production is advantageous to the cancer cell in driving replication, but it also chronically damages the mitochondria and the mtPTP. The ROS-oxidized mtPTP is particularly prone to activation by decreases in mitochondrial inner membrane potential (ΔP). Activation of the mtPTP, in turn, results in increased mitochondrial ROS production (Cai et al. 2000), possibly due in part to the redirection of electrons borne by cytochrome c away from complex IV and to the mitochondrial inner membrane-bound p66^{Shc} to generate H_2O_2 (Giorgio et al. 2005). In the mitochondria, the ANTs are particularly sensitive to inactivation by ROS, at least in *Drosophila* (Yan and Sohal 1998). These various aspects of mitochondrial permeability transition now suggest an explanation for the inhibition of mitochondrial ATP hydrolysis in cancer cells following addition of uncoupler (Pedersen 1978). Because of their chronic exposure to ROS, the cancer cell mtPTPs would be hypersensitive to changes in ΔP. When uncoupler is added, the mtPTP is activated, mitochondrial ROS production increases, and the ANTs are oxidized and inactivated. With ATP–ADP exchange blocked, the ATP synthase is deprived of substrate, and ATP hydrolysis stops. However, if ATP is added before the uncoupler, the ATP would stabilize the mtPTP, blocking increased ROS production, and preserving ADP–ATP exchange and thus ATP hydrolysis.

In conclusion, the application of the mitochondrial paradigm for metabolic and degenerative diseases and aging to cancer permits us to rationalize many perplexing features of cancer biology. Moreover, it refocuses the study of cancer mitochondrial metabolism away from gross dysfunction of OXPHOS and to the interplay between the mitochondrial ROS production and the mitochondrial regulation of apoptosis. Hence, Warburg's observations can now be explained, and with this explanation, new avenues for the treatment and prevention of cancer through drugs that control mitochondrial ROS are suggested.

ACKNOWLEDGMENTS

The author thanks Ms M.T. Lott for her assistance with this manuscript. This work has been supported by National Institutes of Health grants NS21328, AG13154, NS41650, AG24373, TW01366, and HL64017 and by an Ellison Senior Scholar Award.

REFERENCES

Achanta G., Sasaki R., Feng L., Carew J.S., Lu W., Pelicano H., Keating M.J., and Huang P. 2005. Novel role of p53 in maintaining mitochondrial genetic stability through interaction with DNA Pol gamma. *EMBO J.* **24:** 3482.

Alonso A., Martin P., Albarran C., Aquilera B., Garcia O., Guzman A., Oliva H., and Sancho M. 1997. Detection of somatic mutations in the mitochondrial DNA control region of colorectal and gastric tumors by heteroduplex and single-strand conformation analysis. *Electrophoresis* **18:** 682.

Aoki M., Batista O., Bellacosa A., Tsichlis P., and Vogt P.K. 1998. The akt kinase: Molecular determinants of oncogenicity. *Proc. Natl. Acad. Sci.* **95:** 14950.

Astuti D., Latif F., Dallol A., Dahia P.L., Douglas F., George E., Skoldberg F., Husebye E.S., Eng C., and Maher E.R. 2001. Gene mutations in the succinate dehydrogenase subunit SDHB cause susceptibility to familial pheochromocytoma and to familial paraganglioma. *Am. J. Hum. Genet.* **69:** 49.

Baysal B.E., Ferrell R.E., Willett-Brozick J.E., Lawrence E.C., Myssiorek D., Bosch A., van der Mey A., Taschner P.E., Rubinstein W.S., Myers E.N., Richard C.W., Cornelisse C.J., Devilee P., and Devlin B. 2000. Mutations in SDHD, a mitochondrial complex II gene, in hereditary paraganglioma. *Science* **287:** 848.

Bellacosa A., Testa J.R., Staal S.P., and Tsichlis P.N. 1991. A retroviral oncogene, akt, encoding a serine-threonine kinase containing an SH2-like region. *Science* **254:** 274.

Bianchi M.S., Bianchi N.O., and Bailliet G. 1995. Mitochondrial DNA mutations in normal and tumor tissues from breast cancer patients. *Cytogenet. Cell Genet.* **71:** 99.

Birnbaum M.J. 2004. On the InterAktion between hexokinase and the mitochondrion. *Dev. Cell* **7:** 781.

Bourgeron T., Rustin P., Chretien D., Birch-Machin M., Bourgeois M., Viegas-Pequignot E., Munnich A., and Rotig A. 1995. Mutation of a nuclear succinate dehydrogenase gene results in mitochondrial respiratory chain deficiency. *Nat. Genet.* **11:** 144.

Brandon M., Baldi P., and Wallace D.C. 2006. Mitochondrial

mutations in cancer. *Oncogene* (in press).

Brazil D.P., Yang Z.Z., and Hemmings B.A. 2004. Advances in protein kinase B signalling: AKTion on multiple fronts. *Trends Biochem. Sci.* **29:** 233.

Brockington M., Sweeney M.G., Hammans S.R., Morgan-Hughes J.A., and Harding A.E. 1993. A tandem duplication in the D-loop of human mitochondrial DNA is associated with deletions in mitochondrial myopathies. *Nat. Genet.* **4:** 67.

Bustamante E. and Pedersen P.L. 1977. High aerobic glycolysis of rat hepatoma cells in culture: Role of mitochondrial hexokinase. *Proc. Natl. Acad. Sci.* **74:** 3735.

Cai J., Wallace D.C., Zhivotovsky B., and Jones D.P. 2000. Separation of cytochrome c-dependent caspase activation from thiol-disulfide redox change in cells lacking mitochondrial DNA. *Free Radic. Biol. Med.* **29:** 334.

Cann R.L., Stoneking M., and Wilson A.C. 1987. Mitochondrial DNA and human evolution. *Nature* **325:** 31.

Canter J.A., Kallianpur A.R., Parl F.F., and Millikan R.C. 2005. Mitochondrial DNA G10398A polymorphism and invasive breast cancer in African-American women. *Cancer Res.* **65:** 8028.

Chen J.Z., Gokden N., Greene G.F., Green B., and Kadlubar F.F. 2003. Simultaneous generation of multiple mitochondrial DNA mutations in human prostate tumors suggests mitochondrial hyper-mutagenesis. *Carcinogenesis* **24:** 1481.

Chen J.Z., Gokden N., Greene G.F., Mukunyadzi P., and Kadlubar F.F. 2002. Extensive somatic mitochondrial mutations in primary prostate cancer using laser capture microdissection. *Cancer Res.* **62:** 6470.

Chinnery P.F., Samuels D.C., Elson J., and Turnbull D.M. 2002. Accumulation of mitochondrial DNA mutations in ageing, cancer, and mitochondrial disease: Is there a common mechanism? *Lancet* **360:** 1323.

Clayton D.A., Davis R.W., and Vinograd J. 1970. Homology and structural relationships between the dimeric and monomeric circular forms of mitochondrial DNA from human leukemic leukocytes. *J. Mol. Biol.* **47:** 137.

Copeland W.C., Wachsman J.T., Johnson F.M., and Penta J.S. 2002. Mitochondrial DNA alterations in cancer. *Cancer Investig.* **20:** 557.

Evans A.R., Limp-Foster M., and Kelley M.R. 2000. Going APE over ref-1. *Mutat. Res.* **461:** 83.

Fliss M.S., Usadel H., Caballero O.L., Wu L., Buta M.R., Eleff S.M., Jen J., and Sidransky D. 2000. Facile detection of mitochondrial DNA mutations in tumors and bodily fluids. *Science* **287:** 2017.

Gatenby R.A. and Gillies R.J. 2004. Why do cancers have high aerobic glycolysis? *Nat. Rev. Cancer* **4:** 891.

Giorgio M., Migliaccio E., Orsini F., Paolucci D., Moroni M., Contursi C., Pelliccia G., Luzi L., Minucci S., Marcaccio M., Pinton P., Rizzuto R., Bernardi P., Paolucci F., and Pelicci P.G. 2005. Electron transfer between cytochrome c and p66Shc generates reactive oxygen species that trigger mitochondrial apoptosis. *Cell* **122:** 221.

Glaichenhaus N., Leopold P., and Cuzin F. 1986. Increased levels of mitochondrial gene expression in rat fibroblast cells immortalized or transformed by viral and cellular oncogenes. *EMBO J.* **5:** 1261.

Goel A., Mathupala S.P., and Pedersen P.L. 2003. Glucose metabolism in cancer. Evidence that demethylation events play a role in activating type II hexokinase gene expression. *J. Biol. Chem.* **278:** 15333.

Gottlob K., Majewski N., Kennedy S., Kandel E., Robey R.B., and Hay N. 2001. Inhibition of early apoptotic events by Akt/PKB is dependent on the first committed step of glycolysis and mitochondrial hexokinase. *Genes Dev.* **15:** 1406.

Habano W., Sugai T., Yoshida T., and Nakamura S. 1999. Mitochondrial gene mutation, but not large-scale deletion, is a feature of colorectal carcinomas with mitochondrial microsatellite instability. *Int. J. Cancer* **83:** 625.

Harrison D.E. and Archer J.R. 1987. Genetic differences in effects of food restriction on aging in mice. *J. Nutr.* **117:** 376.

Herrmann P.C., Gillespie J.W., Charboneau L., Bichsel V.E., Paweletz C.P., Calvert V.S., Kohn E.C., Emmert-Buck M.R.,

Liotta L.A., and Petricoin E.F., III. 2003. Mitochondrial proteome: altered cytochrome c oxidase subunit levels in prostate cancer. *Proteomics* **3:** 1801.

Holt I.J., Harding A.E., and Morgan-Hughes J.A. 1988. Deletions of muscle mitochondrial DNA in patients with mitochondrial myopathies. *Nature* **331:** 717.

Holt I.J., Harding A.E., Petty R.K., and Morgan-Hughes J.A. 1990. A new mitochondrial disease associated with mitochondrial DNA heteroplasmy. *Am. J. Hum. Genet.* **46:** 428.

Horton T.M., Petros J.A., Heddi A., Shoffner J., Kaufman A.E., Graham S.D., Jr., Gramlich T., and Wallace D.C. 1996. Novel mitochondrial DNA deletion found in a renal cell carcinoma. *Genes Chromosomes Cancer* **15:** 95.

Ishii N., Fujii M., Hartman P.S., Tsuda M., Yasuda K., Senoo-Matsuda N., Yanase S., Ayusawa D., and Suzuki K. 1998. A mutation in succinate dehydrogenase cytochrome b causes oxidative stress and ageing in nematodes. *Nature* **394:** 694.

Jeronimo C., Nomoto S., Caballero O.L., Usadel H., Henrique R., Varzim G., Oliveira J., Lopes C., Fliss M.S., and Sidransky D. 2001. Mitochondrial mutations in early stage prostate cancer and bodily fluids. *Oncogene* **20:** 5195.

Johnson M.J., Wallace D.C., Ferris S.D., Rattazzi M.C., and Cavalli-Sforza L.L. 1983. Radiation of human mitochondria DNA types analyzed by restriction endonuclease cleavage patterns. *J. Mol. Evol.* **19:** 255.

Kelley M.R. and Parsons S.H. 2001. Redox regulation of the DNA repair function of the human AP endonuclease Ape1/ref-1. *Antioxid. Redox Signal.* **3:** 671.

Khogali S.S., Mayosi B.M., Beattie J.M., McKenna W.J., Watkins H., and Poulton J. 2001. A common mitochondrial DNA variant associated with susceptibility to dilated cardiomyopathy in two different populations. *Lancet* **357:** 1265.

Kirches E., Krause G., Warich-Kirches M., Weis S., Schneider T., Meyer-Puttlitz B., Mawrin C., and Dietzmann K. 2001. High frequency of mitochondrial DNA mutations in glioblastoma multiforme identified by direct sequence comparison to blood samples. *Int. J. Cancer* **93:** 534.

Kokoszka J.E., Waymire K.G., Levy S.E., Sligh J.E., Cai J., Jones D.P., MacGregor G.R., and Wallace D.C. 2004. The ADP/ATP translocator is not essential for the mitochondrial permeability transition pore. *Nature* **427:** 461.

Krieg R.C., Knuechel R., Schiffmann E., Liotta L.A., Petricoin E.F., III, and Herrmann P.C. 2004. Mitochondrial proteome: Cancer-altered metabolism associated with cytochrome c oxidase subunit level variation. *Proteomics* **4:** 2789.

Kujoth G.C., Hiona A., Pugh T.D., Someya S., Panzer K., Wohlgemuth S.E., Hofer T., Seo A.Y., Sullivan R., Jobling W.A., Morrow J.D., Van Remmen H., Sedivy J.M., Yamasoba T., Tanokura M., Weindruch R., Leeuwenburgh C., and Prolla T.A. 2005. Mitochondrial DNA mutations, oxidative stress, and apoptosis in mammalian aging. *Science* **309:** 481.

Kurtz A., Lueth M., Kluwe L., Zhang T., Foster R., Mautner V.F., Hartmann M., Tan D.J., Martuza R.L., Friedrich R.E., Driever P.H., and Wong L.J. 2004. Somatic mitochondrial DNA mutations in neurofibromatosis type 1-associated tumors. *Mol. Cancer Res.* **2:** 433.

LaBiche R.A., Demars M., and Nicolson G.L. 1992. Transcripts of the mitochondrial gene ND5 are overexpressed in highly metastatic murine large cell lymphoma cells. *In Vivo* **6:** 317.

LaBiche R.A., Yoshida M., Gallick G.E., Irimura T., Robberson D.L., Klostergaard J., and Nicolson G.L. 1988. Gene expression and tumor cell escape from host effector mechanisms in murine large cell lymphoma. *J. Cell. Biochem.* **36:** 393.

Lee H.C., Li S.H., Lin J.C., Wu C.C., Yeh D.C., and Wei Y.H. 2004. Somatic mutations in the D-loop and decrease in the copy number of mitochondrial DNA in human hepatocellular carcinoma. *Mutat. Res.* **547:** 71.

Lee M.G. and Pedersen P.L. 2003. Glucose metabolism in cancer: Importance of transcription factor-DNA interactions within a short segment of the proximal region of the type II hexokinase promoter. *J. Biol. Chem.* **278:** 41047.

Lehtonen R., Kiuru M., Vanharanta S., Sjoberg J., Aaltonen L.M., Aittomaki K., Arola J., Butzow R., Eng C., Husgafvel-Pursiainen K., Isola J., Jarvinen H., Koivisto P., Mecklin J.P.,

Peltomaki P., Salovaara R., Wasenius V.M., Karhu A., Launonen V., Nupponen N.N., and Aaltonen L.A. 2004. Biallelic inactivation of fumarate hydratase (FH) occurs in nonsyndromic uterine leiomyomas but is rare in other tumors. *Am. J. Pathol.* **164:** 17.

Liu V.W., Shi H.H., Cheung A.N., Chiu P.M., Leung T.W., Nagley P., Wong L.C., and Ngan H.Y. 2001. High incidence of somatic mitochondrial DNA mutations in human ovarian carcinomas. *Cancer Res.* **61:** 5998.

Liu V.W., Wang Y., Yang H.J., Tsang P.C., Ng T.Y., Wong L.C., Nagley P., and Ngan H.Y. 2003. Mitochondrial DNA variant 16189T>C is associated with susceptibility to endometrial cancer. *Hum. Mutat.* **22:** 173.

Majewski N., Nogueira V., Robey R.B., and Hay N. 2004a. Akt inhibits apoptosis downstream of BID cleavage via a glucose-dependent mechanism involving mitochondrial hexokinases. *Mol. Cell. Biol.* **24:** 730.

Majewski N., Nogueira V., Bhaskar P., Coy P.E., Skeen J.E., Gottlob K., Chandel N.S., Thompson C.B., Robey R.B., and Hay N. 2004b. Hexokinase-mitochondria interaction mediated by Akt is required to inhibit apoptosis in the presence or absence of Bax and Bak. *Mol. Cell* **16:** 819.

Masoro E.J. 1993. Dietary restriction and aging. *J. Am. Geriatr. Soc.* **41:** 994.

Masoro E.J., McCarter R.J., Katz M.S., and McMahan C.A. 1992. Dietary restriction alters characteristics of glucose fuel use (erratum in *J. Gerontol.* [1993] **48:** B73). *J. Gerontol.* **47:** B202.

Mathupala S.P., Heese C., and Pedersen P.L. 1997a. Glucose catabolism in cancer cells. The type II hexokinase promoter contains functionally active response elements for the tumor suppressor p53. *J. Biol. Chem.* **272:** 22776.

Mathupala S.P., Rempel A., and Pedersen P.L. 1997b. Aberrant glycolytic metabolism of cancer cells: A remarkable coordination of genetic, transcriptional, post-translational, and mutational events that lead to a critical role for type II hexokinase. *J. Bioenerg. Biomembr.* **29:** 339.

———. 2001. Glucose catabolism in cancer cells: Identification and characterization of a marked activation response of the type II hexokinase gene to hypoxic conditions. *J. Biol. Chem.* **276:** 43407.

Mattiazzi M., Vijayvergiya C., Gajewski C.D., DeVivo D.C., Lenaz G., Wiedmann M., and Manfredi G. 2004. The mtDNA T8993G (NARP) mutation results in an impairment of oxidative phosphorylation that can be improved by antioxidants. *Hum. Mol. Genet.* **13:** 869.

Maximo V., Soares P., Lima J., Cameselle-Teijeiro J., and Sobrinho-Simoes M. 2002. Mitochondrial DNA somatic mutations (point mutations and large deletions) and mitochondrial DNA variants in human thyroid pathology: A study with emphasis on Hurthle cell tumors. *Am. J. Pathol.* **160:** 1857.

McCarter R.J. and Palmer J. 1992. Energy metabolism and aging: A lifelong study of Fischer 344 rats. *Am. J. Physiol.* **263:** E448.

McCord J.M. 2000. The evolution of free radicals and oxidative stress. *Am. J. Med. Genet.* **108:** 652.

Melov S., Ravenscroft J., Malik S., Gill M.S., Walker D.W., Clayton P.E., Wallace D.C., Malfroy B., Doctrow S.R., and Lithgow G.J. 2000. Extension of life-span with superoxide dismutase/catalase mimetics. *Science* **289:** 1567.

Merriwether D.A., Clark A.G., Ballinger S.W., Schurr T.G., Soodyall H., Jenkins T., Sherry S.T., and Wallace D.C. 1991. The structure of human mitochondrial DNA variation. *J. Mol. Evol.* **33:** 543.

Mishmar D., Ruiz-Pesini E.E., Golik P., Macaulay V., Clark A.G., Hosseini S., Brandon M., Easley K., Chen E., Brown M.D., Sukernik R.I., Olckers A., and Wallace D.C. 2003. Natural selection shaped regional mtDNA variation in humans. *Proc. Natl. Acad. Sci.* **100:** 171.

Niemann S. and Muller U. 2000. Mutations in SDHC cause autosomal dominant paraganglioma, type 3. *Nat. Genet.* **26:** 268.

Nomoto S., Yamashita K., Koshikawa K., Nakao A., and Sidransky D. 2002. Mitochondrial D-loop mutations as clonal markers in multicentric hepatocellular carcinoma and plasma. *Clin. Cancer Res.* **8:** 481.

Parrella P., Xiao Y., Fliss M., Sanchez-Cespedes M., Mazzarelli

P., Rinaldi M., Nicol T., Gabrielson E., Cuomo C., Cohen D., Pandit S., Spencer M., Rabitti C., Fazio V.M., and Sidransky D. 2001. Detection of mitochondrial DNA mutations in primary breast cancer and fine-needle aspirates. *Cancer Res.* **61:** 7623.

Pedersen P.L. 1978. Tumor mitochondria and the bioenergetics of cancer cells. *Prog. Exp. Tumor Res.* **22:** 190.

Pedersen P.L., Mathupala S., Rempel A., Geschwind J.F., and Ko Y.H. 2002. Mitochondrial bound type II hexokinase: A key player in the growth and survival of many cancers and an ideal prospect for therapeutic intervention. *Biochim. Biophys. Acta* **1555:** 14.

Petros J.A., Baumann A.K., Ruiz-Pesini E., Amin M.B., Sun C.Q., Hall J., Lim S., Issa M.M., Flanders W.D., Hosseini S.H., Marshall F.F., and Wallace D.C. 2005. mtDNA mutations increase tumorigenicity in prostate cancer. *Proc. Natl. Acad. Sci.* **102:** 719.

Polyak K., Li Y., Zhu H., Lengauer C., Willson J.K., Markowitz S.D., Trush M.A., Kinzler K.W., and Vogelstein B. 1998. Somatic mutations of the mitochondrial genome in human colorectal tumours. *Nat. Genet.* **20:** 291.

Poulton J. 1998. Does a common mitochondrial DNA polymorphism underlie susceptibility to diabetes and the thrifty genotype? *Trends Genet.* **14:** 387.

Poulton J., Brown M.S., Cooper A., Marchington D.R., and Phillips D.I. 1998. A common mitochondrial DNA variant is associated with insulin resistance in adult life. *Diabetologia* **41:** 54.

Ruiz-Pesini E., Mishmar D., Brandon M., Procaccio V., and Wallace D.C. 2004. Effects of purifying and adaptive selection on regional variation in human mtDNA. *Science* **303:** 223.

Schriner S.E., Linford N.J., Martin G.M., Treuting P., Ogburn C.E., Emond M., Coskun P.E., Ladiges W., Wolf N., Van Remmen H., Wallace D.C., and Rabinovitch P.S. 2005. Extension of murine life span by overexpression of catalase targeted to the mitochondria. *Science* **308:** 1909.

Senoo-Matsuda N., Yasuda K., Tsuda M., Ohkubo T., Yoshimura S., Nakazawa H., Hartman P.S., and Ishii N. 2001. A defect in the cytochrome b large subunit in complex II causes both superoxide anion overproduction and abnormal energy metabolism in *Caenorhabditis elegans*. *J. Biol. Chem.* **276:** 41553.

Shoffner J.M., Lott M.T., Lezza A.M., Seibel P., Ballinger S.W., and Wallace D.C. 1990. Myoclonic epilepsy and ragged-red fiber disease (MERRF) is associated with a mitochondrial DNA tRNA[Lys] mutation. *Cell* **61:** 931.

Sohal R.S., Ku H.H., Agarwal S., Forster M.J., and Lal H. 1994. Oxidative damage, mitochondrial oxidant generation and antioxidant defenses during aging and in response to food restriction in the mouse. *Mech. Ageing Dev.* **74:** 121.

Taira M., Yoshida E., Kobayashi M., Yaginuma K., and Koike K. 1983. Tumor-associated mutations of rat mitochondrial transfer RNA genes. *Nucleic Acids Res.* **11:** 1635.

Testa J.R. and Bellacosa A. 2001. AKT plays a central role in tumorigenesis. *Proc. Natl. Acad. Sci.* **98:** 10983.

Tong B.C., Ha P.K., Dhir K., Xing M., Westra W.H., Sidransky D., and Califano J. 2003. Mitochondrial DNA alterations in thyroid cancer. *J. Surg. Oncol.* **82:** 170.

Torroni A., Stepien G., Hodge J.A., and Wallace D.C. 1990. Neoplastic transformation is associated with coordinate induction of nuclear and cytoplasmic oxidative phosphorylation genes. *J. Biol. Chem.* **265:** 20589.

Torroni A., Lott M.T., Cabell M.F., Chen Y., Laverge L., and Wallace D.C. 1994. MtDNA and the origin of Caucasians. Identification of ancient Caucasian-specific haplogroups, one of which is prone to a recurrent somatic duplication in the D-loop region. *Am. J. Hum. Genet.* **55:** 760.

Trifunovic A., Wredenberg A., Falkenberg M., Spelbrink J.N., Rovio A.T., Bruder C.E., Bohlooly Y.M., Gidlof S., Oldfors A., Wibom R., Tornell J., Jacobs H.T., and Larsson N.G. 2004. Premature ageing in mice expressing defective mitochondrial DNA polymerase. *Nature* **429:** 417.

Trounce I., Neill S., and Wallace D.C. 1994. Cytoplasmic trans-fer of the mtDNA nt 8993 TG (ATP6) point mutation associated with Leigh syndrome into mtDNA-less cells demonstrates cosegregation with a decrease in state III respiration and ADP/O ratio. *Proc. Natl. Acad. Sci.* **91:** 8334.

———. 1995. Rescue of mitochondrial DNAs (mtDNA) from young and old human and mouse brain by fusion of synaptosomes with rho[0] cultured cells. *Am. J. Hum. Genet.* **57:** A252.

Trounce I.A., Kim Y.L., Jun A.S., and Wallace D.C. 1996. Assessment of mitochondrial oxidative phosphorylation in patient muscle biopsies, lymphoblasts, and transmitochondrial cell lines. *Methods Enzymol.* **264:** 484.

Van Remmen H., Ikeno Y., Hamilton M., Pahlavani M., Wolf N., Thorpe S.R., Alderson N.L., Baynes J.W., Epstein C.J., Huang T.T., Nelson J., Strong R., and Richardson A. 2003. Life-long reduction in MnSOD activity results in increased DNA damage and higher incidence of cancer but does not accelerate aging. *Physiol. Genomics* **16:** 29.

Vanharanta S., Buchta M., McWhinney S.R., Virta S.K., Peczkowska M., Morrison C.D., Lehtonen R., Januszewicz A., Jarvinen H., Juhola M., Mecklin J.P., Pukkala E., Herva R., Kiuru M., Nupponen N.N., Aaltonen L.A., Neumann H.P., and Eng C. 2004. Early-onset renal cell carcinoma as a novel extraparaganglial component of SDHB-associated heritable paraganglioma. *Am. J. Hum. Genet.* **74:** 153.

Wallace D.C. 1992. Mitochondrial genetics: A paradigm for aging and degenerative diseases? *Science* **256:** 628.

———. 2005. A mitochondrial paradigm of metabolic and degenerative diseases, aging, and cancer: A dawn for evolutionary medicine. *Annu. Rev. Genet.* **39:** 359.

Wallace D.C. and Lott M.T. 2002. Mitochondrial genes in degenerative diseases, cancer and aging. In *Emery and Rimoin's principles and practice of medical genetics* (ed. D.L. Rimoin et al.), p. 299. Churchill Livingstone, London, United Kingdom.

Wallace D.C., Brown M.D., and Lott M.T. 1999. Mitochondrial DNA variation in human evolution and disease. *Gene* **238:** 211.

Wallace D.C., Singh G., Lott M.T., Hodge J.A., Schurr T.G., Lezza A.M., Elsas L.J., and Nikoskelainen E.K. 1988a. Mitochondrial DNA mutation associated with Leber's hereditary optic neuropathy. *Science* **242:** 1427.

Wallace D.C., Zheng X., Lott M.T., Shoffner J.M., Hodge J.A., Kelley R.I., Epstein C.M., and Hopkins L.C. 1988b. Familial mitochondrial encephalomyopathy (MERRF): Genetic, pathophysiological, and biochemical characterization of a mitochondrial DNA disease. *Cell* **55:** 601.

Warburg O.H. 1931. *The metabolism of tumours.* R.R. Smith, New York, New York.

Wu C.W., Yin P.H., Hung W.Y., Li A.F., Li S.H., Chi C.W., Wei Y.H., and Lee H.C. 2005. Mitochondrial DNA mutations and mitochondrial DNA depletion in gastric cancer. *Genes Chromosomes Cancer* **44:** 19.

Xu Y., Krishnan A., Wan X.S., Majima H., Yeh C.C., Ludewig G., Kasarskis E.J., and St. Clair D.K. 1999. Mutations in the promoter reveal a cause for the reduced expression of the human manganese superoxide dismutase gene in cancer cells. *Oncogene* **18:** 93.

Yan L.J. and Sohal R.S. 1998. Mitochondrial adenine nucleotide translocase is modified oxidatively during aging. *Proc. Natl. Acad. Sci.* **95:** 12896.

Yanagihara M., Katano M., Takahashi-Sasaki N., Kimata K., Taira K., and Andoh T. 2005. Ribozymes targeting serine/threonine kinase Akt1 sensitize cells to anticancer drugs. *Cancer Sci.* **96:** 620.

Yeh J.J., Lunetta K.L., van Orsouw N.J., Moore F.D., Jr., Mutter G.L., Vijg J., Dahia P.L., and Eng C. 2000. Somatic mitochondrial DNA (mtDNA) mutations in papillary thyroid carcinomas and differential mtDNA sequence variants in cases with thyroid tumours. *Oncogene* **19:** 2060.

Yoneyama H., Hara T., Kato Y., Yamori T., Matsuura E.T., and Koike K. 2005. Nucleotide sequence variation is frequent in the mitochondrial DNA displacement loop region of individual human tumor cells. *Mol. Cancer Res.* **3:** 14.

Induction of Complete Regressions of Oncogene-induced Breast Tumors in Mice

R. Benezra,* E. Henke,* A. Ciarrocchi,* M. Ruzinova,* D. Solit,¶ N. Rosen,†
D. Nolan,¶ V. Mittal,¶ and P. de Candia*

Departments of *Cancer Biology and Genetics, †Experimental Therapeutics, and ¶Medicine,
Memorial Sloan-Kettering Cancer Center, New York 10021; ¶Cold Spring Harbor Laboratory,
Cold Spring Harbor, New York 11724

Over the past decade, mouse models of cancer have come to resemble human disease much more closely than simple subcutaneous or orthotopic systems. Intervention strategies that work on these new model systems are more likely to have an impact clinically. We have shown recently that antiangiogenic stress imposed by loss of Id protein in endothelial progenitor cells results in dramatic central necrosis in breast tumors initiated in mice by overexpression of the her2/neu oncogene. Tumor cells remain viable at the periphery, perhaps via the hypoxic response pathway which allows the lesions to expand. Inhibition of this pathway by the inactivation of the Hif-1α chaperone Hsp90 in combination with antiangiogenic stress leads to the first reported complete regression of these aggressive breast tumors.

Over the past 20 years, we have learned more about the molecular events leading to cancer than we have in all time preceding. Detailed descriptions of the signaling pathways that have gone awry in the tumor cell and the tumor microenvironment have increased our understanding of the cancer process in dramatic ways. Even a decade ago, at the last Cold Spring Harbor Symposium that focused on cancer, the progress we have seen to date in exploiting this information for the development of targeted therapeutics could not have even been wistfully imagined. As we trumpet our success with Gleevec, for example (see Sawyers, this volume), in managing chronic myelogenous leukemia by inhibiting the enzyme (bcr-abl) that causes it, we are reminded by the lay press and public, perhaps justifiably so, that far too many more people are still dying of cancer than one might have hoped, given the enormous investment we have made in controlling cancer over the past century. But there is one point which is generally overlooked. We as cancer biologists are excited less by the progress made to date than by the rate of increase of new and profound discoveries that are now being made. Although we recognize with deep sadness that we cannot immediately translate this work to help those around us who are suffering from this disease, we sense with profound anticipation that our current work will affect the lives and health of generations to come. We are indeed in the midst of a revolution in cancer biology that only the most myopic among us can possibly fail to see.

How do we speed the translation of our new-found knowledge into effective, nontoxic cancer therapies? One thing that has become abundantly clear is that physiologically relevant mouse models of human cancer, in which oncogenes are overexpressed or tumor suppressor genes are inactivated in adult animals, hold great promise in exploring the mechanistic basis of cancer initiation and progression, as well as therapeutic approaches likely to be meaningful clinically. It is one thing to cure a mouse of a tumor grown under the skin or even orthotopically, but

quite another to eliminate aggressive spontaneous tumors in these animals. As Tyler Jacks so poignantly stated after showing a slide of an aggressive K-ras-induced lung tumor, "Cure this."

We have taken up this challenge by trying to induce complete regressions of mammary tumors in mice that result from overexpression of the her2/neu oncogene (Guy et al. 1992), an oncogene that is overexpressed in approximately 30% of human breast cancers. The lesions arise in these mice with about a 4-month latency and appear as multifocal, dense cellular masses which kill their host within about 7–8 months with close to 100% penetrance. A variety of chemotherapeutic approaches have at best delayed the time to progression of these tumors, with no complete regressions reported to date (Sacco et al. 1996; Shah et al. 1999; Anisimov et al. 2002; Manor et al. 2003).

The strategy we have taken to treat these mice is based on our analysis of Id protein loss in the vessels of tumor xenografts. The Id proteins are a set of four highly related proteins (called Id1–4) which act as naturally occurring dominant negative antagonists of basic helix-loop-helix (bHLH) transcription factors (Ruzinova and Benezra 2003; Perk et al. 2005). They contain the HLH dimerization motif but are missing the basic region which contacts DNA; therefore, heterodimers between Ids and bHLH proteins fail to bind DNA or to activate transcription (see Fig. 1). The Id proteins are expressed at high levels through mid-gestation in a broad but complex spatio-temporal pattern and are dramatically down-regulated late in development and postnatally (Jen et al. 1996, 1997). By and large, their expression is enriched in highly proliferative, undifferentiated cells in various cell lineages, and their loss is associated with alteration in cell fate, often toward a fully differentiated postmitotic state (although there are exceptions). The expression pattern and biochemical activity of Id1 and Id3 are nearly identical, and indeed, only when copies of both Id1 and Id3 are disrupted in animals do the most severe phenotypes mani-

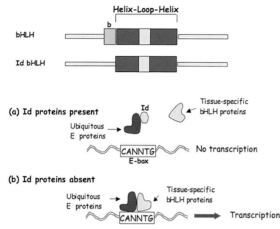

Figure 1. Mechanism of Id action. The Id proteins act as naturally occurring dominant negative antagonists of the basic helix-loop-helix (bHLH) transcription factor family. Id proteins contain the HLH dimerization motif but lack the basic region that contacts DNA. Heterodimers between Id and other members of the family therefore fail to bind DNA. The preferred targets of the Id proteins in the cell are the ubiquitously expressed E proteins, which are themselves obligate heterodimerizing partners of tissue-specific bHLH proteins such as MyoD and NeuroD. Thus, by sequestering E proteins, Id can control tissue-specific gene expression in multiple cell lineages using the same biochemical mechanism. For more detailed review, see Ruzinova and Benezra (2003) and Perk et al. (2005).

fest: premature neural differentiation, hemorrhage in the forebrain, ventricular-septal cardiac defects, and embryonic lethality (Lyden et al. 1999; Fraidenraich et al. 2004). The hemorrhage in the forebrain turned out to be a defect in angiogenesis, and this led us to test whether postnatal tumor angiogenesis was affected in adult animals missing 1–3 copies of the Id1,3 pair. Indeed, reduced Id dosages led to a profound defect in tumor an-

giogenesis in subcutaneous tumors initiated with either B6Rv2 lymphoma cells or a breast cancer cell line (Lyden et al. 1999). These effects were associated with the appearance of stunted and occluded blood vessels and an increase in hemorrhage in these tumors. Lewis lung carcinoma cells, however, produced subcutaneous lesions that continued to expand in the reduced Id backgrounds despite the loss of vascular integrity and an increase in hemorrhage and necrosis. Remarkably, however, despite the growth of the primary lesion, metastasis was dramatically reduced in the Id knockout strains, clearly indicating a difference in Id-dependence in the growth of xenografts and metastatic lesions.

We went on to show that the defect in the animals with reduced Id dosages could be traced to failure to mobilize endothelial cell progenitors to the site of the tumor (Lyden et al. 2001). Id1 levels rise in the bone marrow in response to VEGF, and this expression appears to be essential for the migration of EPCs from the marrow into the periphery and to the site of the tumor. The Id-dependent steps in this pathway are not yet known. Once at the site of the tumor, Id appears to be required for the maintenance of expression of genes involved in a promigratory pathway that may be essential for the formation of a functional vascular network. Integrins α6 and β4, FGFR1, MMP2, and laminin 5 have been observed to be significantly down-regulated in Id-deficient endothelial cells at the site of the tumor (Ruzinova et al. 2003). FGFR1 activated by FGF2 up-regulates and enhances secretion of MMP2. MMP2 in turn converts laminin 5 in a proteolytic fragment, which engages α6 β4 integrins, stimulating the endothelial cell migration (see Fig. 2) (Klein et al. 1993; Giannelli et al. 1997; Pfeifer et al. 2000). Inhibition of single components of the described pathway in matrigel plug assays is sufficient to partially phenocopy Id loss, thereby adding functional significance to the array results. Importantly, this model has received support from

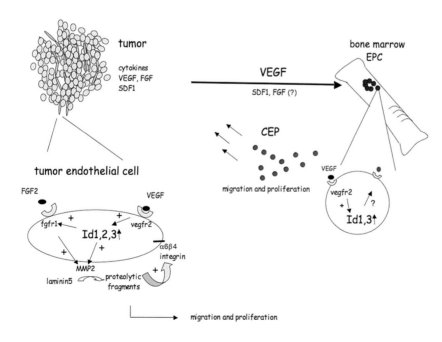

Figure 2. Id proteins in peripheral and bone marrow-derived endothelial cells. In the periphery, Ids are required for maintaining the expression of Fgfr1, MMP2, laminin 5, and α6β4 integrin, which form a promigratory network. This network depends on the engagement of α6β4 integrin with an MMP2 cleavage product of laminin 5. In the bone marrow, Ids are required for the mobilization and proliferation of endothelial progenitor cells (EPCs) which enter the bloodstream as circulating endothelial progenitors (CEP) and migrate to the site of the tumor. Id1 and Id3 in the bone marrow are up-regulated in response to VEGF, and this up-regulation is required for mobilization. The downstream consequences of Id expression in the bone marrow are still not well understood. (Reproduced, with permission, from Perk et al. 2005 [©Macmillan Magazines;].)

an independent genetic analysis where it was shown that hypomorphic mutations in β4 integrin also lead to impaired angiogenesis (Nikolopoulos et al. 2004).

To determine whether Id loss is worth pursuing clinically, it was important to monitor the effects of Id loss on tumors other than xenografts. Tumors that arise as a result of the overexpression of oncogenes or loss of tumor suppressor genes are much more similar pathophysiologically to human disease than tumors that arise from the inoculation of tumor cells subcutaneously. In addition, xenografts have been "cured" with therapeutic approaches that have not fared well in the clinic. However, if a spontaneous tumor model can be brought into complete remission with a treatment regimen, it seems likely that such treatments will have a higher chance of being effective in the clinic. This paper details our success at bringing an aggressive her2/neu-induced mammary carcinoma into complete remission with a combination of Id loss and targeting of the Hsp90 stress response pathway.

THE CROSS

To determine whether a reduction in Id1 or Id3 expression prevents or alters the rate of spontaneous mammary tumor formation in *neu* transgenic mice, we bred mice overexpressing the her2/neu oncogene (YD allele) in the mammary epithelia (using the mouse mammary tumor virus long terminal repeat [MMTV-LTR]) with Id1$^{-/-}$Id3$^{+/-}$ mice. HER2/*neu* encodes a transmembrane tyrosine kinase that is commonly amplified in human breast tumors. Amplification of HER2 correlates with a poor clinical prognosis in breast cancer patients (Slamon et al. 1987), and anti-Her2 antibodies have therapeutic utility in this disease (Slamon et al. 2001; Baselga et al. 2002; Vogel et al. 2002). Mice expressing *neu* under the transcriptional control of the MMTV-LTR develop mammary tumors after a prolonged latency (Guy et al. 1992). YD mice express a *neu* receptor with a 12-amino acid deletion in the extracellular domain that leads to its constitutive dimerization and activation. In addition, four of the five tyrosine phosphorylation sites have been mutated to phenylalanine in the YD *neu* protein, which retains only the fourth ("D") site that binds to Shc when phosphorylated. These mice demonstrate accelerated formation of multifocal solid comedo-type tumors with low metastatic potential (Dankort et al. 2001). Throughout this paper we refer to the Id-deficient populations as missing one, two, or three copies of Id genes, and we do not distinguish between Id1 and Id3. This simplification is possible because no phenotypic differences were observed among Id1- and Id3-deficient mice. Id wild-type, YD *neu* mice developed their first mammary lesion with a mean latency of 193 days (*n* = 34) (de Candia et al. 2003). In Id-deficient mice, tumor onset was not delayed (mean tumor latency of 170 days [*n* = 82], 159 days [*n* = 67], and 178 days [*n* = 23]) in mice missing one, two, or three copies of Id1 or Id3 (de Candia et al. 2003).

Tumor-bearing mice were sacrificed 8 weeks after detection of the first lesion. At sacrifice, tumors were classified as solid if more than 90% of the tumor volume was

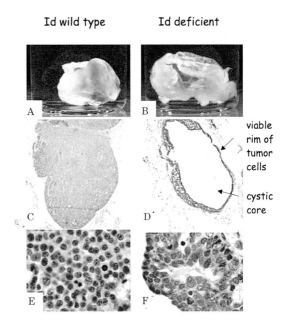

Id wild type   Id deficient

viable
rim of
tumor
cells

cystic
core

Figure 3. Mammary tumors arising in YD *neu* Id-deficient mice were cystic with a small rim of viable cells surrounding an acellular core. (*A,B*) Tumors dissected from a YD *neu* Id1$^{+/+}$Id3$^{+/+}$ mouse (*a*) and from a YD *neu* Id1$^{-/-}$Id3$^{+/-}$ mouse (*B*). (*C,E*) H&E staining of the YD *neu* Id1$^{+/+}$Id3$^{+/+}$ tumor seen in *A*. (*D,F*) H&E staining of the YD *neu* Id1$^{-/-}$Id3$^{+/-}$ tumor seen in *b*. (Reprinted, with permission, from de Candia et al. 2003 [©National Academy of Sciences].)

grossly viable, and cystic if more than 90% of the tumor volume consisted of necrotic or cystic components. Heterogeneous tumors were those that did not meet the criteria for either solid or cystic. The majority of tumors that developed in the Id wild-type mice were entirely solid (53%), with only minimal gross evidence of necrosis. In a subset of Id wild-type tumors, heterogeneous (23.5%) or cystic (23.5%) architecture was observed. In the Id-deficient mice, a significantly larger proportion of tumors were cystic in appearance (64.5%, 56.5%, and 63%, respectively, in the mice deficient in one, two, or three copies of Id).

On histological examination, the cystic lesions in Id-deficient mice consisted of a narrow rim of viable tumor cells surrounding a core of hemorrhagic fluid (Fig. 3). The morphology of the tumor cells in the viable component of the cystic lesions was similar to that observed in solid tumors. In both instances, the tumor cells were anaplastic with a complete loss of glandular morphology, a high nuclear/cytoplasmic ratio, and frequent signs of extracellular matrix invasion. Importantly, this type of "hollowing-out" of the central portion of a tumor has been observed in another antiangiogenic setting: A synovial sarcoma patient treated with the monoclonal antibody against VEGF-A (Avastin/Bevicizumab) shows a response remarkably similar to that observed in the mammary tumors developing in the reduced Id background (D. D'Adamo, pers. comm.). Increased central necrosis of a solid tumor in response to antiangiogenic stress may prove to be a general phenomenon both in animal models and in the clinic.

Abnormal Vascularization of Id-deficient Tumors

We visualized YD *neu* tumor infiltrating vessels by performing in situ hybridization with a marker for tumor endothelium, angiopoietin 2 (Maisonpierre et al. 1997). In cystic tumors, vessels were present in the adjacent extracellular matrix, but only very sporadically inside the thin rim of tumor cells (data not shown). As above, a subset of tumors in the Id-deficient background were solid. In these tumors, we observed abnormal vascularization: Tumor vessels were dilated and twisted and had significantly more anastomoses as compared to their Id wild-type counterparts (de Candia et al. 2003). This pattern has also been observed in the blood vessels of Id1$^{-/-}$Id3$^{-/-}$ embryos, and more recently in lymphoid lesions of PTEN$^{+/-}$Id1$^{-/-}$ animals (Ruzinova and Benezra 2003).

We believe the effects of Id1 and Id3 loss are primarily on the vasculature, since Id1,3 expression, as monitored by antibodies monospecific for Id1 or Id3 and showing no staining in the appropriate Id knockout animals, is confined to the vasculature (de Candia et al. 2003). Indeed, human samples also show little Id1 protein staining in approximately 50 tumor samples of all stages and grades. Rare positive cells in any of these lesions cannot be ruled out, however.

Evidence of Hypoxia in Small Id-deficient Tumors

HIF-1 (hypoxia-inducible factor 1) is a heterodimeric transcription factor regulated by oxygen concentration. The HIF-1α component of the heterodimer cannot be detected in normoxic cells given its continuous degradation via ubiquitination, while it is strongly induced by hypoxia (Huang et al. 1998). We analyzed the expression of HIF-1α by immunohistochemistry in Id wild-type and -deficient YD *neu* tumors. When we stained small lesions (<0.5 cm diameter) in which the formation of a cystic cavity had not yet occurred, we observed that none (0/12) of wild-type lesions expressed Hif-1α, while 50% (6/12) of the Id-deficient lesions showed a strong induction of Hif-1α (de Candia et al. 2003). Thus, small tumors in Id-deficient mice seem to be hypoxic as compared to tumors that arise in wild-type background. Once the solid or cystic lesions became larger (>1.5 cm diameter) Hif-1α was consistently expressed in association with areas of necrosis in Id wild-type and -deficient mice. Interestingly, in the large cystic tumors, the cells in the rim did not express Hif-1α. Thus, these cells do not seem to be hypoxic.

INTERPRETATION AND STRATEGY

The similarity between the effects of Avastin on a solid tumor and loss of Id, i.e. an increase in central necrosis surrounded by a viable rim of cells, leads one to believe that this may be a general consequence of antiangiogenic stress and therefore worthy of further investigation. Indeed, as reported in this volume, another anti-VEGF strategy known as the VEGF trap, which employs a soluble VEGF receptor fragment to sequester free VEGF in the periphery, also leads to a similar effect (see Yancopoulos, this volume). This leads to the next obvious question of how to inhibit the viable rim of cells and to effect a more complete regression of these lesions.

Oncologists have noted that killing the central core of a tumor with chemotherapeutics is more difficult than hitting the rim. Perhaps then a combination of chemotherapy plus antiangiogenic stress would show synergistic effects in eradicating the her2/neu-driven breast tumors. But what agent to choose? It seemed reasonable to assume that the dramatic up-regulation of Hif-1α we observed in the early lesions in the Id knockout backgrounds was an important "bypass" step being utilized by the viable rim to recruit or co-opt local vessels. Targeting this step seemed like a good choice. Fortunately, we had at our disposal a compound called 17-AAG, a derivative of geldanamycin which, by inhibiting the chaperone Hsp90, leads to the degradation of client proteins, one of which is Hif-1α (Mabjeesh et al. 2002). Another protein that is rapidly turned over after Hsp90 inhibition is her2/neu, the oncogene driving the growth of the lesion in the first place. Although the effects on other Hsp90 client proteins could clearly have other unwanted effects, we were encouraged that 17-AAG had been reported as having some antitumor effects on its own in other settings (Neckers 2002; Solit et al. 2002). We proposed therefore that combination of Id loss and administration of 17-AAG to inhibit the Hif-1α bypass pathway would be a more effective strategy than either treatment alone in the management of the transgene-induced mammary carcinomas.

INDUCTION OF COMPLETE REGRESSIONS

YD mice in an Id wild-type or knockout background were treated with 17 mg/kg 17-AAG for 3 consecutive days each week for 8 weeks. Following 8 weeks of therapy, the treatment in Id wild-type mice caused only a modest growth inhibition of 48% (mean tumor volume of 2270 mm^3 in vehicle-treated mice vs. 1189 mm^3 in 17-AAG-treated, $p = 0.09$). The growth inhibitory activity of 17-AAG was dramatically enhanced to 96% inhibition in Id-deficient mice (mean tumor volume of 3863 mm^3 in vehicle-treated mice vs. 138 mm^3 in 17-AAG-treated, $p = 0.0002$) (Fig. 4). With discontinuation of 17-AAG, tumor progression was observed in all mice (Fig. 4), indicating that the effect of the therapy was cytostatic and not cytotoxic in this particular regimen (see also Conclusions).

In wild-type or Id-deficient solid tumors removed from vehicle-alone-treated mice and from Id wild-type 17-AAG-treated unresponsive mice, the viable portion of the tumors consisted of homogeneous sheets of tumor cells (de Candia et al. 2003). Cells in the centers were typically quiescent while those at the periphery demonstrated a high proliferative index. Apoptotic cells were infrequent and scattered without clear pattern (not shown). In the EPL (vehicle-alone)-treated cystic tumors, the cells composing the viable rim were similarly homogeneous and possessed a high proliferative index (data not shown). In contrast, in 7 of 11 17-AAG-treated tumors, a glandular morphology was observed (4 of 4 Id-deficient tumors and 3 of 7 Id wild-type tumors). These tumors had a lower nuclear to cytoplasmic ratio, an absence of mitotic figures, and a low proliferative index. Together then, these results

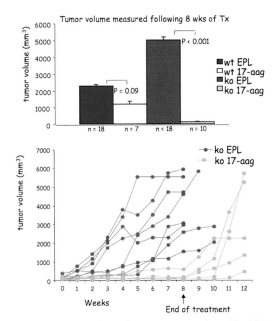

Figure 4. Induction of complete tumor regressions. (*Top*) Mean tumor volume in Id wild-type or Id-deficient animals following 8 weeks of treatment with 17-AAG 75 mg/kg or EPL vehicle only as control. 17-AAG was significantly more effective in YD *neu* Id-deficient mice (two copies missing) than in Id wt mice. Error bars, S.E. (*Bottom*) Following discontinuation of treatment, tumor regrowth was observed in all mice (each line represents change in tumor volume over time of an individual YD *neu* Id-deficient mouse treated with 17-AAG or EPL vehicle only as control). (Reprinted, with permission, from de Candia et al. 2003 [©National Academy of Sciences].)

suggest that 17-AAG has an effect on the differentiation status of the cell, regardless of the Id genotype, but that the consequence of this effect, in addition to any effect due to inhibition of the Hif-1α bypass pathway, leads to more profound growth inhibition when antiangiogenic stress is imposed on the system by loss of Id expression.

CONCLUSIONS

It has been several decades since the Judah Folkman hypothesis, elegant in its simplicity: Tumors should not be able to grow beyond a very limited size if the microvessel density is held low enough, and therefore, antiangiogenic stress should be an effective anticancer strategy. This notion, coupled with the known genetic stability of the targeted endothelial cells, led the way for the development of the new generation of antiangiogenic therapies that are now working their way into the clinic. It is important to note that this strategy went through the so-called "glitter-to-ashes" syndrome familiar to many of us in which early clinical stumbles in a novel area lead the lay press to conclude that this will never work. The technology is perceived as another example of scientists overselling their own ideas or findings, and droves begin jumping off the bandwagon. But this is just when the serious science begins. Indeed, the resurrection of the antiangiogenic approach is in full force with the recent approval of Avastin, shown, in combination with chemotherapy, to extend the lives of patients with advanced colorectal carcinoma.

Avastin will clearly not be the end of the story, however. New targets and new therapeutics are likely to follow based on the exciting science emerging from many laboratories. Indeed, there are indications from a number of preclinical studies that anti-VEGF stress and antiangiogenic stress in general will need to be supplemented with other therapies, since some tumors can find effective bypass pathways when faced with extreme hypoxia. Loss of p53, for example, has been shown to increase the resistance of tumors to antiangiogenic intervention (Yu et al. 2002), presumably by short-circuiting the apoptosis program. Tumors treated with a VEGF trap have severe microvessel density reductions but manage to co-opt local vessels at the periphery. Thus, as one might have expected on the basis of the treatment of other complex diseases, combination therapies targeting multiple points of vulnerability (the vasculature, the cell, and perhaps other components of the stroma) will be most effective in controlling cancer in human populations.

We have been modeling the effects of antiangiogenic intervention using mouse models of human cancer. As has become abundantly clear, mouse models in which oncogenes or tumor suppressor genes are misregulated (either constitutively through development or acutely in adult animals) generate cancers that are pathophysiologically very similar to human disease and are therefore more likely than subcutaneous tumors to accurately predict the course of any given intervention. We have shown that genetic inactivation of members of a gene family (Ids) essential for the mobilization, recruitment, and maturation of endothelial cells at the site of a tumor leads to severe antiangiogenic stress. The consequence of such stress on breast tumors induced by constitutive overexpression of the her2/neu oncogene in the mammary epithelia is a dramatic increase in hypoxia, which is followed by the cystification of the core of lesion but survival of a viable rim of cells at the periphery of the tumor. Subcutaneous breast tumors, on the other hand, show complete regressions in the Id-reduced background. It should be noted, however, that the Lewis lung carcinoma cells injected subcutaneously did show an ability to expand despite extensive hypoxia and necrosis, the first indication of an operational bypass pathway for tumors faced with Id reductions in the endothelium. In other spontaneous tumor model systems, we have shown that in response to reduced Id dosages, some cancers completely regress (intrauterine tumors in Pten[+/−] animals) (Ruzinova et al. 2003) and some tumors show effects that are tumor-grade-dependent (prostate tumors in TRAMP mice) (Li et al. 2004).

How do we treat the tumors that respond to antiangiogenic stress but continue to expand around the centrally necrotic core? The dramatic increase in Hif-1α staining in the early breast lesions in the Id1 knockout mice suggested that the Hif-1α hypoxia response pathway may be the mechanism of bypass. Hsp90 has been shown to be required for the proper folding and stability of Hif-1α (as well as other proteins, including her2/neu). Administration of the Hsp90 inhibitor (17-AAG) to the MMTV-her2/neu Id knockout mice (but not mice with normal tumor angiogenesis) led to the complete regression of these aggressive breast lesions. To our knowledge, this is the first complete remission ever induced in these animals. Importantly, however, when 17-AAG is removed after 8 weeks of treatment, the tumors reappear and begin growing rapidly, indicating that the therapy is cytostatic and not cytotoxic. Whether more prolonged administration of the drug to the Id knockout animals ever leads to a permanent "cure" is worthy of exploration. In any event, these animals should provide a valuable model for tumor dormancy, a problem of great clinical importance.

In summary, physiologically relevant mouse models of cancer will be important predictors of clinical efficacy of various targeted strategies. Biologists have spent the last 20 years defining the important targets in the cancer cell and its microenvironment. Through the use of spontaneous mouse tumor models, we will learn how to hit these targets effectively.

ACKNOWLEDGMENTS

This work was supported by grants from the National Institutes of Health (R.B., V.M.), American-Italian Cancer Foundation (P.d.C., A.C.), Goodwin Experimental Therapeutics (E.H., R.B.), and the Breast Cancer Research Foundation (R.B.).

REFERENCES

Anisimov V.N., Khavinsov V., Alimova I.N., Provintsiali M., Manchini R., and Francheski K. 2002. Epithalon inhibits tumor growth and expression of HER-2/neu oncogene in breast tumors in transgenic mice characterized by accelerated aging. *Bull. Exp. Biol. Med.* **133:** 167.

Baselga J., Rischin D., Ranson M., Calvert H., Raymond E., Kieback D.G., Kaye S.B., Gianni L., Harris A., Bjork T., Averbuch S.D., Feyereislova A., Swaisland H., Rojo F., and Albanell J. 2002. Phase I safety, pharmacokinetic, and pharmacodynamic trial of ZD1839, a selective oral epidermal growth factor receptor tyrosine kinase inhibitor, in patients with five selected solid tumor types. *J. Clin. Oncol.* **20:** 4292.

Dankort D., Maslikowski B., Warner N., Kanno N., Kim H., Wang Z., Moran M.F., Oshima R.G., Cardiff R.D., and Muller W.J. 2001. Grb2 and Shc adapter proteins play distinct roles in Neu (ErbB-2)-induced mammary tumorigenesis: Implications for human breast cancer. *Mol. Cell. Biol.* **21:** 1540.

de Candia P., Solit D.B., Giri D., Brogi E., Siegel P.M., Olshen A.B., Muller W.J., Rosen N., and Benezra R. 2003. Angiogenesis impairment in Id-deficient mice cooperates with an Hsp90 inhibitor to completely suppress HER2/neu-dependent breast tumors. *Proc. Natl. Acad. Sci.* **100:** 12337.

Fraidenraich D., Stillwell E., Romero E., Wilkes D., Manova K., Basson C.T., and Benezra R. 2004. Rescue of cardiac defects in id knockout embryos by injection of embryonic stem cells. *Science* **306:** 247.

Giannelli G., Falk-Marzillier J., Schiraldi O., Stetler-Stevenson W.G., and Quaranta V. 1997. Induction of cell migration by matrix metalloprotease-2 cleavage of laminin-5. *Science* **277:** 225.

Guy C.T., Webster M.A., Schaller M., Parsons T.J., Cardiff R.D., and Muller W.J. 1992. Expression of the neu protooncogene in the mammary epithelium of transgenic mice induces metastatic disease. *Proc. Natl. Acad. Sci.* **89:** 10578.

Huang L.E., Gu J., Schau M., and Bunn H.F. 1998. Regulation of hypoxia-inducible factor 1alpha is mediated by an O2-dependent degradation domain via the ubiquitin-proteasome pathway. *Proc. Natl. Acad. Sci.* **95:** 7987.

Jen Y., Manova K., and Benezra R. 1996. Expression patterns of Id1, Id2, and Id3 are highly related but distinct from that of Id4 during mouse embryogenesis. *Dev. Dyn.* **207:** 235.
———. 1997. Each member of the Id gene family exhibits a unique expression pattern in mouse gastrulation and neurogenesis. *Dev. Dyn.* **208:** 92.

Klein S., Giancotti F.G., Presta M., Albelda S.M., Buck C.A., and Rifkin D.B. 1993. Basic fibroblast growth factor modulates integrin expression in microvascular endothelial cells. *Mol. Biol. Cell* **4:** 973.

Li H., Gerald W.L., and Benezra R. 2004. Utilization of bone marrow-derived endothelial cell precursors in spontaneous prostate tumors varies with tumor grade. *Cancer Res.* **64:** 6137.

Lyden D., Young A.Z., Zagzag D., Yan W., Gerald W., O'Reilly R., Bader B.L., Hynes R.O., Zhuang Y., Manova K., and Benezra R. 1999. Id1 and Id3 are required for neurogenesis, angiogenesis and vascularization of tumour xenografts. *Nature* **401:** 670.

Lyden D., Hattori K., Dias S., Costa C., Blaikie P., Butros L., Chadburn A., Heissig B., Marks W., Witte L., Wu Y., Hicklin D., Zhu Z., Hackett N.R., Crystal R.G., Moore M.A., Hajjar K.A., Manova K., Benezra R., and Rafii S. 2001. Impaired recruitment of bone-marrow-derived endothelial and hematopoietic precursor cells blocks tumor angiogenesis and growth. *Nat. Med.* **7:** 1194.

Mabjeesh N.J., Post D.E., Willard M.T., Kaur B., Van Meir E.G., Simons J.W., and Zhong H. 2002. Geldanamycin induces degradation of hypoxia-inducible factor 1alpha protein via the proteosome pathway in prostate cancer cells. *Cancer Res.* **62:** 2478.

Maisonpierre P.C., Suri C., Jones P.F., Bartunkova S., Wiegand S.J., Radziejewski C., Compton D., McClain J., Aldrich T.H., Papadopoulos N., Daly T.J., Davis S., Sato T.N., and Yancopoulos G.D. 1997. Angiopoietin-2, a natural antagonist for Tie2 that disrupts in vivo angiogenesis. *Science* **277:** 55.

Manor D., Shmidt E.N., Budhu A., Flesken-Nikitin A., Zgola M., Page R., Nikitin A.Y., and Noy N. 2003. Mammary carcinoma suppression by cellular retinoic acid binding protein-II. *Cancer Res.* **63:** 4426.

Neckers L. 2002. Heat shock protein 90 inhibition by 17-allyl-amino-17- demethoxygeldanamycin: A novel therapeutic approach for treating hormone-refractory prostate cancer. *Clin. Cancer Res.* **8:** 962.

Nikolopoulos S.N., Blaikie P., Yoshioka T., Guo W., and Giancotti F.G. 2004. Integrin beta4 signaling promotes tumor angiogenesis. *Cancer Cell* **6:** 471.

Perk J., Iavarone I., and Benezra R. 2005. The Id family of HLH proteins in cancer. *Nat. Rev. Cancer* **5:** 603.

Pfeifer A., Kessler T., Silletti S., Cheresh D.A., and Verma I.M. 2000. Suppression of angiogenesis by lentiviral delivery of PEX, a noncatalytic fragment of matrix metalloproteinase 2. *Proc. Natl. Acad. Sci.* **97:** 12227.

Ruzinova M.B. and Benezra R. 2003. Id proteins in development, cell cycle and cancer. *Trends Cell Biol.* **13:** 410.

Ruzinova M.B., Schoer R.A., Gerald W., Egan J.E., Pandolfi P.P., Rafii S., Manova K., Mittal V., and Benezra R. 2003. Effect of angiogenesis inhibition by Id loss and the contribution of bone-marrow-derived endothelial cells in spontaneous murine tumors. *Cancer Cell* **4:** 277.

Sacco M.G., Benedetti S., Duflot-Dancer A., Mesnil M., Bagnasco L., Strina D., Fasolo V., Villa A., Macchi P., Faranda S., Vezzoni P., and Finocchiaro G. 1996. Partial regression, yet incomplete eradication of mammary tumors in transgenic mice by retrovirally mediated HSVtk transfer 'in vivo'. *Gene Ther.* **3:** 1151.

Shah N., Antony T., Haddad S., Amenta P., Shirahata A., Thomas T.J., and Thomas T. 1999. Antitumor effects of bis(ethyl)polyamine analogs on mammary tumor development in FVB/NTgN (MMTVneu) transgenic mice. *Cancer Lett.* **146:** 15.

Slamon D.J., Clark G.M., Wong S.G., Levin W.J., Ullrich A., and McGuire W.L. 1987. Human breast cancer: Correlation of relapse and survival with amplification of the HER-2/neu oncogene. *Science* **235:** 177.

Slamon D.J., Leyland-Jones B., Shak S., Fuchs H., Paton V., Bajamonde A., Fleming T., Eiermann W., Wolter J., Pegram M., Baselga J., and Norton L. 2001. Use of chemotherapy plus a monoclonal antibody against HER2 for metastatic breast cancer that overexpresses HER2. *N. Engl. J. Med.* **344:** 783.

Solit D.B., Zheng F.F., Drobnjak M., Munster P.N., Higgins B., Verbel D., Heller G., Tong W., Cordon-Cardo C., Agus D.B., Scher H.I., and Rosen N. 2002. 17-Allylamino-17-demethoxygeldanamycin induces the degradation of androgen receptor and HER-2/neu and inhibits the growth of prostate cancer xenografts. *Clin. Cancer Res.* **8:** 986.

Vogel C.L., Cobleigh M.A., Tripathy D., Gutheil J.C., Harris L.N., Fehrenbacher L., Slamon D.J., Murphy M., Novotny W.F., Burchmore M., Shak S., Stewart S.J., and Press M. 2002. Efficacy and safety of trastuzumab as a single agent in first-line treatment of HER2-overexpressing metastatic breast cancer. *J. Clin. Oncol.* **20:** 719.

Yu J.L., Rak J.W., Coomber B.L., Hicklin D.J., and Kerbel R.S. 2002. Effect of p53 status on tumor response to antiangiogenic therapy. *Science* **295:** 1526.

The Fibroblastic Coconspirator in Cancer Progression

M. Egeblad, L.E. Littlepage, and Z. Werb

Department of Anatomy, and Comprehensive Cancer Center, University of California,
San Francisco, California 94143-0452

A remarkable change has occurred in the thinking about epithelial-derived cancer in recent years: From almost entirely focusing on oncogenes and tumor suppressor genes has come the realization that the tumor microenvironment is a coconspirator in the carcinogenic process. Many types of stromal cells, including fibroblasts, adipocytes, macrophages, mast cells, and cells of the vascular system, are crucial contributors to epithelial carcinogenesis. Here, we focus on the fibroblast's role in cancer progression and the molecules involved in the communications between the fibroblasts and the cancer cells, including fibroblast secreted protein 1 (FSP-1 or S100A4), transforming growth factor β (TGF-β), the chemokine CXCL-12 (stromal derived factor 1 α, SDF-1α), type I collagen, and matrix metalloproteinase 13 (MMP-13).

It is now accepted that the stromal microenvironment contributes to tumorigenesis in cancers of epithelial origin. The mutation that initiates the carcinoma occurs in the epithelium, but events that promote tumor progression involve the stroma. In fact, in some cases, the trigger for neoplastic progression may even come from signals within the stromal microenvironment (for review, see Radisky et al. 2001; Bhowmick et al. 2004a). The stromal microenvironment consists of several cell types (fibroblasts, macrophages, vascular components, and inflammatory cells of the innate and acquired immune response), as well as the extracellular matrix (ECM) that they elaborate and all the molecules that are concentrated and immobilized on it. All of these components communicate with each other and with the neoplastic cells to contribute to the aberrant tumor organ.

A classic example of a stromal signal that can trigger neoplasms is chronic inflammation. Epidemiological evidence supporting an association of inflammation with cancer comes from studies showing a relationship between inflammatory bowel disease and colon cancer, between *Helicobacter pylori* infection of the stomach and stomach cancer, and between hepatitis C infection and liver cancer (for review, see Coussens and Werb 2002). Experimental evidence for the link between inflammation and stromal promotion of cancer comes from the studies on two-stage carcinogenesis, in which mutagens do not produce tumors, but require the application of tumor promoters, such as phorbol esters, which can occur long after carcinogen exposure. The tumor promoters trigger an inflammatory response and generate an aberrant tumor-promoting stroma. Another process that can generate tumor-promoting stroma experimentally is irradiation. Irradiation of the mammary gland induces nonreversible changes in the stroma that contribute to neoplasia: Nontransformed mammary epithelial cells injected into irradiated mammary stromal fat pads have greatly increased tumor growth compared to those injected into the contralateral, nonirradiated mammary fat pads (Barcellos-Hoff and Ravani 2000). Similar results have been obtained when comparing nonirradiated fibroblasts with

irradiated fibroblasts, where only the latter stimulates invasiveness of pancreatic cancer (Ohuchida et al. 2004).

Here we discuss the role of the fibroblastic component of the tumor stroma in stimulating neoplastic progression.

FIBROBLASTS INFLUENCE TUMOR PROGRESSION

The fibroblast is one of several cell types involved in stromal regulation of cancer. The fibroblast is capable of adapting to tissue injury, and during wound healing it changes its phenotype to become "reactive." The reactive fibroblast is also known as a myofibroblast—a cell type that shares properties with both fibroblasts and the smooth muscle cells. In addition to wound healing, neoplasia represents another situation where reactive fibroblasts are observed. The reactive fibroblasts observed during neoplasia are often referred to as carcinoma-associated fibroblasts (CAFs). The CAFs differ from normal fibroblasts by abnormally high expression of smooth muscle actin and increased expression of proteolytic enzymes and ECM proteins, such as tenascin.

The importance of the CAFs in epithelial carcinogenesis has been established in recombination experiments: When immortalized, nontumorigenic human prostate epithelial cells were mixed with fibroblasts from human prostate carcinomas grafted to immune-deficient animals, the epithelial cells developed into large carcinomas. In contrast, mixing the epithelial cells with fibroblasts from a normal prostate gland did not result in carcinomas (Olumi et al. 1999).

FIBROBLAST-SECRETED PROTEIN 1 STIMULATES EPITHELIAL CANCER PROGRESSION

The recombination experiments illustrate the effects of CAFs on epithelial carcinogenesis, but only recently have some of the molecules responsible for these effects been identified. However, most of these molecules are not exclusively expressed by the CAFs in the carcinomas. An example is fibroblast-secreted protein (FSP1, also called S100A4 or mts1), which is expressed in both CAFs and carcinoma cells during tumor progression (Ambartsumian et al. 1996), and possibly also by macrophages (Inoue et al. 2005). FSP1 is a calcium-binding protein with both intracellular and extracellular protein-binding partners. Intracellularly, it interacts with and possibly inactivates p53. FSP1 also interacts with non-muscle myosin heavy chain, actin filaments, and non-muscle tropomyosin, thereby potentially influencing the cytoskeleton and regulating cell motility (for review, see Helfman et al. 2005). The extracellular binding partners of FSP1 are largely unknown, with the exception of Annexin II. FSP1 binds to this coreceptor for the serine proteinase plasminogen, which results in increased activation of plasminogen (Semov et al. 2005). FSP1 is proangiogenic, and this is possibly mediated either by the activation of plasminogen or through the transcriptional up-regulation of matrix metalloproteinase (MMP) 13 (Schmidt-Hansen et al. 2004). Both of these proteinases are thought to play a role in endothelial cell invasion.

Compelling evidence exists for FSP as a crucial CAF-expressed factor regulating metastasis: Carcinoma cells that are metastatic when injected into wild-type mice are less likely to form tumors and do not metastasize at all when injected into *Fsp1*$^{-/-}$ mice. Coinjection of *Fsp1*$^{+/+}$ fibroblasts with the tumor cells restores tumor development and metastasis in the *Fsp1*$^{-/-}$ animals, whereas coinjection with *Fsp1*$^{-/-}$ fibroblasts does not (Grum-Schwensen et al. 2005). This suggests that FSP1, when secreted by the fibroblasts, alters the stromal microenvironment, making it more favorable for tumor progression. This could be through the regulation of angiogenesis and inflammation: Tumors forming after coinjection of carcinoma cells with *Fsp1*$^{-/-}$ cells had significantly decreased numbers of infiltrating macrophages, smooth muscle actin-expressing myofibroblasts, and CD31-positive endothelial cells compared to tumors developing after coinjection with *Fsp1*$^{+/+}$ cells (Grum-Schwensen et al. 2005).

As mentioned, FSP1 is also up-regulated in metastatic carcinoma cells, and this can result in the fibroblastic phenotype of the carcinoma cells known as epithelial-to-mesenchymal transition (EMT). EMT has been proposed to be the mechanism responsible for the metastatic phenotype induced by FSP1 (Xue et al. 2003). If FSP1 mainly exerts its tumor-promoting function as a secreted protein, the cellular source of its secretion might not be important. It is possible that FSP1 can be an important factor that induces angiogenesis, inflammation, and EMT, depending on which cell type it acts on rather than which cell type secretes it.

CXCL12 STIMULATES EPITHELIAL CANCER PROGRESSION THROUGH EFFECTS ON CANCER CELLS AND ENDOTHELIAL CELLS

The CXC chemokine CXCL12 (also known as stromal cell-derived factor 1 α, SDF-1α) is another important factor secreted by CAFs (Orimo et al. 2005). CXCL12 acts through several mechanisms: It acts directly on the mammary carcinoma cells stimulating proliferation through

the CXCL12 receptor CXCR4. CXCL12 has also been proposed to stimulate metastasis to the lung and to lymph nodes through high expression of the chemokine at these organ sites, resulting in homing of the cancer cells, which express the CXCL12 receptor, to these organs (Muller et al. 2001). In addition to direct actions on the tumor cells, CXCL12 secretion by CAFs leads to recruitment of endothelial cell precursors to the growing tumor, thereby promoting angiogenesis (Orimo et al. 2005). As mentioned above, there is a strong link between stromal changes, inflammation, and carcinoma progression also when it comes to the effects mediated by the fibroblasts. So far, the functions of CAF-secreted CXCL12 have only been studied using xenograft models employing immune-compromised mice, which makes it impossible to address direct interactions between CAFs and leukocytes mediated by CXCL12. However, CXCL12 is a well-established chemoattractant for leukocytes, and it is thus very likely that CXCL12 would have additional effects acting through leukocytes if studied in the context of a full cellular immune response.

TGF-β HAS BOTH CANCER-PROMOTING AND -INHIBITING EFFECTS, DEPENDING ON WHICH CELL TYPE IT ACTS ON

TGF-β is one of the key players involved in the communications between CAFs and carcinoma cells, but again is expressed by multiple cell types including the stromal fibroblasts, the inflammatory cells, and carcinoma cells (Bhowmick and Moses 2005). Whereas FSP1 and CXCL12 clearly are CAF-secreted promoters of carcinogenesis, TGF-β is a factor with much more complicated effects on tumorigenesis. TGF-β is immune-suppressive when acting on inflammatory cells, thereby promoting carcinogenesis through inhibition of the immune response against the neoplasm. However, when acting on the epithelium, TGF-β is growth-inhibiting and thus inhibits carcinogenesis until the carcinoma cells overcome the growth-suppressive effects of TGF-β, and TGF-β becomes a stimulator of metastasis (for review, see Bhowmick and Moses 2005). Several groups have shown that TGF-β1 can induce differentiation of resting fibroblasts into myofibroblasts in culture (for review, see Elenbaas and Weinberg 2001). Furthermore, increased secretion of TGF-β in irradiated mammary stroma has been suggested as part of the mechanism by which irradiated stroma stimulates tumorigenesis (Barcellos-Hoff and Ravani 2000). Finally, overexpression of TGF-β by fibroblasts stimulates neoplastic growth of human breast epithelium in vivo (Kuperwasser et al. 2004). Thus, TGF-β is a key player in both the generation of a reactive stroma and its action. The actions of TGF-β are clearly cell-type-specific: When the TGF-β receptor II is genetically removed from fibroblasts in mice, rendering these fibroblasts unresponsive to TGF-β signaling, the mice develop neoplasias and carcinomas without any further genetic manipulations of the epithelium (Bhowmick et al. 2004b). However, ablation of the TGF-β receptor II in epithelial cells inhibits tumor progression (Forrester et al. 2005). These results suggest that TGF-β acting on the fibroblasts normally protects the epithelium from developing into carcinomas, whereas TGF-β secreted by CAFs and acting on the epithelium promotes carcinogenesis.

TYPE I COLLAGEN AND CANCER PROGRESSION

In carcinoma, the CAFs are largely responsible for the desmoplastic response, which is a strong stromal response characterized by pronounced changes in the ECM, including increased amounts of collagens, fibronectins, proteoglycans, and glycosaminoglycans (Elenbaas and Weinberg 2001). Many carcinomas, including human breast cancer, show a remarkable up-regulation of fibrillar collagen and collagen-associated proteins. In fact, some of the changes in the composition of the ECM may occur before the carcinoma evolves: High mammographic breast density is a strong predisposing factor for the development of sporadic breast cancer and confers a risk of about 4 relative to women with fatty breasts (Vacek and Geller 2004). Mammographic density is reflective of a changed stromal microenvironment, including increased amounts of collagen (Guo et al. 2001). Since many stromal effects on normal development and tumor development of the mammary gland are shared (Wiseman and Werb 2002), we have undertaken studies to determine the role of type I collagen metabolism in the developing mammary gland. Type I collagen is one of the classic substrates of the MMPs, a family of proteolytic enzymes identified as modifiers of mammary carcinogenesis (for review, see Egeblad and Werb 2002). We found that cleavage of collagen by MMPs is an important step in normal development of the mammary gland (M. Egeblad et al., in prep.). Whether type I collagen metabolism also plays a role in mammary carcinoma remains to be determined. However, it is noteworthy that the presence of collagen-dense fibrotic foci within mammary carcinomas is correlated with an adverse prognosis (Hasebe et al. 2001) and that increased expression of collagen type I is associated with increased risk of metastasis and decreased survival in many human cancers, including breast, lung, and prostate cancers (Ramaswamy et al. 2003).

How collagen contributes to the development and progression of cancer is not known. However, it is known that cancer cells are influenced by the ECM. For example, the sensitivity of cancer cells to apoptotic stimuli is regulated by interactions between integrin receptors on the cancer cells and proteins in the ECM (Weaver et al. 2002). Furthermore, malignant transformation of the breast is associated with dramatic changes in gland tension that include increased ECM stiffness, elevated compression forces, and high tensional resistance stresses. These changes perturb tissue morphogenesis and facilitate tumor invasion (Paszek and Weaver 2004). Interestingly, overexpression of lysyl oxidase-related protein-1 (LOR-1), a protein that is involved in the cross-linking and thereby stabilization of the collagen fibers, results in the formation of very dense collagen fibers surrounding the tumors (Akiri et al. 2003). However, rather than preventing invasion through the encapsulation of the carci-

noma, the LOR-1-overexpressing cells become highly invasive (Akiri et al. 2003).

In addition to any direct effects on the cancer cells, collagen may play a role in the regulation of leukocyte behavior within tumors. In mouse mammary tumors, we found high expression levels of collagen in areas of leukocytes. Indeed, the literature suggests cross-talk between the collagenous stroma and the infiltrating leukocytes in tumors: Macrophages and dendritic cells become activated and secrete chemokines in response to binding to type I collagen (Matsuyama et al. 2004). Vice versa, leukocytes produce the ECM protein, SPARC, which determines stroma and collagen deposition in carcinomas. In the absence of leukocyte-produced SPARC, tumor growth is reduced and large areas of necrosis and impaired vascularization are observed (Sangaletti et al. 2003).

REMODELING OF THE TUMOR MICROENVIRONMENT BY MMPs

The remodeling of the stromal microenvironment (e.g., the cleavage of type I collagen) is mediated in part by secreted proteinases, including the MMPs (Egeblad and Werb 2002). Among the more than 24 MMPs, MMP-13 caught our attention because of the cells that express it and because of its substrates: MMP-13 is expressed by CAF-like cells in human breast cancer (Nielsen et al. 2001), and in vitro, breast cancer cells can stimulate fibroblasts to secrete MMP-13 (Uria et al. 1997). However, MMP-13 may also be expressed by lymphocytes (Willmroth et al. 1998; Wahlgren et al. 2001). Several proteins are known to be substrates for MMP-13 in vitro, including TGF-β, CXCL12, and type I collagen (Egeblad and Werb 2002). Latent TGF-β is cleaved and activated by MMP-13 (D'Angelo et al. 2001), CXCL12 is cleaved and inactivated by MMP-13 (McQuibban et al. 2001), and type I collagen is cleaved into specific fragments by MMP-13. Thus, MMP-13 is a factor secreted by CAFs that may regulate the activity of other factors secreted by or acting on the CAFs, complicating the interpretation of the role of the individual factors in carcinogenesis. In addition to the examples with MMP-13 and its CAF-secreted substrates, TGF-β1 can up-regulate the CXCL12 receptor CXCR4 (Chen et al. 2005), TGF-β1 and type I collagen can stimulate FSP-1 protein expression (Okada et al. 1997), and FSP1 can stimulate endothelial cells to up-regulate the expression of MMP-13 (Schmidt-Hansen et al. 2004). Thus, stromal factors and stromal cells are coconspirators and may act both additively and synergistically, or may repress each other's functions (Fig. 1).

WHAT IS A CAF?

Although we are now starting to understand what molecules are secreted by CAFs and what their functions are, we know surprisingly little about what the tumor-promoting CAFs themselves are and what distinguishes them from the normal fibroblasts. Like true fibroblasts, CAFs express vimentin. However, they also express α-smooth muscle actin and can contract collagen gels in vitro, thereby resembling myofibroblasts. Thus, the ori-

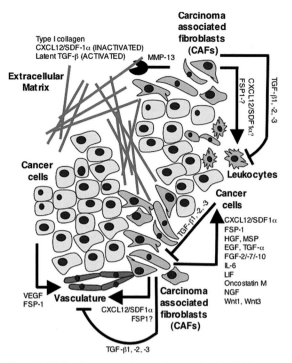

Type I collagen
CXCL12/SDF-1α (INACTIVATED)
Latent TGF-β (ACTIVATED)
MMP-13

Carcinoma
associated
fibroblasts
(CAFs)

CXCL12/SDF1α?
FSP1-?
TGF-β1, -2, -3

Extracellular
Matrix

Leukocytes

Cancer
cells

Cancer
cells

CXCL12/SDF1α
FSP-1
HGF, MSP
EGF, TGF-α
FGF-2/-7/-10
IL-6
LIF
Oncostatin M
NGF
Wnt1, Wnt3

TGF-β1, -2, -3

VEGF
FSP-1

Vasculature

CXCL12/SDF1α
FSP1?

Carcinoma
associated
fibroblasts
(CAFs)

TGF-β1, -2, -3

Figure 1. Molecular coconspirators of stromal-epithelial interactions during tumorigenesis. The cells in the tumor tissue communicate during tumor progression through the secretion of growth factors, chemokines, and cytokines. Shown here are examples of modulators of tumorigenesis that are secreted by one cell type and act on another through activation (*arrows*), inactivation (*blocked lines*), or proteolytic cleavage (*chewing symbol*).

gin of these cells is unclear. They could be derived from fibroblasts or fibroblast precursors and change into CAFs through stimulation by the carcinoma cells. Indeed, it has been shown that when normal fibroblasts are cocultured with carcinoma cells, the fibroblasts undergo a myofibroblastic conversion (Ronnov-Jessen et al. 1995).

Interestingly, the CAFs maintain their ability to stimulate tumor progression through several cell passages but show no evidence of genetic alterations and senesce normally in culture (Orimo et al. 2005). Thus, this would suggest a nonreversible epigenetic change of the fibroblasts. However, the CAFs' ability to stimulate carcinogenesis, even after having been cultured for several generations without further stimulation from the cancer cells, makes it tempting to speculate that the CAFs are an expanded population of an early developmental precursor initially present in the normal precancerous mammary gland, a population that first expands in response to signals from the cancer cells. Data from Schor and coworkers (Schor et al. 1994) suggest that cells with CAF-like properties are present before tumors evolve: When fibroblasts were isolated from breast tissue from patients undergoing surgery for either benign mammary gland lesions or cancer, it was found that the cancer patients' fibroblasts were more motile than the fibroblasts from the patients with benign lesions, even though the fibroblasts were isolated in normal tissue, away from the cancer or the benign lesion. In a subset of the breast cancer patients, they even isolated fibroblasts from the skin that were abnormally motile.

These data therefore suggest that the presence of fibroblasts with CAF-like properties predisposes for the development of cancer, and they raise the question as to whether this is through germ-line mutations that determine fibroblast behavior. Indeed, the premalignant hamartomatous lesions of juvenile polyposis coli, which arise from germ-line mutations in the SMAD4 gene, are largely fibroblastic in nature, and thus a mutation in the stromal compartment initiates the development of the premalignant lesions that eventually lead to colon cancer (Howe et al. 1998; Kinzler and Vogelstein 1998; Vogelstein and Kinzler 2004). Data suggest that the stroma also can be the target of somatic mutations and that, at least in some cases, the mutations found in the fibroblastic cells and the carcinoma cells are different (Moinfar et al. 2000; Kurose et al. 2002). This strongly suggests that the CAFs are not derived from the carcinoma cells, e.g., by EMT, but rather that the mutations have arisen independently in the two cell populations. However, in other cases, CAFs may in fact be derived from carcinoma cells that have undergone EMT. Indeed, immortal fibroblast-like cells that had the same X-inactivation pattern as the epithelial carcinoma cells in the tumor have been isolated from human breast cancer (Petersen et al. 2003). The cells were not tumorigenic by themselves but behaved like CAFs, stimulating epithelial carcinoma cell activation of MMPs in vitro and tumor growth in vivo (Petersen et al. 2003).

CONCLUSIONS AND PERSPECTIVE

It appears that tumors have developed multiple different ways to ensure that CAF-like cells are present in the tumor organ: CAFs may be an expanded precursor cell population, epigenetically changed fibroblasts, mutated fibroblasts, or even epithelial cells that have undergone EMT. Why have the tumors developed so many different ways of recruiting CAFs? Do the CAFs arise as a part of a defense mechanism against the tumor—an attempt to encapsulate the tumors—or do the cancer cells recruit the CAFs (by either of the mechanisms mentioned above) because the communications between the cancer cells and the CAFs are crucial for the tumor progression? These are some of the important questions to be addressed in the future.

The molecular basis for the influence of fibroblast-like cells, the CAFs, on epithelial cancers is emerging, and genes expressed by the stromal cells in the tumors are promising prognostic predictors in human breast cancer (West et al. 2005). Whereas a normal stroma may protect the epithelium from tumorigenesis, an aberrant stroma can initiate tumorigenesis (Olumi et al. 1999; Bhowmick et al. 2004b; Kuperwasser et al. 2004; Ohuchida et al. 2004). Stunningly, restoration of normal microenvironmental signaling can reverse the malignant phenotype in vitro even though the tumor cells retain all their mutations (Weaver et al. 1997). In vivo, malignant mouse teratocarcinoma cells, propagated for 8 years as ascites tumors, when injected into blastocysts, remarkably contributed to multiple cell types in the mice that developed normally with no teratocarcinomas (Mintz and Illmensee 1975).

The ability of the CAFs to regulate epithelial carcinogenesis makes them potential drug targets. However, we are still far from developing strategies to restore aberrant signaling between the fibroblasts and the epithelium in carcinomas. Nevertheless, a few drugs that target the stromal influence on carcinogenesis (e.g., angiogenesis inhibitors) are showing significant effects on cancer patient survival, proving that targeting the stroma is a feasible direction for cancer treatment (Joyce 2005). The complex signaling network within the cancer cells has long been studied and targeted for drug development. The complex signaling between the cells in the tumor tissue is now taking off.

ACKNOWLEDGMENTS

This work was supported by grants from the National Cancer Institute (CA57621, CA58207, and CA10537), a fellowship from the Danish Medical Research Council to M.E., and a Ruth L. Kirschstein National Research Service Award from the National Institutes of Health (F32 CA103534) to L.E.L.

REFERENCES

Akiri G., Sabo E., Dafni H., Vadasz Z., Kartvelishvily Y., Gan N., Kessler O., Cohen T., Resnick M., Neeman M., and Neufeld G. 2003. Lysyl oxidase-related protein-1 promotes tumor fibrosis and tumor progression in vivo. *Cancer Res.* **63:** 1657.

Ambartsumian N.S., Grigorian M.S., Larsen I.F., Karlstrom O., Sidenius N., Rygaard J., Georgiev G., and Lukanidin E. 1996. Metastasis of mammary carcinomas in GRS/A hybrid mice transgenic for the mts1 gene. *Oncogene* **13:** 1621.

Barcellos-Hoff M.H. and Ravani S.A. 2000. Irradiated mammary gland stroma promotes the expression of tumorigenic potential by unirradiated epithelial cells. *Cancer Res.* **60:** 1254.

Bhowmick N.A. and Moses H.L. 2005. Tumor-stroma interactions. *Curr. Opin. Genet. Dev.* **15:** 97.

Bhowmick N.A., Neilson E.G., and Moses H.L. 2004a. Stromal fibroblasts in cancer initiation and progression. *Nature* **432:** 332.

Bhowmick N.A., Chytil A., Plieth D., Gorska A.E., Dumont N., Shappell S., Washington M.K., Neilson E.G., and Moses H.L. 2004b. TGF-beta signaling in fibroblasts modulates the oncogenic potential of adjacent epithelia. *Science* **303:** 848.

Chen S., Tuttle D.L., Oshier J.T., Knot H.J., Streit W.J., Goodenow M.M., and Harrison J.K. 2005. Transforming growth factor-beta1 increases CXCR4 expression, stromal-derived factor-1alpha-stimulated signalling and human immunodeficiency virus-1 entry in human monocyte-derived macrophages. *Immunology* **114:** 565.

Coussens L.M. and Werb Z. 2002. Inflammation and cancer. *Nature* **420:** 860.

D'Angelo M., Billings P.C., Pacifici M., Leboy P.S., and Kirsch T. 2001. Authentic matrix vesicles contain active metalloproteases (MMP). A role for matrix vesicle-associated MMP-13 in activation of transforming growth factor-beta. *J. Biol. Chem.* **276:** 11347.

Egeblad M. and Werb Z. 2002. New functions for the matrix metalloproteinases in cancer progression. *Nat. Rev. Cancer* **2:** 161.

Elenbaas B. and Weinberg R.A. 2001. Heterotypic signaling between epithelial tumor cells and fibroblasts in carcinoma formation. *Exp. Cell Res.* **264:** 169.

Forrester E., Chytil A., Bierie B., Aakre M., Gorska A.E., Sharif-Afshar A.R., Muller W.J., and Moses H.L. 2005. Effect of conditional knockout of the type II TGF-beta receptor gene in mammary epithelia on mammary gland development and polyomavirus middle T antigen induced tumor formation and

metastasis. *Cancer Res.* **65:** 2296.

Grum-Schwensen B., Klingelhofer J., Berg C.H., El-Naaman C., Grigorian M., Lukanidin E., and Ambartsumian N. 2005. Suppression of tumor development and metastasis formation in mice lacking the S100A4(mts1) gene. *Cancer Res.* **65:** 3772.

Guo Y.P., Martin L.J., Hanna W., Banerjee D., Miller N., Fishell E., Khokha R., and Boyd N.F. 2001. Growth factors and stromal matrix proteins associated with mammographic densities. *Cancer Epidemiol. Biomark. Prev.* **10:** 243.

Hasebe T., Sasaki S., Imoto S., and Ochiai A. 2001. Highly proliferative fibroblasts forming fibrotic focus govern metastasis of invasive ductal carcinoma of the breast. *Mod. Pathol.* **14:** 325.

Helfman D.M., Kim E.J., Lukanidin E., and Grigorian M. 2005. The metastasis associated protein S100A4: Role in tumour progression and metastasis. *Br. J. Cancer* **92:** 1955.

Howe J.R., Roth S., Ringold J.C., Summers R.W., Jarvinen H.J., Sistonen P., Tomlinson I.P., Houlston R.S., Bevan S., Mitros F.A., Stone E.M., and Aaltonen L.A. 1998. Mutations in the SMAD4/DPC4 gene in juvenile polyposis. *Science* **280:** 1086.

Inoue T., Plieth D., Venkov C.D., Xu C., and Neilson E.G. 2005. Antibodies against macrophages that overlap in specificity with fibroblasts. *Kidney Int.* **67:** 2488.

Joyce J.A. 2005. Therapeutic targeting of the tumor microenvironment. *Cancer Cell* **7:** 513.

Kinzler K.W. and Vogelstein B. 1998. Landscaping the cancer terrain. *Science* **280:** 1036.

Kuperwasser C., Chavarria T., Wu M., Magrane G., Gray J.W., Carey L., Richardson A., and Weinberg R.A. 2004. Reconstruction of functionally normal and malignant human breast tissues in mice. *Proc. Natl. Acad. Sci.* **101:** 4966.

Kurose K., Gilley K., Matsumoto S., Watson P.H., Zhou X.P., and Eng C. 2002. Frequent somatic mutations in PTEN and TP53 are mutually exclusive in the stroma of breast carcinomas. *Nat. Genet.* **32:** 355.

Matsuyama W., Wang L., Farrar W.L., Faure M., and Yoshimura T. 2004. Activation of discoidin domain receptor 1 isoform b with collagen up-regulates chemokine production in human macrophages: Role of p38 mitogen-activated protein kinase and NF-kappa B. *J. Immunol.* **172:** 2332.

McQuibban G.A., Butler G.S., Gong J.H., Bendall L., Power C., Clark-Lewis I., and Overall C.M. 2001. Matrix metalloproteinase activity inactivates the CXC chemokine stromal cell-derived factor-1. *J. Biol. Chem.* **276:** 43503.

Mintz B. and Illmensee K. 1975. Normal genetically mosaic mice produced from malignant teratocarcinoma cells. *Proc. Natl. Acad. Sci.* **72:** 3585.

Moinfar F., Man Y.G., Arnould L., Bratthauer G.L., Ratschek M., and Tavassoli F.A. 2000. Concurrent and independent genetic alterations in the stromal and epithelial cells of mammary carcinoma: Implications for tumorigenesis. *Cancer Res.* **60:** 2562.

Muller A., Homey B., Soto H., Ge N., Catron D., Buchanan M.E., McClanahan T., Murphy E., Yuan W., Wagner S.N., Barrera J.L., Mohar A., Verastegui E., and Zlotnik A. 2001. Involvement of chemokine receptors in breast cancer metastasis. *Nature* **410:** 50.

Nielsen B.S., Rank F., Lopez J.M., Balbin M., Vizoso F., Lund L.R., Dano K., and Lopez-Otin C. 2001. Collagenase-3 expression in breast myofibroblasts as a molecular marker of transition of ductal carcinoma in situ lesions to invasive ductal carcinomas. *Cancer Res.* **61:** 7091.

Ohuchida K., Mizumoto K., Murakami M., Qian L.W., Sato N., Nagai E., Matsumoto K., Nakamura T., and Tanaka M. 2004. Radiation to stromal fibroblasts increases invasiveness of pancreatic cancer cells through tumor-stromal interactions. *Cancer Res.* **64:** 3215.

Okada H., Danoff T.M., Kalluri R., and Neilson E.G. 1997. Early role of Fsp1 in epithelial-mesenchymal transformation. *Am. J. Physiol.* **273:** F563.

Olumi A.F., Grossfeld G.D., Hayward S.W., Carroll P.R., Tlsty T.D., and Cunha G.R. 1999. Carcinoma-associated fibroblasts direct tumor progression of initiated human prostatic epithelium. *Cancer Res.* **59:** 5002.

Orimo A., Gupta P.B., Sgroi D.C., Arenzana-Seisdedos F., Delaunay T., Naeem R., Carey V.J., Richardson A.L., and Weinberg R.A. 2005. Stromal fibroblasts present in invasive human breast carcinomas promote tumor growth and angiogenesis through elevated SDF-1/CXCL12 secretion. *Cell* **121:** 335.

Paszek M.J. and Weaver V.M. 2004. The tension mounts: Mechanics meets morphogenesis and malignancy. *J. Mammary Gland Biol. Neoplasia* **9:** 325.

Petersen O.W., Nielsen H.L., Gudjonsson T., Villadsen R., Rank F., Niebuhr E., Bissell M.J., and Ronnov-Jessen L. 2003. Epithelial to mesenchymal transition in human breast cancer can provide a nonmalignant stroma. *Am. J. Pathol.* **162:** 391.

Radisky D., Hagios C., and Bissell M.J. 2001. Tumors are unique organs defined by abnormal signaling and context. *Semin. Cancer Biol.* **11:** 87.

Ramaswamy S., Ross K.N., Lander E.S., and Golub T.R. 2003. A molecular signature of metastasis in primary solid tumors. *Nat. Genet.* **33:** 49.

Ronnov-Jessen L., Petersen O.W., Koteliansky V.E., and Bissell M.J. 1995. The origin of the myofibroblasts in breast cancer. Recapitulation of tumor environment in culture unravels diversity and implicates converted fibroblasts and recruited smooth muscle cells. *J. Clin. Invest.* **95:** 859.

Sangaletti S., Stoppacciaro A., Guiducci C., Torrisi M.R., and Colombo M.P. 2003. Leukocyte, rather than tumor-produced SPARC, determines stroma and collagen type IV deposition in mammary carcinoma. *J. Exp. Med.* **198:** 1475.

Schmidt-Hansen B., Ornas D., Grigorian M., Klingelhofer J., Tulchinsky E., Lukanidin E., and Ambartsumian N. 2004. Extracellular S100A4(mts1) stimulates invasive growth of mouse endothelial cells and modulates MMP-13 matrix metalloproteinase activity. *Oncogene* **23:** 5487.

Schor A.M., Rushton G., Ferguson J.E., Howell A., Redford J., and Schor S.L. 1994. Phenotypic heterogeneity in breast fibroblasts: Functional anomaly in fibroblasts from histologically normal tissue adjacent to carcinoma. *Int. J. Cancer* **59:** 25.

Semov A., Moreno M.J., Onichtchenko A., Abulrob A., Ball M., Ekiel I., Pietrzynski G., Stanimirovic D., and Alakhov V. 2005. Metastasis-associated protein S100A4 induces angiogenesis through interaction with Annexin II and accelerated plasmin formation. *J. Biol. Chem.* **280:** 20833.

Uria J.A., Stahle-Backdahl M., Seiki M., Fueyo A., and Lopez-Otin C. 1997. Regulation of collagenase-3 expression in human breast carcinomas is mediated by stromal-epithelial cell interactions. *Cancer Res.* **57:** 4882.

Vacek P.M. and Geller B.M. 2004. A prospective study of breast cancer risk using routine mammographic breast density measurements. *Cancer Epidemiol. Biomark. Prev* **13:** 715.

Vogelstein B. and Kinzler K.W. 2004. Cancer genes and the pathways they control. *Nat. Med.* **10:** 789.

Wahlgren J., Maisi P., Sorsa T., Sutinen M., Tervahartiala T., Pirila E., Teronen O., Hietanen J., Tjaderhane L., and Salo T. 2001. Expression and induction of collagenases (MMP-8 and -13) in plasma cells associated with bone-destructive lesions. *J. Pathol.* **194:** 217.

Weaver V.M., Petersen O.W., Wang F., Larabell C.A., Briand P., Damsky C., and Bissell M.J. 1997. Reversion of the malignant phenotype of human breast cells in three-dimensional culture and in vivo by integrin blocking antibodies. *J. Cell Biol.* **137:** 231.

Weaver V.M., Lelievre S., Lakins J.N., Chrenek M.A., Jones J.C., Giancotti F., Werb Z., and Bissell M.J. 2002. β4 Integrin-dependent formation of polarized three-dimensional architecture confers resistance to apoptosis in normal and malignant mammary epithelium. *Cancer Cell* **2:** 205.

West R.B., Nuyten D.S., Subramanian S., Nielsen T.O., Corless C.L., Rubin B.P., Montgomery K., Zhu S., Patel R., Hernandez-Boussard T., Goldblum J.R., Brown P.O., van de Vijver M., and van de Rijn M. 2005. Determination of stromal signatures in breast carcinoma. *PLoS Biol.* **3:** e187.

Willmroth F., Peter H.H., and Conca W. 1998. A matrix metalloproteinase gene expressed in human T lymphocytes is identical with collagenase 3 from breast carcinomas. *Immunobiology* **198:** 375.

Wiseman B.S. and Werb Z. 2002. Stromal effects on mammary gland development and breast cancer. *Science* **296:** 1046.

Xue C., Plieth D., Venkov C., Xu C., and Neilson E.G. 2003. The gatekeeper effect of epithelial-mesenchymal transition regulates the frequency of breast cancer metastasis. *Cancer Res.* **63:** 3386.

Is Oncogene Addiction Angiogenesis-dependent?

J. FOLKMAN AND S. RYEOM

The Vascular Biology Program, Department of Surgery, Children's Hospital and Harvard Medical School, Boston, Massachusetts 02115

Does an activated oncogene that initiates tumor growth need to remain activated to maintain the cancer phenotype? This question has been answered affirmatively by experiments in which doxycycline-regulated oncogene activation induces growth of large tumors that regress completely upon oncogene inactivation—a phenomenon called oncogene addiction. We assemble here the evidence that oncogene addiction is angiogenesis-dependent. Although activated oncogenes increase tumor cell proliferation and decrease their apoptosis, these activities are not sufficient to expand tumor mass beyond a microscopic size. Oncogenes must also induce tumor angiogenesis for expansion of tumor mass. We propose experiments to validate the "endothelial centric" hypothesis of oncogene addiction.

Rapid tumor growth in mice can be induced by implantation of tumor cells driven by an oncogene (i.e., *myc* or *ras*) under the control of a doxycycline-regulated promoter. Upon inactivation of the oncogene, tumors undergo rapid regression (Chin et al. 1999; Felsher and Bishop 1999; Brandvold et al. 2000; Jain et al. 2002; Karlsson et al. 2003; Shachaf et al. 2004). This phenomenon has been called "oncogene addiction," to indicate the need for "continued activity of a specific oncogene to maintain the cancer phenotype" (Weinstein 2002).

Growth of a tumor and maintenance of tumor mass have been thought to depend on increased tumor cell proliferation and decreased tumor cell apoptosis, both of which are oncogene-driven. However, other experimental evidence reveals that cancer cells arising from oncogene transformation of normal cells are not inherently harmful to the host (Achilles et al. 2001; Folkman and Kalluri 2004). In fact, cancer cells can remain as a microscopic-sized dormant tumor (in situ carcinoma in humans) until the dormant tumor switches to the angiogenic phenotype and is permitted to *expand its tumor mass*. In virtually all animal and human cancers, it is the expanding tumor mass that can potentially invade, metastasize, and eventually kill the host—not the microscopic dormant tumor. In humans, only the expanding tumor mass is potentially symptomatic and detectable by conventional imaging methods—not the microscopic dormant tumor.

In animals, expansion of tumor mass induced by an activated oncogene, and regression of tumor mass following inactivation of an oncogene, both appear as seamless processes. Once oncogene activation has occurred, tumor growth is assumed to be inevitable, and after an oncogene has been inactivated, tumor regression is believed to be virtually automatic.

We assemble here evidence that *angiogenesis* is a critical event in oncogene addiction. There is considerable evidence to suggest that, unless an activated oncogene can trigger the switch to the angiogenic phenotype, growth of tumor mass cannot occur. We further propose that tumor regression following oncogene inactivation *may be pre-*vented by deletion of an endogenous angiogenesis inhibitor engendered by oncogene inactivation. We propose, in other words, that increased tumor cell proliferation and decreased tumor cell apoptosis mediated by oncogene activation are necessary, but not sufficient to expand tumor mass. These events must be followed by sustained angiogenesis. Furthermore, tumor regression after inactivation of a specific oncogene may also require potent inhibition of angiogenesis. Although these ideas are based on an experimental model of a single angiogenesis inhibitor, it is likely that more than one endogenous angiogenesis inhibitor is operating during oncogene activation and inactivation in humans. For the purpose of organizing the data presented here, we use the term "endothelial centric" hypothesis of oncogene addiction.

EXPERIMENTAL ONCOGENE ADDICTION

Since the discovery of oncogenes and tumor suppressor genes, a fundamental question has emerged. Does the activation of an oncogene necessary for the initial development of a tumor continue to be required to maintain the cancer phenotype of that tumor (Weinstein 2002)? Chin et al. (1999) addressed this question by an elegant experiment in which the continued presence of the activated oncogene H-Ras^{V12G} was necessary not only to cause growth of a melanoma, but also to maintain the tumor. Doxycycline-inducible H-Ras^{V12G} melanomas were grown in mice lacking the tumor suppressor INK4a. Withdrawal of doxycycline down-regulated H-Ras^{V12G} and resulted in rapid tumor regression. Histological analysis during the initial stages of regression revealed marked apoptosis in host-derived vascular endothelial cells and in tumor cells. Furthermore, Felsher and Bishop (1999) showed that transgenic mice which conditionally expressed the *myc* proto-oncogene in hematopoietic cells developed T-cell lymphomas and acute myeloid leukemias. When the Myc transgene was inactivated, tumors regressed (Fig. 1). There was precipitate arrest of tumor cell proliferation followed by differentiation and apoptosis of tumor cells. In an osteogenic sarcoma model,

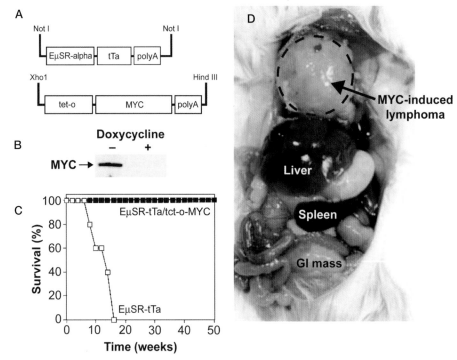

Figure 1. Conditional transgenic model for myc-induced tumorigenesis. (*A*) Tetracycline regulatory system constructs. (*B*) Mice transgenic for both EµSR-tTA nd tet-o-MYC conditionally express MYC protein in splenic lymphocytes. Western analysis was performed on spleen lymphocytes from transgenic mice in the absence (–) or the presence (+) of doxycycline in drinking water. Similar results were seen in four independent experiments. (*C*) Survival curves for transgenic mice. (▫) Mice transgenic for EµSR-tTA and tet-o-MYC; (■) mice transgenic for EµSR-tTA and tet-o-MYC with doxycycline treatment or either EµSR-tTA or tet-o-MYC alone. $n = 20$ animals per group. (*D*) Deceased animals had an enlarged thymus, spleen, liver, and mesenteric lymph nodes. (Reprinted, with permission, from Felsher and Bishop 1999.)

even brief loss of Myc for only 10 days resulted in sustained tumor regression with differentiation of osteocytes that formed histologically normal bone. Subsequent reactivation of Myc did not restore the cells' malignant properties, but induced apoptosis. Other examples have been reported that demonstrate the need for sustained activation of an oncogene for maintenance of the cancer phenotype (Weinstein 2002; Giuriato et al. 2003). In these reports, the cancer phenotype is represented by measurable or visible tumor mass, up to 1 cm^3 or more.

The rapid regrowth of tumor in most reports of reactivation of an oncogene raises a second fundamental question. The rapid regrowth of tumor starting from a few "differentiated" residual tumor cells after tumor regression seems too brief a time for gene mutations to drive these cells through the classic events of tumorigenesis, which include initiation, promotion, transformation, and progression. However, epigenetic, non-mutational events could effect rapid changes in gene expression. Those genes that control the ability of tumor cells to switch to the angiogenic phenotype (Hanahan and Folkman 1996) appear capable of changing their expression rapidly enough to account for the rapid regression of tumors following inactivation of a specific oncogene, and the rapid regrowth of tumor mass after reactivation of the oncogene. The switching of angiogenesis "on" and "off" is a good candidate for a process that could swiftly mediate the growth and regression of large tumor masses.

EXPANSION OF TUMOR MASS IS ANGIOGENESIS-DEPENDENT

Since 1971, when it was first proposed that tumor growth is angiogenesis-dependent, numerous experiments have provided biological and pharmacological evidence for this concept, as well as formal genetic proof (for review, see Folkman 2000; Folkman et al. 2006; see also Kim et al. 1993; O'Reilly et al. 1994, 1997). A summary of these studies reveals that most solid tumors can form microscopic tumors up to approximately 1 mm^3 without the need to recruit new blood vessels. However, further expansion of tumor mass beyond that size requires angiogenesis. Microscopic tumors incapable of switching to this angiogenic phenotype, i.e., non-angiogenic tumors, remain dormant indefinitely.

Tumor dormancy due to blocked angiogenesis is defined as a nonexpanding microscopic tumor, in which proliferation of tumor cells is balanced by apoptosis (Holmgren et al. 1995). (There are other types of tumor dormancy induced by hormone withdrawal, or by immunity, or by tumor cells in G_0.)

The most compelling evidence for the angiogenic switch in human tumors is revealed by separating non-angiogenic tumor cells and angiogenic tumor cells from human tumors obtained from the operating room or from human tumor cell lines (obtained from the American Tissue Culture Collection) (Achilles et al. 2001; Udagawa et al.

2002; Almog et al. 2006; Naumov et al. 2006). Non-an-giogenic tumor cells have been found in virtually every tu-mor so far examined by us, including human breast cancer, colon cancer, osteosarcoma, and liposarcoma. They can make up to ~20% of the tumor cell population in human tu-mors. Non-angiogenic tumor cells have similar prolifera-tion rates and similar karyotypes as angiogenic tumor cells. They differ markedly in their expression of positive and negative angiogenesis regulatory proteins. For exam-ple, non-angiogenic tumor cells often express the angio-genesis inhibitor thrombospondin-1 at high levels and VEGF at moderate levels. In contrast, angiogenic tumor cells express low levels of thrombospondin-1 and in-creased levels of VEGF. These experiments are relevant to oncogene dependence, because they demonstrate a mech-anism by which microscopic dormant tumors can suddenly and rapidly switch to an expanding tumor mass. For ex-ample, non-angiogenic tumor cells from human liposar-coma, when implanted into SCID immunodeficient mice and observed by luciferase bioluminescence, remain mi-croscopic and dormant at <1 mm diameter for a median of 133 days ± 2–3 weeks, at which time virtually 100% of these non-angiogenic dormant tumors become angiogenic and grow exponentially to large tumor masses of >1–2 cm^3 (Fig. 2) (Almog et al. 2006; Naumov et al. 2006). Be-fore the angiogenic switch, the microscopic dormant tu-mors are harmless to the host, analogous to the tumors with an inactivated oncogene. After the angiogenic switch, the tumors are lethal to the mice, analogous to tumors with an activated oncogene. In other types of human tumors, the time to the angiogenic switch is different, but just as pre-dictable. The percentage of non-angiogenic tumors that switch to the angiogenic phenotype is also predictable but differs in other tumors. For example, in a human breast cancer cell line (MDA-MB-436), approximately 80% switch at a median of 60 days. Those that don't become an-giogenic remain harmless through the remainder of the host's life. In another breast cancer (MDA-MB-415), the angiogenic switch occurs after 1 year. Transfection of a non-angiogenic tumor (i.e., osteosarcoma) with Ras will induce the angiogenic switch in virtually all tumors within 2–3 weeks (Udagawa et al. 2002).

DISSOCIATION OF THE TUMOR CELL PROLIFERATIVE INDUCING FUNCTION FROM THE ANGIOGENESIS INDUCING FUNCTION OF ONCOGENES

A common argument against angiogenesis dependence of tumor growth is that angiogenesis could simply be a secondary event that follows tumor cell proliferation. The argument goes that any oncogene activation, or in fact, any therapy that arrested tumor cell proliferation, would also arrest angiogenesis.

However, repeated studies show that tumor cell prolif-eration and angiogenesis can operate independently from each other. As discussed above, non-angiogenic and an-giogenic human tumors have similar proliferation rates. In another study, tumor cells were treated with ionizing irra-diation to render them incapable of cell division and were then implanted into the rabbit cornea; these cells still in-duced angiogenesis similar to nonirradiated tumor cells (Auerbach et al. 1975). A third demonstration of the dis-sociation of tumor cell proliferation and angiogenesis came from experiments with the SV40 large-T oncogene. When wild-type endothelial cells were transformed by the SV40-T oncogene, the resulting neoplastic cells displayed significantly increased proliferation and decreased apopto-sis, as well as the other hallmarks of transformation in vitro (Arbiser et al. 1997). Furthermore, they formed micro-scopic, non-angiogenic, dormant tumors in vivo. These tu-mors were visible under low-power magnification and re-mained harmless throughout the life of the host. However, when the cells were transfected with a second oncogene, Ras, they switched to the angiogenic phenotype, VEGF expression and secretion increased, metalloproteinases-2 and -9 increased, tissue inhibitor of metalloproteinase-2 (TIMP-2) decreased, and fatal angiosarcomas developed.

Watnick et al. demonstrated that relatively low levels of H-ras in combination with the SV40 early region and hTERT result in the transformed phenotype of primary human breast and kidney epithelial cells (Volpert and Alani 2003; Watnick et al. 2003). These cells formed small dormant tumors in nude mice and were limited in further growth because of their inability to induce a vas-

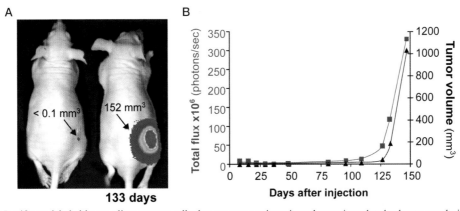

Figure 2. (*A*) Luciferase-labeled human liposarcoma cells that are non-angiogenic and were inoculated subcutaneously in SCID mice. Mouse on the left bears a non-angiogenic dormant tumor that is undetectable by gross examination. In the mouse on the right, the tumor has become angiogenic and is growing rapidly. (*B*) Squares represent bioluminescence. Triangles represent palpable tumor. The tumor became palpable (~50–100 mm^3) approximately 23 days after the significant increase in bioluminescence. (Modified from Almog et al. 2006.)

cular supply. This state of tumor dormancy could be overcome by expressing higher levels of *ras* which suppressed production of the angiogenesis inhibitor, thrombospondin-1. Higher levels of Ras did not significantly increase expression of VEGF.

ACTIVATION OF MULTIPLE ONCOGENES POTENTIATES TUMOR ANGIOGENESIS

Additional supporting evidence for the "endothelial centric" hypothesis of oncogene addiction was reported for human prostate cancer. After a tumor has already become angiogenic and capable of steady growth in mice, its angiogenic activity can be increased further by introducing another oncogene. The human prostate cancers PC-3 and DU-145 were transfected with the oncogene *bcl-2*. VEGF expression was significantly increased by 2.3-fold, and microvessel density was also significantly increased by 2-fold (Fig. 3) (Fernandez et al. 2001). Tumors derived from PC-3-bcl-2-transfected cells grew at approximately twice the rate of tumors derived from control tumor cells. Growth of human prostate cancer (PC-3) was completely suppressed in mice treated with mitomycin C, which blocked tumor cell proliferation. In contrast, prostate cancers transfected with *bcl-2* were protected against tumor cell apoptosis induced by mitomycin C and therefore were completely resistant to this chemotherapeutic agent (Fig. 4). However, when bcl-2-transfected prostate cancer that was resistant to mitomycin C was treated by an angiogenesis inhibitor, TNP-470, tumor growth was completely suppressed. TNP-470 is a synthetic analog of fumagillin (Satchi-Fainaro et al. 2004), inhibits endothelial cell proliferation at 3 logs lower than the concentration necessary to inhibit prolifer-

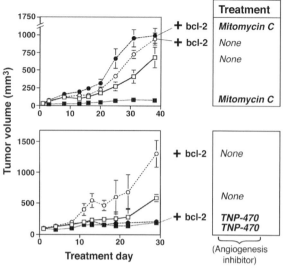

Figure 4. Treatment of human prostate cancer (PC3) in SCID mice, with the angiogenesis inhibitor TNP-470 or the chemotherapeutic agent mitomycin C. Tumors derived from the injection of PC3-neo or PC3-*bcl-2* were treated with (*A*) TNP-470 (30 mg/kg every other day subcutaneously) or (*B*) mitomycin C 1 mg/kg once a week by intraperitoneal injection. (□) PC3-neo tumors, untreated; (■) PC3-neo tumors, treated; (○) PC3-bcl-2 tumors, untreated; and (●) PC3-bcl-2 tumors, treated. For each group of tumors, the average volume for five tumors is plotted. Bars, 95% confidence intervals. (Reprinted, with permission, from Fernandez et al. 2001.)

ation of tumor cells or fibroblasts, and does not inhibit proliferation of the prostate cancer cells. Therefore, *oncogene activation (of bcl-2) can be counteracted by blocking angiogenesis, even in a tumor resistant to cytotoxic chemotherapy.* In other words, in this experiment, oncogene activation decreased tumor cell apoptosis sufficiently to make the resulting tumor resistant to cytotoxic chemotherapy. In contrast, the increased tumor angiogenesis mediated by oncogene activation could still be completely overridden by nontoxic doses of a broad-spectrum angiogenesis inhibitor.

OVEREXPRESSION OF AN ENDOGENOUS ANGIOGENESIS INHIBITOR CAN COUNTERACT HIGH TUMOR CELL PROLIFERATION AND SUPPRESS TUMOR GROWTH IN VIVO

There exists additional evidence demonstrating that expansion of tumor mass can vary directly with angiogenesis while tumor cell proliferation remains relatively constant. When the endogenous angiogenesis inhibitors thrombospondin-1 and/or thrombospondin-2 were transfected into a human squamous cell carcinoma (Streit et al. 1999), tumor cells expressed incremental levels of thrombospondin-1 or a combination of thrombospondin-1 and -2. These cells formed a tumor mass the volume of which varied inversely with thrombospondin-1 expression, and independently of tumor cell proliferation rate (Fig. 5). Increasing thrombospondin-1 expression proportionally decreased tumor angiogenesis and tumor mass, *without* affecting tumor cell proliferation.

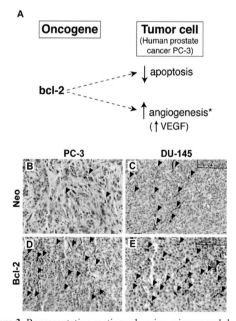

Figure 3. Representative sections showing microvessel density in human prostate cancer in SCID mice. (*A*) PC3-neo cells. (*B*) PC3-bcl-2 cells. (*C*) DU-145 neo cells. (*D*) DU-145-bcl-2 cells. Tumors arising from these stably transfected cells were fixed and stained with anti-CD31 antibody to detect blood vessels. Magnification, 113x. Bars, 60 μm. (Reprinted, with permission, from Fernandez et al. 2001.)

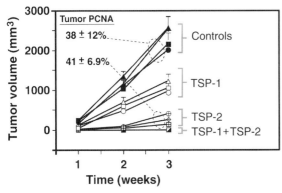

Figure 5. Stable thrombospondin-1 (TSP-1) overexpression in human squamous cell carcinoma cells (A431). Clones expressing increasing levels of TSP-1 significantly inhibited intradermal tumor growth in proportion to TSP-1 expression (i.e., suppressed angiogenesis). Combined overexpression of TSP-1 and TSP-2 completely prevented tumor formation. The largest tumors (controls) had no TSP-1 expression. (Reprinted, with permission, from Streit et al. 1999.)

Table 1. Impact of Oncogenes or Potential Oncogenes on Angiogenesis Regulatory Proteins

Oncogene	Implicated pro-angiogenic activity
K-ras, H-ras	VEGV up-regulation, TSP-1 down-regulation
v-src	VEGV up-regulation, TSP-1 down-regulation
c-myb	TSP-2 down-regulation
N-myc	angiogenic properties in neuroblastoma
c-myc	angiogenic properties in epidermis
HER-2	VEGF up-regulation
EGFR	VEGF, bFGF, IL-8 up-regulation
PyMT	TSP-1 down-regulation
c-fos	VEGF expression
trkB	VEGF down-regulation
HPV-16	secretion of VEGF and IFN-α
v-p3k	VEGF production and angiogenesis
ODC	novel angiogenic factor
PTTG1	VEGF and bFGF up-regulation
E2a-Pbx1	induction of mouse angiogenin-3
bcl-2	VEGF up-regulation*

Data from Rak et al. (2000) and *Fernandez et al. (2001).

ONCOGENE ACTIVATION CAN DIRECTLY INCREASE ANGIOGENESIS ACTIVITY OF A TUMOR

Whereas oncogenes were initially discovered by their ability to increase cell proliferation in vitro, it has only recently been recognized that a major function of oncogenes is to increase tumor angiogenesis. Activated oncogenes can increase angiogenesis either by increasing tumor cell expression of a positive regulator of angiogenesis such as VEGF, or bFGF, or by suppressing expression of an endogenous angiogenesis inhibitor such as thrombospondin-1, or both. Rak et al. (2000) published a series of 15 different oncogenes (Table 1). The list of oncogenes in Table 1 illustrates the extreme heterogeneity of tissues and receptors that are regulated by a relatively small set of pro-angiogenic and anti-angiogenic molecules. The list of oncogenes that regulate angiogenesis continues to grow. Angiogenesis was reported to be an early event in the generation of *myc*-induced lymphomas (Brandvold et al. 2000). In developing embryos, c-*myc* is partially responsible for expression of VEGF during vasculogenesis and is also required for the proper expression of angiopoietin-1 and angiopoietin-2 (Baudino et al. 2002). Furthermore, c-*myc* null embryonic stem cells are dramatically impaired in their ability to form tumors in immune-compromised mice, and the small tumors that sometimes develop are poorly vascularized. Watnick et al. (2003) have demonstrated that in transformed human epithelial cells, the switch to the angiogenic phenotype is mediated by oncogenic Ras suppression of thrombospondin-1. They further show that Ras-dependent repression of thrombospondin-1 is itself dependent on c-*myc* function, and that this myc function is dependent on phosphorylation of the Myc protein rather than the absolute expression level of *myc*. Myc phosphorylation is shown to be mediated through ras signaling via phosphatidyl inositol-3 kinase. Therefore, two oncogenes cooperate to turn on angiogenesis in a tumor cell by suppressing an endogenous angiogenesis inhibitor.

Thrombospondin-1 is only one of at least 28 known endogenous angiogenesis inhibitors that have been discovered in the circulation or in extracellular matrix during the past 20 years (Folkman 2004; Nyberg et al. 2005). It is not clear which of these are possibly down-regulated by oncogenes during the switch to the angiogenic phenotype in tumors. However, when endostatin or tumstatin is knocked out, tumor angiogenesis is significantly increased and tumors grow 200–300% faster. The rate of tumor growth is significantly increased in mice lacking both angiogenesis inhibitors endostatin and tumstatin (Sudhakar et al. 2003).

INACTIVATION OF THE c-*myc* ONCOGENE INCREASES THROMBOSPONDIN-1 EXPRESSION

Another finding by Watnick et al. (2003) addresses the question of the mechanism of the rapid regression of a tumor when an oncogene such as *Myc* is inactivated. In human breast cancer cells, Myc was regulated by the tamoxifen promoter. When the tamoxifen promoter was turned on by estrogen, *Myc* was inactivated and thrombospondin-1 expression was increased (Fig. 6).

In a collaboration with Dean Felsher's lab, Ryeom and Folkman showed that in Myc-induced lymphoma from the Felsher lab (Felsher and Bishop 1999), thrombospondin-1 was suppressed throughout the growing tumor and its stroma. However, thrombospondin-1 was

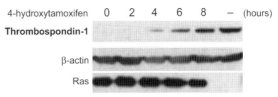

Figure 6. Myc regulation of thrombospondin-1 in human breast cancer cells. Myc is regulated by the tamoxifen promoter in human breast cancer cells. When the tamoxifen promoter is turned on by estrogen, Myc is inactivated and thrombospondin-1 expression is increased. However, upstream molecules are less affected, such as Ras. The loading control is β-actin.

MYC-activation induces a growing lymphoma.

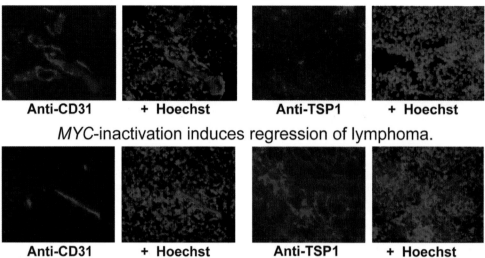

MYC-inactivation induces regression of lymphoma.

Figure 7. Immunohistochemical microsections of a c-myc-activated lymphoma in a mouse. (*Upper left panels*) Tumor blood vessels stained with anti-CD31 antibody. Intense neovascularization in the tumor bed. Lumens are open. (*Upper right panels*) Antibody to thrombospondin-1 shows only sparse thrombospondin-1 in the tumor bed. There is residual thrombospondin-1 in the blood vessels. (*Lower left panels*) Regresson of microvessels in the tumor bed after myc inactivation. Vessels are narrow and closed. (*Lower right panels*) Abundantly increased thrombospondin-1 has appeared in the tumor bed (S. Giuriato et al., unpubl.).

present in the blood and therefore was visualized in the microvasculature lumen (S. Giuriato et al., unpubl.). Inactivation of c-*myc* led to tumor regression, which was associated with a dramatic increase in thrombospondin-1 expression throughout the tumor and its stroma (Fig. 7).

TUMOR REGRESSION FROM INACTIVATION OF AN ONCOGENE IS PRECEDED BY IMPAIRMENT OF VASCULAR FUNCTION

In the tumor model developed by Chin et al. (1999) in which melanoma develops as a result of activation of H-*ras*, neovascularization was assessed by in vivo real-time magnetic resonance imaging (Tang et al. 2005). When ras was inactivated, the resulting tumor regression was preceded by impairment of vascular function. This correlated with activation of apoptosis in host-derived endothelial cells as well as in tumor cells. The real-time in vivo imaging provided evidence that loss of vascular integrity upon inactivation of Ras is an active process rather than a consequence of loss of tumor cell viability.

CONCLUSIONS

Taken together, the evidence assembled here indicates that continuous oncogene activation is necessary to maintain tumor angiogenesis. The angiogenic inducing function of certain oncogenes may operate independently of an oncogene's pro-proliferative effect or antiapoptotic effect on tumor cells.

Activated oncogenes may mediate angiogenesis by upregulating angiogenic proteins (i.e., VEGF) and by downregulating endogenous angiogenesis inhibitors (i.e., thrombospondin-1). A tumor producing high levels of VEGF may not be able to switch to the angiogenic phenotype un-

til there has occurred a significant decreased expression of one or more endogenous angiogenesis inhibitors. Tumor cells driven by activated oncogenes may also regulate pro-angiogenic or antiangiogenic proteins expressed by stromal fibroblasts and/or by vascular endothelium.

Inactivation of an oncogene in a tumor leads to downregulation of pro-angiogenic proteins (i.e., VEGF), upregulation of antiangiogenic proteins (i.e., thrombospondin-1), and rapid vascular regression followed by tumor regression. Oncogene activation can be countered by therapeutic blockade of angiogenesis, even in a tumor that has become resistant to chemotherapy from overexpression of an oncogene such as *bcl-2*. This finding may be important in determining a mechanism for how regressed tumors can escape addiction to a specific oncogene and resume growth (Giuriato and Felsher 2003). Giuriato and Felsher suggest that loss of p53 function could be one explanation. In fact, p53 suppresses angiogenesis by at least four mechanisms: up-regulation of thrombospondin-1 expression (Dameron et al. 1994); degradation of hypoxia inducible factor-1 (Ravi et al. 2000); suppression of VEGF expression (Zhang et al. 2000); and suppression of bFGF-binding protein expression (Sherif et al. 2001). Therefore, as Giuriato and Felsher (2003) emphasize, the loss of p53 function could impede the shutdown of angiogenesis and permit escape of tumor from addiction to a specific oncogene. The list of different angiogenic regulatory molecules that oncogenes encode (Table 1) suggests that tumor escape may not require new mutations, but could simply result from the expansion of a subpopulation of tumor cells that express a different angiogenic protein, bFGF instead of VEGF, for example.

If this phenomenon can be demonstrated in mouse

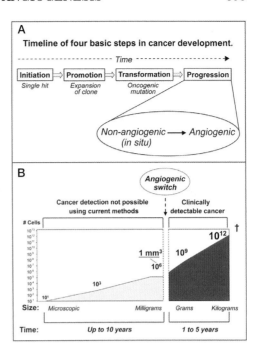

Figure 8. (*A*) Diagram of four classic steps in tumorigenesis relative to the timing of the switch to the angiogenic phenotype during "progression." The switch to the angiogenic phenotype occurs at the stage of microscopic in situ cancer, but is a relatively rare event. By comparing the incidence of in situ cancers found in different organs in autopsies of individuals who died of trauma, but who had no cancer during their lifetime, to the incidence of diagnosed cancer, we estimate that only 1 out of ~600–700 in situ cancers undergo the angiogenic switch. (*B*) Diagram to illustrate that by the time a tumor is first diagnosed, it has been growing for several years undetected. The switch to the angiogenic phenotype when a tumor is at ~1 mm^3 or less may be among the last barriers that a tumor must overcome before it is potentially lethal. The majority of microscopic sized, in situ cancers don't succeed in becoming angiogenic and remain harmless to the host. If anti-oncogene therapy and/or antiangiogenic therapy could be administered before or soon after the angiogenic switch (e.g., guided by accurate biomarkers), human cancer could possibly be treated before symptoms, or before detection by conventional imaging methods. (*A,* Modified from Folkman et al. 2006.)

models and if it is found to operate in human tumors in patients, it could explain the occasional escape of tumors from responding to currently available angiogenesis inhibitors after prolonged use (months to more than a year). Most of the angiogenesis inhibitors approved by the FDA to date, and most of those in clinical trials, target only VEGF or its receptors. However, human prostate cancer can express at least four angiogenic proteins, including VEGF, bFGF, interleukin-8, and platelet-derived growth factor (PDGF) (Uehara 2003). Advanced stages of breast cancer can express up to six pro-angiogenic proteins (Relf et al. 1997). In advanced stages of neuroblastoma, up to seven angiogenic proteins are highly expressed (Eggert et al. 2000). If these findings extend to other human cancers, as survival increases, it is likely that residual tumors in a given patient could express redundant angiogenic factors (Folkman 2006). Such tumors could become refractory to an angiogenesis inhibitor that blocks a single angiogenic factor. This potential problem could be circumvented by (1) employing combinations of angiogenesis inhibitors or by (2) combining angiogenesis inhibitors with antiangiogenic chemotherapy (metronomic chemotherapy) (Browder et al. 2000; Klement et al. 2000; Kerbel and Kamen 2004) or by (3) employing broad-spectrum angiogenesis inhibitors that have little or no toxicity, such as endostatin (Folkman 2006) or Caplostatin (Satchi-Fainaro et al. 2005). It is likely that long-term, broad-spectrum antiangiogenic therapy may be desirable to facilitate a goal of "converting cancer to a chronic manageable disease" (Ezzell 1998).

The studies reported here also suggest that antiangiogenic therapy could possibly bypass the problem of a tumor's escape from oncogene addiction, because blockade of angiogenesis blocks tumor growth downstream of oncogene activation (Fig. 8).

HOW COULD THE ANGIOGENESIS DEPENDENCE OF ONCOGENE ADDICTION BE FORMALLY PROVED IN THE FUTURE?

We have provided indirect evidence that angiogenesis is a requirement for an activated oncogene to induce an expanding tumor mass (including metastasis) (Fig. 9). To provide formal genetic proof of this concept, an oncogene-activated tumor could have the expression of an endogenous angiogenesis inhibitor knocked out, such as thrombospondin-1. These tumors could then be grown in a host null for thrombospondin-1 expression. This model would test whether tumor regression requires either tumor cell production, or host production of angiogenesis inhibitors. The expected outcome could be that oncogene activation would increase tumor growth in the thrombospondin-1 null host as compared to a wild-type tumor in a wild-type host. Therefore, oncogene inactivation could result in a tumor that would

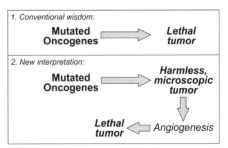

Figure 9. Illustration of the "endothelial centric" view of oncogene addiction. Mutated (activated) oncogenes can transform normal cells to cancer cells, which can grow to a limited microscopic size, i.e., in situ carcinoma. Such a microscopic tumor may remain non-angiogenic, dormant, and harmless, until it can switch to the angiogenic phenotype, after which tumor mass can expand.

not regress or would regress very slowly. To determine whether this prediction holds up, these experiments are in progress in a collaborative effort between the Felsher and Folkman labs.

ACKNOWLEDGMENTS

We thank Randolph Watnick for insightful discussions. This work is supported by The Breast Cancer Research Foundation, National Institutes of Health grants RO1 CA064481 and PO1 CA45548 (J.F.), and an Innovator Award from the Department of Defense W81XWH-04-1-0316.

REFERENCES

Achilles E.G., Fernandez A., Allred E.N., Kisker O., Udagawa T., Beecken W.D., Flynn E., and Folkman J. 2001. Heterogeneity of angiogenic activity in a human liposarcoma: A proposed mechanism for "no take" of human tumors in mice. *J. Natl. Cancer Inst.* **93:** 1075.

Almog N., Henke V., Flores L., Hlatky L., Kung A., Wright R.D., Berger R., Hutchinson L., Naumov G., Bender E., Akslen L., Achilles E.G., and Folkman J. 2006. Prolonged dormancy of human liposarcoma is associated with impaired tumor angiogenesis. *FASEB J.* (in press).

Arbiser J.L., Moses M.A., Fernandez C.A., Ghiso N., Cao Y., Klauber N., Frank D., Brownlee M., Flynn E., Parangi S., Byers H.R., and Folkman J. 1997. Oncogenic H-ras stimulates tumor angiogenesis by two distinct pathways. *Proc. Natl. Acad. Sci.* **94:** 861.

Auerbach R., Arensman R., Kubai L., and Folkman J. 1975. Tumor-induced angiogenesis: Lack of inhibition by irradiation. *Int. J. Cancer* **15:** 241.

Baudino T.A., McKay C., Pendeville-Samain H., Nilsson J.A., Maclean K.H., White E.L., Davis A.C., Ihle J.N., and Cleveland J.L. 2002. c-Myc is essential for vasculogenesis and angiogenesis during development and tumor progression. *Genes Dev.* **16:** 2530.

Brandvold K.A., Neiman P., and Ruddell A. 2000. Angiogenesis is an early event in the generation of myc-induced lymphomas. *Oncogene* **19:** 2780.

Browder T., Butterfield C.E., Kraling B.M., Shi B., Marshall B., O'Reilly M.S., and Folkman J. 2000. Antiangiogenic scheduling of chemotherapy improves efficacy against experimental drug-resistant cancer. *Cancer Res.* **60:** 1878.

Chin L., Tam A., Pomerantz J., Wong M., Holash J., Bardeesy N., Shen Q., O'Hagan R., Pantginis J., Zhou H., Horner J.W., Cordon-Cardo C., Yancopoulos G.D., and DePinho R.A. 1999. Essential role for oncogenic Ras in tumour maintenance. *Nature* **400:** 468.

Dameron K.M., Volpert O.V., Tainsky M.A., and Bouck N. 1994. Control of angiogenesis in fibroblasts by p53 regulation of thrombospondin-1. *Science* **265:** 1582.

Eggert A., Ikegaki N., Kwiatkowski J., Zhao H., Brodeur G.M., and Himelstein B.P. 2000. High-level expression of angiogenic factors is associated with advanced tumor stage in human neuroblastomas. *Clin. Cancer Res.* **6:** 1900.

Ezzell C. 1998. Starving tumors of their lifeblood. *Sci. Am.* **279:** 33.

Felsher D.W. and Bishop J.M. 1999. Reversible tumorigenesis by MYC in hematopoietic lineages. *Mol. Cell* **4:** 199.

Fernandez A., Udagawa T., Schwesinger C., Beecken W., Achilles-Gerte E., McDonnell T., and D'Amato R. 2001. Angiogenic potential of prostate carcinoma cells overexpressing Bcl-2. *J. Natl. Cancer Inst.* **93:** 208.

Folkman J. 2000. Tumor angiogenesis. In *Cancer medicine,* 5th edition (ed. J.F. Holland et al.), p. 132. B.C. Decker, Hamilton, Ontario, Canada.

———. 2004. Endogenous angiogenesis inhibitors. *Acta Pathol.*

Microbiol. Immunol. Scand. **112:** 496.

———. 2006. Antiangiogenesis in cancer therapy—endostatin and its mechanisms of action. *Exp. Cell Res.* **312:** 594.

Folkman J. and Kalluri R. 2004. Cancer without disease. *Nature* **427:** 787.

Folkman J., Heymach J., and Kalluri R. 2006. Tumor angiogenesis. In *Cancer medicine,* 6th edition (ed. D.W. Kufe et al.), p. 157. B.C. Decker, Hamilton, Ontario, Canada.

———. 2004. Cancer without disease. *Nature* **427:** 787.

Giuriato S. and Felsher D.W. 2003. How cancers escape their oncogene habit. *Cell Cycle* **2:** 329.

Hanahan D. and Folkman J. 1996. Patterns and emerging mechanisms of the angiogenic switch during tumorigenesis. *Cell* **86:** 353.

Holmgren L., O'Reilly M.S., and Folkman J. 1995. Dormancy of micrometastases: Balanced proliferation and apoptosis in the presence of angiogenesis suppression. *Nat. Med.* **1:** 149.

Jain M., Arvanitis C., Chu K., Dewey W., Leonhardt E., Trinh M., Sundberg C.D., Bishop J.M., and Felsher D.W. 2002. Sustained loss of a neoplastic phenotype by brief inactivation of MYC. *Science* **297:** 102.

Karlsson A., Giuriato S., Tang F., Fung-Weier J., Levan G., and Felsher D.W. 2003. Genomically complex lymphomas undergo sustained tumor regression upon MYC inactivation unless they acquire novel chromosomal translocations. *Blood* **101:** 2797.

Kerbel R.S. and Kamen B.A. 2004. The anti-angiogenic basis of metronomic chemotherapy. *Nat. Rev. Cancer* **4:** 423.

Kim K.J., Li B., Winer J., Armanini M., Gillett H.S., and Ferrara N. 1993. Inhibition of vascular endothelial growth factor-induced angiogenesis suppresses tumour growth in vivo. *Nature* **362:** 841.

Klement G., Baruchel S., Rak J., Man S., Clark K., Hicklin D.J., Bohlen P., and Kerbel R. 2000. Continuous low-dose therapy with vinblastine and VEGF receptor-2 antibody induces sustained tumor regression without overt toxicity. *J. Clin. Invest.* **105:** R15.

Naumov G.N., Bender E., Zurakowski D., Kang S.-Y., Sampson D., Flynn E., Watnick R.S., Straume O., Akslen L.A., Folkman J., and Almog N. 2006. A model of human tumor dormancy: An angiogenic switch from the nonangiogenic phenotype. *J. Natl. Cancer Inst.* **98:** 316.

Nyberg P., Xie L., and Kalluri R. 2005. Endogenous inhibitors of angiogenesis. *Cancer Res.* **65:** 3967.

O'Reilly M.S., Boehm T., Shing Y., Fukai N., Vasios G., Lane W.S., Flynn E., Birkhead J.R., Olsen B.R., and Folkman J. 1997. Endostatin: An endogenous inhibitor of angiogenesis and tumor growth. *Cell* **88:** 277.

O'Reilly M.S., Holmgren L., Shing Y., Chen C., Rosenthal R.A., Moses M., Lane W.S., Cao Y., Sage E.H., and Folkman J. 1994. Angiostatin: A novel angiogenesis inhibitor that mediates the suppression of metastases by a Lewis lung carcinoma. *Cell* **79:** 315.

Rak J., Yu J.L., Klement G., and Kerbel R.S. 2000. Oncogenes and angiogenesis: Signaling three-dimensional tumor growth. *J. Investig. Dermatol. Symp. Proc.* **5:** 24.

Ravi R., Mookerjee B., Bhujwalla Z.M., Sutter C.H., Artemov D., Zeng Q., Dillehay L.E., Madan A., Semenza G.L., and Bedi A. 2000. Regulation of tumor angiogenesis by p53-induced degradation of hypoxia-inducible factor 1alpha. *Genes Dev.* **14:** 34.

Relf M., LeJeune S., Scott P.A., Fox S., Smith K., Leek R., Moghaddam A., Whitehouse R., Bicknell R., and Harris A.L. 1997. Expression of the angiogenic factors vascular endothelial cell growth factor, acidic and basic fibroblast growth factor, tumor growth factor beta-1, platelet-derived endothelial cell growth factor, placenta growth factor, and pleiotrophin in human primary breast cancer and its relation to angiogenesis. *Cancer Res.* **57:** 963.

Satchi-Fainaro R., Puder M., Davies J.W., Tran H.T., Sampson D.A., Greene A.K., Corfas G., and Folkman J. 2004. Targeting angiogenesis with a conjugate of HPMA copolymer and TNP-470. *Nat. Med.* **10:** 255.

Satchi-Fainaro R., Mamluk R., Wang L., Short S.M., Nagy J.A.,

Feng D., Dvorak A.M., Dvorak H.F., Puder M., Mukhopadhyay D., and Folkman J. 2005. Inhibition of vessel permeability by TNP-470 and its polymer conjugate, caplostatin. *Cancer Cell* **7:** 251.

Shachaf C.M., Kopelman A.M., Arvanitis C., Karlsson A., Beer S., Mandl S., Bachmann M.H., Borowsky A.D., Ruebner B., Cardiff R.D., Yang Q., Bishop J.M., Contag C.H., and Felsher D.W. 2004. MYC inactivation uncovers pluripotent differentiation and tumour dormancy in hepatocellular cancer. *Nature* **431:** 1112.

Sherif Z.A., Nakai S., Pirollo K.F., Rait A., and Chang E.H. 2001. Downmodulation of bFGF-binding protein expression following restoration of p53 function. *Cancer Gene Ther.* **8:** 771.

Streit M., Riccardi L., Velasco P., Brown L.F., Hawighorst T., Bornstein P., and Detmar M. 1999. Thrombospondin-2: A potent endogenous inhibitor of tumor growth and angiogenesis. *Proc. Natl. Acad. Sci.* **96:** 14888.

Sudhakar A., Sugimoto H., Yang C., Lively J., Zeisberg M., and Kalluri R. 2003. Human tumstatin and human endostatin exhibit distinct antiangiogenic activities mediated by alpha v beta 3 and alpha 5 beta 1 integrins. *Proc. Natl. Acad. Sci.* **100:** 4766.

Tang Y., Kim M., Carrasco D., Kung A.L., Chin L., and Weissleder R. 2005. *In vivo* assessment of Ras-dependent maintenance of tumor angiogenesis by real-time magnetic resonance imaging. *Cancer Res.* **65:** 8324.

Udagawa T., Fernandez A., Achilles E.G., Folkman J., and D'Amato R.J. 2002. Persistence of microscopic human cancers in mice: Alterations in the angiogenic balance accompanies loss of tumor dormancy. *FASEB J.* **16:** 1361.

Uehara H. 2003. Angiogenesis of prostate cancer and antiangiogenic therapy. *J. Med. Invest.* **50:** 146.

Volpert O. and Alani R. M. 2003. Wiring the angiogenic switch: Ras, Myc, and Thrombospondin-1. *Cancer Cell* **3:** 199.

Watnick R.S., Cheng Y.-N., Rangarajan A., Ince T.A., and Weinberg R.A. 2003. Ras modulates Myc activity to repress thrombospondin-1 expression and increase tumor angiogenesis. *Cancer Cell* **3:** 219.

Weinstein I.B. 2002. Addiction to oncogenes: The Achilles heal of cancer. *Science* **297:** 63.

Zhang L., Yu D., Hu M., Xiong S., Lang A., Ellis L.M., and Pollock R.E. 2000. Wild-type p53 suppresses angiogenesis in human leiomyosarcoma and synovial sarcoma by transcriptional suppression of vascular endothelial growth factor expression. *Cancer Res.* **60:** 3655.

Structural Basis for the Functions of Endogenous Angiogenesis Inhibitors

M.A. GRANT[†] AND R. KALLURI[*‡]

[*]Center for Matrix Biology and Department of Medicine, Beth Israel Deaconess Medical Center and Harvard Medical School; [†]Division of Molecular and Vascular Medicine, Beth Israel Deaconess Medical Center, Boston, Massachusetts 02215; [‡]Department of Biological Chemistry and Molecular Pharmacology and Harvard–MIT Division of Health Sciences and Technology, Harvard Medical School, Boston, Massachusetts 02115

Tipping the angiogenic balance between pro- and antiangiogenic stimuli to favor vasculature induction and enhanced angiogenesis is a key event in the growth and progression of tumors. Recently, we demonstrated that the genetic loss of normal physiological levels of individual endogenous inhibitors of angiogenesis leads to a change in the balance between proangiogenic stimulators and their inhibitors, thus favoring enhanced angiogensis and increased tumor growth. Therefore, these endogenous angiogenesis inhibitors provide a physiological threshold against the induction of angiogenesis. The antiangiogenic activities of endostatin, tumstatin, and thrombospondin-1 are evaluated and correlated with their three-dimensional structure and active sites, deriving a structural basis for their activities. Collectively, structural analysis of all three inhibitors demonstrates that the active antiangiogenic sites on these molecules are exposed on the surface and available to bind their putative integrin receptors on proliferating endothelial cells.

The development of new blood vessels (neovasculature) from preexisting blood vessels is generally referred to as angiogenesis (Folkman 1972). In adult mammals, the vasculature remains quiescent, except in tissues involved in wound repair and the female reproductive system, which undergo transient neovascularization to grow new capillaries (Folkman and Shing 1992). Quiescence depends on the delicate local balance between endogenous angiogenic stimulators and inhibitors. Tipping the balance between pro- and antiangiogenic stimuli to sufficiently "turn on" the angiogenic phenotype requires upregulation of proangiogenic factors and simultaneous down-regulation of angiogenic inhibitors (Fig. 1) (Folkman 1995; Hanahan and Folkman 1996; Colorado et al. 2000; Bergers and Benjamin 2003). Induction of the "proangiogenic switch" enables endothelial cells to de-

grade the local basement membrane, change morphology, proliferate, invade the surrounding stromal tissue, form microtubes, sprout new capillaries, and reconstitute new basement membrane (Dvorak et al. 1995; Folkman 1995; Hanahan and Folkman 1996; Yancopoulos et al. 2000)— all essential processes in the growth of new blood vessels.

Uncontrolled neovascularization is associated with a number of pathological disorders, including diabetic retinopathy, psoriasis, rheumatoid arthritis, as well as cancer growth and metastasis. The growth of solid tumors, beyond a few cubic millimeters in size, and tumor metastasis are dependent on angiogenesis (Folkman 1995; Hanahan and Folkman 1996). The angiogenic switch involving conversion of quiescent endothelial cells to an active proangiogenic phenotype is a key early event in tumor progression. Therefore, antiangiogenic

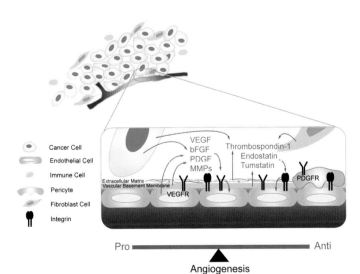

Figure 1. Schematic illustration of the proangiogenic switch favoring tumor vasculature growth and progression. The onset of the angiogenic switch is regulated by a shift in the balance of negative (*red*) and positive (*blue*) regulators of angiogenesis. The positive regulators are most commonly growth factors, which stimulate endothelial cell migration and proliferation. Negative regulators of angiogenesis include components or protein fragments of the extracellular matrix and vascular basement membrane, which inhibit endothelial cell migration and protein synthesis, and induce apoptosis.

targeting of tumor vasculature could limit tumor expansion and be an efficient therapy for cancer progression (Folkman 1971). Clues for potential antiangiogenic targeting of tumor vasculature may arguably lie in a better understanding of the structure and function of physiologically active, endogenous antiangiogenic molecules.

Endogenous inhibitors of angiogenesis include various antiangiogenic peptides, hormone metabolites, and apoptosis stimulators (Fig. 1) (for review, see Folkman 1995; Cao 2001; Nyberg et al. 2005). Currently, nearly 30 different protein and small-molecule inhibitors are known to exist in the body that function as inhibitors of angiogenesis (Nyberg et al. 2005). Like angiogenic stimulators, endogenous inhibitors influence one or more processes during angiogenesis. They are known to antagonize the angiogenic activity induced by growth factors or to inhibit the proteolytic activity of angiogenic proteinases, endothelial cell proliferation, migration, or microtube formation. In addition, whereas some angiogenic inhibitors affect a variety of cell types, others specifically inhibit the growing population of endothelial cells in new blood vessels. An essential source of endogenous inhibitors of angiogenesis is the vascular basement membrane surrounding endothelial cells (VBM) (Fig. 1). VBM are specialized extracellular matrix organized as thin, ultrastructure layers to provide a supporting scaffold for epithelial and endothelial cells (Paulsson 1992). It is well demonstrated that VBM not only provide mechanical support, but also influence cellular behavior such as differentiation, proliferation, and migration of various cells, including endothelial cells during the sprouting of new capillaries. They play an important role in regulating angiogenesis (Tsilibary et al. 1990; Paulsson 1992; Madri 1997; Darland and D'Amore 1999; Colorado et al. 2000). A series of potent endogenous antiangiogenic factors have been described, of which many are fragments of naturally occurring extracellular matrix (ECM) and basement membrane (BM) proteins (for review, see Cao 2001; Folkman 2004; Nyberg et al. 2005). Thus, molecules that are needed to assemble BM to maintain the integrity of blood vessels, under different circumstances, can have antiangiogenic activities.

On the opposing side of the angiogenic switch (Fig. 1), stimulators of angiogenesis include growth factors, such as vascular endothelial growth factor (VEGF), fibroblast growth factor (FGF), and hypoxic conditions that activate hypoxia-inducible factor-1, as well as angiogenic oncogenes, such as Ras and Myc, and tumor suppressors, such as p53 and PTEN that are secreted or produced by a variety of cell types and aid in the development of the tumor vasculature. In tumors, the angiogenic phenotype is characterized by expression of proangiogenic proteins such as VEGF, basic fibroblast growth factor (bFGF), interleukin-8 (IL-8), placenta-like growth factor (PlGF), transforming growth factor-β (TGF-β), PDGF, and others (Relf et al. 1997; Carmeliet et al. 1998; Fukumura et al. 1998; Rak et al. 2000; Yu et al. 2002; Pore et al. 2003; Watnick et al. 2003).

To initiate angiogenesis, endothelial cells have to break down the surrounding BM via secretion of proteolytic en-zymes. Although metalloproteinases play critical proangiogenic roles in this BM degradation, they also generate specific proteolytic fragments of BM proteins that have antiangiogenic activities and, thus, contribute to the down-regulation of angiogenesis. One such endogenous inhibitor of angiogenesis is endostatin, a 20-kD proteolyzed fragment of the heparan sulfate proteoglycan collagen XVIII, which was identified as an endogenous angiogenic inhibitor and is currently in clinical trials (Schellens and Ratain 2002; Thomas et al. 2003). Another important matrix-derived inhibitor of angiogenesis, tumstatin, is a 28-kD proteolyzed fragment of the NC1 domain of the α3 chain of type IV collagen and has demonstrated antiangiogenic and antitumor activities (Maeshima et al. 2000a,b, 2001a,b; Hamano et al. 2003; Pasco et al. 2004; Sund et al. 2005). In addition to matrix-derived angiogenesis inhibitors, several naturally occurring angiogenic antagonists have been identified (for review, see Carpizo and Iruela-Arispe 2000; Cao 2001; Bergers and Benjamin 2003; Nyberg et al. 2005). One such factor, thrombospondin-1 (TSP-1), was identified as one of the first inhibitors to be produced by normal fibroblast cells (Good et al. 1990).

The in vitro and in vivo antiangiogenic activities of endostatin, tumstatin, and TSP-1 have been the subject of intense study. The availability of putative three-dimensional structures of these endogenous inhibitors of angiogenesis provides molecular insight into their important mechanisms of action. Here we describe the antiangiogenic activities of full-length endostatin, tumstatin, and TSP-1, and regions within these factors that exhibit antiangiogenic activity as peptides isolated from their folded-parent proteins, and examine the molecular structure and surface expression of these naturally occurring antagonist subdomains.

ENDOSTATIN

Endostatin is a 20-kD fragment from the carboxy-terminal non-collagenous domain 1 (NC1) of collagen XVIII (O'Reilly et al. 1997; Sasaki et al. 1998). Collagen XVIII belongs to a subfamily of collagens, the multiplexin family, which have a domain organization that differs from other known collagen types in that non-triple-helical regions interrupt the triple-helical domains (Fig. 2). Collagen XVIII is ubiquitous and highly conserved among vertebrates, *Caenorhabditis elegans*, and *Drosophila*. It is a triple-helical hybrid molecule bearing several heparan sulfate side chains, and a major proteoglycan of endothelial and epithelial BM (Halfter et al. 1998; Musso et al. 2001). The carboxy-terminal NC1 of collagen XVIII includes a trimerization region and a hinge region that provides protease-sensitive sites and antiangiogenic fragments, such as endostatin. Physiological proteolytic cleavage of endostatin from the NC1 of collagen XVIII occurs through the activities of several enzymes, including pancreatic elastase-like enzyme (Wen et al. 1999), cathepsin (Felbor et al. 2000), and matrix metalloproteinases (MMP), for example, MMP-7 (Coussens et al. 2002; Egeblad and Werb 2002).

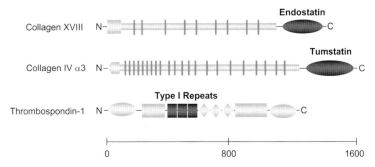

Figure 2. Schematic representation of the domain structure of endogenous angiogenesis inhibitors. The structural domains of endogenous inhibitors of angiogenesis at the focus of this review, namely the non-collagenous (NC1) domains from the α1 chain of type XVIII collagen and the α3 chain of collagen IV, and the type 1 repeats (TSRs) from thrombospondin-1 (TSP-1), are highlighted in black; all other protein domains are shown in gray. The collagens and TSP-1 are represented as monomers for simplicity, yet are known to form trimers. The collagen α chain NC1 domains provide antiangiogenic fragments endostatin and tumstatin, respectively.

Antiangiogenic Activity of Endostatin

Endostatin was first isolated from the conditioned media of nonmetastatic mouse hemangioendothelioma cells as an inhibitor of endothelial proliferation, angiogenesis, and tumor growth in mice (O'Reilly et al. 1997) and later characterized in mice (Standker et al. 1997). The current hypothesis surrounding endogenous endostatin activity is that during endothelial activation, the production of proteolytic enzymes from the BM leads to a release of antiangiogenic fragments to serve as local inhibitors of angiogenesis (Fig. 1). Recombinant endostatin potently blocks angiogenesis and suppresses primary tumor growth in experimental animal models (Table 1). Endostatin interferes with FGF-2-induced signal transduction, inhibiting cell migration (Dixelius et al. 2002), and induces apoptosis (Dhanabal et al. 1999) and cell-cycle arrest (Hanai et al. 2002a), leading to reduced vascularization of tumors (O'Reilly et al. 1997). Endostatin also suppresses growth factor expression, predominantly VEGF (Hajitou et al. 2002), and blocks VEGF receptor-2 (VEGF-R2), via direct interactions (Kim et al. 2002). Endostatin rapidly down-regulates many genes in growing endothelial cells and several signaling pathways in human microvascular endothelium associated with proangiogenic processes (Fig. 3) (Abdollahi et al. 2004). In addition, endostatin can induce Src-dependent disassembly of the actin cytoskeleton (Wickstrom et al. 2002, 2004) and inhibit Wnt signaling (Hanai et al. 2002b). Genetic loss of normal physiological levels of endostatin enhances angiogenesis and increases tumor growth 2- to 3-fold in a mechanism dependent on α5β1 integrin (Sund et al. 2005). Additionally, tumor growth in transgenic mice overproducing endostatin in endothelial cells, a 1.6-fold increase in circulating levels, is 3-fold slower than growth in wild-type mice. Together, these findings suggest that physiological levels of endostatin serve as a source of endothelial-specific tumor suppressor.

Endostatin's Mechanism(s) of Action

Endostatin binds to many endothelial cell-surface proteins, including heparan sulfate proteoglycans, glypicans, VEGF-R2, and α5 and αV containing integrins (Table 1). Endostatin lacks RGD sequences known to bind integrins, and specific integrin-binding sites have not been identified yet. Human endostatin binding to α5β1 integrin leads to the inhibition of focal adhesion kinase/c-Raf/MEK1/2/p38/ERK1 mitogen-activated protein kinase pathway (Fig. 3) (Sudhakar et al. 2003). Endostatin also induces clustering of α5β1 integrin associated with actin stress fibers and colocalization of caveolin-1 (Cav1) to activate phosphatase-dependent Src family kinases (Wickstrom et al. 2002). Recently, endostatin activity was linked

Table 1. Endogenous Angiogenesis Inhibitors

Endogenous inhibitor (MW)	Parent protein	Domain	Receptors	Antiangiogenic effects
Endostatin (20 kD)	α1 chain of type XVIII collagen	NC1 domain	α5β1 integrin, proteoglycans, VEGFR2, tropomyosin	inhibits EC proliferation, migration, induces apoptosis, suppresses tumor growth
Tumstatin (28 kD)	α3 chain of type IV collagen	NC1 domain	αVβ3 integrin α6β1 integrin	inhibits EC proliferation, induces apoptosis, suppresses tumor growth
Thrombospondin-1 (40 kD)	thrombospondin-1 (TSR)	type 1 repeats	CD36, CD47, αβ1 integrin αVβ3 integrin αVβ5 integrin	inhibits EC proliferation, induces apoptosis, induces cell adhesion, suppresses tumor growth, activates TGF-β

(NC1) Non-collagenous domain; (VEGFR2) vascular endothelial growth factor receptor-2; (EC) endothelial cell; (TGF-β) transforming growth factor β.

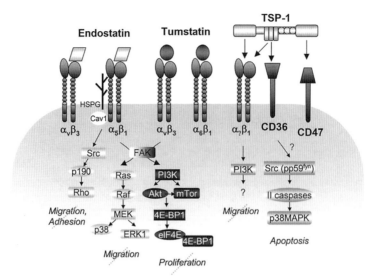

Figure 3. Schematic of the downstream signaling effects of interactions between human endogenous angiogenic inhibitors and their associated cell surface receptors. The effects of endostatin through α5β1 integrin include inhibition of focal adhesion kinase and Src-family kinase phosphorylation to down-regulate key processes in endothelial cell migration and adhesion. The effects of tumstatin are mediated by αVβ3 integrin and include inhibition of focal adhesion kinase phosphorylation that affects signaling through phosphatidylinositol 3-kinase (PI3K), the serine/threonine kinase Akt, mammalian target of rapamycin (mTOR), and eukaryotic translation initiation factor (eIF4E) complexes leading to decreased protein synthesis and endothelial cell proliferation. The effects of thrombospondin-1 (TSP-1) via interaction between the type 1 repeat (TSR) sequence motifs and CD36 induce apoptosis through regulation of the signaling pathway from Src kinase pp59[fyn] to mitogen-activated protein kinase (p38MAPK).

to E-selectin expression on endothelial cells (Yu et al. 2004). Clearly, more studies are needed to elucidate the exact antiangiogenic mechanisms of endostatin.

Three-Dimensional Structure of Endostatin

The crystal structure of recombinant mouse endostatin has been determined at 1.5 Å resolution and reveals a compact fold, similar to the C-type lectin carbohydrate-recognition domain and the hyaluronan-binding link module (Hohenester et al. 1998, 2000). The subsequent crystal structure of human endostatin revealed a zinc-binding site in the amino terminus of endostatin at pH 8.5 (Ding et al. 1998) that is coordinated through H132, H134, H142, and D207, and thus, is likely to serve a role in endostatin structure and not catalytic function (Fig. 4). Interestingly, the antiangiogenic activity of recombinant endostatin was reported to require zinc binding (Boehm et al. 1998); however, subsequent studies failed to show an effect of zinc binding on the inhibition of endothelial cell migration by endostatin (Yamaguchi et al. 1999). Surface arginine residues in endostatin have been suggested to act as binding sites for heparin and heparan sulfate (Hohenester et al. 1998; Sasaki et al. 1999).

A very recent report shows that the entire antitumor and antimigration activities of endostatin are mimicked by a 27-amino-acid peptide (hP1) corresponding to the amino-terminal domain of human endostatin (Fig. 4), and are dependent on the three zinc-binding histidines in the amino-terminal domain (Tjin Tham Sjin et al. 2005). Also recently, an arginine-rich sequence motif (ES-2, IVRRADRAAVP) of human endostatin (Fig. 4) was shown to bind endothelial cell surface β1 integrin and to

heparin, and inhibit endothelial cell migration and tube formation (Wickstrom et al. 2004). It is likely, then, that endostatin has several biological functions mediated by different regions of the protein. Interestingly, examination of the known human endostatin structure reveals that the integrin/heparin-binding sequence (ES-2) and the amino-terminal antiangiogenic sequence (hP1) of endostatin are adjacent to one another in the tertiary structure (Fig. 4). Thus, although these two sites of endostatin activity are discontinuous in primary sequence, together they form a continuous "antiangiogenic active face" on the globular structure of endostatin, where the histidine-dependent zinc-binding site within the most amino-terminal strand neighbors the arginine-rich, surface-exposed, receptor-binding motif to potentially coordinate heparin-dependent and heparin-independent mechanisms of the antiangiogenic action associated with endostatin.

TUMSTATIN

The entire 28-kD fragment of the carboxy-terminal globular non-collagenous (NC1) domain of the α3 chain of type IV collagen was named tumstatin (Fig. 2) (Maeshima et al. 2000a,b). This proteolyzed collagen fragment is likely liberated from the basement membranes of the kidney, lung, and testis, which contain abundant amounts of the α3 chain containing type IV collagen. VBM organization is dependent on the assembly of a type IV collagen network, which is believed to occur through the carboxy-terminal NC1 domain (Madri and Pratt 1986; Tsilibary et al. 1990; Zhang et al. 1994; Timpl 1996; Madri 1997; Zeisberg et al. 2001). Type IV collagen is one of the major macromolecular constituents of all mam-

A   NC1 domain of human type XVIII collagen α1-chain

PPA**HSHRDFQPVLHLVALNSPLSGG**MRGIRGADFQCFQQARAVG
LAGTFRAFLSSRLQDLYS**IVRRADRAAVP**IVNLKDELLFPSWEA
LFSGSEGPLKPGARIFSFDGKDVLRHPTWPQKSVWHGSDPNGRR
LTESYCETWRTEAPSATGQASSLLGGRLLGQSAASCHHAYIVLC
IENSFMTASK

B

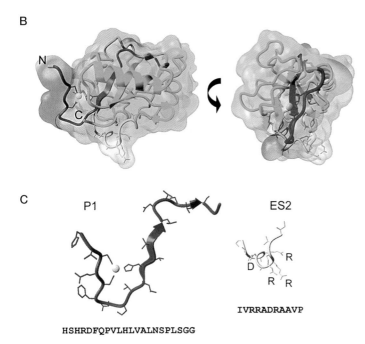

C   P1   ES2

IVRRADRAAVP

HSHRDFQPVLHLVALNSPLSGG

Figure 4. The structure of human endostatin. (*A*) Primary sequence of the proteolytic fragment endostatin from the non-collagenous domain (NC1) of the α1 chain of human collagen XVIII. (*B*) Three-dimensional structure, front and side view, of human endostatin from X-ray crystallographic data (Protein Data Bank ID 1bnl). The regions of endostatin corresponding to antiangiogenic active fragments hP1 and ES2 are rendered in magenta and yellow, respectively, and the remainder of the endostatin backbone is colored green. (*C*) The antiangiogenic active fragments of endostatin, hP1 and ES2, are shown as they exist folded in the intact endostatin structure, with side chains labeled by single-letter amino acid code.

malian basement membranes, including VBM, and is expressed as six distinct α chains, α1–α6 (Hudson et al. 1993; Prockop and Kivirikko 1995). These α chains are assembled into triple helices that further form a network to provide a scaffold for other BM macromolecules. The α1 and α2 chain isoforms are ubiquitously present in human VBM, whereas the other four isoforms exhibit restricted distributions (Hudson et al. 1993; Kalluri et al. 1997). Type IV collagen promotes cell adhesion, migration, differentiation, and growth, while playing a crucial role in angiogenesis (Madri and Pratt 1986; Ingber and Folkman 1988; Madri 1997; Haas and Madri 1999). The non-collagenous NC1 domains of type IV collagen have been implicated as important for the assembly of type IV collagen and also other functions that regulate cell behavior directly (Furcht 1984, 1986; Herbst et al. 1988; Tsilibary et al. 1988, 1990; Chelberg et al. 1990; Cameron et al. 1991; Miles et al. 1995; Zeisberg et al. 2001).

Antiangiogenic and Antitumor Activity of Tumstatin

The full-length endogenous α3 chain NC1 domain fragment, tumstatin, and tumstatin fragments containing residues 54–132 and 74–98, inhibit the formation of new blood vessels in Matrigel plug assays, suppress tumor growth of renal cell and prostate carcinomas in xenograft mouse models, and induce apoptosis of endothelial cells (Table 1) (Maeshima et al. 2000a,b, 2001a,b), specifically by inhibiting protein synthesis in vascular endothelial cells in an integrin-dependent manner leading to endothelial cell-specific apoptosis (Fig. 3) (Maeshima et al. 2002). Overexpression of tumstatin by tumor cells inhibits their invasive properties in a mouse melanoma model (Pasco et al. 2004). Absence of normal physiological levels of tumstatin circulating in the blood facilitates pathological angiogenesis and increased tumor growth (Hamano et al. 2003; Sund et al. 2005). Mice genetically deficient in collagen IV α3 chain show accelerated tumor growth and vascularization, and supplementing these mice with recombinant tumstatin at normal physiological levels abolishes the increased rate of tumor growth. These studies provide compelling evidence for the role of tumstatin as an endogenous inhibitor of angiogenesis and tumor suppressor functioning at physiological levels.

The in vitro activity of tumstatin was evaluated using recombinant human protein produced in bacteria and tumstatin-derived synthetic peptides. Recombinant tumstatin inhibits proliferation of endothelial cells, causes G_1 arrest of growth-factor-stimulated endothelial cells, and induces apoptosis of proliferating endothelial cells via regulation of caspase 3 (Maeshima et al. 2000a,b, 2001a,b). Synthetic peptide derived from the α3 chain of the NC1 domain of type IV collagen, residues 183–205, has been shown to inhibit the proliferation of melanoma and other epithelial tumor cell lines in vitro (Monboisse et al. 1994; Han et al. 1997) and bind to the CD47/αvβ3 integrin complex (Fig. 3) (Shahan et al. 1999a,b, 2000). This interaction appears to stimulate focal adhesion kinase (FAK) and phosphatidylinositol 3-kinase (PI3K) phosphorylation (Pasco et al. 2000). The 183-205 peptide does not affect endothelial cells, but rather demonstrates an anti-melanoma cell activity (Maeshima et al. 2000b). Specifically, the 183-205 fragment of tumstatin binds both endothelial and melanoma cells but only inhibits the proliferation of melanoma cells (Shahan et al. 1999b; Maeshima et al. 2000b; Floquet et al. 2004).

In contrast to this anti-melanoma activity, the antiangiogenic activity of tumstatin was localized to residues 54–132 (tum-5) using deletion mutagenesis (Maeshima et al. 2000b, 2001a; Petitclerc et al. 2000). Tumstatin fragment 54-132 binds both endothelial cells and melanoma cells, but only inhibits the proliferation of endothelial cells, with no effect on tumor cell proliferation. The antiangiogenic site was further defined using overlapping synthetic peptides to a 25-amino-acid region comprising residues 74–98, namely the T7 tumstatin peptide (Maeshima et al. 2001b). The 54-132 tumstatin fragment inhibits the activation of FAK/PI3K/protein kinase B (PKB)/mammalian target of rapamycin (mTOR) signaling and inactivates eukaryotic initiation factor 4E protein (eIF4E), leading to inhibition of cap-dependent protein synthesis (Fig. 3) (Maeshima et al. 2002). Thus, two separate tumstatin activities, one antiangiogenic and the other antitumor cell, have been localized to distinct regions of the tumstatin molecule.

Tumstatin's Mechanism(s) of Activity

Tumstatin has two binding sites for αvβ3 integrin, one in the amino-terminal end of the molecule (residues 54–132) that is associated with antiangiogenic activity, and the other in the carboxy-terminal end (residues 185–203) that is associated with antitumor cell activity (Shahan et al. 1999b; Maeshima et al. 2000b; Floquet et al. 2004). The presence of cyclic RGD peptides does not compete for the αVβ3 integrin-dependent activity of tumstatin, suggesting unique αVβ3 integrin-mediated mechanisms governing these two distinct antiangiogenic and antitumor activities (Maeshima et al. 2000a). αVβ3 integrin was been identified as a receptor for tumstatin (Maeshima et al. 2000a, 2001b), and tumstatin fails to suppress neovascularization of Matrigel plugs in β3 integrin-deficient mice (Hynes 2002; Reynolds et al. 2002). Tumstatin has also been shown to interact with α6β1 integrin; however, the downstream consequences of such interaction have yet to be determined.

Three-Dimensional Homology Modeled Structure of Tumstatin

From crystallographic data it has been shown that the NC1 domains of type IV collagen α1 and α2 chains (α1[IV]NC1 and α2[IV]NC1) are folded virtually identically, and their topologies very closely resemble one another (Than et al. 2002). Based on the high sequence identity between all type IV collagen NC1 domains, the NC1

domain of type IV collagen α3 chain (α3[IV]NC1) is expected to fold with the same topology as the α1(IV)NC1. Therefore, by aligning the α3(IV)NC1 and α1(IV)NC1 sequences and using the known $[(\alpha1)_2\alpha2]_2$ NC1 hexamer structure (Protein Data Base ID 1LI1), a backbone homology α3(IV)NC1 structure has been made (Fig. 5).

In analyzing the α-chain (IV)NC1 alignments and the backbone α3(IV)NC1 homology structure, we have determined that the two distinct regions of tumstatin that exhibit antiangiogenic (T7) and antitumor cell (185–203) activities share partial sequence and structural homology, unidentified as of yet. Seven residues in the amino terminus of the 185–203 sequence align with carboxy-terminal residues in the T7 peptide (Fig. 5). The NC1 domain is composed of two homologous subdomains, and the T7 peptide and the 185–203 sequences are partially homologous regions between the NC1 subdomains (Than et al. 2002). In a recent report, a shorter peptide corresponding to residues 185–191 (CNYYSNS) shared the same inhibitory properties in a mouse melanoma model as the 185–203 sequence (Floquet et al. 2004). The inhibitory effects were conformation-dependent, and residues YSNS, which form a β turn, were crucial for activity. Interestingly, the analogous residues in T7, the sequence SRND, appear to form a β-turn structure in the homology model of α3(IV)NC1 (Fig. 5). Monoclonal antibodies against the αV and β3 integrin subunits were used to determine that the 185-203 peptide binds directly to the β3 subunit (Pasco et al. 2000). Therefore, the β turns located in these regions likely expose tumstatin residues within the turn for interaction and/or provide a recognizable structural ligand for interaction with the β3 integrin subunit. One might also conclude that the distinct activities identified for the T7 and 185–203 peptides are determined by residues, unique to each peptide, that flank the common β-turn structures.

THROMBOSPONDIN

Thrombospondin-1 (TSP-1) was identified as one of the first endogenous angiogenesis inhibitors discovered in normal fibroblast cell cultures (Good et al. 1990). Thrombospondins (TSPs) are multimeric, calcium-binding, modular glycoproteins that modulate ECM structure and cell behavior (for review, see Adams 1997, 2001; Tucker 2004). The best-characterized TSP of the 5 known proteins is TSP-1, which functions in platelet aggregation, inflammation, and regulation of angiogenesis by inducing cell attachment, cell motility, cell proliferation, apoptosis, extracellular protease activation, and growth factor inhibition (Table 1) (for review, see Adams 2001). TSP-1 forms homotrimers, and each TSP subunit contains multiple domains and a coiled-coil oligomerization region. The common feature of all TSPs is a cassette of domains around 650 amino acids in length containing a variable number of type 2 calcium-binding EGF-like domains that are contiguous with seven TSP type 3 repeat regions and a globular carboxyl terminus (Fig. 2). Unique to TSP-1 and TSP-2 are the procollagen domain and distinctive type 1 repeat domains (TSRs), which have specific functions in signaling inhibition of angiogenesis by

A

NC1 domain of human type IV collagen α3-chain

```
WTTRGFVFTRHSQTTAIPSCPEGTVPLYSGFSFLFVQGNQRAHGQDLGTLG
SCLQRFTTMPFLFCNVNDVCNFASRNDYSYWLSTPALMPMNMAPITGRALE
PYISRCTVCEGPAIAIAVHSQTTDIPPCPHGWISLWKGFSFIMFTSAGSEG
TGQALASPGSCLEEFRASPFLECHGRGTCNYYSNSYSFWLASLNPERMFRK
PIPSTVKAGELEKIISRCQVCMKKR
```

B

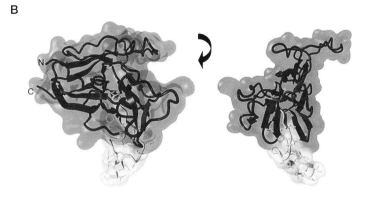

C

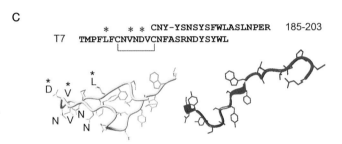

Figure 5. Homology-based model of tumstatin. (*A*) Primary sequence of the proteolytic fragment tumstatin, the entire non-collagenous domain (NC1) of the α3 chain of human collagen IV. (*B*) Homology-based three-dimensional model of tumstatin, shown in front and side views, based on the known trimer structure ([α1]₂α2) of the homologous α1 and α2 chain NC1 domains of human type IV collagen from X-ray crystallographic data and homology modeling. The structures of the ([α1]₂α2)₂ NC1 hexamers from human placenta basement membranes (Protein Data Bank ID 1LI1) were rendered using the molecular graphics visualization program YASARA (YASARA Biosciences) and analyzed to generate modeled structures using the molecular graphics software InsightII (Accelrys). The regions of tumstatin corresponding to antiangiogenic active fragments T7 and the 183-205 sequence are rendered yellow and magenta, respectively, and the remainder of the tumstatin backbone is colored blue. (*C*) The antiangiogenic active fragments of tumstatin, shown as they exist folded in the intact homology tumstatin model, with side chains labeled by single-letter amino acid code.

binding to CD36 and supporting attachment of varied cell types. TSPs appear to function at the cell surface to bring together membrane proteins and cytokines that regulate ECM structure and cellular phenotype. Known binding partners of TSPs include integrins, the integrin-associated protein CD47, CD36, proteoglycans, and the growth factors TGF-β and PDGF (Fig. 3).

TSPs are expressed in most adult tissues; however, TSP-1 and TSP-2 are highly expressed by stromal fibroblasts, tumor-associated endothelial cells, and tumor cells (Fig. 1) (Brown et al. 1999; Hawighorst et al. 2001). TSP-1 expression increases in response to growth factors PDGF, bFGF, and TGF-β, as well as heat shock and hypoxia. TSP-1 is secreted into the extra- and pericellular matrix by a multitude of different cell types including platelets; megakaryocytes; chondrocytes; osteocytes; epithelial, endothelial, and stromal cells (for review, see Carpizo and Iruela-Arispe 2000); as well as cancer cells, where loss of TSP-1 expression by tumor cells contributes to the angiogenic phenotype (Jimenez and Volpert 2001; Volpert et al. 2002; Watnick et al. 2003).

Antiangiogenic Activity of Thrombospondin-1

TSP-1 was the first protein to be identified as a naturally occurring inhibitor of angiogenesis (Good et al. 1990). TSP-1 has been shown to inhibit tumor growth and metastasis, identifying it as a potent inhibitor of in vivo neovascularization and tumorigenesis. In addition, expression of TSP-1 has been inversely correlated with tumor progression in breast and lung carcinomas and melanomas (Zabrenetzky et al. 1994; Streit et al. 1999; Rodriguez-Manzaneque et al. 2001). Collective in vivo studies evaluating the effects of TSP-1 on tumor growth have shown that TSP-1 acts to inhibit tumor growth via antiangiogenic mechanisms, and analysis of the tumors and tumor vasculature indicates that the observed antitumor effect of TSP-1 occurs through an inhibition of angiogenesis rather than a direct effect on tumor cells (Weinstat-Saslow et al. 1994; Zabrenetzky et al. 1994; Campbell et al. 1998; Bleuel et al. 1999; Streit et al. 1999). Genetic approaches to assess the functions of TSP-1 have been performed by targeted gene disruption. To evaluate the importance of TSP-1 for the progression of naturally arising tumors, TSP-1-deficient mice were crossed with p53-deficient mice, resulting in decreased survival. Furthermore, TSP-1-deficient mice showed faster tumor growth with increased vascular density (Lawler et al. 2001; Sund et al. 2005). Additionally, in tumstatin/TSP-1 double-knockout mice, tumors grow twofold faster compared with either tumstatin- or TSP-1-deficient mice. Both results strongly suggest that physiological levels of host-derived factors from the tumor microenvironment serve as endogenous inhibitors of angiogenesis and suppress tumor growth.

The Mechanisms of Thrombospondin-1 Antiangiogenic Activity

Since the initial observation that TSP-1 activates TGF-β, fusion proteins and peptide fragments of TSP-1 have been used to determine the molecular basis of this interaction. Fusion protein and synthetic peptides have shown that the WSHWSPW sequence in the second TSR binds to TGF-β, and the RFK sequence at the carboxyl terminus of the first TSR activates TGF-β (Schultz-Cherry et al. 1995). Nascent TGF-β is proteolytically processed into mature TGF-β and a latency-associated peptide (LAP). The RFK sequence of TSP-1 has been shown to interact to displace LAP and make TGF-β accessible for activity (Ribeiro et al. 1999).

Peptides from the procollagen domain and TSR domains have been shown to inhibit angiogenesis in the corneal pocket assay (Tolsma et al. 1993). Synthetic peptides of the second TSR exhibited antitumor effects that were mediated by an antiangiogenic mechanism (Guo et al. 1997). Using similar approaches, two subdomains within the TSR repeats were identified with antiangiogenic properties: (1) the tryptophan-rich sequence, described above in interactions with TGF-β, from TSR2 and 3 is an inhibitor of angiogenesis in the CAM assay, and (2) the CSVTCG sequence from TSR2 interacts with CD36, specifically, to inhibit angiogenesis (Iruela-Arispe et al. 1999). Interestingly, using larger peptides encompassing these sequences, the antiangiogenic activity of the Trp-rich sequence region was restricted to FGF-2-induced neovascularization, whereas the CD36-binding region's antiangiogenic activity was maintained in both FGF-2- and VEGF-induced neovascularization. It was previously shown that the Trp-rich region prevents FGF-2 binding to endothelial cells, and together these studies suggest that distinct TSP-1 antiangiogenic mechanisms may be growth-factor-dependent (Carpizo and Iruela-Arispe 2000).

CD36, a class B scavenger receptor, has been implicated as the cell surface receptor that mediates the action of TSP-1 on endothelial cells, initially through the CSVTCG motif from TSR2 (Dawson et al. 1997). Subsequently, a secondary binding motif within TSP-1, GVQXR, was shown to bind CD36 and to mediate the migratory inhibition action of TSP-1 (Dawson et al. 1997). Recently, the downstream intracellular interactions involving CD36 have been determined and reveal that TSP-1 induces apoptotic CD36-dependent mechanisms that activate Src-family tyrosine kinase pp59[fyn], group II caspases, and p38MAPK (Jimenez et al. 2000). A direct link between CD36 receptor and pp59[fyn] activation has yet to be determined.

Three-Dimensional Structures of Thrombospondin-1 Repeat Domains

The three-dimensional structure of TSR domains 2 and 3 from human TSP-1 has been determined by X-ray crystallography (Fig. 6) (Tan et al. 2002). The structure (Fig. 6) shows that each TSR folds into a long, thin, stranded domain composed of three antiparallel strands, the first without regular β-strand structure, and the second two with. Intervening loops between the strands are prominently solvent-exposed, and the structures are stabilized by cross-strand disulfide bridging between pairs of cysteines. Two of the active binding site sequences in TSR2, specifically WSHWSPWS and GVITRIR, which are both implicated in antiangiogenic effects that inhibit VEGF- or FGF-2-induced angiogenesis, can be mapped to exposed regions on the first and second strands of TSR2 (Fig. 6) and contribute side chains to a single positively charged groove on the same face of TSR2 (Tan et al. 2002; Lawler and Detmar 2004). The TSR represents a novel domain fold whereby interdigitating side-chain stacking of Cys, Trp, and Arg forms the core structure. In light of the complex core TSR structure, it is intriguing that isolated peptides from either of the interdigitating strands in the TSR2 domain have antiangiogenic inhibitory activities (Tolsma et al. 1993; Dawson et al. 1999; Iruela-Arispe et al. 1999; Jimenez et al. 2000). Recently, two designed, structurally modified fragments from the TSR2 domain of TSP-1 were shown to increase apoptosis in endothelial cells, block neovascularization in mouse Matrigel plug models, inhibit tumor growth in mouse lung carcinoma models, inhibit melanoma metastases, and block the growth of implanted human carcinoma in nude mice (Dawson et al. 1999; Reiher et al. 2002; Haviv et al. 2005). These molecules, which are now in phase II clinical trials, serve as important examples to demonstrate the potential that exists in small, peptide antiangiogenic therapy design that is based on the functional and structural data of endogenous proteins.

SUMMARY

An examination of the structural features and functional activities of the endogenous inhibitors of angiogenesis—endostatin, tumstatin, and TSP-1—amplifies a recurrent theme, that is, the exposed surfaces of naturally occurring endogenous antiangiogenic factors possess multiple, adjacent receptor- or protein-binding sites, often with distinct functional activities. Most of the motifs implicated in cell surface receptor binding by these endogenous factors are novel sequence- or conformation-dependent motifs for interaction. Interestingly, studies using peptide fragments of all three of these inhibitors demonstrate that these small sequence motifs maintain their potent functional activities apart from the structural constraints of their full-length parent molecules. It remains, then, of great interest to more fully elucidate the unique molecular structures inherent in these factors, their receptor-binding sites, and their mechanisms of action, in order to gain insight into their structure/function necessary to facilitate ongoing efforts to develop potent antiangiogenic cancer therapies targeting tumor vasculature.

ACKNOWLEDGMENTS

This work was supported by National Institutes of Health grants DK55001, DK62987, and AA13913, and by funds from the Center for Matrix Biology at the Beth

A   Thrombospondin-1 TSR2 Domain

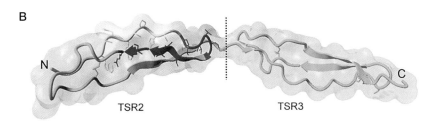

N-KRFKQDGG**WSHWSPWS**S<u>CSVTCG</u>D<u>**GVITRIR**</u>-
LCNSPSPQMNGKPCEGEARETKACKKDACPI-C

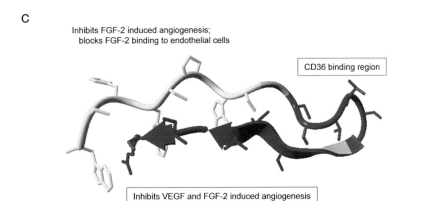

Figure 6. The structure of TSP-1 repeats 2,3 (TSR) of TSP-1. (*A*) Primary sequence of the second type 1 repeat (TSR2) domain of human TSP-1. Regions of TSR2 that have demonstrated antiangiogenic activity are underlined/bolded. (*B*) Three-dimensional structure of TSR2 and TSR3 from human TSP-1 from X-ray crystallographic data (Protein Data Bank ID 1LSL). Regions of the structure corresponding to the antiangiogenic active sequences are rendered using the same color as the underlining in *A*. The remainder of the TSR2 and TSR3 structure is colored cyan. (*C*) Enlarged image of the backbone secondary structure and side chain positions of adjacent antiangiogenic active sequences that comprise the strands and connective turn of a single positively charged groove on the surface of TSR2.

Israel Deaconess Medical Center. M.G. is funded by an An American Heart Association grant 05030348N.

REFERENCES

Abdollahi A., Hahnfeldt P., Maercker C., Grone H.J., Debus J., Ansorge W., Folkman J., Hlatky L., and Huber P.E. 2004. Endostatin's antiangiogenic signaling network. *Mol. Cell* **13:** 649.

Adams J.C. 1997. Thrombospondin-1. *Int. J. Biochem. Cell Biol.* **29:** 861.

———. 2001. Thrombospondins: Multifunctional regulators of cell interactions. *Annu. Rev. Cell Dev. Biol.* **17:** 25.

Bergers G. and Benjamin L.E. 2003. Tumorigenesis and the angiogenic switch. *Nat. Rev. Cancer* **3:** 401.

Bleuel K., Popp S., Fusenig N.E., Stanbridge E.J., and Boukamp P. 1999. Tumor suppression in human skin carcinoma cells by chromosome 15 transfer or thrombospondin-1 overexpression through halted tumor vascularization. *Proc. Natl. Acad. Sci.* **96:** 2065.

Boehm T., O'Reilly M.S., Keough K., Shiloach J., Shapiro R., and Folkman J. 1998. Zinc-binding of endostatin is essential for its antiangiogenic activity. *Biochem. Biophys. Res. Commun.* **252:** 190.

Brown L.F., Guidi A.J., Schnitt S.J., Van De Water L., Iruela-Arispe M.L., Yeo T.K., Tognazzi K., and Dvorak H.F. 1999. Vascular stroma formation in carcinoma in situ, invasive carcinoma, and metastatic carcinoma of the breast. *Clin. Cancer Res.* **5:** 1041.

Cameron J.D., Skubitz A.P., and Furcht L.T. 1991. Type IV collagen and corneal epithelial adhesion and migration. Effects of type IV collagen fragments and synthetic peptides on rabbit corneal epithelial cell adhesion and migration in vitro. *Invest. Ophthalmol. Vis. Sci.* **32:** 2766.

Campbell S.C., Volpert O.V., Ivanovich M., and Bouck N.P. 1998. Molecular mediators of angiogenesis in bladder cancer. *Cancer Res.* **58:** 1298.

Cao Y. 2001. Endogenous angiogenesis inhibitors and their therapeutic implications. *Int. J. Biochem. Cell Biol.* **33:** 357.

Carmeliet P., Dor Y., Herbert J.M., Fukumura D., Brusselmans K., Dewerchin M., Neeman M., Bono F., Abramovitch R., Maxwell P., Koch C.J., Ratcliffe P., Moons L., Jain R.K., Collen D., and Keshert E. 1998. Role of HIF-1alpha in hypoxia-mediated apoptosis, cell proliferation and tumour angiogenesis. *Nature* **394:** 485.

Carpizo D. and Iruela-Arispe M.L. 2000. Endogenous regulators of angiogenesis—Emphasis on proteins with thrombospondin-type I motifs. *Cancer Metastasis Rev.* **19:** 159.

Chelberg M.K., McCarthy J.B., Skubitz A.P., Furcht L.T., and

Tsilibary E.C. 1990. Characterization of a synthetic peptide from type IV collagen that promotes melanoma cell adhesion, spreading, and motility. *J. Cell Biol.* **111:** 261.

Colorado P.C., Torre A., Kamphaus G., Maeshima Y., Hopfer H., Takahashi K., Volk R., Zamborsky E.D., Herman S., Sarkar P.K., Ericksen M.B., Dhanabal M., Simons M., Post M., Kufe D.W., Weichselbaum R.R., Sukhatme V.P., and Kalluri R. 2000. Anti-angiogenic cues from vascular basement membrane collagen. *Cancer Res.* **60:** 2520.

Coussens L.M., Fingleton B., and Matrisian L.M. 2002. Matrix metalloproteinase inhibitors and cancer: Trials and tribulations. *Science* **295:** 2387.

Darland D.C. and D'Amore P.A. 1999. Blood vessel maturation: Vascular development comes of age. *J. Clin. Invest.* **103:** 157.

Dawson D.W., Pearce S.F., Zhong R., Silverstein R.L., Frazier W.A., and Bouck N.P. 1997. CD36 mediates the in vitro inhibitory effects of thrombospondin-1 on endothelial cells. *J. Cell Biol.* **138:** 707.

Dawson D.W., Volpert O.V., Pearce S.F., Schneider A.J., Silverstein R.L., Henkin J., and Bouck N.P. 1999. Three distinct D-amino acid substitutions confer potent antiangiogenic activity on an inactive peptide derived from a thrombospondin-1 type 1 repeat. *Mol. Pharmacol.* **55:** 332.

Dhanabal M., Ramchandran R., Waterman M.J., Lu H., Knebelmann B., Segal M., and Sukhatme V.P. 1999. Endostatin induces endothelial cell apoptosis. *J. Biol. Chem.* **274:** 11721.

Ding Y.H., Javaherian K., Lo K.M., Chopra R., Boehm T., Lanciotti J., Harris B.A., Li Y., Shapiro R., Hohenester E., Timpl R., Folkman J., and Wiley D.C. 1998. Zinc-dependent dimers observed in crystals of human endostatin. *Proc. Natl. Acad. Sci.* **95:** 10443.

Dixelius J., Cross M., Matsumoto T., Sasaki T., Timpl R., and Claesson-Welsh L. 2002. Endostatin regulates endothelial cell adhesion and cytoskeletal organization. *Cancer Res.* **62:** 1944.

Dvorak H.F., Brown L.F., Detmar M., and Dvorak A.M. 1995. Vascular permeability factor/vascular endothelial growth factor, microvascular hyperpermeability, and angiogenesis. *Am. J. Pathol.* **146:** 1029.

Egeblad M., and Werb Z. 2002. New functions for the matrix metalloproteinases in cancer progression. *Nat. Rev. Cancer* **2:** 161.

Felbor U., Dreier L., Bryant R.A., Ploegh H.L., Olsen B.R., and Mothes W. 2000. Secreted cathepsin L generates endostatin from collagen XVIII. *EMBO J.* **19:** 1187.

Floquet N., Pasco S., Ramont L., Derreumaux P., Laronze J.Y., Nuzillard J.M., Maquart F.X., Alix A.J., and Monboisse J.C. 2004. The antitumor properties of the alpha3(IV)-(185-203) peptide from the NC1 domain of type IV collagen (tumstatin) are conformation-dependent. *J. Biol. Chem.* **279:** 2091.

Folkman J. 1971. Tumor angiogenesis: Therapeutic implications. *N. Engl. J. Med.* **285:** 1182.

———. 1972. Anti-angiogenesis: New concept for therapy of solid tumors. *Ann. Surg.* **175:** 409.

———. 1995. Angiogenesis in cancer, vascular, rheumatoid and other disease. *Nat. Med.* **1:** 27.

———. 2004. Endogenous angiogenesis inhibitors. *APMIS* **112:** 496.

Folkman J. and Shing Y. 1992. Angiogenesis. *J. Biol. Chem.* **267:** 10931.

Fukumura D., Xavier R., Sugiura T., Chen Y., Park E.C., Lu N., Selig M., Nielsen G., Taksir T., Jain R.K., and Seed B. 1998. Tumor induction of VEGF promoter activity in stromal cells. *Cell* **94:** 715.

Furcht L.T. 1984. Role of cell adhesion molecules in promoting migration of normal and malignant cells. *Prog. Clin. Biol. Res.* **149:** 15.

———. 1986. Critical factors controlling angiogenesis: Cell products, cell matrix, and growth factors. *Lab. Invest.* **55:** 505.

Good D.J., Polverini P.J., Rastinejad F., Le Beau M.M., Lemons R.S., Frazier W.A., and Bouck N.P. 1990. A tumor suppressor-dependent inhibitor of angiogenesis is immunologically and functionally indistinguishable from a fragment of throm-

bospondin. *Proc. Natl. Acad. Sci.* **87:** 6624.

Guo N.H., Krutzsch H.C., Inman J.K., Shannon C.S., and Roberts D.D. 1997. Antiproliferative and antitumor activities of D-reverse peptides derived from the second type-1 repeat of thrombospondin-1. *J. Pept. Res.* **50:** 210.

Haas T.L. and Madri J.A. 1999. Extracellular matrix-driven matrix metalloproteinase production in endothelial cells: Implications for angiogenesis. *Trends Cardiovasc. Med.* **9:** 70.

Hajitou A., Grignet C., Devy L., Berndt S., Blacher S., Deroanne C.F., Bajou K., Fong T., Chiang Y., Foidart J.M., and Noel A. 2002. The antitumoral effect of endostatin and angiostatin is associated with a down-regulation of vascular endothelial growth factor expression in tumor cells. *FASEB J.* **16:** 1802.

Halfter W., Dong S., Schurer B., and Cole G.J. 1998. Collagen XVIII is a basement membrane heparan sulfate proteoglycan. *J. Biol. Chem.* **273:** 25404.

Hamano Y., Zeisberg M., Sugimoto H., Lively J.C., Maeshima Y., Yang C., Hynes R.O., Werb Z., Sudhakar A., and Kalluri R. 2003. Physiological levels of tumstatin, a fragment of collagen IV alpha3 chain, are generated by MMP-9 proteolysis and suppress angiogenesis via alphaV beta3 integrin. *Cancer Cell* **3:** 589.

Han J., Ohno N., Pasco S., Monboisse J.C., Borel J.P., and Kefalides N.A. 1997. A cell binding domain from the alpha3 chain of type IV collagen inhibits proliferation of melanoma cells. *J. Biol. Chem.* **272:** 20395.

Hanahan D. and Folkman J. 1996. Patterns and emerging mechanisms of the angiogenic switch during tumorigenesis. *Cell* **86:** 353.

Hanai J., Dhanabal M., Karumanchi S.A., Albanese C., Waterman M., Chan B., Ramchandran R., Pestell R., and Sukhatme V.P. 2002a. Endostatin causes G1 arrest of endothelial cells through inhibition of cyclin D1. *J. Biol. Chem.* **277:** 16464.

Hanai J., Gloy J., Karumanchi S.A., Kale S., Tang J., Hu G., Chan B., Ramchandran R., Jha V., Sukhatme V.P., and Sokol S. 2002b. Endostatin is a potential inhibitor of Wnt signaling. *J. Cell Biol.* **158:** 529.

Haviv F., Bradley M.F., Kalvin D.M., Schneider A.J., Davidson D.J., Majest S.M., McKay L.M., Haskell C.J., Bell R.L., Nguyen B., Marsh K.C., Surber B.W., Uchic J.T. Ferrero J., Wang Y.C., Leal J., Record R.D., Hodde J., Badylak S.F., Lesniewski R.R., and Henkin J. 2005. Thrombospondin-1 mimetic peptide inhibitors of angiogenesis and tumor growth: Design, synthesis, and optimization of pharmacokinetics and biological activities. *J. Med. Chem.* **48:** 2838.

Hawighorst T., Velasco P., Streit M., Hong Y.K., Kyriakides T.R., Brown L.F., Bornstein P., and Detmar M. 2001. Thrombospondin-2 plays a protective role in multistep carcinogenesis: A novel host anti-tumor defense mechanism. *EMBO J.* **20:** 2631.

Herbst T.J., McCarthy J.B., Tsilibary E.C., and Furcht L.T. 1988. Differential effects of laminin, intact type IV collagen, and specific domains of type IV collagen on endothelial cell adhesion and migration. *J. Cell Biol.* **106:** 1365.

Hohenester E., Sasaki T., Mann K., and Timpl R. 2000. Variable zinc coordination in endostatin. *J. Mol. Biol.* **297:** 1.

Hohenester E., Sasaki T., Olsen B.R., and Timpl R. 1998. Crystal structure of the angiogenesis inhibitor endostatin at 1.5 Å resolution. *EMBO J.* **17:** 1656.

Hudson B.G., Reeders S.T., and Tryggvason K. 1993. Type IV collagen: Structure, gene organization, and role in human diseases. Molecular basis of Goodpasture and Alport syndromes and diffuse leiomyomatosis. *J. Biol. Chem.* **268:** 26033.

Hynes R.O. 2002. A reevaluation of integrins as regulators of angiogenesis. *Nat. Med.* **8:** 918.

Ingber D. and Folkman J. 1988. Inhibition of angiogenesis through modulation of collagen metabolism. *Lab. Invest.* **59:** 44.

Iruela-Arispe M.L., Lombardo M., Krutzsch H.C., Lawler J., and Roberts D.D. 1999. Inhibition of angiogenesis by thrombospondin-1 is mediated by 2 independent regions within the type 1 repeats. *Circulation* **100:** 1423.

Jimenez B. and Volpert O.V. 2001. Mechanistic insights on the inhibition of tumor angiogenesis. *J. Mol. Med.* **78:** 663.

Jimenez B., Volpert O.V., Crawford S.E., Febbraio M., Silverstein R.L., and Bouck N. 2000. Signals leading to apoptosis-dependent inhibition of neovascularization by thrombospondin-1. *Nat. Med.* **6:** 41.

Kalluri R., Shield C.F., Todd P., Hudson B.G., and Neilson E.G. 1997. Isoform switching of type IV collagen is developmentally arrested in X-linked Alport syndrome leading to increased susceptibility of renal basement membranes to endoproteolysis. *J. Clin. Invest.* **99:** 2470.

Kim Y.M., Hwang S., Pyun B.J., Kim T.Y., Lee S.T., Gho Y.S., and Kwon Y.G. 2002. Endostatin blocks vascular endothelial growth factor-mediated signaling via direct interaction with KDR/Flk-1. *J. Biol. Chem.* **277:** 27872.

Lawler J. and Detmar M. 2004. Tumor progression: The effects of thrombospondin-1 and -2. *Int. J. Biochem. Cell Biol.* **36:** 1038.

Lawler J., Miao W.M., Duquette M., Bouck N., Bronson R.T., and Hynes R.O. 2001. Thrombospondin-1 gene expression affects survival and tumor spectrum of p53-deficient mice. *Am. J. Pathol.* **159:** 1949.

Madri J.A. 1997. Extracellular matrix modulation of vascular cell behaviour. *Transpl. Immunol.* **5:** 179.

Madri J.A. and Pratt B.M. 1986. Endothelial cell-matrix interactions: In vitro models of angiogenesis. *J. Histochem. Cytochem.* **34:** 85.

Maeshima Y., Colorado P.C., and Kalluri R. 2000a. Two RGD-independent alpha vbeta 3 integrin binding sites on tumstatin regulate distinct anti-tumor properties. *J. Biol. Chem.* **275:** 23745.

Maeshima Y., Manfredi M., Reimer C., Holthaus K.A., Hopfer H., Chandamuri B.R., Kharbanda S., and Kalluri R. 2001a. Identification of the anti-angiogenic site within vascular basement membrane-derived tumstatin. *J. Biol. Chem.* **276:** 15240.

Maeshima Y., Sudhakar A., Lively J.C., Ueki K., Kharbanda S., Kahn C.R., Sonenberg N., Hynes R.O., and Kalluri R. 2002. Tumstatin, an endothelial cell-specific inhibitor of protein synthesis. *Science* **295:** 140.

Maeshima Y., Colorado P.C., Torre A., Holthaus K.A., Grunkemeyer J.A., Ericksen M.B., Hopfer H., Xiao Y., Stillman I.E., and Kalluri R. 2000b. Distinct antitumor properties of a type IV collagen domain derived from basement membrane. *J. Biol. Chem.* **275:** 21340.

Maeshima Y., Yerramalla U.L., Dhanabal M., Holthaus K.A., Barbashov S., Kharbanda S., Reimer C., Manfredi M., Dickerson W.M., and Kalluri R. 2001b. Extracellular matrix-derived peptide binds to alpha(v)beta(3) integrin and inhibits angiogenesis. *J. Biol. Chem.* **276:** 31959.

Miles A.J., Knutson J.R., Skubitz A.P., Furcht L.T., McCarthy J.B., and Fields G.B. 1995. A peptide model of basement membrane collagen alpha 1 (IV) 531-543 binds the alpha 3 beta 1 integrin. *J. Biol. Chem.* **270:** 29047.

Monboisse J.C., Garnotel R., Bellon G., Ohno N., Perreau C., Borel J.P., and Kefalides N.A. 1994. The alpha 3 chain of type IV collagen prevents activation of human polymorphonuclear leukocytes. *J. Biol. Chem.* **269:** 25475.

Musso O., Theret N., Heljasvaara R., Rehn M., Turlin B., Campion J.P., Pihlajaniemi T., and Clement B. 2001. Tumor hepatocytes and basement membrane-producing cells specifically express two different forms of the endostatin precursor, collagen XVIII, in human liver cancers. *Hepatology* **33:** 868.

Nyberg P., Xie L., and Kalluri R. 2005. Endogenous inhibitors of angiogenesis. *Cancer Res.* **65:** 3967.

O'Reilly M.S., Boehm T., Shing Y., Fukai N., Vasios G., Lane W.S., Flynn E., Birkhead J.R., Olsen B.R., and Folkman J. 1997. Endostatin: An endogenous inhibitor of angiogenesis and tumor growth. *Cell* **88:** 277.

Pasco S., Monboisse J.C., and Kieffer N. 2000. The alpha 3(IV)185-206 peptide from noncollagenous domain 1 of type IV collagen interacts with a novel binding site on the beta 3 subunit of integrin alpha Vbeta 3 and stimulates focal adhesion kinase and phosphatidylinositol 3-kinase phosphorylation. *J. Biol. Chem.* **275:** 32999.

Pasco S., Ramont L., Venteo L., Pluot M., Maquart F.X., and Monboisse J.C. 2004. In vivo overexpression of tumstatin domains by tumor cells inhibits their invasive properties in a mouse melanoma model. *Exp. Cell Res.* **301:** 251.

Paulsson M. 1992. Basement membrane proteins: Structure, assembly, and cellular interactions. *Crit. Rev. Biochem. Mol. Biol.* **27:** 93.

Petitclerc E., Boutaud A., Prestayko A., Xu J., Sado Y., Ninomiya Y., Sarras M.P., Jr., Hudson B.G., and Brooks P.C. 2000. New functions for non-collagenous domains of human collagen type IV. Novel integrin ligands inhibiting angiogenesis and tumor growth in vivo. *J. Biol. Chem.* **275:** 8051.

Pore N., Liu S., Haas-Kogan D.A., O'Rourke D.M., and Maity A. 2003. PTEN mutation and epidermal growth factor receptor activation regulate vascular endothelial growth factor (VEGF) mRNA expression in human glioblastoma cells by transactivating the proximal VEGF promoter. *Cancer Res.* **63:** 236.

Prockop D.J. and Kivirikko K.I. 1995. Collagens: Molecular biology, diseases, and potentials for therapy. *Annu. Rev. Biochem.* **64:** 403.

Rak J., Mitsuhashi Y., Sheehan C., Tamir A., Viloria-Petit A., Filmus J., Mansour S.J., Ahn N.G., and Kerbel R.S. 2000. Oncogenes and tumor angiogenesis: Differential modes of vascular endothelial growth factor up-regulation in ras-transformed epithelial cells and fibroblasts. *Cancer Res.* **60:** 490.

Reiher F.K., Volpert O.V., Jimenez B., Crawford S.E., Dinney C.P., Henkin J., Haviv F., Bouck N.P., and Campbell S.C. 2002. Inhibition of tumor growth by systemic treatment with thrombospondin-1 peptide mimetics. *Int. J. Cancer* **98:** 682.

Relf M., LeJeune S., Scott P.A., Fox S., Smith K., Leek R., Moghaddam A., Whitehouse R., Bicknell R., and Harris A.L. 1997. Expression of the angiogenic factors vascular endothelial cell growth factor, acidic and basic fibroblast growth factor, tumor growth factor beta-1, platelet-derived endothelial cell growth factor, placenta growth factor, and pleiotrophin in human primary breast cancer and its relation to angiogenesis. *Cancer Res.* **57:** 963.

Reynolds L.E., Wyder L., Lively J.C., Taverna D., Robinson S.D., Huang X., Sheppard D., Hynes R.O., and Hodivala-Dilke K.M. 2002. Enhanced pathological angiogenesis in mice lacking beta3 integrin or beta3 and beta5 integrins. *Nat. Med.* **8:** 27.

Ribeiro S.M., Poczatek M., Schultz-Cherry S., Villain M., and Murphy-Ullrich J.E. 1999. The activation sequence of thrombospondin-1 interacts with the latency-associated peptide to regulate activation of latent transforming growth factor-beta. *J. Biol. Chem.* **274:** 13586.

Rodriguez-Manzaneque J.C., Lane T.F., Ortega M.A., Hynes R.O., Lawler J., and Iruela-Arispe M.L. 2001. Thrombospondin-1 suppresses spontaneous tumor growth and inhibits activation of matrix metalloproteinase-9 and mobilization of vascular endothelial growth factor. *Proc. Natl. Acad. Sci.* **98:** 12485.

Sasaki T., Fukai N., Mann K., Gohring W., Olsen B.R., and Timpl R. 1998. Structure, function and tissue forms of the C-terminal globular domain of collagen XVIII containing the angiogenesis inhibitor endostatin. *EMBO J.* **17:** 4249.

Sasaki T., Larsson H., Kreuger J., Salmivirta M., Claesson-Welsh L., Lindahl U., Hohenester E., and Timpl R. 1999. Structural basis and potential role of heparin/heparan sulfate binding to the angiogenesis inhibitor endostatin. *EMBO J.* **18:** 6240.

Schellens J.H. and Ratain M.J. 2002. Endostatin: Are the 2 years up yet? *J. Clin. Oncol.* **20:** 3758.

Schultz-Cherry S., Chen H., Mosher D.F., Misenheimer T.M., Krutzsch H.C., Roberts D.D., and Murphy-Ullrich J.E. 1995. Regulation of transforming growth factor-beta activation by discrete sequences of thrombospondin 1. *J. Biol. Chem.* **270:** 7304.

Shahan T.A., Fawzi A., Bellon G., Monboisse J.C., and Kefalides N.A. 2000. Regulation of tumor cell chemotaxis by type IV collagen is mediated by a Ca(2+)-dependent mechanism requiring CD47 and the integrin alpha(V)beta(3). *J. Biol. Chem.* **275:** 4796.

Shahan T.A., Ohno N., Pasco S., Borel J.P., Monboisse J.C., and

Kefalides N.A. 1999a. Inhibition of tumor cell proliferation by type IV collagen requires increased levels of cAMP. *Connect. Tissue Res.* **40:** 221.

Shahan T.A., Ziaie Z., Pasco S., Fawzi A., Bellon G., Monboisse J.C., and Kefalides N.A. 1999b. Identification of CD47/integrin-associated protein and alpha(v)beta3 as two receptors for the alpha3(IV) chain of type IV collagen on tumor cells. *Cancer Res.* **59:** 4584.

Standker L., Schrader M., Kanse S.M., Jurgens M., Forssmann W.G., and Preissner K.T. 1997. Isolation and characterization of the circulating form of human endostatin. *FEBS Lett.* **420:** 129.

Streit M., Velasco P., Brown L.F., Skobe M., Richard L., Riccardi L., Lawler J., and Detmar M. 1999. Overexpression of thrombospondin-1 decreases angiogenesis and inhibits the growth of human cutaneous squamous cell carcinomas. *Am. J. Pathol.* **155:** 441.

Sudhakar A., Sugimoto H., Yang C., Lively J., Zeisberg M., and Kalluri R. 2003. Human tumstatin and human endostatin exhibit distinct antiangiogenic activities mediated by alpha v beta 3 and alpha 5 beta 1 integrins. *Proc. Natl. Acad. Sci.* **100:** 4766.

Sund M., Hamano Y., Sugimoto H., Sudhakar A., Soubasakos M., Yerramalla U., Benjamin L.E., Lawler J., Kieran M., Shah A., and Kalluri R. 2005. Function of endogenous inhibitors of angiogenesis as endothelium-specific tumor suppressors. *Proc. Natl. Acad. Sci.* **102:** 2934.

Tan K., Duquette M., Liu J.H., Dong Y., Zhang R., Joachimiak A., Lawler J., and Wang J.H. 2002. Crystal structure of the TSP-1 type 1 repeats: A novel layered fold and its biological implication. *J. Cell Biol.* **159:** 373.

Than M.E., Henrich S., Huber R., Ries A., Mann K., Kuhn K., Timpl R., Bourenkov G.P., Bartunik H.D., and Bode W. 2002. The 1.9-A crystal structure of the noncollagenous (NC1) domain of human placenta collagen IV shows stabilization via a novel type of covalent Met-Lys cross-link. *Proc. Natl. Acad. Sci.* **99:** 6607.

Thomas J.P., Arzoomanian R.Z., Alberti D., Marnocha R., Lee F., Friedl A., Tutsch K., Dresen A., Geiger P., Pluda J., Fogler W., Schiller J.H., and Wilding G. 2003. Phase I pharmacokinetic and pharmacodynamic study of recombinant human endostatin in patients with advanced solid tumors. *J. Clin. Oncol.* **21:** 223.

Timpl R. 1996. Macromolecular organization of basement membranes. *Curr. Opin. Cell Biol.* **8:** 618.

Tjin Tham Sjin, R.M., Satchi-Fainaro R., Birsner A.E., Ramanujam V.M., Folkman J., and Javaherian K. 2005. A 27-amino-acid synthetic peptide corresponding to the NH2-terminal zinc-binding domain of endostatin is responsible for its antitumor activity. *Cancer Res.* **65:** 3656.

Tolsma S.S., Volpert O.V., Good D.J., Frazier W.A., Polverini P.J., and Bouck N. 1993. Peptides derived from two separate domains of the matrix protein thrombospondin-1 have anti-angiogenic activity. *J. Cell Biol.* **122:** 497.

Tsilibary E.C., Koliakos G.G., Charonis A.S., Vogel A.M., Reger L.A., and Furcht L.T. 1988. Heparin type IV collagen interactions: Equilibrium binding and inhibition of type IV collagen self-assembly. *J. Biol. Chem.* **263:** 19112.

Tsilibary E.C., Reger L.A., Vogel A.M., Koliakos G.G., Anderson S.S., Charonis A.S., Alegre J.N., and Furcht L.T. 1990. Identification of a multifunctional, cell-binding peptide sequence from the a1(NC1) of type IV collagen. *J. Cell Biol.* **111:** 1583.

Tucker R.P. 2004. The thrombospondin type 1 repeat superfamily. *Int. J. Biochem. Cell Biol.* **36:** 969.

Volpert O.V., Pili R., Sikder H.A., Nelius T., Zaichuk T., Morris C., Shiflett C.B., Devlin M.K., Conant K., and Alani R.M. 2002. Id1 regulates angiogenesis through transcriptional repression of thrombospondin-1. *Cancer Cell* **2:** 473.

Watnick R.S., Cheng Y.N., Rangarajan A., Ince T.A., and Weinberg R.A. 2003. Ras modulates Myc activity to repress thrombospondin-1 expression and increase tumor angiogenesis. *Cancer Cell* **3:** 219.

Weinstat-Saslow D.L., Zabrenetzky V.S., VanHoutte K., Frazier W.A., Roberts D.D., and Steeg P.S. 1994. Transfection of thrombospondin 1 complementary DNA into a human breast carcinoma cell line reduces primary tumor growth, metastatic potential, and angiogenesis. *Cancer Res.* **54:** 6504.

Wen W., Moses M.A., Wiederschain D., Arbiser J.L., and Folkman J. 1999. The generation of endostatin is mediated by elastase. *Cancer Res.* **59:** 6052.

Wickstrom S.A., Alitalo K., and Keski-Oja J. 2002. Endostatin associates with integrin alpha5beta1 and caveolin-1, and activates Src via a tyrosyl phosphatase-dependent pathway in human endothelial cells. *Cancer Res.* **62:** 5580.

———. 2004. An endostatin-derived peptide interacts with integrins and regulates actin cytoskeleton and migration of endothelial cells. *J. Biol. Chem.* **279:** 20178.

Yamaguchi N., Anand-Apte B., Lee M., Sasaki T., Fukai N., Shapiro R., Que I., Lowik C., Timpl R., and Olsen B.R. 1999. Endostatin inhibits VEGF-induced endothelial cell migration and tumor growth independently of zinc binding. *EMBO J.* **18:** 4414.

Yancopoulos G.D., Davis S., Gale N.W., Rudge J.S., Wiegand S.J., and Holash J. 2000. Vascular-specific growth factors and blood vessel formation. *Nature* **407:** 242.

Yu J.L., Rak J.W., Coomber B.L., Hicklin D.J., and Kerbel R.S. 2002. Effect of p53 status on tumor response to antiangiogenic therapy. *Science* **295:** 1526.

Yu Y., Moulton K.S., Khan M.K., Vineberg S., Boye E., Davis V.M., O'Donnell P.E., Bischoff J., and Milstone D.S. 2004. E-selectin is required for the antiangiogenic activity of endostatin. *Proc. Natl. Acad. Sci.* **101:** 8005.

Zabrenetzky V., Harris C.C., Steeg P.S., and Roberts D.D. 1994. Expression of the extracellular matrix molecule thrombospondin inversely correlates with malignant progression in melanoma, lung and breast carcinoma cell lines. *Int. J. Cancer* **59:** 191.

Zeisberg M., Bonner G., Maeshima Y., Colorado P., Muller G.A., Strutz F., and Kalluri R. 2001. Renal fibrosis: Collagen composition and assembly regulates epithelial-mesenchymal transdifferentiation. *Am. J. Pathol.* **159:** 1313.

Zhang X., Hudson B.G., and Sarras M.P., Jr. 1994. Hydra cell aggregate development is blocked by selective fragments of fibronectin and type IV collagen. *Dev. Biol.* **164:** 10.

VEGF Trap as a Novel Antiangiogenic Treatment Currently in Clinical Trials for Cancer and Eye Diseases, and VelociGene®-based Discovery of the Next Generation of Angiogenesis Targets

J.S. Rudge, G. Thurston, S. Davis, N. Papadopoulos, N. Gale,
S.J. Wiegand, and G.D. Yancopoulos
Regneron Pharmaceuticals, Inc., Tarrytown, New York 10591

The concept that tumors can be controlled by directly targeting their vascular supply has finally come of age, because clinical trials using a humanized monoclonal antibody that blocks VEGF have demonstrated exciting efficacy in cancer patients, as well as in vascular eye diseases that can lead to blindness. However, data suggest that these current regimens may not provide complete VEGF inhibition and, thus, that the maximum therapeutic potential of VEGF blockade has not yet been achieved. We describe the status of a very potent and high-affinity VEGF blocker, termed the VEGF Trap, that may provide the opportunity to maximize the potential of VEGF blockade in cancer as well as in vascular eye diseases. We also describe use of the VEGF Trap as a research tool, when coupled to high-throughput mouse genetics approaches such as *VelociGene®* that can be exploited in strategies to discover and validate the next generation of angiogenesis targets.

The concept that tumors can be controlled by directly targeting their vascular supply has finally come of age. The first antiangiogenesis approach to be validated in human cancer patients involves blocking vascular endothelial growth factor (VEGF-A). In this regard, the most advanced clinical data have been generated with a humanized monoclonal antibody termed bevacizumab (Avastin) that directly binds and blocks all isoforms of VEGF-A (Ferrara et al. 2004). Despite the promising data achieved to date, dose-response studies suggest that higher doses of bevacizumab may provide even greater benefit (Yang et al. 2003; Yang 2004), implying that current bevacizumab regimens may not provide optimal VEGF inhibition and thus may not have yet demonstrated the maximum potential of VEGF blockade in cancer. In addition to the promise of anti-VEGF approaches in cancer, blocking VEGF-A has also been impressive in maintaining and improving vision in wet age-related macular degeneration (AMD), a disease marked by leaky and proliferating vessels which distort the retina, and these data suggest that VEGF blockade may provide benefit in other eye diseases involving vascular leak and proliferation (Bergsland 2004). Efficacy in wet AMD has most notably been achieved using a modified fragment of the bevacizumab antibody, termed ranibizumab (Lucentis), delivered via monthly intraocular injections (Brown et al. 2006; Heier et al. 2006).

In this paper, we focus on the development and status of a novel VEGF-blocking agent, termed the VEGF Trap, that retains many of the advantages of a blocking antibody but may offer further potential (Holash et al. 2002). The VEGF Trap consists of portions of VEGF receptors that have been fused to the constant region of an antibody, resulting in a fully human biologic with exceedingly high affinity that blocks not only all isoforms of VEGF-A, but also related VEGF family members such as placental growth factor (PlGF). The VEGF Trap also displays extended pharmacological half-life, allowing long-term as well as very high affinity blockade. The VEGF Trap has performed impressively in extensive animal studies of cancer and eye diseases, and initial clinical trials appear promising. The VEGF Trap may provide the opportunity to explore the potential of more complete VEGF blockade in cancer, as well as the opportunity for more complete blockade and even longer-interval dosing regimens in eye diseases. To conclude this paper, we describe how the VEGF Trap can be used as a research tool in efforts to discover and validate the next generation of targets in the field of angiogenesis.

DISCOVERY OF VEGF AND ITS REQUISITE ROLES DURING NORMAL DEVELOPMENT AND IN DISEASE SETTINGS

Initial studies by Dvorak and his colleagues (Senger et al. 1986; Dvorak et al. 1999) identified a protein in tumor ascites fluid that was capable of inducing vascular leak and permeability, which they termed vascular permeability factor (VPF). Independent efforts by Ferrara and his colleagues to identify secreted factors that could promote tumor angiogenesis led to the discovery of a protein in bovine pituitary follicular cell conditioned medium with mitogenic properties for endothelial cells which they termed vascular endothelial cell growth factor (VEGF) (Ferrara and Henzel 1989; Leung et al. 1989). Upon sequencing and further studies, this VEGF protein was unexpectedly found to correspond to the VPF previously identified by the Dvorak lab. These findings set the stage for a concerted effort to define the role of VEGF/VPF (hereon VEGF) in cancer angiogenesis as well as other settings of vascular disease, which have led to the realization that both of its initially realized actions—i.e., promoting vascular permeability and vascular growth—appear critical to understanding its roles during normal biology and in disease.

Approximately two decades of intensive investigation by numerous laboratories has revealed a great deal about VEGF and its actions. It is now clear that VEGF is perhaps the most critical vascular regulator during normal development as well as in many disease states, and moreover, that its dosage must be exquisitely regulated in a spatial and temporal manner to avoid vascular disaster. Disruption of both VEGF alleles in developing mice, which ablates all VEGF production, results in complete failure to develop even a primordial vasculature, demonstrating that VEGF is absolutely essential for the earliest stages of blood vessel development. Still more remarkably, disruption of even a single VEGF allele in developing mice, which decreases VEGF levels by half, also results in embryonic lethality due to severe vascular abnormalities (Carmeliet et al. 1996; Ferrara et al. 1996), demonstrating the need for exquisite regulation of VEGF levels to form normal vessels. Reciprocally, modest increases in VEGF levels during development also lead to vascular disaster and lethality (Miquerol et al. 2000). VEGF continues to be critical during early postnatal growth and development, as evidenced by the lethality and major growth disturbances caused by conditional disruption of the VEGF gene or by administration of VEGF blockers (Ravindranath et al. 1992; Carmeliet et al. 1996; Ferrara et al. 1996, 1998; Gerber et al. 1999a; Ryan et al. 1999; Fraser et al. 2000; Zimmermann et al. 2001; Hazzard et al. 2002; Eremina et al. 2003). However, VEGF blockade in older animals is much less traumatic, affecting only those structures that continue to depend on ongoing vascular remodeling, such as occurs in bone growth plates or during remodeling of the female reproductive organs (Ferrara et al. 1998; Gerber et al. 1999a,b). As discussed in greater detail below, vascular remodeling is absolutely required in a variety of pathological settings, such as during tumor growth, providing major therapeutic opportunities for VEGF blockade in the adult setting in which such blockade can be tolerated.

VEGF ISOFORMS, VEGF FAMILY MEMBERS, AND VEGF RECEPTORS

Further study of the gene encoding human VEGF revealed eight exons separated by seven introns, which results in the generation of four isoforms of increasing size—$VEGF_{121}$, $VEGF_{165}$, $VEGF_{189}$, and $VEGF_{206}$ (subscripts refer to number of amino acids comprising the isoform, with the VEGF isoforms varying in length at their carboxyl termini). The main purpose of these isoforms appears to relate to their bioavailability such that the 121 isoform is diffusible, whereas the higher-molecular-weight isoforms remain bound to the extracellular matrix, requiring cleavage to be released (Houck et al. 1992; Park et al. 1993; Keyt et al. 1996).

Because of the discovery of additional members of the VEGF family, VEGF is now often referred to as VEGF-A. Other members of the VEGF family were identified based on their homology with VEGF, as well as their ability to interact with a related set of cell-surface receptors (Eriksson and Alitalo 1999; see below). The first VEGF relative to be identified is PlGF, and until recently, little was known about its normal function (Maglione et al. 1991). Whereas mice lacking PlGF appear to undergo normal vascular development, recent findings indicate that adult mice lacking PlGF exhibit deficiencies in certain models of adult vascular remodeling, including in tumors and eye disease models, raising the interesting possibility that the activity of PlGF may be limited to these settings and that blockade of PlGF may provide enhanced efficacy when combined with VEGF blockade (Persico et al. 1999; Carmeliet 2000). Little is known about VEGF-B, and mice lacking VEGF-B are overtly healthy and fertile. VEGF-C and D seem to play more critical roles in the lymphatic vasculature than in the blood vasculature, showing specificity for a VEGF receptor (see below) expressed on this vasculature; administration of both of these factors leads to lymphatic vessel hyperplasia (Joukov et al. 1996; Orlandini et al. 1996; Olofsson et al. 1999).

Following rapidly on the heels of the discovery of VEGF came the identification of two closely related high-affinity receptors for VEGF—FLT1 (FMS-like tyrosine kinase) now termed VEGFR1 (de Vries et al. 1992), and KDR or Flk1, now termed VEGFR2 (Shibuya et al. 1990; Terman et al. 1992; Millauer et al. 1993). These high-affinity receptors share features of many other growth factor receptors, in that they contain an extracellular domain which binds and is dimerized by ligand, and a cytoplasmic tyrosine kinase domain that can be regulated upon binding of ligand to the extracellular domain. VEGFR2 seems to be the receptor which mediates the major growth and permeability actions of VEGF, whereas VEGFR1 may have a negative role, either by acting as a decoy receptor or by suppressing signaling through VEGFR2. Thus, mice engineered to lack VEGFR2 fail to develop a vasculature and have very few endothelial cells (Shalaby et al. 1995), phenocopying mice lacking VEGF, whereas mice lacking VEGFR1 seem to have excess formation of endothelial cells that abnormally coalesce into disorganized tubules (Fong et al. 1995). Mice engineered to express only a truncated form of VEGFR1, lacking its kinase domain, appear rather normal, consistent with the notion that the primary role of VEGFR1 may be that of a decoy receptor (Hiratsuka et al. 1998), and supporting only a minor role for the cytoplasmic kinase domain. The third member of this receptor family, initially called Flt-4 and now termed VEGFR3, does not bind to VEGF-A nor PlGF, and instead binds to VEGF-C and VEGF-D and seems to mediate the actions of these latter two factors on the lymphatic vasculature (Taipale et al. 1999).

In addition to these primary receptors, a number of potential accessory receptors for the VEGFs have been identified, although the requisite roles of these receptors in mediating VEGF responses have not been clearly elucidated. These potential accessory receptors include the neuropilins (Soker et al. 1998).

ROLE OF VEGF IN TUMOR ANGIOGENESIS SUPPORTS CONCEPT OF BLOCKING VEGF AS AN ANTITUMOR STRATEGY

One area of intense study after the discovery of VEGF was the analysis of VEGF expression levels in different tumor types using in situ hybridization. VEGF was found to be expressed in a number of different tumors such as renal, gastrointestinal, breast, ovarian, pancreatic, and lung, but the variability in expression across the tumor and between different tumor types made the simple correlation between VEGF and severity of the cancer impossible (Yoshiji et al. 1996; Sowter et al. 1997; Volm et al. 1997; Ellis et al. 1998; Tomisawa et al. 1999). However, out of these studies came the interesting finding that one tumor type, renal cell carcinoma, had particularly high VEGF expression which correlated with inactivation of the von Hippel Lindau locus, resulting in loss of control of the tumor's oxygen sensor, hypoxia-inducible factor (HIF) (Iliopoulos et al. 1996; Lonser et al. 2003). The up-regulation of VEGF in an attempt to reoxygenate the tumor through revascularization led to the belief that this tumor may either be highly sensitive to anti-VEGF therapy or highly refractory. Fortunately, the former seems to be the case (Yang et al. 2003).

Concomitant with the analysis of human tumors for VEGF expression came the development of animal models of cancer where the hypothesis that VEGF was required for tumor vasculature, and thus tumor growth, could be tested. In 1993, 4 years after their discovery of VEGF, Ferrara and colleagues demonstrated that a mouse monoclonal antibody to human VEGF (A.4.6.1) could inhibit the growth of several human tumor types in nude mice with inhibition ranging from 70% to more than 90% (Kim et al. 1993). Subsequent to this observation, a number of laboratories using different strategies to inhibit VEGF signaling have shown to a greater or lesser extent that inhibition of VEGF can have a major impact on tumor growth in mice. In addition to numerous studies using the VEGF-blocking antibody, other strategies to block VEGF in tumor models included blocking antibodies targeting VEGFR2 (Prewett et al. 1999), soluble VEGF receptors acting as circulating decoys to capture VEGF and preventing it from binding cell-surface receptors (Ferrara et al. 1998; Gerber et al. 1999a,b; Liang et al. 2006), dominant-negative VEGF receptors expressed at high levels on tumor surfaces, small-molecule inhibitors of VEGF receptor kinases and other kinases (Smith et al. 2004), antisense oligonucleotides targeting VEGF, and VEGF siRNA (Grunweller and Hartmann 2005; Lu et al. 2005).

As the number of studies increased comparing the different modes of inhibiting VEGF, it became apparent that blocking tumor-derived VEGF without blocking stromal VEGF was not as efficacious, implicating stromal VEGF as a crucial player in tumor growth and angiogenesis. Thus, antibodies such as A.4.6.1 which only block human VEGF did not fare as well in blocking human tumor growth in immunocompromised mice as reagents blocking both tumor and host stroma-derived VEGF (Gerber et al. 2000; Liang et al. 2006).

DEVELOPMENT OF VEGF TRAP

The clinical promise of initial anti-VEGF approaches highlighted the need to optimize blockade of this pathway. Early studies indicated that one of the most effective ways to block the VEGF signaling pathway is to prevent VEGF from binding to its endogenous receptors by administering soluble decoy receptors (Ferrara et al. 1998; Gerber et al. 1999b). In particular, a soluble decoy receptor created by fusing the first three immunoglobulin-like (Ig) domains of VEGFR1 to the constant region (Fc portion) of human IgG1 resulted in a forced homodimer that acted as a very high affinity blocking reagent with 5–20 picomolar binding affinity for VEGF, and in tumor experiments this VEGFR1-Fc reagent was efficacious at approximately 500-fold lower concentration than a similar VEGFR2-Fc construct (Kuo et al. 2001). Despite its high affinity, the VEGFR1-Fc was not a feasible clinical candidate because of its poor pharmacokinetic profile; in rodent studies, this protein had to be administered frequently and at very high doses to achieve efficacious levels. In addition, this agent appeared to have nonspecific toxicity effects that did not seem to be accounted for by its blocking of VEGF (Kuo et al. 2001). We decided to exploit our Trap technology platform (Economides et al. 2003), which involves defining and fusing minimal binding units from different receptor components to generate chimeric fusion proteins that act as high-affinity soluble blockers, in an attempt to create a potent and well-behaved Trap for VEGF. The result was a chimeric fusion protein containing a modified domain 2 of VEGFR1 and the third Ig domain of VEGFR2 fused to the Fc region of human IgG1, resulting in a fully human protein that we term VEGF Trap (Holash et al. 2002). This reagent has the advantage of being fully human and thus potentially non-immunogenic, as well as being substantially smaller than previous fusion proteins and antibodies, raising the possibility that it might allow improved tissue and tumor penetration. In addition, this VEGF Trap had greatly improved pharmacological bioavailability as compared to the initial VEGFR1-Fc reagent, exhibiting about a 300-fold increase in the maximum concentration achieved in the circulation (i.e., C_{max}), as well as about a 1000-fold increase in total circulation exposure (i.e., AUC) (Holash et al. 2002). Importantly, the affinity of VEGF Trap binding to both mouse and human VEGF isoforms (0.58 pM, 0.46 pM) was superior to that of the parental VEGFR1-Fc (~ 5–20 pM) (Holash et al. 2002). In addition, the VEGF Trap also bound PlGF with high affinity (1.8 pM).

To determine whether the improved pharmacological bioavailabity and high-affinity binding of VEGF Trap translated into superior performance in vivo, we first used a short-term and quantitative in vivo model of VEGF activity in which a single dose of VEGF induces a stereotypic reduction in blood pressure. In this acute assay model, we found that equivalent doses of VEGF Trap were indeed far superior to that of the parental VEGFR1-Fc (Holash et al. 2002).

VEGF TRAP EXHIBITS IMPRESSIVE EFFICACY IN PRECLINICAL TUMOR MODELS

On the basis of the above evidence suggesting that the VEGF Trap was a potent VEGF blocker that was efficacious in vivo, we moved to evaluate the VEGF Trap in tumor models. Initial studies confirmed the remarkable efficacy of the VEGF Trap. Not only did the VEGF Trap blunt tumor growth in the early models, but it could completely block tumor angiogenesis in many cases, resulting in completely avascular tumors (Holash et al. 2002). These initial studies inspired exploration of the VEGF Trap in multiple tumor models, in the laboratories of many different investigators, with impressive results in almost every case. In addition to its activity in multiple subcutaneous models of melanoma, glioma, and rhabdomyosarcoma tumors (Holash et al. 2002), the VEGF Trap has been shown to work in multiple pancreatic cancer models (Fukasawa and Korc 2004), Wilms' tumor (Huang et al. 2003), Ewing's sarcoma (Dalal et al. 2005), glioblastoma (Wachsberger et al. 2005), and models of ovarian cancer as well as associated malignant ascites (Hu et al. 2005).

In addition to the above published studies, recent unpublished temporal studies indicate that vascular regression can be seen in most tumors within hours of VEGF Trap treatment, resulting in marked and widespread hypoxia within the tumors. In addition, transcription profiling studies during these temporal studies have revealed a set of endothelial-specific genes that are rapidly and profoundly regulated in response to VEGF Trap treatment. Further studies on some of these genes have led to their identification as potential targets for new antiangiogenesis therapies (see below).

In summary, animal tumor studies have indicated that treatment with VEGF Trap effectively inhibited tumor growth of a wide variety of murine, rat, and human tumor cell lines implanted either subcutaneously or orthotopically in mice. VEGF Trap treatment inhibited the growth of tumors representing a variety of tumor types, including melanoma, glioma, rhabdomyosarcoma, ovarian, pancreatic, renal, and mammary tumor tissue, with a broad therapeutic index. Growth of small established tumors was also inhibited. Histological analysis indicated that treatment with VEGF Trap resulted in the formation of largely avascular and necrotic tumors, demonstrating that tumor-induced angiogenesis was blocked. VEGF Trap was also active in blocking tumor growth in similar animal tumor models in combination with paclitaxel, docetaxel, or radiation, and was synergistic with 5-fluorouracil. VEGF Trap as a single agent and in combination with paclitaxel also prevented the formation of ascites in mouse tumor models (Byrne et al. 2003; Hu et al. 2005).

VEGF TRAP IN CLINICAL TRIALS FOR CANCER

The above results in animal tumor models supported the exploration of the VEGF Trap in human studies. Initial clinical studies are promising (Dupont et al. 2005;

Mulay et al. 2006; Rixe et al. 2006) in that the VEGF Trap as a single agent has resulted in objective radiographic responses in several advanced cancer patients suffering from multiply treated chemotherapy-refractory disease, as well as long-term stable disease in patients. Similar data are being generated in patients treated with VEGF Trap in combination with various chemotherapeutic agents. The VEGF Trap is now entering an assortment of additional exploratory as well as potentially pivotal efficacy studies, both as a single agent and in combination with chemotherapy.

VEGF TRAP EXHIBITS IMPRESSIVE EFFICACY IN PRECLINICAL MODELS OF VASCULAR EYE DISEASES

In addition to the role for VEGF in tumor angiogenesis, a variety of studies have indicated that VEGF may play a key pathological role in vascular eye diseases, in particular in diabetic edema and retinopathy settings, and in age-related macular degeneration (AMD), which are leading causes of vision loss and blindness. In these diseases, excess VEGF is thought to result in vascular leak that contributes to abnormal swelling of the retina and resulting vision impairment, as well as in the abnormal growth of choroidal and retinal vessels that can destroy normal retinal architecture. Consistent with these possibilities, the VEGF Trap has demonstrated impressive efficacy in an assortment of animal models of these eye diseases.

Preclinical studies in rodents have shown that VEGF Trap can inhibit choroidal (Saishin et al. 2003) and corneal (Wiegand et al. 2003) neovascularization, as well as suppress vascular leak into the retina (Qaum et al. 2001), and that the VEGF Trap can also promote the survival of corneal transplants by inhibiting associated neovascularization (Cursiefen et al. 2004). In addition, in a primate model of AMD, in which choroidal neovascular lesions and vascular leak are induced by using a laser to create small lesions in the retinas of adult cynomolgus macaques, both systemically and intravitreally delivered VEGF Trap not only prevented development of vascular leak and neovascular membranes when administered prior to laser lesion, but also induced regression when administered after lesions had developed (Wiegand et al. 2005). These preclinical results support a role for VEGF blockade, and in particular for local delivery of the VEGF Trap, in multiple vascular eye diseases ranging from AMD and diabetic eye diseases to corneal injury and transplantation.

VEGF TRAP IN CLINICAL TRIALS FOR VASCULAR EYE DISEASES

The above results in animal models have supported the exploration of the VEGF Trap in human studies of vascular eye diseases. Initial clinical studies in human patients suffering from both AMD and diabetic edema and retinopathy appear quite promising, with evidence in early trials that the VEGF Trap can rapidly and impressively decrease retinal swelling, and that these changes can be associated with improvement in visual acuity (Nguygen et al. 2006; Shah et al. 2006). The VEGF Trap is now entering more advanced clinical trials in vascular eye diseases.

THE NEXT GENERATION OF ANGIOGENESIS TARGETS: ANGIOPOIETINS AND Dll4

Despite the promise of anti-VEGF approaches in general, and that of the VEGF Trap in particular, it is clear both from animal studies and from the emerging human trials that tumors display varying degrees of responsivity to VEGF blockade. Whereas some tumors might show marked regression and/or very long term stabilization, other tumors can continue to grow even in the face of anti-VEGF treatments. The realization that some tumors can be relatively resistant to anti-VEGF approaches raises the need for additional antiangiogenesis approaches that might be useful in such settings. Toward this end, as noted above, we performed transcriptional profiling screens to identify endothelial-specific targets that are markedly regulated either by VEGF blockade or by excess VEGF activity, reasoning that such targets might prove interesting as new antiangiogenesis targets. Confirming the potential of such a screen, one target that was "rediscovered" via such screens was Angiopoietin-2. We had previously independently identified the Angiopoietins as key new angiogenic regulators that seemed to work in tandem with the VEGFs (Davis et al. 1996; Suri et al. 1996; Maisonpierre et al. 1997; Valenzuela et al. 1999; Yancopoulos et al. 2000; Gale et al. 2002), and moreover, obtained substantial data that Angiopoietin-2 in particular was specifically induced in tumor vasculature and that it was important for tumor angiogenesis (Holash et al. 1999); a recent study employing Angiopoietin-2-blocking antibodies confirmed notable antitumor effects (Oliner et al. 2004). On the basis of the confidence in these transcriptional profiling screens engendered by the reidentification of Angiopoietin-2, we explored additional potential targets identified by the screens. Among these targets we have reported the identification of Delta-like ligand 4 (Dll4) (a ligand for the Notch family of receptors) as a gene that is markedly and specifically induced in tumor vasculature (Gale et al. 2004). Moreover, Dll4 is strikingly up-regulated in VEGF-overexpressing tumors and down-regulated in tumors by VEGF blockade. Using VelociGene® technology, which provides a high-throughput approach to create mouse mutants for genes of interest (Valenzuela et al. 2003), we found that mice lacking Dll4 exhibit profound vascular defects early in development (Gale et al. 2004). Remarkably, and as previously seen only for VEGF (see above), deletion of even just one of the two Dll4 alleles in developing embryos resulted in embryonic lethality due to vascular defects (Gale et al. 2004). All this evidence for a critical role for Dll4 in normal as well as tumor angiogenesis provided a rationale to develop blockers for Dll4. Recent testing in tumor models indicates that Dll4 may indeed prove to be an important new antiangiogenesis target, either alone or in combination with the VEGF Trap, or in settings of relative resistance to anti-VEGF therapies.

In addition, the success with this screen in terms of yielding Dll4 as an exciting new antiangiogenesis target has led us to rigorously pursue several additional similarly identified targets.

SUMMARY

In summary, using our Trap technology platform (Economides et al. 2003), we have created the VEGF Trap, a very potent VEGF blocking agent with excellent pharmacological properties. This drug has proven to be highly efficacious in a number of diverse preclinical models. It dramatically inhibits the growth of a variety of types of tumors and can even cause frank tumor regression in some settings. In other preclinical cancer models, we have found that combination of VEGF Trap with a cytotoxic agent can result in potency far greater than that of either single agent. Furthermore, the VEGF Trap is also very effective in animal models of vascular eye diseases. The impressive efficacy in preclinical models of cancer and eye diseases provided a rationale for advancement of the VEGF Trap into clinical trials, where it is producing promising initial results in both cancer and eye diseases.

In addition to its potential therapeutic value in cancer and vascular eye diseases, the VEGF Trap is also an invaluable research tool. Transcription profiling screens using VEGF Trap have allowed a number of strategies designed to identify new antiangiogenesis targets. It is hoped that these strategies are helping to identify the next generation of antiangiogenesis targets, which may work either alone or in combination with the VEGF Trap, or in settings of relative resistance to anti-VEGF therapies.

ACKNOWLEDGMENTS

The authors gratefully acknowledge the substantial contributions of our colleagues at Regeneron, in particular, Jocelyn Holash, Susan D. Croll, Lillian Ho, Michelle Russell, Patricia Boland, Ray Leidich, Donna Hylton, Shelly Jiang, Sarah Nandor, Alexander Adler, Hua Jiang, Elena Burova, Irene Noguera, Ella Ioffe, Tammy Huang, Czeslaw Radziejewski, Calvin Lin, Jingtai Cao, Kevin Bailey, James Fandl, Tom Daly, Eric Furfine, Jesse Cedarbaum, and Neil Stahl. In addition, we acknowledge our collaborators on VEGF Trap studies, including Jessica Kandel, Darrell Yamashiro, Robert Jaffe, Donald McDonald, Murray Korc, Phyllis Wachsberger, Adam Dicker, Tony Adamis, C. Cursiefen, J.W. Streilein, and Peter Campochiaro. We regret if we have omitted key contributors.

REFERENCES

Bergsland E.K. 2004. Update on clinical trials targeting vascular endothelial growth factor in cancer. *Am. J. Health Syst. Pharm.* **1:** 61 (21 suppl. 5): S12–20. Review.

Brown D.M. et al. IOVS 2006. **47:** ARVO E-Abstract 2963.

Byrne A.T., Ross L., Holash J., Nakanishi M., Hu L., Hofmann J.I., Yancopoulos G.D., and Jaffe R.B. 2003. Vascular endothelial growth factor-trap decreases tumor burden, inhibits ascites, and causes dramatic vascular remodeling in an ovarian cancer model. *Clin. Cancer Res.* **9:** 5721.

Carmeliet P. 2000. Mechanisms of angiogenesis and arteriogenesis. *Nat. Med.* **6**: 389.

Carmeliet P., Ferreira V., Breier G., Pollefeyt S., Kieckens L., Gertsenstein M., Fahrig M., Vandenhoeck A., Harpal K., Eberhardt C., Declercq C., Pawling J., Moons L., Collen D., Risau W., and Nagy A. 1996. Abnormal blood vessel development and lethality in embryos lacking a single VEGF allele. *Nature* **380**: 435.

Cursiefen C., Cao J., Chen L., Liu Y., Maruyama K., Jackson D., Kruse F.E., Wiegand S.J., Dana M.R., and Streilein J.W. 2004. Inhibition of hemangiogenesis and lymphangiogenesis after normal-risk corneal transplantation by neutralizing VEGF promotes graft survival. *Invest. Ophthalmol. Vis. Sci.* **45**: 2666.

Dalal S., Berry A.M., Cullinane C.J., Mangham D.C., Grimer R., Lewis I.J., Johnston C., Laurence V., and Burchill S.A. 2005. Vascular endothelial growth factor: A therapeutic target for tumors of the Ewing's sarcoma family. *Clin. Cancer Res.* **11**: 2364.

Davis S., Aldrich T.H., Jones P.F., Acheson A., Compton D.L., Jain V., Ryan T.E., Bruno J., Radziejewski C., Maisonpierre P.C., and Yancopoulos G.D. 1996. Isolation of angiopoietin-1, a ligand for the TIE2 receptor, by secretion-trap expression cloning. *Cell* **87**: 1161.

de Vries C., Escobedo J.A., Ueno H., Houck K., Ferrara N., and Williams L.T. 1992. The fms-like tyrosine kinase, a receptor for vascular endothelial growth factor. *Science* **255**: 989.

Dupont J., Rothenberg M.L., Spriggs D.R., Cedarbaum J.M., Furfine E.S., Cohen D.P., Dancy I., Lee H., Cooper W., and Lockhart A.C. 2005. Safety and pharmacokinetics of intravenous VEGF Trap in a phase I clinical trial of patients with advanced solid tumors. *Proc. Am. Soc. Clin. Oncol.* **23**: 3029.

Dvorak H.F., Nagy J.A., Feng D., Brown L.F., and Dvorak A.M. 1999. Vascular permeability factor/vascular endothelial growth factor and the significance of microvascular hyperpermeability in angiogenesis. *Curr. Top. Microbiol. Immunol.* **237**: 97.

Economides A.N., Carpenter L.R., Rudge J.S., Wong V., Koehler-Stec E.M., Hartnett C., Pyles E.A., Xu X., Daly T.J., Young M.R., Fandl J.P., Lee F., Carver S., McNay J., Bailey K., Ramakanth S., Hutabarat R., Huang T.T., Radziejewski C., Yancopoulos G.D., and Stahl N. 2003. Cytokine traps: Multi-component, high-affinity blockers of cytokine action. *Nat. Med.* **9**: 47.

Ellis L.M., Takahashi Y., Fenoglio C.J., Cleary K.R., Bucana C.D., and Evans D.B. 1998. Vessel counts and vascular endothelial growth factor expression in pancreatic adenocarcinoma. *Eur. J. Cancer* **34**: 337.

Eremina V., Sood M., Haigh J., Nagy A., Lajoie G., Ferrara N., Gerber H.P., Kikkawa Y., Miner J.H., and Quaggin S.E. 2003. Glomerular-specific alterations of VEGF-A expression lead to distinct congenital and acquired renal diseases. *J. Clin. Invest.* **111**: 707.

Eriksson U. and Alitalo K. 1999. Structure, expression and receptor-binding properties of novel vascular endothelial growth factors. *Curr. Top. Microbiol. Immunol.* **237**: 41.

Ferrara N. and Henzel W.J. 1989. Pituitary follicular cells secrete a novel heparin-binding growth factor specific for vascular endothelial cells. *Biochem. Biophys. Res. Commun.* **161**: 851.

Ferrara N., Hillan K.J., Gerber H.P., and Novotny W. 2004. Discovery and development of bevacizumab, an anti-VEGF antibody for treating cancer. *Nat. Rev. Drug Discov.* **3**: 391.

Ferrara N., Carver-Moore K., Chen H., Dowd M., Lu L., O'Shea K.S., Powell-Braxton L., Hillan K.J., and Moore M.W. 1996. Heterozygous embryonic lethality induced by targeted inactivation of the VEGF gene. *Nature* **380**: 439.

Ferrara N., Chen H., Davis-Smyth T., Gerber H.P., Nguyen T.N., Peers D., Chisholm V., Hillan K.J., and Schwall R.H. 1998. Vascular endothelial growth factor is essential for corpus luteum angiogenesis. *Nat. Med.* **4**: 336.

Fong G.H., Rossant J., Gertsenstein M., and Breitman M.L. 1995. Role of the Flt-1 receptor tyrosine kinase in regulating the assembly of vascular endothelium. *Nature* **376**: 66.

Fraser H.M., Dickson S.E., Lunn S.F., Wulff C., Morris K.D., Carroll V.A., and Bicknell R. 2000. Suppression of luteal angiogenesis in the primate after neutralization of vascular endothelial growth factor. *Endocrinology* **141**: 995.

Fukasawa M. and Korc M. 2004. Vascular endothelial growth factor-trap suppresses tumorigenicity of multiple pancreatic cancer cell lines. *Clin. Cancer Res.* **10**: 3327.

Gale N.W., Thurston G., Davis S., Wiegand S.J., Holash J., Rudge J.S., and Yancopoulos G.D. 2002. Complementary and coordinated roles of the VEGFs and angiopoietins during normal and pathologic vascular formation. *Cold Spring Harbor Symp. Quant. Biol.* **67**: 267.

Gale N.W., Dominguez M.G., Noguera I., Pan L., Hughes V., Valenzuela D.M., Murphy A.J., Adams N.C., Lin H.C., Holash J., Thurston G., and Yancopoulos G.D. 2004. Haploinsufficiency of delta-like 4 ligand results in embryonic lethality due to major defects in arterial and vascular development. *Proc. Natl. Acad. Sci.* **101**: 15949.

Gerber H.P., Kowalski J., Sherman D., Eberhard D.A., and Ferrara N. 2000. Complete inhibition of rhabdomyosarcoma xenograft growth and neovascularization requires blockade of both tumor and host vascular endothelial growth factor. *Cancer Res.* **60**: 6253.

Gerber H.P., Vu T.H., Ryan A.M., Kowalski J., Werb Z., and Ferrara N. 1999a. VEGF couples hypertrophic cartilage remodeling, ossification and angiogenesis during endochondral bone formation. *Nat. Med.* **5**: 623.

Gerber H.P., Hillan K.J., Ryan A.M., Kowalski J., Keller G.A., Rangell L., Wright B.D., Radtke F., Aguet M., and Ferrara N. 1999b. VEGF is required for growth and survival in neonatal mice. *Development* **126**: 1149.

Grunweller A. and Hartmann R.K. 2005. RNA interference as a gene-specific approach for molecular medicine. *Curr. Med. Chem.* **12**: 3143.

Hazzard T.M., Xu F., and Stouffer R.L. 2002. Injection of soluble vascular endothelial growth factor receptor 1 into the preovulatory follicle disrupts ovulation and subsequent luteal function in rhesus monkeys. *Biol. Reprod.* **67**: 1305.

Heier J.S. et al. IOVS. 2006. **47**: ARVO E-Abstract 2959.

Hiratsuka S., Minowa O., Kuno J., Noda T., and Shibuya M. 1998. Flt-1 lacking the tyrosine kinase domain is sufficient for normal development and angiogenesis in mice. *Proc. Natl. Acad. Sci.* **95**: 9349.

Holash J., Maisonpierre P.C., Compton D., Boland P., Alexander C.R., Zagzag D., Yancopoulos G.D., and Wiegand S.J. 1999. Vessel cooption, regression, and growth in tumors mediated by angiopoietins and VEGF. *Science* **284**: 1994.

Holash J., Davis S., Papadopoulos N., Croll S.D., Ho L., Russell M., Boland P., Leidich R., Hylton D., Burova E., Ioffe E., Huang T., Radziejewski C., Bailey K., Fandl J.P., Daly T., Wiegand S.J., Yancopoulos G.D., and Rudge J.S. 2002. VEGF-Trap: A VEGF blocker with potent antitumor effects. *Proc. Natl. Acad. Sci.* **99**: 11393.

Houck K.A., Leung D.W., Rowland A.M., Winer J., and Ferrara N. 1992. Dual regulation of vascular endothelial growth factor bioavailability by genetic and proteolytic mechanisms. *J. Biol. Chem.* **267**: 26031.

Hu L., Hofmann J., Holash J., Yancopoulos G.D., Sood A.K., and Jaffe R.B. 2005. Vascular endothelial growth factor trap combined with paclitaxel strikingly inhibits tumor and ascites, prolonging survival in a human ovarian cancer model. *Clin. Cancer Res.* **11**: 6966.

Huang J., Frischer J.S., Serur A., Kadenhe A., Yokoi A., McCrudden K.W., New T., O'Toole K., Zabski S., Rudge J.S., Holash J., Yancopoulos G.D., Yamashiro D.J., and Kandel J.J. 2003. Regression of established tumors and metastases by potent vascular endothelial growth factor blockade. *Proc. Natl. Acad. Sci.* **100**: 7785.

Iliopoulos O., Levy A.P., Jiang C., Kaelin W.G., Jr., and Goldberg M.A. 1996. Negative regulation of hypoxia-inducible genes by the von Hippel-Lindau protein. *Proc. Natl. Acad. Sci.* **93**: 10595.

Joukov V., Pajusola K., Kaipainen A., Chilov D., Lahtinen I., Kukk E., Saksela O., Kalkkinen N., and Alitalo K. 1996. A novel vascular endothelial growth factor, VEGF-C, is a ligand for the Flt4 (VEGFR-3) and KDR (VEGFR-2) receptor tyrosine kinases. *EMBO J.* **15:** 1751.

Keyt B.A., Berleau L.T., Nguyen H.V., Chen H., Heinsohn H., Vandlen R., and Ferrara N. 1996. The carboxyl-terminal domain (111-165) of vascular endothelial growth factor is critical for its mitogenic potency. *J. Biol. Chem.* **271:** 7788.

Kim K.J., Li B., Winer J., Armanini M., Gillett N., Phillips H.S., and Ferrara N. 1993. Inhibition of vascular endothelial growth factor-induced angiogenesis suppresses tumour growth in vivo. *Nature* **362:** 841.

Kuo C.J., Farnebo F., Yu E.Y., Christofferson R., Swearingen R.A., Carter R., von Recum H.A., Yuan J., Kamihara J., Flynn E., D'Amato R., Folkman J., and Mulligan R.C. 2001. Comparative evaluation of the antitumor activity of antiangiogenic proteins delivered by gene transfer. *Proc. Natl. Acad. Sci.* **98:** 4605.

Leung D.W., Cachianes G., Kuang W.J., Goeddel D.V., and Ferrara N. 1989. Vascular endothelial growth factor is a secreted angiogenic mitogen. *Science* **246:** 1306.

Liang W.C., Wu X., Peale F.V., Lee C.V., Meng Y.G., Gutierrez J., Fu L., Malik A.K., Gerber H.P., Ferrara N., and Fuh G. 2006. Cross-species vascular endothelial growth factor (VEGF)-blocking antibodies completely inhibit the growth of human tumor xenografts and measure the contribution of stromal VEGF. *J. Biol. Chem.* **281:** 951.

Lonser R.R., Glenn G.M., Walther M., Chew E.Y., Libutti S.K., Linehan W.M., and Oldfield E.H. 2003. von Hippel-Lindau disease. *Lancet* **361:** 2059.

Lu P.Y., Xie F.Y., and Woodle M.C. 2005. Modulation of angiogenesis with siRNA inhibitors for novel therapeutics. *Trends Mol. Med.* **11:** 104.

Maglione D., Guerriero V., Viglietto G., Delli-Bovi P., and Persico M.G. 1991. Isolation of a human placenta cDNA coding for a protein related to the vascular permeability factor. *Proc. Natl. Acad. Sci.* **88:** 9267.

Maisonpierre P.C., Suri C., Jones P.F., Bartunkova S., Wiegand S.J., Radziejewski C., Compton D., McClain J., Aldrich T.H., Papadopoulos N., Daly T.J., Davis S., Sato T.N., and Yancopoulos G.D. 1997. Angiopoietin-2, a natural antagonist for Tie2 that disrupts in vivo angiogenesis. *Science* **277:** 55.

Millauer B., Wizigmann-Voos S., Schnurch H., Martinez R., Moller N.P., Risau W., and Ullrich A. 1993. High affinity VEGF binding and developmental expression suggest Flk-1 as a major regulator of vasculogenesis and angiogenesis. *Cell* **72:** 835.

Miquerol L., Langille B.L., and Nagy A. 2000. Embryonic development is disrupted by modest increases in vascular endothelial growth factor gene expression. *Development* **127:** 3941.

Mulay M., Limentani S.A., Carroll M., Furfine E.S., Cohen D.P., and Rosen L.S. 2006. Safety and pharmacokinetics of intravenous VEGF Trap plus FOLFOX4 in a combination phase I clinical trial of patients with advanced solid tumors. *Proc. Am. Soc. Clin. Oncol.* **24:** (Abstr.).

Nguyen Q.D. et al. IOVS 2006. **47:** ARVO E-Abstract 2144.

Oliner J., Min H., Leal J., Yu D., Rao S., You E., Tang X., Kim H., Meyer S., Han S.J., Hawkins N., Rosenfeld R., Davy E., Graham K., Jacobsen F., Stevenson S., Ho J., Chen Q., Hartmann T., Michaels M., Kelley M., Li L., Sitney K., Martin F., Sun J.R., Zhang N., Lu J., Estrada J., Kumar R., Coxon A., Kaufman J., Pretorius J., Scully S., Cattley R., Payton M., Coats S., Nguyen L., Desilva B., Ndifor A., Hayward I., Radinsky R., Boone T., and Kendall R. 2004. Suppression of angiogenesis and tumor growth by selective inhibition of angiopoietin-2. *Cancer Cell* **6:** 507.

Olofsson B., Jeltsch M., Eriksson U., and Alitalo K. 1999. Current biology of VEGF-B and VEGF-C. *Curr. Opin. Biotechnol.* **10:** 528.

Orlandini M., Marconcini L., Ferruzzi R., and Oliviero S. 1996. Identification of a c-fos-induced gene that is related to the

platelet-derived growth factor/vascular endothelial growth factor family. *Proc. Natl. Acad. Sci.* **93:** 11675.

Park J.E., Keller G.A., and Ferrara N. 1993. The vascular endothelial growth factor (VEGF) isoforms: Differential deposition into the subepithelial extracellular matrix and bioactivity of extracellular matrix-bound VEGF. *Mol. Biol. Cell* **4:** 1317.

Persico M.G., Vincenti V., and DiPalma T. 1999. Structure, expression and receptor-binding properties of placenta growth factor (PlGF). *Curr. Top. Microbiol. Immunol.* **237:** 31.

Prewett M., Huber J., Li Y., Santiago A., O'Connor W., King K., Overholser J., Hooper A., Pytowski B., Witte L., Bohlen P., and Hicklin D.J. 1999. Antivascular endothelial growth factor receptor (fetal liver kinase 1) monoclonal antibody inhibits tumor angiogenesis and growth of several mouse and human tumors. *Cancer Res.* **59:** 5209.

Qaum T., Xu Q., Joussen A.M., Clemens M.W., Qin W., Miyamoto K., Hassessian H., Wiegand S.J., Rudge J., Yancopoulos G.D., and Adamis A.P. 2001. VEGF-initiated blood-retinal barrier breakdown in early diabetes. *Invest. Ophthalmol. Vis. Sci.* **42:** 2408.

Ravindranath N., Little-Ihrig L., Phillips H.S., Ferrara N., and Zeleznik A.J. 1992. Vascular endothelial growth factor messenger ribonucleic acid expression in the primate ovary. *Endocrinology* **131:** 254.

Rixe O., Verslype C., Meric J.B., Tejpar S., Bloch J., Crabbe M., Khayat D., Furfine E.S., Assadourian S., and Van Cutsem E. 2006. Safety and pharmacokinetics of intravenous VEGF Trap plus irinotecan, 5-fluorouracil, and leucovorin (I-LV5FU2) in a combination phase I clinical trial of patients with advanced solid tumors. *Proc. Am. Soc. Clin. Oncol.* **24:** (Abstr.).

Ryan A.M., Eppler D.B., Hagler K.E., Bruner R.H., Thomford P.J., Hall R.L., Shopp G.M., and O'Neill C.A. 1999. Preclinical safety evaluation of rhuMAbVEGF, an antiangiogenic humanized monoclonal antibody. *Toxicol. Pathol.* **27:** 78.

Saishin Y., Saishin Y., Takahashi K., Lima e Silva R., Hylton D., Rudge J.S., Wiegand S.J., and Campochiaro P.A. 2003. VEGF-TRAP(R1R2) suppresses choroidal neovascularization and VEGF-induced breakdown of the blood-retinal barrier. *J. Cell. Physiol.* **195:** 241.

Senger D.R., Perruzzi C.A., Feder J., and Dvorak H.F. 1986. A highly conserved vascular permeability factor secreted by a variety of human and rodent tumor cell lines. *Cancer Res* **46:** 5629.

Shah S.M., Nguyen Q.D., Harriprisad S., Chu K., Holekamp N., Buskey J., Nadler D., Cedarbaum J., and Campochiaro P.A. 2006. A double-masked, placebo-controlled, safety, and tolerability study of intravenous VEGF trap in patients with diabetic macular edema. *Invest. Ophthalmol. Vis. Sci.* **47:** (Abstr.).

Shalaby F., Rossant J., Yamaguchi T.P., Gertsenstein M., Wu X.F., Breitman M.L., and Schuh A.C. 1995. Failure of blood-island formation and vasculogenesis in Flk-1-deficient mice. *Nature* **376:** 62.

Shibuya M., Yamaguchi S., Yamane A., Ikeda T., Tojo A., Matsushime H., and Sato M. 1990. Nucleotide sequence and expression of a novel human receptor-type tyrosine kinase gene (flt) closely related to the fms family. *Oncogene* **5:** 519.

Smith J.K., Mamoon N.M., and Duhe R.J. 2004. Emerging roles of targeted small molecule protein-tyrosine kinase inhibitors in cancer therapy. *Oncol. Res.* **14:** 175.

Soker S., Takashima S., Miao H.Q., Neufeld G., and Klagsbrun M. 1998. Neuropilin-1 is expressed by endothelial and tumor cells as an isoform-specific receptor for vascular endothelial growth factor. *Cell* **92:** 735.

Sowter H.M., Corps A.N., Evans A.L., Clark D.E., Charnock-Jones D.S., and Smith S.K. 1997. Expression and localization of the vascular endothelial growth factor family in ovarian epithelial tumors. *Lab. Invest.* **77:** 607.

Suri C., Jones P.F., Patan S., Bartunkova S., Maisonpierre P.C., Davis S., Sato T.N., and Yancopoulos G.D. 1996. Requisite role of angiopoietin-1, a ligand for the TIE2 receptor, during embryonic angiogenesis. *Cell* **87:** 1171.

Taipale J., Makinen T., Arighi E., Kukk E., Karkkainen M., and Alitalo K. 1999. Vascular endothelial growth factor receptor-3. *Curr. Top. Microbiol. Immunol.* **237:** 85.

Terman B.I., Dougher-Vermazen M., Carrion M.E., Dimitrov D., Armellino D.C., Gospodarowicz D., and Bohlen P. 1992. Identification of the KDR tyrosine kinase as a receptor for vascular endothelial cell growth factor. *Biochem. Biophys. Res. Commun.* **187:** 1579.

Tomisawa M., Tokunaga T., Oshika Y., Tsuchida T., Fukushima Y., Sato H., Kijima H., Yamazaki H., Ueyama Y., Tamaoki N., and Nakamura M. 1999. Expression pattern of vascular endothelial growth factor isoform is closely correlated with tumour stage and vascularisation in renal cell carcinoma. *Eur. J. Cancer* **35:** 133.

Valenzuela D.M., Griffiths J.A., Rojas J., Aldrich T.H., Jones P.F., Zhou H., McClain J., Copeland N.G., Gilbert D.J., Jenkins N.A., Huang T., Papadopoulos N., Maisonpierre P.C., Davis S., and Yancopoulos G.D. 1999. Angiopoietins 3 and 4: Diverging gene counterparts in mice and humans. *Proc. Natl. Acad. Sci.* **96:** 1904.

Valenzuela D.M., Murphy A.J., Frendewey D., Gale N.W., Economides A.N., Auerbach W., Poueymirou W.T., Adams N.C., Rojas J., Yasenchak J., Chernomorsky R., Boucher M., Elsasser A.L., Esau L., Zheng J., Griffiths J.A., Wang X., Su H., Xue Y., Dominguez M.G., Noguera I., Torres R., Macdonald L.E., Stewart A.F., DeChiara T.M., and Yancopoulos G.D. 2003. High-throughput engineering of the mouse genome coupled with high-resolution expression analysis. *Nat. Biotechnol.* **21:** 652.

Volm M., Koomagi R., and Mattern J. 1997. Prognostic value of vascular endothelial growth factor and its receptor Flt-1 in squamous cell lung cancer. *Int. J. Cancer* **74:** 64.

Wachsberger P., Burd R., Marrero N., Rossetti D., Strickler T.,

Yancopoulos G., Holash J., and Dicker A. 2005. Improvement of fractionated radiation therapy by combination with a VEGF blocker, VEGF Trap. *Annual Meeting of the Radiation Research Society*, Denver, Colorado. (Abstr. PP189).

Wiegand S., Cao J., Renard R., Rudge J., and Yancopoulos G. 2003. Long-lasting inhibition of corneal neovascularization following systemic administration of the VEGF Trap. *Invest. Ophthalmol. Vis. Sci.* **44:** (E-Abstr. 829).

Wiegand S.J., Zimmer E., Nork T.M., Miller P.E., Christian B.J., Miller J.M., Cao J., Cedarbaum J., Yancopoulos G.D., and Furfine E. 2005. VEGF Trap both prevents experimental choroidal neovascularization and causes regression of established lesions in non-human primates. *Invest. Ophthalmol. Vis. Sci.* **46:** (E-Abstr. 1411).

Yancopoulos G.D., Davis S., Gale N.W., Rudge J.S., Wiegand S.J., and Holash J. 2000. Vascular-specific growth factors and blood vessel formation. *Nature* **407:** 242.

Yang J.C. 2004. Bevacizumab for patients with metastatic renal cancer: An update. *Clin. Cancer Res.* **10:** 6367S.

Yang J.C., Haworth L., Sherry R.M., Hwu P., Schwartzentruber D.J., Topalian S.L., Steinberg S.M., Chen H.X., and Rosenberg S.A. 2003. A randomized trial of bevacizumab, an antivascular endothelial growth factor antibody, for metastatic renal cancer. *N. Engl. J. Med.* **349:** 427.

Yoshiji H., Gomez D.E., Shibuya M., and Thorgeirsson U.P. 1996. Expression of vascular endothelial growth factor, its receptor, and other angiogenic factors in human breast cancer. *Cancer Res.* **56:** 2013.

Zimmermann R.C., Xiao E., Husami N., Sauer M.V., Lobo R., Kitajewski J., and Ferin M. 2001. Short-term administration of antivascular endothelial growth factor antibody in the late follicular phase delays follicular development in the rhesus monkey. *J. Clin. Endocrinol. Metab.* **86:** 768.

Molecular Targeted Therapy of Lung Cancer: EGFR Mutations and Response to EGFR Inhibitors

D.A. Haber, D.W. Bell, R. Sordella, E.L. Kwak, N. Godin-Heymann,
S.V. Sharma, T.J. Lynch, and J. Settleman
*Massachusetts General Hospital Cancer Center and Harvard Medical School,
Charlestown, Massachusetts 02129*

Somatic mutations within the kinase domain of the epidermal growth factor receptor (EGFR) are present in approximately 10% of non-small-cell lung cancer (NSCLC), with an increased frequency in adenocarcinomas arising in nonsmokers, women, and individuals of Asian ethnicity. These mutations lead to altered downstream signaling by the receptor and appear to define a subset of NSCLC characterized by "oncogene addiction" to the EGFR pathway, which displays dramatic responses to the reversible tyrosine kinase inhibitors gefitinib and erlotinib. The rapid acquisition of drug resistance in most cases, either through mutation of the "gateway" residue in the EGFR kinase domain or by alternative mechanisms, appears to limit the impact on patient survival. Irreversible inhibitors of EGFR display continued effectiveness in vitro against cells with acquired resistance and are now undergoing genotype-directed clinical trials. The molecular and clinical insights derived from targeting EGFR in NSCLC offer important lessons for the broader application of targeted therapeutic agents in solid tumors.

Lung cancer remains the leading cause of cancer-related deaths in the U.S., and although advances in chemotherapy for advanced disease have resulted in improved survival, the duration of responses is limited and the associated toxicity is high. The advent of molecular targeted therapy, specifically the development of small-molecule inhibitors of the epidermal growth factor receptor (EGFR), has recently provided new therapeutic options for the most common lung tumor histology, non-small-cell lung cancer (NSCLC). These orally administered agents, gefitinib (Iressa) and erlotinib (Tarceva), are well tolerated and have been shown to have dramatic efficacy in a subset of NSCLC. Here we discuss the finding that activating somatic mutations in EGFR appear to define a biological subset of NSCLC susceptible to inhibition of this pathway.

CLINICAL TRIALS OF GEFITINIB IN NSCLC

Gefitinib was the first small-molecule inhibitor of EGFR developed for clinical application (Wakeling et al. 2002). It was modeled after imatinib (Gleevec), which inhibits the ABL, C-KIT, and platelet-derived growth factor receptor (PDGFR) kinases, and is effective in the treatment of chronic myeloid leukemia (CML) and gastrointestinal stromal tumor (GIST). Like imatinib, gefitinib and erlotinib, the two clinically approved agents targeting EGFR, act as competitive (i.e., reversible) inhibitors for binding to the ATP pocket of the kinase. Despite the expression of EGFR in most epithelial cancers, initial clinical trials of gefitinib were discouraging, with the exception of NSCLC, where it was shown to induce partial responses (PR) in approximately 10% of cases (Kris et al. 2003). These responses were notable in that they were exceptionally rapid and profound, and they were more frequently observed in cases with specific clinical characteristics: adenocarci-

nomas (often with bronchioalveolar differentiation), and tumors arising in nonsmokers, women, and patients of East Asian ethnic background (Table 1). Whereas the average duration of a PR was 6–7 months before the disease recurred, rare patients had sustained responses lasting up to 3 years. Our own interest in exploring the genetic basis for this dramatic difference in drug response was triggered by such a case.

EGFR MUTATIONS IN GEFITINIB-RESPONSIVE NSCLC

By analogy with the imatinib-responsive diseases CML and GIST, which harbor the BCR-ABL translocation or activating C-KIT mutations, respectively, we reasoned that cases of NSCLC with dramatic responses to gefitinib might harbor genetic alterations affecting the target receptor, EGFR. EGFR overexpression was not

Table 1. Clinical Predictors of Gefitinib Responses in Lung Cancer (NSCLC)

Overall response rate	10–20%
Median duration of response	7 months (range 4.4 to > 18.6)
Clinical predictors of response	
nonsmokers	29.4%
smokers	4.6%
female	17.5%
male	5.1%
Japan	20%
U.S./Europe	10%
histology	adenocarcinoma (bronchioalveolar) > others

Adapted from FDA Approval Summary: *Clinical Cancer Research* (2004) 10: 1212.

linked to gefitinib response in clinical trials, nor did we find evidence of specific in-frame deletions affecting the EGFR extracellular domain, which had been previously reported in glioblastomas (so-called EGFR vIII mutation). Instead, we observed point mutations and small in-frame deletions within the intracellular kinase domain of EGFR (Lynch et al. 2004). Initial cases available for analysis were derived from 275 patients with chemotherapy-refractory NSCLC, who had been treated with single agent gefitinib over a 3-year period at Massachusetts General Hospital. Of these, 25 patients (9%) were noted to have a dramatic response to gefitinib, and tumor specimens were available for analysis from nine of these cases. Of note, all tumor specimens had been collected at the time of initial diagnosis, typically preceding multiple rounds of chemotherapy treatment, and eventual therapy with gefitinib. Eight of the nine gefitinib-responsive tumors were found to harbor an EGFR kinase domain mutation, whereas none of seven nonresponders had a mutation ($p < 0.001$) (Fig. 1). Coincident with our report, another group from Dana Farber Cancer Institute described EGFR mutations in all five patients with gefitinib-responsive NSCLC (Paez et al. 2004). A third group at Memorial Sloan Kettering Cancer Center described a similar frequency of EGFR mutations in patients with both gefitinib- and erlotinib-responsive NSCLC (Pao et al. 2005). From these reports and subsequent reports from additional research laboratories, it appears that approximately 80% of NSCLC cases identified on the basis of dramatic responses to EGFR inhibitors harbor such mutations, compared with 6% of nonresponders. The overall frequency of EGFR kinase domain mutations in unselected cases of NSCLC is approximately 10% in the U.S. and Europe. Remarkably, the frequency of these mutations is increased in cases with adenocarcinoma (especially adenocarcinomas with areas of bronchioalveolar differentiation), in women, nonsmokers, and patients of Asian origin—consistent with the clinically determined indicators of drug-responsive cancers.

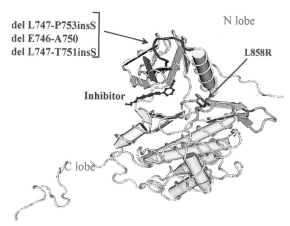

Figure 1. Representative structure of the EGFR ATP pocket, denoting the position of the recurrent in-frame nested deletions and the L858R missense mutation (shown in *red*), which together comprise ~90% of activating mutations associated with gefitinib responsiveness. The inhibitor is shown in blue. (Adapted from Lynch et al. 2004.)

PREDICTIVE VALUE OF EGFR MUTATIONS

Although the majority of NSCLC identified by virtue of a dramatic clinical response to gefitinib or erlotinib harbor EGFR mutations, not all cases with such mutations demonstrate a potent drug response. To address the predictive value of EGFR mutations, we analyzed clinical specimens collected as part of the original "IDEAL" clinical trials, in which gefitinib was administered to chemotherapy-refractory NSCLC patients, and which led to the first identification of subsets with dramatic responses and specific clinical characteristics. As is common with such retrospective analyses, only a fraction of tumor specimens were recovered, and only a subset of those contained sufficient tumor material for molecular analysis. Nonetheless, we were able to analyze approximately 30% of the cases in these large international trials and to confirm that clinical characteristics of cases analyzed were comparable with those of the entire cohort (Bell et al. 2005). Gefitinib responses were found in 46% of EGFR mutant NSCLC, compared with 10% of cases with wild-type EGFR ($p = 0.005$). Most responses were transient (~7 months' duration), and no survival difference was observed between responsive and nonresponsive cases. These results are consistent with other reports (Han et al. 2005; Mitsudomi et al. 2005) that, in aggregate, identify drug responses in 40–80% of EGFR mutant cases. Our results differ from a recent publication in which only 16% of EGFR mutant tumors were found to respond to erlotinib (Tsao et al. 2005), but that study included large numbers of novel unconfirmed sequence variants identified in a "single pass" sequencing of PCR products. In contrast, EGFR mutations identified in drug responders constitute a small number of well-defined recurrent mutations within the kinase domain (see below); we and other investigators have found that PCR amplification of EGFR from small amounts of formalin-fixed, paraffin-embedded specimens can result in a significant number of sequence variants which are not reproducible in duplicate analysis, and can therefore be considered PCR artifacts. Such findings highlight the importance of establishing uniformly high quality DNA sequencing methods for analyzing tumor specimens in order to derive a consensus conclusion regarding the relationship between tumor genotypes and clinical outcomes across multiple clinical centers.

Nonetheless, it is evident that not all NSCLC with EGFR kinase mutations are responsive to treatment with EGFR inhibitors. It is possible that additional genetic lesions in nonresponsive cases may have relieved the "dependence" of these EGFR-mutant tumors on signaling through the EGFR pathway. Supporting that hypothesis is the recent observation that absence of immunoreactivity for PTEN protein expression may identify brain tumors with the EGFR vIII mutation that progress on erlotinib, whereas those expressing wild-type PTEN together with EGFR vIII show a modest response (Mellinghoff et al. 2005). PTEN suppresses the AKT survival pathway, a key effector of EGFR signaling, and hence, PTEN inactivation might compensate for reduced EGFR signaling. However, in our analysis of NSCLC cases with EGFR kinase mutations that did not respond to gefitinib, we did not observe an increased frequency of PTEN mutations, nor did we detect mutations in other pathways that modulate EGFR signaling or general apoptotic signals (Bell et al. 2005). Modulators of gefitinib response in EGFR mutant NSCLC thus remain to be identified. Another critical consideration is that retrospective analyses typically involve only a fraction of tumor specimens collected at the time of initial diagnosis, whereas gefitinib or erlotinib therapy is administered up to 1–2 years later, following multiple courses of chemotherapy. The true predictive value of EGFR mutations will need to be assessed in prospective clinical trials, in which EGFR status is assessed at the time of drug therapy.

The dramatic responses to gefitinib and erlotinib observed in a subset of NSCLC have not been associated with a commensurate improvement in overall survival for the cohort of patients treated with these agents. For erlotinib, but not gefitinib, a moderate improvement in overall survival for all treated patients appears to be driven by disease stabilization in a larger fraction of cases, not specifically by the subset of cases with EGFR mutations and dramatic responses (Shepherd et al. 2005). Although subtle pharmacological differences between these drugs or differences in the composition of clinical cohorts may have contributed to this difference between the two tyrosine kinase inhibitors, this distinction may also have resulted from the higher dosing level chosen for erlotinib in these clinical trials.

Given the relatively high prevalence of EGFR mutations in NSCLC in East Asia, a number of trials conducted in Korea and Japan have provided the most compelling data for a survival advantage (up to 2 years) in EGFR-mutant cases treated with gefitinib (Han et al. 2005; Mitsudomi et al. 2005). In U.S. and European trials, no survival difference was evident in the relatively smaller subset of EGFR mutant cases, despite an increased drug response in such cases. This may reflect the relatively rapid acquisition of drug resistance in many cases with initially responsive disease (see below).

EGFR MUTATIONS AND EGFR AMPLIFICATION

Amplification of the EGFR gene is relatively common in malignant gliomas, where it is often associated with the EGFR vIII mutation. Despite the frequency of this genetic abnormality in EGFR, gliomas exhibit very modest responses to either gefitinib or erlotinib. These observations suggest either that gliomas are less dependent than NSCLC on EGFR signaling, or alternatively, that kinase mutations lead to qualitative differences in these signals, which underlie much of the drug response in NSCLC (see below). In NSCLC, amplification of EGFR, involving either wild-type alleles or alleles harboring a kinase mutation, has also been reported. Some studies have used FISH analysis to grade tumors as having a range of abnormalities, from low-grade nonspecific aneuploidy to high levels of specific EGFR amplification, leading to the conclusion that high-level aneuploidy and/or EGFR amplification, together with increased EGFR protein expression measured by immunohistochemistry, provide a predictive index of susceptibility to EGFR inhibitors (Hirsch et al. 2005). In our analysis of the IDEAL clinical trials, we measured EGFR amplification by quantitative PCR (qPCR), using control probes selected to exclude aneuploidy (Bell et al. 2005). Only 7% of NSCLC were found to have significant EGFR amplification using this approach, compared with ~30% reported using FISH analysis, presumably reflecting the lower frequency of high-level amplification measured across the entire tumor specimen, compared with individual cell analysis using FISH. Most EGFR amplification detected by qPCR reflected amplification of the wild-type allele, although some cases had amplification of a mutant allele. EGFR amplification as measured by qPCR was predictive of gefitinib responsiveness, although not as strongly as EGFR mutations. Remarkably, however, the characteristics of NSCLC with EGFR amplification differed markedly from those with kinase domain mutations (Table 2). EGFR mutations were more common in adenocarcinomas and tumors arising in women and nonsmokers, all of which are characteristics previously identified in NSCLC tumors with dramatic responses to this agent. In striking contrast, tumors with EGFR amplification were indistinguishable from the entire cohort, being more common in men and in smokers, and not being associated with a specific histological type (Bell et al. 2005). Furthermore, EGFR mutations were more commonly observed in tumors from younger patients, whereas amplification predominated in tumors from older patients. Taken together, these observations suggest that although both markers may denote alterations in EGFR signaling that are directly relevant to tumor growth and drug response, they appear to arise in distinct subsets of NSCLC. Additional studies are needed in which tumor samples are prospectively collected at the time of drug treatment for a meaningful comparison of EGFR mutations and amplification (or both) as predictors of drug response.

Table 2. EGFR Mutations and Amplification Define Distinct Patient Subgroups

Characteristics	Mutation frequency (%)	p value	Amplification frequency (%)	p value
Nonsmoker	25.5	0.0004	6.3	0.82
	7.7		8.1	
Adenocarcinoma/BAC	17.4	0.0001	6.9	0.74
	5.1		7.8	
Age < 64 years	14.3	0.031	6.6	0.0009
> 64 years	6.8		18.5	

Adapted from Bell et al. 2005.

FUNCTIONAL PROPERTIES OF MUTANT EGFR

The EGFR kinase domain mutations identified in gefitinib-responsive NSCLC are clustered around the ATP-binding pocket, which constitutes the drug-binding site (Fig. 1) (Lynch et al. 2004; Paez et al. 2004; Pao et al. 2005). Large-scale tumor genotyping studies have now shown that approximately 80–90% of mutations consist either of small, nested in-frame deletions, centered around the LREA motif in the kinase domain, or the L858R missense mutation in the activation loop. In comparing NSCLC tumor cell lines with either a deletion mutation or L858R with comparable NSCLC cell lines expressing wild-type EGFR, we observed that cells with mutant EGFR displayed increased proliferation when cultured in the absence of serum but in the presence of exogenous EGF (Sordella et al. 2004). Thus, these mutations may mediate ligand-dependent proliferation. Consistent with this model, immunohistochemical analysis of primary NSCLCs with mutant EGFR shows expression of its two ligands, EGF and TGF-α, in tumor cells themselves, but not in the reactive stroma (Riemenschneider et al. 2005). Taken together, these observations suggest that somatic EGFR mutations arise in NSCLC cells that express EGFR ligands, thus enhancing a potential autocrine growth loop.

To dissect the effect of EGFR mutations on downstream signaling pathways, we undertook a series of experiments, including transient transfection of EGFR-expression plasmids into Cos-7 cells, which express low levels of endogenous EGFR; stable transfection of these plasmids into nontransformed mouse mammary epithelial cells, expression of endogenous erb-B family members; and comparison of established lung carcinoma cell lines of bronchioalveolar histology, either expressing wild-type EGFR or the in-frame deletion or L858R mutants (Sordella et al. 2004). Our findings were consistent across these different cell types and are summarized as follows: (1) Neither EGFR mutation enhances ligand-independent EGFR signaling; however, they lead to a 2- to 3-fold increase in both the magnitude and duration of EGFR autophosphorylation following exposure to the ligand EGF. (2) The pattern of EGFR autophosphorylation differs between wild-type and mutant receptors, with Tyr-992 and Tyr-1068 phosphorylation specifically increased in the mutants. EGFR Tyr-845 is specifically autophosphorylated to high levels by L858R, but not the deletion mutant. The total level of receptor autophosphorylation is unaltered between wild type and mutant, suggesting the importance of these qualitative differences in ligand-mediated activation. (3) Activation of mutant EGFR selectively enhances activation of downstream pathways. Specifically, activation of AKT and STAT pathways is dramatically increased following phosphorylation of the mutant receptors, whereas activation of the ERK pathway is, if anything, reduced compared with the wild-type EGFR (Sordella et al. 2004). Taken together, these observations suggest that mutant EGFRs selectively activate survival or antiapoptotic pathways (STAT, AKT), whereas the wild-type receptor is relatively more potent in triggering proliferative signals (ERK) (Fig. 2).

ONCOGENE ADDICTION AND GEFITINIB RESPONSE

The signaling differences evident between wild-type and mutant EGFR are correlated with enhanced sensitivity to tyrosine kinase inhibition. Treatment of some NSCLC cell lines harboring mutant EGFR with gefitinib demonstrates a 50- to 100-fold increase in drug sensitiv-

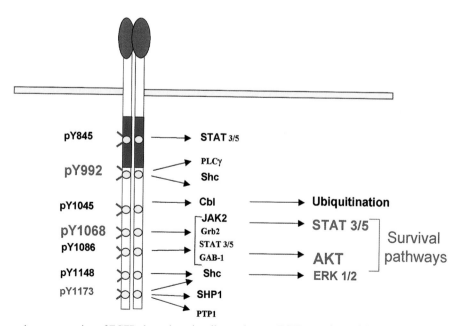

Figure 2. Schematic representation of EGFR-dependent signaling pathways. EGFR tyrosine residues shown in red are preferentially autophosphorylated following EGF stimulation of the mutant receptors. The AKT and STAT pathways are preferentially activated by the mutant receptors. (Adapted from Sordella et al. 2004.)

ity, compared with cell lines expressing the wild-type receptor. More significantly, the importance of mutant EGFR signaling can be demonstrated using siRNA strategies. Thus, in NSCLC cells with wild-type EGFR, knockdown of the receptor using siRNA has minimal impact on cellular proliferation. In contrast, in cells with mutant EGFR, a comparable knockdown triggers widespread apoptosis (Sordella et al. 2004). Furthermore, in cells expressing the deletion mutation, transfection of an siRNA construct specifically targeting this mutant mRNA triggers cell death, whereas in comparable cells with the L858R mutation, siRNA targeting that specific missense mutation has the same effect. These observations suggest a model in which expression of the mutant allele is itself required for cell survival, with apoptosis initiated following withdrawal of these survival signals, either following treatment with gefitinib or EGFR siRNA. Such a scenario has been proposed to underlie oncogene addiction, a phenomenon according to which cancer cells harboring multiple genetic lesions may nonetheless display exquisite dependency on a single oncogenic stimulus, in whose absence they undergo cell death or growth arrest (Weinstein 2002). On the basis of data using temperature-sensitive oncogene mutants, we have proposed that cells need not be dependent on a persistent oncogenic stimulus per se, but rather that the abrupt withdrawal of signaling from such a critical pathway may lead to a transient imbalance between downstream apoptotic and antiapoptotic signals, thus triggering rapid cell death. We refer to this mechanism as "oncogenic shock" (Sharma et al. 2006). Experimental validation of the oncogenic shock model will be important in a number of model systems, since it predicts that following the transient signaling imbalance which arises upon acute inactivation of an oncogene, cancers may adapt to loss of the oncogenic signal and thus acquire independence from the oncogene. As drug combination regimens emerge, involving concomitant use of targeted and classic chemotherapeutic agents, understanding the mechanistic basis of oncogene addiction will be essential to ensuring an enhancement, rather than a suppression, of drug response.

ENHANCED INHIBITION OF MUTANT EGFR BY GEFITINIB

The arguments presented above support a biological dependence mechanism by which the mutant EGFR identifies a tumor in which EGFR signals are critical for cell survival. In addition to this mechanism, we have also observed that mutant EGFRs display an approximately 10-fold increased sensitivity to gefitinib-mediated inhibition. This is evident in transiently transfected Cos-7 cells, as well as in cell lines stably expressing wild-type or mutant EGFR (Lynch et al. 2004). Although it is difficult to extrapolate such in vitro results to the clinical setting, it is of interest that the measured trough plasma concentrations achievable at clinically recommended gefitinib dosage are predicted to completely abrogate signaling by mutant EGFR, but not by wild-type receptor. These results raise the possibility that, in addition to altering downstream signaling pathways, the EGFR mutations may struc-

turally alter the ATP pocket in such a way as to enhance binding by inhibitors and further increase the drug response.

ACQUIRED RESISTANCE TO GEFITINIB: THE T790M MUTATION

Rare patients with NSCLC harboring EGFR mutations may sustain prolonged clinical responses, but in most cases, an initial dramatic response to gefitinib is followed by tumor regrowth within about 6 months. Two groups have independently reported the presence of a secondary somatic EGFR mutation in such cases (Pao et al. 2004; Kobayashi et al. 2005), and to date, approximately 50% of tumors with acquired drug resistance appear to harbor the same missense mutation, T790M. Remarkably, this mutation affects the homologous residue within the catalytic site of the ABL kinase domain targeted by the T315I mutation, frequently observed in imatinib-resistant CML. This so-called "gatekeeper" residue appears to modulate access of small-molecule inhibitors to the catalytic site. In our own studies, we also identified the T790M mutation in independent metastatic lesions, which had recurred after an initial response in two patients whose primary tumor harbored an activating EGFR mutation (Kwak et al. 2005). Surprisingly, however, the abundance of this drug resistance mutation was considerably lower than would be expected if it were the sole mechanism underlying acquired resistance. In the first patient, the wild-type and initial somatic activating EGFR mutation were present in a 1:1 ratio, as expected for a heterozygous mutation. However, the secondary drug resistance somatic mutation T790M was only observed at a 1:5 ratio to the wild-type allele. In the second case, where 4 independent liver metastases were analyzed, no T790M alleles were detected in an analysis of uncloned PCR products, but the mutation was detected at low levels in 2 of the 4 tumors following analysis of cloned PCR products (ranging in frequency from 1/55 to 2/48 PCR-derived clones). Again, the first somatic mutation in all metastases was still present in the expected 1:1 ratio with the wild-type allele. No EGFR amplification was evident. We conclude that the T790M mutation is a "hot spot" for secondary mutations linked to acquired drug resistance but that other mechanisms are also likely to play a role in tumor recurrence. We note that even in cases with a dramatic response to gefitinib, only a partial response is achievable, and hence, the number of persistent tumor cells is very high. The acquisition of drug resistance in such cases is not a clonal process: We therefore hypothesize that a combination of mechanisms, some genetic (like T790M), others potentially epigenetic, may contribute to tumor regrowth following an initial response to gefitinib or erlotinib.

ALTERED EGFR TRAFFICKING AND IN VITRO DRUG RESISTANCE

To model the acquisition of resistance to gefitinib in NSCLC cells with activating EGFR mutations, we treated cell lines with the drug in vitro and selected multiple independent drug-resistant clones (Kwak et al. 2005). The T790M mutation was not observed in this setting, nor was amplification of the mutant EGFR. However, 50- to 100-fold resistance was readily achieved and appeared to be stable in the absence of drug selection. Analysis of receptor trafficking, using visualization of immunofluorescent-tagged EGF in whole cells, as well as immunoblotting analysis of membrane-bound receptor using biotin-labeled ligand, revealed a consistent increase in receptor internalization following treatment with ligand. The mechanism underlying this alteration remains to be elucidated, and its clinical relevance cannot be readily ascertained in the absence of molecular markers that can be studied in clinical specimens. Nonetheless, these findings raise the possibility that epigenetic mechanisms may direct altered internalization of the receptor. Dissociation of gefitinib from the receptor is likely within the lower pH of endosomes, possibly leading to persistent downstream signaling. We note that gefitinib-resistant clones display persistent sensitivity to siRNA targeting EGFR, indicating that they remain "addicted" to EGFR signaling and appear not to have acquired additional genetic lesions in downstream effectors (Kwak et al. 2005).

IRREVERSIBLE EGFR INHIBITORS: CIRCUMVENTING ACQUIRED DRUG RESISTANCE

Both gefitinib and erlotinib are reversible inhibitors of EGFR that compete with ATP for binding to the catalytic pocket. Irreversible inhibitors of EGFR were initially developed to address potential pharmacodynamic concerns associated with competitive binding to the receptor. These agents, including EKB 569 (targeting EGFR) and HKI 272 (targeting both EGFR and erb-B2), made by Wyeth Pharmaceuticals, are similar in overall structure to the reversible inhibitors but differ in the presence of a so-called "Michael acceptor" which can form a covalent bond with Cys-773 within the catalytic pocket of the receptor (Rabindran et al. 2004). Our initial studies of these irreversible inhibitors indicated that they shared the selective killing of EGFR-mutant NSCLC cell lines and were comparable with reversible inhibitors in their relative effects on these cells versus those with wild-type EGFR. However, irreversible inhibitors demonstrated persistent activity against EGFR-mutant cells that had acquired resistance to gefitinib or erlotinib, either through expression of the secondary T790M mutation, or through apparent alterations in receptor internalization (Kwak et al. 2005). In both models, gefitinib was no longer effective in suppressing EGFR-mediated signaling or in cell killing, whereas the irreversible inhibitors showed persistent activity (Fig. 3). We presume that the improved reaction kinetics provided by the irreversible inhibition are sufficient to circumvent reduced drug binding due to the T790M mutation, as well as the potential dissociation of the drug–receptor complex resulting from altered internalization. Furthermore, we note that in marked contrast to reversible inhibitors, NSCLC cell lines with acquired resistance to irreversible inhibitors cannot be readily established in cell culture. Taken together, these observations have led to the initiation of clinical trials of HKI 272 in patients with EGFR-mutant NSCLC that have acquired resistance to gefitinib and/or erlotinib. Should such trials prove encouraging, these "second-generation" EGFR inhibitors may warrant clinical testing in the initial treatment of patients with EGFR-mutant NSCLC.

Clinical studies are needed to test the effectiveness of irreversible EGFR kinase inhibitors predicted by in vitro studies. However, these observations raise the possibility that such covalent drug binding may prove important in targeting transmembrane growth factor receptor kinases, for which multiple mechanisms of drug resistance appear to be a common feature. Even for cytoplasmic kinases, such as ABL, the gatekeeper residue (codon 315 of BCR-

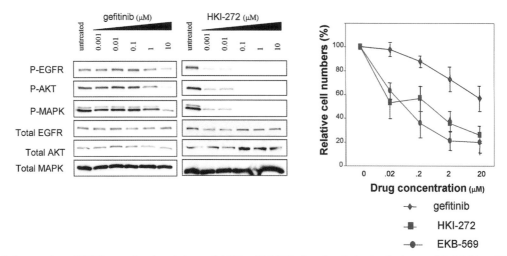

Figure 3. Suppression of EGFR autophosphorylation and AKT and MAPK phosphorylation by the irreversible inhibitor HKI 272 in cells that have an activating sensitizing EGFR mutation, but which have acquired resistance to gefitinib in culture. Failure of gefitinib to suppress EGFR, AKT, and MAPK phosphorylation is demonstrated (*left panel*). Cell killing induced by HKI 272 in these gefitinib-resistant cell lines is shown (*right panel*). (Adapted from Kwak et al. 2005.)

ABL) appears to be a hot spot for imatinib resistance, for which current second-generation ABL inhibitors targeting the open rather than closed configuration of the kinase have not proven effective (Shah et al. 2004). The effect of irreversible EGFR inhibitors in circumventing mutations affecting the analogous gatekeeper residue in EGFR offers hope that a similar strategy, if feasible, may hold some promise for refractory BCR-ABL mutations as well. By analogy with EGFR, the potential benefits of using irreversible inhibitors in targeting oncogenic kinases may not be evident initially, since both reversible and irreversible inhibitors may share comparable efficacy against previously untreated cells. As drug resistance emerges, however, irreversible inhibitors may prove capable of inducing longer-lasting responses. Whereas the toxicity profile of EKB 569 and HKI 272 appears minimal, this may not be true for other small molecules with such reactive side chains. Taken together, our in vitro observations raise the possibility that irreversible kinase inhibitors may offer advantages that need to be tested in clinical trials.

CONCLUDING REMARKS

Much remains to be understood with respect to targeting EGFR in NSCLC, but some lessons may be drawn, with potential implications for the treatment of lung cancer, as well as other cancers that may be targeted by "molecular therapeutics." In NSCLC, a relatively small number of somatic mutations capable of activating the kinase activity of EGFR are correlated with dramatic clinical responses to inhibitors of this pathway. Mutational analysis of EGFR is now commercially available, which will facilitate prospective genotype-directed studies of drug response. High-level EGFR amplification may also be associated with responsiveness to kinase inhibitors, and together with mutational activation, illustrates the importance of genetic alterations as molecular markers of drug response. Other genetic or epigenetic factors that modulate drug response are likely but remain to be identified. Despite their dramatic nature, the drug responses associated with EGFR-mutant tumors are unlikely to have a major effect in improving survival unless acquired drug resistance can be overcome. Ongoing clinical trials of irreversible EGFR inhibitors, which appear effective in vitro, may address this critical issue.

The concept that common epithelial malignancies may comprise multiple genetically defined subclasses, and that dramatic clinical responses to any given targeted therapy may be limited to a relatively small subset, is likely to have significant implications for the development and testing of these novel agents. The cost of early-phase clinical trials may be significantly reduced if tumor genotyping can select a subset with a high probability of drug susceptibility. Reliable preclinical approaches to defining such drug-responsive tumor types need to be developed, and these may include a combination of nucleotide sequencing and in vitro functional analyses. The nature of early-phase studies themselves may evolve, as traditional dose escalation "Phase I toxicity studies" may

become less relevant, given the minimal toxicity of these agents and the need to define appropriate dosing based on responsiveness in susceptible tumors, rather than limiting toxicity in nonresponsive cases. Although the potentially reduced costs of drug development associated with targeted clinical testing may be encouraging, concern has been raised about reduced financial incentives for pharmaceutical companies considering designing new drugs for smaller market shares. Nonetheless, the development of truly effective cancer therapies, as demonstrated by the success of Gleevec in the treatment of CML, provides an inspiring model for the application of targeted therapies in epithelial tumors.

ACKNOWLEDGMENTS

We are grateful to all the members of the Center for Molecular Therapeutics, Center for Cancer Risk Analysis, and Center for Thoracic Oncology of the Massachusetts General Hospital Cancer Center for their ongoing commitment and collaboration. This work was supported by grants from the National Institutes of Health, the Doris Duke Charitable Foundation, the National Foundation for Cancer Research, the Sandler Family Foundation, the V Foundation, the Saltonstall Foundation, and Sue's Fund for lung cancer research at Massachusetts General Hospital.

REFERENCES

Bell D.W., Lynch T.J., Haserlat S.M., Harris P.L., Okimoto R.A., Brannigan B.W., Sgroi D.C., Muir B., Riemenschneider M.J., Iacona R.B., Krebs A.D., Johnson D.H., Giaccone G., Herbst R.S., Manegold C., Fukuoka M., Kris M.G., Baselga J., Ochs J.S., and Haber D.A. 2005. Epidermal growth factor receptor mutations and gene amplification in non-small-cell lung cancer: Molecular analysis of the IDEAL/INTACT gefitinib trials. J. Clin. Oncol. 23: 8081.
Han S.W., Kim T.Y., Hwang P.G., Jeong S., Kim J., Choi I.S., Oh D.Y., Kim J.H., Kim D.W., Chung D.H., Im S.A., Kim Y.T., Lee J.S., Heo D.S., Bang Y.J., and Kim N.K. 2005. Predictive and prognostic impact of epidermal growth factor receptor mutation in non-small-cell lung cancer patients treated with gefitinib. J. Clin. Oncol. 23: 2493.
Hirsch F.R., Varella-Garcia M., McCoy J., West H., Xavier A.C., Gumerlock P., Bunn P.A., Jr., Franklin W.A., Crowley J., and Gandara D.R. (Southwest Oncology Group). 2005. Increased epidermal growth factor receptor gene copy number detected by fluorescence in situ hybridization associates with increased sensitivity to gefitinib in patients with bronchioloalveolar carcinoma subtypes: A Southwest Oncology Group Study. J. Clin. Oncol. 23: 6838.
Kobayashi S., Boggon T.J., Dayaram T., Janne P.A., Kocher O., Meyerson M., Johnson B.E., Eck M.J., Tenen D.G., and Halmos B. 2005. EGFR mutation and resistance of non-small-cell lung cancer to gefitinib. N. Engl. J. Med. 352: 786.
Kris M.G., Natale R.B., Herbst R.S., Lynch T.J., Jr., Prager D., Belani C.P., Schiller J.H., Kelly K., Spiridonidis H., Sandler A., Albain K.S., Cella D., Wolf M.K., Averbuch S.D., Ochs J.J., and Kay A.C. 2003. Efficacy of gefitinib, an inhibitor of the epidermal growth factor receptor tyrosine kinase, in symptomatic patients with non-small cell lung cancer: A randomized trial. J. Am. Med. Assoc. 290: 2149.
Kwak E.L., Sordella R., Bell D.W., Godin-Heymann N., Okimoto R.A., Brannigan B.W., Harris P.L., Driscoll D.R., Fidias P., Lynch T.J., Rabindran S.K., McGinnis J.P., Wissner A., Sharma S.V., Isselbacher K.J., Settleman J., and Haber D.A. 2005. Irreversible inhibitors of the EGF receptor may circum-

vent acquired resistance to gefitinib. *Proc. Natl. Acad. Sci.* **102:** 7665.

Lynch T.J., Bell D.W., Sordella R., Gurubhagavatula S., Okimoto R.A., Brannigan B.W., Harris P.L., Haserlat S.M., Supko J.G., Haluska F.G., Louis D.N., Christiani D.C., Settleman J., and Haber D.A. 2004. Activating mutations in the epidermal growth factor receptor underlying responsiveness of non-small-cell lung cancer to gefitinib. *N. Engl. J. Med.* **350:** 2129.

Mellinghoff I.K., Wang M.Y., Vivanco I., Haas-Kogan D.A., Zhu S., Dia E.Q., Lu K.V., Yoshimoto K., Huang J.H., Chute D.J., Riggs B.L., Horvath S., Liau L.M., Cavenee W.K., Rao P.N., Beroukhim R., Peck T.C., Lee J.C., Sellers W.R., Stokoe D., Prados M., Cloughesy T.F., Sawyers C.L., and Mischel P.S. 2005. Molecular determinants of the response of glioblastomas to EGFR kinase inhibitors. *N. Engl. J. Med.* **353:** 2012.

Mitsudomi T., Kosaka T., Endoh H., Horio Y., Hida T., Mori S., Hatooka S., Shinoda M., Takahashi T., and Yatabe Y. 2005. Mutations of the epidermal growth factor receptor gene predict prolonged survival after gefitinib treatment in patients with non-small-cell lung cancer with postoperative recurrence. *J. Clin. Oncol.* **23:** 2513.

Paez J.G., Janne P.A., Lee J.C., Tracy S., Greulich H., Gabriel S., Herman P., Kaye F.J., Lindeman N., Boggon T.J., Naoki K., Sasaki H., Fujii Y., Eck M.J., Sellers W.R., Johnson B.E., and Meyerson M. 2004. EGFR mutations in lung cancer: Correlation with clinical response to gefitinib therapy. *Science* **304:** 1497.

Pao W., Miller V.A., Politi K.A., Riely G.J., Somwar R., Zakowski M.F., Kris M.G., and Varmus H. 2005. Acquired resistance of lung adenocarcinomas to gefitinib or erlotinib is associated with a second mutation in the EGFR kinase domain. *PloS Med.* **3:** e73.

Pao W., Miller V., Zakowski M., Doherty J., Politi K., Sarkaria I., Singh B., Heelan R., Rusch V., Fulton L., Mardis E., Kupfer D., Wilson R., Kris M., and Varmus H. 2004. EGF receptor gene mutations are common in lung cancers from "never smokers" and are associated with sensitivity of tumors to gefitinib and erlotinib. *Proc. Natl. Acad. Sci.* **101:** 13306.

Rabindran S.K., Discafani C.M., Rosfjord E.C., Baxter M., Floyd M.B., Golas J., Hallett W.A., Johnson B.D., Nilakantan R., Overbeek E., Reich M.F., Shen R., Shi X., Tsou H.R., Wang Y.F., and Wissner A. 2004. Antitumor activity of HKI-272, an orally active, irreversible inhibitor of the HER-2 tyrosine kinase. *Cancer Res.* **64:** 3958.

Riemenschneider M.J., Bell D.W., Haber D.A., and Louis D.N. 2005. Pulmonary adenocarcinomas with mutant epidermal growth factor receptors. *N. Engl. J. Med.* **352:** 1724.

Shah N.P., Tran C., Lee F.Y., Chen P., Norris D., and Sawyers C.L. 2004. Overriding imatinib resistance with a novel ABL kinase inhibitor. *Science* **305:** 399.

Sharma S.V., Fischbach M.A., Haber D.A., and Settleman J. 2006. Oncogenic shock: Explaining oncogene addiction through differential signal attenuation. *Clin. Cancer Res.* (in press).

Shepherd F.A., Rodrigues Pereira J., Ciuleanu T., Tan E.H., Hirsh V., Thongprasert S., Campos D., Maoleekoonpiroj S., Smylie M., Martins R., van Kooten M., Dediu M., Findlay B., Tu D., Johnston D., Bezjak A., Clark G., Santabarbara P., and Seymour L. (National Cancer Institute of Canada Clinical Trials Group). 2005. Erlotinib in previously treated non-small-cell lung cancer. *N. Engl. J. Med.* **353:** 123.

Sordella R., Bell D.W., Haber D.A., and Settleman J. 2004. Gefitinib-sensitizing EGFR mutations in lung cancer activate anti-apoptotic pathways. *Science* **305:** 1163.

Tsao M.S., Sakurada A., Cutz J.C., Zhu C.Q., Kamel-Reid S., Squire J., Lorimer I., Zhang T., Liu N., Daneshmand M., Marrano P., da Cunha Santos G., Lagarde A., Richardson F., Seymour L., Whitehead M., Ding K., Pater J., and Shepherd F.A. 2005. Erlotinib in lung cancer: Molecular and clinical predictors of outcome. *N. Engl. J. Med.* **353:** 133.

Wakeling A.E., Guy S.P., Woodburn J.R., Ashton S.E., Curry B.J., Barker A.J., and Gibson K.H. 2002. ZD1839 (Iressa): An orally active inhibitor of epidermal growth factor signaling with potential for cancer therapy. *Cancer Res.* **62:** 5749.

Weinstein I.B. 2002. Cancer. Addiction to oncogenes—The Achilles heal of cancer. *Science* **297:** 63.

Aberrant Gene Silencing in Tumor Progression: Implications for Control of Cancer

S.B. BAYLIN* AND W.Y. CHEN[†]

*The Sidney Kimmel Comprehensive Cancer Center at Johns Hopkins, Baltimore, Maryland 21231;
[†]City of Hope/Beckman Research Institute, Duarte, California 91010

Although it is clear that genetic alterations are critical for the initiation and maintenance of human cancer, it is also becoming evident that epigenetic changes may be essential for the development of these diseases as well. The best studied of these latter processes is heritable transcriptional repression of genes associated with aberrant DNA hypermethylation of their promoters. Herein we review how very early occurrence of these gene silencing events may contribute to loss of key gene functions which result in disruption of cell regulatory pathways that may contribute to abnormal cell population expansion. These altered regulatory events may then provide a setting where mutations in the same disrupted pathways may be readily selected and serve to lock tumor progression into place. This hypothesis has potential impact on means to prevent and control cancer and for the use of epigenetic markers for cancer risk assessment and early diagnosis.

It is apparent, from work outlined in multiple papers in this volume, that cancer is a disease driven not only by genetic, but also by epigenetic changes. All types of human cancers have broad shifts in chromatin patterns, as compared to the normal cells from which they derive, and these abnormalities potentially contribute to heritable increases and decreases in gene expression (Jones and Laird 1999; Jones and Baylin 2002; Herman and Baylin 2003). This paper focuses on the decreases that provide an alternative mechanism to gene mutations for deriving loss of tumor suppressor gene function (Jones and Laird 1999; Jones and Baylin 2002; Herman and Baylin 2003). Although the molecular determinants for this loss of gene expression are still being elucidated, the best-understood component, at present, is an abnormal increase in DNA methylation involving CpG islands in gene promoters and which is associated with the transcriptional repression of involved genes (Jones and Laird 1999; Jones and Baylin 2002; Herman and Baylin 2003). This brief review outlines how such epigenetically silenced genes are being discovered and how the consequences of the lost gene expression for tumor progression are being outlined. Understanding of the position of the lost gene function in tumor progression is a particular focus, as is definition of the abnormalities of cell control pathways that ensue. Finally, current understanding of the molecular events in chromatin regulation of cancer epigenetic gene silencing that may initiate and maintain the abnormal gene transcriptional repression is examined.

EPIGENETIC GENE SILENCING IN CANCER

The shifts in DNA methylation that occur in tumor cells and the promoter-localized increases that accompany abnormal decreases in gene transcription are outlined in this volume by J. Herman and T. Tlsty. Briefly, despite widespread losses of DNA methylation in regions where this DNA modification should normally be present, local gains of methylation are simultaneously found in CpG islands in the promoter regions of a growing list of genes in all cancer types (Jones and Laird 1999; Jones and Baylin 2002; Herman and Baylin 2003). The association of this local promoter change with loss of gene function important for tumor development has at least three historical phases. First, the concept gained attention as promoter DNA hypermethylation began to be associated with well-recognized tumor suppressor genes which, when mutated in the germ line of families, lead to inherited forms of cancer. Almost half of such genes, which can be mutated in tumors of somatic cell origin, have now been well characterized to also be inactivated in this setting by epigenetic gene silencing (Jones and Laird 1999; Jones and Baylin 2002; Herman and Baylin 2003).

Second, the recognition of epigenetic silencing of the above genes has led to a host of candidate tumor suppressor genes being associated with this type of loss of function in cancer. Such genes are generally recognized when searches for mutations fail to find such genetic changes and loss of expression of the genes in question is documented at the level of mRNA transcripts. At least 30 such genes, involving a widespread distribution over many chromosomes in cancer cells, have now been defined (Jones and Laird 1999; Jones and Baylin 2002; Herman and Baylin 2003). This group of genes, as discussed below, presents a challenge for discovering the true importance of the associated transcriptional silencing for tumor progression steps.

The third groups of genes are those being discovered through a growing list of technologies designed to randomly screen cancer genomes for all types of epigenetic abnormalities, including those associated with promoter hypermethylation and transcriptional silencing. These techniques include hybridization chip procedures for detection of CpG island methylation, methylation-sensitive restriction-enzyme-based production of DNA fragments representing alterations in patterns of DNA methylation, and expression microarray approaches to detect re-expression of abnormally silenced genes when the chromatin events mediating transcriptional repression are pharmacologically reversed (Akama et al. 1997; Huang et al. 1999; Toyota et al. 1999; Costello et al. 2000; Salem et al. 2000; Suzuki et al. 2002; Yamashita et al. 2002; Shi et al. 2003; Ushijima 2005; Yu et al. 2005). Again, the major challenge when such searches identify promoter hypermethylated genes is to elucidate the true importance of the loss of gene expression for tumor development.

Several important themes have emerged from all of the above gene discoveries that are beginning to alter our view of cancer as a disease strictly arising through genetic changes. First, more loss of tumor-suppressor-like gene function may occur in cancer via epigenetically mediated heritable transcription repression events than via frank gene mutations (Jones and Laird 1999; Jones and Baylin 2002; Herman and Baylin 2003). Thus, multiple genes are now being described in which mutations have not been observed but abnormal gene silencing is frequent in multiple cancer types (Jones and Laird 1999; Jones and Baylin 2002; Herman and Baylin 2003). Second, all major cellular control pathways which, when disrupted, contribute to tumorigenesis (Hanahan and Weinberg 2000), have now been shown to be involved with epigenetically mediated gene silencing (Jones and Laird 1999; Jones and Baylin 2002; Herman and Baylin 2003). Third, as expanded upon below, many abnormal gene silencing events may arise early in tumor progression, and specifically in preinvasive stages, and these may act to facilitate abnormal expansion of stem/progenitor-like cells in which subsequent genetic and epigenetic abnormalities arise and foster tumor progression (Kiyono et al. 1998; Romanov et al. 2001; Jones and Baylin 2002; Herman and Baylin 2003; Chen et al. 2004; Suzuki et al. 2004).

POSITION AND FUNCTION OF EPIGENETIC GENE SILENCING IN TUMOR PROGRESSION

In the best-characterized genes that are abnormally epigenetically silenced in cancer, there has been emphasis, through careful comparison of normal and abnormal tissues, on understanding the timing during tumor progression for onset of promoter hypermethylation and loss of gene function. From these studies, there is a growing list of such genes that appear to lose transcription very early during neoplastic development, often at precancerous stages of tumor progression (Belinsky et al. 1997, 1998; Kiyono et al. 1998; Nuovo et al. 1999; Jones and Baylin 2002; Herman and Baylin 2003; Holst et al. 2003; Chen et al. 2004; Suzuki et al. 2004). In addition, a possibly emerging theme is that such loss of gene function might be one mechanism through which neoplastic cells may become, somewhat in terms of a concept derived by Weinstein (2002), "addicted" to certain oncogenic driving pathways. A striking example of these concepts (Suzuki et al. 2004), outlined in Figure 1, is the appearance in very early lesions at risk for progression to colon cancer, atypical crypt foci (ACF), of abnormal promoter methylation in the *SFRP*s (secreted frizzled related proteins). These genes encode a family of proteins with ability to antagonize activation of the Wnt pathway at the level of cell membrane Wnt–Wnt ligand interaction (Finch et al. 1997; Melkonyan et al. 1997; Rattner et al. 1997). This hypermethylation, and associated gene silencing, were found to be present in one or more of the *SFRP*s, and usually multiple ones, in virtually all primary colon cancers examined (Suzuki et al. 2004). In a series of biology studies with cultured colon cancer cells, it

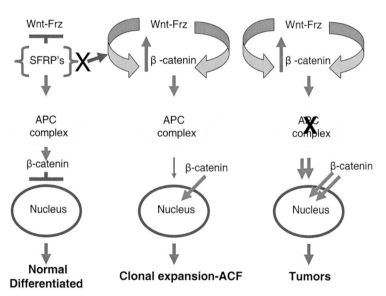

Figure 1. Model depicting how epigenetic gene silencing, very early in the preinvasive stages of colon tumor evolution, as discussed in the text, can "addict" cells to overactivity of the Wnt pathway, even in the absence of downstream mutations. In the far left panel, normal expression of the SFRPs, as colon epithelial cells differentiate, blunts interaction of Wnt with the receptor Frz and thus helps to down-regulate the pathway. This leads to low cytoplasmic levels of the key downstream transcriptional initiator of Wnt pathway activation, β-catenin. This control cooperates with a properly functioning APC tumor suppressor complex that facilitates phosphorylation of β-catenin, which renders it susceptible to cytoplasmic degradation and prevents high levels of this protein from reaching the nucleus. Abnormal epigenetic silencing of the SFRPs (*large X, left panel*) leads (*red arrow*) to (*middle panel*) Wnt–Frz interaction, activation of the pathway (*large blue arrows*), increased cytoplasmic levels of β-catenin (*green arrow* at *top* of *middle panel*), and partial overriding of the APC complex leading to some increase in levels of this protein in the nucleus and abnormal, preinvasive, expansion of colon epithelial precursor cells (atypical crypt foci or ACF). A mutation (*large X, right panel*) in APC, other members of the complex, or an activating mutation of β-catenin, leads to further constitutive Wnt pathway activity via crippling of function of the APC complex. Thus, further increases in nuclear β-catenin and resultant progression to invasive tumors are selected for.

emerged that replacement of SFRPs in cells with absent expression blocked Wnt pathway-driven transcriptional activity and caused apoptosis (Suzuki et al. 2004). This occurred even in cells harboring the key mutations in downstream Wnt pathway genes that activate the pathway intracellularly and are thought to be the very early, or "gatekeeper," steps in colon cancer evolution (Kinzler and Vogelstein 1997; Gregorieff and Clevers 2005).

The picture that emerges from these studies of the SFRPs is that loss of these proteins early in colon cancer development leads to abnormal constitutive activation at the ligand level of the key developmental Wnt pathway that has the ability to abnormally expand stem/progenitor cells in the colon (Kinzler and Vogelstein 1997; Gregorieff and Clevers 2005). These cells, which would be, in essence, addicted to overactivity of the Wnt pathway, would be primed for readily selecting mutations in downstream Wnt pathway genes, which most commonly occur in the APC tumor suppressor gene, which would drive the Wnt pathway harder and facilitate tumor progression (Fig. 1). The above-mentioned cell biology of the SFRPs in colon cancer cells shows how this selection could occur. APC mutations cripple the intracellular complex that normally leads, in the cytoplasm, to phosphorylation and degradation of β-catenin, which otherwise can go to the nucleus and mediate the transcriptional events central to the activated Wnt pathway (Kinzler and Vogelstein 1997; Gregorieff and Clevers 2005). Such complex crippling, however, may depend for function on the levels of β-catenin presented to the complex; active Wnt ligand at the membrane, facilitated by loss of SFRPs, leads to elevation of intracellular levels of this protein (Kinzler and Vogelstein 1997; Suzuki et al. 2004; Gregorieff and Clevers 2005). In early preinvasive colon lesions, such SFRP loss may lead to enough constitutive increases in β-catenin to partially overwhelm even an intact APC complex, leading to early progenitor cell expansion. This SFRP loss also leads to increased levels of β-catenin in those colon tumors harboring activating mutations in this protein. In summary (Fig. 1), epigenetically mediated loss of the SFRPs may drive colon cancer progression from the earliest to latest stages by selecting for, and facilitating, definitive mutations in the Wnt pathway. The question may even be raised, albeit a heretical one, whether the mutations in Wnt pathway genes would even result in clonal cell expansion without the "epigenetic gatekeeper" role of loss of function in genes such as the *SFRPs* (Fig. 2).

The role of epigenetic gene silencing in early cancer development has also become apparent in data emerging from comparing primary human tumor analyses to animal models of epigenetic gene silencing. Such animal models are going to be increasingly utilized to determine the true role of genes discovered to be silenced in tumors in association with promoter methylation, but for which no significant incidence of mutations is found. Mouse knockout studies of such genes can be used to test the consequences for the role of the genes in processes such as embryonic and mature tissue development plus the consequences of loss of function for tumorigenesis. We have taken such an approach for a gene, HIC1 (Hypermethylated-in-Cancer

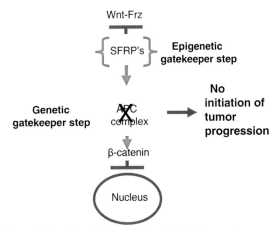

Figure 2. Model predicting, as described in the text, how a mutation in APC would not, without the epigenetic inactivation of the SFRPs or related proteins, begin to drive tumor progression.

1), which was discovered in a random search approach for hypermethylated genes possibly residing in a chromosome 17p region frequently deleted in multiple human cancer types (Wales et al. 1995). This region is distal to the tumor suppressor gene *p53* and is often deleted independent of deletion and/or mutations of *p53*. Interestingly, HIC1, which is hypermethylated early, in preinvasive stages of cancers such as breast (Fujii et al. 1998) and colon (Wales et al. 1995), is also a transcription activation target of p53 (Wales et al. 1995; Guerardel et al. 2000). The constitutive homozygous knockout of Hic-1 is lethal (Carter et al. 2000), but the heterozygotes get late-onset tumors in which the wild-type allele is universally retained and hypermethylated (Chen et al. 2003). Interestingly, there is a gender-associated tumor spectrum in which male mice get predominantly epithelial cancers and females get lymphomas and soft-tissue sarcomas (Chen et al. 2003).

The possible addiction of cells to pathways disrupted by the epigenetic silencing of HIC1 is apparent in the fact that this protein is involved in modulating activity of the powerful tumor suppressor, p53. This interaction may be viewed in two ways. First, crossing of Hic-1 heterozygous mice with p53 heterozygotes markedly modulates the time of appearance, virulence, and tumor spectrum as compared to either of the heterozygotes alone (Chen et al. 2004). Thus, both male and female double heterozygotes get new tumor types for the strain of mice studied, including osteosarcomas, breast tumors, and ovarian tumors (Chen et al. 2004). Again, the wild-type allele of *Hic-1* is almost always retained and hypermethylated, whereas the wild-type allele of *p53* is virtually always deleted (Chen et al. 2004). It appears that the epigenetic milieu, in this case epigenetic inactivation of Hic-1, determines the location, spectrum, and virulence of tumors induced even by genetic inactivation of the powerful tumor suppressor, p53 (Fig. 3).

Second, from a mechanistic standpoint in terms of one way in which HIC1 appears to function as a tumor suppressor, our recent data show that epigenetic loss of this

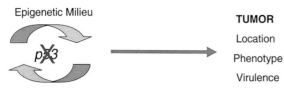

Figure 3. Model predicting, as described in the text, how mutations in the powerful tumor suppressor gene, *p53*, will drive tumorgenicity in directions determined by the epigenetic milieu.

protein leads to disruption of a complex network involving the key stress-sensing protein, SIRT1 (Frye 1999; Luo et al. 2001; Vaziri et al. 2001; Nemoto et al. 2004), and p53. SIRT1, a member of the class III family of sirtuins (Frye 1999; Vaziri et al. 2001), has p53 as one of its targets (Luo et al. 2001; Vaziri et al. 2001; Langley et al. 2002). Deactylation of p53 down-regulates the transcriptional function of this protein (Luo et al. 2001; Vaziri et al. 2001; Langley et al. 2002). We have recently found that HIC1 is a direct transcriptional repressor of SIRT1 and also complexes with SIRT1—both proteins are localized to the SIRT1 promoter (Chen et al. 2005). With epigenetic inactivation of HIC1, SIRT1 levels increase and acetylation of p53 is lost during DNA damage (Chen et al. 2005). This leads, in HIC1-deficient cells, to decreased p53 function and diminution of cell apoptotic response to DNA damage (Chen et al. 2005), providing a potential early oncogenic stimulus to cells. Again, this loss of HIC1 and diminished p53 function may drive cells down a pathway favorable for selection of genetic inactivation of p53, which then locks cells farther into tumor progression.

It appears evident from the examples provided above that the early role of epigenetic silencing, especially in the abnormal expansion of stem/progenitor cells which can precede and set the risk for cancer development, merits intensive continued investigation. The concept is that the likelihood of progression to frank malignancy or the virulence course of a particular tumor depends not only on given gene mutations, but also on the milieu of epigenetic alterations in which they occur. It must be remembered that these epigenetic changes may be ongoing not only in tumor cells or their precursors but also, as recently suggested (Hu et al. 2005), in stromal cells surrounding the neoplastic cells. Recent data have re-emphasized the importance of stromal cell abnormalities in contributing significantly to tumor progression (Tlsty 2001; Orimo et al. 2005). This concept of an epigenetic milieu of epigenetic abnormalities determining the course of tumor development has profound implications for prevention and therapeutic approaches to cancer, and for molecular strategies aimed at marker development for cancer risk assessment, early diagnosis, and prognosis prediction.

MOLECULAR STEPS IN ESTABLISHING AND MAINTAINING ABNORMAL HERITABLE TRANSCRIPTIONAL REPRESSION IN CANCER

There are no more important biological questions concerning epigenetically mediated loss of gene function in cancer than determining the molecular steps that establish and maintain the abnormal memory patterns during tumor development. We have come to understand much more about the latter than about the former, although both areas must undergo extensive clarification through ongoing research efforts.

With respect to causing initiation of the process of abnormal promoter methylation and associated silencing of tumor suppressor genes, we only have emerging clues. Certainly, there is building contribution to answering this question from the unraveling of molecular steps that cause gene promoters to be marked for silencing and maintained in a stably silent state. Critical to such silencing are studies of chromatin remodeling complexes, the histone modifications that separate active from inactive gene states, and the series of polycomb complexes under study from model organisms to man (Jenuwein and Allis 2001; Kouzarides 2002; Peters et al. 2003; Lund and van Lohuizen 2004). Particularly for the polycomb groups, we know that key components such as the protein Bmi1, complexes such as PRC4 which contains the histone methyltransferase, EZH2, and its partners, are increased in stem/progenitor cells and tumor cells that have properties of such cells (Varambally et al. 2002; Kirmizis et al. 2003; Kleer et al. 2003; Kuzmichev et al. 2005). Few specific targets for these silencing complexes, particularly in normal or neoplastic mammalian cells, are known. One key tumor suppressor gene that is frequently hypermethylated and silenced in cancer, *p16*, is a known indirect or direct target of Bmi1 (Lessard et al. 1999; Lund and van Lohuizen 2004), but the precise link as to how such targeting may be translated into the very stable silencing associated with promoter DNA methylation, or as to how and when such methylation appears during tumor development, is not known.

One emerging concept is that the course of epigenetic silencing of tumor suppressor genes may be a progressive one during tumor evolution in which degrees of silencing precede the imposition of abnormal DNA methylation on the promoter (Jones and Baylin 2002; Bachman et al. 2003). This concept encompasses key data, from model organisms to man, indicating that certain histone methylation marks, such as methylation of lysines 9 and 27 of histone H3 (methyl-K9-H3 and methyl-K27-H3), may be essential for recruiting DNA methylation (Selker et al. 1987; Bell et al. 1991; Tamaru and Selker 2001, 2003; Jackson et al. 2002; Johnson et al. 2002; Plath et al. 2003; Cao and Zhang 2004). Data from a study by Rauscher and colleagues (Ayyanathan et al. 2003), as we have reviewed (Fahrner and Baylin 2003), may be most relevant to the process under discussion. This study indicates that when transcriptional silencing of a promoter is transiently established, a very localized zone of histone transcriptional repression marks, and particularly methyl-K9-H3 and the recruitment of the protein HP1, is placed in and around the binding site for the transcriptional repression complex. If the complex is removed, most clones of cells revert to active transcription of the targeted gene and concomitant loss of the transcriptional repression marks. However, some clones retain the promoter repression marks, have absent or diminished transcription, and with continued growth, cells from such clones evolve very stable transcriptional repression mediated by recruitment of promoter DNA methylation. It is possible that these dynamics derived in an experimental cell model system are highly pertinent to the dynamics ongoing in natural tumor progression which lead to abnormal heritable transcriptional silencing of genes.

With respect to maintenance of heritable silencing of tumor suppressor genes in tumor cells, we know much more than how the process is established (for review, see Jones and Baylin 2002; Herman and Baylin 2003). We, and other investigators, have established that the promoters of such silenced genes have localization of classic transcriptional silencing marks which include, in addition to CpG island methylation, presence of deactylated K9-H3 and K14- H3 and methyl-K9-H3. In turn, key activating marks, including methyl-K4-H3 and acetyl-K9 and K14-H3, are absent in such genes but are present to the virtual exclusion of the repressive marks when the same genes are expressed in a cancer cell (Fahrner et al. 2002; Ghoshal et al. 2002; Koizume et al. 2002; Nguyen et al. 2002; Bachman et al. 2003; Kondo et al. 2003). In this layering of transcriptionally repressive chromatin, the DNA methylation appears to be quite dominant; this is an important point with respect to selection during tumor progression of the most stably silenced state. The clearest example of this point is that some degree of DNA demethylation of the promoter must be achieved before transcription can be restored and key transcriptional activation marks, such as acetyl K9-H3 and K14-H3 and methyl-K9-H3, appear and repression marks, such as deacetylated K9-H3 and K-14-H3 and methyl-K9-H3, decrease (Fahrner et al. 2002; Nguyen et al. 2002). This fits with earlier observations that cancer cell treatment with class 1 histone deactylase (HDAC) inhibitors fails to transcriptionally activate densely promoter-DNA-methylated tumor suppressor genes but will synergize with DNA demethylating agents to do so (Cameron et al. 1999). Despite all of these observations, however, our knowledge of all the molecular events that mediate maintenance of the abnormally heritable silencing state of cancer cells, and their hierarchical relationships to one another, is almost assuredly quite incomplete. This critical aspect of the epigenetic abnormalities in tumor progression thus merits intense investigation. It also has profound implications for the translational quest to target reversal of epigenetic gene silencing as a means for cancer prevention and treatment.

CONCLUSIONS

This paper has stressed the point that a series of epigenetic, as well as genetic, alterations are ongoing throughout the initiation and maintenance phases of human tumor progression. In terms of the former, although a complex array of chromatin patterns are altered during tumor evolution, the best understood, at present, is an abnormal heritable transcriptional repression of proven or candidate tumor suppressor genes. This repression is mediated by a layering of chromatin changes at the level of histone modifications upon which DNA methylation is imposed as the step that tightly locks the silencing in. Many of the gene silencing events appear to occur at very early stages of neoplastic progression and even serve as "epigenetic gatekeeper steps," or an epigenetic milieu, without which key tumor suppressor mutations might not be able to play their full roles in fostering tumor evolution. These epigenetic steps may addict cells to oncogenic stimuli from abnormal signal transduction pathway activation or partial crippling of tumor suppressor genes lying downstream from abnormally silenced genes. Understanding the molecular events that initiate and maintain this heritable gene silencing may allow it to be targeted for reversal in strategies aimed at the prevention and treatment of cancer. The component of abnormal promoter DNA methylation is also providing a promising molecular marker strategy for cancer risk assessment, early detection, and gauging of prognosis.

ACKNOWLEDGMENTS

This study is supported by grants from the National Cancer Institute (CA043318) and National Institutes of Environmental Health Sciences (ES11858). We thank Kathy Bender for her help with the manuscript preparation.

REFERENCES

Akama T.O., Okazaki Y., Ito M., Okuizumi H., Konno H., Muramatsu M., Plass C., Held W.A., and Hayashizaki Y. 1997. Restriction landmark genomic scanning (RLGS-M)-based genome-wide scanning of mouse liver tumors for alterations in DNA methylation status. *Cancer Res.* **57**: 3294.

Ayyanathan K., Lechner M.S., Bell P., Maul G.G., Schultz D.C., Yamada Y., Tanaka K., Torigoe K., and Rauscher F.J., III. 2003. Regulated recruitment of HP1 to a euchromatic gene induces mitotically heritable, epigenetic gene silencing: A mammalian cell culture model of gene variegation. *Genes Dev.* **17**: 1855.

Bachman K.E., Park B.H., Rhee I., Rajagopalan H., Herman J.G., Baylin S.B., Kinzler K.W., and Vogelstein B. 2003. Histone modifications and silencing prior to DNA methylation of a tumor suppressor gene. *Cancer Cell* **3**: 89.

Belinsky S.A., Swafford D.S., Middleton S.K., Kennedy C.H., and Tesfaigzi J. 1997. Deletion and differential expression of p16INK4a in mouse lung tumors. *Carcinogenesis* **18**: 115.

Belinsky S.A., Nikula K.J., Palmisano W.A., Michels R., Saccomanno G., Gabrielson E., Baylin S.B., and Herman J.G. 1998. Aberrant methylation of p16(INK4a) is an early event in lung cancer and a potential biomarker for early diagnosis. *Proc. Natl. Acad. Sci.* **95**: 11891.

Bell M.V., Hirst M.C., Nakahori Y., MacKinnon R.N., Roche A., Flint T.J., Jacobs P.A., Tommerup N., Tranebjaerg L., and Froster-Iskenius U., et al. 1991. Physical mapping across the fragile X: Hypermethylation and clinical expression of the fragile X syndrome. *Cell* **64**: 861.

Cameron E.E., Bachman K.E., Myohanen S., Herman J.G., and Baylin S.B. 1999. Synergy of demethylation and histone deacetylase inhibition in the re-expression of genes silenced in cancer. *Nat. Genet.* **21**: 103.

Cao R. and Zhang Y. 2004. The functions of E(Z)/EZH2-mediated methylation of lysine 27 in histone H3. *Curr. Opin. Genet. Dev.* **14**: 155.

Carter M.G., Johns M.A., Zeng X., Zhou L., Zink M.C., Mankowski J.L., Donovan D.M., and Baylin S.B. 2000. Mice deficient in the candidate tumor suppressor gene Hic1 exhibit developmental defects of structures affected in the Miller-Dieker syndrome. *Hum. Mol. Genet.* **9:** 413.

Chen W.Y., Wang D.H., Chiu Yen R.W., Luo J., Gu W., and Baylin S.B. 2005. Tumor suppressor HIC1 directly regulates SIRT1 and modulates p53 dependent apoptotic DNA damage responses. *Cell* (in press).

Chen W.Y., Zeng X., Carter M.G., Morrell C.N., Chiu Yen R.W., Esteller M., Watkins D.N., Herman J.G., Mankowski J.L., and Baylin S.B. 2003. Heterozygous disruption of Hic1 predisposes mice to a gender-dependent spectrum of malignant tumors. *Nat. Genet.* **33:** 197.

Chen W., Cooper T.K., Zahnow C.A., Overholtzer M., Zhao Z., Ladanyi M., Karp J.E., Gokgoz N., Wunder J.S., Andrulis I.L., Levine A.J., Mankowski J.L., and Baylin S.B. 2004. Epigenetic and genetic loss of Hic1 function accentuates the role of p53 in tumorigenesis. *Cancer Cell* **6:** 387.

Costello J.F., Fruhwald M.C., Smiraglia D.J., Rush L.J., Robertson G.P., Gao X., Wright F.A., Feramisco J.D., Peltomaki P., Lang J.C., Schuller D.E., Yu L., Bloomfield C.D., Caligiuri M.A., Yates A., Nishikawa R., Su Huang H., Petrelli N.J., Zhang X., O'Dorisio M.S., Held W.A., Cavenee W.K., and Plass C. 2000. Aberrant CpG-island methylation has non-random and tumour-type-specific patterns. *Nat. Genet.* **24:** 132.

Fahrner J.A. and Baylin S.B. 2003. Heterochromatin: Stable and unstable invasions at home and abroad. *Genes Dev.* **17:** 1805.

Fahrner J.A., Eguchi S., Herman J.G., and Baylin S.B. 2002. Dependence of histone modifications and gene expression on DNA hypermethylation in cancer. *Cancer Res.* **62:** 7213.

Finch P.W., He X., Kelley M.J., Uren A., Schaudies R.P., Popescu N.C., Rudikoff S., Aaronson S.A., Varmus H.E., and Rubin J.S. 1997. Purification and molecular cloning of a secreted, Frizzled-related antagonist of Wnt action. *Proc. Natl. Acad. Sci.* **94:** 6770.

Frye R.A. 1999. Characterization of five human cDNAs with homology to the yeast SIR2 gene: Sir2-like proteins (sirtuins) metabolize NAD and may have protein ADP-ribosyltransferase activity. *Biochem. Biophys. Res. Commun.* **260:** 273.

Fujii H., Biel M.A., Zhou W., Weitzman S.A., Baylin S.B., and Gabrielson E. 1998. Methylation of the HIC-1 candidate tumor suppressor gene in human breast cancer. *Oncogene* **16:** 2159.

Ghoshal K., Datta J., Majumder S., Bai S., Dong X., Parthun M., and Jacob S.T. 2002. Inhibitors of histone deacetylase and DNA methyltransferase synergistically activate the methylated metallothionein I promoter by activating the transcription factor MTF-1 and forming an open chromatin structure. *Mol. Cell. Biol.* **22:** 8302.

Gregorieff A. and Clevers H. 2005. Wnt signaling in the intestinal epithelium: From endoderm to cancer. *Genes Dev.* **19:** 877.

Guerardel C., Deltour S., Pinte S., Monte D., Begue A., Godwin A.K., and Leprince D. 2000. Identification in the human candidate tumor suppressor gene HIC-1 of a new major alternative TATA-less promoter positively regulated by p53. *J. Biol. Chem.* **276:** 3078.

Hanahan D. and Weinberg R.A. 2000. The hallmarks of cancer. *Cell* **100:** 57.

Herman J.G. and Baylin S.B. 2003. Gene silencing in cancer in association with promoter hypermethylation. *N. Engl. J. Med.* **349:** 2042.

Holst C.R., Nuovo G.J., Esteller M., Chew K., Baylin S.B., Herman J.G., and Tlsty T.D. 2003. Methylation of p16(INK4a) promoters occurs in vivo in histologically normal human mammary epithelia. *Cancer Res.* **63:** 1596.

Hu M., Yao J., Cai L., Bachman K.E., van den Brule F., Velculescu V., and Polyak K. 2005. Distinct epigenetic changes in the stromal cells of breast cancers. *Nat. Genet.* **37:** 899.

Huang T.H., Perry M.R., and Laux D.E. 1999. Methylation profiling of CpG islands in human breast cancer cells. *Hum. Mol. Genet.* **8:** 459.

Jackson J.P., Lindroth A.M., Cao X., and Jacobsen S.E. 2002. Control of CpNpG DNA methylation by the KRYPTONITE histone H3 methyltransferase. *Nature* **416:** 556.

Jenuwein T. and Allis C.D. 2001. Translating the histone code. *Science* **293:** 1074.

Johnson L., Cao X., and Jacobsen S. 2002. Interplay between two epigenetic marks. DNA methylation and histone H3 lysine 9 methylation. *Curr. Biol.* **12:** 1360.

Jones P.A. and Baylin S.B. 2002. The fundamental role of epigenetic events in cancer. *Nat. Rev. Genet.* **3:** 415.

Jones P.A. and Laird P.W. 1999. Cancer epigenetics comes of age. *Nat. Genet.* **21:** 163.

Kinzler K.W. and Vogelstein B. 1997. Cancer-susceptibility genes. Gatekeepers and caretakers. *Nature* **386:** 761.

Kirmizis A., Bartley S.M., and Farnham P.J. 2003. Identification of the polycomb group protein SU(Z)12 as a potential molecular target for human cancer therapy. *Mol. Cancer Ther.* **2:** 113.

Kiyono T., Foster S.A., Koop J.I., McDougall J.K., Galloway D.A., and Klingelhutz A.J. 1998. Both Rb/p16INK4a inactivation and telomerase activity are required to immortalize human epithelial cells. *Nature* **396:** 84.

Kleer C.G., Cao Q., Varambally S., Shen R., Ota I., Tomlins S.A., Ghosh D., Sewalt R.G., Otte A.P., Hayes D.F., Sabel M.S., Livant D., Weiss S.J., Rubin M.A., and Chinnaiyan A.M. 2003. EZH2 is a marker of aggressive breast cancer and promotes neoplastic transformation of breast epithelial cells. *Proc. Natl. Acad. Sci.* **100:** 11606.

Koizume S., Tachibana K., Sekiya T., Hirohashi S., and Shiraishi M. 2002. Heterogeneity in the modification and involvement of chromatin components of the CpG island of the silenced human CDH1 gene in cancer cells. *Nucleic Acids Res.* **30:** 4770.

Kondo Y., Shen L., and Issa J.P. 2003. Critical role of histone methylation in tumor suppressor gene silencing in colorectal cancer. *Mol. Cell. Biol.* **23:** 206.

Kouzarides T. 2002. Histone methylation in transcriptional control. *Curr. Opin. Genet. Dev.* **12:** 198.

Kuzmichev A., Margueron R., Vaquero A., Preissner T.S., Scher M., Kirmizis A., Ouyang X., Brockdorff N., Abate-Shen C., Farnham P., and Reinberg D. 2005. Composition and histone substrates of polycomb repressive group complexes change during cellular differentiation. *Proc. Natl. Acad. Sci.* **102:** 1859.

Langley E., Pearson M., Faretta M., Bauer U.M., Frye R.A., Minucci S., Pelicci P.G., and Kouzarides T. 2002. Human SIR2 deacetylates p53 and antagonizes PML/p53-induced cellular senescence. *EMBO J.* **21:** 2383.

Lessard J., Schumacher A., Thorsteinsdottir U., van Lohuizen M., Magnuson T., and Sauvageau G. 1999. Functional antagonism of the Polycomb-Group genes eed and Bmi1 in hemopoietic cell proliferation. *Genes Dev.* **13:** 2691.

Lund A.H. and van Lohuizen M. 2004. Polycomb complexes and silencing mechanisms. *Curr. Opin. Cell Biol.* **16:** 239.

Luo J., Nikolaev A.Y., Imai S., Chen D., Su F., Shiloh A., Guarente L., and Gu W. 2001. Negative control of p53 by Sir2alpha promotes cell survival under stress. *Cell* **107:** 137.

Melkonyan H.S., Chang W.C., Shapiro J.P., Mahadevappa M., Fitzpatrick P.A., Kiefer M.C., Tomei L.D., and Umansky S.R. 1997. SARPs: A family of secreted apoptosis-related proteins. *Proc. Natl. Acad. Sci.* **94:** 13636.

Nemoto S., Fergusson M.M., and Finkel T. 2004. Nutrient availability regulates SIRT1 through a forkhead-dependent pathway. *Science* **306:** 2105.

Nguyen C.T., Weisenberger D.J., Velicescu M., Gonzales F.A., Lin J.C., Liang G., and Jones P.A. 2002. Histone H3-lysine 9 methylation is associated with aberrant gene silencing in cancer cells and is rapidly reversed by 5-aza-2'-deoxycytidine. *Cancer Res.* **62:** 6456.

Nuovo G.J., Plaia T.W., Belinsky S.A., Baylin S.B., and Herman J.G. 1999. In situ detection of the hypermethylation-induced inactivation of the p16 gene as an early event in oncogenesis. *Proc. Natl. Acad. Sci.* **96:** 12754.

Orimo A., Gupta P.B., Sgroi D.C., Arenzana-Seisdedos F., Delaunay T., Naeem R., Carey V.J., Richardson A.L., and Weinberg R.A. 2005. Stromal fibroblasts present in invasive human breast carcinomas promote tumor growth and angiogenesis through elevated SDF-1/CXCL12 secretion. *Cell* **121:** 335.

Peters A.H., Kubicek S., Mechtler K., O'Sullivan R.J., Derijck A.A., Perez-Burgos L., Kohlmaier A., Opravil S., Tachibana M., Shinkai Y., Martens J.H., and Jenuwein T. 2003. Partitioning and plasticity of repressive histone methylation states in mammalian chromatin. *Mol. Cell* **12:** 1577.

Plath K., Fang J., Mlynarczyk-Evans S.K., Cao R., Worringer K.A., Wang H., de la Cruz C.C., Otte A.P., Panning B., and Zhang Y. 2003. Role of histone H3 lysine 27 methylation in X inactivation. *Science* **300:** 131.

Rattner A., Hsieh J.C., Smallwood P.M., Gilbert D.J., Copeland N.G., Jenkins N.A., and Nathans J. 1997. A family of secreted proteins contains homology to the cysteine-rich ligand-binding domain of frizzled receptors. *Proc. Natl. Acad. Sci.* **94:** 2859.

Romanov S.R., Kozakiewicz B.K., Holst C.R., Stampfer M.R., Haupt L.M., and Tlsty T.D. 2001. Normal human mammary epithelial cells spontaneously escape senescence and acquire genomic changes. *Nature* **409:** 633.

Salem C.E., Markl I.D., Bender C.M., Gonzales F.A., Jones P.A., and Liang G. 2000. PAX6 methylation and ectopic expression in human tumor cells. *Int. J. Cancer* **87:** 179.

Selker E.U., Jensen B.C., and Richardson G.A. 1987. A portable signal causing faithful DNA methylation de novo in *Neurospora crassa*. *Science* **238:** 48.

Shi H., Wei S.H., Leu Y.W., Rahmatpanah F., Liu J.C., Yan P.S., Nephew K.P., and Huang T.H. 2003. Triple analysis of the cancer epigenome: An integrated microarray system for assessing gene expression, DNA methylation, and histone acetylation. *Cancer Res.* **63:** 2164.

Suzuki H., Gabrielson E., Chen W., Anbazhagan R., van Engeland M., Weijenberg M.P., Herman J.G., and Baylin S.B. 2002. A genomic screen for genes upregulated by demethylation and histone deacetylase inhibition in human colorectal cancer. *Nat. Genet.* **31:** 141.

Suzuki H., Watkins D.N., Jair K.W., Schuebel K.E., Markowitz S.D., Dong Chen W., Pretlow T.P., Yang B., Akiyama Y., Van Engeland M., Toyota M., Tokino T., Hinoda Y., Imai K., Herman J.G., and Baylin S.B. 2004. Epigenetic inactivation of SFRP genes allows constitutive WNT signaling in colorectal cancer. *Nat. Genet.* **36:** 417.

Tamaru H. and Selker E.U. 2001. A histone H3 methyltransferase controls DNA methylation in *Neurospora crassa*. *Nature* **414:** 277.

———. 2003. Synthesis of signals for de novo DNA methylation in *Neurospora crassa*. *Mol. Cell. Biol.* **23:** 2379.

Tlsty T.D. 2001. Stromal cells can contribute oncogenic signals. *Semin. Cancer Biol.* **11:** 97.

Toyota M., Ho C., Ahuja N., Jair K.W., Li Q., Ohe-Toyota M., Baylin S.B., and Issa J.P. 1999. Identification of differentially methylated sequences in colorectal cancer by methylated CpG island amplification. *Cancer Res.* **59:** 2307.

Ushijima T. 2005. Detection and interpretation of altered methylation patterns in cancer cells. *Nat. Rev. Cancer* **5:** 223.

Varambally S., Dhanasekaran S.M., Zhou M., Barrette T.R., Kumar-Sinha C., Sanda M.G., Ghosh D., Pienta K.J., Sewalt R.G., Otte A.P., Rubin M.A., and Chinnaiyan A.M. 2002. The polycomb group protein EZH2 is involved in progression of prostate cancer. *Nature* **419:** 624.

Vaziri H., Dessain S.K., Ng Eaton E., Imai S.I., Frye R.A., Pandita T.K., Guarente L., and Weinberg R.A. 2001. hSIR2(SIRT1) functions as an NAD-dependent p53 deacetylase. *Cell* **107:** 149.

Wales M.M., Biel M.A., el Deiry W., Nelkin B.D., Issa J.P., Cavenee W.K., Kuerbitz S.J., and Baylin S.B. 1995. p53 activates expression of HIC-1, a new candidate tumour suppressor gene on 17p13.3. *Nat. Med.* **1:** 570.

Weinstein I.B. 2002. Cancer. Addiction to oncogenes—The Achilles heal of cancer. *Science* **297:** 63.

Yamashita K., Upadhyay S., Osada M., Hoque M.O., Xiao Y., Mori M., Sato F., Meltzer S.J., and Sidransky D. 2002. Pharmacologic unmasking of epigenetically silenced tumor suppressor genes in esophageal squamous cell carcinoma. *Cancer Cell* **2:** 485.

Yu L., Liu C., Vandeusen J., Becknell B., Dai Z., Wu Y.Z., Raval A., Liu T.H., Ding W., Mao C., Liu S., Smith L.T., Lee S., Rassenti L., Marcucci G., Byrd J., Caligiuri M.A., and Plass C. 2005. Global assessment of promoter methylation in a mouse model of cancer identifies ID4 as a putative tumor-suppressor gene in human leukemia. *Nat. Genet.* **37:** 265.

Dissecting Cancer Pathways and Vulnerabilities with RNAi

T.F. WESTBROOK, F. STEGMEIER, AND S.J. ELLEDGE

Howard Hughes Medical Institute, Department of Genetics, Harvard Partners Center for Genetics and Genomics, Harvard Medical School, Boston, Massachusetts 02115

The latest generation of molecular-targeted cancer therapeutics has bolstered the notion that a better understanding of the networks governing cancer pathogenesis can be translated into substantial clinical benefits. However, functional annotation exists for only a small proportion of genes in the human genome, raising the likelihood that many cancer-relevant genes and potential drug targets await identification. Unbiased genetic screens in invertebrate organisms have provided substantial insights into signaling networks underlying many cellular and organismal processes. However, such approaches in mammalian cells have been limited by the lack of genetic tools. The emergence of RNA interference (RNAi) as a mechanism to suppress gene expression has revolutionized genetics in mammalian cells and has begun to facilitate decoding of gene functions on a genome scale. Here, we discuss the application of such RNAi-based genetic approaches to elucidating cancer-signaling networks and uncovering cancer vulnerabilities.

Tumorigenesis is a multistep process during which incipient cancer cells acquire a myriad of genetic and epigenetic alterations. Such alterations confer numerous changes in cell behavior, including inappropriate survival and proliferation (Hanahan and Weinberg 2000). However, the genetic perturbations underlying these aberrant cell behaviors are concealed by the complex instability of most cancer cell genomes. As a consequence, the goal of identifying genes promoting (oncogenes) and restraining (tumor suppressors) tumorigenesis has proved challenging. Much of our understanding of cancer cell biology has been derived from biochemical and reverse genetic approaches in which a gene of interest is interrogated for its relationships to other gene products and its roles in various cellular processes. This approach has yielded significant insight into select signaling networks and provided a molecular basis for much of cancer biology. However, the majority of this insight has been directed to a relatively small proportion of genes in the human genome, raising the likelihood that many genes underlying cancer cell phenotypes and, thus, potential drug targets have yet to be identified. Forward genetic approaches offer a plausible solution to this challenge, allowing one to elucidate genes underlying a given phenotype without a priori knowledge of its biochemical functions. Indeed, the unbiased genetic screens applied in yeast, worms, and flies have often provided entry points into studies of cancer-related phenomena that have been recalcitrant to other approaches. Until recently, mammalian cells have been refractory to loss-of-function genetic approaches due to the lack of time- and cost-efficient tools to create recessive, defined perturbations in somatic cells. The discovery of RNA interference (RNAi) and the subsequent exploitation of this biological phenomenon as a means to manipulate gene expression have begun to revolutionize mammalian genetics (Paddison and Hannon 2002; Brummelkamp and Bernards 2003; Hannon and Rossi 2004). This perspective focuses on how emerging RNAi-based genetic strategies could be used to delineate the genetic networks that govern tumorigenesis and rapidly identify promising molecular targets for cancer therapy.

RNAi is a gene regulatory pathway that is triggered in response to dsRNA molecules (Hannon 2002; Dykxhoorn et al. 2003). Since its formal description in *Caenorhabditis elegans* by Fire and colleagues (Fire et al. 1998), RNAi has been linked to gene-silencing phenomena in evolutionarily diverse organisms. RNA triggers have been shown to suppress gene expression by a variety of mechanisms, including mRNA degradation, loss of protein translation, and transcriptional silencing (Meister and Tuschl 2004). Although the complexities of these phenomena are far from understood, the hallmark of RNAi is the cleavage of dsRNA into 21- to 22-nucleotide molecules, or small interfering RNAs (siRNAs), by an RNase III enzyme, Dicer (Bernstein et al. 2001). These cleavage products are unwound and incorporated into an RNA-induced silencing complex (RISC), which utilizes the siRNA to identify homologous sequences within cognate mRNAs and degrade the mRNA (via the ribonuclease Ago2) or suppress translation from the mRNA template (Hannon 2002; Dykxhoorn et al. 2003).

Since its discovery, RNAi has become a common tool for loss-of-function studies in invertebrates (*Drosophila melanogaster* and *C. elegans*) in which gene-specific silencing is induced by the introduction of long dsRNAs. However, the use of such long dsRNA as an RNAi trigger is not plausible in mammalian somatic cells due to the PKR- and interferon-mediated responses to long-dsRNA molecules, which induce sequence-independent degradation of mRNAs and global repression of protein synthesis (Minks et al. 1979; Manche et al. 1992; Stark et al. 1998). Tuschl and colleagues circumvented this nonspecific toxicity by demonstrating that chemically synthesized siRNAs were sufficient to target complementary mRNAs for destruction but did not elicit the interferon response (Elbashir et al. 2001). Since this watershed event, the use of RNAi as a tool to decipher gene function has become commonplace in mammalian cell biology. As our understanding of RNAi biochemistry has evolved, so have the methods by which this endogenous pathway of gene regulation is harnessed for studying mutant phenotypes (Paddison and Hannon 2002; Brummelkamp and Bernards 2003; Hannon and Rossi 2004). siRNAs can be transfected directly into target cells, enabling studies of transient phenotypes that can be assayed in cells amenable to transfection. Alternatively, silencing triggers can be encoded genetically by small inverted repeats that express short hairpin RNAs (shRNAs) (Brummelkamp et al. 2002; Paddison et al. 2002; Sui et al. 2002; Yu et al. 2002). These shRNA transcripts form a stem loop structure that is processed by endogenous nuclease(s) into RNAs that can be incorporated into RISC. The design of these shRNAs was based on the discovery of endogenous triggers of the RNAi machinery, called small temporal RNAs or microRNAs (miRNAs) (Grishok et al. 2001; Hutvagner et al. 2001; Ketting et al. 2001). Initially, shRNAs were expressed from polymerase III (pol III) promoters such as U6 or H1 (Brummelkamp et al. 2002; Paddison et al. 2002; Sui et al. 2002; Yu et al. 2002), because of the precisely defined initiation and termination sequences for pol III. However, increasing knowledge of miRNA biogenesis has allowed flexibility in promoter usage as well as design of silencing triggers that more closely mimic endogenous miRNA transcripts (discussed below), presumably allowing more efficient processing of the targeting sequence. Importantly, shRNAs and miRNAs can be stably expressed from plasmid, retroviral, or lentiviral contexts, thus allowing long-term analyses of mutant phenotypes.

The ease of delivery and efficiency of sequence-specific gene silencing elicited by dsRNAs has facilitated genome-scale screens for modifiers of several cellular and organismal phenotypes in invertebrates (see, e.g., Ashrafi et al. 2003; Lee et al. 2003; Boutros et al. 2004; Baeg et al. 2005; DasGupta et al. 2005; Sieburth et al. 2005). In contrast, RNAi has predominantly been used in mammalian cells as a reverse genetic tool to eliminate specific gene function. However, large collections of array-format siRNA libraries have been generated, and, more recently, retrovirus-encoded shRNA libraries targeting the human and mouse genomes have been developed (Berns et al. 2004; Paddison et al. 2004; Silva et al. 2005), ushering in a new era of forward-genetic screening in mammalian systems. The advantages of these different formats for RNAi-mediated gene discovery have been reviewed in depth (Silva et al. 2004; Willingham et al. 2004). We discuss the impact these new functional genetic tools will have on cancer biology and drug target discovery.

DELINEATING CANCER-RELEVANT PATHWAYS AND DRUG TARGETS

The majority of traditional chemotherapies were discovered based on their ability to kill rapidly proliferating cancer cells. Unfortunately, these therapies inhibit gene products and cellular processes that are required in rapidly dividing normal tissues (e.g., hematopoietic), resulting in a delicate balance between killing cancer cells

and toxicity to the patient. The most recent generation of so-called targeted cancer drugs is designed to inactivate the very oncogenic lesions that contribute to the aberrant survival and proliferation of tumor cells, and has yielded remarkable success in some malignancies (Slamon et al. 1989; Druker et al. 1996; Druker 2002; Lynch et al. 2004; Paez et al. 2004; Sordella et al. 2004). The potential of these molecular-targeted therapies is embedded in the emerging concept of "oncogene addiction," or oncogene dependence (Weinstein 2002), which suggests that cancer cells are genetically or epigenetically reprogrammed upon suffering an oncogenic lesion such that the initiating lesion is required for maintenance of tumor cell phenotype(s). Support for such a concept comes from both in vitro and in vivo experiments. For instance, numerous studies have utilized conditional mouse models of cancer to explore oncogene dependence. In many of these models, expression of the initiating oncogene was required for tumor maintenance, with tumor cells undergoing differentiation, arrest, and/or apoptosis upon removal of the initial oncogenic stimulus (Jonkers and Berns 2002, 2004). Observations from the clinic also support the concept of oncogene dependence. Imatinib has been used to inhibit the aberrant signaling from BCR-ABL, c-KIT, and PDGFRA in the treatment of chronic myelogenous leukemia (CML), gastrointestinal stromal tumor (GIST), and hypereosinophilic syndrome (HES), respectively (Druker et al. 1996, 2001; Tuveson et al. 2001; Demetri et al. 2002; Cools et al. 2003). Notably, many patients suffering relapsed CML have incurred resistance mutations in the BCR-ABL fusion, corroborating the role of this lesion in disease maintenance (Gorre et al. 2001). Since the landmark success of imatinib, other molecular-targeted therapies have demonstrated efficacy, with trastuzumab (Her2/neu-blocking antibody) used to treat breast cancers with HER2/neu amplification/overexpression and gefitinib used to target non-small-cell lung cancers (NSCLC) with mutant EGFR (Slamon et al. 1989; Lynch et al. 2004; Paez et al. 2004; Sordella et al. 2004). Whereas these experimental and clinical observations support the concept of oncogene addiction, the underlying mechanisms by which cancer cells become dependent on such perturbations remain unclear. Nonetheless, the concept of oncogene dependence invokes an important vulnerability of cancer cells: novel gene–gene interactions that do not exist in counterpart normal cells. Consequently, identifying the genetic and epigenetic perturbations that contribute to tumor genesis and exploring the unique genetic relationships that result from these lesions are central goals in cancer biology.

IDENTIFYING MODULATORS OF KNOWN CANCER PATHWAYS

A plethora of genetic and epigenetic lesions have been implicated in cancer initiation and progression. Some of these lesions are highly represented in human cancers (e.g., p53, Rb). Indeed, it has been hypothesized that the function of a few key oncogenes and tumor suppressors must be dysregulated, either by direct insult or by alterations in upstream and downstream regulators, in all cancer types. Therefore, delineating the networks that regulate these key cancer pathways represents a promising approach to identifying new regulators of tumorigenesis. Recently, several forward genetic screens have incorporated this strategy in the context of *Drosophila* and mammalian tissue culture cells. Such screens have often relied on reporter constructs in which a promoter of interest is linked to a gene encoding a fluorescent or luminescent protein (e.g., GFP, firefly luciferase), with regulators of the reporter isolated by fluctuations in fluorescence or luminescence intensity. For instance, one can identify pathways that regulate transcription of a gene of interest by linking regulatory sequences from its promoter to a reporter gene. We have applied this strategy to identify repressors of hTERT gene transcription (Lin and Elledge 2003). hTERT is the catalytic subunit of the telomerase enzyme, and its activity is absent from most somatic tissues but is up-regulated in >90% of human cancers. Because amplification and translocations of hTERT are not observed in cancer, we surmised that pathways responsible for repressing hTERT transcription might be dysregulated during tumor genesis and thus represent tumor suppressor activities. Supporting this hypothesis, an antagonist of oncogenic Myc signaling (MAD1), an effector of the TGF-β tumor suppressor pathway (SIP1), and a bona fide tumor suppressor (MENIN) were all identified as repressors of hTERT transcription in this screen. Whereas this screen employed a retroviral mutagenesis strategy, application of RNAi-based libraries in a similar context will undoubtedly elucidate new pathways controlling hTERT expression.

Some oncogenes and tumor suppressors have already been organized into well-characterized pathways, and several groups have recently performed RNAi-based screens to identify new modulators of these critical pathways using synthetic promoter elements that drive transcription in response to pathway activation. The Hedgehog (Hh) and Wnt-Wingless signaling pathways play crucial roles in development, stem-cell homeostasis, and tumorigenesis (Nybakken and Perrimon 2002; Logan and Nusse 2004). Using an array-format library of dsRNA directed against the *Drosophila* genome, Perrimon and colleagues performed a screen for modulators of a Wnt-responsive luciferase reporter (DasGupta et al. 2005). This screen isolated most of the known elements of the Wnt pathway. In addition, a plethora of novel positive and negative regulators of Wnt signaling were identified, underscoring the complexity of the genetic networks that may impinge on Wnt-dependent processes. In a similar strategy, the Beachy laboratory screened for components of the Hh pathway using a Hh-responsive reporter (Lum et al. 2003). Again, both known and previously unrecognized regulators of Hh signaling were isolated. Furthermore, two components of the Wnt pathway were identified as modulators of Hh signaling, providing potential nodes of cross talk and/or co-regulation between these two pathways.

Similar approaches to identifying new modulators of cancer-relevant pathways have been applied in mammalian cells, although predominantly with smaller RNAi libraries directed against gene families. Using an shRNA

library targeting deubiquitinating enzymes (DUBs), the Bernards and D'Andrea laboratories identified a negative regulator (USP1) of the monoubiquitination of the Fanconi anemia complementation group D2 protein, or FANCD2 (Nijman et al. 2005). Fanconi anemia is a recessive genetic disorder characterized by genomic instability, hypersensitivity to DNA-crosslinking agents, and a predisposition to a variety of malignancies (D'Andrea 2003). FANCD2 monoubiquitination is hypothesized to be a critical regulatory event in the Fanconi anemia pathway (Meetei et al. 2003), and USP1 was found to antagonize this event (Nijman et al. 2005). Using the same DUB-shRNA library and an NF-κB-responsive reporter, Bernards and colleagues also identified an antagonist of NF-κB signaling, the familial cylindromatosis tumor suppressor (CYLD) (Brummelkamp et al. 2003). Loss of CYLD confers benign tumors arising from sweat glands (cylindromas) of the head and neck. Intriguingly, pharmacological inhibition of NF-κB led to regression of cylindromas, suggesting that aberrant activation of the NF-κB pathway may contribute to the pathogenesis of this disease. Schultz and colleagues performed a similar screen for modulators of NF-κB signaling, employing a much larger siRNA library targeting approximately 8000 human genes (Zheng et al. 2004). In addition to several established components of the NF-κB pathway, > 90 genes were implicated in NF-κB signaling, although future study is needed to determine the specificity of these effects.

IDENTIFYING NOVEL CANCER PATHWAYS

The above approaches will undoubtedly serve to illuminate networks that impinge upon and transduce the effects of those genes already heavily implicated in human tumorigenesis. However, cancer cells exhibit complex phenotypes, including altered responses to mitogenic and cytostatic signals, resistance to programmed cell death, immortalization, neoangiogenesis, and invasion and metastasis (Hanahan and Weinberg 2000), for which our knowledge of the underlying molecular mechanisms is far from complete. Genetic screens in model organisms have been instrumental in advancing our understanding of cell proliferation, apoptosis, migration, and the developmental programs that regulate these cell behaviors in vivo. Furthermore, traditional genetic screens in *C. elegans* and *Drosophila* have recently been complemented with systematic genome-scale RNAi-based screens for genes that regulate cellular or organismal phenotypes such as viability, proliferation, longevity, and fat storage (Ashrafi et al. 2003; Lee et al. 2003; Boutros et al. 2004; Hamilton et al. 2005). Yet, some cancer phenotypes (e.g., neoangiogenesis) cannot be studied in these model organisms, and the components and/or wiring of several mammalian oncogene/tumor suppressor pathways are not conserved in these organisms. Therefore, dissecting cancer cell phenotypes by means of forward genetic screens in mammalian cells is an important approach toward our understanding of cancer biology and therapeutic design.

Forward genetics has already been used with some success in mammalian cancer biology in the form of gain-of-function screens. For instance, the human Ras oncogene was cloned as a transforming activity by transfecting mouse fibroblasts with genomic DNA fragments from a human bladder cancer (Goldfarb et al. 1982; Shih and Weinberg 1982). More recently, retroviral cDNA libraries have been used to probe such phenotypes as cellular senescence and anoikis (Peeper et al. 2002; Shvarts et al. 2002; Douma et al. 2004). Although large collections of mammalian siRNA and shRNA libraries have only recently been described (Berns et al. 2004; Paddison et al. 2004; Silva et al. 2005), successful application of these reagents in loss-of-function screens has already begun to emerge. Cooke and colleagues provided the first example of such a success in their siRNA-based screen for modulators of TRAIL-induced apoptosis (Aza-Blanc et al. 2003). TRAIL is a member of the tumor necrosis factor (TNF) superfamily, and this ligand has gained attention because of its ability to induce apoptosis in a tumor-cell-specific fashion (Ashkenazi and Dixit 1999). Using an array-based platform of chemically synthesized siRNAs targeting 510 human genes (enriched for human kinases), Aza-Blanc et al. identified several known mediators of TRAIL-induced death, previously uncharacterized genes that affect TRAIL activity, as well as genes that synthetically interact with the TRAIL pathway (see below). More recently, siRNA collections have also been used to isolate genes required for cell proliferation and viability in vitro (Kittler et al. 2004; MacKeigan et al. 2005).

In addition to these array-format siRNA-based screens, retrovirus-encoded human shRNA libraries have been employed as pooled collections. Such libraries enable stable loss-of-function genetic selections, and use in a pooled format circumvents the prohibitive cost and labor involved in array-format genome-scale screens (for review, see Silva et al. 2004; Willingham et al. 2004). Bernards and colleagues used this strategy to identify new antagonists of the p53 pathway (Berns et al. 2004). Human fibroblasts were engineered with a temperature-sensitive allele of SV40 LT, enabling limitless replicative potential at the permissive temperature. Culturing these cells at the nonpermissive temperature elicits a p53-dependent arrest, allowing shRNAs that enabled proliferation under this selective pressure to be isolated. In addition to p53 itself, five candidate genes were identified. Reduced expression of each candidate prevented p53-dependent induction of the CDK-inhibitor p21^{CIP1} and proliferative arrest, suggesting that these genes antagonize p53 function on some level. Determining the role(s) of these modifiers of in vitro culture-based cellular mortality in other p53-dependent processes (including tumor suppression) will be an important avenue for future study.

Pooled shRNA libraries have also been employed in an in vitro screen for candidate tumor suppressors (Westbrook et al. 2005). Using a pre-transformed cell line engineered from primary human mammary epithelial cells (HMECs), we isolated shRNAs that elicited anchorage-independent proliferation, a common phenotype of cancer cells. In the context of this system, previously characterized regulators of cell proliferation and survival were identified, including two bona fide human tumor suppressors: PTEN and TGFBR2 (Vivanco and Sawyers 2002; Siegel and Massague 2003). REST/NRSF, a transcriptional repressor of neural genes (Chong et al. 1995; Schoenherr and Anderson 1995), was also isolated as a suppressor of epithelial cell transformation. The unanticipated role for REST as a human tumor suppressor was supported by both human genetic evidence and observations implicating REST as an antagonist of PI3K signaling, a pathway with well-established roles in cancer. Although it was not unexpected that modifiers of PI3K signaling may be isolated (hyperactivation of PI3K can transform HMECs in this genetic context), the implication that REST function may be perturbed in human cancer provides a potential mechanism for the aberrant expression of neural genes observed in many epithelial cancers.

Unanticipated insights into cancer biology like the one above underscore the potential of unbiased genetic screens in dissecting cancer-related processes. In vitro models of many of these processes, including survival, growth-factor dependency, anoikis, invasion, migration, and 3-dimensional organization, already exist in some forms and will surely be exploited as platforms for genetic screens and selections. Indeed, our ability to explore these phenomena should be limited only by our ability to faithfully recapitulate these phenotypes in vitro or to devise forward genetic approaches to investigate them in vivo. Performing in vivo screens offers substantial promise to investigating complex biological processes for which we have a poor understanding of the cellular attributes that culminate in the phenotype. For instance, metastasis is a multistep process requiring invasion, intravasation, survival in circulation, extravasation, and survival and proliferation at a distant site (Chambers et al. 2002). Genetic screens in the context of experimental and orthotopic models of metastasis would potentially identify modulators of metastasis without prior knowledge of the selective pressures faced by cancer cells. The Hynes, Massague, and Weinberg laboratories have already used in vivo selection of rare metastatic variants from human cancer cell lines in combination with transcriptional profiling to identify groups of genes whose altered expression correlates with metastatic activity (Clark et al. 2000; Kang et al. 2003; Yang et al. 2004; Minn et al. 2005). A subset of these genes has been found to contribute to the metastatic phenotype and is predictive of metastatic occurrence in patients (Minn et al. 2005). Applying RNAi-based libraries to such experimental designs may enable the identification of gene sets that play a role in metastasis without relying on altered gene expression of these modulators. Similar unbiased genetic screens could also be used to interrogate mechanisms of oncogene addiction and chemoresistance in already established mouse models.

DISCOVERING CANCER VULNERABILITIES: SYNTHETIC LETHAL SCREENS

Establishing the gene networks that regulate known oncogenes and tumor suppressors and elucidating additional networks that govern cancer cell phenotypes will provide new targets to explore for cancer therapeutics. As mentioned above, current targeted cancer therapies are predominantly based on the principles of oncogene addiction. These therapies take advantage of the fact that tumor cells have greater sensitivity to pharmacological inhibition of their dysregulated signaling pathways than their untransformed counterparts. Thus, these targeted therapies exhibit enhanced tumor-selective killing relative to conventional chemotherapeutics by taking advantage of this genetic dependency. The ideal therapeutic target is a protein that is only essential in tumor cells but not normal cells. This type of genetic interaction, where a mutation alone is compatible with viability, but in combination with another lesion leads to death, is referred to as synthetic lethality.

Screening for synthetic lethal gene interactions has been commonly used to dissect signaling pathways and phenotypes in model organisms (for review, see Guarente 1993). Identifying target genes that exhibit synthetic lethality with cancer-associated mutations promises to be fertile ground for cancer therapeutics. Such synthetic lethal interactions are particularly appealing for molecular lesions that are not "druggable" (e.g., loss-of-function mutations in tumor suppressors) or are essential to normal physiological processes. For instance, inhibitors of mTOR have been described to be selectively toxic to $PTEN^{-/-}$ tumors (as well as $PTEN^{-/-}$ isogenic MEFs) at concentrations that do not affect the viability of $PTEN^{+/+}$ cells, indicating that loss of mTOR activity is synthetically lethal with PTEN dysfunction (Neshat et al. 2001). Likewise, elevated expression of the MYC oncogene in human fibroblasts and cancer cells confers hypersensitivity to agonists of the death receptor DR5 (including the TRAIL ligand, discussed above) (Wang et al. 2004), providing an attractive therapeutic opportunity for the vast number of human cancers that exhibit MYC overexpression. These synthetic lethal interactions have been rationalized based on their connections in biochemical pathways. Recently, Ashworth and colleagues described an unexpected sensitivity of cells lacking the tumor suppressors $BRCA1^{-/-}$ or $BRCA2^{-/-}$ to inhibition of Poly(ADP-ribose) polymerase (PARP) (Farmer et al. 2005). This sensitivity was postulated to result from dysfunction in two complementary pathways of DNA repair: base excision repair (PARP) and double-strand-break repair by homologous recombination (BRCA1, BRCA2). Collectively, these synthetic lethal interactions emphasize the idea that the oncogenic lesions of cancer cells expose unique vulnerabilities and thus provide novel therapeutic opportunities.

These successes of exploiting synthetic lethality for specific tumor cell killing were discovered, at least in part, by hypothesis-driven experiments. However, this candidate gene approach is severely limited by our incomplete understanding of mammalian signaling networks as well as its inherent low-throughput nature. Instead, high-throughput chemical and genetic screening methods enable the unbiased identification of synthetic interactions with cancer genes. Proof-of-principle chemical screens for synthetic lethality have already emerged. Kinzler and colleagues identified compounds that exhibited selective toxicity toward a colon cancer cell line harboring an endogenous activating mutation of K-Ras but not toward an isogenic derivative in which the K-Ras mutant was deleted (Torrance et al. 2001). Using a similar approach, Fantin et al. (2002) isolated a compound that inhibits the proliferation of mouse and human breast cancer cells overexpressing HER2/neu. Stockwell and colleagues identified compounds that selectively kill engineered tumorigenic cells but not their isogenic counterparts (Dolma et al. 2003). In addition to a novel compound, this strategy uncovered several current anticancer therapies that exhibit genotypic specificity, suggesting that the efficacy of some current therapies may be improved when administered to patients respective of tumor genotypes.

Whereas these screens underscore the potential for identifying vulnerabilities specific to cancer cells, the utility of chemical-based screens is hampered by the often difficult endeavor of drug-target identification. In contrast, the application of RNAi to such loss-of-function synthetic lethality screens offers the potential to interrogate gene–gene interactions and rapidly identify candidate targets. Identifying synthetic lethal interactions in mammalian cells has already been demonstrated with an array-format siRNA library. In a screen for modifiers of TRAIL-induced killing (discussed above), Cooke and colleagues identified siRNAs that inhibited (ex. MYC) or enhanced (AKT1) TRAIL-mediated cell death (Aza-Blanc et al. 2003). Validating this screen, the synthetic lethal interaction between ectopic MYC expression and TRAIL signaling was discovered independently by Quon and coworkers (Wang et al. 2004).

As discussed above, applying genome-wide array-based siRNA screens in mammalian cells is not amenable to use in most individual laboratories. Alternatively, large collections of retrovirus-encoded shRNA libraries could be applied as pools in synthetic lethality screens. However, this strategy has two essential requirements: (1) the capability to track individual shRNA fitness in complex populations, and (2) an shRNA expression system that yields high-penetrance loss of function.

To monitor the relative abundance of shRNAs within a pooled population, we and other investigators have proposed the use of a DNA-bar-coding strategy that has been previously applied in *Escherichia coli* and subsequently in the *Saccharomyces cerevisiae* gene-knockout collections (Hensel et al. 1995; Shoemaker et al. 1996; Winzeler et al. 1999; Giaever et al. 2002). Adapted to shRNA libraries, this approach relies on a random 60-nucleotide DNA sequence that is unique to each individual shRNA expression vector (Paddison et al. 2004). A parallel approach relies on the shRNA-encoding gene itself as the bar code identifier (Berns et al. 2004). By PCR amplification of the integrated bar codes from cell populations, one can measure bar code abundance by hybridization to custom microarrays on which the complementary sequences have been printed (Fig. 1). As such, the fitness of cells expressing a given shRNA can be followed by measuring the relative abundance of the linked bar code sequences under control and experimental conditions. We have recently demonstrated the first successful application of this approach in mammalian cells

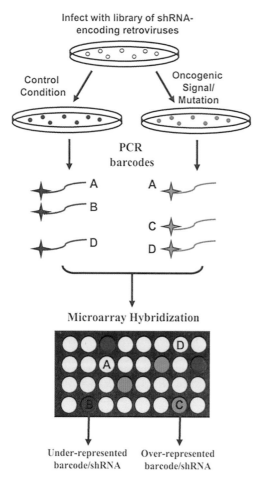

Infect with library of shRNA-
encoding retroviruses

Control
Condition

Oncogenic
Signal/
Mutation

PCR
barcodes

A
B

D

A

C

D

Microarray Hybridization

Under-represented
barcode/shRNA

Over-represented
barcode/shRNA

Figure 1. Schematic representation of pooled strategy for using molecular bar codes to track shRNAs in complex populations. Target cells are infected with a retroviral shRNA library, with each shRNA-expressing virus also encoding a unique 60-bp sequence, or molecular bar code. Infected cells are exposed to control or experimental conditions (e.g., oncogene or tumor suppressor lesion). Bar codes are PCR-amplified from the resulting populations and transcribed, incorporating fluorescent nucleotides. cRNA is used to hybridize to complementary bar codes printed on a custom microarray, thus quantitating the relative changes in any given bar code between the two populations. Individual bar codes are represented by A, B, C, and D, with B and C representing bar codes with lower and higher fitness, respectively, in the presence of the experimental condition.

(Westbrook et al. 2005). To identify candidate tumor suppressors (discussed above), we screened for shRNAs that elicited anchorage-independent proliferation in pre-transformed HMECs. Resultant anchorage-independent colonies were pooled and assessed for the enrichment of bar codes linked to the individual shRNAs. Sequencing of individual proviral shRNAs and bar codes confirmed the efficacy of the bar code microarrays in identifying the corresponding shRNA population, thus validating this approach in the context of enrichment screens. However, the use of the bar code approach to measure the loss of shRNAs from a complex population of cells is more challenging and has not yet been demonstrated.

Although several technical and biological factors may affect the use of pooled shRNA collections in synthetic

lethality screens, the most confounding issue regards the penetrance of shRNA-mediated silencing. The application of bar-coding strategies requires the shRNA-expressing retroviruses to be present as single integrants. However, expression of transgenes from retroviral constructs has been shown to be highly variable, depending on the genomic context of integration, suggesting that the efficacy of any given shRNA would also vary across a population of independent integrants. Indeed, although several systems for shRNA expression have been generated, these systems have typically relied on multiple integrations per cell to achieve knockdown of a gene of interest in pooled populations (Wiznerowicz and Trono 2003; Malphettes and Fussenegger 2004; Tiscornia et al. 2004; Ventura et al. 2004; Zhou et al. 2005), indicating that current shRNA expression systems are inadequate for bar-code-based synthetic lethal screens.

Recent studies suggest that this obstacle to synthetic lethality screens might be overcome with a new shRNA expression vector design. This lentiviral system incorporates two novel features that, together, confer high-penetrance knockdown of a given target gene from single-copy proviral shRNA transgenes (Dickins et al. 2005; Silva et al. 2005; Stegmeier et al. 2005). First, the shRNA sequence is embedded within the context of miR30 (Silva et al. 2005), a naturally occurring microRNA transcript whose biogenesis has been previously characterized (Cullen 2004). Cullen and colleagues have shown that artificial sequences inserted within this transcript can effectively reduce the levels of a synthetic target mRNA containing the appropriate complementary sequence (Zeng et al. 2002). We have exploited this observation by embedding libraries of shRNAs directed against human and mouse genes into a miR30 context (Fig. 2). In a direct comparison of vectors encoding simple shRNA transcripts with pSM2, transient transfection experiments indicate that the miR30 context significantly improves the expression of the mature siRNA sequence as well as consequent knockdown of target mRNAs (Silva et al. 2005). However, single-copy integration of the synthetic miR30-shRNA transgene is still not sufficient to elicit robust target mRNA knockdown when expressed from the pol III promoters (e.g., U6, H1) that are typically used to transcribe artificial shRNAs (Stegmeier et al. 2005). Fortuitously, we have discovered that the synthetic miR30-shRNA elicits significantly improved knockdown of a target gene when transcribed from the cytomegalovirus (CMV) promoter (Fig. 2). This is in agreement with recent reports that endogenous microRNAs are transcribed predominantly by pol II (Cai et al. 2004). Interestingly, target mRNA knockdown is substantially higher when sequences are inserted between the CMV promoter and the miR30-shRNA, suggesting that spacing parameters may contribute to the synthetic miRNA processing or function (Fig. 2) (Stegmeier et al. 2005). This observation enabled us to incorporate various genes encoding fluorescent proteins or antibiotic-resistance markers upstream of the miRNA-shRNA, thus allowing one to track or select populations of cells that express the miRNA-shRNA transcript. Most importantly, single-copy integration of this lentiviral vector system elicits highly pene-

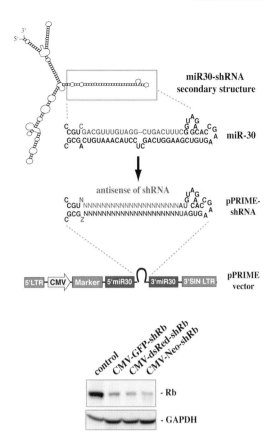

Figure 2. Pol II-driven miR30-embedded shRNAs effectively silence target gene expression at single copy. Schematic representation of an shRNA sequence incorporated into miR30 within the pPRIME vector (*P*otent *R*NA *I*nterference using *M*icroRNA *E*xpression). Secondary structure of the miR30-shRNA hybrid is shown as predicted by RNAFOLD (http://rna.tbi.univie.ac.at/cgi-bin/RNAfold.cgi). The pPRIME vector series incorporates genes encoding antibiotic-resistance markers or fluorescent proteins within the same transcript as the miR30-shRNA. In the bottom panel, the tumor suppressor Rb was targeted with an shRNA expressed from three different pPRIME derivatives. Cells were infected at an moi of <0.3, and transduced cells were isolated by Neomycin selection or fluorescence-activated cell sorting. Approximately 1 week post-infection, cell lysates were analyzed for Rb expression by western blot.

trant knockdown of the target gene, as measured in pooled populations and individual clones (Fig. 2) (Stegmeier et al. 2005). This innovation, coupled with the bar-coding strategy, will facilitate the use of shRNA libraries in genome-scale loss-of-function screens. In particular, these advances should foster the use of synthetic lethal approaches to study a variety of biological processes in addition to cancer biology.

FUTURE DIRECTIONS OR CONCLUSIONS

Since President Nixon declared war on cancer in 1971, we have made significant progress in deciphering the molecular lesions that contribute to tumor formation. However, the therapeutic options for treating most cancers is still a frustrating and often futile exercise. Traditional chemotherapeutics (such as DNA-damaging and anti-mitotic agents) are often plagued by tremendous side effects due to their inability to discriminantly kill cancer over normal proliferative tissues. However, the recent successes of targeted molecular therapy (such as Imatinib and Herceptin) present good examples of how our increased molecular understanding of aberrant cancer cell signaling can lead to more efficient therapies. Importantly, these targeted drugs illustrate that many genetic changes within cancer cells will create vulnerabilities that can be exploited for the development of more specific therapies. One promising way to reveal such vulnerabilities is to search for synthetic lethal interactions with the tumor-specific lesions. The synthetic lethal approach has not been exploited in the past because there were no robust methods for systematically identifying synthetic lethal genes. However, recent advances in chemical genetics and RNAi technology will undoubtedly facilitate the discovery of promising new drug targets and perhaps help us to finally win the war on cancer.

ACKNOWLEDGMENTS

We acknowledge members of the Elledge and Hannon laboratories and all those whose work was not cited due to constraints of space and scope.

REFERENCES

Ashkenazi A. and Dixit V.M. 1999. Apoptosis control by death and decoy receptors. *Curr. Opin. Cell Biol.* **11**: 255.

Ashrafi K., Chang F.Y., Watts J.L., Fraser A.G., Kamath R.S., Ahringer J., and Ruvkun G. 2003. Genome-wide RNAi analysis of *Caenorhabditis elegans* fat regulatory genes. *Nature* **421**: 268.

Aza-Blanc P., Cooper C.L., Wagner K., Batalov S., Deveraux Q.L., and Cooke M.P. 2003. Identification of modulators of TRAIL-induced apoptosis via RNAi-based phenotypic screening. *Mol. Cell* **12**: 627.

Baeg G.H., Zhou R., and Perrimon N. 2005. Genome-wide RNAi analysis of JAK/STAT signaling components in *Drosophila*. *Genes Dev.* **19**: 1861.

Berns K., Hijmans E.M., Mullenders J., Brummelkamp T.R., Velds A., Heimerikx M., Kerkhoven R.M., Madiredjo M., Nijkamp W., Weigelt B., Agami R., Ge W., Cavet G., Linsley P.S., Beijersbergen R.L., and Bernards R. 2004. A large-scale RNAi screen in human cells identifies new components of the p53 pathway. *Nature* **428**: 431.

Bernstein E., Caudy A.A., Hammond S.M., and Hannon G.J. 2001. Role for a bidentate ribonuclease in the initiation step of RNA interference. *Nature* **409**: 363.

Boutros M., Kiger A.A., Armknecht S., Kerr K., Hild M., Koch B., Haas S.A., Consortium H.F., Paro R., and Perrimon N. 2004. Genome-wide RNAi analysis of growth and viability in *Drosophila* cells. *Science* **303**: 832.

Brummelkamp T.R. and Bernards R. 2003. New tools for functional mammalian cancer genetics. *Nat. Rev. Cancer* **3**: 781.

Brummelkamp T.R., Bernards R., and Agami R. 2002. A system for stable expression of short interfering RNAs in mammalian cells. *Science* **296**: 550.

Brummelkamp T.R., Nijman S.M., Dirac A.M., and Bernards R. 2003. Loss of the cylindromatosis tumour suppressor inhibits apoptosis by activating NF-kappaB. *Nature* **424**: 797.

Cai X., Hagedorn C.H., and Cullen B.R. 2004. Human micro RNAs are processed from capped, polyadenylated transcripts that can also function as mRNAs. *RNA* **10**: 1957.

Chambers A.F., Groom A.C., and MacDonald I.C. 2002. Dissemination and growth of cancer cells in metastatic sites. *Nat. Rev. Cancer* **2**: 563.

Chong J.A., Tapia-Ramirez J., Kim S., Toledo-Aral J.J., Zheng

Y., Boutros M.C., Altshuller Y.M., Frohman M.A., Kraner S.D., and Mandel G. 1995. REST: A mammalian silencer protein that restricts sodium channel gene expression to neurons. *Cell* **80:** 949.

Clark E.A., Golub T.R., Lander E.S., and Hynes R.O. 2000. Genomic analysis of metastasis reveals an essential role for RhoC. *Nature* **406:** 532.

Cools J., DeAngelo D.J., Gotlib J., Stover E.H., Legare R.D., Cortes J., Kutok J., Clark J., Galinsky I., Griffin J.D., Cross N.C., Tefferi A., Malone J., Alam R., Schrier S.L., Schmid J., Rose M., Vandenberghe P., Verhoef G., Boogaerts M., Wlodarska I., Kantarjian H., Marynen P., Coutre S.E., Stone R., and Gilliland D.G. 2003. A tyrosine kinase created by fusion of the PDGFRA and FIP1L1 genes as a therapeutic target of imatinib in idiopathic hypereosinophilic syndrome. *N. Engl. J. Med.* **348:** 1201.

Cullen B.R. 2004. Transcription and processing of human microRNA precursors. *Mol. Cell* **16:** 861.

D'Andrea A. 2003. Fanconi anemia. *Curr. Biol.* **13:** R546.

DasGupta R., Kaykas A., Moon R.T., and Perrimon N. 2005. Functional genomic analysis of the Wnt-wingless signaling pathway. *Science* **308:** 826.

Demetri G.D., von Mehren M., Blanke C.D., Van den Abbeele A.D., Eisenberg B., Roberts P.J., Heinrich M.C., Tuveson D.A., Singer S., Janicek M., Fletcher J.A., Silverman S.G., Silberman S.L., Capdeville R., Kiese B., Peng B., Dimitrijevic S., Druker B.J., Corless C., Fletcher C.D., and Joensuu H. 2002. Efficacy and safety of imatinib mesylate in advanced gastrointestinal stromal tumors. *N. Engl. J. Med.* **347:** 472.

Dickins R.A., Hemann M.T., Zilfou J.T., Simpson D.R., Ibarra I., Hannon G.J., and Lowe S.W. 2005. Probing tumor phenotypes using stable and regulated synthetic microRNA precursors. *Nat. Genet.* **37:** 1289.

Dolma S., Lessnick S.L., Hahn W.C., and Stockwell B.R. 2003. Identification of genotype-selective antitumor agents using synthetic lethal chemical screening in engineered human tumor cells. *Cancer Cell* **3:** 285.

Douma S., Van Laar T., Zevenhoven J., Meuwissen R., Van Garderen E., and Peeper D.S. 2004. Suppression of anoikis and induction of metastasis by the neurotrophic receptor TrkB. *Nature* **430:** 1034.

Druker B.J. 2002. STI571 (Gleevec) as a paradigm for cancer therapy. *Trends Mol. Med.* **8:** S14.

Druker B.J., Tamura S., Buchdunger E., Ohno S., Segal G.M., Fanning S., Zimmermann J., and Lydon N.B. 1996. Effects of a selective inhibitor of the Abl tyrosine kinase on the growth of Bcr-Abl positive cells. *Nat. Med.* **2:** 561.

Druker B.J., Talpaz M., Resta D.J., Peng B., Buchdunger E., Ford J.M., Lydon N.B., Kantarjian H., Capdeville R., Ohno-Jones S., and Sawyers C.L. 2001. Efficacy and safety of a specific inhibitor of the BCR-ABL tyrosine kinase in chronic myeloid leukemia. *N. Engl. J. Med.* **344:** 1031.

Dykxhoorn D.M., Novina C.D., and Sharp P.A. 2003. Killing the messenger: Short RNAs that silence gene expression. *Nat. Rev. Mol. Cell Biol.* **4:** 457.

Elbashir S.M., Harborth J., Lendeckel W., Yalcin A., Weber K., and Tuschl T. 2001. Duplexes of 21-nucleotide RNAs mediate RNA interference in cultured mammalian cells. *Nature* **411:** 494.

Fantin V.R., Berardi M.J., Scorrano L., Korsmeyer S.J., and Leder P. 2002. A novel mitochondriotoxic small molecule that selectively inhibits tumor cell growth. *Cancer Cell* **2:** 29.

Farmer H., McCabe N., Lord C.J., Tutt A.N., Johnson D.A., Richardson T.B., Santarosa M., Dillon K.J., Hickson I., Knights C., Martin N.M., Jackson S.P., Smith G.C., and Ashworth A. 2005. Targeting the DNA repair defect in BRCA mutant cells as a therapeutic strategy. *Nature* **434:** 917.

Fire A., Xu S., Montgomery M.K., Kostas S.A., Driver S.E., and Mello C.C. 1998. Potent and specific genetic interference by double-stranded RNA in *Caenorhabditis elegans*. *Nature* **391:** 806.

Giaever G., Chu A.M., Ni L., Connelly C., Riles L., Veronneau S., Dow S., Lucau-Danila A., Anderson K., Andre B., Arkin A.P., Astromoff A., El-Bakkoury M., Bangham R., Benito R.,

Brachat S., Campanaro S., Curtiss M., Davis K., Deutschbauer A., Entian K.D., Flaherty P., Foury F., Garfinkel D.J., and Gerstein M., et al. 2002. Functional profiling of the *Saccharomyces cerevisiae* genome. *Nature* **418:** 387.

Goldfarb M., Shimizu K., Perucho M., and Wigler M. 1982. Isolation and preliminary characterization of a human transforming gene from T24 bladder carcinoma cells. *Nature* **296:** 404.

Gorre M.E., Mohammed M., Ellwood K., Hsu N., Paquette R., Rao P.N., and Sawyers C.L. 2001. Clinical resistance to STI-571 cancer therapy caused by BCR-ABL gene mutation or amplification. *Science* **293:** 876.

Grishok A., Pasquinelli A.E., Conte D., Li N., Parrish S., Ha I., Baillie D.L., Fire A., Ruvkun G., and Mello C.C. 2001. Genes and mechanisms related to RNA interference regulate expression of the small temporal RNAs that control *C. elegans* developmental timing. *Cell* **106:** 23.

Guarente L. 1993. Synthetic enhancement in gene interaction: A genetic tool come of age. *Trends Genet.* **9:** 362.

Hamilton B., Dong Y., Shindo M., Liu W., Odell I., Ruvkun G., and Lee S.S. 2005. A systematic RNAi screen for longevity genes in *C. elegans*. *Genes Dev.* **19:** 1544.

Hanahan D. and Weinberg R.A. 2000. The hallmarks of cancer. *Cell* **100:** 57.

Hannon G.J. 2002. RNA interference. *Nature* **418:** 244.

Hannon G.J. and Rossi J.J. 2004. Unlocking the potential of the human genome with RNA interference. *Nature* **431:** 371.

Hensel M., Shea J.E., Gleeson C., Jones M.D., Dalton E., and Holden D.W. 1995. Simultaneous identification of bacterial virulence genes by negative selection. *Science* **269:** 400.

Hutvagner G., McLachlan J., Pasquinelli A.E., Balint E., Tuschl T., and Zamore P.D. 2001. A cellular function for the RNA-interference enzyme Dicer in the maturation of the let-7 small temporal RNA. *Science* **293:** 834.

Jonkers J. and Berns A. 2002. Conditional mouse models of sporadic cancer. *Nat. Rev. Cancer* **2:** 251.

———. 2004. Oncogene addiction: Sometimes a temporary slavery. *Cancer Cell* **6:** 535.

Kang Y., Siegel P.M., Shu W., Drobnjak M., Kakonen S.M., Cordon-Cardo C., Guise T.A., and Massague J. 2003. A multigenic program mediating breast cancer metastasis to bone. *Cancer Cell* **3:** 537.

Ketting R.F., Fischer S.E., Bernstein E., Sijen T., Hannon G.J., and Plasterk R.H. 2001. Dicer functions in RNA interference and in synthesis of small RNA involved in developmental timing in *C. elegans*. *Genes Dev.* **15:** 2654.

Kittler R., Putz G., Pelletier L., Poser I., Heninger A.K., Drechsel D., Fischer S., Konstantinova I., Habermann B., Grabner H., Yaspo M.L., Himmelbauer H., Korn B., Neugebauer K., Pisabarro M.T., and Buchholz F. 2004. An endoribonuclease-prepared siRNA screen in human cells identifies genes essential for cell division. *Nature* **432:** 1036.

Lee S.S., Lee R.Y., Fraser A.G., Kamath R.S., Ahringer J., and Ruvkun G. 2003. A systematic RNAi screen identifies a critical role for mitochondria in *C. elegans* longevity. *Nat. Genet.* **33:** 40.

Lin S.Y. and Elledge S.J. 2003. Multiple tumor suppressor pathways negatively regulate telomerase. *Cell* **113:** 881.

Logan C.Y. and Nusse R. 2004. The Wnt signaling pathway in development and disease. *Annu. Rev. Cell Dev. Biol.* **20:** 781.

Lum L., Yao S., Mozer B., Rovescalli A., Von Kessler D., Nirenberg M., and Beachy P.A. 2003. Identification of Hedgehog pathway components by RNAi in *Drosophila* cultured cells. *Science* **299:** 2039.

Lynch T.J., Bell D.W., Sordella R., Gurubhagavatula S., Okimoto R.A., Brannigan B.W., Harris P.L., Haserlat S.M., Supko J.G., Haluska F.G., Louis D.N., Christiani D.C., Settleman J., and Haber D.A. 2004. Activating mutations in the epidermal growth factor receptor underlying responsiveness of non-small-cell lung cancer to gefitinib. *N. Engl. J. Med.* **350:** 2129.

MacKeigan J.P., Murphy L.O., and Blenis J. 2005. Sensitized RNAi screen of human kinases and phosphatases identifies new regulators of apoptosis and chemoresistance. *Nat. Cell Biol.* **7:** 591.

Malphettes L. and Fussenegger M. 2004. Macrolide- and tetra-cycline-adjustable siRNA-mediated gene silencing in mammalian cells using polymerase II-dependent promoter derivatives. *Biotechnol. Bioeng.* **88:** 417.

Manche L., Green S.R., Schmedt C., and Mathews M.B. 1992. Interactions between double-stranded RNA regulators and the protein kinase DAI. *Mol. Cell. Biol.* **12:** 5238.

Meetei A.R., de Winter J.P., Medhurst A.L., Wallisch M., Waisfisz Q., van de Vrugt H.J., Oostra A.B., Yan Z., Ling C., Bishop C.E., Hoatlin M.E., Joenje H., and Wang W. 2003. A novel ubiquitin ligase is deficient in Fanconi anemia. *Nat. Genet.* **35:** 165.

Meister G. and Tuschl T. 2004. Mechanisms of gene silencing by double-stranded RNA. *Nature* **431:** 343.

Minks M.A., West D.K., Benvin S., and Baglioni C. 1979. Structural requirements of double-stranded RNA for the activation of 2′,5′-oligo(A) polymerase and protein kinase of interferon-treated HeLa cells. *J. Biol. Chem.* **254:** 10180.

Minn A.J., Gupta G.P., Siegel P.M., Bos P.D., Shu W., Giri D.D., Viale A., Olshen A.B., Gerald W.L., and Massague J. 2005. Genes that mediate breast cancer metastasis to lung. *Nature* **436:** 518.

Neshat M.S., Mellinghoff I.K., Tran C., Stiles B., Thomas G., Petersen R., Frost P., Gibbons J.J., Wu H., and Sawyers C.L. 2001. Enhanced sensitivity of PTEN-deficient tumors to inhibition of FRAP/mTOR. *Proc. Natl. Acad. Sci.* **98:** 10314.

Nijman S.M., Huang T.T., Dirac A.M., Brummelkamp T.R., Kerkhoven R.M., D'Andrea A.D., and Bernards R. 2005. The deubiquitinating enzyme USP1 regulates the Fanconi anemia pathway. *Mol. Cell* **17:** 331.

Nybakken K. and Perrimon N. 2002. Hedgehog signal transduction: Recent findings. *Curr. Opin. Genet. Dev.* **12:** 503.

Paddison P.J. and Hannon G.J. 2002. RNA interference: The new somatic cell genetics? *Cancer Cell* **2:** 17.

Paddison P.J., Caudy A.A., Bernstein E., Hannon G.J., and Conklin DS. 2002. Short hairpin RNAs (shRNAs) induce sequence-specific silencing in mammalian cells. *Genes Dev.* **16:** 948.

Paddison P.J., Silva J.M., Conklin D.S., Schlabach M., Li M., Aruleba S., Balija V., O'Shaughnessy A., Gnoj L., Scobie K., Chang K., Westbrook T., Cleary M., Sachidanandam R., McCombie W.R., Elledge S.J., and Hannon G.J. 2004. A resource for large-scale RNA-interference-based screens in mammals. *Nature* **428:** 427.

Paez J.G., Janne P.A., Lee J.C., Tracy S., Greulich H., Gabriel S., Herman P., Kaye F.J., Lindeman N., Boggon T.J., Naoki K., Sasaki H., Fujii Y., Eck M.J., Sellers W.R., Johnson B.E., and Meyerson M. 2004. EGFR mutations in lung cancer: Correlation with clinical response to gefitinib therapy. *Science* **304:** 1497.

Peeper D.S., Shvarts A., Brummelkamp T., Douma S., Koh E.Y., Daley G.Q., and Bernards R. 2002. A functional screen identifies hDRIL1 as an oncogene that rescues RAS-induced senescence. *Nat. Cell Biol.* **4:** 148.

Schoenherr C.J. and Anderson D.J. 1995. The neuron-restrictive silencer factor (NRSF): A coordinate repressor of multiple neuron-specific genes. *Science* **267:** 1360.

Shih C. and Weinberg R.A. 1982. Isolation of a transforming sequence from a human bladder carcinoma cell line. *Cell* **29:** 161.

Shoemaker D.D., Lashkari D.A., Morris D., Mittmann M., and Davis R.W. 1996. Quantitative phenotypic analysis of yeast deletion mutants using a highly parallel molecular bar-coding strategy. *Nat. Genet.* **14:** 450.

Shvarts A., Brummelkamp T.R., Scheeren F., Koh E., Daley G.Q., Spits H., and Bernards R. 2002. A senescence rescue screen identifies BCL6 as an inhibitor of anti-proliferative p19(ARF)-p53 signaling. *Genes Dev.* **16:** 681.

Sieburth D., Ch'ng Q., Dybbs M., Tavazoie M., Kennedy S., Wang D., Dupuy D., Rual J.F., Hill D.E., Vidal M., Ruvkun G., and Kaplan J.M. 2005. Systematic analysis of genes required for synapse structure and function. *Nature* **436:** 510.

Siegel P.M. and Massague J. 2003. Cytostatic and apoptotic actions of TGF-beta in homeostasis and cancer. *Nat. Rev. Cancer* **3:** 807.

Silva J., Chang K., Hannon G.J., and Rivas F.V. 2004. RNA-interference-based functional genomics in mammalian cells: Reverse genetics coming of age. *Oncogene* **23:** 8401.

Silva J.M., Li M.Z., Chang K., Ge W., Golding M.C., Rickles R.J., Siolas D., Hu G., Paddison P.J., Schlabach M.R., Sheth N., Bradshaw J., Burchard J., Kulkarni A., Cavet G., Sachidanandam R., McCombie W.R., Cleary M.A., Elledge S.J., and Hannon G.J. 2005. Second-generation shRNA libraries covering the mouse and human genomes. *Nat. Genet.* **37:** 1281.

Slamon D.J., Godolphin W., Jones L.A., Holt J.A., Wong S.G., Keith D.E., Levin W.J., Stuart S.G., Udove J., and Ullrich A., et al. 1989. Studies of the HER-2/neu proto-oncogene in human breast and ovarian cancer. *Science* **244:** 707.

Sordella R., Bell D.W., Haber D.A., and Settleman J. 2004. Gefitinib-sensitizing EGFR mutations in lung cancer activate anti-apoptotic pathways. *Science* **305:** 1163.

Stark G.R., Kerr I.M., Williams B.R., Silverman R.H., and Schreiber R.D. 1998. How cells respond to interferons. *Annu. Rev. Biochem.* **67:** 227.

Stegmeier F., Hu G., Rickles R.J., Hannon G.J., and Elledge S.J. 2005. A lentiviral microRNA-based system for single-copy polymerase II-regulated RNA interference in mammalian cells. *Proc. Natl. Acad. Sci.* **102:** 13212.

Sui G., Soohoo C., Affar el B., Gay F., Shi Y., and Forrester W.C. 2002. A DNA vector-based RNAi technology to suppress gene expression in mammalian cells. *Proc. Natl. Acad. Sci.* **99:** 5515.

Tiscornia G., Tergaonkar V., Galimi F., and Verma I.M. 2004. CRE recombinase-inducible RNA interference mediated by lentiviral vectors. *Proc. Natl. Acad. Sci.* **101:** 7347.

Torrance C.J., Agrawal V., Vogelstein B., and Kinzler K.W. 2001. Use of isogenic human cancer cells for high-throughput screening and drug discovery. *Nat. Biotechnol.* **19:** 940.

Tuveson D.A., Willis N.A., Jacks T., Griffin J.D., Singer S., Fletcher C.D., Fletcher J.A., and Demetri G.D. 2001. STI571 inactivation of the gastrointestinal stromal tumor c-KIT oncoprotein: Biological and clinical implications. *Oncogene* **20:** 5054.

Ventura A., Meissner A., Dillon C.P., McManus M., Sharp P.A., Van Parijs L., Jaenisch R., and Jacks T. 2004. Cre-lox-regulated conditional RNA interference from transgenes. *Proc. Natl. Acad. Sci.* **101:** 10380.

Vivanco I. and Sawyers C.L. 2002. The phosphatidylinositol 3-kinase AKT pathway in human cancer. *Nat. Rev. Cancer* **2:** 489.

Wang Y., Engels I.H., Knee D.A., Nasoff M., Deveraux Q.L., and Quon K.C. 2004. Synthetic lethal targeting of MYC by activation of the DR5 death receptor pathway. *Cancer Cell* **5:** 501.

Weinstein I.B. 2002. Cancer. Addiction to oncogenes: The Achilles heal of cancer. *Science* **297:** 63.

Westbrook T.F., Martin E.S., Schlabach M.R., Leng Y., Liang A.C., Feng B., Zhao J.J., Roberts T.M., Mandel G., Hannon G.J., Depinho R.A., Chin L., and Elledge S.J. 2005. A genetic screen for candidate tumor suppressors identifies REST. *Cell* **121:** 837.

Willingham A.T., Deveraux Q.L., Hampton G.M., and Aza-Blanc P. 2004. RNAi and HTS: Exploring cancer by systematic loss-of-function. *Oncogene* **23:** 8392.

Winzeler E.A., Shoemaker D.D., Astromoff A., Liang H., Anderson K., Andre B., Bangham R., Benito R., Boeke J.D., Bussey H., Chu A.M., Connelly C., Davis K., Dietrich F., Dow S.W., El Bakkoury M., Foury F., Friend S.H., Gentalen E., Giaever G., Hegemann J.H., Jones T., Laub M., Liao H., and R.W. Davis, et al. 1999. Functional characterization of the *S. cerevisiae* genome by gene deletion and parallel analysis. *Science* **285:** 901.

Wiznerowicz M. and Trono D. 2003. Conditional suppression of cellular genes: Lentivirus vector-mediated drug-inducible RNA interference. *J. Virol.* **77:** 8957.

Yang J., Mani S.A., Donaher J.L., Ramaswamy S., Itzykson R.A., Come C., Savagner P., Gitelman I., Richardson A., and Weinberg RA. 2004. Twist, a master regulator of morphogenesis, plays an essential role in tumor metastasis. *Cell* **117:** 927.

Yu J.Y., DeRuiter S.L., and Turner D.L. 2002. RNA interference by expression of short-interfering RNAs and hairpin RNAs in mammalian cells. *Proc. Natl. Acad. Sci.* **99:** 6047.

Zeng Y., Wagner E.J., and Cullen B.R. 2002. Both natural and designed micro RNAs can inhibit the expression of cognate mRNAs when expressed in human cells. *Mol. Cell* **9:** 1327.

Zheng L., Liu J., Batalov S., Zhou D., Orth A., Ding S., and Schultz P.G. 2004. An approach to genomewide screens of expressed small interfering RNAs in mammalian cells. *Proc. Natl. Acad. Sci.* **101:** 135.

Zhou H., Xia X.G., and Xu Z. 2005. An RNA polymerase II construct synthesizes short-hairpin RNA with a quantitative indicator and mediates highly efficient RNAi. *Nucleic Acids Res.* **33:** e62.

Emerging Approaches in Molecular Profiling Affecting Oncology Drug Discovery

S.H. FRIEND

Merck Research Laboratories, West Point, Pennsylvania 19486; Rosetta Inpharmatics, LLC, a wholly owned subsidiary of Merck & Co., Inc., Seattle, Washington 98109

The purpose of this paper is to provide some perspectives on whether we are at a tipping point in understanding oncology and oncology drug discovery. It describes how model organisms have prepared us for more efficient drug discovery, lessons that are in use today. It provides examples of the emerging integration of biomarkers in patient care. It also details how over the next several years the processes of carrying out target identification and identifying responders to drugs will become more and more similar. In conclusion, a discussion is provided about who can do what to link the various components of this information-rich drug discovery process together.

If we turn the clock back to 1995, we find already increased numbers of specific molecular targets. Several lines of evidence were able to show specific mechanisms of actions surrounding specific targeted therapies, and there was an emerging understanding of the specific risks that came from genetic alterations. Despite this, there was minimal knowledge on why any of the existing therapies in cancer were working in specific patients. In 1995 I was fortunate to have an in-depth discussion with Harold Varmus, who was eloquent in pointing out the difference between probing the pathophysiology of disease and trying to change therapeutic options for patients. The outcome of this discussion was a remarkable year in which I took a sabbatical going in and out of pharmaceutical companies with the express purpose of better understanding the diversity and how large pharma and biotech companies carried out drug discovery. Four main lessons came out of this year. First, it was clear that the methods used in a general sense to identify the right targets were primarily narrowly chosen. Such efforts were mainly guided by interest in specific genes that had been in vogue. Second, the efforts needed to move early compounds through to drugs required primarily brute force to optimize the on-target effects of these compounds. This required the significant use of resources, not only time, but also cost. Third, the ability in oncology to identify the right subpopulations for the right drugs is done primarily empirically. As is well known in the drug discovery world, it is not uncommon for more than ten clinical trials to be performed in oncology before a respectable signal of response can be found. The last lesson was that the critical design for combination therapies that are the basis of much of the therapy given to patients currently is one of "trial and error." Coming out of this sabbatical year, it was easy to commit to more efficient drug discovery. At this time, I was fortunate to link up with Lee Hartwell, who was a key proponent for the use of genetics to more rationally design drugs. Thus began a period of collaboration of work based initially in yeast to develop models

to increase the probability of success in developing drugs. The outcome of this work involves the nonbiased detection of targets and the nonbiased identification of individuals who might be likely to respond.

Working with Lee Hartwell, it became evident that in the long run the most valuable tool to help guide drug discovery might be an "ideal detector" that allowed one to simultaneously monitor the function of all proteins within a given cell. To develop such a detector, one would need tens of thousands of independent reporters to detect changes within the cell. Second, it would be important to build a large database of known patterns. And third, one would need to be able to compare unknown patterns to large compendia of known patterns. The most obvious technology available at the time to carry this out was provided by the gene expression arrays that were beginning to be commonly used in the mid-1990s. The early experiments that we carried out to understand the limits of this method involved developing probes that could detect the levels of each of the genes in the yeast, *Saccharomyces cerevisiae*. It also required building a compendium of knockout strains of yeast that were knocked out either as single copies of mutants, or mutants where both alleles of any given gene were knocked out. By linking a large international consortium of yeast laboratories, it was possible to build this compendium of mutants and then to profile hundreds of mutants to compile compound and mutant yeast profiles. As shown in Figure 1, drugs such as lovastatin clustered with gene disruptions such as hmg1/2 and drug signatures of the compound tunicamycin were closely linked to the signature for the disruption of the gas1 gene. This work, carried out by Tim Hughes and others at Rosetta Inpharmatics, showed that many of the boundary conditions inside a simple organism were sufficient to "decode" the mechanism of action related to drugs by comparing it to known genetic alterations (Hughes et al. 2000).

A more difficult test of the compendium approach was to determine whether it was possible to use expression pro-

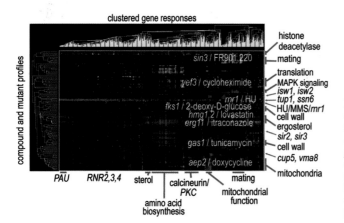

Figure 1. Two-dimensional agglomerative hierarchical clustering of 127 experiments and 568 genes, selected to include only experiments with 2 or more genes up- or down-regulated greater than threefold, and significant at $p \leq 0.01$; and only genes that are up- or down-regulated at greater than threefold, and at $p \leq 0.01$, in 2 or more experiments. (*PAU*) *PAU* gene family; (*S/C*) stress and carbohydrate metabolism; (*AA*) amino acid biosynthesis; (*PKC*) responsive to protein kinase C. (Reprinted, with permission, from Hughes et al. 2000 [© Elsevier].)

files in various mutant cells to build signaling pathways. An article published by Chris Roberts and coworkers in 2000 showed that combining genetics and expression profiling allowed one to reveal MAPK pathway cross talk. These early experiments gave strong evidence that under some conditions, the diversity of information captured from yeast was able to inform the mechanism of action of compounds (Roberts et al. 2000).

At the same time, it was possible to answer other questions related to the context specificity of cancer drugs by doing other experiments in yeast. In particular, we were interested in determining whether it was possible to delineate the mechanisms of action of compounds by looking at the effects that compounds had in strains of yeast particular genetic mutations. Work published by Phillip Szankasi, Chris Roberts, Andrew Murray, and others in 1997 showed the ability to determine the mechanism of different commonly used chemotherapeutic agents by this strategy. Two examples are worth noting. Treating strains of yeast with a large range of mutations in various pathways showed a high sensitivity to cisplatin in yeast that had defects in the genes rad6 and rad18 that controlled the pathway for repairing the damage to cisplatin. Similarly, experiments looking at the sensitivity of various mutant strains to mitoxantrone showed a high degree of sensitivity when yeast had defects in rad50, rad51, and rad52 that made up the double-strand-break repair pathway (Hartwell and Weinert 1989).

The other question answered in yeast was whether one could carry out nonbiased genome-wide screens to identify druggable targets that could selectively kill cells harboring defects found in human tumors. During the years 1996–1998, a large group of scientists including Eric Foss, Chris Roberts, Julian Simon, John Lamb, Jenya Kroll, and Brian Thornton at the Seattle Project based at the Fred Hutchinson Cancer Research Center began to carry out synthetic lethal screens. One of these started with a defect in mismatched repair by knocking out the mlh1 gene. This screen revealed that alterations in polymerase δ, polymerase ε, and rnr1 were all synthetic lethal with defects in mlh1. A second screen was designed around defects in the

ATM pathway used as the primary mutation disruption of the mec1 gene. In the mec1 synthetic lethal screen, it was possible to show synthetic lethal alleles that ranged from rnr1, rnr2, and rnr4 through cdc8, cdc17, and cdc21. This screen also identified PRI1 (DNA primates subunit) and rad27, which is a 5′ flap endonuclease.

All of the above experiments involved with profiling known and unknown patterns, searching for mechanisms of action using known drugs and specific mutations, and finally, the synthetic lethal screens, were carried out in yeast because the organism was genetically valuable and its complete sequence was known. These experiments helped determine the boundary conditions for the mammalian experiments we carry out today, but they only gave distant clues as to the specific realities of such pathways in human systems. The transition from work in yeast model systems to experiments in man represented one of the major missions of Rosetta Inpharmatics. The rest of the experiments to be described here involve more recent efforts to carry out similar experiments in mammalian cells.

Some of the early experiments that identified differences in the behavior of human tumors came from a large collaboration set up with Rene Bernards and Laura Van't Veer at the Netherlands Cancer Institute. Working with samples that had been carefully collected over many years and their accompanying medical records, it was possible to delineate patients with breast cancer who had progressed to distant metastasis rapidly as opposed to another set of patients who had had prolonged survival without distant metastasis. In 2002, we published gene signatures that allowed us to distinguish these different sets of patients using full genome expression profiling (Van't Veer et al. 2002). This work and similar experiments by many other investigators have enabled scientists to routinely search for expression profiles that can be linked to the natural history of various cancers and, more importantly, to identify the response to particular drugs. The early concept of building a compendium of known patterns to identify the biology of unknown samples has become commonplace in many oncology treatment protocols. Some of the more exciting recent work has involved a closer linkage between specific clinical parameters and molecular signatures. One example that we recently published involved identifying a set of patients who had high levels of estrogen receptors in their breast cancers but who had an extremely poor outcome that could be predicted by monitoring expression profiling (Dai et al. 2005). It is likely that this combination of clinical and molecular profiling clues will be commonly integrated so that the right patient is able to get the right drug at the right time.

The counterpart to the original unbiased full-genome screens that were carried out in yeast have also been carried out in mammalian systems. Working with a number of investigators at Cold Spring Harbor Laboratory, at the Salk Institute, and at biotech companies such as Alnylam, we have developed siRNA oligos and shRNA vectors to disrupt the expression of specific genes in mouse and human cells. The siRNA libraries that we have been using involve developing pools of siRNAs that in each well have three different siRNAs for a particular gene. We have developed such siRNA pools for 22,116 human genes, and we also have developed siRNAs that inhibit over 200 micro RNAs. Within the Automated Biotechnology Center in North Wales, Pennsylvania at Merck Research Laboratories and at Rosetta Inpharmatics in Seattle, Washington, we have developed automated robotics capabilities that allow us to carry out primary synthetic lethal screens over a period of weeks. These fully automated siRNA synthetic lethal screens involve plating cells on day 1, transfecting siRNAs on day 2, treating the cells with drugs and adding sensitizers the next day, and following the growth of various cells. We have found that it is necessary to have highly consistent transfection efficiencies. We have found it important to have a consistent sensitization of reference genes in the presence of sensitizer agents. We also have found it important to test for siRNA library integrity again using internal controls. As shown in Figure 2, it is possible to carry out a gemcitabine siRNA high-throughput screen in HeLa cells according to the methods just mentioned. It was helpful to identify primary hits at both low and high concentrations of gemcitabine and also to look for the overlap of genes that sensitize both low and high concentrations of gemcitabine. These selective primary hits were then retested, and a subset of confirmed primary hits was obtained. Thirty-two genes were found to confirm as primary hits at low concentrations of gemcitabine; 180 genes were confirmed to hit at high concentrations of gemcitabine. More importantly, 127 genes were confirmed to produce synthetic lethality with gemcitabine at both low and high concentrations. Preliminary analysis of the confirmed hits from the HeLa cell gemcitabine screen indicated enrichment of genes in a number of different pathways. We have found genes that are involved with microtubule spindle and centrosome assembly. Preliminary analysis also suggests genes involved with proteosome stability and RNA metabolism.

By carrying out synthetic lethal screens with both compounds and RNAs, we have identified situations where both siRNAs and small molecular combinations will sensitize cells that are either wild-type or defective for the

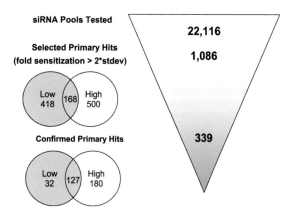

Figure 2. Summary of the HeLa/gemcitabine siRNA high-throughput screen results. Selected hits are highlighted where there is a sensitization greater than two standard deviations.

p53 gene. For the primary screens involving the compounds, we began with approximately 1.5 million compounds, and by filtering those for confirmed hits and for hits that exhibited greater than 1.5-fold sensitivity for p53 cells, we still retained over 1000 compounds. By selecting for compounds that exhibited the greatest dose-dependent effect, this set of genes was able to be down-selected to 11 compounds. Possibly the most interesting conclusion from these experiments has come from taking these sensitizing compounds and testing them in panels of cell lines from diverse tissues, all of which have been rendered as matched pairs, either having wild-type or disrupted p53 using shRNA vectors to disrupt the p53 status. Such studies have shown that compounds which may provide sensitization in one cell type that is defective for p53 will sometimes be able to provide an increased sensitivity across other cell lines of diverse tissues; whereas other compounds seem to have more limited sensitization that is restricted to particular cell lines. We consider this an important result because it more closely approximates the diversity that is likely to be found in actual patients. In summary, we think that the combination of unbiased syn-

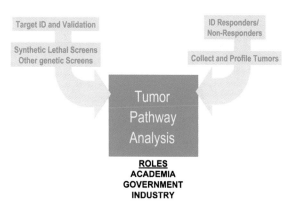

Figure 3. Tumor pathway analysis: Benefit of combining the efforts to identify and validate targets with the information used to identify responders.

thetic lethal screens to define targets, and unbiased synthetic lethal screens to define compounds, will be valuable, not only for identifying new targets for cancer therapies, but also in better identifying which patients these compounds are most likely to work in.

Over the next 5–10 years, significant work is needed to take these preliminary unbiased screens for new targets and powerful methods for identifying responders in order to affect drug discovery. The good news is that many of these methods are now ready to be used in the broader clinical environment. At the same time, significant issues still need to be worked out related to the roles academia, government, and industry can take in order to most efficiently integrate these new technologies into active patient care. Until recently, the early work in drug discovery involved with identifying targets and validating those targets has been seen as quite separate from the work that is being done by clinicians to collect and profile tumors. As shown in Figure 3, many of the methods that have been used for target ID and validation using profiling and synthetic lethal screens are likely in the future to be used to identify responders and nonresponders. The reason for this is that at the heart of the identification of new targets, and of patients who respond to drugs, is the need for a better understanding of tumor pathway analysis. The major limitation in achieving both these goals is likely to be the tools that are needed to interrogate the information generated by these diverse biological methods.

ACKNOWLEDGMENTS

We thank Drs. Peter Linsley, Steven Bartz, Aimee Jackson, Michele Cleary, Priya Kunapuli, Namjin Chung, Marc Ferrer, and Berta Strulovici.

REFERENCES

Dai H., van't Veer L., Lamb J., He Y.D., Mao M., Fine B.M., Bernards R., van de Vijver M., Deutsch P., Sachs A., Stoughton R., and Friend S.H. 2005. A cell proliferation signature is a marker of extremely poor outcome in a subpopulation of breast cancer patients. *Cancer Res.* **65:** 4059.

Hartwell L.H. and Weinert T.A. 1989. Checkpoints: Controls that ensure the order of cell cycle events. *Science* **246:** 629.

Hughes T.R., Marton M.J., Jones A.R., Roberts C.J., Stoughton R., Armour C.D., Bennett H.A., Coffey H., Dai H., He Y.D., Kidd M.J., King A.M., Meyer M.R., Slade D., Lum P.Y., Stepaniants S.B., Shoemaker D.D., Gachotte D., Chakraburtty K., Simon J., Bard M., and Friend S.H. 2000. Functional discovery via a compendium of expression profiles. *Cell* **102:** 109.

Roberts C.J., Nelson B., Marton M.J., Stoughton R., Meyer M.R., Bennett H.A., He Y., Dai H., Walker W., Hughes T., Tyers M., Boone C., and Friend S.H. 2000. Signaling and circuitry of multiple MAPK pathways revealed by a matrix of global gene expression profiles. *Science* **287:** 873.

Van't Veer L.J., Dai H., Van de Vijver M.J., He Y.D., Hart A.A.M., Mao M., Peterse H.L., Van der Kooy K., Marton M.J., Witteveen A.T., Schreiber G.J., Kerkhoven R.M., Roberts C.J., Linsley P.S., Bernards R., and Friend S.H. 2002. Gene expression profiling predicts clinical outcome of breast cancer. *Nature* **415:** 530.

Screens Using RNAi and cDNA Expression as Surrogates for Genetics in Mammalian Tissue Culture Cells

J. Pearlberg, S. Degot, W. Endege, J. Park, J. Davies, E. Gelfand, J. Sawyer,
A. Conery, J. Doench, W. Li, L. Gonzalez, F.M. Boyce, L. Brizuela,
J. LaBaer, D. Grueneberg, and E. Harlow
*Department of Biological Chemistry and Molecular Pharmacology, Harvard Medical School,
Boston, Massachusetts 02115*

We have developed methods for the automation of transfection-grade DNA preparation, high-throughput retroviral preparation, and highly parallel phenotypic screens to establish approaches that will allow investigators to examine in an unbiased manner the roles of proteins in mammalian cells. These methods have been used to raise or lower the levels of individual kinases in individual micro-well cultures either by cDNA or short hairpin RNA expression and will allow investigators to treat mammalian cells in culture in manners that are analogous to genetic screens in yeast. Our proof-of-principle experiments have been performed in human cells using repositories that represent over 75% of the protein, nucleotide, carbohydrate, lipid, and amino acid kinases in the human genome. These initial experiments have demonstrated the feasibility of two general types of screens. We have performed phenotypic screens to identify proteins with specific roles in a chosen function and genetic interaction screens to establish epistatic relations between different proteins. The results suggest that any phenotype that can be scored by a robust assay in tissue culture is amenable to these types of screens and that interactions between mammalian proteins can be established. These results point to the near-term goal of establishing comprehensive, unbiased screens that will allow queries on the roles of all human proteins.

Genetic screens in model organisms have proven to be one of the most important discovery platforms of the last century. Forward genetics using unbiased mutagenesis screens has identified key components of physiological events in a wide array of biological systems (see, e.g., Hartwell et al. 1970, 1974; Hafen et al. 1987; Simon et al. 1991; Nurse et al. 1998; Moon et al. 2004). In many cases, the genes identified in one model organism have led to the identification of related processes in other species not amenable to mutagenesis screens. This has been particularly true in mammalian cells where genetic approaches have been unavailable or difficult. For example, genetic studies in model organisms have proven to be an especially powerful way to find and decipher the function of oncogenes and tumor suppressor genes important in cancer development (Jacks et al. 1994; Forsburg 2001; Xie and Abbruzzese 2003).

Here we describe our approach to genetic screens in mammalian tissue culture cells. Our efforts are animated by the emergence of RNAi technology as well as novel expression vectors, which make it possible to raise or lower the level of a specific protein within essentially any cell that can grow in culture and to study phenotypic changes (Brizuela et al. 2002; Brummelkamp et al. 2002; Hannon 2002; Carpenter and Sabatini 2004; Hannon and Rossi 2004; Paddison et al. 2004; Pearlberg and LaBaer 2004; Rual et al. 2004; Park et al. 2005; Moffat and Sabatini 2006). These tools, when combined with robotic and bioinformatic support platforms, enable these experiments to be performed in a highly parallel high-throughput format. Although changing the levels of a targeted protein is not equivalent to mutagenizing a host cell, expression screens offer a number of advantages in study-

ing biological functions. First, the gene under study is known from the onset of the experiment, so no further work is needed to identify and to clone the gene in which a mutation has occurred. Second, the availability of expression RNAi or cDNA vectors facilitates the examination of similar phenotypic changes in a broad range of cells. Third, having the expression sequences in hand provides the tools for immediate biochemical studies, the setting in which most protein function is revealed. Although RNAi and cDNA expression studies do not replace genetic screens, they represent an important avenue for functional studies in mammalian cells.

The ultimate objective for construction of large repositories of sequence-verified cDNAs for open reading frames (ORFs) and RNAi expression vectors will be to cover the entire human proteome. Screens using these large repositories promise to approach the goal of a comprehensive interrogation of the biochemical activities that underlie all cell processes. In the work described here, we have focused on a smaller subset of the proteome, the human kinases. The kinase protein family was chosen for several reasons. First, the kinases are known to play important roles in many or most of the cell decision processes (Hunter 2000). Second, they are frequently mutated in human cancer (Davies et al. 2002; Bardelli et al. 2003; Lynch et al. 2004; Paez et al. 2004). Third, kinases are a common target for drug development, and it is clear that specific small-molecule inhibitors of key kinases can revert characteristics of the tumor cell (Carter et al. 1992; Cobleigh et al. 1999; Druker et al. 2001; Cunningham et al. 2004; see Workman, this volume). Fourth, many laboratories, including our own, have extensive experience in the study of kinase activities and so will be able to follow up leads from many screens in an expeditious manner. Finally, although kinase activities have been studied heavily, our knowledge of them is still incomplete. For the work described here, we have been studying protein, nucleotide, carbohydrate, lipid, and amino acid kinases.

In the proof-of-principle studies discussed below, we have learned how to make and use RNAi and cDNA vectors for parallel screens of human cells. This work includes everything from the establishment of robotic procedures for DNA preparation to high-throughput retrovirus production to robust assay development. We show that biological phenotypes of many types can be screened for changes and that shRNA and cDNA expression can be used in combination to look for genetic interactions and to establish epistatic relationships. Importantly, we also have devoted considerable effort to establish methods that allow screens to be performed in a cost-effective manner which will allow these types of assays to be done by many laboratories. Our findings argue that high-throughput functional screens will be an important tool for studying biological activities and promise that comprehensive screens of the entire proteome can be achieved in the near future.

MATERIALS AND METHODS

Construction of retroviral vectors. pJP1520 was constructed in two steps: The gene encoding the puromycin-*N*-acetyl transferase (PAC) gene was amplified in a PCR and cloned downstream of the 5′ long terminal repeat (LTR) as an NcoI and NotI fragment, creating pJP1519. Next, a fragment was amplified from pLPLNCX (BD Clontech) that comprised the cytomegalovirus (CMV) promoter as well as the loxP recombinational cloning cassette and was then imported into pJP1519 as a NotI and SalI fragment, creating pJP1520. pJP1563, 1564, and 1565 were constructed by removing the PAC gene and replacing it with the blasticidin deaminase (BSDR), hygromycin phosphotransferase (hph), or neomycin phosphotransferase (Neo) genes, respectively. The construction of the epitope-tagged retroviral vectors was performed with a series of PCRs such that overlapping fragments generated fusions of the appropriate epitope tag (either amino- or carboxy-terminal) in the appropriate reading frame.

Recombinational cloning. Purification of Cre recombinase: The coding sequence of Cre recombinase was cloned into the PET28b expression vector (Novagen) so that it contained an amino-terminal 6xHis tag. Next, BL21DE3pLysS cells were transformed with this construct and bacterial lysates were prepared from 1 liter of culture. The mixture was then passed over a Ni^{++} affinity column (Qiagen), the column was washed, and Cre was eluted with imidazole. The eluate was then dialyzed overnight with two changes of medium. From this, approximately 30 ml of active enzyme was generated. All Cre reactions were performed with 200 ng of donor and acceptor vectors, and 1 μl of enzyme. After 30 minutes at 37°C, the reactions were stopped by incubating at 70°C for 10 minutes. 5 μl was then used to transform *Escherichia coli*. Competent cells were prepared according to the

method of Inoue et al. (1990). After transformation, cells were plated on LB agar plates containing 100 μg/ml ampicillin, 34 μg/ml chloramphenicol, and 7% sucrose. Colonies were picked the following day and grown in Terrific Broth (TB) containing the same selection cocktail. Plasmid DNA was prepared, and an XbaI diagnostic digestion was performed.

Preparation of plasmid DNA. 1.2 ml of TB with antibiotics was inoculated in 96-well culture blocks and grown overnight in a Multitron shaker. The cells were pelleted, and a standard alkaline lysis was performed. This lysate, in a volume of 850 μl, was cleared by passage via centrifugation through a 96-well 25-μ pore size filter plate (Whatman). The filtrate was then loaded onto the anion exchange (AIEX) resin plate. The AIEX plates are prepared in advance by pouring (either as slurry or powder) resin into a 25-μ filter plate. The mixture is spun at low speed for 3 minutes. The resin is then washed, and a high-salt elution step is performed. The DNA is then precipitated by the addition of an equal volume of isopropanol and the DNA is pelleted by centrifugation, washed with 70% ethanol, and dried. The pellet is resuspended in 100 μl of TE (10 mM Tris, pH 8; 1 mM EDTA), and DNA is quantitated using the Hoechest Dye H33258. The DNA concentration was normalized to 5 μg/μl and stored at –20°C.

Generation of virus. Generation of Moloney murine leukemia virus (MMLV): 293T cells were seeded at a density of 65,000 cells per well in a volume of 100 μl in 96-well plates. The following day, cells in each well were transfected with100 ng of MMLV retroviral vector, 75 ng of a gag-pol expression construct, and 50 ng of a vesicular stomatitis virus G (VSVG) expression construct using Fugene 6 transfection reagent according to the manufacturer's suggestions (Roche). The plates were immediately centrifuged for 30 minutes at 2000 rpm and then placed in a 37°C tissue culture incubator. The following morning, medium was removed and 200 μl of fresh medium was added. The plates were then placed in a 32°C tissue culture incubator, and medium was harvested, stored at 4°C, and replenished daily for 1 week. At the end of the collection period, the viral supernatants for each daily collection were aliquoted in 100-μl volumes and stored in 96-well plates at –20°C.

Generation of lentivirus: 293T cells were seeded in 96-well plates at a density of 55,000 cells per well in a volume of 100 μl. The following day, cells in each well were transfected with 100 ng of lentiviral vector, 100 ng of a gag-pol-rev expression plasmid, and 20 ng of a VSVG expression plasmid, using Fugene 6 transfection reagent according to the manufacturer's suggestions (Roche). The plates were immediately centrifuged for 30 minutes at 2000 rpm and then placed in a 37°C tissue culture incubator. Viral supernatant was collected (200 μl) twice daily for 3 days starting the day following transfection. At the end of the collection period, the virus was aliquoted and stored at –20°C.

Viral infections: All viral infections were performed the day after plating cells. From 3 μl to 10 μl of thawed viral supernatant (either MMLV or lentivirus) was added to each well in the presence of 8 μg/ml polybrene. The plates were spun for 30 minutes at 2250 rpm and then placed in a 37°C tissue culture incubator. The following day, the medium was removed and fresh medium was added.

Growth and proliferation assays. For the cell outgrowth assay in SKBR3 cells, cells were infected with either lentivirus or MMLV and 24 hours postinfection were treated with 1 μM Iressa (provided by Astra Zeneca). After 2 weeks, the wells were visually inspected, and those wells in which the cells displayed obvious growth were scored as positive. For quantitative proliferation assays, after approximately 4 days of either drug treatment or infection, a one-tenth volume of a Resazurin stock solution (stock 150 mg/liter, prepared in PBS) was added to the well. After 4–12 hours, a fluorometric reading was performed in a TECAN plate reader set to an excitation wavelength of 535 nm and an emission wavelength of 590 nm.

Scoring of kinases. *Essential kinases:* Each duplicate data point was taken in average and then measured against the average value for the entire experiment. Those data points whose value was less than 50% of the average for the experiment were designated as essential kinases.

Drug-sensitizing kinases: In this case, to score as a hit, the effect of the shRNA itself, in the absence of drug, was taken into account. In the absence of drug, the Resazurin value for a given well was required to be at least 75% of the average for the entire no-drug-treatment arm of the experiment. Those shRNAs that passed this test were then analyzed in the context of the drug-treatment arm of the experiment. To score as a hit, the Resazurin value was required to be at most 50% of the average for the entire drug-treatment arm of the experiment.

RESULTS

To begin the development of high-throughput functional screens, we have made several fundamental decisions about acceptable technical approaches. Two goals are particularly important to our strategy. First, we have chosen to use viral vectors to ensure easy and efficient transduction of expression constructs. Transfection of siRNAs themselves, shRNA vectors, or cDNA vectors is possible, but this greatly limits the types of cells that can be studied, and adjusting expression levels is extremely difficult. In addition, expression vectors of all types are easily shared and, consequently, compared across labs and experimental systems. Second, we have devised methods that allow each construct to be tested independently. Pooling strategies are powerful in many settings, but they are not suitable for screens in which the phenotypic readout comprises some aspect of a growth defect, such as cell cycle arrest. An additional limitation relates to working with pooled libraries. Since the starting library is a mixture of species, the precise identity of a clone that scores positive in a screen is anonymous: It must then be determined by retrieving that clone from the cell and sequencing the insert. Moreover, it is possible to extract additional information from a genetic screen from those clones that fail to elicit the phenotype in question only

when the identity of all clones is known prior to executing the experiment.

There have been two major stages to developing high-throughput functional screens in our lab. The first stage centered on the development of methods and techniques to produce large numbers of expression clones with sufficient ease and of adequate quality to use in parallel screening assays. Another goal of these technical approaches has been to produce these reagents at low enough cost to make screening assays possible for most academic research labs. The second stage has been the development of tissue culture methods and screening assays to utilize these reagents. Both of these stages have been completed successfully; a brief outline of our strategy and results is presented below.

Stage 1: Expression Clones

The basis of this system rests on the ability to effectively transfer a gene (or knockdown shRNA) to a variety of cell types. This process must be efficient, reliable, generalizable, selectable, and, preferably, trackable. To this end, a retroviral vector with the appropriate markers fulfills these requirements and makes this an ideal method for high-throughput gene delivery. An additional feature that makes this strategy for gene transfer attractive is that the manipulations required to produce retroviral stocks do not involve multiple complicated steps, making the adaptation to a high-throughput scale of operation possible.

The viral vector employed for our shRNA experiments is a lentiviral design developed by a collaborative group of investigators, collectively known as the RNAi Consortium (TRC) (http://www.broad.mit.edu/genome_bio/trc/). The TRC generously provided the shRNA constructs used here prior to publication. In this system, the shRNA is expressed from the human U6 promoter, downstream from which resides an expression cassette for the PAC gene between the LTR elements, so that transduced cells can be selected for upon the addition of puromycin. The expression cassette is designed so that the processed duplex RNA is 21 nucleotides in length. As is the case with other shRNA libraries, this clone collection is degenerate, with approximately 4–5 shRNAs, each targeted to a specific gene (Moffat et al. 2006). The shRNA set in our possession designed to target roughly 450 kinases numbers some 2500 discrete clones.

In our laboratory, we have generated a Moloney retroviral cDNA expression vector with recombinational cloning elements and have validated its stability during cloning manipulations. We have also performed functional validation studies in mammalian cells to ensure that the retroviral and expression elements work as intended. We went to some length to characterize this vector prior to implementing it into our cloning and experimental pipelines because it would be used for the expression of thousands of cDNAs in the course of our work, as we describe in some detail here. This vector was designed to accommodate the Creator recombinational cloning system, based on cre recombinase, developed by BD Clontech (http://www.clontech.com/clontech/index.shtml). This design took advantage of the cDNA repository developed by the Harvard Institute of

452   PEARLBERG ET AL.

Proteomics (HIP www.hip.harvard.edu). HIP's founding principle was to create and distribute a catalogued collection of full-length, sequence-verified cDNA clones, available for use in a wide variety of settings.

As of this writing, HIP has generated approximately 5500 full human cDNAs, all of which have been sequence-verified. These gene ORFs have been cloned into a master recombinational cloning vector, which facilitates transfer into a variety of expression vectors. From this collection, we have focused our interest on the complement of human kinases. From among the many Moloney retroviral vectors we tested, we found that the vector pMMPf2 (provided by Richard Mulligan of The Harvard Gene Therapy Initiative, Harvard Medical School, http://hgti.med.harvard.edu) proved to be the most stable and least prone to rearrangements in E. coli during cloning manipulations. Therefore, we decided to incorporate the features necessary for our experiments into this vector. pMMPf2 is a Type C gammaretrovirus vector whose LTRs comprise elements of both MMLV and murine proliferative sarcoma virus. As with other retroviral vectors used for gene delivery, the gag, pol, and env genes have been removed. We have modified this vector in the following ways: PAC, which confers resistance to puromycin, was inserted as an NcoI and NotI fragment downstream of the 5′LTR. Growing cells in the presence of puromycin will allow selection of those cells that have been successfully infected. In a second step, a loxP recombinational expression cassette, compatible with the Creator recombinational cloning system as used at HIP, was amplified in a PCR and introduced as a NotI and XhoI fragment between the LTRs, just downstream

from the PAC gene, generating the plasmid, pJP1520 (Fig. 1A). We have tested pJP1520 to ensure that it is stable during procedures performed in E. coli and that it remains stable during subsequent propagation. For reasons that remain obscure, pJP1520 has performed remarkably better than other vector constructs in tests for arrangements of the various selection and expression elements that we required. These tests included the isolation of multiple independent isolates with transferred expression ORFs and long-term culture. Other vectors showed significantly increased levels of recombination in E. coli. Of note, pJP1520 showed almost no recombinations, even when these procedures were carried out in the recA-positive bacterial strain MM294.

To complement pJP1520, three additional Moloney retroviral vectors, each with a different selectable marker (that for hygromycin, blasticidin, or G418 [neomycin]), have been constructed. An additional series of vectors, also based on pJP1520, was designed so that either an amino- or carboxy-terminal epitope tag (either flag, myc, HA, or taptag) is appended to the ORF after recombinational transfer (Fig. 1B). We anticipate that these vectors will prove useful in a variety of settings.

To date, we have transferred over 500 full-length kinase cDNAs generated by HIP into pJP1520 as well as its blasticidin-markered sibling, pJP1563. The initial cloning of these kinases, as well as their recombinational transfer, was performed in 96-well format. For these cloning operations, we use Cre recombinase that we have made in our laboratory; it performs as well as any commercial source we have tested and is substantially cheaper. In addition, we do not use commercially prepared competent cells. We

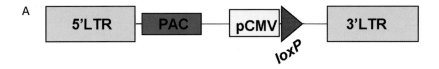

Name	Resistance Marker	Epitope Tag (position)
pJP1520	puromycin	none
pJP1563	blasticidin	none
pJP1564	Hygromycin	none
pJP1565	Neomycin	none
pJP1536	puromycin	3xFlag (N-ter)
pJP1537	puromycin	Myc (N-ter)
pJP1538	puromycin	HA (N-ter)
pJP1539	puromycin	TAP-tag (N-ter)
pJP1540	puromycin	3xFlag (C-ter)
pJP1541	puromycin	Myc (C-ter)
pJP1542	puromycin	HA (C-ter)
pJP1543	puromycin	TAP-tag (C-ter)

Figure 1. Retroviral expression vectors with recombinational cloning elements. (*A*) Schematic drawing of the relevant elements of the pJP1520 vector. Included in the diagram are the LTR elements, a 600-bp fragment of the human CMV immediate-early enhancer/promoter, the PAC gene, and the 34-bp loxP element. (*B*) Retroviral vectors derived from pJP1520.

have found that competent cells prepared in-house are as efficient as any commercial source and provide a remarkable cost savings. Each kinase cDNA ORF is sequence-verified after it is cloned into the master recombinational cloning vector. All cloning steps are tracked with a laboratory information management system (LIMS). After the transfer reaction into either of the two Moloney retroviral vectors, a restriction digestion is performed to assess the success of the reaction. We have found that on first pass, we achieve a success transfer rate of approximately 90%. All of our clones are stored as glycerol stocks in a Biobank robotic freezer storage system.

Stage 1: High-Throughput Generation of Transfection-grade DNA

Perhaps the single most challenging step we have faced is the conversion of a glycerol stock into highly transfectable plasmid DNA. Although a number of high-throughput plasmid DNA preparation kits are available from commercial vendors, we have found them to be expensive, and they deliver DNA that shows low rates of transfection compared to other sources. Therefore, we have developed our own methods, based on standard alkaline lysis, to prepare plasmid DNA of sufficient purity for transfection of mammalian cells (Fig. 2A). A few key points of the DNA preparation methods are highlighted here, and the details of these methods and protocols will

be published elsewhere. Typically, we grow cultures in a 96-well culture block in a volume of 1–1.5 ml of TB per well. Then a standard alkaline lysis step is performed, and the lysates are cleared by passage through a filter plate. In our experience, either centrifugation or a vacuum can be applied at this step. We then tested a number of anion exchange resins and found two that worked well: the weak DEAE anion exchanger, Nucleobond, and the strong QAE anion exchanger, cholestyramine. Nucleobond, developed by Machery Nagel, is the resin used by Qiagen in their Maxiprep kits. The cholestyramine resin binds plasmid DNA exceptionally well under our conditions, and we have found it to be an inexpensive reagent that works well. We load either of the resins into the wells of a 96-well filter plate and perform the wash and elution steps either by vacuum or by centrifugation. We have tested a variety of methods to then remove the salt from the eluate. We currently use alcohol precipitation as the method of choice. We have found that the transfection efficiency of the plasmid DNA prepared by our high-throughput miniprep methods is equal to that of plasmid DNA prepared with a Qiagen Maxiprep kit (Fig. 2B). From a 1-ml culture, our yields are typically in excess of 10 μg. This provides enough DNA for 200 transfections. Without robotic assistance, 12 plates—corresponding to 1200 minipreps—can be processed in a day by one person. With robotics, this scale can be increased five- to tenfold.

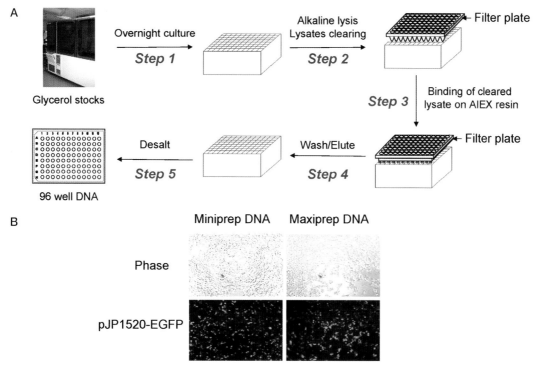

Figure 2. Work flow for high-throughput minipreps. (*A*) Simplified scheme of DNA minipreps. All of the shRNA and cDNA expression clones glycerol stock are stored in Thermo Electron Biobank freezer system. From these glycerol stocks, bacteria are grown overnight in 1.2 ml of TB medium (Step 1). After pelleting, an alkaline lysis step is performed and the supernatant is cleared by centrifugation through a filter plate (Step 2). The cleared lysates are then loaded on a second filter plate containing an AIEX resin (Step 3). After a wash step, DNA is eluted (Step 4). The transfection-quality miniprep DNA is then obtained by a final desalting step (Step 5). (*B*) Comparison of in-house miniprep transfection efficiency to Qiagen Maxiprep DNA. 100 ng of pJP1520 DNA obtained using either our miniprep protocol or Qiagen Maxiprep was transfected in 293T cells. 48 hours later, the transfection efficiency was assessed by GFP expression.

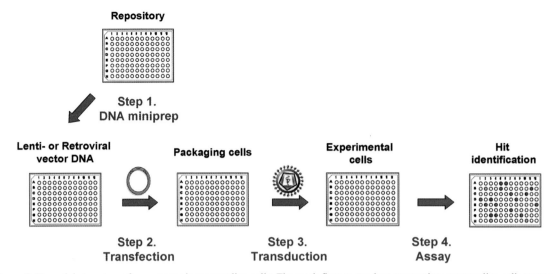

Figure 3. Essential steps to perform screens in mammalian cells. The work flow to conduct screens into mammalian cells starts with the conversion of bacterial glycerol stocks from the repository into DNA using our 96-well miniprep DNA protocol. After normalization of DNA concentration, 293T cells are co-transfected with the DNAs of interest, the packaging constructs (Gag/pol and Gag/pol/rev for the MMLV retrovirus and lentivirus, respectively), and VSVG protein to produce pseudotyped viruses. These viruses are then used to transduce the experimental cell line in 96-well or 384-well format.

Stage 1: High-Throughput Generation of Retrovirus Stocks

From the high-quality plasmid DNA we have in hand, we are able to generate high-titer virus. The work flow is shown in Figure 3. Transfections are performed in 96-well format, and viral supernatant is collected, aliquoted, and frozen. The transfection and all downstream liquid-handling steps are performed robotically with a Sciclone ALH3000 robot (Caliper Life Sciences). Procedurally, the generation of lentivirus and MMLV retrovirus is very similar in our laboratory, and we have spent some effort to optimize each system. Starting from 100 ng of viral vector DNA, we typically generate roughly 0.8 ml of lentivirus and 1.5 ml of MMLV retrovirus. Using test viruses that express the enhanced green fluorescent protein (EGFP), we have determined by flow cytometry that the titer of the lentivirus is slightly below 10^7 per ml. For the MMLV retrovirus, it is approximately 10^6 per ml. Since our screens are performed for the most part in 384-well plates, with approximately 400–800 cells per well, we find that we can use 3–5 µl of virus per well. For both the lentiviral and MMLV platforms, we pseudotype our virus with the VSVG protein, which imparts a broad degree of flexibility to our experimental system. As a biosafety precaution, our Sciclone robot is surrounded by a custom laminar flow hood (Flow Sciences), with an airflow system that generates negative pressure. With these methods, virus production is robust, and the limiting factor in the production of screening reagents is the DNA preparation.

As we have developed and refined the methods described above to generate virus, we have also in parallel begun to perform some pilot genetic screens. Here we present some examples of the types of screens we have developed. Because the data sets generated by these approaches are large, the detailed findings of these screens will be presented elsewhere.

Stage 2: Identification of Essential Kinases in Lung Cancer Cell Lines

To begin to develop a framework to understand key signaling molecules and their attendant pathways in lung cancer tumor cell lines, we initiated a series of screens designed to identify the set of essential kinases in a number of non-small-cell lung cancer cell lines. The results of these experiments from four such cell lines (A549, NCI-H23, NCI-H358, NCI-1299) are discussed here. These efforts utilized the lentiviral shRNA library described above. As mentioned previously, approximately 450 kinases were interrogated, and with a library degeneracy of 4 or 5 shRNA hairpins targeted to each kinase. This corresponds to roughly 2500 discrete lentiviral shRNA clones from which plasmid DNA was prepared and virus was generated. For these experiments, lentiviruses were prepared in 96-well format and were then used to transduce the lung tumor cell lines in 384-well format. Each infection was performed in quadruplicate, and then half of the wells were treated with puromycin selection and half were not. The cells were then grown for 4 days, and a proliferation assay was performed. The puromycin selection allowed us to define in a general sense the efficiency of viral transduction. In the scatter plot shown in Figure 4, those wells treated with puromycin were plotted against their untreated counterparts, and the results indicate that the viral infections worked well. From the set of wells not treated with puromycin we were able to determine those shRNA molecules that inhibited proliferation, i.e., identify essential kinases. As shown in Table 1, roughly 50–100 essential kinases were identified from each of four cell lines tested. In total, from among the four cell lines tested, 177 essential kinases were found. Roughly 60% of those essential kinases were not shared across the cell lines tested. A small number of kinases (8) was found to be essential in all four cell lines (Fig. 5). In 10% of the cases when an

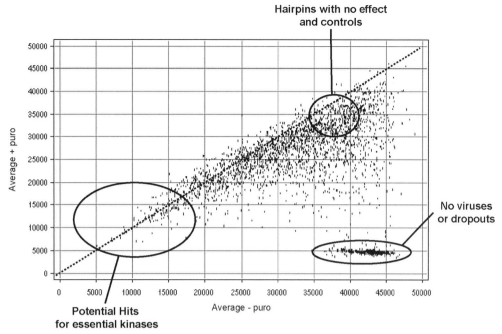

Figure 4. Scatter plot of data points from essential kinase screen in NCI-H23 lung cancer cell line. In each experiment, infection was performed in quadruplicate. From among the quadruplicate wells, two wells received puromycin and two did not, and after several days, cell proliferation was assayed. The duplicate points for each condition were averaged and plotted against each other. The x and y axes represent the raw Resazurin values from the fluorometric readings. This scatter plot shows the correlation between the two conditions (presence or absence of puromycin). An r of 1 is indicated by the dashed black line. Hits are identified as indicated in the figure and described in Materials and Methods.

shRNA scored as a hit, additional hairpins targeted to different regions of that gene also scored positive. It is our expectation that as more cell lines are tested in this manner, we may be able to determine those kinases whose expression is required by a broad spectrum (or perhaps all) of tumor lines. In addition, we may be able to discern patterns based on tissue histology or the presence of particular genetic alterations (e.g., mutations in EGFR or Kras).

Stage 2: Genetic Modifier Screens

A second type of assay, also based on the same phenotypic readout, is a genetic modifier screen designed to identify those kinases whose expression levels modify the response of tumor cell lines to various chemotherapeutics. These pilot efforts have been initiated in a set of breast cancer and lung cancer cell lines, and various subsets of our shRNA set as well as our cDNA set have been used for these experiments. Our initial studies began with the breast cancer cell line SKBR3. This cell line displays moderate sensitivity to the EGFR inhibitor Iressa, with an IC$_{50}$ of approximately 1 μM (data not shown). In this case, a small screen in which approximately 250 kinases, prepared as retrovirus and overexpressing individual kinases as described above, were examined to determine which conferred increased resistance to Iressa. Here we employed a simple yet robust assay in which we determined those wells in which there was obvious cell growth after a period of 2 weeks (Fig. 6). Of the kinases tested, about 12 enabled this cell line to grow in the presence of 1 μM—and in some cases 10 μM — Iressa for several weeks. It is worth noting that a number of those kinases that scored positive in this assay bear an obvious relationship to the action of EGFR and the EGFR pathway. For example, Her2, ErbB3, and Akt all render SKBR3 cells resistant to Iressa (shown as Wells B10, C3, and E9, respectively, in Fig. 6). In addition, we have identified a number of kinases with no obvious relationship to EGFR or the EGFR pathway that increase the resistance of SKBR3 cells to Iressa.

In a similar vein, we also identified particular kinases that when underexpressed, via shRNA-mediated knockdown, render SKBR3 cells resistant to Iressa. In this pilot

Table 1. Overview of Essential Kinase Screens in Four Different Lung Cancer Cell Lines

Cell line	A549	NCI-H23	NCI-H358	NCI-H1299
Histological type	adenocarcinoma	non-small-cell carcinoma	adenocarcinoma	large-cell carcinoma
Total number hairpins scoring	115	81	82	50
triplicate hairpins for the same gene	5	3	1	0
duplicate hairpins for the same gene	9	7	8	4
Total number of different genes	93	69	70	46

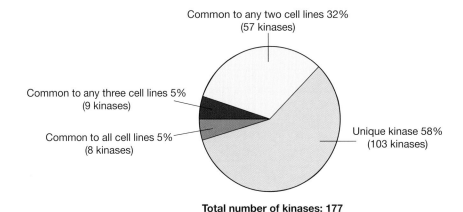

Total number of kinases: 177

Figure 5. Essential kinases shared among four cell lines.

experiment, a few hundred shRNA clones, corresponding to roughly 100 genes, were assayed and scored as described above. In this scenario, the shRNA cassette was introduced into SKBR3 cells via lentiviral infection. As was the case for the cDNA expression experiments described above, after infection, the cells were grown in the presence of 1 μM Iressa for 2 weeks. Roughly 10 kinases, when targeted for knockdown, allow SKBR3 cells to grow in these conditions (for examples, see Fig. 6). In a few cases, two shRNA clones, each corresponding to a different region of the same gene, that conferred resistance to Iressa were identified. Since the set of kinases targeted in this small shRNA experiment for the most part did not overlap those kinases tested in our cDNA expression experiment above, we are unable to determine whether in the case where shRNA renders a cell resistant to our test drug, there is a corresponding cDNA that renders the cell sensitive. We

anticipate that as our test sets become more complete, we will encounter examples of this. Since it is known that GSK3B, at least in some contexts, antagonizes the action of Akt, it is interesting that GSK3B scores when targeted for knockdown, given that Akt when overexpressed scores similarly (shown as Well A5 in Fig. 6). As of this writing, we have not determined the degree of knockdown elicited by the shRNA clones used in our experiments. These efforts are ongoing, and as we accrue information regarding the efficacy of knockdown by particular shRNA clones in our possession, we shall eliminate from our experiments those clones that are not effective. In addition, this information will impart additional meaning to those clones that do not score despite the fact that they result in mRNA knockdown.

We have also performed a similar series of experiments with our cDNA expression clones in a set of non-

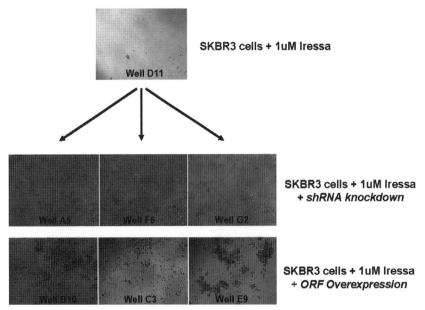

Figure 6. Modulation of Iressa sensitivity. SKBR3 cells were cultured in the presence of 1 μM Iressa for 2 weeks (*top photograph*). Cells rendered resistant to 1 μM Iressa by either shRNA knockdown or cDNA overexpression of particular kinases (*bottom photographs*).

small-cell lung cancer lines. In some cases, the starting cell line, such as HCC827 or H1650, displayed inherent sensitivity to Iressa. Therefore, these two lines were used to identify kinases that, when overexpressed, increased resistance to Iressa. As was the case with SKBR3 cells, a number of kinases relating to EGFR and its downstream effectors, such as Akt, ErbB3, and HER2, scored in either or both of these cell lines. In addition, a small number of kinases, whose relation to EGFR remains obscure, or at best tenuous, were identified. The fact that in these pilot screens we identify kinases whose properties obviously relate to the action of the drug as well as those do not provide a measure of confidence that our screening system will uncover novel proteins whose function is physiologically relevant to the action of Iressa (or for that matter, any other test drug).

Stage 2: Genetic Suppression

One of the most powerful experiments that can be undertaken with our approach is that of genetic suppression. Thus, we attempted the following simple experiment. From some of our initial shRNA studies, we identified ErbB3 as an essential kinase in a number of our cell lines. We were then interested in identifying those kinases that when overexpressed would rescue—or suppress—the phenotype elicited by either of two ErbB3 shRNA knockdown cassettes (Fig. 7). This experiment took advantage of the various selectable markers carried by our viral vectors. In this case, HeLa cells were seeded in 96-well plates and the cells were transduced with virus (based on pJP1563), so that the cells in each well were engineered to overexpress an individual kinase (roughly 250 kinases

were surveyed). The cells were then put into blasticidin selection. The day after, either of the two ErbB3 shRNA cassettes was introduced into the cells via lentiviral transduction. Puromycin selection was then instituted. Ordinarily, knockdown of ErbB3 would result in death of HeLa cells. From among the 250 kinases that were overexpressed, we identified one kinase, MAP3K14, that overcame the killing mediated by ErbB3 knockdown. This result argues that this line of experimentation will allow us to establish genetic relationships among genes and pathways much in the same way as has been done in yeast and other model organisms for the past several decades.

DISCUSSION

Experiments with mammalian tissue culture cells have proven to be an excellent system for biochemical studies. Methods to lyse cells, purify components, and reassemble cellular processes in a test tube have led to major advances in our understanding of DNA synthesis, transcription, translation, and many other key aspects of cell physiology. Similarly, affinity methods to rapidly purify individual proteins and examine the isolated proteins for changes in association and modifications have been a staple of building signal transduction pathways and understanding many aspects of regulation. Imaging methods provide ever-higher resolution of the spatial and temporal location of proteins. One approach that has been missing from the tools used to study mammalian cells in culture is any process that resembles genetics. Mutagenesis screens allow researchers to identify key genes in an unbiased manner and can approach comprehensive coverage of the entire genome. The availability of comprehensive li-

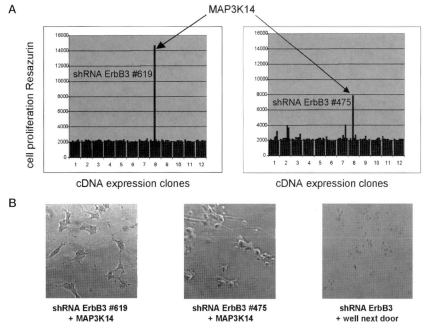

Figure 7. Example of genetic suppression. (*A*) Map3K14 rescue of ErbB3 shRNA-mediated killing of HeLa cells. From among 250 kinases tested, Map3K14 was found to suppress the growth defect elicited by either of two ErbB3 shRNA knockdown cassettes (shRNA ErbB3 #475 or shRNA ErbB3 #619) in HeLa cells. Cell growth was determined using a Resazurin-based proliferation assay. (*B*) Cell images were collected by phase-contrast microscopy.

braries of shRNAs and cDNA expression vectors will allow screens that approach the characteristics of genetic screens. With these tools, the levels of a particular protein can be raised or lowered within a target cell in assay formats that closely resemble genetic mutation screens.

It is worth noting that although the comparison to genetics helps one understand how to use and plan experiments using expression screens, there are true differences between these approaches. Mutagenesis in theory can hit any gene or regulatory sequence. High-throughput functional screens only interrogate the proteins represented in the repository. This collection is increasing but is still short of comprehensive, and in the proof-of-principle work described here, we have examined only the kinase protein family. Mutations can change the function of a protein in many fashions, including loss of function and gain of function. High-throughput screens rely on differences caused by increasing or decreasing the levels of a particular protein. Importantly, mutations directly affect only the altered protein, whereas expression of shRNAs or cDNAs can have effects off target. It is now well understood that shRNAs can affect mRNAs that are not the designed target, and high levels of proteins expressed from cDNAs can lead to unexpected protein–protein associations that can act as dominant interfering interactions. Both shRNA and cDNA off-target effects can be eliminated in secondary screens by use of multiple hairpins to the same target in the case of shRNAs, and by mapping the effector regions for cDNAs. The use of high-throughput functional screens has several advantages over mutagenesis. The most important is that from the completion of the screen the exact protein under study is known. Mutagenesis commonly requires the mapping and cloning of the lesion before the gene in question can be identified. All of these facts distinguish the use of expression screens from classic mutagenesis. However, like mutagenesis, the goal of functional screens is to pinpoint a gene or protein that can serve as a starting point for more detailed experimentation. High-throughput functional screens now open this experimental door for investigation of tissue culture cells.

A reasonable goal for the next several years will be to build shRNAs and cDNAs for every protein in human cells. As these reagent-building projects progress, and as these tools get used in screens, extensive analysis of their actions can be assembled and used to refine the reagent set with the goal of having a validated reagent set. With these developments, the genetic information gleaned from the sequencing efforts of the last decade can be converted into powerful reagents that will allow each protein to be tested for its role in chosen cellular processes.

What types of assay formats and strategies can be approached with high-throughput functional screens? We have chosen to approach the development of these reagents with three general goals. First, we have sought to develop methods that will allow each protein to be tested separately. Other investigators have shown the value of using pools of clones. Pooling strategies are cost- and labor-efficient but often limit assay design

methods. Testing each clone individually allows more types of screens to be available for assay, promotes validation of each reagent, and leads to the possibility to record and share the effects of each clone. Our second approach has been to develop methods that lower the cost of screens. We have done this by avoiding commercial kits and relying on component plastics, resins, and chemicals. We have found these methods to greatly lower the costs of doing screens, and in many cases, we have produced methods that are superior to equivalent commercial products. Finally, we have developed methods that utilize viral infections as a method to induce both cDNA and shRNA constructs. At present, our favored vectors are all retrovirus-based, but other viral vectors will likely be valuable as well. These approaches have led us to believe that essentially any characteristic of a cell can be explored using high-throughput function screens as long as a robust assay format can be designed.

ACKNOWLEDGMENTS

The authors are deeply indebted to W. Hahn, N. Hacohen, D. Root, D. Sabatini, E. Lander, and all members of the RNAi Consortium for providing a portion of their RNAi repository prior to publication; to Jeng Shin-Lee and R. Mulligan for advice on retroviral cloning and preparation and for access to the retroviral backbone pMMPf2. In addition, the authors thank Lance K. Ching for excellent technical assistance, as well as all of the members of the Harvard Institute of Proteomics for their comments and recommendations. This work was supported in part by a sponsored research agreement from Astra Zeneca.

REFERENCES

Bardelli A., Parsons D.W., Silliman N., Ptak J., Szabo S., Saha S., Markowitz S., Willson J.K., Parmigiani G., Kinzler K.W., Vogelstein B., and Velculescu V.E. 2003. Mutational analysis of the tyrosine kinome in colorectal cancers. *Science* **300:** 949.
Brizuela L., Richardson A., Marsischky G., and LaBaer J. 2002. The FLEXGene repository: Exploiting the fruits of the genome projects by creating a needed resource to face the challenges of the post-genomic era. *Arch. Med. Res.* **33:** 318.
Brummelkamp T.R., Bernards R., and Agami R. 2002. A system for stable expression of short interfering RNAs in mammalian cells. *Science* **296:** 550.
Carpenter A.E. and Sabatini D.M. 2004. Systematic genome-wide screens of gene function. *Nat. Rev. Genet.* **5:** 11.
Carter P., Presta L., Gorman C.M., Ridgway J.B., Henner D., Wong W.L., Rowland A.M., Kotts C., Carver M.E., and Shepard H.M. 1992. Humanization of an anti-p185HER2 antibody for human cancer therapy. *Proc. Natl. Acad. Sci.* **89:** 4285.
Cobleigh M.A., Vogel C.L., Tripathy D., Robert N.J., Scholl S., Fehrenbacher L., Wolter J.M., Paton V., Shak S., Lieberman G., and Slamon D.J. 1999. Multinational study of the efficacy and safety of humanized anti-HER2 monoclonal antibody in women who have HER2-overexpressing metastatic breast cancer that has progressed after chemotherapy for metastatic disease. *J. Clin. Oncol.* **17:** 2639.
Cunningham D., Humblet Y., Siena S., Khayat D., Bleiberg H., Santoro A., Bets D., Mueser M., Harstrick A., Verslype C., Chau I., and Van Cutsem E. 2004. Cetuximab monotherapy and cetuximab plus irinotecan in irinotecan-refractory metastatic colorectal cancer. *N. Engl. J. Med.* **351:** 337.
Davies H., Bignell G.R., Cox C., Stephens P., Edkins S., Clegg

S., Teague J., Woffendin H., Garnett M.J., Bottomley W., Davis N., Dicks E., Ewing R., Floyd Y., Gray K., Hall S., Hawes R., Hughes J., Kosmidou V., Menzies A., Mould C., Parker A., Stevens C., Watt S., and Hooper S., et al. 2002. Mutations of the BRAF gene in human cancer. *Nature* **417:** 949.

Druker B.J., Talpaz M., Resta D.J., Peng B., Buchdunger E., Ford J.M., Lydon N.B., Kantarjian H., Capdeville R., Ohno-Jones S., and Sawyers C.L. 2001. Efficacy and safety of a specific inhibitor of the BCR-ABL tyrosine kinase in chronic myeloid leukemia. *N. Engl. J. Med.* **344:** 1031.

Forsburg S.L. 2001. The art and design of genetic screens: Yeast. *Nat. Rev. Genet.* **2:** 659.

Hafen E., Basler K., Edstroem J.E., and Rubin G.M. 1987. Sevenless, a cell-specific homeotic gene of *Drosophila*, encodes a putative transmembrane receptor with a tyrosine kinase domain. *Science* **236:** 55.

Hannon G.J. 2002. RNA interference. *Nature* **418:** 244.

Hannon G.J. and Rossi J.J. 2004. Unlocking the potential of the human genome with RNA interference. *Nature* **431:** 371.

Hartwell L.H., Culotti J., and Reid B. 1970. Genetic control of the cell-division cycle in yeast. I. Detection of mutants. *Proc. Natl. Acad. Sci.* **66:** 352.

Hartwell L.H., Culotti J., Pringle J.R., and Reid B.J. 1974. Genetic control of the cell division cycle in yeast. *Science* **183:** 46.

Hunter T. 2000. Signaling—2000 and beyond. *Cell* **100:** 113.

Inoue H., H. Nojima, and H. Okayama. 1990. High efficiency transformation of *Escherichia coli* with plasmids. *Gene* **96:** 23.

Jacks T., Remington L., Williams B.O., Schmitt E.M., Halachmi S., Bronson R.T., and Weinberg R.A. 1994. Tumor spectrum analysis in p53-mutant mice. *Curr. Biol.* **4:** 1.

Lynch T.J., Bell D.W., Sordella R., Gurubhagavatula S., Okimoto R.A., Brannigan B.W., Harris P.L., Haserlat S.M., Supko J.G., Haluska F.G., Louis D.N., Christiani D.C., Settleman J., and Haber D.A.. 2004. Activating mutations in the epidermal growth factor receptor underlying responsiveness of non-small-cell lung cancer to gefitinib. *N. Engl. J. Med.* **350:** 2129.

Moffat J. and Sabatini D.M. 2006. Building mammalian signalling pathways with RNAi screens. *Nat. Rev. Mol. Cell Biol.* **7:** 177.

Moffat J. Grueneberg D.A., Yang X., Kim S.Y., Kloepfer A.M., Hinkle G., Piqani B., Eisenhaure T.M., Luo B., Grenier J.K., Carpenter A.E., Foo S.Y., Stewart S.A., Stockwell B.R., Hacohen N., Hahn W.C. Lander E.S., Sabatini D.M., and Root D.E. 2006. A lentiviral RNAi library for human and mouse genes applied to an arrayed viral high-content screen. *Cell* **124:** 1283.

Moon R.T., Kohn A.D., De Ferrari G.V., and Kaykas A.. 2004. WNT and beta-catenin signalling: Diseases and therapies. *Nat. Rev. Genet.* **5:** 691.

Nurse P., Masui Y., and Hartwell L.. 1998. Understanding the cell cycle. *Nat. Med.* **4:** 1103.

Paddison P.J., Caudy A.A., Sachidanandam R., and Hannon G.J. 2004. Short hairpin activated gene silencing in mammalian cells. *Methods Mol. Biol.* **265:** 85.

Paez J.G., Janne P.A., Lee J.C., Tracy S., Greulich H., Gabriel S., Herman P., Kaye F.J., Lindeman N., Boggon T.J., Naoki K., Sasaki H., Fujii Y., Eck M.J., Sellers W.R., Johnson B.E., and Meyerson M.. 2004. EGFR mutations in lung cancer: Correlation with clinical response to gefitinib therapy. *Science* **304:** 1497.

Park J., Hu Y., Murthy T.V., F. Vannberg, Shen B., Rolfs A., Hutti J.E., Cantley L.C., LaBaer J., E. Harlow, and L. Brizuela. 2005. Building a human kinase gene repository: Bioinformatics, molecular cloning, and functional validation. *Proc. Natl. Acad. Sci.* **102:** 8114.

Pearlberg J. and LaBaer J. 2004. Protein expression clone repositories for functional proteomics. *Curr. Opin. Chem. Biol.* **8:** 98.

Rual J.F., Hirozane-Kishikawa T., Hao T., Bertin N., Li S., Dricot A., Li N., Rosenberg J., Lamesch P., Vidalain P.O., Clingsmith T.R., Hartley J.L., Esposito D., Cheo D., Moore T., Simmons B., Sequerra R., Bosak S., Doucette-Stamm L., Le Peuch C., Vandenhaute J., Cusick M.E., Albala J.S., Hill D.E., and Vidal M. 2004. Human ORFeome version 1.1: A platform for reverse proteomics. *Genome Res.* **14:** 2128.

Simon M.A., Bowtell D.D., Dodson G.S., Laverty T.R., and Rubin G.M. 1991. Ras1 and a putative guanine nucleotide exchange factor perform crucial steps in signaling by the sevenless protein tyrosine kinase. *Cell* **67:** 701.

Xie K. and Abbruzzese J.L. 2003. Developmental biology informs cancer: The emerging role of the hedgehog signaling pathway in upper gastrointestinal cancers. *Cancer Cell* **4:** 245.

Cancer Targets in the Ras Pathway

P. Rodriguez-Viciana, O. Tetsu, K. Oda, J. Okada, K. Rauen,
and F. McCormick
Cancer Research Institute, University of California San Francisco Comprehensive Cancer Center,
San Francisco, California 94115

Ras proteins play a direct causal role in human cancer and in other diseases. Mutant H-Ras, N-Ras, and K-Ras occur in varying frequencies in different tumor types, for reasons that are not known. Other members of the Ras superfamily may also contribute to cancer. Mutations also occur in downstream pathways, notably B-Raf, PTEN, and PI 3′ kinase: These pathways interact at multiple points, including cyclin D1, and act synergistically. In some cases mutations in Ras and effectors are mutually exclusive; in other cases, they coexist. Drugs blocking elements of the pathway are in different stages of clinical development. One of these, the Raf kinase/VEGF-R2 inhibitor Sorafenib, has already been approved for treatment of renal cancer and is being tested in other indications. However, therapeutic targets in the Ras pathway have not yet been fully validated as bona fide targets.

Mutant Ras proteins play a direct causal role in human cancer. Oncogenic mutant Ras proteins are resistant to down-regulation by GTPase activating proteins, and therefore remain in their active, GTP-bound state persistently (Bourne et al. 1991). Table 1 summarizes the frequency with which Ras mutations have been detected in primary human tumors and cancer-derived cell lines, using data from the Sanger Center COSMIC database www.sanger.ac.uk/genetics/CGP/cosmic/.

Although all three Ras genes, H-Ras, N-Ras, and K-Ras, occur in varying frequencies in different tumor types, K-Ras is the form that is causally involved in the major cancers that afflict humans most frequently. The reasons for these differences have not been determined. The simplest interpretation is that these frequencies reflect levels of expression of proto-oncogenic forms and therefore reflect the relative contributions each protein makes to signal output. In support of this, mice lacking both H-Ras

Table 1. Ras Pathway Mutations in Human Cancer

	% Positive samples						
	EGF-R	HRAS	NRAS	KRAS	BRAF	PIK	PTEN
Breast	1	1	0	5	1	27	3
Large intestine	0	1	2	31	15	24	9
Lung	18	0	1	19	2	2	7
Prostate	0	6	0	8	0	0	13
Autonomic ganglia	0	0	8	3	1	0	2
Biliary tract	—	0	1	33	15	0	0
Bone	0	2	0	1	0	0	2
CNS	0	0	2	3	5	5	19
Cervix	0	10	2	9	0	0	6
Adrenal gland	—	1	5	0	0	0	0
Endometrium	—	1	0	14	1	50	34
Eye	—	0	0	31	2	0	0
Heam/lymphoid	—	0	12	4	2	0	4
Kidney	—	0	0	1	15	0	4
Liver	1	0	10	9	3	18	4
Esophagus	—	1	0	2	3	0	1
Ovary	0	0	3	18	16	6	5
Pancreas	0	0	2	60	4	0	2
Salivary gland	—	20	0	2	0	0	27
Skin	0	6	16	2	44	0	13
Small intestine	0	0	25	26	4	0	0
Soft tissue	0	8	7	14	4	6	4
Stomach	0	4	2	6	1	6	6
Testis	0	0	4	5	0	0	0
Thyroid	—	5	7	4	27	0	3
Urinary tract	—	12	3	4	0	11	6

These data were collected from the Sanger Center COSMIC database, December 2005 release. Frequencies of mutation in the four most common cancers are shown in the first four rows.

and N-Ras are viable (Esteban et al. 2001), whereas mice lacking K-Ras are not (Johnson et al. 1997). However, we have found that all three Ras proteins are usually expressed within the same cell, at approximately the same level, suggesting that the three Ras proteins may have different functions which may be selected for during tumorigenesis in a tissue-specific fashion.

The first half of H-, K-, and N-Ras, which includes the switch 1 and 2 domains that are involved in interaction with effectors, are identical. Consistent with this, we have not found any difference in the ability of the three Ras proteins to interact with a comprehensive list of effectors. On the other hand, Ras proteins differ at the carboxyl terminus, a region involved in membrane localization, and indeed, H-, K-, and N-Ras have been found in different microdomains of the plasma membrane, as well as in different endomembrane compartments. Although the biological consequences of this differential localization are not yet clear, it is possible that the Ras proteins recruit their effectors and signal from different membrane compartments, and differences may be related to their characteristic mutational spectrum (Rodriguez-Viciana et al. 2004).

Recently, constitutional activating mutations in H-ras were detected in patients suffering from Costello syndrome, a complex developmental disorder characterized by craniofacial abnormalities, developmental delays, and a predisposition to neoplasia (Aoki et al. 2005; Estep et al. 2006; Gripp et al. 2006; Kerr et al. 2006). 34G to A transitions occur in 91% of affected individuals: This mutation was characterized previously as an activating allele of moderate transforming activity in focus-forming assays and occurs in human cancers. Less frequent mutations include 35G to C also in codon 12, and 37G to T at codon 13. In one case, it was possible to demonstrate loss of the normal H-Ras allele in a tumor that developed in a child suffering from this syndrome. Further analysis of biological and genetic attributes of this syndrome and related disorders may be informative in understanding specific functions of H-Ras in human development. Constitutional activating mutations have also been reported in the K-Ras gene in Noonan syndrome, a condition related to Costello syndrome (Schubbert et al. 2006). In these cases, K-Ras is activated by a mutation that is not fully transforming and is, in fact, partially sensitive to downregulation by GAP. Thus, individuals with fully activated H-Ras show a similar (although not identical) phenotype to those with a weak activated allele of K-Ras, confirming the suggestion that K-Ras is a more potent oncogene in vivo. Interestingly, part of the Ras pathway is activated by mutation in another syndrome, cardio-facial-cutaneous syndrome: In these individuals, activating mutations in B-Raf, MEK1, and MEK2 appear to be the cause of the disease (Rodriguez-Viciana et al. 2006). Interestingly, the mutations that activate B-Raf are generally not found in cancers, and indeed, these affected individuals are not cancer-prone. In addition, activating mutations in MEK1 and MEK2 have not been found in human cancers, although they appear to be fully active by preliminary biochemical analysis.

Structures of Ras proteins have been solved in several states: inactive, GDP-bound; active, bound to GppNHp

(nonhydrolyzable GTP analog), position-12 mutant versions, complexes with exchange factors, GAPs, and effectors (Wittinghofer and Pai 1991). Despite this wealth of information, strategies for identifying Ras inhibitors have not been forthcoming. Considering the extremely high affinity of Ras proteins for GTP (K_d, 1 pM) it seems unlikely that competitive inhibitors could be identified. Screens for small molecules that restore GTP hydrolysis of GTP bound to Ras failed to identify lead compounds, and analysis of high-resolution structures of mutant proteins suggested that this approach was doomed to fail. Activating substitutions were thought to present a steric block to GTP hydrolysis by preventing attack of γ-phosphate by a water molecule. This view has been revised recently: The structure of Ras bound in a transition state complexed with GDP.AlF4 and GAP suggests failure to hydrolyze GTP is the result of displacement of critical catalytic residues from GAP (the "arginine finger") rather than steric block. Consistent with this, a GTP analog in which an amino group is covalently attached to the γ-phosphate is hydrolyzed efficiently by mutant Ras proteins (Ahmadian et al. 1999). Whether this presents an opportunity for therapeutic intervention remains to be seen. Meanwhile, most approaches to blocking Ras activity depend on inhibition of downstream effectors rather than Ras itself. Considerable efforts expended on blocking Ras processing through farnesyl transferase were thwarted by the existence of a "back-up" modification that enables K-Ras to remain active through geranylgeranyl modification instead of farnesylation. However, several inhibitors have been developed extensively and tested in clinical trials. Since H-Ras is not geranylgeranylated in the absence of a farnesyl group, it is inhibited effectively by these compounds. Furthermore, H-Ras appears to be dispensable in normal tissues, at least in mice, suggesting that diseases driven by activated H-Ras would likely respond to these inhibitors without significant side effects on normal tissue.

INCREASING COMPLEXITY OF Ras SIGNALING

It was established in 1984 that Raf function was required for Ras transformation, and a direct interaction of Ras and Raf and mechanisms of Ras-dependent Raf activation were described in 1992 and thereafter. Very soon, however, it became apparent that Ras can also interact with and activate other effectors, including class I PI 3′-kinase (PI3′K) and RalGEFs. Furthermore, Ras effectors were shown to act synergistically, implying that the full transforming potential of Ras depends on simultaneous activation of interacting downstream effector pathways (Fig. 1). Other Ras effectors identified from two-hybrid screens and other approaches include AF-6, RIN, PLCε, Nore1/Rassf5, IMP, and many others that await characterization (Rodriguez-Viciana et al. 2004). Analysis of mutations in human tumors has validated both the Raf and PI3′K pathways as crucial Ras effectors in human tumorigenesis (see below). However, data from a variety of experimental systems, including knock-out mice deficient for other effectors such as RalGDS, PLCε, and

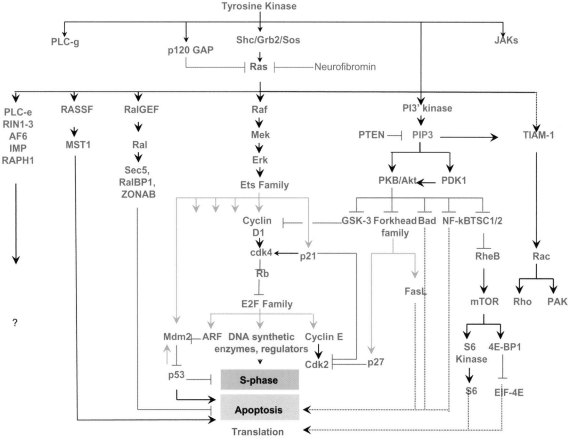

Figure 1. Signaling pathways downstream of Ras.

Tiam1, suggest that other effectors will likely make an important contribution to Ras-induced tumor formation. Activated Ras has been implicated in many of the properties of the malignant phenotype (i.e., uncontrolled proliferation, survival, invasion, and metastasis). It is likely that different effector pathways (or combinations of them) will contribute differentially to the various aspects of tumor biology in different cell types as well as during different stages of tumor progression.

In addition to the prototypic Ras proteins (H-, K-, and N-Ras), the Ras family includes other closely related GTPases that share many of the biochemical and biological properties of Ras, including the ability to behave as oncogenes (Fig. 2). In particular, members of the R-Ras subgroup of the Ras family, which includes R-Ras, TC21/R-Ras2, and M-Ras/R-Ras3, have a high degree of overlap in their ability to interact with and regulate many of Ras known effectors. For example, H-, N-, and K-Ras, R-Ras, TC21, and M-Ras have similar abilities to activate the RalGEF family of effectors and the p110α and γ isoforms of class I PI3K. H-, N-, and K-Ras, on the other hand, are the strongest at interacting with and activating Raf kinases. R-Ras and TC21, however, are the only GTPases that can activate the p110δ PI3K (Rodriguez-Viciana et al. 2004). Individual GTPases have specific blueprints of effector interactions, and their signaling and biological properties should be considered in the context of the full spectrum of their many effector interactions.

With their ability to activate both the Raf and PI3K pathways, the R-Ras subgroup of Ras family GTPases may play a role in human cancer. In our hands, an activated L81 M-Ras mutant is as potent an oncogene as active Ras in a variety of classic transformation assays, and mutations in TC21 have already been found in a handful of human tumors (Rodriguez-Viciana et al. 2004). Determination of whether mutational activation of these GTPases is a rare or frequent way of deregulating the Ras pathway in tumors with wild-type Ras will have to await a comprehensive genetic analysis of human tumors, as has already been performed for other gene families. We have analyzed M-Ras sequences in a panel of 60 breast cancer cell lines and have so far failed to detect activating mutations in this gene (J. Gray and F. McCormick, unpubl.). A further degree of complexity is illustrated by our observation that, in some cases, Ras family GTPases can cross-talk to each other and cooperate in the activation of the same effector pathway. M-Ras, when activated, can target a phosphatase holoenzyme complex made up of Shoc2 and the catalytic subunit of protein phosphatase 1 to remove a negative regulatory phosphate group from Raf kinase molecules complexed with active Ras proteins, thereby further stimulating Raf-specific activity (Fig. 3). Importantly, Shoc2 function is essential for ERK activity in tumor cells with mutant Ras, and therefore, the Shoc2-PP1C holoenzyme represents an additional target for pharmacological inhibition of the ERK pathway (P.

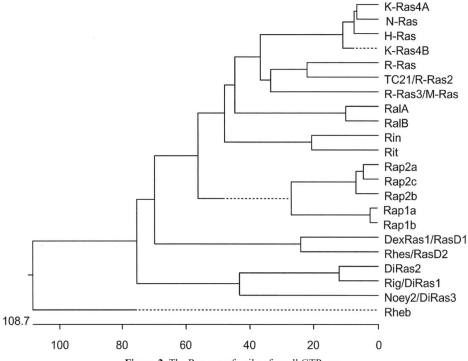

Figure 2. The Ras superfamily of small GTPases.

Rodriguez-Viciana and F. McCormick, in prep.). Clearly, a better understanding of the many effector pathways regulated by Ras and its closely related GTPases will likely lead to the identification of novel targets of therapeutic intervention in human cancer.

CANCER GENETICS AND RAS EFFECTORS

Until recently, the PI 3′K pathway appeared to be the more critical Ras effector pathway in human cancer, based on the observation that mutations occur frequently in major regulators of this pathway, including PI3′K itself and the lipid phosphate PTEN. Activating mutations in Akt2, PDK1, and PAK4 have also been reported at lower frequency. In 2002, frequent activation of B-Raf was reported in many types of human cancer, most notably malignant melanoma (Davies et al. 2002). This discovery confirmed the importance of the MAPK pathway in cancer and encouraged development of drugs that target enzymes in the pathway. In addition, the coexistence of mutations in the Ras pathway in human tumors has led to new insights relating to signal cross-talk and codependence. For example, activating mutations in N-Ras are mutually exclusive with muta-

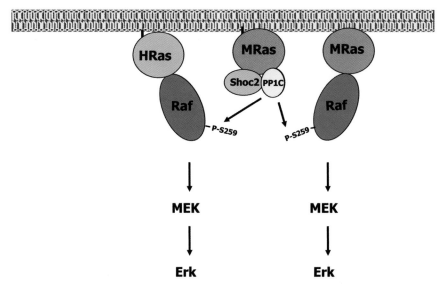

Figure 3. Model for the action of R-Ras3 (M-Ras) on Raf kinase, through recruitment of SHOC-2/PP1C complexes to the plasma membrane.

tions in PTEN in this disease, and also with mutations in B-Raf. This suggests that both major Ras effector arms need to be activated to sustain the malignant phenotype, and that the combined effect of activated MAPK and PI3′K can be achieved by a single mutation in N-Ras, or two independent mutations in B-Raf and PTEN. These two pathways may converge at several key points: For example, p27 expression is increased by hyperactivation of MAPK, potentially leading to growth arrest. However, the PI3′K pathway targets p27 for degradation. These observations suggest an obvious molecular basis for coactivation of these pathways. Another point of intersection may be cyclin D1. Transcription of cyclin D1 is regulated by the MAPK pathway, but cyclin D1 protein is stabilized by the PI3′K pathway; high levels of cyclin D1 protein obviously need inputs from both signaling pathways. Consistent with a role for cyclin D1 in malignant melanoma, this gene is amplified in rare forms of melanoma in which Ras, B-Raf, and PTEN are wild type (Bastian et al. 2001).

Transcriptional regulation of cyclin D1 involves several different types of transcription factors such as AP-1/c-Jun (Albanese et al. 1995; Bakiri et al. 2000), CREB (Tetsu and McCormick 1999), NF-κB (Guttridge et al. 1999; Hinz et al. 1999), and c-Ets (Albanese et al. 1995; Tetsu and McCormick 1999). In addition, we showed that cyclin D1 is a major transcriptional target of the APC/β-catenin/TCF signaling pathway (Tetsu and McCormick 1999; Hulit et al. 2004; Lepourcelet et al. 2004). Increased expression of cyclin D1 protein therefore depends on hyperactive signals from a number of pathways. Stabilization of the protein through activation of the PI3′K pathway has also been reported, suggesting that signals both from the RAF/MEK/ERK pathway, leading to transcriptional activation, and from the PI3′K pathway, leading to posttranscriptional activation, may be necessary: A similar situation has been described for Mdm2, in which the RAF/MEK/ERK pathway increases transcription, and the PI3′K pathway leads to stabilization.

In contrast to the relatively simple relationship between Ras and its major effectors in melanoma, mutations in K-Ras, PTEN, and PI3′K coexist in other types of cancer: Mutations in K-Ras and PI3′K often coexist in colon cancer, for example. We have analyzed mutations in the *PIK3CA* gene in 66 endometrial carcinoma patients. We identified coexistence of *PTEN* and *PIK3CA* mutations in 26% (17/66) of patients (Oda et al. 2005). Tumors with *PTEN* mutation showed a tendency to carry *PIK3CA* mutation more frequently (17/37 = 46%) than tumors without *PTEN* mutation (7/29 = 24%), although statistical significance was not reached ($p = 0.078$ in Fisher's exact test). Subsequently, we evaluated the relationship between *PIK3CA* mutation and other clinicopathological factors. There was no evidence of an association of *PIK3CA* mutations with histological grade, FIGO stage, lymph node metastasis, and ER/PgR status. These data are in striking contrast to those of breast carcinoma, showing that *PIK3CA* mutations correlate with expression of hormone receptors and node metastasis, and are mutually exclusive with loss of PTEN expression. However, 2/8 (25%) *PTEN* mutant breast carcinomas also

possessed *PIK3CA* mutations, suggesting that coexistence of *PTEN/PIK3CA* mutations could occur in other tumors as well (Oda et al. 2005).

Coexistence of mutations in both *PTEN* and *PIK3CA* may imply that more than one input activating the PI3K/Akt pathway is required to completely activate this pathway in endometrial cancers, but not in melanoma. In breast carcinoma, *PIK3CA* mutations correlate with ErbB2 overexpression, suggesting that another activating event may be necessary to fully activate the PI3K pathway. Alternatively, either PTEN or p110α may possess additional function(s) distinct from the PI3K pathway.

DEVELOPMENT OF SORAFENIB/NEXAVAR, A Raf KINASE INHIBITOR

In 1992, the drug discovery group at ONYX Pharmaceuticals screened a library of compounds for inhibitors of Raf-1 kinase activity. As a source of active kinase for this screen, Raf-1 was expressed in Sf9 cells using baculovirus vectors. The protein had been engineered with an epitope tag to facilitate purification, and cells were co-infected with a vector expressing v-src to activate Raf-1 kinase. A compound that was selective for Raf-1 was identified and a medicinal chemistry program was initiated to identify derivatives with improved properties. The compound shown in Figure 4, first referred to as BAY43-9006, then Sorafenib, entered Phase I clinical trials in 2000. At that time, it was assumed that inhibition of Raf kinase in cancer cells would reverse aspects of the transformed phenotype. This assumption was based on experimental systems in which Raf kinase was inhibited using microinjected antibodies or dominant negative constructs. These approaches suggested that Raf kinase is an appropriate target for intervention, but did not predict side effects through Raf inhibition in normal tissue, and did not predict the consequences of blocking Ras in cancers in vivo. Furthermore, it was not clear whether Raf kinase is activated in tumors that do not harbor oncogenic Ras alleles. For these reasons, Phase I trials were launched for all types of cancers, without bias toward cancers with high frequencies of Ras mutation. During these trials, stabilization of disease was noted in patients suffering from renal cell carcinoma, a disease with no obvious association with activated Raf kinase. At this time, the specificity of Sorafenib/Nexavar was scrutinized, and a potent effect on VEGF-R2 was observed: This may well account for clinical effects in renal cell carcinoma, since this disease is associated with activated VEGF signaling through loss of the VHL tumor suppressor (Wilhelm et al. 2004). After completion in 2005 of a successful Phase III trial, in which a significant improvement in time to progression was reported, Nexavar was approved in the U.S. for treatment of metastatic renal cell carcinoma (Fig. 5).

In 2002, existence of BRAF mutations in human cancers was first reported. Activation frequencies approaching 70% were detected in malignant melanoma, and significant frequencies in several other human cancers (Davies et al. 2002). On the basis of these discoveries,

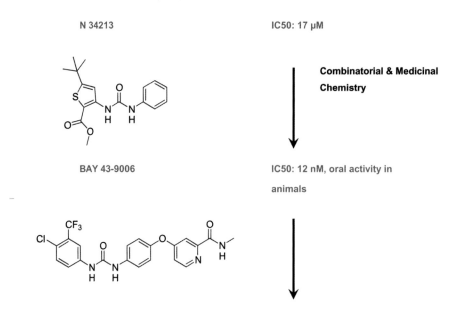

N 34213   IC50: 17 µM

                                           Combinatorial & Medicinal
                                           Chemistry

BAY 43-9006   IC50: 12 nM, oral activity in

                                           animals

                                           Phase I clinical trials, July 2000

Figure 4. Structure of the lead compound identified in a screen for Raf kinase inhibitors, and structure of Sorafenib.

clinical trials were initiated in which Nexavar was tested in patients suffering from malignant melanoma. To date, little clinical activity has been observed as a single agent, however, even though the drug appeared to hit the target effectively, i.e., MEK phosphorylation was blocked significantly. Lack of efficacy could be because (1) late-stage melanomas may no longer be Raf-dependent; (2) Raf inhibition causes growth arrest, but not apoptosis; or (3) the drug is not potent enough. Relating perhaps to the second point, BRAF mutations frequently coexist with PTEN mutations, as described above. Loss of PTEN has been reported to render other targeted therapies ineffective, presumably because cells in which PI3′K has been up-regulated are more difficult to kill. Nevertheless, Nexavar is currently being tested in combination therapies and as a single agent in multiple disease indications. However, the clinical value of blocking the Ras or Raf pathway remains uncertain.

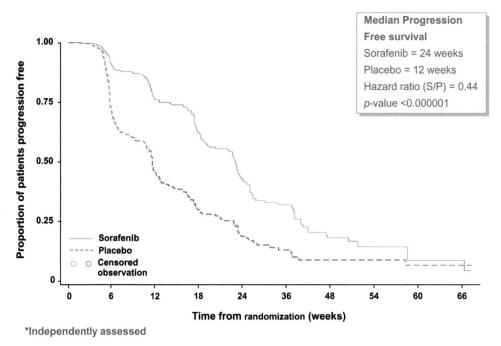

Median Progression Free survival
Sorafenib = 24 weeks
Placebo = 12 weeks
Hazard ratio (S/P) = 0.44
p-value <0.000001

*Independently assessed

Figure 5. Increased survival in patients treated with Sorafenib/Nexavar as an orally active single agent, in patients suffering from renal cell carcinoma.

CONCLUSIONS

Ras proteins and their downstream effectors play direct causal roles in human cancer. Analysis of mutations in these pathways reveals that the MAPK pathway and the PI3K pathways are activated frequently in cancers, in addition to K-Ras, and, to a lesser degree, N-Ras and H-Ras. To date, only one drug (Nexavar) targeting the Ras pathway has been approved for cancer treatment, but a number of others are under development. The clinical value of targeting these pathways remains unclear, since Nexavar was approved for treatment of renal cell cancer based, most likely, on its activity against VEGF-R2 rather than Raf kinase. However, we expect that single agents and combinations of agents targeting key enzymes in these pathways will play a powerful role in cancer treatment in the future, and that their successful clinical development will depend on a clear understanding of the complexities of the entire Ras pathway.

REFERENCES

Ahmadian M.R., Zor T., Vogt D., Kabsch W., Selinger Z., Wittinghofer A., and Scheffzek K. 1999. Guanosine triphosphatase stimulation of oncogenic Ras mutants. *Proc. Natl. Acad. Sci.* **96:** 7065.

Albanese C., Johnson J., Watanabe G., Eklund N., Vu D., Arnold A., and Pestell R.G. 1995. Transforming p21ras mutants and c-Ets-2 activate the cyclin D1 promoter through distinguishable regions. *J. Biol. Chem.* **270:** 23589.

Aoki Y., Niihori T., Kawame H., Kurosawa K., Ohashi H., Tanaka Y., Filocamo M., Kato K., Suzuki Y., Kure S., and Matsubara Y. 2005. Germline mutations in HRAS proto-oncogene cause Costello syndrome. *Nat. Genet.* **37:** 1038.

Bakiri L., Lallemand D., Bossy-Wetzel E., and Yaniv M. 2000. Cell cycle-dependent variations in c-Jun and JunB phosphorylation: A role in the control of cyclin D1 expression. *EMBO J.* **19:** 2056.

Bastian B.C., LeBoit P.E., and Pinkel D. 2001. Genomic approaches to skin cancer diagnosis. *Arch. Dermatol.* **137:** 1507.

Bourne H.R., Sanders D.A., and McCormick F. 1991. The GTPase superfamily: Conserved structure and molecular mechanism. *Nature* **349:** 117.

Davies H., Bignell G.R., Cox C., Stephens P., Edkins S., Clegg S., Teague J., Woffendin H., Garnett M.J., Bottomley W., Davis N., Dicks E., Ewing R., Floyd Y., Gray K., Hall S., Hawes R., Hughes J., Kosmidou V., Menzies A., Mould C., Parker A., Stevens C., Watt S., Hooper S., Wilson R., Jayatilake H., Gusterson B.A., Cooper C., Shipley J., Hargrave D., Pritchard-Jones K., Maitland N., Chevenix-Trench G., Riggins G.J., Bigner D.D., Palmieri G., Cossu A., Flanagan A., Nicholson A., Ho J.W., Leung S.Y., Yuen S.T., Weber B.L., Seigler H.F., Darrow T.L., Paterson H., Marais R., Marshall C.J., Wooster R., Stratton M.R., and Futreal P.A. 2002. Mutations of the BRAF gene in human cancer. *Nature* **417:** 949.

Esteban L.M., Vicario-Abejon C., Fernandez-Salguero P., Fernandez-Medarde A., Swaminathan N., Yienger K., Lopez E., Malumbres M., McKay R., Ward J.M., Pellicer A., and Santos E. 2001. Targeted genomic disruption of H-ras and N-ras, individually or in combination, reveals the dispensability of both loci for mouse growth and development. *Mol. Cell. Biol.* **21:** 1444.

Estep A.L., Tidyman W.E., Teitell M.A., Cotter P.D., and Rauen K.A. 2006. HRAS mutations in Costello syndrome: Detection of constitutional activating mutations in codon 12 and 13 and loss of wild-type allele in malignancy. *Am. J. Med. Genet. A* **140:** 8.

Gripp K.W., Lin A.E., Stabley D.L., Nicholson L., Scott C.I., Jr., Doyle D., Aoki Y., Matsubara Y., Zackai E.H., Lapunzina P., Gonzalez-Meneses A., Holbrook J., Agresta C.A., Gonzalez I.L., and Sol-Church K. 2006. HRAS mutation analysis in Costello syndrome: Genotype and phenotype correlation. *Am. J. Med. Genet. A* **140:** 1.

Guttridge D.C., Albanese C., Reuther J.Y., Pestell R.G., and Baldwin A.S., Jr. 1999. NF-kappaB controls cell growth and differentiation through transcriptional regulation of cyclin D1. *Mol. Cell. Biol.* **19:** 5785.

Hinz M., Krappmann D., Eichten A., Heder A., Scheidereit C., and Strauss M. 1999. NF-kappaB function in growth control: Regulation of cyclin D1 expression and G0/G1-to-S-phase transition. *Mol. Cell. Biol.* **19:** 2690.

Hulit J., Wang C., Li Z., Albanese C., Rao M., Di Vizio D., Shah S., Byers S.W., Mahmood R., Augenlicht L.H., Russell R., and Pestell R.G. 2004. Cyclin D1 genetic heterozygosity regulates colonic epithelial cell differentiation and tumor number in ApcMin mice. *Mol. Cell. Biol.* **24:** 7598.

Johnson L., Greenbaum D., Cichowski K., Mercer K., Murphy E., Schmitt E., Bronson R.T., Umanoff H., Edelmann W., Kucherlapati R., and Jacks T. 1997. K-ras is an essential gene in the mouse with partial functional overlap with N-ras. *Genes. Dev.* **11:** 2468.

Kerr B., Delrue M-A., Sigaudy S., Perveen R., Marche M., Burgelin I., Stef M., Tang B., Eden T., O'Sullivan J., De Sandre-Giovannoli A., Reardon W., Brewer C., Bennett C., Quarrell O., McCann E., Donnai D., Stewart F., Hennekam R., Cave H., Verloes A., Philip N., Lacombe D., Levy N., Arveiler B., and Black G. 2006. Genotype-phenotype correlation in Costello syndrome; HRAS mutation analysis in 43 cases. *J. Med. Genet.* (in press).

Lepourcelet M., Chen Y.N., France D.S., Wang H., Crews P., Petersen F., Bruseo C., Wood A.W., and Shivdasani R.A. 2004. Small-molecule antagonists of the oncogenic Tcf/beta-catenin protein complex. *Cancer Cell* **5:** 91.

Oda K., Stokoe D., Taketani Y., and McCormick F. 2005. High frequency of coexistent mutations of PIK3CA and PTEN genes in endometrial carcinoma. *Cancer Res.* **65:** 10669.

Rodriguez-Viciana P., Sabatier C., and McCormick F. 2004. Signaling specificity by Ras family GTPases is determined by the full spectrum of effectors they regulate. *Mol. Cell. Biol.* **24:** 4943.

Rodriguez-Viciana P., Tetsu O., Tidyman W.E., Estep A.L., Conger B.A., Santa Cruz M., McCormick F., and Rauen K.A. 2006. Germline mutations in genes within the MAPK pathway cause cardio-facio-cutaneous syndrome. *Science* **311:** 1287.

Schubbert S., Zenker M., Rowe S.L., Boll S., Klein C., Bollag G., van der Burgt I., Musante L., Kalscheuer V., Wehner L.E., Nguyen H., West B., Zhang K.Y., Sistermans E., Rauch A., Niemeyer C.M., Shannon K., and Kratz C.P. 2006. Germline KRAS mutations cause Noonan syndrome. *Nat. Genet.* **38:** 331.

Tetsu O. and McCormick F. 1999. Beta-catenin regulates expression of cyclin D1 in colon carcinoma cells. *Nature* **398:** 422.

Wilhelm S.M., Carter C., Tang L., Wilkie D., McNabola A., Rong H., Chen C., Zhang X., Vincent P., McHugh M., Cao Y., Shujath J., Gawlak S., Eveleigh D., Rowley B., Liu L., Adnane L., Lynch M., Auclair D., Taylor I., Gedrich R., Voznesensky A., Riedl B., Post L.E., Bollag G., and Trail P.A. 2004. BAY 43-9006 exhibits broad spectrum oral antitumor activity and targets the RAF/MEK/ERK pathway and receptor tyrosine kinases involved in tumor progression and angiogenesis. *Cancer Res.* **64:** 7099.

Wittinghofer A. and Pai E.F. 1991. The structure of Ras protein: A model for a universal molecular switch. *Trends Biochem. Sci.* **16:** 382.

Subversion of the Bcl-2 Life/Death Switch in Cancer Development and Therapy

J.M. Adams, D.C.S. Huang, A. Strasser, S. Willis, L. Chen, A. Wei, M. Van Delft,
J.I. Fletcher, H. Puthalakath, J. Kuroda, E.M. Michalak, P.N. Kelly,
P. Bouillet, A. Villunger,* L. O'Reilly, M.L. Bath, D.P. Smith,
A. Egle, A.W. Harris, M. Hinds, P. Colman, and S. Cory

The Walter and Eliza Hall Institute of Medical Research, Melbourne, Victoria, Australia 3050

The Bcl-2 protein family, which largely determines commitment to apoptosis, has central roles in tumorigenesis and chemoresistance. Its three factions of interacting proteins include the BH3-only proteins (e.g., Bim, Puma, Bad, Noxa), which transduce diverse cytotoxic signals to the mammalian pro-survival proteins (Bcl-2, Bcl-x_L, Bcl-w, Mcl-1, A-1), whereas Bax and Bak, when freed from pro-survival constraint, provoke the mitochondrial permeabilization that triggers apoptosis. We have discovered unexpected specificity in their interactions. Only Bim and Puma, which mediate multiple cytotoxic signals, engage all the pro-survival proteins. Noxa and Bad instead bind subsets and cooperate in killing, indicating that apoptosis requires neutralization of different pro-survival subsets. Furthermore, Mcl-1 and Bcl-x_L, but not Bcl-2, directly sequester Bak in healthy cells, and Bak is freed only when BH3-only proteins neutralize both its guards. BH3-only proteins such as Bim are tumor suppressors and mediate many of the cytotoxic signals from anticancer agents. Hence, compounds mimicking them may prove valuable for therapy. Indeed, the recently described ABT-737 is a promising "BH3 mimetic" of Bad. We find that, like Bad, ABT-737 kills cells efficiently only if Mcl-1 is absent or down-regulated. Thus, manipulation of apoptosis by targeting the Bcl-2 family has exciting potential for cancer treatment.

In 1988, the *bcl-2* gene, which had been identified earlier as a novel gene translocated in follicular lymphoma to an immunoglobulin locus, was shown to act by preventing cell death rather than by driving cell proliferation (Vaux et al. 1988). This discovery engendered the now widely accepted concept that impairment of apoptosis is a central step in the development of cancer (Hanahan and Weinberg 2000). The apoptotic defect can, as in follicular lymphoma, be due to overexpression of Bcl-2, but more commonly results from mutations that ablate function of the p53 tumor suppressor, which acts upstream of Bcl-2. Particularly pertinent to this paper, it is now recognized that the resulting defects in apoptotic signaling reduce the efficacy of conventional cytotoxic therapy for cancer. Nevertheless, since the core apoptotic machinery remains intact in tumors, the cancer cell does remain vulnerable to many cytotoxic signals. Indeed, paradoxically, the multiple aberrations in the cell cycle circuitry and control of differentiation of the tumor cell probably render it more vulnerable than its normal counterpart. Hence, improved understanding of apoptotic pathways should lead to more rational and more effective ways to treat cancer, including the prospect of directly engaging the apoptotic machinery by targeting Bcl-2 and its close relatives (Cory and Adams 2002, 2005; Cory et al. 2003).

The cell's decision to commit suicide in response to developmental cues, to physiological signals such as cytokine deprivation, and to diverse forms of intracellular stress, including those imposed by chemotherapeutic agents and radiation, is primarily determined by the Bcl-2 family of interacting proteins (Cory and Adams 2002; Cory et al. 2003; Danial and Korsmeyer 2004). These proteins are thought to control this "intrinsic" pathway to death primarily by regulating the integrity of intracellular membranes, including the outer membrane of the mitochondrion. When that membrane is permeabilized, apoptogenic proteins such as cytochrome *c* leach out and provoke the scaffold protein Apaf-1 to assemble with pro-caspase-9 into the "apoptosome," which then processes the effector caspases (-3, -6, and -7) that cleave numerous proteins to mediate cell demolition. Bcl-2 has much less impact on the separate "extrinsic" apoptotic pathway from death receptors such as TNF or Fas; that pathway leads to activation of initiator caspase-8, which can bypass the mitochondrion in many cell types by direct activation of the effector caspases (Strasser et al. 1995, 2000; Huang et al. 1999).

In mammals, the propensity of cells to undergo suicide is set primarily by the interactions of three factions of the Bcl-2 family (Cory and Adams 2002; Cory et al. 2003). The five pro-survival proteins (Bcl-2, Bcl-x_L, Bcl-w, Mcl-1, and A1) are opposed by two pro-apoptotic groups. Members of the first group, Bax and Bak, are structurally similar to Bcl-2 and bear three "BH" (*Bcl-2 Homology*) domains, whereas the diverse members of the other group share with each other and the rest of the family only the ~16-amino-acid-residue BH3 interaction domain. When activated by a cytotoxic signal, these "BH3-only proteins," which include Bim, Puma, Noxa, Bid, Bik, Hrk, Bad, and Bmf, engage pro-survival relatives by inserting the BH3 domain into a hydrophobic groove on their surface. The resulting neutralization of pro-survival function

---

*Present address: The Innsbruck Medical University, Biocenter, Division of Pathophysiology, Innsbruck, Austria.

somehow allows Bax and Bak to oligomerize in the mitochondrial outer membrane and thereby provoke its permeabilization.

We are exploring how the interaction of different Bcl-2 family members triggers the cell death switch, how this protein family regulates tissue homeostasis, how disruption of that regulation promotes tumorigenesis, and how impaired apoptosis affects cancer therapy. We briefly review these issues here and emphasize our recent findings on the roles of BH3-only proteins in transmission of specific death signals, evidence for specificity in interaction of family members, and our new model for the regulation of Bak. Finally, we discuss recent findings that highlight the therapeutic prospects for targeting the Bcl-2 family with small molecules.

BH3-ONLY MEDIATORS OF CYTOTOXIC SIGNALS

As reviewed elsewhere (Huang and Strasser 2000; Bouillet and Strasser 2002; Puthalakath and Strasser 2002; Strasser 2005), the BH3-only proteins are sensors and transducers of multiple cytotoxic insults. Presumably, their multiplicity has evolved to allow exquisite control over cell death. For example, Bim and Bmf are regulated in part by sequestration to the cytoskeleton. Thus, Bim can be sequestered by dynein motor complexes to the microtubules (Puthalakath et al. 1999), and Bmf by the myosin V complex to the actin cytoskeleton (Puthalakath et al. 2001). Interestingly, Bim is unleashed in response to paclitaxel (Taxol), which affects microtubules, whereas Bmf can be activated by loss of cell attachment to the matrix (anoikis) (Puthalakath et al. 2001) and by treatment with HDAC inhibitors (Zhang et al. 2005). Thus, certain BH3-only proteins seem to represent sentinels positioned to register stress to specific subcellular compartments. To enable responses to other cytotoxic cues, however, these proteins are controlled in multiple ways. Bim, for example, can be regulated at the transcriptional level, by phosphorylation and by protein turnover (Bouillet and Strasser 2002; Puthalakath and Strasser 2002; Akiyama et al. 2003).

Disruption of the genes encoding BH3-only proteins has provided important insights into their physiological functions. Mice deficient in Bim have been particularly informative. Their defects have revealed that Bim is critical for removing superfluous hematopoietic cells, for apoptosis induced by cytokine deprivation, and for prevention of autoimmunity (Bouillet et al. 1999). Indeed, Bim has proven to be crucial in eliminating lymphocytes that recognize self-antigens, including both developing T cells in the thymus (Bouillet et al. 2002) and B cells emerging in the bone marrow (Enders et al. 2003). Remarkably, Bim is also required to eliminate activated peripheral T cells (Hildeman et al. 2002), to terminate immune responses (Pellegrini et al. 2003), and to ensure the normal death of granulocytes (Villunger et al. 2003a) and osteoclasts (Akiyama et al. 2003).

We think that tissue homeostasis is regulated largely by the balance between BH3-only proteins and Bcl-2 pro-survival family members. As reviewed elsewhere (Marsden and Strasser 2003; Strasser 2005), cytokines are major reg-

ulators of cell survival in vivo, and it is notable that the lymphopenia provoked by loss of the interleukin-7 receptor can be overcome by either overexpression of Bcl-2 (Maraskovsky et al. 1997) or loss of Bim (Pellegrini et al. 2004). Furthermore, excess leukocytes are found in mice that either overexpress Bcl-2 in the hematopoietic compartment (Ogilvy et al. 1999) or lack Bim (Bouillet et al. 1999). These findings suggested that Bim might be a dominant antagonist of Bcl-2 during hematopoiesis. Since loss of Bcl-2 had been shown to produce attrition in several cell compartments (Veis et al. 1993), including lymphocytes, we tested whether concomitant loss of Bim would compensate. Indeed, the degenerative disorders provoked by Bcl-2 loss, including a fatal polycystic kidney disease, were precluded by loss of even one allele of Bim, and lymphocyte numbers were restored (Bouillet et al. 2001).

The apoptosis provoked by DNA damage requires the p53 tumor suppressor, and this is thought to be a key component of its tumor suppressor function (Vousden and Lu 2002). A number of the targets of this transcription factor had been implicated in apoptosis, but it was unclear which was required, or indeed whether any single one could mediate this function. Two genes induced by p53, *noxa* and *puma* (*bbc3*), attracted our attention because they were known to encode BH3-only proteins. We tested their roles by knocking out each of the genes. In cells from mice with either *noxa* or *puma* disrupted, we observed decreased DNA damage-induced apoptosis in fibroblasts, and loss of Puma greatly protected lymphocytes from cell death after genotoxic damage (Villunger et al. 2003b). Remarkably, Puma-deficient lymphocytes proved nearly as refractory to DNA damage as those lacking p53 itself (Jeffers et al. 2003; Villunger et al. 2003b). Hence, the apoptosis of lymphocytes after DNA damage is accounted for almost exclusively by the transcriptional activation of Puma. Noxa appears to have an analogous, albeit more restricted, role in other cell types such as fibroblasts (Shibue et al. 2003; Villunger et al. 2003b).

Such findings have led us to propose that most, if not all, cytotoxic responses are mediated through one or more BH3-only protein (Fig. 1). Thus, specific cytotoxic responses are impaired in cells from mice lacking Bid (Yin et al. 1999), Bim (Bouillet et al. 1999, 2002; Hildeman et al. 2002; Enders et al. 2003; Pellegrini et al. 2003; Villunger et al. 2003a, 2004), Noxa (Shibue et al. 2003; Villunger et al. 2003b), and Puma (Jeffers et al. 2003; Villunger et al. 2003b). For example, deficiency of Bim protects lymphocytes against cytokine withdrawal, paclitaxel, and deregulated calcium flux and gives a small but significant reduction in apoptosis induced by γ-radiation or glucocorticoids but has no impact on apoptosis triggered by phorbol esters (Bouillet et al. 1999). In contrast, loss of Puma protects lymphoid cells against DNA damage, phorbol ester, glucocorticoids, and cytokine withdrawal but has no impact on apoptosis induced by calcium flux (Jeffers et al. 2003; Villunger et al. 2003b). Due to the varying expression patterns of these proteins, however, the cell types in which they carry out essential functions may well differ. Accordingly, Bim plays a more critical role in hematopoietic cells (Bouillet et al. 1999) than in neurons, where it is also expressed (Putcha et al. 2001).

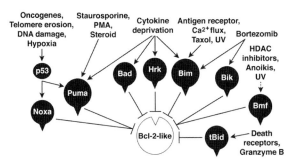

Figure 1. Cytotoxic signals conveyed by different BH3-only proteins. The indicated roles of Bim, Puma, Noxa, Bad, and Bid are based on impairment of the specific cytotoxic signals in cells from mice with a knockout of the corresponding gene. The inferred roles for the others are based on other types of data, such as increased expression in cells subjected to that stimulus. The "beak" on the BH3-only molecules denotes the BH3 domain. It should be noted that the involvement of specific BH3-only proteins varies somewhat in different cell types. For example, Hrk expression is restricted to neuronal cells.

The BH3-only proteins have been generally assumed to interact promiscuously with all the pro-survival proteins, but recently we have unexpectedly found that most exhibit notable selectivity (Chen et al. 2005). Quantitative analysis using an optical biosensor to determine the affinity of various BH3 peptides for the five Bcl-2-like proteins revealed that the interactions varied more than 10,000-fold in affinity. Bim and Puma avidly engaged all five pro-survival proteins, but the other BH3-only proteins showed preferences. Most strikingly, Bad bound tightly to Bcl-2, Bcl-x$_L$, and Bcl-w but not to Mcl-1 or A1, whereas Noxa instead bound only Mcl-1 and A1 (Fig. 2A).

Importantly, the binding data correlated with pro-apoptotic activity. Bim and Puma, which bind all the pro-survival proteins, potently induced apoptosis, whereas ones

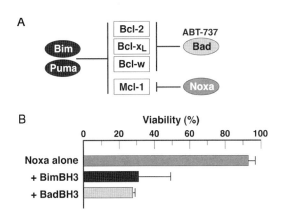

Figure 2. Specificity in the association of BH3-only proteins with pro-survival family members and the consequences for pro-apoptotic activity. (*A*) Different BH3-only proteins interact with particular subsets of the pro-survival proteins (Chen et al. 2005). The BH3 mimetic ABT-737 has a binding profile similar to that of Bad (see text). (*B*) Noxa and Bad exhibit synergy in killing fibroblasts. Each on its own has only weak killing activity, but the combination of Noxa, which interacts only with Mcl-1 in fibroblasts (where A1 is not expressed), and Bad, which neutralizes only Bcl-2, Bcl-x$_L$, and Bcl-w, is as potent as Bim. This synergy suggests that killing requires neutralization of more than one subset of the pro-survival proteins. A likely explanation is that both Mcl-1 and Bcl-x$_L$ can prevent Bak activation (see Fig. 4).

that bind only a subset of them (e.g., Bad, Noxa) were considerably weaker killers (Chen et al. 2005). This finding probably explains why cells that lack Bim or Puma exhibit much more marked defects in apoptosis than cells lacking one of the other BH3-only proteins (Fig. 1). Notably, however, Bad and Noxa, which bind complementary targets, cooperated to induce potent killing (Fig. 2B). We therefore think that apoptosis usually requires neutralizing more than one type of pro-survival protein.

The basis for binding specificity of specific BH3 domains is becoming clearer as more structures of these proteins emerge, such as a high-resolution view of Bim bound to Bcl-x$_L$ (Liu et al. 2003) and the structures we have determined for Bcl-w (Hinds et al. 2003) and Mcl-1 (Day et al. 2005). Consideration of these structures allowed us to identify two mutations to the Noxa BH3 peptide that greatly increased its binding to Bcl-x$_L$ (Chen et al. 2005). Such findings have significant implications for the search for BH3 mimetic drugs (see below).

SEQUESTRATION MODEL FOR Bak REGULATION

Activation of Bax or Bak is essential for apoptosis in most if not all cells (Lindsten et al. 2000), and both clearly act downstream of the BH3-only proteins (Cheng et al. 2001; Zong et al. 2001), but how the pro-survival proteins prevent activation of Bak and Bax has remained controversial (Adams 2003). Although Bax and Bak have largely redundant function, their regulation must differ significantly, because Bak resides in the mitochondrial membrane of healthy cells, whereas Bax is cytosolic prior to a death signal, probably because in healthy cells its hydrophobic carboxy-terminal membrane anchor is buried within a surface groove (Suzuki et al. 2000).

We have recently explored the activation of Bak and have proposed that Bak is normally sequestered by two specific pro-survival Bcl-2 family members (Willis et al. 2005). Importantly, in healthy cells we found that Bak associates directly with both Mcl-1 and Bcl-x$_L$, but not with Bcl-2, Bcl-w, or A1 (Willis et al. 2005). The interaction requires the BH3 of Bak (Fig. 3), so that domain presum-

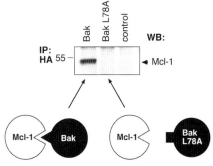

Figure 3. Bak binds to Mcl-1 via its BH3 domain. Replacement of a critical conserved leucine residue in the Bak BH3 by alanine (L78A) eliminates binding to Mcl-1 (Willis et al. 2005). Wild-type Bak and the L78A mutant, both tagged with the HA epitope, were immunoprecipitated (IP) from transfected cells, or control untransfected cells, and a western blot (WB) was performed with an Mcl-1 antibody.

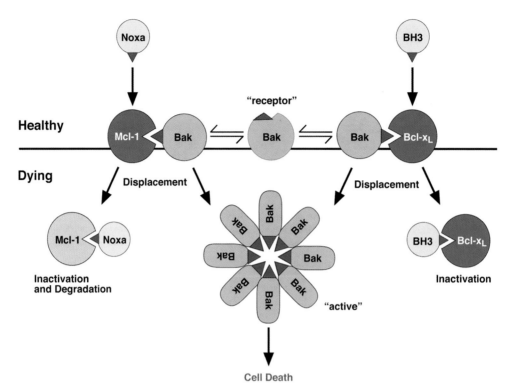

Figure 4. Model for the regulation of Bak. The essence of the model (Willis et al. 2005) is that, in healthy cells, at least a portion of Bak exists in the mitochondrial outer membrane in a form bound to Mcl-1 and Bcl-x$_L$, via the BH3 (*red beak*) of Bak. Bak can be released for death duty only by BH3-only proteins that engage both Mcl-1 (e.g., Noxa) and Bcl-x$_L$ (e.g., Bad). Bak may then aggregate into a form (as yet unknown) that permeabilizes the mitochondrial outer membrane, provoking release of apoptogenic proteins such as cytochrome *c* that induce caspase activation. We speculate that some of the Bak molecules may normally remain in a "receptor" conformer to account for the observation that Bak oligomerization also requires the Bak BH3 domain (Willis et al. 2005). (Reprinted, with permission, from Willis et al. 2005.)

ably fits into the groove on Mcl-1 and Bcl-x$_L$. Indeed, a Bak BH3 peptide binds avidly to both of these pro-survival proteins but not to the others (Willis et al. 2005). When cytotoxic signals activate BH3-only proteins that can engage both Mcl-1 and Bcl-x$_L$, the BH3-only proteins displace Bak (Fig. 4). Accordingly, Noxa can bind to Mcl-1 and displace Bak, but Bak-mediated cell death also requires neutralization of Bcl-x$_L$ by other BH3-only proteins, such as Bad. Hence, Noxa can kill mouse embryonic fibroblasts lacking Bcl-xL but not those lacking Bcl-2 (Willis et al. 2005).

We were intrigued to find that Noxa not only displaces Mcl-1 from Bak, but also triggers Mcl-1 degradation in a proteasome-dependent manner (Willis et al. 2005). Interestingly, Mcl-1 degradation in response to genotypic damage apparently also involves a newly described ubiquitin E3 ligase (denoted Mule for *M*cl-1 *u*biquitin *l*igase *E*3) (Zhong et al. 2005). Notably, Mule possesses a BH3 domain similar to Bak, allowing its specific association with Mcl-1 and not other Bcl-2 family members. At present, it is unclear whether Mule acts downstream of Noxa, perhaps displacing Mcl-1 from Noxa, or whether Noxa and Mule instead lie on two independent pathways to Mcl-1 destruction by the proteasome.

Our observations suggest that Bak is held in check solely by Mcl-1 and Bcl-x$_L$ and induces apoptosis if, and only if, released from both its guards (Fig. 4). Once freed

from them, Bak may spontaneously associate with itself to induce the damage to intracellular membranes that elicits cell death. The mechanism by which Bak (or Bax) aggregates in the membrane is not known, but we found that it required the Bak BH3 domain (Willis et al. 2005). That observation may mean that a key step in the oligomerization of Bak (and perhaps also of Bax) is formation of Bak–Bak homodimers in which a Bak molecule with an exposed BH3 domain has inserted it into the groove on another molecule of Bak that retains a "receptor" conformation (Fig. 4).

THE Bcl-2 FAMILY IN TUMORIGENESIS

As reviewed elsewhere (Cory and Adams 2002; Cory et al. 2003), pro-survival family members such as Bcl-2 and Bcl-x$_L$ are overexpressed in many human tumors, and transgenic mouse models have provided compelling direct evidence that their overexpression contributes to neoplasia. Overexpression of Bcl-2 in the B-lymphocyte compartment, for example, was shown over a decade ago to provoke a marked expansion of nonproliferating B cells (McDonnell et al. 1989; Strasser et al. 1991), and tumors developed rapidly when a cooperating oncogene such as c-*myc* was coexpressed (Strasser et al. 1990). The tumors provoked by Bcl-2 alone arose only after a protracted period and comprised pre-B lymphomas and plasmacytomas, many of which exhibited c-*myc* translocations (McDonnell and Korsmeyer 1991; Strasser et al. 1993).

Given the original link of translocated human *BCL2* with follicular lymphoma, it was surprising that the Ig enhancer-driven *BCL2* transgene did not yield that tumor type. Recently, however, mice bearing a transgene that imposed overexpression of Bcl-2 throughout the hematopoietic compartment (Ogilvy et al. 1999) have yielded the first animal model of follicular lymphoma (Egle et al. 2004b). Intriguingly, these B-lymphoid tumors were preceded by grossly enlarged germinal centers, development of which required help from the expanded pool of CD4 T cells produced by this transgene. As these mice are also subject to autoimmune disease, it seems likely that antigenic or autoimmune stimulation through the B-cell antigen receptor plays a critical role in development of the tumors. It is therefore tempting to think that antigenic stimulation also has a role in human follicular lymphoma, as some other evidence has previously suggested (Zelenetz et al. 1992).

Since Bcl-2 pro-survival family members are oncoproteins, we wanted to determine whether their BH3-only antagonists can act as tumor suppressors. Bim was of particular interest because it is a major antagonist of Bcl-2 in the lymphoid compartment (Bouillet et al. 2001). Since overexpression of Bcl-2 markedly increases the rate of tumor development in our well-studied Eμ-*myc* transgenic mice (Strasser et al. 1990), we tested whether loss of Bim would act similarly. Indeed, loss of even a single allele of Bim accelerated tumorigenesis (Egle et al. 2004a). Because the acceleration primarily reflected leukemia of mature B cells, the tumor suppressor role of Bim may be confined to particular stages of development. Pertinently, homozygous deletions of the human *BIM* locus have now been found in a significant fraction of human mantle cell lymphomas (Tagawa et al. 2005).

Significantly, Bim appears to act as a tumor suppressor by mediating the apoptosis induced by Myc under suboptimal growth conditions. In lymphocytes, overexpressed Myc appears to lower the threshold for apoptosis by reducing levels of Bcl-x_L and Bcl-2 while elevating those of Bim (Egle et al. 2004a). Thus, Bim deficiency presumably contributes to oncogenesis by allowing more B-lineage cells to survive in the face of overexpressed Myc, just as does loss of p53 in cells that retain Bim. Accordingly, most of the tumors from the Bim-deficient cells retained p53 function, whereas most of those arising in Bim-proficient cells have lost p53 function.

To better gauge how oncogene activation affects cell survival and tumorigenesis in different cell lineages, we have characterized transgenic mouse strains with Myc expressed in most hematopoietic cells (Smith et al. 2005). Surprisingly, the type of tumors that arise depends on the level of Myc (D.P. Smith et al., in prep.).

IMPLICATIONS OF APOPTOTIC REGULATION FOR CYTOTOXIC THERAPY

Cytotoxic therapy for cancer will undoubtedly benefit from a deeper understanding of how the Bcl-2 family is regulated, in particular from insights into the critical roles of specific BH3-only proteins in the responses to different chemotherapeutic agents (Fig. 1). For example, recent evidence indicates that the apoptosis induced in chronic myeloid leukemia cells by Gleevec (imatinib) relies in part on Bim (Kuribara et al. 2004). Indeed, we find that both Bim and Bad have critical roles in this response (J. Kuroda and A. Strasser, unpubl.).

A striking illustration of the way in which understanding of apoptotic mechanisms could affect future treatment strategies emerged from a recent collaborative study with Eileen White and colleagues. Just as we had reported with lymphocytes (Bouillet et al. 1999), the sensitivity of epithelial carcinoma cells to paclitaxel (Taxol) proved to require Bim (Tan et al. 2005). If the tumor cells contained an activated Ras oncogene, however, the cells were rendered refractory to paclitaxel, because excess Ras activity caused Bim to be targeted for proteasomal degradation. Nevertheless, Bim levels and sensitivity to paclitaxel could both be restored by addition of the clinically relevant proteasome inhibitor bortezomib (PS-341). These results provide a rational basis for combining paclitaxel and bortezomib in therapy, particularly in cells where the Ras pathway is active (Tan et al. 2005).

In the killing of some human cancer cell lines, bortezomib also exhibits synergy with TRAIL, a ligand for certain death receptors. A study with Andrew Kraft and colleagues revealed the likely basis for the synergy: Bortezomib provokes higher levels of Bik and/or Bim in the various lines, apparently by inhibiting their degradation (Nikrad et al. 2005). These findings indicate that combination chemotherapy may soon have a more rational foundation.

THERAPEUTIC POTENTIAL OF "BH3 MIMETICS"

As discussed elsewhere (Baell and Huang 2002; Cory et al. 2003; Cory and Adams 2005), because abnormalities in cancer cells, such as p53 mutations, disturb the transduction of cytotoxic signals to the Bcl-2 family (i.e., prevent Puma/Noxa induction), an anticancer drug that mimicked a BH3-only protein should be efficacious (Fig. 5). Two of our findings are pertinent to the design of such BH3 mimetics. First, our demonstration (Chen et al. 2005) of preferential binding by certain BH3 domains (Fig. 2A) suggests that it should eventually be feasible to target a specific Bcl-2-like protein, such as one needed to maintain a particular tumor type, or at least a subset of the pro-survival proteins. The specificity should increase the therapeutic index of a BH3 mimetic by reducing deleterious effects on normal tissues. Second, our evidence (Willis et al. 2005) that only Mcl-1 and Bcl-x_L guard Bak (Fig. 4) suggests that targeting these pro-survival proteins may be particularly effective, even in tumors that greatly overexpress Bcl-2. In view of the frequent overexpression of Bcl-2 in cancer cells, that could be a significant advantage.

Development of a small-molecule inhibitor of a protein–protein interaction is very challenging. As reviewed elsewhere (Baell and Huang 2002; Cory et al. 2003), several putative BH3 mimetics have been reported, but most

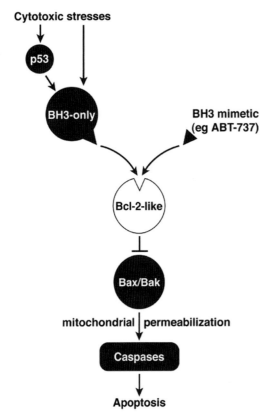

Figure 5. The potential of BH3 mimetic drugs. The action of many conventional cytotoxic drugs is blunted by mutations in tumor cells, such as those that prevent p53 function. Because the core apoptotic machinery remains intact in most tumors, engaging the pro-survival proteins in a fashion akin to their natural antagonists should prove an effective way to kill tumor cells.

ples, but also small-cell lung carcinoma (SCLC). Most strikingly, with xenografts of two different SCLC lines, ABT-737 at the highest dose tested induced stable regression of the tumors in 77% of the mice (Oltersdorf et al. 2005). Remarkably, the drug was tolerated well, the only adverse effects noted being some drop in lymphocytes and platelets.

In view of the considerable promise of ABT-737, we have been studying its mode of action (A. Wei et al., in prep.). As expected for an authentic BH3 mimetic, its ability to kill fibroblasts requires Bax or Bak. Its pro-apoptotic activity on wild-type fibroblasts, however, was relatively weak. Since the binding of ABT-737 to pro-survival proteins closely resembles that of Bad (Fig. 2A), we tested whether Noxa would augment killing by ABT-737, as it does with Bad (Fig. 2B), by engaging Mcl-1 and promoting its degradation (Willis et al. 2005). Indeed, fibroblasts overexpressing Noxa became far more sensitive to ABT-737. Furthermore, the enhanced activity was clearly mediated by the inactivation of Mcl-1, because RNAi against Mcl-1 as well as Noxa overexpression rendered two human tumor cell lines far more sensitive to ABT-737, as shown in Figure 6 for the breast cancer cell line MCF-7.

Because the level of Mcl-1 in hematopoietic cells is tightly regulated by cytokines, we tested whether cytokine deprivation would also augment killing by ABT-737. The test employed a cytokine-dependent myeloid cell line, FDC-P1, engineered to overexpress Bcl-2. Indeed, the starved cells were far more sensitive to the drug, despite the presence of abundant Bcl-2, which protects the untreated cells from death on cytokine deprivation. A likely explanation for the increased sensitivity is that the

of these compounds bind to their target with only micromolar affinity, whereas BH3 peptides bind with nanomolar affinity (Chen et al. 2005). That raises significant questions about their specificity. Since BH3-only proteins require either Bax or Bak to kill cells (Cheng et al. 2001; Zong et al. 2001), a true BH3 mimetic should not kill cells lacking both Bax and Bak. We find, however, that several compounds inferred to be BH3 mimetics but having low affinity for their putative targets kill $bax^{-/-}bak^{-/-}$ fibroblasts as readily as wild-type fibroblasts (A. Wei et al., in prep.). Hence, these compounds kill cells in a nonspecific manner.

As discussed further elsewhere (Cory and Adams 2005), strong proof of principle that BH3 mimetics have promise for cancer therapy has come very recently from Abbott Laboratories (Oltersdorf et al. 2005). By structure-based design with Bcl-x_L as a target, Oltersdorf et al. have developed a compound, denoted ABT-737, with high (low nM) affinity for Bcl-x_L, Bcl-2, and Bcl-w, albeit very poor affinity for Mcl-1 and A1. With many tumor cell lines, they report that ABT-737 displays strong synergy in inducing apoptosis with conventional chemotherapeutic agents, as well as γ-radiation. Moreover, as a single agent, ABT-737 kills tumor cells of certain types; intriguingly, the susceptible cells include not only follicular lymphoma and chronic lymphocytic leukemia sam-

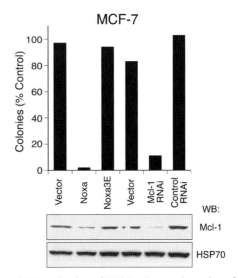

Figure 6. Neutralization of Mcl-1 enhances the action of BH3 mimetic ABT-737. MCF-7 breast carcinoma cells were infected with retroviruses expressing Noxa, which inactivates Mcl-1 and triggers its degradation (Willis et al. 2005), an inactive mutant of Noxa that does not bind Mcl-1 (Noxa3E), a siRNA against Mcl-1, or appropriate controls. The cells were then treated with ABT-737 (1 μM), and colonies were counted 7 days later. The western blot (WB) shows the reduced level of Mcl-1 produced by Noxa and the Mcl-1 RNAi.

cytokine deprivation both lowered the level of Mcl-1 and elevated that of Bim.

Since killing by ABT-737, like that by Bad, is greatly augmented if Mcl-1 is neutralized by Noxa or eliminated by RNAi, ABT-737 may prove most effective as a single agent in tumors with low or negligible levels of Mcl-1. Furthermore, its synergy with various chemotherapeutic agents and radiation probably reflects down-regulation of Mcl-1 by these agents (Cuconati et al. 2003; Nijhawan et al. 2003). In view of the results discussed above, the cytotoxic action of ABT-737 may be mediated preferentially through release of Bak (Fig. 4).

CONCLUSIONS

Impaired apoptosis is a central step in tumorigenesis. Although loss of p53 function is the most frequent cause, the Bcl-2 family probably contributes directly or indirectly in a significant proportion of human tumors. Over-expression of the pro-survival proteins, particularly Bcl-2, is frequent, and in some cell types, loss of a BH3-only antagonist such as Bim can have a similar effect. Gain of Bcl-2 or loss of Bim is tumorigenic in part because both counter the cell death impetus resulting from oncogene activation, such as constitutive Myc expression.

The eight or more BH3-only proteins appear to be the essential transducers of most cell death signals, including those elicited by most conventional cytotoxic agents (Fig. 1). Hence, better understanding of their specific roles and the complex ways they are regulated is likely to provide a more rational foundation for therapy, particularly combination chemotherapy, which remains highly empirical.

The interaction of BH3-only proteins with the pro-survival proteins exhibits more specificity than has generally been expected (Chen et al. 2005). Bim and Puma bind promiscuously to all the pro-survival proteins, and this may well account for their greater pro-apoptotic activity and the more marked apoptotic defects observed upon knockout of their genes (Fig. 1). The other BH3-only proteins, however, bind preferentially to different subsets, with Bad and Noxa engaging complementary groups (Fig. 2A). Since they also exhibit synergy in cell killing (Fig. 2B), we have suggested that commitment to apoptosis requires neutralization of more than one subset of the pro-survival proteins (Chen et al. 2005).

Insight into the issue of how the pro-survival family members regulate commitment to apoptosis has come from our studies on Bak regulation (Willis et al. 2005). To our surprise, Bak appears to be kept under control by only two of its pro-survival counterparts, Bcl-x$_L$ and Mcl-1, and Bcl-2 seems to have no role in guarding it (Fig. 4). In healthy cells, Bak molecules associate with these guardians via the Bak BH3 (Fig. 3). In our model, if both Bcl-x$_L$ and Mcl-1 are inactivated, Bak may spontaneously aggregate and trigger damage to the outer mitochondrial membrane and probably other membranes (Fig. 4). As yet, we do not know whether Bax is regulated somewhat similarly.

The recently developed BH3 mimetic ABT-737 (Oltersdorf et al. 2005), along with findings with certain constrained BH3 peptides (Walensky et al. 2004), has provided strong proof of principle that triggering apoptosis of tumor cells by directly engaging the pro-survival proteins (Fig. 5) represents a promising new approach to cancer therapy (Cory and Adams 2005). The binding profile of ABT-737 mimics that of Bad (Fig. 2A). Accordingly, we found that although the drug mediated Bax/Bak-dependent apoptosis, its potency was limited unless Mcl-1 was down-regulated (Fig. 6). Hence, we surmise that ABT-737 will prove most efficacious as a single agent in tumors in which Mcl-1 is low or absent. Its killing action is markedly enhanced, however, by treatments that provoke Mcl-1 down-regulation, such as exposure to conventional cytotoxic agents or cytokine deprivation. Thus, it may well prove efficacious on a wider range of tumors in combination with agents that down-regulate Mcl-1. The success of ABT-737 in preclinical mouse models (Oltersdorf et al. 2005) suggests that for many tumors the Bcl-2-guarded gateway to cell death is the Achilles' heel. Hence, BH3 mimetics seem destined to be valuable new weapons in the war on cancer.

ACKNOWLEDGMENTS

Our research is supported by a program grant from the National Health and Medical Research Council, a Specialized Center of Research grant from the Leukemia and Lymphoma Society, and project grants from the National Cancer Institute (CA43540 and CA80188). We thank Saul Rosenberg, Alex Shoemaker, and Steve Elmore from Abbott Laboratories for ABT-737 samples and for communicating their findings with it prior to publication.

REFERENCES

Adams J.M. 2003. Ways of dying: Multiple pathways to apoptosis. *Genes Dev.* **17:** 2481.

Akiyama T., Bouillet P., Miyazaki T., Kadono Y., Chikuda H., Chung U.I., Fukuda A., Hikita A., Seto H., Okada T., Inaba T., Sanjay A., Baron R., Kawaguchi H., Oda H., Nakamura K., Strasser A., and Tanaka S. 2003. Regulation of osteoclast apoptosis by ubiquitylation of proapoptotic BH3-only Bcl-2 family member Bim. *EMBO J.* **22:** 6653.

Baell J.B. and Huang D.C.S. 2002. Prospects for targeting the Bcl-2 family of proteins to develop novel cytotoxic drugs. *Biochem. Pharmacol.* **64:** 851.

Bouillet P. and Strasser A. 2002. BH3-only proteins—Evolutionarily conserved pro-apoptotic Bcl-2 family members essential for initiating programmed cell death. *J. Cell Sci.* **115:** 1567.

Bouillet P., Cory S., Zhang L.-C., Strasser A., and Adams J.M. 2001. Degenerative disorders caused by Bcl-2 deficiency are prevented by loss of its BH3-only antagonist Bim. *Dev. Cell* **1:** 645.

Bouillet P., Metcalf D., Huang D.C.S., Tarlinton D.M., Kay T.W.H., Köntgen F., Adams J.M., and Strasser A. 1999. Proapoptotic Bcl-2 relative Bim required for certain apoptotic responses, leukocyte homeostasis, and to preclude autoimmunity. *Science* **286:** 1735.

Bouillet P., Purton J.F., Godfrey D.I., Zhang L.-C., Coultas L., Puthalakath H., Pellegrini M., Cory S., Adams J.M., and Strasser A. 2002. BH3-only Bcl-2 family member Bim is required for apoptosis of autoreactive thymocytes. *Nature* **415:** 922.

Chen L., Willis S.N., Wei A., Smith B.J., Fletcher J.I., Hinds M.G., Colman P.M., Day C.L., Adams J.M., and Huang D.C.S. 2005. Differential targeting of pro-survival Bcl-2 proteins by their BH3-only ligands allows complementary apoptotic function. *Mol. Cell* 17: 393.

Cheng E.H., Wei M.C., Weiler S., Flavell R.A., Mak T.W., Lindsten T., and Korsmeyer S.J. 2001. BCL-2, BCL-x$_L$ sequester BH3 domain-only molecules preventing BAX- and BAK-mediated mitochondrial apoptosis. *Mol. Cell* 8: 705.

Cory S. and Adams J.M. 2002. The Bcl2 family: Regulators of the cellular life-or-death switch. *Nat. Rev. Cancer* 2: 647.

———. 2005. Killing cancer cells by flipping the Bcl-2/Bax switch. *Cancer Cell* 8: 5.

Cory S., Huang D.C.S., and Adams J.M. 2003. The Bcl-2 family: Roles in cell survival and oncogenesis. *Oncogene* 22: 8590.

Cuconati A., Mukherjee C., Perez D., and White E. 2003. DNA damage response and MCL-1 destruction initiate apoptosis in adenovirus-infected cells. *Genes Dev.* 17: 2922.

Danial N.N. and Korsmeyer S.J. 2004. Cell death: Critical control points. *Cell* 116: 205.

Day C.L., Chen L., Richardson S.J., Harrison P.J., Huang D.C.S., and Hinds M.G. 2005. Solution structure of prosurvival Mcl-1 and characterization of its binding by proapoptotic BH3-only ligands. *J. Biol. Chem.* 280: 4738.

Egle A., Harris A.W., Bouillet P., and Cory S. 2004a. Bim is a suppressor of Myc-induced mouse B cell leukemia. *Proc. Natl. Acad. Sci.* 101: 6164.

Egle A., Harris A.W., Bath M.L., O'Reilly L., and Cory S. 2004b. VavP-*Bcl2* transgenic mice develop follicular lymphoma preceded by germinal center hyperplasia. *Blood* 103: 2276.

Enders A., Bouillet P., Puthalakath H., Xu Y., Tarlinton D.M., and Strasser A. 2003. Loss of the pro-apoptotic BH3-only Bcl-2 family member Bim inhibits BCR stimulation-induced apoptosis and deletion of autoreactive B cells. *J. Exp. Med.* 198: 1119.

Hanahan D. and Weinberg R.A. 2000. The hallmarks of cancer. *Cell* 100: 57.

Hildeman D.A., Zhu Y., Mitchell T.C., Bouillet P., Strasser A., Kappler J., and Marrack P. 2002. Activated T cell death in vivo mediated by pro-apoptotic Bcl-2 family member, Bim. *Immunity* 16: 759.

Hinds M.G., Lackmann M., Skea G.L., Harrison P.J., Huang D.C.S., and Day C.L. 2003. The structure of Bcl-w reveals a role for the C-terminal residues in modulating biological activity. *EMBO J.* 22: 1497.

Huang D.C. and Strasser A. 2000. BH3-only proteins—Essential initiators of apoptotic cell death. *Cell* 103: 839.

Huang D.C., Hahne M., Schroeter M., Frei K., Fontana A., Villunger A., Newton K., Tschopp J., and Strasser A. 1999. Activation of Fas by FasL induces apoptosis by a mechanism that cannot be blocked by Bcl-2 or Bcl-x$_L$. *Proc. Natl. Acad. Sci.* 96: 14871.

Jeffers J.R., Parganas E., Lee Y., Yang C., Wang J., Brennan J., MacLean K.H., Han J., Chittenden T., Ihle J.N., McKinnon P.J., Cleveland J.L., and Zambetti G.P. 2003. Puma is an essential mediator of p53-dependent and -independent apoptotic pathways. *Cancer Cell* 4: 321.

Kuribara R., Honda H., Matsui H., Shinjyo T., Inukai T., Sugita K., Nakazawa S., Hirai H., Ozawa K., and Inaba T. 2004. Roles of Bim in apoptosis of normal and Bcr-Abl-expressing hematopoietic progenitor. *Mol. Cell. Biol.* 24: 6172.

Lindsten T., Ross A.J., King A., Zong W., Rathmell J.C., Shiels H.A., Ulrich E., Waymire K.G., Mahar P., Frauwirth K., Chen Y., Wei M., Eng V.M., Adelman D.M., Simon M.C., Ma A., Golden J.A., Evan G., Korsmeyer S.J., MacGregor G.R., and Thompson C.B. 2000. The combined functions of proapoptotic Bcl-2 family members Bak and Bax are essential for normal development of multiple tissues. *Mol. Cell* 6: 1389.

Liu X., Dai S., Zhu Y., Marrack P., and Kappler J.W. 2003. The structure of a Bcl-x$_L$/Bim fragment complex: Implications for Bim function. *Immunity* 19: 341.

Maraskovsky E., O'Reilly L.A., Teepe M., Corcoran L.M., Peschon J.J., and Strasser A. 1997. Bcl-2 can rescue T lymphocyte development in interleukin-7 receptor-deficient mice but not in mutant *rag-1$^{-/-}$* mice. *Cell* 89: 1011.

Marsden V. and Strasser A. 2003. Control of apoptosis in the immune system: Bcl-2, BH3-only proteins and more. *Annu. Rev.*

Immunol. 21: 71.

McDonnell T.J. and Korsmeyer S.J. 1991. Progression from lymphoid hyperplasia to high-grade malignant lymphoma in mice transgenic for the t(14;18). *Nature* 349: 254.

McDonnell T.J., Deane N., Platt F.M., Nuñez G., Jaeger U., McKearn J.P., and Korsmeyer S.J. 1989. *bcl*-2-immunoglobulin transgenic mice demonstrate extended B cell survival and follicular lymphoproliferation. *Cell* 57: 79.

Nijhawan D., Fang M., Traer E., Zhong Q., Gao W., Du F., and Wang X. 2003. Elimination of Mcl-1 is required for the initiation of apoptosis following ultraviolet irradiation. *Genes Dev.* 17: 1475.

Nikrad M., Johnson T., Puthalalath H., Coultas L., Adams J., and Kraft A.S. 2005. The proteasome inhibitor bortezomib sensitizes cells to killing by death receptor ligand TRAIL via BH3-only proteins Bik and Bim. *Mol. Cancer Ther.* 4: 443.

Ogilvy S., Metcalf D., Print C.G., Bath M.L., Harris A.W., and Adams J.M. 1999. Constitutive bcl-2 expression throughout the hematopoietic compartment affects multiple lineages and enhances progenitor cell survival. *Proc. Natl. Acad. Sci.* 96: 14943.

Oltersdorf T., Elmore S.W., Shoemaker A.R., Armstrong R.C., Augeri D.J., Belli B.A., Bruncko M., Deckwerth T.L., Dinges J., Hajduk P.J., Joseph M.K., Kitada S., Korsmeyer S.J., Kunzer A.R., Letai A., Li C., Mitten M.J., Nettesheim D.G., Ng S., Nimmer P.M., O'Connor J.M., Oleksijew A., Petros A.M., Reed J.C., Shen W., Tahir S.K., Thompson C.B., Tomaselli K.J., Wang B., Wendt M.D., Zhang H., Fesik S.W., and Rosenberg S.H. 2005. An inhibitor of Bcl-2 family proteins induces regression of solid tumours. *Nature* 435: 677.

Pellegrini M., Belz G., Bouillet P., and Strasser A. 2003. Shut down of an acute T cell immune response to viral infection is mediated by the pro-apoptotic Bcl-2 homology 3-only protein Bim. *Proc. Natl. Acad. Sci.* 100: 14175.

Pellegrini M., Bouillet P., Robati M., Belz G.T., Davey G.M., and Strasser A. 2004. Loss of Bim increases T cell production and function in interleukin 7 receptor-deficient mice. *J. Exp. Med.* 200: 1189.

Putcha G.V., Moulder K.L., Golden J.P., Bouillet P., Adams J.M., Strasser A., and Johnson E.M.J. 2001. Induction of Bim, a proapoptotic BH3-only Bcl-2 family member, is critical for neuronal apoptosis. *Neuron* 29: 615.

Puthalakath H. and Strasser A. 2002. Keeping killers on a tight leash: Transcriptional and post-translational control of the pro-apoptotic activity of BH3-only proteins. *Cell Death Differ.* 9: 505.

Puthalakath H., Huang D.C.S., O'Reilly L.A., King S.M., and Strasser A. 1999. The pro-apoptotic activity of the Bcl-2 family member Bim is regulated by interaction with the dynein motor complex. *Mol. Cell* 3: 287.

Puthalakath H., Villunger A., O'Reilly L.A., Beaumont J.G., Coultas L., Cheney R.E., Huang D.C.S., and Strasser A. 2001. Bmf: A pro-apoptotic BH3-only protein regulated by interaction with the myosin V actin motor complex, activated by anoikis. *Science* 293: 1829.

Shibue T., Takeda K., Oda E., Tanaka H., Murasawa H., Takaoka A., Morishita Y., Akira S., Taniguchi T., and Tanaka N. 2003. Integral role of Noxa in p53-mediated apoptotic response. *Genes Dev.* 17: 2233.

Smith D.P., Bath M.L., Harris A.W., and Cory S. 2005. T-cell lymphomas mask slower developing B-lymphoid and myeloid tumors in transgenic mice with broad hematopoietic expression of MYC. *Oncogene* 24: 3544.

Strasser A. 2005. The role of BH3-only proteins in the immune system. *Nat. Rev. Immunol.* 5: 189.

Strasser A., Harris A.W., and Cory S. 1993. Eμ-*bcl*-2 transgene facilitates spontaneous transformation of early pre-B and immunoglobulin-secreting cells but not T cells. *Oncogene* 8: 1.

Strasser A., O'Connor L., and Dixit V.M. 2000. Apoptosis signaling. *Annu. Rev. Biochem.* 69: 217.

Strasser A., Harris A.W., Bath M.L., and Cory S. 1990. Novel primitive lymphoid tumours induced in transgenic mice by cooperation between *myc* and *bcl*-2. *Nature* 348: 331.

Strasser A., Harris A.W., Huang D.C.S., Krammer P.H., and

Cory S. 1995. Bcl-2 and Fas/APO-1 regulate distinct pathways to lymphocyte apoptosis. *EMBO J.* **14:** 6136.

Strasser A., Whittingham S., Vaux D.L., Bath M.L., Adams J.M., Cory S., and Harris A.W. 1991. Enforced *BCL2* expression in B-lymphoid cells prolongs antibody responses and elicits autoimmune disease. *Proc. Natl. Acad. Sci.* **88:** 8661.

Suzuki M., Youle R.J., and Tjandra N. 2000. Structure of Bax: Coregulation of dimer formation and intracellular localization. *Cell* **103:** 645.

Tagawa H., Karnan S., Suzuki R., Matsuo K., Zhang X., Ota A., Morishima Y., Nakamura S., and Seto M. 2005. Genome-wide array-based CGH for mantle cell lymphoma: Identification of homozygous deletions of the proapoptotic gene BIM. *Oncogene* **24:** 1348.

Tan T.T., Degenhardt K., Nelson D.A., Beaudoin B., Nieves-Neira W., Bouillet P., Villunger A., Adams J.M., and White E. 2005. Key roles of BIM-driven apoptosis in epithelial tumors and rational chemotherapy. *Cancer Cell* **7:** 227.

Vaux D.L., Cory S., and Adams J.M. 1988. *Bcl*-2 gene promotes haemopoietic cell survival and cooperates with c-*myc* to immortalize pre-B cells. *Nature* **335:** 440.

Veis D.J., Sorenson C.M., Shutter J.R., and Korsmeyer S.J. 1993. Bcl-2-deficient mice demonstrate fulminant lymphoid apoptosis, polycystic kidneys, and hypopigmented hair. *Cell* **75:** 229.

Villunger A., Scott C., Bouillet P., and Strasser A. 2003a. Essential role for the BH3-only protein Bim but redundant roles for Bax, Bcl-2, and Bcl-w in the control of granulocyte survival. *Blood* **101:** 2393.

Villunger A., Michalak E.M., Coultas L., Müllauer F., Böck G., Ausserlechner M.J., Adams J.M., and Strasser A. 2003b. p53- and drug-induced apoptotic responses mediated by BH3-only proteins Puma and Noxa. *Science* **302:** 1036.

Villunger A., Marsden V.S., Zhan Y., Erlacher M., Lew A.M., Bouillet P., Berzins S., Godfrey D.I., Heath W.R., and Strasser A. 2004. Negative selection of semimature CD4(+)8(-)HSA+ thymocytes requires the BH3-only protein Bim but is independent of death receptor signaling. *Proc. Natl. Acad. Sci.* **101:** 7052.

Vousden K.H. and Lu X. 2002. Live or let die: The cell's response to p53. *Nat. Rev. Cancer* **2:** 594.

Walensky L.D., Kung A.L., Escher I., Malia T.J., Barbuto S., Wright R.D., Wagner G., Verdine G.L., and Korsmeyer S.J. 2004. Activation of apoptosis in vivo by a hydrocarbon-stapled BH3 helix. *Science* **305:** 1466.

Willis S.N., Chen L., Dewson G., Wei A., Naik E., Fletcher J.I., Adams J.M., and Huang D.C. 2005. Pro-apoptotic Bak is sequestered by Mc1 and Bcl-xL, but not Bcl-2, until displaced by BH3-only proteins. *Genes Dev.* **19:** 1294.

Yin X.-M., Wang K., Gross A., Zhao Y., Zinkel S., Klocke B., Roth K.A., and Korsmeyer S.J. 1999. Bid-deficient mice are resistant to Fas-induced hepatocellular apoptosis. *Nature* **400:** 886.

Zelenetz A.D., Chen T.T., and Levy R. 1992. Clonal expansion in follicular lymphoma occurs subsequent to antigenic selection. *J. Exp. Med.* **176:** 1137.

Zhang Y., Adachi M., Kawamura R., and Imai K. 2005. Bmf is a possible mediator in histone deacetylase inhibitors FK228 and CBHA-induced apoptosis. *Cell Death Differ.* (in press).

Zhong Q., Gao W., Du F., and Wang X. 2005. Mule/ARF-BP1, a BH3-only E3 ubiquitin ligase, catalyzes the polyubiquitination of Mcl-1 and regulates apoptosis. *Cell* **121:** 1085.

Zong W.X., Lindsten T., Ross A.J., MacGregor G.R., and Thompson C.B. 2001. BH3-only proteins that bind pro-survival Bcl-2 family members fail to induce apoptosis in the absence of Bax and Bak. *Genes Dev.* **15:** 1481.

Making Progress through Molecular Attacks on Cancer

C.L. SAWYERS

Howard Hughes Medical Institute, Departments of Medicine, Medical and Molecular Pharmacology and Urology, UCLA, Los Angeles, California 90095

The success of kinase inhibitor therapy in chronic myeloid leukemia (CML) has validated the long-held thesis in the cancer research community that a precise molecular understanding of cancer can directly affect cancer therapy. Now that several years have passed since the approval of imatinib/Gleevec for CML treatment, we have a greater appreciation for the challenges involved in effectively deploying these agents in the clinic. In this paper, I review recent events in the treatment of CML and highlight early applications of kinase inhibitor therapy to other diseases such as glioblastoma. I conclude with a vision that it may be possible, through analysis of tumor proteins secreted into serum, to track distinct molecular features of various cancers in order to select appropriate molecularly targeted therapy and measure treatment response. This new science of cancer biomarkers could radically transform the conduct of clinical trials and speed the evaluation of new molecularly targeted agents.

TUMORS WITH KINASE MUTATIONS ARE KINASE-DEPENDENT AND RESPOND TO KINASE INHIBITORS

A central theme that has emerged from this work is the notion of "kinase-dependent" cancer; i.e., those cancers whose growth is driven by a specific kinase or set of kinases (Sawyers 2003). By definition, such cancers should respond (shrink) when exposed to an inhibitor that effectively blocks the enzymatic activity of the responsible kinase. Although CML serves as a paradigm, it is unique in that essentially all patients with clinical CML share a common molecular abnormality, activation of the ABL tyrosine kinase by chromosome translocation. It is perhaps more instructive to consider other diseases where only subsets of patients respond to these drugs. Examples include gastrointestinal stromal tumors (GIST), chronic myelomonocytic leukemia (CMML), hypereosinophilic syndrome (HES), and bronchoalveolar lung cancer. In each of these cases, clinical sensitivity (defined as objective response or shrinkage, measured radiographically) to a kinase inhibitor has been correlated with a mutation in the gene encoding the target kinase that alters its biological potency, creating an oncogenic allele that drives the growth of that cancer. Table 1 (top) summarizes the mutant kinase target and effective kinase inhibitor for each of these tumors.

Although lung cancer patients with EGFR kinase domain mutations clearly have a greater chance of objective response when treated with inhibitors such as Iressa or Tarceva, there is much debate in the lung cancer community about whether these mutations predict for any long-term clinical benefit to patients, since there appears to be no improvement in survival. One possibility is that drug resistance (and relapse) develops in responders before a survival benefit is realized, in which case a second drug that combats or prevents resistance is needed. In CML, there is strong precedent in support of this view, because the mechanism of resistance to imatinib has been defined and novel ABL kinase inhibitors have been shown to work (Gorre et al. 2001; Shah et al. 2002) (see below). Initial data from several groups, as presented by Dr. Varmus (Varmus et al., this volume) and Dr. Haber (Haber et al., this volume), suggest that the same may be true in lung cancer, since resistance mechanisms are similar and novel inhibitors with efficacy against resistant cells have been described. The long-term data in lung cancer patients treated with EGFR inhibitors are further complicated by the evidence for a small but significant survival benefit to treated patients without known EGFR mutations. Although these data seem paradoxical at present, further molecular characterization of these patients for other mutations or pathway abnormalities is likely to clarify the situation, based on precedent recently established

Table 1. Kinase-driven Cancers with Kinase Mutations

Disease	Kinase	Mechanism	Drug
CML	ABL	fusion protein	Gleevec
GI stromal tumor	KIT	mutation	Gleevec
Hypereosinophilic syndrome	PDGFRα	fusion protein	Gleevec
CMML	PDGFRβ	fusion protein	Gleevec
Lung cancer	EGFR	mutation	Iressa/Tarceva
AML	Flt3	mutation	?
Melanoma	B-Raf	mutation	?
Lung cancer	Her2	mutation	?
Breast cancer, etc.	PI3K (p110α)	mutation	?
Polycythemia vera, ET	JAK2	mutation	?

in glioblastoma (Mellinghoff et al. 2005) (see below).

Assuming the paradigm that mutant kinases predict for kinase dependence continues to hold up, there is great optimism that kinase inhibitors will be effective in other diseases with known kinase mutations. Currently, the list of candidates is not very long (B-Raf in melanoma, Her2 in lung cancer, Flt3 in AML, JAK2 in myeloproliferative disease) (Table 1, bottom), but there is optimism that it will continue to grow with time. Specifically, human cancer kinome resequencing efforts are currently under way and have identified novel kinase mutations in subsets of patients. Although the actual frequency of specific mutations in certain cancers is likely to be low, there is great interest in developing a comprehensive catalog of all kinase (and other gene) mutations found in human cancers. Although the magnitude and cost of such a project are under debate, there is little doubt that discovery of additional kinase mutations could rapidly have clinical impact. Small-molecule inhibitors to mutant kinases can now be readily identified through standard screening approaches, followed by clinical evaluation in patients most likely to respond; i.e., those whose tumors contain mutations in the target kinase.

IMPORTANCE OF TUMOR SUPPRESSOR GENE STATUS IN RESPONSE TO KINASE INHIBITORS

It is important to recognize certain complexities that may influence tumor response to kinase inhibitors, even in tumors with a mutation in the target kinase. Analysis of glioblastoma patients treated with EGFR inhibitors by the UCLA Neurooncology Group (Ingo Mellinghoff, Tim Cloughesy, Paul Mischel) serves as an example. The response rate to the drugs (Iressa or Tarceva) in relapsed glioma is ~15% in phase II studies. Of 49 such patients treated at UCLA, 7 had dramatic, radiographically documented objective responses. Molecular profiling of the EGFR in all these patients revealed that 6 of these 7 patients had mutations in the extracellular domain (called EGFR variant iii). (Of note, no patients had mutations in the EGFR kinase domain, thereby distinguishing this mechanism from that found in lung cancer.) However, 6 of 19 patients who rapidly progressed through EGFR inhibitor therapy also had EGFRviii mutations. The variable that distinguishes these two groups is presence or absence of the PTEN tumor suppressor gene, which was expressed in wild-type form in all of the responding patients but in only 2 of the progressive disease patients with EGFRviii mutations. These data were confirmed in an independent sample set and suggest that molecular assessment of both EGFRviii and PTEN is required to define sensitivity to EGFR inhibitors in glioblastoma patients (Mellinghoff et al. 2005). The broader implication is that future application of patient-tailored kinase inhibitor therapy is likely to require evaluation of a suite of molecular variables for optimal predictive power.

Loss of the PTEN tumor suppressor gene is also of interest for potential therapeutic opportunities because PTEN is a lipid phosphatase that regulates the PI3-kinase

pathway (Vivanco and Sawyers 2002). Tumors lacking PTEN have increased activation of PI3K and downstream effectors such as Akt and mTOR, raising the possibility of dependence on these kinases in the absence of direct mutation of the kinase. We and other workers have demonstrated a synthetic lethal-like relationship between PTEN loss and mTOR in various mouse models treated with the mTOR inhibitor rapamycin, which causes cytostasis or regression of PTEN null tumors (Neshat et al. 2001; Podsypanina et al. 2001; Majumder et al. 2004; Wendel et al. 2004). Based on this work, clinical trials of mTOR inhibitors have been initiated with the goal of assessing response rate in patients with PTEN mutant cancers.

At UCLA we have addressed this question in glioblastoma and in prostate cancer, based on the relatively high frequency of PTEN loss (~40%) in these two diseases. A critical first step in both trials was to establish clinically robust assays of PTEN pathway status to select appropriate patients for these clinical trials. Using immunohistochemistry, we demonstrated that PTEN expression and downstream pathway activation could be measured in formalin-fixed, paraffin-embedded prostate and glioma samples (Choe et al. 2003; Thomas et al. 2004). The second step was to design trials so that PTEN pathway status could be determined from biopsy material and pathway inhibition could be measured using appropriate pharmacodynamic readouts. For these reasons, we used a neoadjuvant clinical design where patients are treated with mTOR inhibitor briefly (1–4 weeks) prior to a planned surgical resection, allowing us to measure pathway status in resected tumor. In both the prostate and the glioma trials, we were successful in defining doses of mTOR inhibitor that inhibit target in tumor cells with minimal side effects. Anti-tumor activity is suggested by changes in proliferation index, but formal efficacy data will require phase II studies.

ACQUIRED RESISTANCE TO KINASE INHIBITORS: MECHANISMS AND POTENTIAL SOLUTIONS

A second issue complicating the success of kinase inhibitor therapy is acquired resistance, defined as disease relapse on continuous therapy after an initial response. First recognized as a significant problem initially in advanced-stage CML patients, acquired resistance also occurs in chronic-phase CML, GIST, HES, and bronchoalveolar lung cancer. The best understanding of resistance mechanisms comes from CML, where >85% of relapsed patients have mutations in the ABL kinase domain that alter drug sensitivity (Shah et al. 2002). Of note, similar mechanisms have been reported for GIST and HES but explored in less detail.

In the case of ABL, 38 different mutations have been reported to date, but 3–4 mutations account for 60–70% of all cases. Insights into how these mutations cause resistance became apparent through the solution by John Kuriyan's group of the co-crystal structure of imatinib bound to ABL (Schindler et al. 2000). Curiously, only a small number of the mutations occur at contact residues where substitution of the new amino acid leads to loss of a hydrogen-bond donor or steric hindrance due to bulkier side chains. Rather, the majority of mutations are at residues that appear, based on structural modeling studies, to alter the conformational flexibility of ABL such that it can no longer achieve the closed, inactive conformation required for optimal imatinib binding (Shah et al. 2002).

These structural studies raise the possibility that a second ABL kinase inhibitor which binds in a less conformation-dependent fashion may have activity against certain imatinib-resistant mutants. We tested this hypothesis using dual SRC/ABL kinase inhibitors that can bind ABL in the active or inactive conformation. One such compound, BMS-354825 (also called dasatinib), blocked the growth of murine hematopoietic cells transformed by all but one imatinib-resistant BCR-ABL mutant in culture and showed anti-leukemic activity in mouse models (Shah et al. 2004). This compound also induced hematologic and cytogenetic remissions in a high fraction of imatinib-resistant CML patients in a phase I trial with minimal side effects (Sawyers et al. 2004, 2005). Phase II studies are currently under way with promising data presented recently with 6 months followup (Guilhot et al. 2005; Hochhaus et al. 2005; Ottmann et al. 2005; Talpaz et al. 2005).

We have also examined potential mechanisms of resistance to BMS-345825 by saturation mutagenesis. Unlike imatinib, resistance occurs almost exclusively through mutations at drug contact residues, presumably due to less conformation-stringent binding requirements. In addition, some mutations were isolated that confer resistance to BMS-354825 but not to imatinib (Burgess et al. 2005). These data provide evidence in favor of either sequential or combination therapy with these two compounds for CML.

NEXT STEPS IN CLINICAL TRIAL DESIGN: THE NEED FOR ACCESSIBLE BIOMARKERS

The neoadjuvant trial designs discussed above for testing mTOR inhibitors in PTEN-null cancers provide a unique opportunity to obtain tumor tissue to make molecular measurements of pathway status, but the requirement for tissue acquisition places significant limitations on patient eligibility. Noninvasive technologies for measuring pathway activation would greatly transform the conduct of clinical trials. Over the past several years, there has been a growing interest in defining serum biomarkers for cancer diagnosis and early detection, based on evidence of distinct patterns of certain serum proteins detected in cancer patients using proteomic technologies. Our group is examining the possibility that distinct sets of proteins secreted by tumor cells with different genetic pathway mutations might be used to measure pathway status in serum. As a first step, we have conducted a whole mouse transcriptome profiling experiment of two genetically engineered mouse prostate cancer models designed to mimic lesions found in human prostate cancer, one with transgenic expression of c-Myc and the other with conditional deletion of PTEN (Ellwood-Yen et al. 2003; Wang

et al. 2003). In preliminary studies conducted with the groups of Hong Wu and Tom Graeber at UCLA, we have defined gene expression signatures that easily distinguish PTEN and Myc-driven cancers, even when the analysis is restricted to genes predicted to encode only secreted proteins. If these predicted proteins are indeed secreted and measurable in serum, one can envision using a suite of serum biomarkers to define the genetic status of a patient's tumor and determine pathway inhibition in response to therapy. Such tools, coupled with advances in probe development for molecular imaging, could transform clinical cancer diagnosis and rapidly allow therapies to be appropriately tailored to the genetic makeup of the tumor. These technological advances are critical for successful application of molecularly targeted therapies on a larger scale against a range of malignancies beyond chronic myeloid leukemia.

ACKNOWLEDGMENTS

I thank many colleagues at UCLA who have contributed to this studies, including Neil Shah, Ingo Mellinghoff, Tim Cloughesy, Paul Mischel, Hong Wu, Tom Graeber, Ron Paquette, Michael Burgess, and John Nicoll. Work in my laboratory is supported by the Howard Hughes Medical Institute, the Leukemia and Lymphoma Society, the National Cancer Institute, and the Doris Duke Charitable Foundation.

REFERENCES

Burgess M.R., Skaggs B.J., Shah N.P., Lee F.Y., and Sawyers C.L. 2005. Comparative analysis of two clinically active BCR-ABL kinase inhibitors reveals the role of conformation-specific binding in resistance. *Proc. Natl. Acad. Sci.* **102:** 3395.

Choe G., Horvath S., Cloughesy T.F., Crosby K., Seligson D., Palotie A., Inge L., Smith B.L., Sawyers C.L., and Mischel P.S. 2003. Analysis of the phosphatidylinositol 3'-kinase signaling pathway in glioblastoma patients in vivo. *Cancer Res.* **63:** 2742.

Ellwood-Yen K., Graeber T.G., Wongvipat J., Iruela-Arispe M.L., Zhang J., Matusik R., Thomas G.V., and Sawyers C.L. 2003. Myc-driven murine prostate cancer shares molecular features with human prostate cancer. *Cancer Cell* **4:** 223.

Gorre M.E., Mohammed M., Ellwood K., Hsu N., Paquette R., Rao P.N., and Sawyers C.L. 2001. Clinical resistance to STI-571 cancer therapy caused by BCR-ABL gene mutation or amplification. *Science* **293:** 876.

Guilhot F., Apperley J.F., Shah N., Kim D.W., Grigg A., Cheng S., Iyer M., and Cortes J. 2005. A phase II study of Dasatinib in patients with accelerated phase chronic myeloid leukemia (CML) who are resistant or intolerant to Imatinib: First results of the CA180005 'START-A' study. *American Society of Hematology 47th Annual Meeting*, Abstract 39.

Hochhaus A., Baccarani M., Sawyers C., Nagler A., Facon T., Goldberg S.L., Cervantes F., Larson R.A., Voi M., Ezzeddine R., and Kantarjian H. 2005. Efficacy of Dasatinib in patients with chronic phase Philadelphia chromosome-positive CML resistant or intolerant to Imatinib: First results of the CA180013 'START-C' phase II study. *American Society of Hematology 47th Annual Meeting,* Abstract 41.

Majumder P.K., Febbo P.G., Bikoff R., Berger R., Xue Q., McMahon L.M., Manola J., Brugarolas J., McDonnell T.J., Golub T.R., Loda M., Lane H.A., and Sellers W.R. 2004. mTOR inhibition reverses Akt-dependent prostate intraepithelial neoplasia through regulation of apoptotic and HIF-1-dependent pathways. *Nat. Med.* **10:** 594.

Mellinghoff I.K., Wang M.Y., Vivanco I., Haas-Kogan D.A., Zhu S., Dia E.Q., Lu K.V., Yoshimoto K., Huang J.H., Chute D.J., Riggs B.L., Horvath S., Liau L.M., Cavenee W.K., Rao P.N., Beroukhim R., Peck T.C., Lee J.C., Sellers W.R., Stokoe D., Prados M., Cloughesy T.F., Sawyers C.L., and Mischel P. 2005. Molecular determinants of the response of glioblastomas to EGFR kinase inhibitors. *N. Engl. J. Med.* **353:** 2012.

Neshat M.S., Mellinghoff I.K., Tran C., Stiles B., Thomas G., Petersen R., Frost P., Gibbons J.J., Wu H., and Sawyers C.L. 2001. Enhanced sensitivity of PTEN deficient tumors to inhibition of FRAP/mTOR. *Proc. Natl. Acad. Sci.* **98:** 10314.

Ottmann O.G., Martinelli G., Dombret H., Kantarjian H., Hochhaus A., Simonsson B., Aloe A., Apanovitch A., and Shah N. 2005. A phase II study of Dasatinib in patients with chronic myeloid leukemia (CML) in lymphoid blast crisis or Philadelphia-chromosome positive acute lymphoblastic leukemia (Ph+ ALL) who are resistant or intolerant to Imatinib: The 'START-L' CA180015 study. *American Society of Hematology 47th Annual Meeting,* Abstract 42.

Podsypanina K., Lee R.T., Politis C., Hennessy I., Crane A., Puc J., Neshat M., Wang H., Yang L., Gibbons J., Frost P., Dreisbach V., Blenis J., Gaciong Z., Fisher P., Sawyers C., Hedrick-Ellenson L., and Parsons R. 2001. An inhibitor of mTOR reduces neoplasia and normalizes p70/S6 kinase activity in Pten+/– mice. *Proc. Natl. Acad. Sci.* **98:** 10320.

Sawyers C.L. 2003. Opportunities and challenges in the development of kinase inhibitor therapy for cancer. *Genes Dev.* **17:** 2998.

Sawyers C.L., Kantarjian H., Shah N., Cortes J., Paquette R., Donato N., Nicoll J., Bleickardt E., Chen T.T., and Talpaz M. 2005. Dasatinib (BMS-354825) in patients with chronic myeloid leukemia (CML) and Philadelphia-chromosome positive acute lymphoblastic leukemia (Ph+ ALL) who are resistant or intolerant to Imatinib: Update of a phase I study. *American Society of Hematology 47th Annual Meeting,* Abstract 38.

Sawyers C.L., Shah N.P., Kantarjian H.M., Donato N., Nicoll J., Bai S.A., Huang F., Clark E., DeCillis A.P., and Talpaz M. 2004. Hematologic and cytogenetic responses in Imatinib-re-sistant chronic phase chronic myeloid leukemia patients treated with the dual SRC/ABL kinase inhibitor BMS-354825: Results from a phase I dose escalation study. *American Society of Hematology 46th Annual Meeting,* Abstract 1.

Schindler T., Bornmann W., Pellicena P., Miller W.T., Clarkson B., and Kuriyan J. 2000. Structural mechanism for STI-571 inhibition of abelson tyrosine kinase. *Science* **289:** 1938.

Shah N.P., Tran C., Lee F.Y., Chen P., Norris D., and Sawyers C.L. 2004. Overriding Imatinib resistance with a novel ABL kinase inhibitor. *Science* **305:** 399.

Shah N.P., Nicoll J.M., Nagar B., Gorre M.E., Paquette R.L., Kuriyan J., and Sawyers C.L. 2002. Multiple BCR-ABL kinase domain mutations confer polyclonal resistance to the tyrosine kinase inhibitor Imatinib (STI571) in chronic phase and blast crisis chronic myeloid leukemia. *Cancer Cell* **2:** 117.

Talpaz M., Rousselot P., Kim D.W., Guilhot F., Corm S., Bleickardt E., Zink R., Rosti G., Coutre S., and Sawyers C. 2005. A phase II study of Dasatinib in patients with chronic myeloid leukemia (CML) in myeloid blast crisis who are resistant or intolerant to Imatinib: First results of the CA180006 'START-B' study. *American Society of Hematology 47th Annual Meeting,* Abstract 40.

Thomas G.V., Horvath S., Smith B.L., Crosby K., Lebel L.A., Schrage M., Said J., De Kernion J., Reiter R.E., and Sawyers C.L. 2004. Antibody-based profiling of the phosphoinositide 3-kinase pathway in clinical prostate cancer. *Clin. Cancer Res.* **10:** 8351.

Vivanco I. and Sawyers C.L. 2002. The phosphatidylinositol 3-kinase AKT pathway in human cancer. *Nat. Rev. Cancer* **2:** 489.

Wang S., Gao J., Lei Q., Rozengurt N., Pritchard C., Jiao J., Thomas G.V., Li G., Roy-Burman P., Nelson P.S., Liu X., and Wu H. 2003. Prostate-specific deletion of the murine Pten tumor suppressor gene leads to metastatic prostate cancer. *Cancer Cell* **4:** 209.

Wendel H.G., De Stanchina E., Fridman J.S., Malina A., Ray S., Kogan S., Cordon-Cardo C., Pelletier J., and Lowe S.W. 2004. Survival signalling by Akt and eIF4E in oncogenesis and cancer therapy. *Nature* **428:** 332.

Predicting Clinical Benefit in Non-Small-Cell Lung Cancer Patients Treated with Epidermal Growth Factor Tyrosine Kinase Inhibitors

L.C. AMLER, A.D. GODDARD, AND K.J. HILLAN

Development Sciences, Genentech, Inc., South San Francisco, California 94080

Erlotinib and gefitinib are small-molecule inhibitors of the epidermal growth factor tyrosine kinase. Erlotinib is approved for the treatment of locally advanced or metastatic non-small-cell lung cancer after failure of at least one prior chemotherapy regimen. Although it is active in unselected patients, clinical characteristics and tumor molecular markers associated with enhanced benefit have been identified. Notably, never-smoker status or a positive EGFR FISH test has been consistently predictive of greater erlotinib benefit. Other markers, such as EGFR mutations and EGFR protein expression, as determined by immunohistochemistry, and KRAS mutation status have not proven to be consistently associated with differential benefit.

The epidermal growth factor receptor (EGFR) is a receptor tyrosine kinase expressed in the majority of non-small-cell lung cancers (NSCLC) (Dazzi et al. 1989; Kaseda et al. 1989). The efficacy of EGFR tyrosine kinase inhibitors (EGFR TKIs) in preclinical tumor models, together with their favorable toxicity profiles, led to their clinical development in NSCLC and other solid tumors (Higgins et al. 2004). Erlotinib and gefitinib are small-molecule inhibitors of the EGFR tyrosine kinase, which showed evidence of antitumor activity in patients with NSCLC as single agents (Lynch et al. 2004b). This activity was recently shown to translate to a significant survival benefit in a randomized phase III trial of erlotinib versus placebo (hazard ratio [HR] = 0.73) in second-/third-line NSCLC (Shepherd et al. 2005), whereas gefitinib failed to demonstrate a significant survival advantage in a trial of similar design (HR = 0.89) (Tamura and Fukuoka 2005).

Erlotinib's survival advantage in second-/third-line lung cancer was observed in an unselected patient population. However, it is possible that some patient subpopulations might derive greater benefit than others. Indeed, one hypothesis would be that patients whose tumors are most dependent on EGFR signaling for growth and survival would derive greatest therapeutic benefit, whereas patients with tumors that are functionally independent of EGFR would not derive benefit. In this review, we examine the molecular and clinical markers that have been shown to be associated with outcome in NSCLC patients treated with EGFR TKIs and we discuss how these are related to tumor dependence on signaling through EGFR.

EGFR MUTATIONS PREDICT FOR RESPONSE FROM EGFR TKI THERAPY, BUT HAVE NOT BEEN ASSOCIATED WITH PROLONGED SURVIVAL

Somatic mutations in the tyrosine kinase domain of EGFR were recently described in tumors of NSCLC patients who showed objective clinical responses (tumor shrinkage) to erlotinib (Pao et al. 2004) and gefitinib (Lynch et al. 2004a; Paez et al. 2004) monotherapy. Patients with EGFR-mutant tumors were more likely to be never-smokers, females, and of Asian ethnicity (Lynch et al. 2004a). The frequency of heterozygous mutations varies according to the population being studied but has been reported to be approximately 10–12% in patients from the United States and 19–26% in patients from Southeast Asia.

The most frequently observed mutations are in exons 19–22 of the EGFR gene, with approximately 90% being either in-frame deletions in exon 19 or a L858R substitution in exon 21 (Pao et al. 2004). Functional analysis of the mutant receptors in cell lines shows evidence of specific gain of function, with elevated ligand-dependent activation of the receptor. Furthermore, the mutants were inhibited by lower concentrations of gefitinib and erlotinib compared with wild-type EGFR (Lynch et al. 2004a; Paez et al. 2004; Pao and Miller 2005). Thus, EGFR mutations appear to define tumors that are dependent on EGFR signaling and that are responsive to EGFR inhibition.

Compared to wild-type EGFR, the mutant EGFR selectively activates the Akt and STAT signaling pathways, which support cell survival, but has no effect on ERK signaling, which induces cell proliferation (Sordella et al. 2004). Consistent with this observation, NSCLC cells expressing mutant EGFR undergo apoptosis upon treatment with EGFR TKIs, suggesting that mutant EGFRs selectively support tumor cell survival, on which NSCLCs become dependent. This could account for the higher frequency of objective tumor responses seen in patients with mutant EGFR-bearing tumors upon treatment with an EGFR TKI.

In a Korean study of 90 consecutive NSCLC patients treated with gefitinib monotherapy, the response rate was 14% (10/73) in EGFR wild type and 65% (11/17) in EGFR mutant tumors, respectively. Of patients who responded, 48% were EGFR wild type and 52% were EGFR mutant (Han et al. 2005). A similar observation has been made in patients who respond to erlotinib (Johnson et al. 2004; Pao et al. 2004).

The impact of EGFR mutations on survival has been analyzed retrospectively in samples from three randomized trials. Two of these were negative trials (TRIBUTE/erlotinib [Eberhard et al. 2005] and INTACT-2/gefitinib [Bell et al. 2005a]), where an EGFR TKI was combined with chemotherapy in first-line lung cancer therapy. In both trials there were increased tumor response rates in patients with EGFR mutant tumors that were in the EGFR TKI treatment arm (statistically significant in TRIBUTE and a trend in INTACT-2). However, there was no evidence of a statistically significant treatment effect of mutation status on either progression-free survival or survival. In both studies, patients with EGFR mutated tumors had a better prognosis, regardless of the therapy arm. In BR.21, a monotherapy trial that showed a positive survival advantage in the overall patient population, EGFR mutation status was associated neither with an overall survival benefit, nor with a better prognosis (Tsao et al. 2005). Interestingly, data from an underpowered, and as yet unconfirmed, study suggest that specific EGFR mutations may have unique clinical characteristics, as EGFR TKI-treated patients with exon-19 deletion mutations had longer median survival than patients with the L858R point mutation (34 months versus 8 months) (Riely et al. 2006). This observation should be considered in future analysis of data from clinical trials.

Some patients with tumors bearing EGFR mutations, who have progressed on erlotinib or gefitinib therapy, have been shown to contain an additional EGFR mutation. This secondary mutation in exon 20 leads to substitution of methionine for threonine at position 790 (T790M) in the kinase domain (Pao et al. 2005a). An analogous mutation (T315I) has been observed in the ABL kinase in association with acquired resistance to imatinib (Branford et al. 2002), suggesting that this may be a common therapy-associated TKI escape mechanism in tumors with activating mutations in the tyrosine kinase domain. The emergence of additional mutations on therapy suggests the tumor is dependent on activation of the EGFR pathway for its survival and growth. Interestingly, susceptibility to inherited NSCLC may be associated with the germ-line transmission of the T790M mutation, suggesting that altered EGFR signaling is also important in the genetic susceptibility to lung cancer (Bell et al. 2005a).

INCREASED EGFR GENE COPY NUMBER APPEARS TO BE THE MOLECULAR MARKER THAT IS MOST POSITIVELY PREDICTIVE FOR EGFR TKI SURVIVAL BENEFIT

EGFR gene copy number has been studied as a predictive marker for patients treated with EGFR inhibitors, on the assumption that increased gene copy number, and/or amplification, indicates tumor dependency on the EGFR pathway (Cappuzzo et al. 2005; Hirsh et al. 2005a). EGFR copy number was assessed by FISH in both BR.21 and ISEL (Hirsh et al. 2005b) and correlated with clinical outcome. Greater survival benefit was seen in the EGFR fluorescence in situ hybridization (FISH)-positive (amplification and high polysomy) patients compared with EGFR FISH-negative patients (Fig. 1). Current information indicates that a positive EGFR FISH test is the best single molecular marker for prediction of clinical benefit of erlotinib monotherapy. Whereas some EGFR FISH-negative patients may respond to erlotinib therapy, a negative EGFR FISH test indicates less likelihood of a clinical benefit. The predictive value of FISH testing is being further assessed prospectively in a number of on-going randomized phase III trials.

EGFR PROTEIN EXPRESSION BY IMMUNOHISTOCHEMISTRY AND CLINICAL BENEFIT

In general, EGFR protein expression by immunohistochemistry (IHC) has not been as reliable a predictor of clinical benefit (Table 1) as FISH. In BR.21 and Tribute, EGFR protein expression was assessed by IHC using the Dako Cytomation EGFR pharmDx™ kit. Univariate analysis of EGFR protein expression in BR.21 showed that survival was prolonged in erlotinib versus the placebo group. However, EGFR IHC positivity was not a statistically significant covariate when a multivariate analysis was performed.

Performance of EGFR IHC is dependent on the antibody used, tissue fixation, and storage time of tissue sections prior to staining (Atkins et al. 2004). The last two variables, fixation and storage time, were not standardized in either study, which could have had an impact on the outcome of the analysis. Control of the key variables that affect perfor-

Table 1. Predictive Value of IHC for a Survival Benefit in BR.21, TRIBUTE, and ISEL

	BR.21	TRIBUTE	ISEL
	Erlotinib monotherapy 2nd / 3rd line	Erlotinib with chemo (CP) 1st line	Gefitinib monotherapy 2nd / 3rd line
Number of subjects	731	1079	1692
Number of patients tested	326 (44.6%)	344 (31.9%)	379 (22.4%)
HR for overall survival	HR for overall survival		
All subjects	0.73 (95% CI = 0.61–0.86)	1.00 (95% CI = 0.86–1.16)	0.86 (95% CI = 0.76–0.99)
IHC positive	0.68 (95% CI = 0.49–0.94)	1.27 (95% CI = 0.95–1.71)	0.77 (95% CI = 0.56–1.08)
IHC negative	0.93 * (95% CI = 0.63–1.36)	1.02 (95% CI = 0.54–1.95)	1.57 (95% CI = 0.86–2.87)

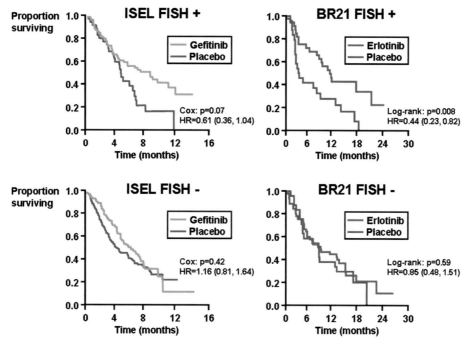

Figure 1. EGFR FISH and survival outcome in patients treated with single agent erlotinib or gefitinib.

mance of EGFR IHC should be incorporated in all ongoing prospective studies that include EGFR IHC testing.

KRAS MUTATIONS, WHICH ARE ASSOCIATED WITH SMOKING HISTORY, SELECT FOR A POPULATION OF PATIENTS THAT DO NOT APPEAR TO BENEFIT FROM EGFR TKI THERAPY

The RAS/MAPK pathway is a major signaling network that links EGFR activation to cell proliferation and survival (Atkins et al. 2004). Mutations in downstream effectors of EGFR signaling could lead to resistance to EGFR inhibitors (Yarden and Sliwkowski 2001; Bianco et al. 2003). In NSCLC, the most frequently reported alteration in EGFR signaling pathways is mutation of the KRAS gene (Huncharek et al. 1999; Nelson et al. 1999; Ahrendt et al. 2001; Broermann et al. 2002; Keller et al. 2002; Rajagopalan et al. 2002; Grossi et al. 2003; She et al. 2003). KRAS mutations occur in approximately 20% of NSCLC, are consistently associated with smoking (Ahrendt et al. 2001), and have been associated with poor prognosis (Graziano et al. 1999; Huncharek et al. 1999; Nelson et al. 1999; Schiller et al. 2001; Broermann et al. 2002; Keller et al. 2002; Rajagopalan et al. 2002; Grossi et al. 2003). Because EGFR and KRAS function sequentially in the MAPK signaling pathway, activating mutations in these two molecules might be functionally redundant. Consistent with this hypothesis, in the large majority of NSCLC tumors examined to date, EGFR and KRAS mutations were mutually exclusive (Eberhard et al. 2005; Tam et al. 2006).

Analysis of response rate in NSCLC patients with either erlotinib or gefitinib suggests that KRAS mutations were associated with a lack of tumor regression (Pao et al. 2005b). Retrospective analysis of tumor tissues from 264 (25%) of the patients in TRIBUTE suggests that patients with KRAS mutant tumors experience worse survival when erlotininib was combined with chemotherapy (HR = 2.06: 95% CI = 1.11–3.80), compared with those treated with chemotherapy alone (HR = 1.05: 95% CI = 0.73–1.50). This negative interaction appears to be related to expression of EGFR, because in patients in whom both EGFR IHC and KRAS mutation status were available, there was a significant association with poor outcome in patients with KRAS mutant tumors that expressed EGFR (Table 2).

Table 2. Association of KRAS Mutations and EGFR IHC with Survival in TRIBUTE

KRAS mutants and EGFR expression by IHC		
	Erlotinib + chemo	Chemo alone
EGFR IHC–		
n	11	9
Median OS (mo) (95% CI)	9.0 (3.4, 12.9)	12.8 (3.3, .)
Log rank P-value	0.5507	
Hazard ratio (95% CI)	1.4 (0.5, 4.3)	
EGFR IHC+		
n	12	20
Median OS (mo) (95% CI)	3.4 (2.1, 4.4)	13.5 (11.1, 15.1)
Log rank *p*-value	<0.001	
Hazard ratio (95% CI)	4.9 (2.1, 11.5)	

Table 3. Summary of Survival Benefit Observed in Never-Smokers Treated with Erlotinib (BR.21 and TRIBUTE) or Gefitinib (ISEL)

	BR.21	TRIBUTE	ISEL
	Erlotinib monotherapy 2nd / 3rd line	Erlotinib with chemo (CP) 1st line	Gefitinib monotherapy 2nd / 3rd line
Number of subjects	731	1079	1692
Number of never-smokers	146 (20.0%)	116 (10.8%)	375 (22%)
HR for overall survival	HR for overall survival		
All subjects	0.73 (95 % CI = 0.61–0.86)	1.00 (95% CI = 0.86–1.16)	0.89 (95% CI = 0.77–1.02)
Never-smokers	0.42 (95% CI = 0.28–0.64)	0.49 (95% CI = 0.28–0.85)	0.67 (95% CI = 0.49–0.92)
Current/former smokers	0.87 (95% CI = 0.71–1.05)	1.11 (95% CI = 0.94–1.29)	0.92 (95% CI = 0.79–1.06)

It is unclear why a negative interaction was observed when erlotinib was administered in combination with chemotherapy in patients whose tumors bore KRAS mutations. It will be important to determine whether this observation is confirmed by retrospective analysis of other randomized controlled trials. Erlotinib has been shown to prolong survival when administered in combination with gemcitabine in pancreatic cancer, a tumor where KRAS mutations are very common.

NEVER-SMOKER STATUS IS CONSISTENTLY PREDICTIVE OF GREATER PATIENT BENEFIT (SURVIVAL AND RESPONSE) FOR ERLOTINIB OR GEFITINIB MONOTHERAPY AND FOR ERLOTINIB IN COMBINATION WITH CHEMOTHERAPY

Lung cancer patients who have never smoked tobacco have consistently shown a benefit from both erlotinib and gefitinib (Table 3). This novel therapeutic observation is unique to EGFR TKIs and has been observed in phase III trials with erlotinib (BR.21) (Shepherd et al. 2005) and gefitinib (ISEL) monotherapy as well as for erlotinib in combination with chemotherapy (TRIBUTE) (Herbst et al. 2005).

Studies have suggested that tumors arising in never-smokers are molecularly and biologically distinct and may be associated with a better prognosis (Sanchez-Cespedes et al. 2001). Never-smokers are more likely to have mutations than smokers in the tyrosine kinase domain of EGFR and almost never harbor mutations in KRAS (Tam et al. 2006). In countries of Southeast Asia, lung cancer is more common in never-smokers than in smokers; thus, racial background, smoking history, and gene mutation status should be considered when designing and interpreting clinical trials in NSCLC with EGFR-TKIs.

SUMMARY AND CONCLUSIONS

Predictive molecular biomarkers for NSCLC patients treated with EGFR TKIs have largely been determined from studies of small case series and retrospective analyses of subsets of patients from randomized trials; in some cases, these were extracted from negative clinical trials. Overall, the predictive data generated to date can be summarized as follows:

1. EGFR mutations predict dramatic tumor shrinkage but have not been shown to be a good marker for the clinically meaningful endpoint of prolonged survival.
2. EGFR protein expression, as determined by IHC, predicts greater treatment benefit in BR.21 but is not a predictor of benefit in TRIBUTE.
3. High EGFR gene copy number may be the single molecular marker that is most predictive for erlotinib monotherapy.
4. KRAS mutations, which are positively associated with smoking history, select for a subset of patients who do not appear to benefit from erlotinib therapy.
5. Never-smoker status is consistently predictive of greater erlotinib benefit (survival and response) for monotherapy and in combination with chemotherapy.

This and other emerging diagnostic information will aid significantly in designing future studies and, ultimately, should help physicians decide which patients will be most likely to benefit from EGFR TKIs.

ACKNOWLEDGMENTS

We thank Dr. Fred R. Hirsch of the University of Colorado Cancer Center for providing and granting permission to reproduce Figure 1.

REFERENCES

Ahrendt S.A., Decker P.A., Alawi E.A., Zhu Yr Y.R., Sanchez-Cespedes M., Yang S.C., Haasler G.B., Kajdacsy-Balla A., Demeure M.J., and Sidransky D. 2001. Cigarette smoking is strongly associated with mutation of the K-ras gene in patients with primary adenocarcinoma of the lung. *Cancer* **92:** 1525.

Atkins D., Reiffen K.A., Tegtmeier C.L., Winther H., Bonato M.S., and Storkel S. 2004. Immunohistochemical detection of EGFR in paraffin-embedded tumor tissues: Variation in staining intensity due to choice of fixative and storage time of tissue sections. *J. Histochem. Cytochem.* **52:** 893.

Bell D.W., Gore I., Okimoto R.A., Godin-Heymann N., Sordella R., Mulloy R., Sharma S.V., Brannigan B.W., Mohapatra G., Settleman J., and Haber D.A. 2005a. Inherited susceptibility to lung cancer may be associated with the T790M drug resistance mutation in EGFR. *Nat. Genet.* **37:** 1315.

Bell D.W., Lynch T.J., Haserlat S.M., Harris P.L., Okimoto R.A., Brannigan B.W., Sgroi D.C., Muir B., Riemenschneider M.J., Iacona R.B., Krebs A.D., Johnson D.H., Giaccone G., Herbst R.S., Manegold C., Fukuoka M., Kris M.G., Baselga J., Ochs J.S., and Haber D.A. 2005b. Epidermal growth factor receptor mutations and gene amplification in non-small-cell lung cancer: Molecular analysis of the IDEAL/INTACT gefitinib trials. *J. Clin. Oncol.* **23:** 8081.

Bianco R., Shin I., Ritter C.A., Yakes F.M., Basso A., Rosen N., Tsurutani J., Dennis P.A., Mills G.B., and Arteaga C.L. 2003. Loss of PTEN/MMAC1/TEP in EGF receptor-expressing tumor cells counteracts the antitumor action of EGFR tyrosine kinase inhibitors. *Oncogene* **22:** 2812.

Branford S., Rudzki Z., Walsh S., Grigg A., Arthur C., Taylor K., Herrmann R., Lynch K.P., and Hughes T.P. 2002. High frequency of point mutations clustered within the adenosine triphosphate-binding region of BCR/ABL in patients with chronic myeloid leukemia or Ph-positive acute lymphoblastic leukemia who develop imatinib (STI571) resistance. *Blood* **99:** 3472.

Broermann P., Junker K., Brandt B.H., Heinecke A., Freitag L., Klinke F., Berdel W.E., and Thomas M. 2002. Trimodality treatment in stage III non small cell lung carcinoma: Prognostic impact of K-ras mutations after neoadjuvant therapy. *Cancer* **94:** 2055.

Cappuzzo F., Hirsch F.R., Rossi E., Bartolini S., Ceresoli G.L., Bemis L., Haney J., Witta S., Danenberg K., Domenichini I., Ludovini V., Magrini E., Gregorc V., Doglioni C., Sidoni A., Tonato M., Franklin W.A., Crino L., Bunn P.A., Jr., and Varella-Garcia M. 2005. Epidermal growth factor receptor gene and protein and gefitinib sensitivity in non-small-cell lung cancer. *J. Natl. Cancer Inst.* **97:** 643.

Dazzi H., Hasleton P.S., Thatcher N., Barnes D.M., Wilkes S., Swindell R., and Lawson R.A. 1989. Expression of epidermal growth factor receptor (EGF-R) in non-small cell lung cancer. Use of archival tissue and correlation of EGF-R with histology, tumour size, node status and survival. *Br. J. Cancer* **5:** 746.

Eberhard D.A., Johnson B.E., Amler L.C., Goddard A.D., Heldens S.L., Herbst R.S., Ince W.L., Janne P.A., Januario T., Johnson D.H., Klein P., Miller V.A., Ostland M.A., Ramies D.A., Sebisanovic D., Stinson J.A., Zhang Y.R., Seshagiri S., and Hillan K.J. 2005. Mutations in the epidermal growth factor receptor and in KRAS are predictive and prognostic indicators in patients with non-small-cell lung cancer treated with chemotherapy alone and in combination with erlotinib. *J. Clin. Oncol.* **23:** 5900.

Graziano S.L., Gamble G.P., Newman N.B., Abbott L.Z., Rooney M., Mookherjee S., Lamb M.L., Kohman L.J., and Poiez B.J. 1999. Prognostic significance of K-ras codon 12 mutations in patients with resected stage I and II non-small-cell lung cancer. *J. Clin. Oncol.* **17:** 668.

Grossi F., Loprevite M., Chiaramondia M., Ceppa P., Pera C., Ratto G.B., Serrano J., Ferrara G.B., Costa R., Boni L., and Ardizzoni A. 2003. Prognostic significance of K-ras, p53, bci-2, PCNA, CD34 in radically resected non-small cell lung cancers. *Eur. J. Cancer* **39:** 1242.

Han S.W., Kim T.Y., Hwang P.G., Jeong S., Kim J., Choi I.S., Oh D.Y., Kim J.H., Kim D.W., Chung D.H., Im S.A., Kim Y.T., Lee J.S., Heo D.S., Bang Y.J., and Kim N.K. 2005. Predictive and prognostic impact of epidermal growth factor receptor mutation in non-small-cell lung cancer patients treated with gefitinib. *J. Clin. Oncol.* **23:** 2493.

Herbst R.S., Prager D., Hermann R., Fehrenbacher L., Johnson B.E., Sandler A., Kris M.G., Tran H.T., Klein P., Li X., Ramies D., Johnson D.H., Miller V.A.; TRIBUTE Investigator Group. 2005. TRIBUTE: A phase III trial of erlotinib hydrochloride (OSI-774) combined with carboplatin and paclitaxel chemotherapy in advanced non-small-cell lung cancer. *J Clin Oncol.* **23:** 5892.

Higgins B., Kolinsky K., Smith M., Beck G., Rashed M., Adames V., Linn M., Wheeldon E., Gand L., Birnboeck H., and Hoffmann G. 2004. Antitumor activity of erlotinib (OSI-774, Tarceva) alone or in combination in human non-small cell lung cancer tumor xenograft models. *Anticancer Drugs* **5:**503.

Hirsch F.R., Varella-Garcia M., and Bunn P.A., et al. 2005a. Molecular analysis of EGFR gene copy number, EGFR expression, and Akt activation in advanced non-small-cell lung cancer (aNSCLC) treated with gefitinib or placebo (ISEL trial). In *17th Annual AACR-NCI-EORTC International Conference on Molecular Targets and Cancer Therapeutics*, Philadelphia, Pennsylvania. Abstract A268.

Hirsch F.R., Varella-Garcia M., McCoy J., West H., Xavier A.C., Gumerlock P., Bunn P.A., Jr., Franklin W.A., Crowley J., Gandara D.R., and Southwest Oncology Group. 2005b. Increased epidermal growth factor receptor gene copy number detected by fluorescence in situ hybridization associates with increased sensitivity to gefitinib in patients with bronchioloalveolar carcinoma subtypes: A Southwest Oncology Group Study. *J. Clin. Oncol.* **23:** 6838.

Huncharek M., Muscat J., and Geschwind J.F. 1999. K-ras oncogene mutation as a prognostic marker in non-small cell lung cancer: A combined analysis of 881 cases. *Carcinogenesis* **20:** 1507.

Johnson B.E., Lucca J., Rabin M.S., Lynch T.J., Ostler P., Skarin A.T., Temel J., Liu G., and Janne P.A. 2004. Preliminary results from a phase II study of the epidermal growth factor receptor tyrosine kinase inhibitor erlotinib in patients >70 years of age with previously untreated advanced non-small cell lung carcinoma. *J. Clin. Oncol.* **22:** 633. (Abstr. 7080.)

Kaseda S., Ueda M., Ozawa S., Ishihara T., Abe O., and Shimizu N. 1989. Expression of epidermal growth factor receptors in four histologic cell types of lung cancer. *J. Surg. Oncol.* **42:** 16.

Keller S.M., Vangel M.G., Adak S., Wagner H., Schiller J.H., Herskovic A., Komaki R., Perry M.C., Marks R.S., Livingston R.B., and Johnson D.H. 2002. The influence of gender on survival and tumor recurrence following adjuvant therapy of completely resected stages II and IIIa non-small cell lung cancer. *Lung Cancer* **37:** 303.

Lynch T.J., Bell D.W., Sordella R., Gurubhagavatula S., Okimoto R.A., Brannigan B.W., Harris P.L., Haserlat S.M., Supko J.G., Haluska F.G., Louis D.N., Christiana D.C., Settleman J., and Haber D.A. 2004a. Activating mutations in the epidermal growth factor receptor underlying responsiveness of non-small-cell lung cancer to gefitinib. *N. Engl. J. Med.* **350:** 2129.

Lynch T.J., Adjei A.A., Bunn P.A., Jr., DuBois R.N., Gandara D.R., Giaccone G., Govindan R., Herbst R.S., Johnson B.E., Khuri F.R., Perez-Soler R., Rosell R., Rowinsky E.K., Sandler A.B., Scagliotti G.V., Schiller J.H., Shapiro G.I., Socinski M.A., and Hart C.S. 2004b. Novel agents in the treatment of lung cancer: Conference summary statement. *Clin. Cancer Res.* **10:** 4199s.

Nelson H.H., Christiani D.C., Mark E.J., Wiencke J.K., Wain J.C., and Kelsey K.T. 1999. Implications and prognostic value of K-ras mutation for early-stage lung cancer in women. *J. Natl. Cancer Inst.* **91:** 2032.

Paez J.G., Janne P.A., Lee J.C., Tracy S., Greulich H., Gabriel S., Herman P., Kaye F.J., Lindeman N., Boggon T.J., Naoki K., Sasaki H., Fujii Y., Eck M.J., Sellers W.R., Johnson B.E., and Meyerson M. 2004. EGFR mutations in lung cancer: Correlation with clinical response to gefitinib therapy. *Science* **304:** 1497.

Pao W. and Miller V.A. 2005. Epidermal growth factor receptor mutations, small-molecule kinase inhibitors, and non-small-cell lung cancer: Current knowledge and future directions. *J. Clin. Oncol.* **23:** 2556.

Pao W., Miller V.A., Politi K.A., Riely G.J., Somwar R., Zakowski M.F., Kris M.G., and Varmus H. 2005a. Acquired resistance of lung adenocarcinomas to gefitinib or erlotinib is associated with a second mutation in the EGFR kinase domain. *PLoS Med.* **2:** e73.

Pao W., Wang T.Y., Riely G.J., Miller V.A., Pan Q., Ladanyi M., Zakowski M.F., Heelan R.T., Kris M.G., and Varmus

H.E. 2005b. KRAS mutations and primary resistance of lung adenocarcinomas to gefitinib or erlotinib. *PLoS Med.* **2:** e17.

Pao W., Miller V., Zakowski M., Doherty J., Politi K., Sarkaria I., Singh B., Heelan R., Rusch V., Fulton L., Mardis E., Kupfer D., Wilson R., Kris M., and Varmus H. 2004. EGF receptor gene mutations are common in lung cancers from "never smokers" and are associated with sensitivity of tumors to gefitinib and erlotinib. *Proc. Natl. Acad. Sci.* **101:** 13306.

Rajagopalan H., Bardelli A., Lengauer C., Kinzler K.W., Vogelstein B., and Velculescu V.E. 2002. Tumorigenesis: RAF/RAS oncogenes and mismatch-repair status. *Nature* **418:** 934.

Riely G.J., Pao W., Pham D., Li A.R., Rizvi N., Venkatraman E.S., Zakowski M.F., Kris M.G., Ladanyi M., and Miller V.A. 2006. Clinical course of patients with non-small cell lung cancer and epidermal growth factor receptor exon 19 and exon 21 mutations treated with gefitinib or erlotinib. *Clin. Cancer Res.* **12:** 839.

Sanchez-Cespedes M., Ahrendt S.A., Piantadosi S., Rosell R., Monzo M., Wu L., Westra W.H., Yang S.C., Jen J., and Sidransky D. 2001. Chromosomal alterations in lung adenocarcinoma from smokers and non-smokers. *Cancer Res.* **61:** 1309.

She Q.B., Solit D., Basso A., and Moasser M.M. 2003. Resistance to gefitinib in PTEN-null HER-overexpressing tumor cells can be overcome through restoration of PTEN function or pharmacologic modulation of constitutive phosphatidylinositol 3'-kinase/Akt pathway signaling. *Clin. Cancer Res.* **9:** 4340.

Shepherd F.A., Rodrigues Pereira J., Ciuleanu T., Tan E.H., Hirsh V., Thongprasert S., Campos D., Maoleekoonpiroj S., Smylie M., Martins R., van Kooten M., Dediu M., Findlay B.,

Tu D., Johnston D., Bezjak A., Clark G., Santabarbara P., and Seymour L. 2005. National Cancer Institute of Canada Clinical Trials Group. Erlotinib in previously treated non-small-cell lung cancer. *N. Engl. J. Med.* **353:** 123.

Schiller J.H., Adak S., Feins R.H., Keller S.M., Fry W.A., Livingston R.B., Hammond M.E., Wolf B., Sabatini L., Jett J., Kohman L., and Johnson D.H. 2001. Lack of prognostic significance of p53 and K-ras mutations in primary resected non-small-cell lung cancer on E4592: A laboratory ancillary study on an Eastern Cooperative Oncology Group prospective randomized trial of postoperative adjuvant therapy. *J. Clin. Oncol.* **19:** 448.

Sordella R., Bell D.W., Haber D.A., and Settleman J. 2004. Gefitinib-sensitizing EGFR mutations in lung cancer activate anti-apoptotic pathways. *Science* **305:** 1163.

Tam I.Y., Chung L.P., Suen W.S., Wang E., Wong M.C., Ho K.K., Lam W.K., Chiu S.W., Girard L., Minna J.D., Gazdar A.F., and Wong M.P. 2006. Distinct epidermal growth factor receptor and KRAS mutation patterns in non-small cell lung cancer patients with different tobacco exposure and clinicopathologic features. *Clin. Cancer Res.* **12:** 1647.

Tamura K. and Fukuoka M. 2005. Gefitinib in non-small cell lung cancer. *Expert Opin. Pharmacother.* **6:** 985.

Tsao M.S., Sakurada A., Cutz J.C., Zhu C.Q., Kamel-Reid S., Squire J., Lorimer I., Zhang T., Liu N., Daneshmand M., Marrano P., da Cunha Santos G., Lagarde A., Richardson F., Seymour L., Whitehead M., Ding K., Pater J., and Shepherd F.A. 2005. Erlotinib in lung cancer: Molecular and clinical predictors of outcome. *N. Engl. J. Med.* **353:** 133.

Yarden Y. and Sliwkowski M.X. 2001. Untangling the ErbB signalling network. *Nat. Rev. Mol Cell. Biol.* **2:** 127.

Exploiting the p53 Pathway for the Diagnosis and Therapy of Human Cancer

D.P. LANE

Institute of Cell and Molecular Biology, Singapore 138673

After 26 years of research and the publication of 38,000 papers, our knowledge of the p53 human tumor suppressor protein is impressive. Over half of all human cancers have mutations in the p53 gene, and the p53 pathway in animal models dramatically regulates the cellular response to ionizing radiation and chemotherapeutic drugs. The ability to translate this knowledge to patient benefit is, however, still in its infancy. The many approaches to determining the status of the p53 pathway in human tumor biopsy samples and the attempts to develop p53-selective therapies are described. A great deal of our knowledge of the p53 system remains incomplete, and the issue of how to best conduct translational research in cancer is debated using the difficulties around the p53 system as an example. The need for a more unified and coordinated approach to critical technological developments and clinical trial protocols is discussed.

Since its original description in 1979 (Lane and Crawford 1979), the p53 protein and the gene that encodes it have been the subject of intense study; over 38,000 papers are identified in Pub Med using p53 as the search term. The reasons for this are the finding that more than half of all human tumors have lost normal p53 gene function by virtue of mutation and the growing understanding of the critical function of p53 as a tumor suppressor (Greenblatt et al. 1994; Vogelstein et al. 2000). In this paper, I discuss the attempts that we and others have made to exploit our growing understanding of the p53 system for the diagnosis and therapy of human cancer. This has been an intense effort, and to date its success is very limited. However, the challenges faced in this task reflect those of translational medicine in general, and the intensity and focus of the p53 effort make it a particularly instructive case history. The considerations in this paper reflect not only on the scientific issues, but also on some of the organizational social and political points raised in Clifton Leaf's article in *Fortune* magazine on why we are losing the war against cancer (Leaf 2004). If we calculate that the scientific funding required to produce the average paper is $100,000 (I suspect quite a conservative estimate), then academic p53 research has consumed $3,800,000,000, and 75 million human cases of cancer with p53 mutations have occurred since its discovery. Yet our certain knowledge of the p53 system is surprisingly incomplete, and internationally, we still have neither effective p53-based therapies nor diagnostics in approved clinical use except in the People's Republic of China.

CERTAIN AND UNCERTAIN KNOWLEDGE ABOUT p53

This huge research effort has produced a great deal of "certain knowledge" about p53. I would define this as a core set of research findings that have been widely tested, reproduced, and accepted, and on which further confirmatory findings have been based. These findings usually lie in three areas: epidemiology, genetics, and structural

and physical protein biochemistry. In all three of these broad areas, our scientific tools seem to be robust and reliable, subject to widely agreed upon and understood standards of proof. The uncertain knowledge about p53 refers to a vast literature of mostly cell-based transfection experiments that are widely discussed but are still to a large extent contradictory or unverified or which, although undoubtedly true in a given experimental context, have an unproven biological significance. Examples of such claims include reports that p53 is an exonuclease (Mummenbrauer et al. 1996), or that p53 binds to cdc2 and tubulin (Maxwell et al. 1991), or closer to home, our own observation that p53 is modified by the Nedd8 ubiquitin-like protein (Xirodimas et al. 2004). I discuss these issues in more detail below, but it should be recognized that observations in this uncertain category can sometimes cross over into the certain knowledge category by virtue of further rigorous experimentation usually involving genetic models. The problem is that so many are left to languish in the uncertain category.

The p53 gene encodes a 393-amino acid protein whose complete crystal structure has not yet been determined. However, we do have crystal (Cho et al. 1994) and NMR-based (Canadillas et al. 2006) structural determinations of the core DNA-binding domain, the amino-terminal Mdm2-binding protein region (Kussie et al. 1996), and the oligomerization domain (Jeffrey et al. 1995; Miller et al. 1996). A large collection of monoclonal antibodies to p53 has been produced and epitope-mapped (Stephen et al. 1995). Thanks principally to the efforts of the Fersht lab, we have a strong understanding of the thermodynamic properties of the DNA-binding domain and the effect of mutations on these properties (Frielder et al. 2003; Veprintsev et al. 2006). Homologs of human p53 are found in all vertebrates studied, but in addition, have also been found in nematode worms and flies, allowing studies of p53 in two genetically amenable species, *Caenorhabditis elegans* (Derry et al. 2001) and *Drosophila melanogaster* (Brodsky et al. 2000; Jin et al. 2000; Ollmann et al. 2000). In addition to p53 itself, two p53-related genes, known as p73 and p63, have been described in some vertebrate species (Moll and Slade 2004). These p53-like proteins share a particular homology with the DNA-binding domain of p53. It is disquieting that many basic questions about the quaternary structure of the p53 protein remain unresolved and the mechanisms of its regulation in vivo are not well understood. In particular, of the many posttranslational modifications of p53 that can be detected in "in vitro" systems, which ones are important in vivo is still unresolved. It is striking that as recently as last year we described that the human p53 gene could encode nine proteins, an observation missed by the field for over 20 years (Bourdon et al. 2005).

The current central theory of p53 action is that it acts as a sequence-specific transcription factor to activate and repress a large number of genes that control cell growth and survival. The p53 response is very tightly controlled by multiple pathways and is induced in response to cellular stress. A huge area of current research is the determination of the precise upstream signals to p53 and the mechanisms by which p53 exerts its tumor suppressor function. A large body of evidence strongly suggests that p53 function is critical in reducing cancer frequency in vertebrates, including man. The human evidence derives from two principal findings, first and most importantly from the studies of the Li-Fraumeni cancer family syndrome (Varley 2003). In the majority of families with this broad familial cancer syndrome, there is genetic linkage to the p53 locus, and the p53 gene is mutated to produce a protein that is nonfunctional in transcription activation assays. The second supportive finding is the very high frequency of somatic mutations in p53 in human cancer (Hainaut et al. 1998). These mutations are often point mis-sense mutations that again result in proteins which have lost transcription activation function. How can one be certain that these mutations are not simply chance occurrences, but rather have significance for the properties of the tumor cell? One biological argument extends from the extensive work in mouse genetic model systems, and the other arises from the case of human cervical cancer, in which p53 mutations do not occur but p53 function appears to be inactivated by the activity of the viral HPV E6 protein that is invariably expressed in these cancers (Mantovani and Banks 2001).

A key control pathway that regulates p53 activity is the function of two negative regulatory proteins, Mdm2 and Mdm4 (Bond et al. 2005a,b). These proteins bind to p53 and inactivate its function as a tumor suppressor. Mdm2 acts as an E3 ligase promoting the degradation of p53, and the inhibition of this activity appears to be a principal route by which p53 levels rise in response to stress signals and the p53 response is initiated. A small protein, p14 Arf, can bind to Mdm2 and block its inhibitory function, thus activating the p53 response. The promoter of the Arf gene is activated in many tumor cells, and the Arf protein accumulates in cells that have lost p53 function (Lowe and Sherr 2003).

QUESTIONS RAISED BY MOUSE MODELS

Mouse genetic models of the p53 pathway have proved to be of enormous value and establish certain key param-

eters of the p53 response. They also provide a critical link between biochemical observations and biological consequences. If I have come to any conclusions from being an active participant and interested observer of the p53 field since its inception, it is to emphasize the importance of these models. The key first finding was that mice which lacked p53 gene expression could mature to adulthood but spontaneously developed cancer at a greatly elevated rate (Donehower et al. 1992). The p53 knockout mouse has emerged as a key tool in the field, but many of the lessons from this model are still not fully absorbed by the community. Here I want to emphasize two of them; the first concerns the phenomenon of haplo-insufficiency and the second relates to issues around the p53 system and tissue culture. When Knudson (2001) developed his two-hit theory to explain the link between the somatic and inherited forms of retinoblastoma, he clarified in a remarkable way our understanding of the genetics of cancer. In this model, tumors occur more frequently in the inherited cases because only one allele of the Rb gene (the remaining wild-type allele) must be lost for the cell to lack all Rb function. Thus, the critical event is a loss of heterozygosity usually achieved by the deletion of a whole chromosome or chromosomal segment from the wild-type allele. In the p53 model, however, an additional complexity has emerged which is clearly seen in the mouse model. When tumors derived from p53 heterozygote mice are examined, loss of heterozygosity is found in only about half the cases examined (Wijnhoven et al. 2001). In the other half of tumors, the wild-type allele is retained. The same phenomena have been described for tumors isolated from Li-Fraumeni patients (Varley et al. 1997). One of the most important early observations made with the p53 knockout mice was their resistance to radiation-induced death. This observation had a critical impact, emphasizing the importance of the genetics of the host response to radiation rather than the precise dose of radiation as a key variable in radiobiology. Studies on thymocytes isolated from p53 null and p53 heterozygote nulls (and later extended to studies on the intestine) established that the apoptotic response to ionizing radiation in mice is p53-dependent and shows cell-autonomous haplo-insufficiency (Clarke et al. 1993; Lowe et al. 1993). Thus, the biological response of cells having two copies of the p53 gene is readily differentiated from the response of those having a single copy of the gene. This finding of haplo-insufficiency has been extended in other mouse genetic studies to the key p53 regulators, p19Arf and Mdm2 (Eischen et al. 2004). The full impact of these observations has not, however, been broadly appreciated by the field. For example, many models of feedback loops of p53 regulation are discussed, since p53 can induce the synthesis of its negative regulators such as Mdm2, Cop 1, and Pirh2, but all of these models fail to appreciate that they are unable to cope with the difference in p53 levels brought about by haplo-insufficiency. The second key finding from the p53 knockout mice concerns the issue of genetic instability in tissue culture. Examination of normal tissues from these mice establishes that they are diploid, yet after even a very brief period in tissue culture, the cells of p53 knockout mice, but not p53 wild-type mice, become extraordinarily aneuploid (Tsukada et al. 1993). Two explanations can be put forward to elucidate this remarkable observation. Either cell culture imposes an extraordinary level of stress on genetic stability compared to in vivo conditions, or in vivo mechanisms exist of great capacity to eliminate aneuploid cells when they arise. Either explanation carries important implications for most studies on p53-controlled genetic instability in cancer, but the issue has not been closely examined. More recently, mouse models have been used to challenge key biochemical observations made about p53 regulation. The carboxyl terminus of p53 contains seven lysine residues, and these are variably subject to modification by acetylation ubiquitination, Sumo, and Nedd8 conjugation. Alteration of these residues has profound effects on the function and regulation of p53 in the normal tissue culture model systems that are largely based on transient transfection. However, when a p53 gene in which six of these seven lysines had been replaced with arginine was used to replace the endogenous gene in a recently developed model, the mouse showed almost completely normal regulation of p53 function, including the critical property of tumor suppression (Krummel et al. 2005). More informative have been studies of the expression and activity of point mutant p53 proteins in the mouse. Since most somatic mutations that occur in human tumors and most Li-Fraumeni families have mutations of this type, these new models more accurately reflect the human situation than do the knockout mice. The new mice establish that the point mutant proteins can act as dominant negatives over wild-type p53 but can also have p53-independent oncogenic function. For example, mouse tumors arising in such mice are more prone to metastasize than are tumors arising in p53 knockout mice (Lang et al. 2004; Olive et al. 2004).

THE ROLE OF p53 IN RESPONSE TO RADIATION AND CHEMOTHERAPY

The clear and striking prediction of the discovery of the importance of the p53 response to ionizing radiation in the mouse models was that human tumors with mutant p53 may be resistant to radiation therapy. This concept was extended, largely through the work of Scott Lowe's team, to other commonly used cytotoxic cancer therapies (Lowe 1995). The mouse results fitted the model well, and it became clear that the p53 response was very important to the therapeutic activity of many of the common anticancer drugs in these models. It has proved hard to extend these findings in a useful way to human cancers, and the reasons for this, which are discussed below, reflect many of the observations made by Leaf (2004).

DIAGNOSTIC USE OF THE p53 PATHWAY

Given that the animal studies described above implied that the presence or absence of p53 mutation may have a profound effect on the behavior and response to therapy of human tumors, it was expected that determining the p53 status of cancers would rapidly acquire major clinical significance (Wallace-Brodeur and Lowe 1999). A recent meta-analysis of such studies in colon cancer has, how-

ever, confirmed anecdotal understanding that this is not the case (Munro et al. 2005). Since p53 mutations are one of the commonest alterations found in human cancers, this can be seen as a massive failure of translational research, and it is well worth analyzing why this might be the case.

Lack of Suitable Samples

Human clinical material is much harder to study than mouse tissue. What is needed are large cohorts of fully consented patients with precisely diagnosed cancers and exact clinical histories, biopsy samples of whose tumors have been stored in suitable conditions to allow analysis. Although such collections are now being made in several centers, it is still a great challenge to obtain them. The service requirements of the surgery and pathology departments, combined with lack of standard operating procedures, result in great and confounding variability of sample type. This is often further troubled by issues of ownership. Clinicians involved in sample collection feel a sense of ownership, whereas science laboratories able to conduct the tests are staffed by scientists on short-term contracts who, after an initial exciting "claim," do not want to be involved in tightly controlled repetitive analysis. These practical and cultural difficulties often conspire to block progress.

Lack of an Agreed Test Method

Broadly, three methods have been used to establish p53 status in human tumors. In the first, antibodies to p53 are used to stain tumor sections. In the second, the p53 gene or its mRNA is amplified from tumor material and examined by either direct sequencing or indirect methods of sequence or function analysis. Finally, in the third method, p53 function is deduced by the analysis of gene expression profile using microarrays. All of these methods have specific technical and theoretical problems, and typing of tumors by one method often contradicts typing by another. Recent in-depth analysis of the different methods, however, suggests that a useful and practical test can be developed.

WHY DO TUMORS STAIN WITH ANTI-p53 ANTIBODIES?

In the 1980s, it was first observed that the level of p53 protein was much higher in some tumor cell lines and some tumor tissue samples than in normal tissues. In the early 1990s, the development and wide distribution of polyclonal and monoclonal antibodies to p53 that worked on conventional paraffin sections motivated an enormous number of studies of p53 staining (Vojtesek et al. 1993). In some senses, the results were remarkable. In many cases, intense nuclear staining of p53 was seen to be confined to obviously neoplastic cells in the section, while the surrounding normal tissue failed to stain. Analysis of the large number of studies has revealed that not all tumors that have mutant p53 will stain, however. This is because some mutations create stop codons so that the complete protein cannot be expressed. Staining can also be variable across sections in a way that seems not to reflect simple difficulties in processing. In general, but not always, point mis-sense mutations give rise to tumors that stain strongly with p53 antibodies. The mechanism behind this staining is still not understood. In tissue culture systems, mutant p53 accumulates to high levels in every cell in the culture due to an extended half-life of the protein compared to that of wild-type p53. Initially, it was thought that the mutation itself directly stabilized the protein. However, the discovery of the Mdm2 protein as an E3 ligase for p53 suggested an alternate explanation. In this feedback model, Mdm2 transcription is regulated by p53, and so, when mutant p53 is present, the Mdm2 protein is not synthesized and so p53 is stable. Indeed, reintroduction of cDNAs encoding Mdm2 into human tumor cells will cause a reduction in mutant p53 levels (Midgley and Lane 1997). Although intellectually very satisfying, this model has also now been shown to be incomplete. Many human tumor cell lines that express high levels of p53 continue to express Mdm2. When mice are made that can only produce mutant p53, the protein is undetectable by immunohistochemistry in their normal tissues, whereas the tumors that these animals develop stain strongly with anti-p53 antibodies. This suggests an as-yet-undefined method by which the activity of Mdm2 is inhibited in tumor cells but not in normal cells. An attractive model is one of "futile signaling" in which the tumor state signals to the p53 pathway to block p53 degradation even though the p53 is mutant and therefore inactive. These complexities mean that the relationship between p53 function and p53 staining is complex. Recently, a method using a panel of antibodies and a standardized staining protocol has been developed, and along with image analysis approaches, deserves further study. A big advantage of such approaches is their low cost and compatibility with service pathology specimens (Nenutil et al. 2005).

SEQUENCING THE p53 GENE

The second approach to p53 analysis depends on sequencing of the p53 gene either from DNA or RNA extracted from the tumor biopsy. This has proved challenging mostly because of the very large number of mutations that have been found in p53, necessitating that all the open reading frames be analyzed. In many cases, some differential annealing strategy is used to help detect and localize mutations. Large databases of human p53 mutations have been collected, and all common mutations have been found to inactivate p53 function in transcription assays (Hainaut et al. 1998). In a clever variant that exploits this fact, rapid methods have been devised to amplify the p53 mRNA and then test the function of the gene the cDNA encodes directly in a yeast-based reporter assay (Ishioka et al. 1993). This approach appears to detect a higher frequency of mutation than direct sequencing and is now being employed in a large European trial. Problems associated with such sequence-based approaches are quality of RNA or DNA extraction, expense and time taken for an exhaustive analysis, and tumor heterogeneity.

A p53-DEPENDENT TRANSCRIPTION PROFILE

A final recent approach has been to look for a transcriptional profile that reflects p53 status. This is an attractive approach, because in theory it should allow a functional stratification of tumors into those in which the p53 pathway is operating and those in which it is not. It makes the assumption that tumors with normal p53 are able to activate transcription of a gene set distinct from those with mutant p53 or absence of p53 function. In a recent analysis using this method to study a well-characterized set of breast cancers whose p53 gene had been sequenced, two important classes of tumors were identified. One group had a normal p53 sequence but did not express the normal p53 gene set; rather, they expressed the mutant p53 gene set. Further analysis showed that in these tumors the mRNA for p53 itself was absent or at very low levels. This suggests a new method to inactivate p53, that of transcriptional silencing, which would explain how using sequence analysis alone could cause tumors to be misclassified. The alternate case was also uncovered, where tumors expressed the normal gene set even though sequence analysis demonstrated the presence of mutant p53. Here, however, the mutations turned out to be unusual and may represent a rare type of bystander mutation that does not abolish function. With this improved classification, a clearer difference was seen both in survival and in the response to therapy between the p53 functional and nonfunctional groups. These results are important, because one model imagined that the reason why p53 status appeared not to influence response to therapy could be that the p53 pathway is ablated in all cancers. In this model, the ablation would be due to the inhibition of other steps in the pathway in those tumors with wild-type p53. The gene expression analysis does not support this view, but instead suggests that human tumors can be distinguished on the basis of their p53 pathway functional status (Miller et al. 2005). The analysis of these studies emphasizes the difficulty of accurate diagnostic studies of gene function in human cancers. Yet without such studies, little progress can be made in accurately determining the role of p53 in the clinic. Imagine, for example, a drug (as discussed below) that would only be active on tumors with wild-type p53. Without an accurate and precise diagnostic, using, for example, only staining for p53 or sequencing, the drug would be given to patients who had no p53 function and therefore would be bound not to respond. This would reduce the chance of such a drug showing efficacy and thus gaining regulatory approval. If such sophisticated testing is going to be essential, a key goal will be the manufacture of a sophisticated lab on a chip that can produce such data with speed and accuracy at the time of biopsy and at low cost. Even then, the results may not show the clear linkage between p53 status and response seen in the animal models because of the genetic heterogeneity of the human population and the larger size, cell number, and generation time, and therefore greater chance for multiple mutation in human tumors rather than mouse models. Indeed, recent studies of polymorphism in the p53 protein sequence (Donehower 2005) and in the Mdm2 promoter (Bond et al. 2004) that can regulate the intensity of the p53 response and affect cancer incidence and aging reveal at least nine genotypes in the human population of varying sensitivity of p53 response.

THERAPEUTIC APPROACHES TO THE p53 PATHWAY

The discovery that mutation of the p53 gene was a frequent and common event in the majority of human cancers has led to great efforts to exploit this fact for therapy. One approach has been to ask how much the presence or absence of p53 function contributes to the response to existing anticancer drugs. As discussed above, these efforts have been of limited success, and it is still unclear whether this is because all such drugs have complex mechanisms of action that involve p53-dependent and -independent pathways or because of failure to accurately type the status of human tumors. Probably both factors are important. Thus, clinically few decisions are made on the basis of p53 status. One system where it has been used is in bladder cancer, where p53 status influences the clinical decision to surgically remove the bladder. Reports suggest that among the commonly used therapies, 5-FU works better in functionally p53 wild-type tumors, whereas the taxanes work best in functionally p53 mutant tumors. One of the most obvious routes to the use of p53 has been in the field of gene therapy. The delivery of the p53 gene using an adenovirus vector has been approved in China, and the treatment is in late-stage clinical trials in the U.S. The preclinical data are very encouraging and the clinical problem appears to be one of consistent delivery. In its approved use, the gene therapy is given as multiple injections along with radiotherapy in the treatment of head and neck cancer. Recent research suggests ways to engineer more active variants of p53 that may help these therapies (Liu et al. 2001). Another therapy based on a defective adenovirus reported to replicate only in cells that lack p53 function has also been adopted for full development in China after early trials in the U.S. The basis for the tumor-selective replication of this virus, however, turns out not to be due to p53, but rather to heat shock protein expression and events linked to nuclear export (O'Shea et al. 2005).

ATTEMPTS TO REACTIVATE MUTANT p53

The ready detection of high intracellular concentrations of mutant p53 proteins in human tumor cells and the finding that those cells retained susceptibility to wild-type p53 gene therapy have prompted the search for p53 reactivating small molecules. Initial work from our laboratory showed that wild-type p53 proteins produced in bacterial expression systems were inactive in DNA-binding assays. Their activity could be recovered, however, by modifications of the carboxy-terminal 30 amino acids of the protein ranging from simple deletion through to phosphorylation or the action of heat shock proteins (Hupp et al. 1992). We were further able to show that some mutant p53 proteins could also be induced to bind in a sequence-specific manner to DNA with similar activators (Hupp et al. 1993). Eventually, this led to the de-

velopment of small peptide activators of p53 which have been shown to be effective in animal models. In an alternate approach, other groups have identified small molecules such as CP31398 (Foster et al. 1999), PRIMA-1 (Bykov et al. 2002), and MIRA-1 (Bykov et al. 2005) that can activate mutant p53 in cell-based assays. The mechanism of action of these small-molecular-weight compounds is still unclear. Work using macromolecular NMR, however, has shown how a small peptide able to bind the DNA-binding domain of mutant p53 proteins can help fold the protein into an active form (Friedler et al. 2002). With the exception of CP31398, all of these compounds have emerged from the academic community rather than the pharmaceutical industry, and the concept of changing protein-folding patterns as a target for drug development is still seen as very challenging. The realization that mutant p53 proteins may show a gain of independent oncogenic function has, however, led to further support for these proposals, as loss of mutant p53 activity may be therapeutically significant.

ACTIVATING WILD-TYPE p53

Since half of all tumors retain the wild-type p53 gene sequence, it has been proposed that finding molecules able to activate the p53 response in tumor cells may be of therapeutic benefit. Two major criticisms have been raised against this proposal. First, many existing therapeutic drugs activate the p53 response and, second, treated tumors will gain resistance via p53 mutation, which is a common event. These criticisms have been countered by the successful development of p53 activating compounds that show efficacy in preclinical models (Vassilev et al. 2004).

BLOCKING THE p53 Mdm2 INTERACTION

The most intensively studied route to the activation of p53 in tumor cells has been in the development of agents that block the p53 Mdm2 interaction. The first suggestions that such an approach may be viable emerged from an antibody microinjection experiment in which the anti-Mdm2 antibody 3G5 was found to cause the accumulation and activation of p53 in human tumor cell lines. In an intense study from my laboratory in collaboration with scientists from Ciba-Geigy (now Novartis), peptide libraries, phage display, and peptide display aptamers were used to validate this target (V. Bottger et al. 1996, 1999; A. Bottger et al. 1997b). The solution of the X-ray structure of a p53 peptide Mdm2 complex (Kussie et al. 1996) confirmed the definition of the p53 Mdm2 interaction, and specific molecules that block the interaction were able to stabilize and activate p53 (A. Bottger et al. 1997a). Recently, after many years of effort, a small-molecule inhibitor of the interaction has been described. The nutlin compound is an effective activator of p53 and can inhibit the growth of p53 wild-type tumors in xenografts. The compound is remarkably specific and establishes that p53 levels are continually regulated by Mdm2 in normal cells and, most importantly, that tumor cells are selectively susceptible to p53-induced death (Vassilev et al. 2004).

PARADOXICAL p53 ACTIVATION BY INHIBITORS OF TRANSCRIPTIONAL ELONGATION

In surveys of molecules that can activate the p53 response, it was apparently paradoxical that agents which inhibit general transcription such as DRB or actinomycin D were very good activators of the p53 response (Berkson et al. 2005). In general, the response to DNA damage is to inhibit transcription, whereas in the case of the p53 pathway, DNA damage induces specific gene expression. These issues have become particularly pertinent as two inhibitors of kinases involved in transcriptional elongation have entered clinical trials as anticancer treatments. The two molecules, R-roscovitine (CYC202 or Seliciclib) and flavopiridol, were originally identified as cyclin-dependent kinase inhibitors that preferentially inhibited the cdk2/cyclin A and cdk2/cyclin E enzymes. Both compounds were found to induce apoptosis in cancer cells, with particular efficacy in B-cell tumors. The mechanism of action was eventually traced to a selective inhibition of transcriptional elongation via inhibition of RNAP II phosphorylation (probably by cdk9/cyclin T) which resulted in the loss of expression of the antiapoptotic protein Mcl1 (Gojo et al. 2002; Alvi et al. 2005; MacCallum et al. 2005; Raje et al. 2005). At the same time, it was clearly established that R-roscovitine (CYC202 or Seliciclib) could induce p53 accumulation and a potent p53-dependent transcriptional response (Kotala et al. 2001). The p53 response, therefore, seems geared to work in the presence of a general shutdown of transcription, and a very recent paper suggests that this may reflect distinct requirements for RNAP II phosphorylation at p53-induced genes which allow them to escape the normal response to DNA damage. Deeper understanding of this transcriptional switch may be of great value in developing selective regulators of transcription (Gomes et al. 2006).

ACTIVATION OF p53 BY INHIBITORS OF NUCLEAR EXPORT, OVERCOMING HPV INHIBITION

The p53 and Mdm2 proteins are both able to shuttle between nucleus and cytoplasm by virtue of active nuclear import and export. The nuclear export inhibitor leptomycin B, which acts by binding to CRM-1, has proved to be an extraordinarily potent inducer of the p53 response. Surprisingly, leptomycin B kills human tumor cells with a high degree of p53 dependence, suggesting that of all the effects of blocking nuclear export, the activation of the p53 response is the major apoptosis-inducing event (Lain et al. 1999; Smart et al. 1999). In comparative studies with the nutlin compounds, leptomycin B is almost as selective, but far more potent. A clear mechanistic distinction can be made, however, as leptomycin is able to activate p53 in HPV-transformed cells where p53 is controlled by the HPV E6 protein (Hietanen et al. 2000). As expected from its target, the nutlin compound is inactive in HPV-transformed cells. Our attempts to introduce leptomycin B into the clinic have met many of the obstacles

described by Leaf (2004), despite the existence of dedicated support for such approaches within the UK. The major obstacles relate to the costs of toxicity testing and GMP manufacture for compounds that are in the public domain. Given the promising activity of the compound in the treatment of HPV-transformed cells and the desperate need for such an agent in the treatment of HPV-induced anogenital lesions, these delays are very frustrating.

CELL-BASED SCREENING FOR NOVEL ACTIVATORS OF THE p53 PATHWAY

The analysis of both R-roscovitine and leptomycin B as activators of the p53 response revealed two new ways that the p53 response might be controlled and underscored the value of "chemical-biology" approaches. We therefore set about establishing a simple cell-based screen for small-molecule activators of the p53 response (Berkson et al. 2005). The screen consists of a reporter cell line in which the endogenous wild-type p53 protein transcriptional activation is measured by a stably integrated β-galactosidase gene under the control of a minimal promoter and a repeated p53-binding site. Careful selection and maintenance of the line allows the screening of tens of thousands of compounds with low background and excellent signals from known inducers such as DNA damage and DRB. Screening of both the NCI diversity set (Berkson et al. 2005) and, more recently, a large commercial library using limited robotics has been remarkably successful. Over 100 hits have been further characterized to eliminate generally toxic compounds or those that induce DNA damage, and a small subgroup of compounds is now entering further development. Excitingly, compounds that show nutlin-like characteristics have already been identified, underscoring the potential value of cell-based screens (S. Lain, pers. comm.).

CONCLUSIONS

The research on the p53 system represents a good case to study key questions about the structure of modern science. Has the way that we manage scientific research in the 21st century speeded or inhibited the expected translational benefit of the major discovery that over half of all human cancers suffer from a common genetic alteration? This question is at the heart of Clifton Leaf's discussion. Why do so many people work on p53? Is it the appropriate distribution of resource? Should fewer people work on p53 and more resource be spent in other areas? Why is so much of p53 science uncertain? One feature of the field has been the clear establishment of a self-organizing p53 "club." Every other year, scientists in the field, without any support from any outside agency, run the p53 international workshop. The next such workshop will be in New York in 2006; the 2004 event was held in New Zealand. This meeting is unique in both its openness and its organization. The field is also distinguished by a high level of collegiality and the ready sharing of reagents and methods, even in the face of commercial pressures. Yet these very strengths also reinforce the investigator-led, publication-driven model that Leaf describes. It is undoubtedly hard to see clearly when one is on the "inside" of such an environment, and retrospect is always the easy way to come to the right conclusions. I would finish then by making two observations. First, the field is not self-critical enough. Despite all of the strictures of peer review, the pressure has not been sufficient to tilt the balance of research toward the more "certain" science. Anecdotally, the surprising and novel claim has a much higher chance of being published than a careful, precise, even dogged, study that can be relied on for perpetuity. Second, there comes a point when certain technological and organizational steps are needed to move a field forward. These are not well supported by current funding structures. It should be possible to design both a trial and a device to definitively answer whether p53 status is important in the treatment of human cancer. The device might be a lab on a chip that can be applied directly to samples in the operating theater. Similarly, it should be possible to define all genes activated and repressed by p53 and all p53-binding sites occupied in chromatin (Wei et al. 2006). It should be possible to catalog all proteins binding to p53 under physiological endogenous conditions, and it should be possible to take p53 activating compounds rapidly into clinical trial. If making these steps reduces the pool of investigator-led research for a time, it would be a worthwhile pause. That time could be used to harvest the existing literature in a more complete manner and to record it in ways to make it properly accessible. We have started in Singapore, with central government funding to attempt to address these issues.

ACKNOWLEDGMENTS

The opinions are my own, the references are illustrative rather than comprehensive. I thank the Cancer Research UK and A*Star, Singapore, for support. I thank the members of my lab past and present for valuable discussions and support, and David Coomber and Chandra Verma in particular for help with this manuscript. I am a Gibb fellow of Cancer Research UK.

REFERENCES

Alvi A.J., Austen B., Weston V.J., Fegan C., MacCallum D., Gianella-Borradori A., Lane D.P., Hubank M., Powell J.E., Wei W., Taylor A.M., Moss P.A., and Stankovic T. 2005. A novel CDK inhibitor, CYC202 (R-roscovitine), overcomes the defect in p53-dependent apoptosis in B-CLL by down-regulation of genes involved in transcription regulation and survival. *Blood* **105:** 4484.

Berkson R.G., Hollick J.J., Westwood N.J., Woods J.A., Lane D.P., and Lain S. 2005. Pilot screening programme for small molecule activators of p53. *Int. J. Cancer.* **115:** 701.

Bond G.L., Hu W., and Levine A. 2005a. A single nucleotide polymorphism in the MDM2 gene: From a molecular and cellular explanation to clinical effect. *Cancer Res.* **65:** 5481.

———. 2005b. MDM2 is a central node in the p53 pathway: 12 years and counting. *Curr. Cancer Drug Targets* **5:** 3.

Bond G.L., Hu W., Bond E.E., Robins H., Lutzker S.G., Arva N.C., Bargonetti J., Bartel F., Taubert H., Wuerl P., Onel K., Yip L., Hwang S.J., Strong L.C., Lozano G., and Levine A.J. 2004. A single nucleotide polymorphism in the MDM2 promoter attenuates the p53 tumor suppressor pathway and accelerates tumor formation in humans. *Cell* **119:** 591.

Bottger A., Bottger V., Sparks A., Liu W.L., Howard S.F., and Lane D.P. 1997b. Design of a synthetic Mdm2-binding mini protein that activates the p53 response in vivo. *Curr. Biol.* **7:** 860.

Bottger A., Bottger V., Garcia-Echeverria C., Chene P., Hochkeppel H.K., Sampson W., Ang K., Howard S.F., Picksley S.M., and Lane D.P. 1997a. Molecular characterization of the hdm2-p53 interaction. *J. Mol. Biol.* **269:** 744.

Bottger V., Bottger A., Garcia-Echeverria C., Ramos Y.F., van der Eb A.J., Jochemsen A.G., and Lane D.P. 1999. Comparative study of the p53-mdm2 and p53-MDMX interfaces. *Oncogene* **18:** 189.

Bottger V., Bottger A., Howard S.F., Picksley S.M., Chene P., Garcia-Echeverria C., Hochkeppel H.K., and Lane D.P. 1996. Identification of novel mdm2 binding peptides by phage display. *Oncogene* **13:** 2141.

Bourdon J.C., Fernandes K., Murray-Zmijewski F., Liu G., Diot A., Xirodimas D.P., Saville M.K, and Lane D.P. 2005. p53 isoforms can regulate p53 transcriptional activity. *Genes Dev.* **19:** 2122.

Brodsky M.H., Nordstrom W., Tsang G., Kwan E., Rubin G.M., and Abrams J.M. 2000. *Drosophila* p53 binds a damage response element at the reaper locus. *Cell* **101:** 103.

Bykov V.J., Issaeva N., Zache N., Shilov A., Hultcrantz M., Bergman J., Selivanova G., and Wiman K.G. 2005. Reactivation of mutant p53 and induction of apoptosis in human tumor cells by maleimide analogs. *J. Biol. Chem.* **280:** 30384.

Bykov V.J., Issaeva N., Shilov A., Hultcrantz M., Pugacheva E., Chumakov P., Bergman J., Wiman K.G., and Selivanova G. 2002. Restoration of the tumor suppressor function to mutant p53 by a low-molecular-weight compound. *Nat. Med.* **8:** 282.

Canadillas J.M., Tidow H., Freund S.M., Rutherford T.J., Ang H.C., and Fersht A.R. 2006. Solution structure of p53 core domain: Structural basis for its instability. *Proc. Natl. Acad. Sci.* **103:** 2109.

Cho Y., Gorina S., Jeffrey P.D., and Pavletich N.P. 1994. Crystal structure of a p53 tumor suppressor-DNA complex: Understanding tumorigenic mutations. *Science* **265:** 346.

Clarke A.R, Purdie C.A, Harrison D.J, Morris R.G, Bird C.C, Hooper M.L, and Wyllie A.H. 1993. Thymocyte apoptosis induced by p53-dependent and independent pathways. *Nature* **362:** 849.

Derry W.B., Putzke A.P., and Rothman J.H. 2001. *Caenorhabditis elegans* p53: Role in apoptosis, meiosis, and stress resistance. *Science* **294:** 591.

Donehower L.A. 2005. p53: Guardian AND suppressor of longevity? *Exp. Gerontol.* **40:** 7.

Donehower L.A., Harvey M., Slagle B.L., McArthur M.J., Montgomery C.A., Jr., Butel J.S., and Bradley A. 1992. Mice deficient for p53 are developmentally normal but susceptible to spontaneous tumours. *Nature* **356:** 215.

Eischen C.M., Alt J.R., and Wang P. 2004. Loss of one allele of ARF rescues Mdm2 haploinsufficiency effects on apoptosis and lymphoma development. *Oncogene* **23:** 8931.

Foster B.A., Coffey H.A., Morin M.J., and Rastinejad F. 1999. Pharmacological rescue of mutant p53 conformation and function. *Science* **286:** 2507.

Friedler A., Veprintsev D.B., Hansson L.O., and Fersht A.R. 2003. Kinetic instability of p53 core domain mutants: Implications for rescue by small molecules. *J. Biol. Chem.* **278:** 24108.

Friedler A., Hansson L.O., Veprintsev D.B., Freund S.M., Rippin T.M., Nikolova P.V., Proctor M.R., Rudiger S., and Fersht A.R. 2002. A peptide that binds and stabilizes p53 core domain: Chaperone strategy for rescue of oncogenic mutants. *Proc. Natl. Acad. Sci.* **99:** 937.

Gojo I., Zhang B., and Fenton R.G. 2002. The cyclin-dependent kinase inhibitor flavopiridol induces apoptosis in multiple myeloma cells through transcriptional repression and down-regulation of Mcl-1. *Clin. Cancer Res.* **8:** 3527.

Gomes N.P., Bjerke G., Llorente B., Szostek S.A., Emerson B.M., and Espinosa J.M. 2006. Gene-specific requirement for P-TEFb activity and RNA polymerase II phosphorylation within the p53 transcriptional program. *Genes Dev.* **20:** 601.

Greenblatt M.S., Bennett W.P., Hollstein M., and Harris C.C. 1994. Mutations in the p53 tumor suppressor gene: Clues to cancer etiology and molecular pathogenesis. *Cancer Res.* **54:** 4855.

Hainaut P., Hernandez T., Robinson A., Rodriguez-Tome P., Flores T., Hollstein M., Harris C.C., and Montesano R. 1998. IARC database of p53 gene mutations in human tumors and cell lines: Updated compilation, revised formats and new visualisation tools. *Nucleic Acids Res.* **26:** 205.

Hietanen S., Lain S., Krausz E., Blattner C., and Lane D.P. 2000. Activation of p53 in cervical carcinoma cells by small molecules. *Proc. Natl. Acad. Sci.* **97:** 8501.

Hupp T.R., Meek D.W., Midgley C.A., and Lane D.P. 1992. Regulation of the specific DNA binding function of p53. *Cell* **71:** 875.

———. 1993. Activation of the cryptic DNA binding function of mutant forms of p53. *Nucleic Acids Res.* **21:** 3167.

Ishioka C., Frebourg T., Yan Y.X., Vidal M., Friend S.H., Schmidt S., and Iggo R. 1993. Screening patients for heterozygous p53 mutations using a functional assay in yeast. *Nat. Genet.* **5:** 124.

Jeffrey P.D., Gorina S., and Pavletich N.P. 1995. Crystal structure of the tetramerization domain of the p53 tumor suppressor at 1.7 angstroms. *Science* **267:** 1498.

Jin S., Martinek S., Joo W.S., Wortman J.R., Mirkovic N., Sali A., Yandell M.D., Pavletich N.P., Young M.W., and Levine A.J. 2000. Identification and characterization of a p53 homologue in *Drosophila melanogaster. Proc. Natl. Acad. Sci.* **97:** 7301.

Kotala V., Uldrijan S., Horky M., Trbusek M., Strnad M., and Vojtesek B. 2001. Potent induction of wild-type p53-dependent transcription in tumour cells by a synthetic inhibitor of cyclin-dependent kinases. *Cell. Mol. Life Sci.* **58:** 1333.

Knudson A.G. 2001. Two genetic hits (more or less) to cancer. *Nat. Rev. Cancer* **1:** 157.

Krummel K.A., Lee C.J., Toledo F., and Wahl G.M. 2005. The C-terminal lysines fine-tune p53 stress responses in a mouse model but are not required for stability control or transactivation. *Proc. Natl. Acad. Sci.* **102:** 10188.

Kussie P.H., Gorina S., Marechal V., Elenbaas B., Moreau J., Levine A.J., and Pavletich N.P. 1996. Structure of the MDM2 oncoprotein bound to the p53 tumor suppressor transactivation domain. *Science* **274:** 948.

Lain S., Midgley C., Sparks A., Lane E.B., and Lane D.P. 1999. An inhibitor of nuclear export activates the p53 response and induces the localization of HDM2 and p53 to U1A-positive nuclear bodies associated with the PODs. *Exp. Cell Res.* **248:** 457.

Lane D.P. and Crawford L.V. 1979. T antigen is bound to a host protein in SV40-transformed cells. *Nature* **278:** 261.

Lang G.A., Iwakuma T., Suh Y.A., Liu G., Rao V.A., Parant J.M., Valentin-Vega Y.A., Terzian T., Caldwell L.C., Strong L.C., El-Naggar A.K., and Lozano G. 2004. Gain of function of a p53 hot spot mutation in a mouse model of Li-Fraumeni syndrome. *Cell* **119:** 861.

Leaf C. 2004. Why we're losing the war on cancer (and how to win it). *Fortune* (March 22, p. 77).

Liu W.L., Midgley C., Stephen C., Saville M., and Lane D.P. 2001. Biological significance of a small highly conserved region in the N terminus of the p53 tumour suppressor protein. *J. Mol. Biol.* **313:** 711.

Lowe S.W. 1995. Cancer therapy and p53. *Curr. Opin. Oncol.* **7:** 547.

Lowe S.W. and Sherr C.J. 2003. Tumor suppression by Ink4a-Arf: Progress and puzzles. *Curr. Opin. Genet. Dev.* **13:** 77.

Lowe S.W., Schmitt E.M., Smith S.W., Osborne B.A., and Jacks T. 1993. p53 is required for radiation-induced apoptosis in mouse thymocytes. *Nature* **362:** 847.

MacCallum D.E., Melville J., Frame S., Watt K., Anderson S., Gianella-Borradori A., Lane D.P., and Green S.R. 2005. Seliciclib (CYC202, R-Roscovitine) induces cell death in multiple myeloma cells by inhibition of RNA polymerase II-dependent transcription and down-regulation of Mcl-1. *Cancer Res.* **65:** 5399.

Mantovani F. and Banks L. 2001. The human papillomavirus E6 protein and its contribution to malignant progression. *Oncogene* **20:** 7874.

Maxwell S.A., Ames S.K., Sawai E.T., Decker G.L., Cook R.G., and Butel J.S. 1991. Simian virus 40 large T antigen and p53 are microtubule-associated proteins in transformed cells. *Cell Growth Differ.* **2:** 115.

Midgley C.A. and Lane D.P. 1997. p53 protein stability in tumour cells is not determined by mutation but is dependent on Mdm2 binding. *Oncogene* **15:** 1179.

Miller L.D., Smeds J., George J., Vega V.B., Vergara L., Ploner A., Pawitan Y., Hall P., Klaar S., Liu E.T., and Bergh J. 2005. An expression signature for p53 status in human breast cancer predicts mutation status, transcriptional effects, and patient survival. *Proc. Natl. Acad. Sci.* **102:** 13550

Miller M., Lubkowski J., Rao J.K., Danishefsky A.T., Omichinski J.G., Sakaguchi K., Sakamoto H., Appella E., Gronenborn A.M., and Clore G.M. 1996. The oligomerization domain of p53: Crystal structure of the trigonal form. *FEBS Lett.* **399:** 166.

Moll U.M. and Slade N. 2004. p63 and p73: Roles in development and tumor formation. *Mol. Cancer Res.* **2:** 371.

Mummenbrauer T., Janus F., Muller B., Wiesmuller L., Deppert W., and Grosse F. 1996. p53 protein exhibits 3′-to-5′ exonuclease activity. *Cell* **85:** 1089.

Munro A.J., Lain S., and Lane D.P. 2005. p53 abnormalities and outcomes in colorectal cancer: A systematic review. *Br. J. Cancer* **92:** 434.

Nenutil R., Smardova J., Pavlova S., Hanzelkova Z., Muller P., Fabian P., Hrstka R., Janotova P., Radina M., Lane D.P., Coates P.J., and Vojtesek B. 2005. Discriminating functional and non-functional p53 in human tumours by p53 and MDM2 immunohistochemistry. *J. Pathol.* **207:** 251.

Olive K.P., Tuveson D.A., Ruhe Z.C., Yin B., Willis N.A., Bronson R.T., Crowley D., and Jacks T. 2004. Mutant p53 gain of function in two mouse models of Li-Fraumeni syndrome. *Cell* **119:** 847.

Ollmann M., Young L.M., Di Como C.J., Karim F., Belvin M., Robertson S., Whittaker K., Demsky M., Fisher W.W., Buchman A., Duyk G., Friedman L., Prives C., and Kopczynski C. 2000. *Drosophila* p53 is a structural and functional homolog of the tumor suppressor p53. *Cell* **101:** 91.

O'Shea C.C., Soria C., Bagus B., and McCormick F. 2005. Heat shock phenocopies E1B-55K late functions and selectively sensitizes refractory tumor cells to ONYX-015 oncolytic viral therapy. *Cancer Cell* **8:** 61.

Raje N., Kumar S., Hideshima T., Roccaro A., Ishitsuka K., Yasui H., Shiraishi N., Chauhan D., Munshi N.C., Green S.R., and Anderson K.C. 2005. Seliciclib (CYC202 or R-roscovitine), a small-molecule cyclin-dependent kinase inhibitor, mediates activity via down-regulation of Mcl-1 in multiple myeloma. *Blood* **106:** 1042.

Smart P., Lane E.B., Lane D.P., Midgley C., Vojtesek B., and Lain S. 1999. Effects on normal fibroblasts and neuroblastoma cells of the activation of the p53 response by the nuclear export inhibitor leptomycin B. *Oncogene* **18:** 7378.

Stephen C.W., Helminen P., and Lane D.P. 1995. Characterisation of epitopes on human p53 using phage-displayed peptide libraries: Insights into antibody-peptide interactions. *J. Mol. Biol.* **248:** 58.

Tsukada T., Tomooka Y., Takai S., Ueda Y., Nishikawa S., Yagi T., Tokunaga T., Takeda N., Suda Y., and Abe S. 1993. Enhanced proliferative potential in culture of cells from p53-deficient mice. *Oncogene* **8:** 3313.

Varley J.M. 2003. Germline TP53 mutations and Li-Fraumeni syndrome. *Hum. Mutat.* **21:** 551.

Varley J.M., Thorncroft M., McGown G., Appleby J., Kelsey A.M., Tricker K.J., Evans D.G., and Birch J.M. 1997. A detailed study of loss of heterozygosity on chromosome 17 in tumours from Li-Fraumeni patients carrying a mutation to the TP53 gene. *Oncogene* **14:** 865.

Vassilev L.T., Vu B.T., Graves B., Carvajal D., Podlaski F., Filipovic Z., Kong N., Kammlott U., Lukacs C., Klein C., Fotouhi N., and Liu E.A. 2004. In vivo activation of the p53 pathway by small-molecule antagonists of MDM2. *Science* **303:** 844.

Veprintsev D.B., Freund S.M., Andreeva A., Rutledge S.E., Tidow H., Canadillas J.M., Blair C.M., and Fersht A.R. 2006.

Core domain interactions in full-length p53 in solution. *Proc. Natl. Acad. Sci.* **103:** 2115.

Vogelstein B., Lane D., and Levine A.J. 2000. Surfing the p53 network. *Nature* **408:** 307.

Vojtesek B., Fisher C.J., Barnes D.M., and Lane D.P. 1993. Comparison between p53 staining in tissue sections and p53 proteins levels measured by an ELISA technique. *Br. J. Cancer* **67:** 1254.

Wallace-Brodeur R.R. and Lowe S.W. 1999. Clinical implications of p53 mutations. *Cell. Mol. Life Sci.* **55:** 64.

Wei C.L., Wu Q., Vega V.B., Chiu K.P., Ng P., Zhang T., Shahab A., Yong H.C., Fu Y., Weng Z., Liu J., Zhao X.D., Chew J.L., Lee Y.L., Kuznetsov V.A., Sung W.K., Miller L.D., Lim B., Liu E.T., Yu Q., Ng H.H., and Ruan Y. 2006. A global map of p53 transcription-factor binding sites in the human genome. *Cell* **124:** 207.

Wijnhoven S.W., Kool H.J., van Teijlingen C.M., van Zeeland A.A., and Vrieling H. 2001. Loss of heterozygosity in somatic cells of the mouse. An important step in cancer initiation? *Mutat. Res.* **473:** 23.

Xirodimas D.P., Saville M.K., Bourdon J.C., Hay R.T., and Lane D.P. 2004. Mdm2-mediated NEDD8 conjugation of p53 inhibits its transcriptional activity. *Cell* **118:** 83.

Drugging the Cancer Kinome: Progress and Challenges in Developing Personalized Molecular Cancer Therapeutics

P. WORKMAN

Cancer Research UK Centre for Cancer Therapeutics, The Institute of Cancer Research,
Haddow Laboratories, Sutton, Surrey SM2 5NG United Kingdom

A major goal of cancer research is to translate our understanding of the causation of malignancy at the level of the genome and biochemical pathways into the development of drugs with improved activity and cancer selectivity. This paper provides a personal perspective of the current status of efforts to achieve this goal, with a particular focus on drugging the cancer kinome. Remarkable progress has been made in this area, but many challenges remain. The value of cancer kinome sequencing is emphasized. Three projects in which the author's laboratory is involved are reviewed in detail. These involve the discovery and development of inhibitors of cyclin-dependent kinases, phosphoinositide 3-kinases, and the Hsp90 molecular chaperone.

THE THERAPEUTIC PROMISE OF CANCER GENOMICS

Just as it is the objective of basic cancer research to understand the fundamental basis of malignancy, so it is the goal of modern molecular therapeutics research to develop drugs that exploit this basic knowledge (Workman and Kaye 2002; Workman 2003a,b; Bronchud et al. 2004). The last five years in particular have seen the translation of our understanding of genomics and molecular biology of cancer into new treatments targeted to pathways responsible for malignancy. In contrast to the drugs developed in the cytotoxic era, the new molecular therapeutics that are being developed in this second golden era of cancer drug development are designed to attack the oncogenic players and pathways that are deranged in cancer: Hence, there is an expectation that these agents will be more efficient and have fewer side effects compared to conventional cytotoxic drugs (Workman 2005).

Although our comprehension of the molecular processes that propel malignancy remains very much incomplete, there is no doubt that the accumulation of genetic and epigenetic abnormalities is critical for cancer progression (Balmain et al. 2003; Vogelstein and Kinzler 2004). These abnormalities in turn produce the hallmark characteristics of cancer, including uncontrolled cell cycle progression and proliferation, inappropriate survival, immortalization, invasion, angiogenesis, and metastasis (Hanahan and Weinberg 2000). It is believed that selection for alterations providing a growth advantage occurs, according to the model of clonal evolution (Nowell 1976). The contribution of various genes to malignant progression is illustrated schematically in Figure 1A, and the exploitation of this knowledge for the development of new therapeutics is depicted alongside in Figure 1B. We now understand very well that the engine of cancer is fueled by the activation oncogenes (which are the "accelerators" of cancer) and the inactivation of tumor suppressor genes (which are the "brakes" on malignancy). In addition, tumor development is encouraged by the mutation and loss of genes involved in DNA repair. Furthermore, the oncogenic process seems to be strongly supported by genes that had been considered previously to play "housekeeping" roles, such as histone deacetylases and the molecular chaperone Hsp90. The ultimate aim must be to identify and understand all of the genes and pathways that are involved in all cancers and to develop drugs that are active in each case.

The choice of molecular targets for cancer drug development is now rooted very firmly in the identification of new cancer genes and the functional pathways that they hijack. High-profile articles in the lay press have helped to fuel public debate about the extent to which the massive investment in cancer research since Richard Nixon's famous "war on cancer" in the 1970s, together with the much-hyped genomic revolution, have already delivered the goods in terms of benefit to patients (Anonymous 2004; Leaf 2004). The clinical activity and regulatory approval of small-molecule drugs like imatinib (Gleevec), gefitinib (Iressa), and erlotinib (Tarceva; see Fig. 2 for structures), and also the therapeutic antibodies trastuzamab (Herceptin), cetuximab (Erbutix), and bevacizumab (Avastin), have provided some reassurance that we are now on the right track. An article published in *Business Week* while the Symposium meeting was in progress argued that "medical care is reaching a tipping point" and pointed to the 400 cancer drugs that are now in clinical trial, many of which are directed to cancer genome targets (Arnst 2005).

In this paper, I provide a personal perspective on drug development based on cancer genomics, with particular emphasis on "drugging the cancer kinome." I summarize the considerable challenges that face us, as well as the remarkable progress that has been made. I start by discussing cancer kinome targets and focus particularly on the impact of human genome and cancer genome sequencing. I then illustrate many of the issues with exam-

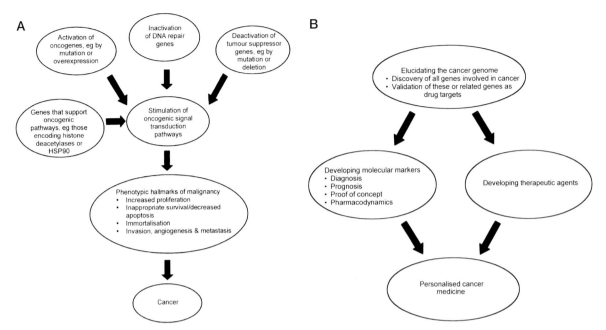

Figure 1. Genomics and contemporary drug development. (*A*) Schematic illustration of how malignancy is initiated and driven by abnormalities in cancer genes. (*B*) Exploitation of the cancer genome for the development of targeted molecular therapeutics and personalized cancer treatment. (Modified from Workman 2005.)

ples from our own recent experience in developing small-molecule inhibitors against three molecular targets, namely cyclin-dependent kinases (CDKs), phosphoinositide 3-kinase (PI3Ks), and the Hsp90 molecular chaperone. The reader is also referred to previous personal views from this author in published interviews (Workman 2001, 2003c).

CANCER KINOME TARGETS

Oncogenic kinases clearly punch above their weight in the league tables of cancer genes. Of the 291 cancer-causing genes identified in a recent census, 27 (6%) encode protein kinase domains, much higher than the 6 (2%) that would be predicted on the basis of random selection (Futreal et al. 2004). The druggability of kinases as a target class is confirmed by the examples listed in the previous section of this paper. As mentioned, both antibody-based and small-molecule approaches to drugging the cancer kinome have been successful. Kinases now represent the most frequently targeted gene classes in cancer and are second only to G-protein-coupled receptors when ranked across all therapeutic areas (Cohen 2002; Hopkins and Groom 2002).

This has stimulated interest to search for new drug targets among the 518 putative kinases in the human genome (Cohen 2002; Manning et al. 2002). The earliest kinase targets represented the results of decades of painstaking biological research. On the basis of a large body of work, we now know that kinases can be activated in cancer by mutation, translocation, amplification, over-expression, and posttranslational modification. The discovery of kinase targets has recently benefited from the availability of the complete human genome sequence (In-

ternational Human Genome Sequencing Consortium 2004) and the application of gene expression profiling by microarray, together with high-throughput mutation detection and high-throughput sequencing approaches (Weir et al. 2004; Workman 2005).

In the first breakthrough made by high-throughput cancer genome sequencing, activating mutations in B-RAF were identified, particularly in melanoma but also in papillary thyroid, serous ovarian, and other cancers (Davies et al. 2002; Garnett and Marais 2004). This discovery immediately stimulated the evaluation in malignant melanoma of sorafenib (formerly known as BAY 43-9006; see Fig. 2), a multi-targeted kinase inhibitor that blocks B-RAF and C-RAF, among others (Wilhelm et al. 2004). Although single-agent activity was disappointing, striking activity has been seen for sorafenib in combination with cytotoxic chemotherapy in melanoma, and this drug is now being evaluated in randomized trials (Danson and Lorrigan 2005). Because of its action on many kinases, it is difficult to evaluate the role of B-RAF inhibition in the activity of sorafenib, and there is therefore interest in identifying more selective B-RAF inhibitors. A high-throughput screen for inhibitors of the most common V600E B-RAF mutant was carried out in our Centre and identified a 3,5, di-substituted pyridine class of inhibitors (Newbatt et al. 2005).

In addition to the genetics, functional and structural biology studies have now fully validated B-RAF as a bona fide oncogene and drug target (Garnett and Marais 2004; Wan et al. 2004). X-ray crystallography studies of mutant B-RAF with sorafenib showed very elegantly how the V600E mutant promotes the active kinase conformation by disrupting the hydrophobic interaction that occurs between the regulatory activation segment and the glycine-

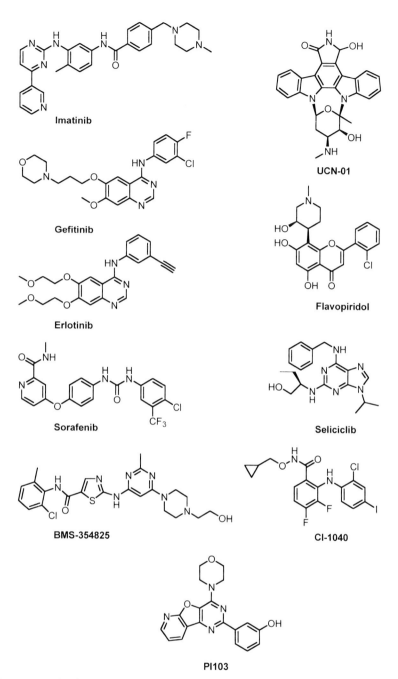

Figure 2. Chemical structures of various representative small-molecule kinase inhibitory drugs. Imatinib (Gleevec) inhibits BCR-ABL, KIT, and PDFGR receptor kinases and is approved for the treatment of chronic myeloid leukemia and gastrointestinal stromal tumors. Gefitinib (Iressa) and erlotinib (Tarceva) inhibit EGFR and are approved in non-small-cell lung cancer. Sorafenib is an inhibitor of VEFGR-2, VEGFR-3, PDGFβ, RAF, and other kinases and shows activity in renal cancer. BMS-354825 is an inhibitor of SRC and BCR-ABL that retains activity in imatinib-resistant mutants of the latter. UCN-01 is the 7-hydroxy derivative of the prototype broad-spectrum kinase inhibitor staurosporine and inhibits CHK1. Flavopiridol is a broad-spectrum CDK inhibitor that has undergone extensive clinical trials. Seliciclib (CYC202, *R*-roscovitine) is a more selective CDK inhibitor with relatively greater potency for CDKs 2, 7, and 9. CI-1040 is a MEK1/2 inhibitor that entered clinical trials; an analog of this agent is now in clinical development. PI103 is a selective inhibitor of the class 1 PI3K isoforms.

rich P loop. Indeed, almost all of the mutations in the B-RAF protein are grouped around these regions, resulting in destabilization of the inactive conformation and stimulation of the enzyme catalytic activity.

Prompted by the success with B-RAF, exon resequencing has been used to probe for somatic mutations in pro-

tein kinases, lipid kinases, and phosphatases. In a systematic study of the kinome of colorectal cancers (Bardelli et al. 2003), somatic mutations were identified in 5/90 tyrosine kinase genes (*NTKR3, FES, KDR, EHA3, and MLK4*), 1/43 tyrosine kinase-like genes (*MLK4*), and one receptor guanylate cyclase gene (*GUCY2F*). Although mutations were common in the kinase domains, suggesting potential activation, further work is required to validate these potential drug targets.

A related study of the phosphatome of colorectal cancers identified mutations in the kinase domains of 6/87 members of this superfamily (*PTPRF, PTPRG, PTPRT, PTPN3, PTPN13,* and *PTPN14*) (Wang et al. 2004). The mutations indicated the potential for inactivation of the phosphatase activity, suggesting that *PRPRT* and others may be tumor suppressor genes. If so, therapeutic exploitation would require identification of the corresponding kinases, since pharmacological resurrection of inactive phosphatases is not currently feasible.

A precedent for such an approach comes from work on *PTEN*, which is well known as the second most common tumor suppressor gene after *p53*. This tumor suppressor gene is implicated in glioblastoma, prostate, and endometrial malignancies (Dahia 2000). *PTEN* encodes a lipid phosphatase that is responsible for reversing the biochemical reactions that produce phosphatidylinositol 3,4 biphosphate and phosphatidylinositol 3,4,5-triphosphate and are catalyzed by the class I PI3Ks. Systematic sequencing of the coding regions of 8 PI3Ks and another 8 PI3K-like genes led to the discovery of mutations only in the *PIK3CA* gene (Samuels et al. 2004). This gene encodes the p110α catalytic subunit, a class 1A PI3K. The mutations suggested likely activation of the kinase. Activation was demonstrated biochemically in one case, and subsequent studies confirmed this and also showed oncogenic activity (Kang et al. 2005). *PI3K3CA* mutations have been found in colorectal, glioblastoma, gastric, and breast cancers (Bachman et al. 2004; Samuels et al. 2004). Together with previous evidence for amplification of *PIK3CA* (Shayesteh et al. 1999) and a wealth of other data, these mutation studies add support for the development of PI3K inhibitors for cancer treatment (Stein and Waterfield 2000; Vivanco and Sawyers 2002; Ward et al. 2003; Drees et al. 2004; Workman 2004a). This is addressed in a later section.

Another externally important example of the value of cancer kinome sequencing is the discovery that activating mutations in the *EGFR* gene can lead to sensitivity of patients with non-small-cell lung cancer to the EGFR inhibitors gefitinib and erlotinib (Lynch et al. 2004; Paez et al. 2004; Pao et al. 2004). Since I was involved in the gefitinib discovery team at Zeneca (now AstraZeneca), this breakthrough was a particularly exciting one to me personally. The results provide evidence in humans that mutant *EGFR* is the major driving oncogene in a subset of non-small-cell lung cancers. It is also reasonable to conclude that mutational activation of *EGFR* in these patients represents an example of "oncogene addiction" (Weinstein 2002), analogous to the role of *BCR-ABL* in chronic myeloid leukemia and mutant *KIT* in gastrointestinal stromal tumors (Sawyers 2003; Druker 2004). Subsequent studies have shown that a second mutation in the catalytic domain can lead to resistance to erlotinib and gefitinib (Kobayashi et al. 2005; Pao et al. 2005). Resistance to imatinib can also be caused by similar mutations in the kinase domain of BCR-ABL (Gorre et al. 2001) and can be overcome by an alternative inhibitor BMS-354825

(see Fig. 2) (Shah et al. 2004). This is likely to be a recurring theme (Daub et al. 2004).

CYCLIN-DEPENDENT KINASE INHIBITORS

Deregulation of cell cycle control proteins by mutation and altered expression is extremely common in human tumors (Sherr 1996, 2000). This led to the idea that small-molecule catalytic inhibitors of CDKs involved in cell cycle regulation could have therapeutic activity in cancer by minimizing the effects of the natural polypeptide inhibitors that are commonly lost in malignancy (Garrett et al. 2003). Inhibition of CDKs would be expected to lead to cell cycle arrest, and there was also evidence that apoptosis might be induced selectively in cancer cells (Chen et al. 1999).

We have collaborated with Cyclacel Limited in the development of the trisubstituted aminopurine CDK inhibitor seliciclib (CYC202; *R*-roscovitine; see Fig. 2). Seliciclib exhibits its highest level of potency against CDK2/cyclin E, but other CDKs are also affected, particularly CDK1 and the transcriptional kinases CDK7 and 9 that phosphorylate RNA polymerase II and thereby regulate gene transcription (Whittaker et al. 2004). It was difficult to predict which molecular effects would be most important for the antitumor activity of seliciclib. In our mechanism of action studies we used western blotting to study effects on candidate proteins and pathways, and we also employed gene expression profiling using our in-house cDNA microarray facility as a non-biased, global approach to explore the mechanism of action of seliciclib and to discover potential biomarkers of drug action.

We showed that treatment of human colon cancer cells with seliciclib in tissue culture resulted in a decrease in phosphorylation of the retinoblastoma protein RB at multiple sites (Whittaker et al. 2004). This was confirmed using an antibody that recognized the hypophosphorylated form at the Ser-608 site. Surprisingly, we also saw an increase in ERK1/2 phosphorylation, but a decrease in FOS protein expression. Furthermore, we saw a reduction in expression of cyclins at both the protein and mRNA levels. In addition, seliciclib caused a decrease in the expression of both the hyperphosphorylated and hypophosphorylated forms of RNA polymerase II, consistent with inhibition of CDKs 7 and 9. Figure 3 shows some of these effects in the HCT116 human colon xenograft in nude mice. No effects are seen on ERK phosphorylation in this model, perhaps because it has a *KRAS* mutation.

Gene expression microarray profiling showed that around 10–15% of genes were either up-regulated or down-regulated by seliciclib (Whittaker et al. 2003 and in prep.). Of particular interest was a systematic pattern of reduced expression at the mRNA level of genes involved in the regulation of mitosis, including those encoding cyclin B2, CDC25C, PLK-1, and Aurora-1. Down-regulation was confirmed at the protein level.

We hypothesized that seliciclib was exerting both direct and indirect effects on cell cycle CDKs (Whittaker et al. 2004). There appears to be a direct effect on CDK2, since inhibition of the phosphorylation of the proposed CDK2 site on RB, Thr-821, was an early response to the

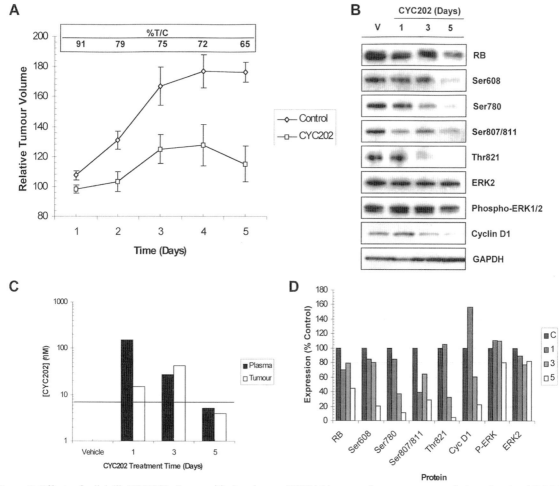

Figure 3. Effects of seliciclib (CYC202, *R*-roscovitine) on human HCT116 human colon cancer xenografts in nude mice. (*A*) Inhibition of tumor growth. (*B*) Inhibition of RB phosphorylation and cyclin D1 expression in the tumor tissue of treated animals. (*C*) Achievement of active drug levels in the tumor tissue. The solid horizontal line indicates the growth inhibitory IC_{50} for the tumor cells in culture. (*D*) Quantitation of the changes in molecular markers (shown in *B*) by microdensitometry. For more details, see Whittaker et al. (2004), from which the data are taken. The pharmacokinetic-pharmacodynamic data constitute a "pharmacologic audit trail" (see Workman 2002, 2003d,e), which is extremely important to establish in rational, mechanism-based new drug development.

drug. Indirect effects on cell cycle CDKs appear to occur via inhibition of CDKs 7 and 9, leading in turn to inhibition of RNA polymerase II and a reduction in the levels of short-lived mRNAs, including those for multiple cyclins. Depletion of multiple cyclins would deliver a combinatorial blockade of several CDKs simultaneously, thereby explaining the decreased phosphorylation of RB at several different sites. Furthermore, antitumor effects may be associated with down-regulation of transcripts and cognate proteins other than cyclins. For example, we proposed that the down-regulation of mitotic control proteins will have profound effects on the cell cycle at the G2M phase. In addition, we (Whittaker et al. 2003 and in prep.) and others (Alvi et al. 2005; MacCallum 2005) have shown that seliciclib reduces the expression of the antiapoptotic protein MCL1. This could contribute to the apoptotic effects of the drug. In addition, down-regulation of MYC expression could provide an explanation for the reported therapeutic effects of the seliciclib analog purvanalol in a MYC-driven transgenic cancer model (Tward et al., this volume).

The combinatorial pharmacological effects of seliciclib discussed above can be seen as an advantage for this CDK inhibitor. This is because various results show that blockade of CDK2 alone appears to be insufficient for cell proliferation, as demonstrated by various molecular strategies in human colon cancer cell lines and also in CDK2 knockout mice (Berthet et al. 2003; Orteaga et al. 2003; Tetsu and McCormick 2003). This example illustrates a general issue of current interest with kinase inhibitors: the value of highly targeted agents versus those with some degree of multi-kinase inhibition.

The mechanistic insights provided by the various mRNA and protein profiling studies (Whittaker et al. 2003 and in prep.; Alvi et al. 2005) suggest potential indications for seliciclib in particular tumor types. Our observations in human colon cancer cell lines, described above, suggest that this may be an area in which therapeutic activity might be sought. Seliciclib is being evaluated clinically in B-cell chronic lymphocytic leukemia and mantle cell lymphoma, where down-regulation of MCL1 and other survival proteins may be advantageous, and also in non-small-cell lung cancer (Guzi 2004). It has recently been shown that melanoma may be an interesting target for seliciclib and related agents, since CDK2 may have a critical role in this cancer linked to its melanocyte-specific transcriptional regulation by MITF (Du et al. 2004).

Another application of the molecular profiling studies described above is the identification of pharmacodynamic biomarkers that can be used to show proof of concept for drug action at the proposed molecular target, as well as to select the optimum drug dose and schedule (Workman 2002, 2003d,e). We have defined pharmacokinetic–pharmacodynamic relationships for seliciclib in a human colon cancer xenograft model, demonstrating, for example, inhibition of RB phosphorylation and a reduction in cyclin expression in this system (Raynaud et al. 2005). Figure 3 shows that these molecular changes are seen when active drug levels are achieved in the tumor tissue and that this is associated in turn with inhibition of tumor growth.

In the search for purine-based CDK inhibitors with the best properties, we have employed the technique of cassette dosing, which allows a higher throughput by the use of compound mixtures, to study the pharmacokinetic properties of over 100 analogs of seliciclib in the mouse (Raynaud et al. 2004). We have also shown that seliciclib is rapidly and extensively converted to the carboxylate metabolite in this species (Nutley et al. 2005), an effect also seen in the phase I clinical trials of the drug carried out at our institution (Benson et al. 2003) and elsewhere (Guzi 2004). On the basis of these studies, we have designed second-generation inhibitors with improved potency and pharmacokinetic/metabolic properties.

PHOSPHOINOSITIDE 3-KINASE INHIBITORS

Earlier in this paper, evidence was reviewed that supports PI3K as a drug target, particularly in cancers that show evidence of up-regulation of, and molecular dependence on, this pathway (Stein and Waterfield 2000; Vivanco and Sawyers 2002; Workman 2004a). In addition to mutation and overexpression of the *PIK3CA* gene that encodes the p110α catalytic subunit, and the loss of the *PTEN* tumor suppressor, other indicators of deregulation of the PI3K pathway include overexpression and mutation of upstream tyrosine kinase receptors; overexpression and activation of the downstream serine-threonine kinase AKT/PKB; mutation and overexpression of the *RAS* family, which can be placed both upstream and downstream of PI3K; and finally, up-regulation of the PI3K-AKT pathway in resistance to EGFR inhibitors (Sordella et al. 2004). Taken together, these multiple molecular abnormalities provide extremely powerful genetic and biochemical validation for PI3K as a drug target. This is supported by evidence from mouse models of cancer, for example, as presented by several speakers at the Symposium meeting.

To date, relatively few PI3K inhibitors have been identified. Moreover, these have considerable limitations, including weak potency, poor PI3K isoform or more general kinase selectivity, very limited stability and/or poor pharmacokinetic/metabolic properties. However, PI3K inhibitors have begun to emerge recently that have more attractive, drug-like properties and potential for therapeutic activity (Stein and Waterfield 2000; Ward et al. 2003; Drees et al. 2004; Workman 2004a). On balance, the available evidence indicates that the class 1A PI3K isoforms p110α and p110β may be the most appropriate to concentrate on initially for cancer therapy. Much of the target validation work has focused on p110α, but siRNA knockdown experiments also suggest that inhibition of p110β could be important (Czauderna et al. 2003).

A collaboration was established involving the Ludwig Institute for Cancer Research at University College London, Cancer Research UK, The Institute of Cancer Research, and the Yamanouchi Pharmaceutical Company. This led to the identification of a series of compounds that have the properties of highly selective and extremely potent inhibitors of the class 1A PI3Ks. We are now developing the pyridofuropyrimidine (PFP) series in collaboration with PIramed Limited.

PI103 (see Fig. 2) is an example of the PFP series that has been studied in depth (Ahmadi et al. 2004; Guillard et al. 2004; Patel et al. 2004; Workman et al. 2004). PI103 exhibited IC_{50} values against recombinant class 1A enzymes p110α, p110β, and p110δ of 2–3 nM, compared to 15 nM for the class 1B isoform p110γ and 3.85 μM for the class III isoform Vps34. In addition, IC_{50} values for PKA and PKC enzymes were >1 μM. PI103 inhibited the proliferation of a wide range of human cancer cell lines in culture. For example, in the case of the PC3 prostate cancer cell line, which is PTEN negative and exhibits high levels of phospho-AKT, 50% growth inhibition was achieved at an exposure concentration of 100 nM for 4 days. PI103 caused a rapid and concentration-dependent inhibition of AKT phosphorylation at both the Ser-473 and Thr-308 sites. In addition, down-regulation of cyclin D1 was seen. A very tight G_1 arrest was the predominant cellular response in cancer cell lines. Apoptosis was also induced in certain lines but, perhaps surprisingly, is not the predominant phenotypic response. We have looked in particular detail at the properties of PI103 in human glioma cell lines, with a view to potential therapeutic evaluation in this setting, among others. Once again, promising growth inhibitory activity was seen, and this was again associated with the molecular marker changes listed in the preceding paragraph. Over and above the effects of PI103 on cancer proliferation, the compound also inhibited both the motility and the invasive properties of tumor and endothelial cells.

Pharmacokinetic studies showed a volume of distribution (Vz) of 150 ml and a clearance (CL) of 120 ml/hr. Inhibition of the growth of human tumor xenografts was seen, including the U87MG glioblastoma. PI103 was also active in the OVCAR3 human cancer xenograft model, and this was associated with a reduction in the phosphorylation of AKT.

Further medicinal chemistry optimization, based on PI103 as a starting point, has resulted in second-generation PI3K inhibitors showing promising pharmacological activity and improved physicochemical properties, including much greater aqueous solubility at physiological pH. At the same time, these second-generation compounds retain high potency and selectivity against p110α, β, and δ, with no inhibitory activity against a panel of 72 kinases representative of the human kinome (Manning et al. 2002) when tested at a concentration of 0.5 μM. This demonstrates a very high degree of kinase selectivity.

The analog PI540 exhibited an aqueous solubility in excess of 100 μM, as compared to 3.5 μM for the earlier lead PI103. In terms of stability in mouse liver microsomes, PI540 was 91% stable at 30 minutes compared to a value of 13% for PI103. CaCo-2 cell permeability studies predicted good cellular uptake properties. No inhibitory activity was noted against the principal form of human cytochrome P450. In addition, PI540 did not inhibit hERG channel activity when assayed using the rubidium efflux method. PI540 exhibited good therapeutic activity in several different human tumor xenograft models, and these included glioblastoma and other cancers that exhibit molecular abnormalities that are likely to be predictive of molecular dependence on the PI3K signaling pathway. Of importance is that this class of inhibitors retains activity against recombinant forms of two of the common p110α mutants that have been reported, and that activity is seen in cell lines reported to harbor these mutations.

Of particular interest with respect to these potent and selective small-molecule inhibitors of PI3K is that they exhibit effects on several of the hallmark traits of malignancy (Hanahan and Weinberg 2000), including proliferation, survival, invasion, metastasis, and angiogenesis. In view of this, PI3K inhibitors may have the potential to deliver stand-alone single-agent therapeutic activity. Alternatively, they may be given in combination with cytotoxics, or with other molecular therapeutics. The optimal combinations will require careful consideration and would ideally be based on rational approaches focused on molecular pathology and pathway dependence (Jackman et al. 2004). Targeted use of PI3K inhibitors in patients with high activity of this pathway, and molecular dependence on it, is a major opportunity to be addressed.

Hsp90 MOLECULAR CHAPERONE INHIBITORS

Understanding the efficient folding of newly synthesized proteins into their unique, functionally active, three-dimensional structures remains a fundamental problem in biology (Dobson and Karplus 1999). Although the native fold is encoded in the amino acid sequence, the successful folding of many proteins in the crowded environment of the cell requires active assistance from a range of molecular chaperones (Bukau et al. 2000; Hartl and Hayer-Hartl 2002; Young et al. 2004). The complex chaperone machinery of the cell, together with the input of metabolic energy, is essential to prevent misfolding and aggregation into nonnative states in which hydrophobic amino acid residues and unstructured regions of the polypeptide backbone are exposed to solvent (Bukau et al. 2000; Hartl and Hayer-Hartl 2002; Young et al. 2004). In certain cases, aggregation can lead to production of fibrillar structures known as amyloid that are associated with many pathological conditions, including Huntington's, Alzheimer's, and other diseases (Dobson 1999; Radford 2000).

In addition to preventing aggregation and encouraging productive de novo folding under normal conditions, the chaperone machinery of the cell is also needed under stress conditions, such as elevated temperatures, when unfolding of native proteins can occur. Many chaperones show increased expression under such conditions and are referred to as stress or heat shock proteins or Hsps (Morimoto 1998; Gething and Sambrook 2000).

A large number of chaperones are involved in the orchestration of native protein folding and the stress response (Bukau et al. 2000; Hartl and Hayer-Hartl 2002; Young et al. 2004). In the mammalian cytosol, nascent chains that emerge from the peptide exit tunnel of the ribosome interact with the nascent-chain-associated complex or NAC (Wang et al. 1995). After this, most small proteins do not require additional chaperones. Longer polypeptide chains interact subsequently with the classic Hsp70s and prefoldin, which, in addition to stabilizing elongating chains, can promote cotranslational and post-translational folding and can also facilitate transfer to downstream chaperones (Deuerling et al. 1999). A fairly restricted group of proteins that are slow in folding and are sensitive to aggregation are dependent on chaperonins, which are large cylindrical double-ring complexes, exemplified by the Group II oligomeric chaperonin of the eukaryotic cytosol known as the TCP-1 ring complex (TriC) or as the chaperonin-containing TCP-1 (CCT) (Bukau et al. 2000; Hartl and Hayer-Hartl 2002; Young et al. 2004). The most abundant substrates for folding by CCT are the cytoskeletal proteins actin and tubulin (Llorca et al. 2000, 2001). It is possible that CCT may play a somewhat broader role, since around 70 proteins can be co-precipitated with it (Thulasiraman et al. 1999) and the von Hippel-Lindau tumor suppressor and WD40-repeat, 7-blade propeller proteins are emerging as substrates (Frydman 2001; Valpuesta et al. 2002).

A particular group of cellular proteins, including many kinases and other signal transduction proteins such as steroid hormone receptors, require the specialized chaperone system based on Hsp90 for their folding, stability, and functional regulation (Buchner 1999; Young et al. 2001; Maloney and Workman 2002; Wegele et al. 2004). A list of Hsp90-interacting proteins is available (http://www.picard.ch/downloads/Hsp90interactors.pdf) and among the known Hsp90 clients is a rogues' gallery of oncogenic proteins (Maloney and Workman 2002; Isaacs et al. 2003). Hsp90 works in close collaboration with other co-chaperones, including Hsp70. Substrate transfer from the Hsp70 family member Hsc70 is mediated by the adapter protein Hop/p60, which binds to the extended carboxy-terminal sequence of the two chaperones via its tetratricopeptide repeat (TPR) domains (Scheufler et al. 2000). In addition to its protein-folding role, Hsp90 is also involved in regulating the transfer of nonnative or misfolded proteins to the ubiquitin-proteasome degradation machinery. The ubiquitin ligase CHIP binds to Hsp90 via an amino-terminal TPR domain, thereby targeting Hsp90 substrates for degradation (Connell et al. 2001; Demand et al. 2001). In addition, CHIP cooperates with BAG-1, which binds to both the proteasome and Hsc70 (Luders et al. 2000). These interactions indicate a key role for the chaperones Hsp90 and Hsc70 in the integration of folding versus proteasomal degradation and hence in protein quality control in the cell.

Molecular chaperones may not, at first sight, be obvious candidates for selection as cancer drug targets. They are not, to our knowledge, subject to mutation or amplification. Interestingly, however, there is an extensive literature indicating that Hsp90 and Hsp70 can be overexpressed in human cancers (Maloney and Workman 2002). Furthermore, the requirement for Hsp90 in the folding, stability, and functional regulation of a celebrity A-list of oncoproteins suggests that inhibition of Hsp90 may provide simultaneous, combinatorial blockade of multiple oncogenic pathways (Workman 2004b) as well as offering a means to modulate all of the hallmark traits of the disease, including unrestricted proliferation and cell cycle progression, inappropriate survival, immortalization, invasion, angiogenesis, and metastasis (Hanahan and Weinberg 2000). In addition, cancer cells are in a stressed state due to the effects of deregulated oncogenes and tumor suppressor genes, together with environmental effects in solid tumors such as hypoxia, acidosis, and nutrient deprivation (Whitesell et al. 2003; Mosser and Morimoto 2004). These factors may lead to greater dependence on Hsp90 and other chaperones in cancer versus normal cells; for example, by driving Hsp90 into a high-affinity, activated superchaperone complex that is much more sensitive to inhibitors (Kamal et al. 2003; Workman 2004c). It is well established that molecular chaperones such as Hsp90, Hsp70, and Hsp27 are overexpressed in various malignancies, and these proteins have been suggested to be of prognostic value in breast, renal, and endometrial cancers (for review, see Jolly and Morimoto 2000; Maloney and Workman 2002). Increased expression of Hsp90 helps the cancer cell to deal with stresses associated with mutation and overexpression of oncogenes as well as microenvironmental challenges present within solid tumors (Whitesell et al. 2003; Mosser and Morimoto 2004). It has been reported that the sensitivity of cancer cells to Hsp90 inhibitors may be due, at least in part, to the engagement of the chaperone within malignant cells in an activated, high-affinity superchaperone complex that is much more sensitive to Hsp90 inhibitors compared to the uncomplexed Hsp90 in normal cells (Kamal et al. 2003; Workman 2004c). This may provide part of the explanation for why Hsp90 inhibitors such as 17-AAG accumulate preferentially in cancer cells and tissues (Egorin et al. 2002; Chiosis et al. 2003a; Workman 2003e).

Of particular importance is that Hsp90 is essential for the stability and function of many oncogenic client proteins, including ERBB2, BCR-ABL, AKT/PKB, C-RAF, CDK4, PLK-1, MET, mutant p53, HIF-1α, estrogen and androgen receptors, and telomerase hTERT (Maloney and Workman 2002; Wegele et al. 2004). Since Hsp90 inhibition drives client protein depletion via the ubiquitin-proteasome pathway (Schulte et al. 1995; Schneider et al. 1996), this will result in the simultaneous combinatorial depletion of multiple oncoproteins, blockade of many

oncogenic pathways, and modulation of all the hallmark traits of cancer (Workman 2004b,c). These combinatorial effects should not only be valuable in treating cancers driven by multiple molecular abnormalities, but should also reduce opportunities for resistance to develop. An additional attractive possibility for selective effects on cancer versus normal cells is that Hsp90 may act as a buffer against the potentially damaging effects of mutations that accumulate during malignant progression, analogous to the role proposed for the chaperone in buffering phenotypic variation in the environment (Rutherford and Lindquist 1998). Thus, Hsp90 inhibitors could deliver a synthetic lethal effect on cancer cells.

Note here that Hsp90 and most of the chaperones discussed above are ATPase enzymes. ATPases are known to be druggable by small molecules and, although current drugs do not act at the ATP site, this presents an important opportunity for drug design, analogous to the successful approach with ATP-mimetics in the kinase area (Chene 2002). However, it is known that natural products of the geldanamycin and radicicol classes exert their anticancer activity by binding at the amino-terminal ATP site of Hsp90 (Roe et al. 1999). This had led to an explosion of interest in Hsp90 inhibitors (Solit et al. 2003; Chiosis et al. 2004; Dymock et al. 2004).

Our interest in developing inhibitors of molecular chaperones for cancer treatment can be envisaged as part of an overall conceptual framework in which we seek to attack cancer cells not only by targeting specific molecular abnormalities, but also by inhibiting critical support functions on which cancer cells appear to be more dependent than normal cells (Workman 2005). These systems include chaperones, chromatin-modifying enzymes such as histone deacetylases, and the proteasome machinery. Molecular chaperones are especially attractive targets because of the growing evidence of their key role in managing the cellular stress associated with oncogenesis and malignant progression (Mosser and Morimoto 2004). The regulatory approval of the proteasome inhibitor bortezomib has established the principle that clinical value can be gained with drugs that interfere with the protein quality machinery of the cell (Adams 2002; Mitsiades et al. 2005). Thus, we hypothesize that there is potential for a new range of drugs that modulate protein folding and degradation in cancer and other diseases.

We carried out one of the initial group of Phase I clinical trials on the first-in-class Hsp90 inhibitor 17-AAG, which is an analog of the natural product geldanamycin (Fig. 4) (Banerji et al. 2005b). This study provided the first proof of concept for Hsp90 inhibition, measured by client protein and heat shock protein expression in the tumor tissue of treated patients, in addition to similar effects on peripheral blood lymphocytes that were also reported by ourselves and other workers (Goetz et al. 2005; Grem et al. 2005). The molecular biomarkers that we selected for use in the trial were based on our own cDNA microarray gene expression and proteomic profiling studies (see below), as well as published literature, and were validated by pharmacokinetic-pharmacodynamic relationships obtained in a human tumor xenograft model (Banerji et al. 2005a; and see below). Analysis by west-

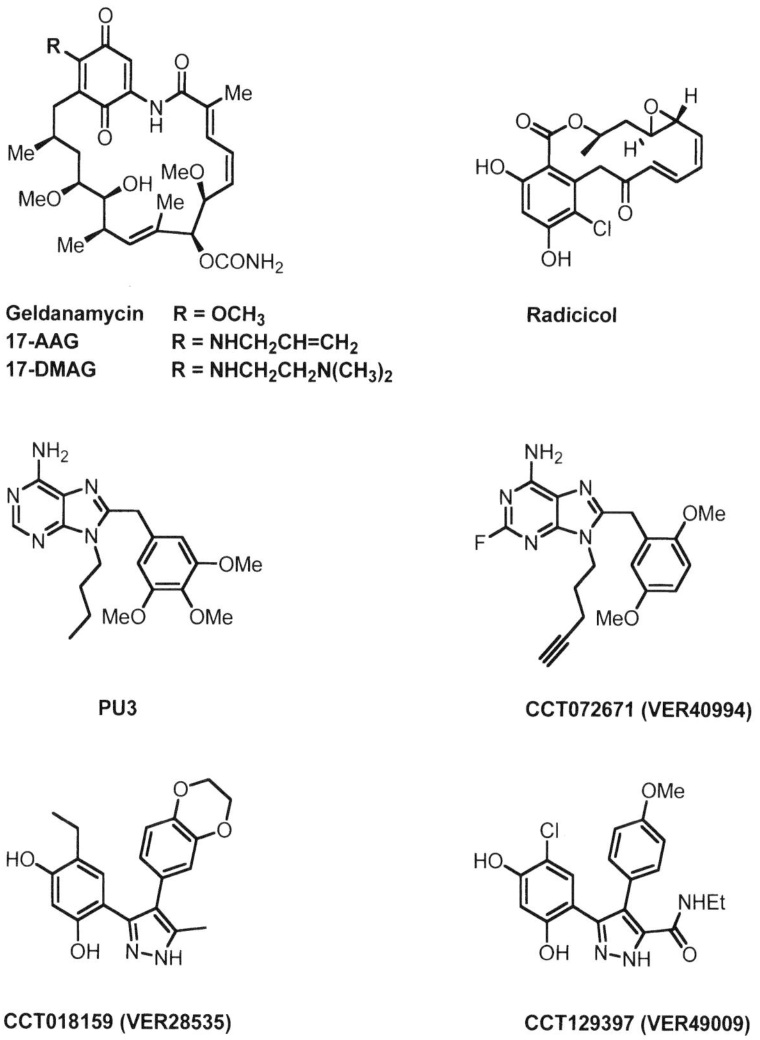

Figure 4. Chemical structures of representative Hsp90 inhibitors. Geldanamycin and radicicol are natural product inhibitors. 17-AAG and 17-DMAG are geldanamycin analogs that are undergoing early clinical trials. PU3 and CCT072671 (VER40994) are examples of purine inhibitors developed by structure-based design. CCT018159 (VER28535) is a 3,4-diarylpyrazole discovered by high-throughput screening, and CCT129397 (VER49009) is a more potent analog designed from the X-ray crystal structure of CCT0180159 bound to Hsp 90.

ern blotting of tumor biopsies obtained at 24 hours after doses of 320 and 450 mg/m²/week showed that Hsp72 was up-regulated in 8/9 patients, the CDK4 client protein was depleted in 8/9 patients, and the C-RAF client protein was depleted in 4/6 patients evaluable for this biomarker. The molecular signature of Hsp90 inhibition was maintained in a single patient studied at 1 and 3 days after dosing but was not seen reproducibly at 5 days. Up-regulation of Hsp72 was demonstrated within the tumor cells by immunohistochemistry in two patients with melanoma. We observed prolonged stable disease for two patients with advanced, metastatic malignant melanoma, leading to a Phase II clinical trial that is now under way at our institution in association with the Royal Free Hospital, London. Mechanistic studies have also been initiated to understand the sensitivity of melanoma cells to 17-AAG (see below).

Our Phase I trial demonstrated that it was feasible, in a once-weekly schedule, to deliver a dose of 17-AAG re-

sulting in potentially therapeutic plasma concentrations, Hsp90 target inhibition in tumor tissue, and possible therapeutic activity. However, the formulation was limiting, leading to clinical trials by ourselves and others with the soluble analog 17-DMAG (Hollingshead et al. 2005) and the search for new Hsp90 inhibitor chemotypes (see below).

We have investigated the detailed molecular and cellular consequences of treating cancer cells with 17-AAG for two major reasons: first, to identify genes and proteins that govern sensitivity to Hsp90 inhibitors; and second, to identify molecular biomarkers of Hsp90 inhibition for potential clinical use (Banerji et al. 2003; Maloney et al. 2003). The cDNA gene expression profiling study that we published with 17-AAG was the first with an Hsp90 inhibitor and one of the first to study global expression changes with any drug (Clarke et al. 2000). Using a 4132 cDNA array, we showed that the expression of genes encoding client proteins was not altered at the mRNA level, whereas genes coding for Hsp72, Hsc70, keratins 8 and 18, and caveolin 1 were deregulated by 17-AAG in human colon cancer cells. We observed cell-line-dependent deregulation of *HSP90β* expression, with the more sensitive HT29 cells showing depletion of the drug target, whereas the more resistant HCT116 cells exhibited induction of *HSP90β*. Thus, we showed that the dynamic regulation of target expression by the drug is likely to be a factor influencing sensitivity to 17-AAG.

We also demonstrated in human colon cancer cell lines that combinatorial inhibition of signal transduction, including blockade of both the RAS-RAF-MEK-ERK1/2 and PI3K-PKB pathways, can lead to cell cycle arrest and apoptosis (Hostein et al. 2001). In the same paper, we showed that the KM12 colon cancer cell line that overexpressed BAG-1 and lacked expression of BAX was unable to undergo apoptosis in response to 17-AAG. We subsequently showed, by comparing the response of HCT116 colon cancer cells in which BAX was knocked out by homologous recombination (Zhang et al. 2000), that this proapoptopic protein is required for apoptosis in response to 17-AAG and that, in its absence, cell death proceeds more slowly and by necrosis (M. Powers et al., unpubl.).

A further detailed study of changes in expression profile in response to 17-AAG was carried out in A2780 human ovarian cancer cells (A. Maloney et al., in prep.). We used both cDNA microarrays and proteomic analysis, the latter in collaboration with Professor Mike Waterfield (Ludwig Institute for Cancer Research, University College London). One of the most important observations was the identification of AHA1, as a stress-regulated cochaperone that activates the essential, inherent ATPase of Hsp90 (Panaretou et al. 2002). We showed that *AHA1* was up-regulated at both the mRNA and protein levels by 17-AAG in human cancer cells. We have subsequently used siRNA to knock down AHA1, and preliminary data show that this sensitizes cells to 17-AAG (J. Holmes et al., unpubl.). Thus, AHA1 expression may potentially affect sensitivity to 17-AAG in patients.

In our mRNA and protein profiling studies in A2780 cells, we used both active Hsp90 inhibitors and an inactive analog to distinguish on-target and off-target effects (A. Maloney et al., in prep.). Expected changes, including the up-regulation of various heat shock proteins, were shown in greater detail than previously, with most effects demonstrated to be on-target, including those involving Hsp70-8, Hsp70-2, Hsp90β (but not Hsp90α), Hsp47, and Hsp27-1. A group of MYC-regulated genes, which we also saw down-regulated in our clinical study of gene expression in rectal cancer patients treated with 5-fluorouracil (Clarke et al. 2003), showed reduced expression and may be an antiproliferative signature. The most novel and interesting discovery was that a group of proteins involved in chromatin regulation, acetylation, and methylation exhibited altered expression in response to 17-AAG. The heterochromatin protein HP1 was up-regulated, whereas both the histone acetyltransferase HAT-1 and the arginine methyltransferase PRMT5 (SKBI/JBP1) were down-regulated by the drug. Total cell acetylation was also decreased by 17-AAG. These results are consistent with an emerging interaction between protein acetylation and Hsp90 function. For example, histone deacetylase inhibitors may inhibit the chaperone by increasing Hsp90 acetylation (Yu et al. 2002). Studies in model organisms (Sangster et al. 2003; Zhao et al. 2005) also illustrate close links between chromatin and Hsp90. Of particular significance, our immunoprecipitation studies showed for the first time that PRMT5 is a binding partner and potential client protein for Hsp90 (A. Maloney et al., in prep.).

Along with *AHA1*, heat shock proteins were the genes most robustly and routinely induced by Hsp90 inhibitors (A. Maloney et al., in prep.). We are carrying out a comprehensive series of experiments to understand the role of Hsp90 and Hsp70 family members in governing sensitivity to Hsp90 inhibitors in cancer cells. This has been challenging because of the potential redundancy involved.

In addition to co-chaperones, we have examined the effects of selected client proteins on cellular sensitivity to Hsp90 inhibitors. ERBB2 is one of the most sensitive and potentially important Hsp90 client proteins (Citri et al. 2004). We created an isogenic model in which ERBB2 was overexpressed and functionally active in ERBB2 negative CH1 ovarian cells. Using this, we showed that ERBB2 overexpression resulted in a fivefold increase in sensitivity to geldanamycin (Smith et al. 2002).

Another important client protein that we have studied is B-RAF. Having observed prolonged stable disease in two melanoma patients in our Phase I trial (Banerji et al. 2005b), we hypothesized that this may be related to the high incidence of *B-RAF* mutation in this disease (Davies et al. 2002) and that mutant B-RAF may be a sensitive client protein. In collaboration with Dr. Richard Marais, we have shown that the most common V600E mutant of B-RAF is an Hsp90 client protein that is much more dependent on the chaperone than the wild type for stability and activity (de Rocha Dias et al. 2005). We also showed that the majority of other mutant forms of B-RAF are very sensitive to 17-AAG-mediated proteasomal degradation. Similar results have been obtained by N. Rosen and colleagues (pers. comm.). The structural determinants for the interaction of client proteins with Hsp90 remain unclear (but see Xu et al. 2005). Our results suggest that it is the adoption of the active conformation, rather than the level of activity, that determines sensitivity to 17-AAG. Our demonstration that mutant B-RAF proteins are hypersensitive to Hsp90 inhibition suggests a possible mechanism for the clinical activity of 17-AAG in melanoma.

The tumor suppressor p53 is a client protein that is depleted by 17-AAG (Kelland et al. 1999). The compound pifithrin α was identified in a screen for suppression of p53-mediated *trans*-activation (Komarov et al. 1999) and subsequently claimed to block "heat shock signaling" (Komarova et al. 2003). However, we identified significant pharmaceutical limitations with pifithrin α and could detect no effects on Hsp90 activity or indeed on p53 function (Walton et al. 2005).

In the search for biomarkers of Hsp90 inhibition, we used a combination of literature information and results from our cDNA microarray gene expression and proteomic profiling (Clarke et al. 2000; A. Maloney et al., in prep.; see above), together with approaches based on magnetic resonance spectroscopy and positron emission tomography. We validated a molecular signature of client protein and heat shock protein changes for 17-AAG in an ovarian cancer xenograft model and established pharmacokinetic-pharmacodynamic relationships (Banerji et al. 2005a) prior to our Phase I trial (see above). We developed novel solid-phase immunoassays to quantify the molecular signature using the TRF-Cellisa approach (Hardcastle et al. 2005). In collaboration with our magnetic resonance spectroscopy and imaging colleagues, we identified magnetic resonance spectroscopic (MRS) PD biomarkers, comprising increases in phosphocholine and phosphomonoester levels for 17-AAG in human colon cancer models (Chung et al. 2003). This MRS signature was distinct from those we have seen with inhibitors of MEK1/2 (Beloueche-Babari et al. 2005), PI3K (M. Beloueche-Babari et al., in prep.) and choline kinase (Al-Saffar et al. 2005). In collaboration with our positron emission tomography collaborators, we have identified radiolabeled choline as a potential marker for Hsp90 inhibition (Liu et al. 2002) as well as radiolabeled annexin V to image apoptosis (Collingridge et al. 2003). Such assays could be used to image PD effects of Hsp90 inhibitors in animal models and patients alongside assays for client protein degradation (Smith-Jones et al. 2004).

We have demonstrated profound effects of geldanamycin and 17-AAG on key aspects of neoangiogenesis (S. Brader et al., in prep.). Together with other studies (de Candia et al. 2003; Kaur et al. 2004), our results suggest that effects on angiogenesis may play a major role in the response to Hsp90 inhibitors in vivo, consistent with the proposed combinatorial action on the hallmarks of cancer (Workman 2004b).

17-AAG continues to show promise as a first-in-class Hsp90 inhibitor. It does, however, have a number of limitations (Workman 2004b), including its poor solubility and cumbersome formulation; relatively weak target potency; reduced activity in the presence of P-glycoprotein and the absence of DT-diaphorase/NQO1 activity (Brunton et al. 1998; Kelland et al. 1999); and low oral bioavailability and metabolism by polymorphic cytochrome P450 CYP3A4 (Egorin et al. 1998). There is, therefore, a strong case for developing improved second-generation inhibitors. We have taken a broad approach to this. We examined a series of 17-AAG analogs available from the U.S. National Cancer Institute; we pursued a structure-based approach to the design of stable and drug-like analogs of radicicol; we explored purine-based inhibitors; and we undertook a high-throughput screening approach to identify novel chemotypes.

We studied structure/activity relationships (SAR) for the various pharmacological activities of 24 geldanamycin analogs, focusing on 17-amino-substituted compounds related to 17-AAG (see Fig. 4), since this motif appeared to confer beneficial therapeutic properties for reasons that were not clear. Previous SAR studies had focused on effects on ERBB2, since the Hsp90 mechanism was not defined at that time (Schnur et al. 1995a,b). Overall, we found that there was a consistent SAR linking in-

hibition of the ATPase activity of recombinant Hsp90, depletion of C-RAF client protein, induction of HSP70, and cancer cell growth inhibition, consistent with primary action at the Hsp90 target (A. Maloney et al., unpubl.). We derived a specific SAR for the potentiation of antiproliferative activity by NQO1/DT-diaphorase that we discovered (Kelland et al. 1999). This effect was restricted to alkyl-substituted 17-amino analogs, and the greatest differential was seen with 17-AAG itself. In the case of 17-DMAG, in which the 17-allylamino moiety is replaced by 17-diethylaminoethylamino (Fig. 4), the "potentiation factor" was reduced from 24 to 5 in the NQO1+/– isogenic pair that we developed (Sharp et al. 2000). This suggests a significant difference from 17-AAG, reducing the risk of a potential resistance mechanism but also decreasing the potential therapeutic advantage in high NQO1-expressing cancers. However, as we noted previously, the NQO1 effect is offset by metabolism to the 17-amino compound which lacks the NQO1 dependence (Kelland et al. 1999). We also characterized the mouse plasma and tissue pharmacokinetics and microsomal metabolism of selected 17-AAG analogs (Smith et al. 2004), incorporating an evaluation of the cassette dosing method that we developed for the CDK inhibitor project (Raynaud et al. 2004).

It remains an intriguing possibility that, as suggested previously (Workman 2004c), reduction of the quinone could be involved in the activity of 17-AAG in the context of the Hsp90 superchaperone complex that was reported to predominate in cancer cells (Kamal et al. 2003). It should be noted that the quinol of 17-AAG is entering clinical trials as a soluble prodrug form (IPI-504; Sydor et al. 2005).

The first series of synthetic drug-like small-molecule Hsp90 inhibitors were the purine analogs designed by Chiosis et al. (2001, 2003b) to mimic the unusual "C-shape" adopted by ADP/ATP in the Hsp90 amino terminus (Prodromou et al. 1997; Stebbins et al. 1997). In collaboration with Vernalis, we determined X-ray co-crystal structures with human HSP90α and β of a lead purine inhibitor PU3 (see Fig. 4) (Wright et al. 2004). We showed that the purine does mimic the adenine of ADP/ADT but, unexpectedly, the trimethoxyphenyl ring induces a conformational change in the loop region capping the ATP site to create a new binding pocket. Crystal structures explained the SAR and allowed the design of more potent analogs, e.g., the 1-pentynyl compound CCT072671 or VER40994 was at least 50 times more active than PU3 (Wright et al. 2004).

We identified the 3,4-diarylpyrazole series in a high-throughput screen of our (then) 53,000 compound collection against the ATPase activity of the full-length recombinant yeast Hsp90 using a malachite green readout (Aherne et al. 2003; Rowlands et al. 2004). Yeast enzyme was used because of its higher ATPase activity, but compounds were confirmed as active against human Hsp90 activated by AHA1 (Panaretou et al. 2002). The initial pyrazole series was exemplified by the μM hit CCT018159 or VER28535 (Fig. 4). The molecular mode of action in cells was confirmed, synthetic routes were developed, and X-ray co-crystal structures obtained with

Professor Pearl explained early SAR and identified optimization opportunities (Cheung et al. 2005). This led to a research collaboration with Vernalis. Structure-based optimization, particularly the introduction of the 5-amide substitution to gain a hydrogen bond interaction with Gly-97 (human), led to potent analogs; this is exemplified by CCT129397 or VER49009, which has nanomolar activity, compares favorably with 17-AAG, and has the required potency and potential to become a clinical candidate (Dymock et al. 2005). In addition, 4-amino derivatives (X. Barril et al., in prep.) with a similar binding mode to CCT129397 or VER49009 and 3-(5-chloro-2,4-dihydroxyphenyl)-pyrazole-4-carboxamides that access interaction via Phe-138 (Brough et al. 2005) were developed. Pyrazoles examined showed a very high degree of selectivity for Hsp90 versus the ATPases of DNA topoisomerase II and Hsp72, as well as a panel of kinases representing the human kinome (Manning et al. 2002). In contrast to 17-AAG, we showed that NQO1 and P-glycoprotein had little effect on sensitivity. We used the SAR and X-ray structures with the 3,4-diarylpyrazole series to design a fluorescent derivative that can be used to measure low-nanomolar IC_{50} values (R. Howes et al., in prep.). These studies illustrate the power of high-throughput screening combined with X-ray crystallography-driven, structure-based design and indicate the considerable therapeutic potential of inhibiting the Hsp90 molecular chaperone.

CONCLUDING REMARKS

Advances in our understanding of the human genome and now the cancer genome are having a major impact on drug development. Our comprehension of the cancer kinome and its exploitation for drug discovery has been especially successful. Drugging the cancer kinome is clearly an achievable goal. Several kinase inhibitors are already approved and many more are in development. Both small-molecule and antibody approaches show great promise.

In this paper, I have mentioned both successes and challenges in developing the more established small-molecule kinase inhibitors, for example, imatinib and the EGFR inhibitors, as well as emerging inhibitors of CDKs and PI3K. Current issues with kinase inhibitors include:

- Selecting patients based on evidence of molecular dependence and oncogene addiction
- The need for biomarkers of drug action for use in intelligent hypothesis-testing, proof-of-concept clinical trials
- The development of resistance through kinase mutations
- The potential need to inhibit multiple kinases to overcome cancers with multiple abnormalities and to prevent the development of resistance
- The difficulty in selecting and developing rational combination treatments

Several of the limitations with kinase inhibitors can be overcome using inhibitors of the Hsp90 molecular chaperone which provide combinatorial knockdown of multiple cancer kinases and other oncoproteins and simultaneous blockade of many oncogenic pathways (Workman 2003f). Prospects for the development of personalized cancer treatments, targeted to the kinome and genome abnormalities of individual human cancers, are very exciting.

ACKNOWLEDGMENTS

Thanks to Dr. Ian Collins and Dr. Vassilios Bavetsias for the chemical structure figures and to many colleagues and collaborators for valuable discussions. Work in the author's laboratory (www.icr.ac.uk/cctherap) is funded by Cancer Research UK Programme Grant Number [CUK] C309/A2187; the author is a Cancer Research UK Life Fellow. Work on CDK, PI3K, and Hsp90 was also funded in part by Cyclacel Limited, PIramed Limited, and Vernalis, respectively.

REFERENCES

Adams J. 2002. Proteasome inhibition: A novel approach to cancer therapy. *Trends Mol. Med.* (suppl.) **8**: S49.

Aherne W., Maloney A., Prodromou C., Rowlands M.G., Hardcastle A., Boxall K., Clarke P., Walton M.I., Pearl L., and Workman P. 2003. Assays for HSP90 and inhibitors. *Methods Mol. Med.* **85**: 149.

Ahmadi K., Alderton W., Chuckowree I., Depledge P., Folkes A., Pergl-Wilson G., Saghir N., Shuttleworth S., Wan N., Raynaud F., Saghir N.S.S., Wan N.C., and Zhyvoloup A. 2004. Identification of potent, selective, soluble and permeable small molecule PI3 kinase inhibitors for the treatment of cancer. Proceedings of the EORTC-NCI-AACR Symposium on Molecular Targets and Cancer Therapeutics (Abstr. 320). *Eur. J. Cancer* **2**: 8. (Suppl.)

Al Saffar N.M.S., Troy H., Ramirez de Molina A., Jackson L.E., Madhu B., Griffths J.R., Leach M.O., Workman P., Lacal J.C., Judson I.R., and Chung Y.-L. 2005. Non-invasive magnetic resonance spectroscopic pharmacodynamic markers of the choline kinase inhibitor MN58b in human carcinoma models. *Cancer Res.* (in press).

Alvi A.J., Austen B., Weston V.J., Fegan C., MacCallum D., Gianella-Borradori A., Lane D.P., Hubank M., Powell J.E., Wei W., Taylor A.M., Moss P.A. and Styankovic T. 2005. A novel CDK inhibitor, CYC202 (R-roscovitine), overcomes the defect in p53-dependent apoptosis in B-CLL by down-regulation of genes involved in transcription regulation and survival. *Blood* **105**: 4484.

Anonymous. 2004. The future of cancer treatment: Up close and personal. *The Economist,* October 16, 2004.

Arnst C. 2005. Biotech, finally. *Business Week,* June 13, 2005.

Bachman K.E., Argani P., Samuels Y., Silliman N., Ptak J., Szabo S., Konishi H., Karakas B., Blair B.G., Lin C., Peters B.A., Velculescu V.E., and Park B.H. 2004. The PI3KCA gene is mutated in a high frequency in human cancers. *Cancer Biol. Ther.* **3**: 772.

Balmain A., Gray J., and Ponder B. 2003. The genetics and genomics of cancer. *Nat. Genet.* **33**: 288.

Banerji U., Judson I., and Workman P. 2003. The clinical applications of heat shock protein inhibitors in cancer—Present and future. *Curr. Cancer Drug Targets* **3**: 385.

Banerji U., Walton M., Raynaud F., Grimshaw R., Kelland L., Valenti M., Judson I., and Workman P. 2005a. Pharmacokinetic-pharmacodynamic relationships for the HSP90 molecular chaperone inhibitors 17-allylamino, 17-demethoxygeldanamycin (17-AAG) in human ovarian cancer models. *Clin. Cancer Res.* **11**: 7023.

Banerji U., O'Donnell A., Scurr M., Pacey S., Stapleton S., Asad Y., Simmons L., Maloney A., Raynaud F., Campbell M., Walton M., Lakhani S., Kaye S., Workman P., and Judson I. 2005b. Phase I pharmacokinetic and pharmacodynamic study of 17-allylamino, 17-demethoxygeldanamycin in patients with advanced malignancies. *J. Clin. Oncol.* **23:** 4152.

Bardelli A., Parsons D.W., Silliman N., Ptak J., Szabo S., Saha S., Markowitz S., Willson J.K., Parmigiani G., Kinzler K.W., Vogelstein B., and Velculescu V.E. 2003. Mutational analysis of the tyrosine kinome in colorectal cancers. *Science* **300:** 949.

Beloueche-Babari M., Jackson L.E., Al-Saffar N.M., Workman P., Leach M.O., and Ronen S.M. 2005. Magnetic resonance spectroscopy monitoring of mitogen-activated protein kinase signaling inhibition. *Cancer Res.* **65:** 3356.

Benson C., White J., Twelves C., O'Donnell A., Cruickshank C., Tan S., Gianella-Borradori A., and Judson I. 2003. A phase I trial of the oral cyclin dependent kinase inhibitor CYC202 in patients with advanced malignancy. *Proc. Am. Soc. Clin. Oncol.* **22:** 209.

Berthet C., Aleem E., Coppola V., Tessarollo L., and Kaldis P. 2003. CDK2 knockout mice are viable. *Curr. Biol.* **13:** 1775.

Bronchud M.H., Foote M.A., Giaccone G, Olopade O., and Workman P., Eds. 2004. *Principles of molecular oncology,* 2nd. edition. Humana Press, Totowa, New Jersey.

Brough P.A., Barril X., Beswick M., Dymock B.W., Drysdale M.J., Wright L., Grant K., Massey A., Surgenor A., and Workman P. 2005. 3-(5-Chloro-3,4-dihydroxyphenyl)-pyrazole-4-carboxamides as inhibitors of the Hsp90 molecular chaperone. *Bioorg. Med. Chem. Lett.* **15:** 5197.

Brunton V.G., Steele G., Lewis A.D., and Workman P. 1998. Geldanamycin-induced cytotoxicity In human colon cancer cell lines: Evidence against the involvement of c-Src or DT-diaphorase. *Cancer Chemother. Pharmacol.* **41:** 417.

Buchner J. 1999. Hsp90 and Co.—A holding for folding. *Trends Biochem. Sci.* **24:** 136.

Bukau B., Deuerling E., Pfund C., and Craig E. 2000. Getting newly synthesised proteins into shape. *Cell* **101:** 119.

Chen Y.N., Sharma S.K., Ramsey T.M., Jiang L., Martin M.S., Baker K., Adams P.D., Bair K.W., and Kaelin W.G., Jr. 1999. Selective killing of transformed cells by cyclin/cyclin dependent kinase 2 antagonists. *Proc. Natl. Acad. Sci.* **96:** 4325.

Chene P. 2002. ATPases as drug targets: Learning from their structure. *Nat. Rev. Drug Discov.* **1:** 665.

Cheung K.M., Matthews T.P., James K., Rowlands M.G., Boxall K.J., Sharp S.Y., Maloney A., Roe S.M., Prodromou C., Pearl L.H., Aherne G.W., McDonald E., and Workman P. 2005. The identification, synthesis, protein crystal structure and *in vitro* biochemical evaluation of a new 3,4-diarylpyrazole class of Hsp90 inhibitors. *Bioorg. Med. Chem. Lett.* **15:** 3338.

Chiosis G., Vilenchik M., Kim J., and Solit D. 2004. Hsp90: The vulnerable chaperone. *Drug Discov. Today* **9:** 881.

Chiosis G., Huezo H., Rosen N., Mimnaugh E., Whitesell L., and Neckers L. 2003a. 17AAG: Low target binding affinity and potent cell activity—Finding an explanation. *Mol. Cancer Ther.* **2:** 123.

Chiosis G., Lucas B., Huezo H., Solit D., Basso A., and Rosen N. 2003b. Development of purine-scaffold small molecule inhibitors of Hsp90. *Curr. Cancer Drug Targets* **3:** 371.

Chiosis G., Timaul M.N., Lucas B., Munster P.N., Zheng F.F., Sepp-Lorenzino L., and Rosen N. 2001. A small molecule designed to bind to the adenine nucleotide pocket of Hsp90 causes Her2 degradation and the growth arrest and differentiation of breast cancer cells. *Chem. Biol.* **8:** 289.

Chung Y.L., Troy H., Banerji U., Jackson L.E., Walton M.I., Stubbs M., Griffiths J.R., Judson I.R., Leach M.O., Workman P., and Ronen S.M. 2003. Magnetic resonance spectroscopic pharmacodynamic markers of the heat shock protein 90 inhibitor 17-allylamino,17-demethoxygeldanamycin (17AAG) in human colon cancer models. *J. Natl. Cancer Inst.* **95:** 1624.

Citri A., Kochupurakkal B.S., and Yarden Y. 2004. The achilles heel of ErbB-2/HER2: Regulation by the Hsp90 chaperone machine and potential for pharmacological intervention. *Cell Cycle* **3:** 51.

Clarke P.A., George M.L., Easdale S., Cunningham D., Swift R.I., Hill M.E., Tait D.M., and Workman P. 2003. Molecular pharmacology of cancer therapy in human colorectal cancer by gene expression profiling. *Cancer Res.* **63:** 6855.

Clarke P.A., Hostein I., Banerji U., Stefano F.D., Maloney A.,

Walton M., Judson I., and Workman P. 2000. Gene expression profiling of colon adenocarcinoma cells following inhibition of signal transduction by 17-allylamino-17-demethoxygeldanamycin, an inhibitor of the HSP90 molecular chaperone. *Oncogene* **19:** 4125.

Cohen P. 2002. Protein kinases—The major drug targets of the twenty-first century? *Nat. Rev. Drug Discov.* **1:** 309.

Collingridge D.R., Glaser M., Osman S., Barthel H., Hutchinson O.C., Luthra S.K., Brady F., Bouchier-Hayes L., Martin S.J., Workman P., Price P., and Aboagye E.O. 2003. *In vitro* selectivity, *in vivo* biodistribution and tumour uptake of annexin V radiolabelled with a positron emitting radioisotope. *Br. J. Cancer* **89:** 1327.

Connell P., Ballinger C.A., Jiang J., Wu Y., Thompson L.J., Hohfeld J., and Patterson C. 2001. The co-chaperone CHIP regulates protein triage decisions mediated by heat-shock proteins. *Nat. Cell Biol.* **3:** 93.

Czauderna F., Fechtner M., Aygun H., Arnold W., Klippel A., Giese K., and Kaufmann J. 2003. Functional studies of the PI(3)-kinase signalling pathway employing synthetic and expressed siRNA. *Nucleic Acids Res.* **31:** 670.

Dahia P.L. 2000. PTEN, a unique tumor suppressor gene. *Endocr. Relat. Cancer* **7:** 115.

Danson S. and Lorigan P. 2005. Improving outcomes in advanced malignant melanoma: Update on systemic therapy. *Drugs* **65:** 733.

Daub H., Specht K., and Ullrich A. 2004. Strategies to overcome resistance to targeted protein kinase inhibitors. *Nat. Rev. Drug Discov.* **3:** 1001.

Davies H., Bignell G.R., Cox C., Stephens P., Edkins S., Clegg S., Teague J., Woffendin H., Garnett M.J., Bottomley W., Davis N., Dicks E., Ewing R., Floyd Y., Gray K., Hall S., Hawes R., Hughes J., Kosmidou V., Menzies A., Mould C., Parker A., Stevens C., Watt S., Hooper S., Wilson R., Jayatilake H., Gusterson B.A., Cooper C., Shipley J., Hargrave D., Pritchard-Jones K., Maitland N., Chenevix-Trench G., Riggins G.J., Bigner D.D., Palmieri G., Cossu A., Flanagan A., Nicholson A., Ho J.W., Leung S.Y., Yuen S.T., Weber B.L., Seigler H.F., Darrow T.L., Paterson H., Marais R., Marshall C.J., Wooster R., Stratton M.R., and Futreal P.A. 2002. Mutations of the BRAF gene in human cancer. *Nature* **417:** 949.

de Candia P., Solit D.B., Giri D., Brogi E., Siegel P.M., Olshen A.B., Muller W.J., Rosen N., and Benezra R. 2003. Angiogenesis impairment in Id-deficient mice cooperates with an Hsp90 inhibitor to completely suppress HER2/neu-dependent breast tumors. *Proc. Natl. Acad. Sci.* **100:** 12337.

Demand J., Alberti S., Patterson C., and Hohfeld J. 2001. Cooperation of a ubiquitin domain protein and an E3 ubiquitin ligase during chaperone/proteasome coupling. *Curr. Biol.* **11:** 1569.

de Rocha Dias S., Friedlos F., Light Y., Springer C., Workman P., and Marais R. 2005. Activated B-RAF is an Hsp90 client protein that is targeted by the anticancer drug 17-AAG. *Cancer Res.* (in press).

Deuerling E., Schulze-Specking A., Tomoyasu T., Mogk A., and Bukau B. 1999. Trigger factor and DnaK cooperate in folding of newly synthesized proteins. *Nature* **400:** 693.

Dobson C.M. 1999. Protein misfolding, evolution and disease. *Trends Biochem. Sci.* **24:** 329.

Dobson C.M. and Karplus M. 1999. The fundamentals of protein folding: Bringing together theory and experiment. *Curr. Opin. Struct. Biol.* **9:** 92.

Drees B.E., Mills G.B., Rommel R., and Prestwich G.D. 2004. Therapeutic potential of phosphoinositide 3 kinase inhibitors. *Expert Opin. Ther. Patents* **14:** 703.

Druker B. 2004. Molecularly targeted therapy: Have the floodgates opened? *Oncologist* **9:** 357.

Du J., Widlund H.R., Horstmann M.A., Ramaswamy S., Ross K., Huber W.E., Nishimura E.K., Golub T.R., and Fisher D.E. 2004. Critical role of CDK2 for melanoma growth linked to its melanocyte-specific transcriptional regulation by MITF. *Cancer Cell* **6:** 565.

Dymock B., Drysdale M., McDonald E., and Workman P. 2004. Inhibitors of Hsp90 and other chaperones for the treatment of cancer. *Expert Opin. Ther. Patents* **14:** 837.

Dymock B.W., Barril X., Brough P.A., Cansfield J.E., Massey A., McDonald E., Hubbard R.E., Surgenor A., Roughley S.D., Webb P., Workman P., Wright L., and Drysdale M.J. 2005. Novel, potent small-molecule inhibitors of the molecular chaperone Hsp90 discovered through structure-based design. *J. Med. Chem.* **48:** 4212.

Egorin M.J., Rosen D.M., Wolff J.H., Callery P.S., Musser S.M., and Eiseman J.L. 1998. Metabolism of 17-(allylamino)-17-demethoxygeldanamycin (NSC 330507) by murine and human hepatic preparations. *Cancer Res.* **58:** 2385.

Egorin M.J., Lagattuta T.F., Hamburger D.R., Covey J.M., White K.D., Musser S.M., and Eiseman J.L. 2002. Pharmacokinetics, tissue distribution, and metabolism of 17-(dimethylaminoethyl-lamino)-17-demethoxygeldanamycin (NSC 707545) in CD2F1 mice and Fischer 344 rats. *Cancer Chemother. Pharmacol.* **49:** 7.

Frydman J. 2001. Folding of newly translated proteins *in vivo*. The role of molecular chaperones. *Annu. Rev. Biochem.* **70:** 603.

Futreal A., Coin L., Marshall M., Down T., Hubbard T., Wooster R., Rahman N., and Stratton M.R. 2004. A census of human cancer genes. *Nat. Rev. Cancer* **4:** 177. (For updates see: www.sanger.ac.uk/genetics/CGP/Census).

Garnett M.J. and Marais R. 2004. Guilty as charged: B-RAF is a human oncogene. *Cancer Cell.* **6:** 313.

Garrett M.D., Walton M.I., McDonald E., Judson I., and Workman P. 2003. The contemporary drug development process: Advances and challenges in preclinical and clinical development. *Prog. Cell Cycle Res.* **5:** 145.

Gething M.J. and Sambrook J. 2000. Protein folding in the cell. *Nature* **355:** 33.

Goetz M.P., Toft D., Reid J., Ames M., Stensgard B., Safgren S., Adjei A.A., Sloan J., Atherton P., Vasile V., Salazaar S., Adjei A., Croghan G., and Erlichman C. 2005. Phase I trial of 17-allylamino-17-demethoxygeldanamycin in patients with advanced cancer. *J. Clin. Oncol.* **23:** 1078.

Gorre M.E., Mohammed M., Ellwood K., Hsu N., Paquette R., Rao P.N., and Sawyers C.L. 2001. Clinical resistance to STI-571 cancer therapy caused by BCR-ABL gene mutation or amplification. *Science* **293:** 876.

Grem J.L., Morrison G., Guo X.D., Agnew E., Takimoto C.H., Thomas R., Szabo E., Grochow L., Grollman F., Hamilton J.M., Neckers L., and Wilson R.H. 2005. Phase I and pharmacologic study of 17-(allylamino)-17-demethoxygeldanamycin in adult patients with solid tumors. *J. Clin. Oncol.* **23:** 1885.

Guillard S., Clarke P.A., te Poele R., Di Stefano F., Raynaud F., and Workman P. 2004. Characterisation of a novel class 1 isoform selective phosphoratidyl-inositol 3-kinase inhibitor in glioma. Proceedings of the EORTC-NCI-AACR Symposium on Molecular Targets and Cancer Therapeutics (Abstr. 379). *Eur. J. Cancer* **2:** 8. (Suppl.)

Guzi T. 2004. CYC-202 Cyclacel. *Curr. Opin. Investig. Drugs* **5:** 1311.

Hanahan D. and Weinberg R. 2000. The hallmarks of cancer. *Cell* **100:** 57.

Hardcastle A., Boxall K., Richards J., Tomlin P., Sharp S., Clarke P., Workman P., and Aherne W. 2005. Solid-phase immunoassays in mechanism-based drug discovery: Their application in the development of inhibitors of the molecular chaperone heat-shock protein 90. *Assay Drug Dev. Technol.* **3:** 273.

Hartl F.U. and Hayer-Hartl M. 2002. Molecular chaperones in the cytosol: From nascent chain to folded protein. *Science* **295:** 1852.

Hollingshead M., Alley M., Burger A.M., Borgel S., Pacula-Cox C., Fiebig H.H., and Sausville E.A. 2005. *In vivo* antitumor efficacy of 17-DMAG (17-dimethylaminoethylamino-17-demethoxygeldanamycin hydrochloride), a water-soluble geldanamycin derivative. *Cancer Chemother. Pharmacol.* **56:** 115.

Hopkins A.L. and Groom C.R. 2002. The druggable genome. *Nat. Rev. Drug Discov.* **1:** 727.

Hostein I., Robertson D., DiStefano F., Workman P., and Clarke P.A. 2001. Inhibition of signal transduction by the HSP90 inhibitor 17-allylamino-17-demethoxygeldanamycin results in

cytostasis and apoptosis. *Cancer Res.* **61:** 4003.

International Human Genome Sequencing Consortium. 2004. Finishing the euchromatic sequence of the human genome. *Nature* **431:** 931.

Isaacs J.S., Xu W., and Neckers L. 2003. Heat shock protein 90 as a molecular target for cancer therapeutics. *Cancer Cell* **3:** 213.

Jackman A.L., Kaye S., and Workman P. 2004. The combination of cytotoxic and molecularly targeted therapies—Can it be done? *Drug Discov. Today: Ther. Strategies* **1:** 445.

Jolly C. and Morimoto R.I. 2000. Role of the heat shock response and molecular chaperones in oncogenesis and cell death. *J. Natl. Cancer Inst.* **92:** 1564.

Kamal A., Thao L., Sensintaffar J., Zhang L., Boehm M.F., Fritz L.C., and Burrows F.J. 2003. A high-affinity conformation of Hsp90 confers tumour selectivity on Hsp90 inhibitors. *Nature* **425:** 407.

Kang S., Bader A.G., and Vogt P.K. 2005. Phosphatidylinositol 3-kinase mutations identified in human cancer are oncogenic. *Proc. Natl. Acad. Sci.* **102:** 802.

Kaur G., Belotti D., Burger A.M., Fisher-Nielson K., Borsotti P., Riccardi E., Thillainathan J., Hollingshead M., Sausville E.A., and Giavazzi R. 2004. Antiangiogenic properties of 17-(dimethylaminoethylamino)-17-demethoxygeldanamycin: An orally bioavailable heat shock protein 90 modulator. *Clin. Cancer Res.* **10:** 4813.

Kelland L.R., Sharp S.Y., Rogers P.M., Myers T.G., and Workman P. 1999. DT-diaphorase expression and tumor cell sensitivity to 17-allylamino, 17-demethoxygeldanamycin, an inhibitor of heat shock protein 90. *J. Natl. Cancer Inst.* **91:** 1940.

Kobayashi S., Boggon T.J., Dayaram T., Janne P.A., Kocher O., Meyerson M., Johnson B.E., Eck M.J., Tenen D.G., and Halmos B. 2005. *EGFR* mutation and resistance of non-small-cell lung cancer to gefitinib. *N. Engl. J. Med.* **352:** 786.

Komarov P.G., Komarova E.A., Kondratov R.V., Christov-Tselkov K., Coon J.S., Chernov M.V., and Gudkov A.V. 1999. A chemical inhibitor of p53 that protects mice from the side effects of cancer therapy. *Science* **285:** 1733.

Komarova E.A., Neznanov N., Komarov P.G., Chernov M.V., Wang K., and Gudkov A.V. 2003. p53 inhibitor pifithrin alpha can suppress heat shock and glucocorticoid signaling pathways. *J. Biol. Chem.* **278:** 15465.

Leaf C. 2004. Why we're losing the war on cancer—And how to win it. *Fortune*, March 12, 2004.

Liu D., Hutchinson O.C., Osman S., Price P., Workman P., and Aboagye E.O. 2002. Use of radiolabelled choline as a pharmacodynamic marker for the signal transduction inhibitor geldanamycin. *Br. J. Cancer* **87:** 783.

Llorca O., Martin-Benito J., Grantham J., Ritco-Vonsovici M., Willison K.R., Carrascosa J.L., and Valpuesta J.M. 2001. The 'sequential allosteric ring' mechanism in the eukaryotic chaperonin-assisted folding of actin and tubulin. *EMBO J.* **20:** 4065.

Llorca O., Martin-Benito J., Ritco-Vonsovici M., Grantham J., Hynes G.M., Willison K.R., Carrascosa J.L., and Valpuesta J.M. 2000. Eukaryotic chaperonin CCT stabilizes actin and tubulin folding intermediates in open quasi-native conformations. *EMBO J.* **19:** 5971.

Luders J., Demand J., and Hohfeld J. 2000. The ubiquitin-related BAG-1 provides a link between the molecular chaperones Hsc70/Hsp70 and the proteasome. *J. Biol. Chem.* **275:** 4613.

Lynch T.J., Bell D.W., Sordella R., Gurubhagavatula S., Okimoto R.A., Brannigan B.W., Harris P.L., Haserlat S.M., Supko J.G., Haluska F.G., Lois D.N., Christiani D.C., Settleman J., and Haber D.A. 2004. Activating mutations in the epidermal growth factor receptor underlying responsiveness of non-small-cell lung cancer to gefitinib. *N. Engl. J. Med.* **350:** 2129.

MacCallum D.E., Melville J.E., Frames S., Watt K., Anderson S., Gianella-Borradori A., Lane D.P., and Green S.R. 2005. Seliciclib (CYC202, R-roscovitine) induces cell death in multiple myeloma cells by inhibition of RNA polymerase II-dependent transcription and down-regulation of Mcl-1. *Cancer Res.* **65:** 5399.

Maloney A. and Workman P. 2002. HSP90 as a new therapeutic

target for cancer therapy: The story unfolds. *Expert Opin. Biol. Ther.* **2:** 3.

Maloney A., Clarke P.A., and Workman P. 2003. Genes and proteins governing the cellular sensitivity to HSP90 inhibitors: A mechanistic perspective. *Curr. Cancer Drug Targets* **3:** 331.

Manning G., Whyte D.B., Martinez R., Hunter T., and Sudarsanam S. 2002. The protein kinase complement of the human genome. *Science* **298:** 1912.

Mitsiades C.S., Mitsiades N., Hideshima T., Richardson P.G., and Anderson K.C. 2005. Proteasome inhibition as a therapeutic strategy for hematologic malignancies. *Expert Rev. Anticancer Ther.* **5:** 465.

Morimoto R.I. 1998. Regulation of the heat shock transcriptional response: Cross talk between family of heat shock factors, molecular chaperones and regulators. *Genes Dev.* **12:** 3788.

Mosser D. and Morimoto R.I. 2004. Molecular chaperones and the stress of oncogenesis. *Oncogene.* **23:** 2907.

Newbatt Y., Burns S., Hayward R., Whittaker S.R., Kirk R., Marshall C.S., Springer C.J., McDonald E., Cancer Genome Project., Marais R., Workman P., and Aherne G.W. 2005. Identification of inhibitors of the kinase activity of oncogenic V600E BRAF in an enzyme cascade high throughput screen. *J. Biomol. Screen.* (in press).

Nowell P.C. 1976. The clonal evolution of tumor cell populations. *Science* **194:** 23.

Nutley B.P., Raynaud F.I., Wilson S.C., Fischer P.M., Hayes A., Goddard P.M., McClue S.J., Jarman M., Lane D.P., and Workman P. 2005. Metabolism and pharmacokinetics of the cyclin-dependent kinase inhibitor R-roscovitine in the mouse. *Mol. Cancer Ther.* **4:** 125.

Orteaga S., Prieto I., Odajima J., Martín A., Dubus P., Sotillo R., Barbero J.L., Malumbres M., and Barbacid M. 2003. Cyclin-dependent kinase 2 is essential for meiosis but not for mitotic cell division in mice. *Nat. Genet.* **35:** 25.

Paez J.G., Jänne P.A., Lee J.C., Tracy S., Greulich H., Gabriel S., Herman P., Kaye F.J., Lindeman N., Boggon T.J., Naoki K., Sasaki H., Fujii Y., Eck M.J., Sellers W.R., Johnson B.E., and Meyerson M. 2004. EGFR mutations in lung cancer: Correlation with clinical response to gefitinib therapy. *Science* **304:** 1497.

Panaretou B., Siligardi G., Meyer P., Maloney A., Sullivan J.K., Singh S., Millson S.H., Clarke P.A., Naaby-Hansen S., Stein R., Cramer R., Mollapour M., Workman P., Piper P.W., Pearl L.H., and Prodromou C. 2002. Activation of the ATPase activity of HSP90 by the stress-regulated cochaperone aha1. *Mol. Cell* **10:** 1307.

Pao W., Miller V.A., Politi K.A., Riely G.J., Somwar R., Zakowski M.F., Kris M.G., and Varmus H. 2005. Acquired resistance of lung adenocarcinomas to gefitinib or erlotinib is associated with a second mutation in the EGFR kinase domain. *PLoS Med.* **2:** e73.

Pao W., Miller V., Zakowski M., Doherty J., Politi K., Sarkaria I., Singh B., Heelan R., Rusch V., Fulton L., Mardis E., Kupfer D., Wilson R., Kris M., and Varmus H. 2004. EGF receptor gene mutations are common in lung cancers from "never smokers" and are associated with sensitivity of tumors to gefitinib and erlotinib. *Proc. Natl. Acad. Sci.* **101:** 13306.

Patel S., Saghir N., Zhyvoloup A., Lensun L., Pergl-Wilson G., Depledge P., Eccles S., Kelland L.R., Clarke P.A., Ahmadi K., Raynaud F.I., Di Stefano F., Workman P., and Alderton W. 2004. Identification of potent selective inhibitors of PI3K as candidate anticancer drugs. *Proc. Am. Assoc. Cancer Res.* (Abstract LB-247).

Prodromou C., Roe S.M., O'Brien R., Ladbury J.E., Piper P.W., and Pearl L.H. 1997. Identification and structural characterization of the ATP/ADP-binding site in the HSP90 molecular chaperone. *Cell* **90:** 65.

Radford S.E. 2000. Protein folding: Progress made and promises ahead. *Trends Biochem. Sci.* **25:** 611.

Raynaud F.I., Fischer P.M., Nutley B.P., Goddard P.M., Lane D.P., and Workman P. 2004. Cassette dosing pharmacokinetcs of a library of 2,6,9-trisubstituted purine CDK2 inhibitors prepared by parallel synthesis. *Mol. Cancer Ther.* **3:** 353.

Raynaud F.I., Whittaker S.R., Fischer P.M., McClue S., Walton

M.I., Barrie S.E., Garrett M.D., Rogers P., Clarke S.J., Kelland L.R., Valenti M., Brunton L., Eccles S., Lane D.P., and Workman P. 2005. In vitro and in vivo pharmacokinetic-pharmacodynamic relationships for the trisubstituted aminopurine cyclin-dependent kinase inhibitors olomoucine, bohemine and CYC202. *Clin. Cancer Res.* **11:** 4875.

Roe S.M., Prodromou C., O'Brien R., Ladbury J.E., Piper P.W., and Pearl L.H. 1999. Structural basis for inhibition of the Hsp90 molecular chaperone by the antitumour antibiotics radicicol and geldanamycin. *J. Med. Chem.* **42:** 260.

Rowlands M.G., Newbatt Y.M., Prodromou C., Pearl L.H., Workman P., and Aherne W. 2004. High-throughput screening assay for inhibitors of heat-shock protein 90 ATPase activity. *Anal. Biochem.* **327:** 176.

Rutherford S.L. and Lindquist S. 1998. HSP90 as a capacitor for morphological evolution. *Nature* **396:** 336.

Samuels Y., Wang Z. Bardelli N., Ptak J., Szabo S., Yan H., Gazder A., Powell S.M., Riggins G.J., Willison J.K., Markowitz S., Kinzler K.W., Vogelstein B., and Velculescu V.E. 2004. High frequency of mutations of the PIK3CA gene in the human cancer. *Science* **23:** 304.

Sangster T.A., Quietsch C., and Lindquist S. 2003. HSP90 and chromatin. Where is the link? *Cell Cycle* **2:** 166.

Sawyers C.L. 2003. Opportunities and challenges in the development of kinase inhibitor therapy for cancer. *Genes Dev.* **17:** 2998.

Scheufler C., Brinker A., Bourenkov G., Pegoraro S., Moroder L., Bartunik H., Hartl F.U., and Moarefi I. 2000. Structure of TPR domain-peptide complexes: Critical elements in the assembly of the Hsp70-Hsp90 multichaperone machine. *Cell* **101:** 199.

Schnieder C., Sepp-Lorenzino L., Nimmesgern E., Ouerfelli O., Danishefsky S., Rosen N., and Hartl F.U. 1996. Pharmacologic shifting of a balance between protein refolding and degradation mediated by HSP90. *Proc. Natl. Acad. Sci.* **93:** 14536.

Schnur R.C., Corman M.L., Gallaschun R.J., Cooper B.A., Dee M.F., Doty J.L., Muzzi M.L., DiOrio C.I., Barbacci E.G., Miller P.E., Pollack V.A., Savage D.M., Sloan D.E., Pustilnik L.R., Moyer J.D., and Moyer M.P. 1995a. ErbB-2 oncogene inhibition by geldanamycin derivatives: Synthesis, mechanism of action, and structure-activity relationships. *J. Med. Chem.* **38:** 3813.

Schnur R.C., Corman M.L., Gallaschun R.J., Cooper B.A., Dee M.F., Doty J.L., Muzzi M.L., Moyer J.D., DiOrio C.I., Barbacci E.G., Miller P.E., O'Brien A.T., Morin M.J., Foster B.A., Pollack V.A., Savage D.M., Sloan D.E., Pustilnik L.R., and Moyer M.P. 1995b. Inhibition of the oncogene product p185erbB-2 *in vitro* and *in vivo* by geldanamycin and dihydrogeldanamycin derivatives. *J. Med. Chem.* **38:** 3806.

Schulte T.W., Blagosklonny M.V., Ingui C., and Neckers L. 1995. Disruption of the Raf-1-HSP90 molecular complex results in destabilization of Raf-1 and loss of Raf-1-Ras association. *J. Biol. Chem.* **270:** 24585.

Shah N.P., Tran C., Lee F.Y., Chen P., Norris D., and Sawyers C.L. 2004. Overriding imatinib resistance with a novel ABL kinase inhibitor. *Science* **305:** 399.

Sharp S.Y., Kelland L.R., Valenti M.R., Brunton L.A., Hobbs S., and Workman P. 2000. Establishment of an isogenic human colon tumor model for NQO1 gene expression: Application to investigate the role of DT-diaphorase in bioreductive drug activation *in vitro* and *in vivo. Mol. Pharmacol.* **58:** 1146.

Shayesteh L., Lu Y., Kuo W.L., Baldocchi R., Godfrey T., Collins C., Pinkel D., Powell B., Mills G.B., and Gray J.W. 1999. PIK3CA is implicated as an oncogene in ovarian cancer. *Nat. Genet.* **21:** 99.

Sherr C.J. 1996. Cancer cell cycles. *Science* **274:** 1672.

———. 2000. The Pezcoller Lecture: Cancer cell cycles revisited. *Cancer Res.* **60:** 3689.

Smith N.F., Hayes A., Nutley B.P., Raynaud F.I., and Workman P. 2004. Evaluation of the cassette dosing approach for assessing the pharmacokinetics of geldanamycin analogues in mice. *Cancer Chemother. Pharmacol.* **54:** 475.

Smith V., Hobbs S., Court W., Eccles S., Workman P., and Kelland L.R. 2002. ErbB2 overexpression in an ovarian cancer cell line confers sensitivity to the HSP90 inhibitor geldanamycin. *Anticancer Res.* **22:** 1993.

Smith-Jones P.M., Solit D.B., Akhurst T., Afroze F., Rosen N., and Larson S.M. 2004. Imaging the pharmacodynamics of HER2 degradation in response to Hsp90 inhibitors. *Nat. Biotechnol.* **22:** 701.

Solit D.B., Scher H.I., and Rosen N. 2003. Hsp90 as a therapeutic target in prostate cancer. *Semin. Oncol.* **30:** 709.

Sordella R., Bell D.W., Haber D.A., and Settleman J. 2004. Gefitinib-sensitizing EGFR mutations in lung cancer activate anti-apoptotic pathways. *Science* **305:** 1163.

Stebbins C.E., Russo A.A., Schneider C., Rosen N., Hartl F.U., and Pavletich N.P. 1997. Crystal structure of an Hsp90-geldanamycin complex: Targeting of a protein chaperone by an antitumor agent. *Cell* **89:** 239.

Stein R. and Waterfield M.D. 2000. PI3-kinase inhibition: A target for drug development? *Mol. Med. Today.* **6:** 347.

Sydor J.R., Pien C.S., Zhang Y., Ali J., Dembski M.S., Ge J., Grenier L., Hudak J., Normant E., Pak R., Patterson J., Pink M., Sang J., Woodward C., Mitsiades C.S., Anderson K.C., Grayzel D.S., Wright J., Tong J.K., Adams J., Palombella V.J., and Barrett J.A. 2005. Anti-tumor activity of a novel, water soluble Hsp90 inhibitor IPI-504 in multiple myeloma. *Proc. Am. Assoc. Cancer Res.* (Abstract 6160).

Tetsu O. and McCormick F. 2003. Proliferation of cancer cells despite CDK2 inhibition. *Cancer Cell* **3:** 233.

Thulasiraman V., Yang C.F., and Frydman J. 1999. *In vivo* newly translated polypeptides are sequestered in a protected folding environment. *EMBO J.* **18:** 85.

Valpuesta J.M., Martin-Benito J., Gomez-Puertas P., Carrascosa J.L., and Willison K.R. 2002. Structure and function of a protein folding machine: The eukaryotic chaperonin CCT. *FEBS Lett.* **529:** 11.

Vivanco I. and Sawyers C.L. 2002. The phosphatidylinositol 3-kinase AKT pathway in human cancer. *Nat. Rev. Cancer* **2:** 489.

Vogelstein B. and Kinzler K.W. 2004. Cancer genes and the pathways they control. *Nat. Med.* **10:** 789.

Walton M.I., Wilson S.C., Hardcastle I.R., Mirza A.R., and Workman P. 2005. An evaluation of the ability of pifithrin-α and -β to inhibit p53 function in two wild type p53 human tumour lines. *Mol Cancer Ther.* **4:** 1369.

Wan T.C., Garnett M.J., Roe S.M., Lee S., Niculescu-Duvaz D., Good V.M., Jones C.M, Marshall C.J., Springer C.J, Barford D., and Marais R. 2004. Mechanism of activation of the RAF-ERK signalling pathway by oncogenic mutations of B-RAF. *Cell* **116:** 855.

Wang S., Sakai H., and Weidmann M. 1995. NAC covers ribosome-associated nascent chains thereby forming a protective environment for regions of nascent chains just emerging from the peptidyl transferase center. *J. Cell Biol.* **130:** 519.

Wang Z., Shen D., Parsons D.W., Bardelli A., Sager J., Szabo S., Ptak J., Silliman N., Peters B.A., van der Hejden M.S., Parmigiani G., Yan H., Wang T.L., Riggins G., Powell S.M., Willison J.K., Markowitz S., Kinzler K.W., Vogelstein B., and Velculescu V.E. 2004. Mutational analysis of the tyrosine phosphatome in colorectal cancers. *Science* **304:** 1164.

Ward S.G., Sotsios Y., Dowden J., Bruce I., and Finan P. 2003. Therapeutic potential of phosphoinositide 3-kinase inhibitors. *Chem. Biol.* **10:** 207.

Wegele H., Muller L., and Buchner J. 2004. Hsp70 and Hsp90—A relay team for protein folding. *Rev. Physiol. Biochem. Pharmacol.* **151:** 1.

Weinstein I.B. 2002. Cancer. Addiction to oncogenes—The Achilles heal of cancer. *Nature* **297:** 63.

Weir B., Zhao X., and Meyerson M. 2004. Somatic alterations in the human cancer genome. *Cancer Cell* **6:** 433.

Whitesell L., Bagatell R., and Falsey R. 2003. The stress response: Implications for the clinical development of Hsp90 inhibitors. *Curr. Cancer Drug Targets* **3:** 349.

Whittaker S.R., Walton M.I., Garrett M.D., and Workman P. 2004. The cyclin-dependent kinase inhibitor CYC202 *(R-*roscovitine) inhibits retinoblastoma protein phosphorylation,

causes loss of cyclin D1 and activates the mitogen-activated protein kinase pathway. *Cancer Res.* **64:** 262.

Whittaker S.R., te Poele R., Walton M.I., Garrett M.D., and Workman P. 2003. Gene expression profiling of the cyclin-dependent kinase inhibitor CYC202 (*R*-roscovitine). *Proc. Am. Assoc. Cancer Res.* (Abstract 3996.)

Wilhelm S.M., Carter C., Tang L., Wilkie D., McNabola A., Rong H., Chen C., Zhang X., Vincent P., McHugh M., Cao Y., Shujath J., Gawlak S., Eveleigh D., Rowley B., Liu L., Adnane L., Lynch M., Auclair D., Taylor I., Gedrich R., Voznesensky A., Riedl B., Post L.E., Bollag G., and Trail P.A. 2004. BAY 43-9006 exhibits broad spectrum oral antitumor activity and targets the RAF/MEK/ERK pathway and receptor tyrosine kinases involved in tumor progression and angiogenesis. *Cancer Res.* **64:** 7099.

Workman P. 2001. Paul Workman—At the cutting edge of drug discovery (interview by Dorothy Bonn). *Lancet Oncol.* **2:** 113.

———. 2002. Challenges of PK/PD measurements in modern drug development. *Eur. J. Cancer* **18:** 2189.

———. 2003a. Strategies for treating cancers caused by multiple genomic abnormalities: From concepts to cures? *Curr. Opin. Investig. Drugs* **12:** 1415.

———. 2003b. The opportunities and challenges of personalized genome-based molecular therapies for cancer: Targets, technologies, and molecular chaperones. *Cancer Chemother. Pharmacol.* (suppl. 1) **52:** S45.

———. 2003c. Paul Workman on the challenges of cancer drug development. Interview by Katherine E. Pestell. *Drug Discov. Today* **8:** 775.

———. 2003d. How much gets there and what does it do?: The need for better pharmacokinetic and pharmacodynamic endpoints in contemporary drug discovery and development. *Curr. Pharm. Des.* **9:** 891.

———. 2003e. Auditing the pharmacological accounts for HSP90 inhibitors. Unfolding the relationship between pharmacokinetics and pharmacodynamics. *Mol. Cancer Ther.* **2:** 131.

———. 2003f. Overview: Translating HSP90 biology into Hsp90 drugs. *Curr. Cancer Drug Targets* **3:** 297.

———. 2004a. Inhibiting the phosphoinositide 3-kinase pathway for cancer treatment. *Biochem. Soc. Trans.* **32:** 393.

———. 2004b. Combinatorial attack on multistep oncogenesis by inhibiting the Hsp90 molecular chaperone. *Cancer Lett.* **206:** 149.

———. 2004c. Altered states: Selectively drugging the HSP90 cancer chaperone. *Trends Mol. Med.* **109:** 47.

———. 2005. Genomics and the second golden era of cancer research. *Mol. BioSystems* **1:** 17.

Workman P. and Kaye S.B. 2002. Translating basic cancer research into new cancer therapeutics. *Trends Mol. Med.* **8:** S1-S8.

Workman P., Raynaud F., Clarke P.A., te Poele R., Eccles S., Kelland L., Di Stefano F., Ahmadi K., Parker P. and Waterfield M. 2004. Pharmacological properties and in vitro and in vivo antitumour activity of the potent and selective PI3 kinase inhibitor PI103. Proceedings of the EORTC-NCI-AACR Symposium on Molecular Targets and Cancer Therapeutics (Abstr. 414A). *Eur. J. Cancer* **2:** 8. (Suppl.)

Wright L., Barril X., Dymock B., Sheridan L., Surgenor A., Beswick M., Drysdale M., Collier A., Massey A., Davies N., Fink A., Fromont C., Aherne W., Boxall K., Sharp S., Workman P., and Hubbard R.E. 2004. Structure-activity relationships in purine-based inhibitor binding to HSP90 isoforms. *Chem. Biol.* **11:** 775.

Xu W., Yuan X., Xiang Z., Mimnaugh E., Marcu M., and Neckers L. 2005. Surface charge and hydrophobicity determine ErbB2 binding to the Hsp90 chaperone complex. *Nat. Struct. Mol. Biol.* **12:** 120.

Young J.C., Moarefi I., and Hartl F.U. 2001. Hsp90: A specialised but essential protein-folding tool. *J. Cell Biol.* **154:** 267.

Young J.C., Agashe V.R., Siegers K., and Hartl F.U. 2004. Pathways of chaperone-mediated protein folding in the cytosol. *Nat. Rev. Mol. Cell Biol.* **5:** 781.

Yu X., Guo Z.S., Marcu M.G., Neckers L., Nguyen D.M., Chen G.A., and Schrump D.S. 2002. Modulation of p53, ErbB1, ErbB2, and Raf-1 expression in lung cancer cells by depsipeptide FR901228. *J. Natl. Cancer Inst.* **94:** 504.

Zhang L., Yu J., Park B.H., Kinzler K.W., and Vogelstein B. 2000. Role of BAX in the apoptotic response to anticancer agents. *Science* **290:** 989.

Zhao R., Davey M., Hsu Y.C., Kaplanek P., Tong A., Parsons A.B., Krogan N., Cagney G., Mai D., Greenblatt J., Boone C., Emili A., and Houry W.A. 2005. Navigating the chaperone network: An integrative map of physical and genetic interactions mediated by the HSP90 chaperone. *Cell* **120:** 715.

Modeling of Protein Signaling Networks in Clinical Proteomics

D.H. Geho, E.F. Petricoin, L.A. Liotta, and R.P. Araujo
Center for Applied Proteomics and Molecular Medicine, Department of Molecular and Microbiology,
George Mason University, Manassas, Virginia 20110

Molecular interactions that underlie pathophysiological states are being elucidated using techniques that profile proteomic endpoints in cellular systems. Within the field of cancer research, protein interaction networks play pivotal roles in the establishment and maintenance of the hallmarks of malignancy, including cell division, invasion, and migration. Multiple complementary tools enable a multifaceted view of how signal protein pathway alterations contribute to pathophysiological states. One pivotal technique is signal pathway profiling of patient tissue specimens. This microanalysis technology provides a proteomic snapshot at one point in time of cells directly procured from the native context of a tumor microenvironment. To study the adaptive patterns of signal pathway events over time, before and after experimental therapy, it is necessary to obtain biopsies from patients before, during, and after therapy. A complementary approach is the profiling of cultured cell lines with and without treatment. Cultured cell models provide the opportunity to study short-term signal changes occurring over minutes to hours. Through this type of system, the effects of particular pharmacological agents may be used to test the effects of signal pathway inhibition or activation on multiple endpoints within a pathway. The complexity of the data generated has necessitated the development of mathematical models for optimal interpretation of interrelated signaling pathways. In combination, clinical proteomic biopsy profiling, tissue culture proteomic profiling, and mathematical modeling synergistically enable a deeper understanding of how protein associations lead to disease states and present new insights into the design of therapeutic regimens.

The drive to create personalized approaches for medical care is underpinned by two attractive, interrelated endpoints: the elucidation of a molecular description for a patient's disease along with an effective and minimally toxic therapeutic regimen. Because of our currently limited understanding of how commonly used therapeutics effect their functions, patients often receive a battery of agents in a cocktail or in succession. Unfortunately, the conventional therapies are successful for only a subset of patients, and responses are often temporary. Moreover, selected therapies may be ineffective for a given patient's disease, thereby exposing the patient to the unwanted symptomatic or pathological side effects caused by the ineffective drug. One approach toward the improvement of therapeutic outcome shifts the therapeutic targets beyond individual molecules to entire networks inside and outside the cell in the context of the tissue microenvironment. Characterization of such molecular network defects that underlie disease states such as cancer will reveal insights into pathophysiology and provide molecular targets for intervention.

A remarkably varied palette of biomolecules, including nucleic acids, proteins, lipids, and carbohydrates, coalesce to form a molecular system in an organism. Although significant effort has been invested in cataloging and studying the nucleic acid content of biological systems, an incomplete picture emerges when only genetic material is used to study a complex system such as a cell or tissue microenvironment. Although DNA is an information archive, proteins perform pivotal structural, synthetic, signaling and recognition functions. Of particular interest in cancer, protein signaling pathways consist of transient networks of proteins that come together and dis-

perse in a dynamic manner (Hunter 2000). In these signaling cascades, one protein binds to another and, in so doing, confers a posttranslational modification such as phosphorylation or cleavage. These subtle molecular changes are excluded from analysis by a genomics-only approach to molecular profiling.

For these reasons, molecular, personalized diagnostics for patients will require high-throughput profiling of the proteomic content within cells of interest. Clinical proteomics is a rapidly evolving discipline that has arisen out of this pressing need to generate molecular portraits of disease. Protein microarrays enable low-abundance proteins to be studied in a reproducible, high-throughput system (MacBeath and Schreiber 2000; Zhu and Snyder 2001; MacBeath 2002; Liotta et al. 2003). With this approach, known protein targets are probed using isoform-specific antibodies. The relative abundance of key proteins can be compared across specimens, providing a method for assessing the activity levels of key nodes within signaling protein pathways.

Because it is a fundamental means of personalizing diagnostics, profiling of actual patient tissues is a central goal of clinical proteomics. As a complementary approach for studying cellular signaling pathways in a rapid, real-time format, proteins extracted from cell culture assays are also being incorporated into protein microarrays. Mathematical modeling is required to organize the large volumes of information emanating from microarray studies, yielding insight into how signaling networks interact in a disease state. These three approaches, taken together, are offering new insights into the pathophysiology and treatment of diseases such as cancer.

PROTEOMIC PROFILING OF PATIENT BIOPSIES

Technological challenges have, until recently, precluded systematic studying of the proteomic information with a patient's tissue specimen. One inherent difficulty in profiling the proteomic content of a tissue is that much important information resides in a population of low-abundance molecules. Whereas nucleic acid research is facilitated by polymerase chain reaction technologies, no comparable intrinsic amplification mechanism has yet been discovered for proteomic studies. Therefore, detection platforms with a high degree of sensitivity are required to glean an accurate picture of a tissue's proteomic profile.

HANDLING OF BIOPSY MATERIAL FOR PROTEOMIC ANALYSIS

For the promise of molecular medicine to be realized fully, the information contained within the biopsy must be translated into a molecular format. Thus, the process of molecular retrieval is central to the quality of information that is generated. When a biopsy is procured, the equivalent of a snapshot of a patient's disease process is obtained. As such, how it is handled determines the amount and quality of information that is derived from the procedure. For clinical proteomics research, immediately after a biopsy is obtained it must be snap-frozen in an embedding medium and then kept at −80°C for long-term storage in order to preserve labile molecules in the sample. For further study, a thin frozen section is made of the tissue. On morphological inspection of the cells within a patient's biopsy specimen, it is apparent that numerous cell types are found within a tissue microenvironment. For example, in cancer specimens, there are not only tumor cells, but also the surrounding cells that contribute to the pathophysiological state. These cells may include nerves, blood vessels, fibroblasts, smooth muscle, lymphocytes, other inflammatory cells, and extravasated red blood cells (Liotta and Kohn 2001). Laser capture microdissection, however, provides a means for isolating a pure cell population from such a heterogeneous cellular environment (Emmert-Buck et al. 1996). Once purified cells from the biopsy are isolated, the protein content of the cells is extracted and can be utilized in profiling technologies such as the protein microarray.

PROTEIN MICROARRAY FORMATS

Two formats for protein microarrays have been implemented (Liotta et al. 2003). One method uses an antibody capture strategy and is called the forward phase array. The capture antibody for an analyte is immobilized onto a substrate, while a second antibody is used to detect a distinct epitope on the same analyte. The requirement of two antibodies in a forward phase array is a marked limitation of this approach, because specific antibodies for two distinct epitopes can be difficult, either because of limited antibody reagents or, alternatively, the analyte may be very small. A more efficient system requires the use of only one antibody per analyte. A format that enables this type of array is called the reverse phase microarray (RPMA). With the RPMA, proteins extracted from cells purified out of human tissues by laser capture microdissection are arrayed directly onto a substrate such as nitrocellulose. The proteins are spotted onto an array using an arraying device, similar to those utilized in genomic array systems (Fig. 1). The heterogeneous proteins from a cellular extract are arrayed directly onto such a

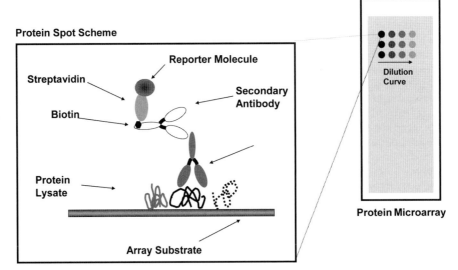

Figure 1. Standard reverse phase microarray. Protein analytes harvested from a purified cell population, obtained either through laser capture microdissection or cells from culture, are treated to extract the proteins contained within. The proteins, also called analytes, are arrayed onto a substrate such as nitrocellulose. Unbound sites on the nitrocellulose are then blocked. The immobilized analytes are probed with an antibody specific for protein endpoint of interest. These can be endpoints such as phosphorylated signaling proteins. The primary antibody is then detected using a secondary antibody specific for the isoform of the primary antibody. This secondary antibody is labeled with a biotin group. The biotin is detected using streptavidin linked to a reporter molecule, such as a quantum dot or horseradish peroxidase.

substrate in a series of dilutions. In the standard RPMA format, a primary antibody specific for a known target protein, such as a phosphorylated isoform of a signaling protein, is incubated on the protein spot. Over a hundred antibodies validated by western blots are currently used to probe targeted analytes within protein extracts. These antibodies provide a means to study growth-regulatory, apoptotic, and cytoskeleton-linked pathways. Bound primary antibody is then detected by a secondary antibody that is biotinylated. As with immunohistochemistry, the secondary antibody is bound by streptavidin linked to a catalyst reporter molecule such as horseradish peroxidase (HRP). Because the proteins of interest are of low abundance, a biotinyl tyramide signal amplification system is used, which significantly enhances the sensitivity of the RPMA (King et al. 1997). After biotinyl tyramide groups are deposited, streptavidin-HRP is applied again followed by enzymatic deposition of a chromagen such as diaminobenzidene (DAB). This sensitive system can detect protein levels approaching attogram amounts. It is estimated that in the range of 1,000–5,000 molecules per spot can be detected using this system. Furthermore, utilization of patient material is maximized using this system, as 10,000 procured human cells allow the production of up to 100 RPMAs.

In an effort to increase the versatility of RPMAs, streptavidin-conjugated quantum dots have been used as an alternative reporter agent for RPMA (Geho et al. 2005). Through this study, it was determined that a pegylated form of the streptavidin–quantum dot bioconjugate was required, as nonpegylated reagent bound nonspecifically to arrayed protein spots. One benefit of this reporter technique is that signals can be detected without amplification when sensitive hyperspectral imaging is employed (Schultz et al. 2001; Huebschman et al. 2002). Another benefit of the quantum dots is their potential to be used in a multiplexed format, since they have narrow emission spectra. The development of a multiplexed format will enable more protein targets, or endpoints, to be detected on a single array surface. Each antibody probe could be linked to a particular type of quantum dot, yielding a characteristic emission spectrum. A further benefit of the quantum dot technology is that these fluorophores are resistant to photobleaching, unlike organic fluorophores, and can be imaged months after the original excitation.

As an additional strategy for increasing the amount of antibody probes that can be used with each slide, a sector array format has also been developed (Espina et al. 2004). This approach requires the engineering of a reservoir system and a matching glass slide with distinct nitrocellulose pads, or sectors. With this type of array, multiple sectors are present on a single array surface, each of which may be incubated with a unique reaction condition. The sector array format significantly increases the amount of information that may be gleaned from a single array slide.

The RPMA allows a target analyte to be compared across various clinical specimens on the same array. This format enables low-abundance endpoints such as phosphorylated, or activated, signaling proteins to be detected among specimens. To perform comparisons, a reference standard can be included in the array (Sheehan et al.

2005). One type of reference standard is a mixture of known analytes such as synthetically produced peptides, with known concentrations. If a source such as peptides is used as the reference standard, the standard is renewable and chemically defined, which enhances its reproducibility. With a reference standard included on each array, the relative abundance of important signaling molecules can be assessed across specimens.

Of particular interest using these techniques has been the profiling of known signaling proteins. An early study using RPMA format demonstrated that pro-survival signaling pathways were key to the development of a cancer invasion front in prostate cancer (Paweletz et al. 2001). Signaling protein studies have been extended to other disease states as well, such as lymphoma and ovarian cancer (Wulfkuhle et al. 2003; Zha et al. 2004; Sheehan et al. 2005). Bioinformatic clustering analyses enable molecular profiles to be grouped according to similarities in protein populations. The RPMA format enables numerous distinct protein endpoints within cells to be measured and compared across disease types and, within disease types, across the spectrum of disease from in situ disease to advanced metastatic disease. Furthermore, the effects of therapeutic interventions on defined molecular endpoints can be monitored using this type of diagnostic system.

PROTEOMIC PROFILING OF TREATED CELLS IN CULTURE

The previously described format employed patient biopsy specimens as the source of the proteomic material for profiling (see Fig. 2). Previous work demonstrated that a significant gulf stands between cells grown in culture and those extracted from disease tissue (Ornstein et

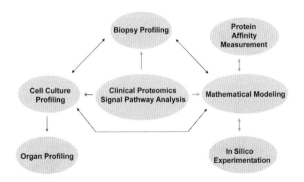

Figure 2. Proteomic signal pathway profiling. Signal pathway profiling is emerging as a multifaceted discipline employing distinct yet complementary tools. Proteomic profiling of biopsy specimens provides unique access to the molecular content of patient material. This enables a personalized molecular portrait to be fashioned. Tissue culture, or higher-order cultures, provide a real-time laboratory for measuring alterations in signaling pathways following treatment with pharmacological agents. Mathematical modeling studies provide a means for understanding complex signaling networks. As models grow in sophistication, theoretical in silico experimentation will provide a means of stratifying molecular targets as potential therapeutic targets.

al. 2000). It is essential, when providing a molecular diagnosis for a patient, to study the cells within their native microenvironment using laser capture microdissection. However, this provides a "snapshot" of the tissue's proteomic activity, frozen in time. To study the kinetics of signaling pathways, an alternative and complementary system is required. Cell culture systems that possess the signaling molecule pathways of interest provide a unique means to measure the response of the pathways to pharmacological perturbation. Using similar protein extraction techniques and RPMA technology, the temporal variations in protein activities in particular pathways can be monitored in a real-time framework. Treatment of cells in culture with defined chemotherapeutic agents also represents a technique for elucidating the mechanism of drug activities. In one case study, a combination therapy comprising carboxyamidotriazole (a voltage-independent calcium channel inhibitor) and a celecoxib analog was shown to have a supra-additive growth inhibition in cell culture conditions (Winters et al. 2005). The RPMA format elucidated the mechanism of the cytotoxic activity; namely, with these two agents the cytotoxicity is effected through the suppression of proliferation and the initiation of apoptosis.

Three-dimensional spatial and temporal fluctuations of heterotypic and homotypic cell physiological functions acting within the architectural setting of an intact tissue or organ affect the activity levels of signaling molecules. To more closely approximate the cellular and molecular complexity of a tissue microenvironment in culture systems, organs or organ fragments may in the future be maintained in tissue reactors for cell signaling assays. Following treatment of the organized tissue with defined agents, the tissue could then be frozen and microdissected, in a manner similar to patient biopsies described above. This scenario will provide a more complex setting for studying cellular signaling pathways. Cells maintained within an organ or tissue context provide a more realistic portrait of molecular events than isolated tissue culture cells because of the presence of three-dimensional architectural elements, comprising stromal cells and extracellular matrix, which surround a cell in such a tissue context. These three-dimensional elements necessarily affect cellular signaling and must be taken into account in order to build more comprehensive models of cellular signaling events.

MATHEMATICAL MODELING IN CLINICAL PROTEOMICS

Notwithstanding the potential of RPMA technology to furnish an array of information on a given tumor's proteomic fingerprint, an important consideration from a translational standpoint is how to organize this information into a coherent picture of the dysfunction of the signal transduction networks, and to use this understanding to develop an effective therapeutic regimen to eradicate the tumor. Indeed, even with the inchoate understanding of intracellular biochemical control prevailing today, it is recognized that a cell has very subtle and complex techniques at its disposal to process biochemical signals (Tyson et al. 2003). Even the simple phosphorylation cycle formed by

a kinase and an opposing phosphatase—a fundamental building block in any network of protein–protein interactions—exhibits important control characteristics through its ability to create an ultrasensitive "switch-like" response to an upstream signal under certain conditions (Goldbeter and Koshland 1981). Moreover, this simple signaling motif generally occurs in a layered structure to form a so-called "kinase cascade," which is itself interconnected with other cascades, and interlaced with manifold control interactions such as feedback and feed-forward loops (Fig. 3). Operating in concert with these mechanisms are still other features such as redundancy and spatiotemporal compartmentalization, which further complicate the processing of biochemical signals.

Thus, in view of the daunting complexity of signaling networks, both topologically and functionally, the effects of a particular therapeutic intervention on particular parts of the cell signaling network, and on the cell's behavior as a whole, may be recondite and unintuitive. Furthermore, the difficulties in understanding intracellular responses to therapeutic regimens are magnified considerably in the context of "combination therapies" (Araujo et al. 2004, 2005)—where multiple nodes in the cell's signaling net-

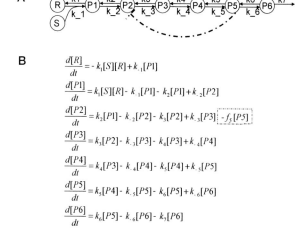

Figure 3. Mathematical modeling of a signaling molecule cascade with feedback inhibition. A simplified model of a hypothetical six-node kinase cascade (adapted from Araujo et al. 2004). (*A*) An extracellular stimulus (S) binds to a free receptor (R) on the cell membrane, leading to the phosphorylation of the first protein (P1) in the cascade. Each protein then phosphorylates the next protein downstream: P1 phosphorylates P2, P2 phosphorylates P3, and so on. Proteins may also be dephosphorylated by phosphatases, giving rise to a reverse reaction between a phosphorylated protein and the preceding upstream protein. Moreover, any given phosphorylated protein may promote or inhibit the phosphorylation of upstream or downstream proteins. A negative feedback loop is shown with a dashed line here as an example, with protein P5 inhibiting the phosphorylation of the upstream protein P2. (*B*) Modeling equations corresponding to the simple network in *A*. Note that these equations are based on the assumption of mass action kinetics, which neglects some of the control subtleties afforded by Michaelis-Menten kinetics. The basic model may be supplemented by feedback loops by making simple additions to the modeling equations. In the example given here, the negative feedback loop shown with a dashed line in *A* is accounted for by the extra term shown with a dashed line surrounding it in *B*. (Adapted from Araujo et al. 2004.)

work are targeted simultaneously—owing to the nonadditive effects of the individual agents. Early modeling studies on even the very simplest mathematical representations of cell signaling networks—with minimal feedback control or ultrasensitive characteristics—reveal that inhibiting a number of serially connected processes in a signaling cascade can produce a supra-additive (synergistic) attenuation of downstream signals in comparison with targeting the same processes individually (Araujo et al. 2005).

For this reason, the development of a successful patient-tailored therapy based on detailed RPMA-obtained information is dependent on the concomitant development of mechanistic mathematical models to bridge the divide between the molecular portrait of an individual patient's aberrant signaling network and an effective treatment. In this manner, the most effective complement of therapeutic targets may be determined, and an in silico drug trial conducted.

FROM PROMISE TO REALITY: THE CHALLENGES AHEAD FOR INDIVIDUALIZED MOLECULAR MEDICINE

Reconciling Static and Dynamic Kinetic Signatures in Signaling Pathways

The union of RPMA analysis of an individual patient's tissue biopsy with mathematical paradigms which interpret this information and point the way to the corresponding most effective therapy promises to be a fecund one, with the potential to revolutionize the treatment of disease. Nevertheless, for this concept to become a reality, the complexity of its implementation must be appreciated, and a clear plan for overcoming current challenges must be formulated.

For individualized molecular-targeted medicine to realize its fullest potential—yielding potent and effective treatment strategies with as little toxicity as possible—there must exist a means to discern the precise nature of the dysfunction in a given signaling network. The cardinal step in reaching this overall goal is identifying the full suite of proteins contributing to the disease and the nature of their aberrant activities (whether they be hyperphosphorylated or overexpressed, for example), a formidable task, in which the RPMA technology has enormous potential.

Nevertheless, the ability to translate this compendium of information into a diagnosis of network dysfunction is dependent on a detailed, a priori knowledge of the architecture of relevant signaling pathways, the kinetics of individual protein–protein interactions, as well as the functional structure of molecular control machinery such as feedback and feed-forward loops. Here, cell culture experiments, along with protein-binding studies, will form an essential backdrop for the tissue biopsy data through their ability to paint a dynamic, *time-dependent* portrait of a signaling network's response to stimulating ligands and/or other perturbations to cytoplasmic or nuclear signaling events.

Moreover, it is worth considering that these time-dependent studies are the experimental counterparts to the mathematical frameworks which assist both in determining kinetic parameters and elucidating network architectures, as well as providing a platform for in silico drug trials. Intracellular signaling is dynamic by its very nature, and the effects of any variations in stimulating signals should be understood in the context of a time-dependent study. Of course, after a period of unchanging conditions in the tissue microenvironment, intracellular protein concentrations may attain steady states in some cases, and in other cases, exhibit sustained oscillations about a "setpoint." On the other hand, should the extracellular milieu exhibit ongoing fluctuations in any properties that influence intracellular events, the processes involved in intracellular communication may constitute a very complex dynamic picture indeed.

Either way, an understanding of the relationship between the *static* picture of intracellular signaling furnished by the RPMA analysis of tissue biopsies and the *dynamic* picture furnished by corresponding cell culture studies and cognate mathematical models must emerge in order to assess the dysfunction of a particular tissue's signaling network, and thus, the true nature of a patient's disease. This reconciliation of paradigms is a complex question that must be addressed before significant advances can be made in this area of research.

Therefore, the goal of individualized therapy is to be pursued on a number of frontiers: high-throughput analysis of tissue biopsy data (via RPMA), the elucidation of the kinetics of intracellular signaling (via cell culture studies in combination with RPMA and mathematical modeling), and mathematical techniques to reconcile "static" tissue biopsy data with "dynamic" descriptions of intracellular signaling. Once the nature of signaling dysfunction is determined in an individual patient, the final frontier consists of identifying the most effective and least toxic strategy for launching an assault on the signaling network to elicit the desired clinical outcome. In the case of a particular cancer, this would usually mean tipping the balance of biochemical signaling events away from cell proliferation and cell survival and in favor of apoptosis.

Combination Therapeutics: Insights from Mathematical Modeling

Beyond the problem of identifying effective mechanisms to selectively modulate aberrantly activated signaling pathways with target-based drugs, a further challenge remains: toxicity. The narrow "therapeutic index" of much of the existing pharmacopoeia means that only a very restricted range of doses produces therapeutic benefit with tolerable toxicity, with doses outside of this range yielding either unacceptable toxicity or insufficient therapeutic benefit. Recent theoretical studies of intracellular signaling have focused on a new concept in the treatment of disease—"network-targeted" combination therapy—which holds the promise of obviating many of these shortcomings. In this new approach, the emphasis is on distributing drug delivery among several targets, rather than concentrating the therapeutic intervention at a single signaling molecule.

Combination therapies afford at least four key benefits in comparison with monotherapies:

1. For a given drug dose at each molecular target (or node), the attenuation of downstream signals is significantly enhanced when a multiplicity of targets is chosen rather than a single target, particularly when the nodes are serially linked (see Fig. 4) (Araujo et al. 2005).

2. The desired response may be produced with lower doses of the necessary agents when multiple nodes are targeted, rather than a single node in isolation (Araujo et al. 2004, 2005). Not only could this property reduce

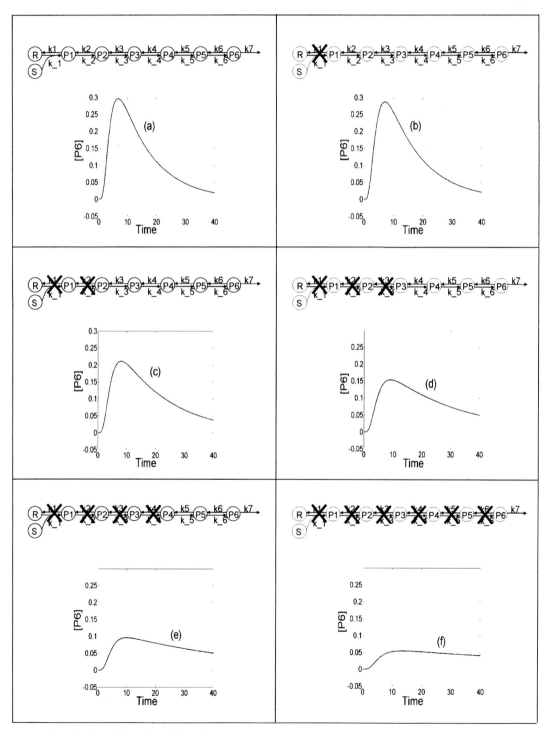

Figure 4. Mathematical modeling of the effects of combination therapy on signaling molecule cascades. The temporal evolution of a biochemical signal in a simple six-node network comprising proteins P1 through P6, in response to the binding of a stimulus, S, to an upstream receptor, R. Case *a* corresponds to an unperturbed network (no drugs). In case *b*, the receptor is targeted with a dose of IC_{50} of an appropriate inhibitor. In cases *c* through *f* a number of nodes are targeted, each with a dose of IC_{50}. As more nodes are added to the treatment program, the output signal progressively diminishes. (Note that the biochemical signal under consideration is the concentration of the most downstream protein, P6.) (Adapted from Araujo et al. 2004.)

the harmful side effects of drugs in current use, but it may impart clinical applicability to a huge compendium of agents which, of themselves, are too toxic at their therapeutically effective doses. This new concept may therefore spawn an enormous new repertoire of molecular-targeted therapeutics for clinical evaluation.

3. The location of target nodes in relation to the local architecture of the signaling network has important implications for the effectiveness of a therapy. Nodes embedded in negative feedback loops may represent very poor targets in some cases (Sauro and Kholodenko 2004), for example, since the automatic control characteristics of this signaling motif have the tendency to constrain the system response to follow a defined set point and resist the effects of any disturbances. Moreover, recent theoretical studies (Araujo et al. 2004) provide circumstantial evidence that receptors, being at the most upstream location in a signaling cascade, may represent quite poor targets. This is an important consideration in view of the number of drugs developed to target receptors (Iressa, Herceptin, Gleevec, etc.). On the other hand, receptors may represent a less complex therapeutic target in comparison with downstream nodes embedded in more complicated network architectures involving inter-pathway cross talk and feedback loops.

4. One of the consequences of the markedly nonlinear relationships between kinetic parameters and concentrations of signaling proteins is the nonadditive attenuation of signals for a multiplicity of target nodes, in comparison with targeting the same nodes individually (Araujo et al. 2005). Signal attenuation may therefore be synergistic, producing an extra inhibition that is not due to an extra dose of drug. We may therefore view this bonus inhibition as entirely nontoxic.

Thus, combination therapeutics, when conducted under the umbrella of an individualized assessment of intracellular signaling dysfunction, should allow much more effective disruption of biochemical signals and better control over overall cell behavior, with much lower drug doses and reduced systemic toxicity.

CONCLUSION

The promise of the integrated coupling of diagnosis with therapeutic intervention represents a new paradigm and will show benefit at multiple points in the biomedical network. For the biomedical researcher, the capability to profile the molecular content of diseased tissue will reveal a more complete understanding of disease pathophysiology. Pathologists will provide an entirely new service by including molecular pathway assessments to accompany their morphological descriptions. For clinicians, a more personalized, detailed molecular understanding of their patient's disease will provide more insight for developing therapeutic plans. Pharmaceutical company drug discovery teams will be able to perform an early assessment of a drug's effectiveness at a signal network level for a given molecular defect. This would provide a cost-effective means for prioritization of high-value therapeutics early in the discovery and

development process. Most importantly, patients will benefit through receiving a unique molecular characterization, resulting in a therapeutic plan that best fits their pathophysiology.

REFERENCES

Araujo R.P., Liotta L.A., and Petricoin E.F. 2004. Network-targeted combination therapy: A new concept in cancer treatment. *Drug Discov Today: Therapeutic Strategies* **1**: 425.

Araujo R.P., Petricoin E.F., and Liotta L.A. 2005. A mathematical model of combination therapy using the EGFR signaling network. *Biosystems* **80**: 57.

Emmert-Buck M.R., Bonner R.F., Smith P.D., Chuaqui R.F., Zhuang Z., Goldstein S.R., Weiss R.A., and Liotta L.A. 1996. Laser capture microdissection. *Science* **274**: 998.

Espina V., Petricoin E.F., Liotta L.A., and Geho D. 2004. Application of sector protein microarrays to clinical samples. *Clin. Proteomics* **1**: 91.

Geho D., Lahar N., Gurnani P., Huebschman M., Herrmann P., Espina V., Shi A., Wulfkuhle J., Garner H., Petricoin E., III, Liotta L.A., and Rosenblatt K.P. 2005. Pegylated, streptavidin-conjugated quantum dots are effective detection elements for reverse-phase protein microarrays. *Bioconjug. Chem.* **16**: 559.

Goldbeter A. and Koshland D.E., Jr. 1981. An amplified sensitivity arising from covalent modification in biological systems. *Proc. Natl. Acad. Sci.* **78**: 6840.

Huebschman M.L., Schultz R.A., and Garner H.R. 2002. Characteristics and capabilities of the hyperspectral imaging microscope. *IEEE Eng. Med. Biol. Mag.* **21**: 104.

Hunter T. 2000. Signaling—2000 and beyond. *Cell* **100**: 113.

King G., Payne S., Walker F., and Murray G.I. 1997. A highly sensitive detection method for immunohistochemistry using biotinylated tyramine. *J. Pathol.* **183**: 237.

Liotta L.A. and Kohn E.C. 2001. The microenvironment of the tumour-host interface. *Nature* **411**: 375.

Liotta L.A., Espina V., Mehta A.I., Calvert V., Rosenblatt K., Geho D., Munson P.J., Young L., Wulfkuhle J., and Petricoin E.F., III. 2003. Protein microarrays: Meeting analytical challenges for clinical applications. *Cancer Cell* **3**: 317.

MacBeath G. 2002. Protein microarrays and proteomics. *Nat. Genet.* (suppl.) **32**: 526.

MacBeath G. and Schreiber S.L. 2000. Printing proteins as microarrays for high throughput function determination. *Science* **289**: 1760.

Ornstein D.K., Gillespie J.W., Paweletz C.P., Duray P.H., Herring J., Vocke C.D., Topalian S.L., Bostwick D.G., Linehan W.M., Petricoin E.F., III, and Emmert-Buck M.R. 2000. Proteomic analysis of laser capture microdissected human prostate cancer and in vitro prostate cell lines. *Electrophoresis* **21**: 2235.

Paweletz, C.P., L. Charboneau, V.E. Bichsel, N.L. Simone, T. Chen, J.W. Gillespie, M.R. Emmert-Buck, M.J. Roth, I.E. Petricoin, and L.A. Liotta. 2001. Reverse phase protein microarrays which capture disease progression show activation of prosurvival pathways at the cancer invasion front. *Oncogene* **20**: 1981.

Sauro H.M. and Kholodenko B.N. 2004. Quantitative analysis of signaling networks. *Prog. Biophys. Mol. Biol.* **86**: 5.

Schultz R.A., Nielsen T., Zavaleta J.R., Ruch R., Wyatt R., and Garner H.R. 2001. Hyperspectral imaging: A novel approach for microscopic analysis. *Cytometry* **43**: 239.

Sheehan K.M., Calvert V.S., Kay E.W., Lu Y., Fishman D., Espina V., Aquino J., Speer R., Araujo R., Mills G.B., Liotta L.A., Petricoin E.F., III, and Wulfkuhle J.D. 2005. Use of reverse phase protein microarrays and reference standard development for molecular network analysis of metastatic ovarian carcinoma. *Mol. Cell. Proteomics* **4**: 346.

Tyson J.J., Chen K.C., and Novak B. 2003. Sniffers, buzzers, toggles and blinkers: Dynamics of regulatory and signaling pathways in the cell. *Curr. Opin. Cell Biol.* **15**: 221.

Winters M.E., Mehta A.I., Petricoin E.F., III, Kohn E.C., and Liotta L.A. 2005. Supra-additive growth inhibition by a celecoxib analogue and carboxyamido-triazole is primarily mediated through apoptosis. *Cancer Res.* **65**: 3853.

Wulfkuhle J.D., Aquino J.A., Calvert V.S., Fishman D.A., Coukos G., Liotta L.A., and Petricoin E.F., III. 2003. Signal pathway profiling of ovarian cancer from human tissue specimens using reverse-phase protein microarrays. *Proteomics* **3**: 2085.

Zha H., Raffeld M., Charboneau L., Pittaluga S., Kwak L.W., Petricoin E., III, Liotta L.A., and Jaffe E.S. 2004. Similarities of prosurvival signals in Bcl-2-positive and Bcl-2-negative follicular lymphomas identified by reverse phase protein microarray. *Lab. Invest.* **84**: 235.

Zhu H. and Snyder M. 2001. Protein arrays and microarrays. *Curr. Opin. Chem. Biol.* **5**: 40.

The Beginning of the End of Frustration

Department of Biology, Howard Hughes Medical Institute, Center for Cancer Research, Massachusetts Institute of Technology, Cambridge, Massachusetts 02139

The 70th Cold Spring Harbor Symposium, entitled "Molecular Approaches to Controlling Cancer," represented a critical and exciting transition in the fields of cancer research and cancer control. After years of successful research into the molecular genetic and cellular defects that underlie the disease, anticancer agents developed on the basis of these insights are now being used regularly in the treatment of cancer patients. Based on the availability of many more experimental drugs, powerful new methods of analysis, accurate models of the disease, and novel insights into cancer-relevant pathways that affect disease initiation and progression, there is considerable reason for optimism in the ability to one day control cancer.

The 70th Cold Spring Harbor Symposium was the fourth in this illustrious series that has focused on cancer. The last time the Symposium was dedicated to this disease and its research sphere was in 1994. My counterpart for that edition was Ed Harlow, who wrote in the introduction of his summary that despite impressive advances in our understanding of the molecular underpinnings of cancer, our ability to treat or otherwise control the disease had not substantially improved. He concluded that it was a "frustrating time" (Harlow 1994).

In the ensuing 11 years, times have changed. The 70th Symposium was held in early June 2005. Entitled "Molecular Approaches to Controlling Cancer," it marked a turning point in this field. After decades of painstaking research aimed at understanding the genes that go awry in the development of cancer and the cellular and physiological processes that are affected in the progression of the disease, the field of molecular oncology is—finally—having an impact on the treatment of patients with cancer. For the more than 500 attendees of the 70th Symposium, the sense of accomplishment was palpable, and there were tangible examples of success. Indeed, in the last half-dozen years, several new anticancer agents, borne from our improved understanding of the molecular biology of cancer, have been approved for use in humans. These agents are changing the lives of cancer patients through prolongation of life, reduced side effects of treatment, and, in some cases, cures.

As reviewed at the Symposium, substantial new progress in the rational development of new drugs for cancer, as well as critical new insights into the biology of the disease, have led to the realistic sense that the control of cancer is within reach. Moreover, with a remarkably powerful new tool kit composed of genomic information and sophisticated methods to interrogate cells and organisms, the pace of discovery has noticeably hastened. The field of cancer science has matured a great deal over the years. One now sees regular examples of the continuum of basic research and clinical investigation, with the latter

increasingly including molecular measurements and other detailed analyses of diseased tissue. This more integrated approach to cancer research, cancer drug development, and clinical investigation is essential to achieve our common goal.

Not surprisingly, the 66 oral presentations and numerous posters at the 70th Symposium covered considerable ground. The papers contained within this volume provide a detailed description of the science described in six days of oral presentations. I do not try to represent them fully here and, instead, only touch on some important themes that emerged over the course of an exhilarating (and exhausting) week. Unfortunately, I will not be able to adequately capture the feeling of hope that emerged from this collection of talks and posters. Suffice it to say that we are witnessing the beginning of the end of frustration.

CHARACTERIZING CANCER DRUG SENSITIVITY AND RESISTANCE

The era of targeted therapies for cancer is now well under way with drugs such as Gleevec, Herceptin, Iressa, Tarceva, Avastin, and others now used widely to treat various tumor types. The efficacy of this new generation of anticancer agents provides the basis for much of the enthusiasm for our ability to effectively counteract the effects of molecular alterations in developing tumors. However, although it is well established when and where these agents should be prescribed in some cases, considerable work remains to completely define the specific molecular context that confers drug sensitivity and resistance. To fully realize the power of personalized medicine for cancer, it will be necessary to match the genotype of the tumor (as well as other associated individual characteristics) to the appropriate agent or agents that have the best chance of eradicating it. In many cases, this will involve the use of targeted anticancer drugs in combination with conventional chemotherapeutics or radiation. Beyond establishing the hallmarks of initial sensitivity, it is also essential that we continue to investigate the mechanisms of acquired drug resistance. As with conventional anticancer agents, the use of targeted agents leads eventually to re-

---

All authors cited here without dates refer to papers in this volume.

sistant tumors and relapse. The mechanisms of resistance are being elucidated in a small number of cases, but this remains a critical area of study.

Two sets of examples illustrate the state of the field in this area. The most completely understood exploration of sensitivity/resistance involves Gleevec and the treatment of chronic myelogenous leukemia (CML). Sawyers and colleagues have demonstrated that leukemias that are initially sensitive to treatment by virtue of the presence of a Bcr-Abl fusion oncoprotein can achieve resistance through Abl kinase domain mutations that affect drug binding. Fortunately, a new class of Abl kinase inhibitors has proven to be effective in treating this category of Gleevec-resistant CML (Sawyers). The use of the epidermal growth factor receptor (EGFR) inhibitors Iressa and Tarceva in the treatment of lung cancer has generated considerable interest and debate in the past year, and several speakers discussed their findings in this area. Whereas it is clear that mutations in EGFR in some forms of non-small-cell lung cancer confer sensitivity to these drugs (Varmus et al.; Thomas et al.), additional data described by Hillan (Amler et al.) and Haber (Haber et al.) indicate that other alterations (including EGFR gene amplification) are associated with sensitivity as well. Moreover, reminiscent of the Gleevec experience, resistance to Iressa/Tarceva appears to be commonplace. One form of resistance is associated with a second-site mutation in EGFR, and this may be amenable to second-generation small-molecule inhibitors (Varmus et al.; Haber et al.). However, based on cell culture models, extragenic mutations can also confer resistance to Iressa/Tarceva (Haber et al.).

Several presentations heralded the next phase of targeted anticancer agents. Ashworth and colleagues have developed a strategy to take advantage of the DNA repair deficiency of cancer cells mutant for BRCA1/2 (Tutt et al.). They have demonstrated that such cells are exquisitely sensitive to inhibition of the DNA repair-associated enzyme PARP, thus revealing a potential therapeutic window for the treatment of BRCA1/2 mutant breast and ovarian cancers. In the very promising area of antiangiogenesis therapy, for which clinical validation has already come from the use of Avastin, additional agents and strategies are rapidly emerging. Yancopolous described the further development of the "VEGF Trap" method of VEGF inhibition, including promising preclinical and early clinical data (Rudge et al.). Moreover, he discussed the importance of understanding the specific context that determines initial tumor responsiveness and resistance to therapy. Benezra and colleagues have substantially advanced the study of Id proteins in establishing and maintaining tumor vasculature, now showing that Id gene mutations coupled with the use of the HSP90 inhibitor 17AAG block tumor development in a mouse model of breast cancer (Benezra et al.). As reviewed by Kaelin, McCormick, Workman, and others (Kaelin; Rodriguez-Viciana et al.; Workman), additional kinase inhibitors are showing promise in different phases of clinical testing. These authors all emphasized the importance of matching the inhibitor to the genetics and biology of

the treated tumor. Finally, Lane and Adams discussed new agents that target key factors in cell death regulation (p53 and the Bcl-2 family), which will broaden the range of therapeutic opportunities (Lane; Adams).

MOUSE MODELS OF CANCER COME OF AGE

A large percentage of the presentations at the 70th Symposium highlighted the use of genetically engineered mouse models of cancer. It is quite clear that thoughtful preclinical testing—of hypotheses as well as anticancer agents—is a key step in refining concepts of how cancers arise and progress and how to best treat them. Multiple presentations illustrated the power of such models in addressing critical questions, such as the cells of origin of cancer (Parada et al.; Kim et al.; Lawson et al.; P. Beachy, unpubl.), mechanisms of tumor progression (Calbó et al.; Tward et al.; Simin et al.; Tonon et al.), modes of cancer drug sensitivity and resistance (Varmus et al.; Zender et al.; Barbacid et al.), key cancer genetics pathways (Sherr et al.; Grisendi and Pandolfi; Tuveson and Hingorani; Evan et al.; Iaquinta et al.; M. Serrano, unpubl.), and how to match the biology of the tumor with its treatment (Benezra et al.; Folkman and Ryeom; D. Hanahan, unpubl.). Also noteworthy was the increasing attention paid to comparative analysis of the tumor development and cancer genetics in humans and in cognate mouse models. The use of these models will undoubtedly refine and, in some cases, define methods of detecting cancer, preventing tumor development and spread, and eliminating advanced disease.

CONSIDERING CANCER IN CONTEXT

Cancer cells develop in the context of normal cells and, throughout their progression to metastasis, have intimate and essential interactions with the cells that surround them. This more tissue-oriented view of cancer is important not only for shaping our thinking about the factors that govern tumor development but also for identifying novel opportunities for intervention. The conceptualization of cancer as an aberrancy of normal development and tissue homeostasis is centuries old; however, the methods to investigate these critical interactions and visualize the many normal cell types that affect incipient cancer cells have been developed rather recently. Numerous speakers focused on the role of cell-cell interactions and non-tumor-cell-autonomous factors that can influence the transformation process and/or participate in tumor progression.

Pioneering work from Bissell and colleagues has emphasized the importance of developmental context and the role of cell–cell and cell–matrix adhesion in determining the response to oncogenic stimuli (Bissell et al.). Thus, the setting in which a cell finds itself—whether it be in two- or three-dimensional structures in culture or in the midst of a tissue in vivo—can have a profound effect on how it manifests its genotype. The use of three-dimensional cell culture models has also been exploited by Brugge and coworkers to explore pathways that stimulate cell proliferation and survival (J. Brugge, unpubl.). This system has yielded a number of important findings that address how cells overcome their contextual signals in the process of tumor initiation. Infiltrating cells of the immune system, vasculature, and other stromal elements represent additional key players in the biology of cancer, and the molecular and cellular mechanisms that underlie their involvement in this process are being realized at an impressive pace (Egeblad et al.; Grant and Kalluri; Rudge et al.; Folkman and Ryeom; Kaelin; P. Gupta et al.; D. Hanahan, unpubl.). As with tumor angiogenesis, many of these interactions may furnish the basis for powerful new anticancer strategies.

The relationship between tissue homeostasis and cancer development has been enhanced further with recent evidence linking tissue stem cells with the early stages of tumorigenesis. For example, as discussed by Morrison (Pardal et al.) and M. van Lohuizen (unpubl.), pathways that are important in stem cell self-renewal are commonly targeted in cancer. In addition, various studies using mouse models of cancer have implicated stem/progenitor cells as the cell of origin of different tumor types (Lawson et al.; Parada et al.; Kim et al.). These studies do not rule out the possibility that more differentiated cells can undergo transformation and participate in tumor initiation as well. However, the inherent properties of stem cells make them particularly attractive targets. Studying the descendants of these abnormal cells in otherwise normal tissue can lead to the identification of cells with features of preneoplasia, as discussed by Tlsty (Berman et al.). The identification of the cell type(s) that seeds tumors is important for our basic understanding of the origins of the process and will certainly have implications for early detection and chemoprevention of cancer.

The vast majority of cancer deaths are attributable to the effects of metastasis, and yet we still know rather little about this process. Recent progress is encouraging, however. As with tumor initiation, close analogies with normal development and the importance of cell–cell interactions are evident regarding metastasis as well. Weinberg and colleagues have performed a series of experiments recently that focus on the transcriptional control of the epithelial–mesenchymal transition (EMT) during metastatic spread (P. Gupta et al.). The EMT occurs during gastrulation and at other developmental stages, and it has been linked to the propensity of tumor cells to migrate, invade, and remodel the extracellular matrix. Massagué has used transcriptional profiling to identify a series of genes that act in concert to influence the tissue destination of tumor cells and their behavior once there (G. Gupta et al.). Given that the metastatic process may initiate very early in tumor progression, the inhibition of metastasis per se will be challenging. However, with greater insight into the biology of metastatic cells, it may be possible to ameliorate the tissue-damaging effects of established metastases.

CANCER RESEARCH IN THE POST-GENOMIC ERA

Another notable change in the nature of cancer research as represented at the 70th Symposium was the reliance on whole-genome analysis. The sequencing of the genomes of humans and many experimental organisms has provided a wealth of new information and a remarkable series of new analytic and experimental tools. Powerful insights into the biology of cancer cells and potential new targets of therapy are emerging from in-depth analysis of the sequence, structure, and expression state of large collections of genes in human tumor cells and those from mouse models (Garraway et al.; Futreal et al.; Thomas et al.; Tonon et al.; Hicks et al.; J. Gray, unpubl.). The epigenetic state of the cancer genome is another rich source of information about gene regulation in tumors, and the pathways that govern chromatin modulation in tumorigenesis are potential targets of therapy (Baylin and Chen; Berman et al.; Herman; Feinberg). Likewise, understanding the mechanisms that govern chromosome integrity and how these processes are subverted in cancer is an essential component of a more integrated view of molecular oncology (de Lange; Galloway et al.; Armanios and Greider; J. Campisi, unpubl.).

The work of Futreal and colleagues at the Wellcome Trust Sanger Institute on the sequencing of the entire protein kinase family in a series of human cancer samples and cell lines engendered considerable discussion. Although it is clear that some somatically acquired mutations can be identified through such methods and that these represent attractive targets for anticancer therapy, for most tumors studied, the frequency of mutation was quite low (Futreal et al.). On the other extreme, a few samples exhibited a remarkably high mutation frequency, perhaps suggesting prior exposure to a powerful mutagen or a defect in one or more DNA repair mechanisms (Futreal et al.). In this context, it would be difficult to distinguish the cancer-relevant mutations from the random mutations. During a special session on the proposed joint National Cancer Institute–National Genome Research Institute effort to sequence large gene collections from selected human tumors, there was a spirited discussion of the likely outcomes given the Sanger Institute experience. Moreover, in times of tightening federal budgets for cancer research, many participants questioned the wisdom of very large scale spending on such an initiative, especially when so many known cancer genes and pathways remain incompletely understood. Still, given the potential for short-term benefit in terms of identifying druggable targets for cancer therapy, it seems prudent to undertake a series of pilot projects involving sequencing up to a few thousand genes from a limited number of well-annotated tumor samples; ideally, these same samples would also be subjected to other forms of genomic analysis. The information gained from these pilot studies would then determine whether a larger-scale effort is warranted.

Genome-scale functional analysis and sophisticated, RNAi-based genetic screens described at the Symposium provided a glimpse into an exciting new direction in cancer research. Using collections of cDNAs (Pearlberg et al.; J. Brugge, unpubl.), shRNA libraries (Westbrook et al.; G. Hannon; R. Bernards; both unpubl.), or combinations of siRNAs and chemotherapeutic drugs (Friend), several speakers discussed the power of large-scale, cell-based screens to modulate cancer phenotypes or pathways. Such screens will also be key to discovering genes and pathways on which cancer cells are specifically dependent, with or without exposure to therapeutic agents.

LOOKING AHEAD

The 70th Cold Spring Harbor Symposium was an inspiring moment in the history of cancer research and cancer care. We are now witnessing the steady approval of molecularly targeted agents for the treatment of the disease. The dramatic improvement in the methods to model cancer and the emerging arsenal of tools and techniques to study tumors with unprecedented precision will yield many more therapeutic agents in the years to come. These same methods—applied to models of the disease and, very importantly, human clinical specimens—will guide the use of the proper agents in individual patients through an understanding of the basis of drug sensitivity and resistance. This process will lead to more durable responses in the clinic and, increasingly, cures for the disease.

Much work remains, and many critical facts await discovery. For example, subjects that were presented in a more limited fashion at the Symposium, such as cancer immunology (J. Allison, unpubl.), cancer cell metabolism (Thompson et al.; Wallace), and the role of microRNAs in cancer (G. Hannon, unpubl.), are likely to be critical for our understanding of cancer progression and treatment. However, unlike 11 years ago when Ed Harlow described the frustrating disparity between advances in cancer research and the state of the art in cancer treatment, the tide is now beginning to turn. It would be irresponsible to put a date on when we will finally conquer cancer in all of its manifestations. However, before the next Cold Spring Harbor Symposium on this topic, many battles will be won, and the end of the war will be well within sight.

REFERENCE

Harlow E. 1994. An introduction to the puzzle. *Cold Spring Harbor Symp. Quant. Biol.* **59:** 709.

Author Index

A

Adams J.M., 469
Aguirre A.J., 11
Alexander J., 51
Amler L.C., 483
Antoniou A., 35
Araujo R.P., 517
Armanios M., 205
Ashworth A., 139
Aslanian A., 309
Azucena, Jr., E.F., 167

B

Barbacid M., 233
Bash R., 283
Bath M.L., 469
Bauer D.E., 357
Baylin S.B., 427
Bell D.W., 419
Benezra R., 375
Berger A., 25
Berman H., 317
Berns A., 225
Beroukhim R., 25
Bertwistle D., 129
Bishop J.M., 217
Bissell M.J., 343
Bond E., 111
Bond G., 111
Bouillet P., 469
Boyce F.M., 449
Brennan C., 11
Brizuela L., 449
Buzzai M., 357

C

Calbó J., 225
Cano F., 275
Cardiff R.D., 283
Chan N., 275
Chen L., 469
Chen T.-H., 73
Chen W.Y., 427
Cheng D., 187
Chin L., 11
Christophorou M., 263
Ciarrocchi A., 375
Codrington R., 275
Colman P., 469
Conery A., 449
Cordón-Cardo C., 149, 251
Cory S., 469
Courtneidge S.A., 167
Crawford Y.G., 317

D

Dansen T., 263
Daser A., 275
Davies J., 449

Davis S., 411
de Candia P., 375
de Lange T., 197
Degot S., 449
den Besten W., 129
DePinho R.A., 11
Ditsworth D., 357
Doench J., 449
Drynan L., 275
Du Y.-C.N., 1
Dubus P., 233
Dunning A., 35

E

Easton D.F., 35
Edgar B.A., 299
Egeblad M., 383
Egholm M., 73
Egle A., 469
Eisenman R.N., 299
Elledge S.J., 435
Endege W., 449
Esposito D., 51
Evan G.I., 263

F

Farmer H., 139
Feinberg A.P., 335
Feng B., 11
Feng W., 73
Feng Z., 111
Feunteun J., 93
Finch A., 263
Fisher D.E., 25
Flemming P., 251
Fletcher J.I., 469
Folkman J., 389
Fordyce C.A., 317
Forster A., 275
Friend S.H., 445
Futreal P.A., 43

G

Gale N., 411
Galloway D.A., 209
Ganesan S., 93
Garraway L.A., 25
Gauthier M.L., 317
Geho D.H., 517
Gelfand E., 449
Gerald W.L., 149
Gewin L.C., 209
Gil G., 111
Goddard A.D., 483
Godin-Heymann N., 419
Gonzalez L., 449
Grandori C., 209
Grant M.A., 399
Greider C.W., 205
Greulich H., 73

Grewal S.S., 299
Grimm J., 241
Grisendi S., 83
Grubor V., 51
Grueneberg D., 449
Gupta G.P., 149
Gupta P.B., 291

H

Haber D.A., 419
Hannon G.J., 251
Harlow E., 449
Harris A.W., 469
Harris S.L., 111
Hartwell K., 291
Hatzivassiliou G., 357
He S., 177
Henke E., 375
Herman J.G., 329
Hicks J., 51
Hill R., 283
Hillan K.J., 483
Hinds M., 469
Hingorani S.R., 65
Hirshfield K., 111
Hu W., 111
Huang D.C.S., 469

I

Iaquinta P.J., 309
Iglehart J.D., 93

J

Jacks T., 241, 525
Jackson E.L., 241
Jackson S.P., 139
Ji H., 11
Jones K.D., 217

K

Kaelin, Jr., W.G., 159
Kalluri R., 399
Kang Y., 149
Kastan M.B., 99
Katzenellenbogen R.A., 209
Kay M.A., 217
Kelly P.N., 469
Kenny P.A., 343
Khatry D.B., 11
Kim C.F.B., 241
Kirsch D.G., 241
Kissil J., 241
Kitagawa R., 99
Knoepfler P.S., 299
Kozakiewicz K., 317
Krasnitz A., 51
Kuo M.-L., 129
Kuroda J., 469

Kwak E.L., 419
Kwon C.-H., 173

L

LaBaer J., 449
Lane D.P., 489
Lane K., 241
Lawlor E.A., 263
Lawson D.A., 187
Lee J.C., 73
Lees J.A., 309
Levine A.J., 111
Li W., 449
Lindsten T., 357
Liotta L.A., 517
Littlepage L.E., 383
Livingston D.M., 93
Lobato N., 275
Lokshin M., 121
Lord C.J., 139
Lowe S.W., 251
Lucito R., 251
Lukacs R., 187
Lum J.J., 357
Lundin P., 51
Luo W., 209
Lynch T.J., 419

M

Malumbres M., 233
Maner S., 51
Mani S., 291
Martín A., 233
Martin E.S., 11
Martin N.M., 139
Martins C., 263
Massagué J., 149
Maulik G., 11
McCabe N., 139
McCarthy K., 283
McCormick F., 461
McDermott K.M., 317
McDougall J.K., 209
Metzler M., 275
Meuwissen R., 225
Meyerson M.L., 25, 73
Michalak E.M., 469
Minn A.J., 149
Miron A., 93
Mittal V., 375
Molofsky A.V., 177
Morrison S.J., 177
Murphy D., 263
Muthuswamy L., 51
Myers H., 209

N

Nam C.-H., 275
Navin N., 51

Nickerson E., 73
Nolan D., 375

O

O'Reilly L., 469
Oda K., 461
Odajima J., 233
Okada J., 461
Olive K.P., 241
Olshen A.B., 149
Orian A., 299
Ortega S., 233

P

Pandolfi P.P., 83
Pannell R., 275
Pao W., 1
Papadopoulos N., 411
Parada L.F., 173
Pardal R., 177
Park J., 449
Parkhurst S.M., 299
Pass I., 167
Pearlberg J., 449
Petricoin E.F., 517
Pharoah P.D.P., 35
Podsypanina K., 1
Politi K., 1
Ponder B.A.J., 35
Powers S., 251
Prescott J., 263
Prives C., 121
Protopopov A., 11
Puthalakath H., 469

R

Rabbitts T., 275
Radisky D.C., 343
Rauen K., 461

Richardson A.L., 93
Riggs M., 51
Rimm D., 25
Ringshausen I., 263
Robins H., 111
Rodriguez S., 275
Rodriguez-Viciana P., 461
Rosen N., 375
Rothberg J.M., 73
Roussel M.F., 129
Rubin M.A., 25
Rudge J.S., 411
Ruzinova M., 375
Ryeom S., 389

S

Santamaría D., 233
Sawyer J., 449
Sawyers C.L., 479
Seals D.F., 167
Sellers W.R., 25, 73
Serganova I., 149
Settleman J., 419
Sharma S.V., 419
Shaw A.T., 241
Sherr C.J., 129
Siegel P.M., 149
Sigaroudinia M., 317
Silver D., 93
Simin K., 283
Simons J., 73
Smith D.P., 469
Smith G.C.M., 139
Solit D., 375
Song Y., 283
Sordella R., 419
Sotillo R., 233
Spector M.S., 251
Stegmeier F., 435
Strasser A., 469
Stratton M.R., 43

Sugimoto M., 129
Sweet-Cordero A., 241

T

Tago K., 129
Tanaka T., 121, 275
Tengs T., 73
Teresky A.K., 111
Tesfay L., 167
Tetsu O., 461
Thomas R.K., 73
Thompson C.B., 357
Thurston G., 411
Tlsty T.D., 317
Tonon G., 11
Troge J., 51
Turner N., 139
Tutt A.N.J., 139
Tuveson D.A., 65
Tward A.D., 217

V

Van Delft M., 469
Van Dyke T., 283
van Montfort E., 225
van Tellingen O., 225
Varmus H., 1
Villunger A., 469

W

Wallace D.C., 363
Wang R., 217
Wang Z.C., 93
Wei A., 469
Weinberg R.A., 291
Weir B.A., 25
Weissleder R., 241
Werb Z., 383

Westbrook T.F., 435
Widlund H., 25
Wiegand S.J., 411
Wigler M., 51
Williams R.T., 129
Willis S., 469
Witte O.N., 187
Wong K.-K., 11
Wooster R., 43
Workman P., 499

X

Xiao A., 283
Xin L., 187
Xu Q., 187
Xue W., 251

Y

Yancopoulos G.D., 411
Yang J., 291
Yang Z., 11
Yant S., 217
Yin C., 283
You M.J., 11
Yu X., 111
Yuza Y., 73

Z

Zender L., 251
Zetterberg A., 51
Zhang J., 317
Zhang Q., 283
Zhang Y., 11
Zhao F., 357
Zhao X., 25
Zhu Y., 173
Zindy F., 129
Zong W.-X., 357

Subject Index

A

17-AAG experimental compound, 378–380, 506–510
ABL tyrosine kinase inhibitors, 479–481. *See also* Imatinib
ABT-737 experimental compound, 469, 474–475
Acute myeloid leukemia (AML), 193
Acute promyelocytic leukemia (APL), 85
Adenocarcinoma
    colorectal, p53 and p73 regulation in, 121–127
    of lung
        cancer stem cells of, 247–248
        EGFR gene mutations in, 3–5, 73–79
        EGFR inhibitor treatment response in, 73–79, 419–425, 483–484
        genomic profile of, 5–6, 11, 16–17, 20
    pancreatic ductal, 17–21, 65–70
    prostatic, mouse models of, 283, 287–289
Adenomatous polyposis coli (APC) gene. *See APC* gene
Adult stem cells. *See* Stem cells, adult
Aflatoxin B1 ingestion, and hepatocellular carcinoma, 251
Aging
    mitochondrial alterations and, 367–370
    tumor suppressors and, 177–182
AKT1 gene and AKT1 protein, in radiation-induced cell death, 114–118
AML (acute myeloid leukemia), 193
Anaerobic glycolysis, in cancer cells, 363
Androgen dependence, in prostate cancer, 192–193
Aneuploid breast tumors, ROMA CGH and FISH analysis of, 51–62
Aneuploidy
    of p53 knockout mouse cells in tissue culture, 490–491
    telomere-related, 200
Angiogenesis
    mechanisms and control of, 399–400
    oncogene addiction and, 389–396
    VEGF in, 411–413
Angiogenesis inhibitors
    endogenous
        overexpression of, and tumor growth suppression, 392–393
        structural basis for functions of, 399–407
    therapeutic use of. *See* Antiangiogenic therapy
Angiopoietins, as target for antiangiogenesis therapy, 415
Animal models. *See* Mouse models

Antiangiogenic therapy. *See also* Angiogenesis inhibitors
    for breast cancer, 375–380
    chemotherapeutic resistance in, 395, 526
    targets for, 411, 414–415
    VEGF Trap as, 411–415
Anti-p53 antibodies, staining of, 491–492
APC gene, and colorectal cancer, 192
Apc gene mutations, *IGF2* loss of imprinting and, 335, 338–339
APL (acute promyelocytic leukemia), 85
Aplastic anemia, telomere shortening and, 205–207
Apoptosis
    Bcl-2 life/death switch and, 469–475, 526
    Perp and *AKT1* polymorphisms and, 111–118
    pVHL and, in hereditary pheochromocytoma, 159, 161–162
    regulation of, 357–361
Arf gene
    activation of expression of, 130–132, 135
    in stem cell self-renewal and cancer cell proliferation, 179–181
Arf tumor suppressor. *See also* p19Arf protein
    p53-dependent and -independent functions of, 129–135
Arf/p53 tumor surveillance network, E2F transcription factor in regulation of, 309–315
Ascl-1 expression, in mouse model of SCLC, 225–231
Association studies, for polygenic inheritance investigations, 35–38
Astrocytoma
    mouse models of, 283–287
    in neurofibromatosis type 1, 173–175
ATM (ataxia telangiectasia mutated) protein
    activation of, 99–102
    in neoplastic proliferation and aging, 181
    phosphorylation of substrates by, 102
    SMC1 substrate of, 102–108
ATP production, in growing cells, 357, 361
Autophagy, and transient growth factor-independent survival of cells, 358–360
Avastin (bevacizumab), 377, 379, 411

B

B23. *See* NPM (nucleophosmin)
Bak regulation, in apoptosis, 471–472, 475
Basal-like breast cancer, inactive X-chromosome abnormalities in, 93–96

Base excision repair pathway, in treatment of breast cancer in *BRCA1/2* carriers, 142
BAY43-9006 experimental compound. *See* Sorafenib
Bcl-2 life/death switch, in tumorigenesis and therapy, 469–475
Bcl-2 proteins, in maintenance of cell survival, 357
Beckwith-Wiedemann syndrome, 335–337
Beta-cells, Myc activation in, 265–267
Bevacizumab (Avastin), 377, 379, 411
BH3 mimetics, therapeutic potential of, 469, 473–475
BH3-only proteins, of Bcl-2 family, and apoptosis, 469–471, 475
Biomarkers of cancer. *See also* Prognostic tools; Screens
    in breast cancer, 317, 324
    clinical proteomics and, 246, 517–523
    loss of genetic imprinting as, 337–340
    in lung cancer, 246
    p53 status as, 491
    predictive of EGFR inhibitor response in NSCLC, 483–486
    serum proteins as, 481
Biopsies, patient, proteomic profiling of, 517–523
B-lymphocyte cell line, EBV-transformed, 111–118
Bmi-1 proto-oncogene and Bmi-1 protein, 177–182
BMS-354825 (dasatinib), 481
bobbed rDNA locus, dMyc association with, 302–304
Bone metastasis of breast cancer, site-specific metastasis genes and, 152–155
B-RAF inhibitors, 500–501
Brain tumors. *See* Astrocytoma; Glioma, malignant
BRCA1 mutant cancer
    cancer therapy strategies for, 139–146, 526
    Xi abnormalities in, 93–96
BRCA1/2 genes
    contribution to breast cancer susceptibility, 35
    epigenetic inactivation of, 330
BRCA1/2 proteins
    deficiency of, and homologous recombination defect, 139–140
    in recruitment of ATM, 106–108
Breakage-fusion-bridge cycles, in dicentric chromosome formation, 199, 201–202
Breast cancer. *See also entries beginning with* Mammary
    aneuploid and diploid, ROMA CGH and FISH analysis of, 51–62
    BRCA1 mutant and sporadic basal-like, Xi abnormalities in, 93–96

531

Breast cancer *(Continued)*
　in *BRCA1/2* carriers
　　carboplatin chemotherapy clinical
　　　trials, 141–142, 146
　　therapeutic strategies for, 139–146,
　　　526
　cellular microenvironment and,
　　343–352
　chemotherapeutic resistance in, and
　　kinase screening in tissue
　　culture, 455–456
　extracellular matrix in tumor induction
　　and progression, 345,
　　349–352
　murine, complete regression in
　　response to antiangiogenic
　　stress, 375–380
　new mutator phenotype, 46
　pathways of tumor progression in, 283
　polygenic inherited predisposition to,
　　35–40
　primary tumorigenicity, and organ-
　　specific metastasis genes,
　　155–156
　resequencing of protein kinase gene
　　family in, 43–48
　site-specific genes in metastasis of,
　　149–158
　tumor progression pathways in, 289
Breast cancer and ovarian cancer
　syndrome, 66
Burkitt's lymphoma, 84

C

Cancer. *See also specific cancer types,*
　e.g., Adenocarcinoma,
　Breast cancer
　biomarkers of. *See* Biomarkers of
　　cancer
　epigenetic changes in, 329–332,
　　335–340, 427–431, 527
　initiation of. *See* Tumorigenesis
　metastasis of. *See* Metastasis
　progression of. *See* Tumor progression
　treatment of. *See* Chemotherapeutic
　　resistance; Therapeutic
　　strategies for cancer;
　　specific drugs and drug
　　classes
Cancer cells
　invasiveness of, Tks5 and, 168–169
　metastasis of. *See* Metastasis
　microenvironment of, 343–352,
　　383–387, 526–527
　nutrient uptake and apoptosis
　　suppression in, 357–361
　proliferation of
　　vs. angiogenesis induction, 391–392
　　proto-oncogene and tumor
　　　suppressor activation and,
　　　177–182
　proteomic profiling of, and
　　personalized therapy,
　　517–523
　RNAi in study of signaling networks
　　in, 435–441
Cancer drug development, progress and
　challenges in, 499–510
Cancer genetics research, history of,
　83–90
Cancer kinome targets, and personalized
　molecular cancer
　therapeutics, 499–510

Cancer risk assessment. *See* Biomarkers
　of cancer
Cancer stem cells
　in lung cancer, 247–248
　telomerase activity in, 205–207
　in tumorigenesis, 193, 225
Cancer stem cell theory, telomerase
　activity and, 205–207
Cancer-signaling networks
　protein-signaling network models,
　　clinical proteomic analysis
　　of, 517–523
　RNAi studies of, 435–441
Carboplatin chemotherapy, in *BRCA1/2*
　mutant breast cancer,
　141–142, 146
Carcinoma. *See also* Adenocarcinoma
　ductal carcinoma in situ, 317, 322–324
　hepatocellular carcinoma, 218–222,
　　251–260
　renal cell carcinoma, 159, 161, 465
　squamous cell carcinoma
　　of esophagus, 332
　　of lung, 11, 16–17, 20
Carcinoma-associated fibroblasts,
　383–387
β-Catenin, 219–220, 222
Cathepsin proteases, as lung cancer
　biomarker, 246
CDH1 gene, epigenetic inactivation of,
　330
Cdk inhibitors, 234, 502–504
Cdk2 kinase, 234, 237–238
Cdk4 kinase, 235–237
Cdk4R24C kinase, mutant, melanoma
　induction by, 235
Cdk6 kinase, genetic analysis of in vivo
　role of, 236–237
Cdks (cyclin-dependent kinases)
　in cell cycle regulation and cancer,
　　233–239
　genetic analysis of in vivo role of,
　　236–238
　phenotypic expression of mutations of,
　　234
cDNA expression, screens using, in
　mammalian tissue culture
　cells, 449–458
Cell cycle, cyclin-dependent kinases in,
　233–239
Cell type of origin, and metastatic
　proclivity, 293
Cell-based screens, for novel p53
　activators, 494
Centromeres, dysfunction of, and genomic
　instability in human cancer,
　321–322
CGH. *See* Comparative genomic
　hybridization
Chemotherapeutic drugs. *See specific*
　drugs and drug classes,
　e.g., Erlotinib, Tyrosine
　kinase inhibitors
Chemotherapeutic resistance
　acquired, to kinase inhibitors, 3, 6,
　　73–79, 480–481, 525–526
　in antiangiogenic therapy, 395, 526
　and kinase screening in breast cancer
　　and NSCLC cells, 455–457
　tissue polarity in regulation of, 349
　in vitro, to gefitinib, 423–424
Chemotherapy. *See* Therapeutic strategies
　for cancer; *specific drugs*
　and drug classes

Choroid plexus epithelial cells, pRb
　pathway inactivation in,
　283–289
Chromatin changes, promoter region
　methylation and, 329–330
Chromosomal translocation in human
　cancer, mouse models
　mimicking, 275–281
Chromosome formation, dicentric,
　breakage-fusion-bridge
　cycles in, 199
Chronic myelogenous leukemia (CML)
　hematopoietic stem cells and, 193
　kinase inhibitor therapy for, 3, 194,
　　419, 479–481, 526
Chronic myelomonocytic leukemia
　(CMML), 479–480
Cip/Kip proteins, in cell cycle regulation,
　234, 237–238
CKI proteins, expression of, in cancer, 233
Clear-cell renal carcinoma, 159, 161
Clinical markers. *See* Biomarkers of
　cancer; Prognostic tools
Clinical proteomics. *See* Proteomics,
　clinical
Clinical trials
　carboplatin chemotherapy, in
　　BRCA1/2 mutant breast
　　cancer, 141–142, 146
　of gefitinib in NSCLC, 419
　of VEGF Trap for cancer and vascular
　　eye diseases, 414–415
CML. *See* Chronic myelogenous leukemia
CMML (chronic myelomonocytic
　leukemia), 479–480
CNS lymphoma, epigenetic silencing in,
　331
Collagen, type 1, and cancer progression,
　385
Colony-forming assays for stem cells, 188
Colorectal adenocarcinoma cell lines, p53
　and p73 regulation in,
　121–127
Colorectal cancer
　adenomatous polyposis coli gene and,
　　192
　epigenetic gene silencing in, 428–429
　loss of genetic imprinting and,
　　337–338
　mouse model for, 338–340
Combination therapy, network-targeted,
　521–522
Comparative genomic hybridization
　(CGH)
　analysis of aneuploid and diploid
　　breast tumors, 51–62
　genetic study of human lung cancer
　　subtypes, 11–22
Competitive repopulation assay for stem
　cells, 188
Costello syndrome, 462
COX-2 (prostaglandin-endoperoxide
　synthase 2), association
　with p16^{Ink4a}
　hypermethylation, 322–324
CpG dinucleotide, methylation of,
　329–332
Cre-expressing lentivirus vectors, T$_{121}$
　induction by, 286–287, 289
Cre-*loxP* recombination system, 275,
　277–279
CT (micro-computed tomography), in
　murine lung cancer
　modeling, 245

CXCL-12 (stromal-cell derived factor 1
    α), 384
CYC202 (seliciclib; *R*-roscovitine),
    502–504
Cyclin-dependent kinase (Cdk) inhibitors,
    234, 502–504
Cyclin-dependent kinases. *See* Cdks
Cyclins, 233–234
Cytotoxic therapy, apoptotic regulation in,
    469, 473–475

D

Darwinian model of tumor progression
    and metastasis, 291–293
Dasatinib (BMS-354825), 481
DCIS. *See* Ductal carcinoma in situ
Delta-like ligand 4, as target for
    antiangiogenesis therapy,
    415
Diagnostics. *See* Biomarkers of cancer;
    Personalized molecular
    cancer therapeutics/
    diagnostics; Prognostic
    tools
Dicentric chromosome formation, breakage-
    fusion-bridge cycles in, 199
Diploid breast tumors, ROMA CGH and
    FISH analysis of, 51–62
dMnt transcription factor, 299–305
dMyc transcription factor, 299–305
DNA alterations, lineage-restricted, in
    human tumors, 27–32
DNA, complementary, expression screens
    using, 449–458
DNA damage response/DNA repair
    ATM-dependent, 99–108
    in *BRCA* mutant cells, 139–146, 526
    telomere dysfunction and, 200–201
DNA methylation, altered, 329–332,
    335–340, 427–431
DNA microarrays, for genotyping, 26–27
DNA, mitochondrial, variations in disease
    and climatic adaptation,
    365–367
DNA repair defects. *See* DNA damage
    response/DNA repair
DNA, ribosomal, *bobbed* locus, dMyc
    association with, 302–304
DNA-bar coding strategy, 439–440
DNA-based genomic studies, 26–27
Drosophila Myc and Mnt transcription
    factors (dMyc; dMnt),
    transcriptional regulation
    by, 299–305
Drug development, progress and
    challenges in, 499–510
Drug discovery, molecular profiling in,
    445–448
Drug resistance. *See* Chemotherapeutic
    resistance
Ductal carcinoma in situ (DCIS),
    epithelial cell p16^Ink4a
    activity in, 317, 322–324
Dyskeratosis congenita, autosomal
    dominant, 205–207

E

E2F transcription factors, in regulation of
    Arf/p53 tumor surveillance
    network, 309–315
E6 oncoprotein of human
    papillomaviruses, 209–213

E6/E6AP complex, 209–213
EBV-transformed human B-lymphocyte
    cell line, 111–118
EGFR gene
    copy number of, and response to
        EGFR inhibitors, 484
    mouse model mutations, 242–243
    mutations of
        in lung adenocarcinoma, 3–5,
            73–79
        in malignant glioma, 421
        in non-small-cell lung cancer, 3–5,
            242–243, 419–425,
            483–484
        and response to EGFR inhibitors,
            73–79, 419–425, 483–484
        T790M, 423
    sequencing of, 502
EGFR inhibitors. *See* Epidermal growth
    factor receptor (EGFR)
    inhibitors
EGFR protein
    amplification of, in malignant glioma,
        421
    expression of, and response to EGFR
        inhibitors, 484–485
    in non-small-cell lung cancer, 3–5,
        242–243, 419–425
EKB 569 experimental compound,
    424–425
Embryonic stem cells, mouse,
    homologous recombination
    techniques in, 275–281
Endocrine signaling
    androgen dependence in prostate
        cancer, 192–193
    in small-cell lung cancer, 226
Endostatin, structure and mechanism of
    action of, 400–402
Endothelial cells, in angiogenesis, 400
Epidermal growth factor receptor. See
    EGFR gene; EGFR protein
Epidermal growth factor receptor (EGFR)
    inhibitors. *See also specific
    drugs*
    clinical response in NSCLC, predictive
        markers for, 483–486
    differential sensitivity to, in lung
        adenocarcinoma, 73–79
    irreversible, 424–425
    lung cancer response to, 3–4, 73–79,
        419–425
    oncogene addiction and, 3–4, 26,
        43–44, 422–423
    resistance to, 3, 419–425, 479–481,
        525–526
Epigenetic silencing
    in cancer and preneoplasia, 329–332
    in tumor progression, 427–431
Epigenetics
    in cancer research, 527
    loss of genetic imprinting in cancer
        causality, 335–340
Epithelial-to-mesenchymal transition
    and cancer cell invasion and
        metastasis, 294–295
    FSP1 and, 384
    metalloproteinases and, 350–351
Erlotinib (Tarceva)
    clinical response in NSCLC
        predictive markers for, 483–486
    resistance to, 242–243, 419–421,
        526
    oncogene addiction and, 3–4, 26, 43

relapse with, and differential
    sensitivity to, 75–77
ER^TAM switch, 265–267, 270–271
Esophageal cancer, 332
Estrogen receptor, modified, in reversible
    switch, 265–267, 270–271
Ews-Erg fusion, and neoplasia induction,
    280
Extracellular matrix, in tumor induction
    and progression, 343–352,
    383–387, 526–527
Extracellular signals, in maintenance of
    cell survival, 357–361

F

Familial atypical multiple mole and
    melanoma syndrome, 66
Fibroblast secreted protein 1, and cancer
    progression, 384
Fibroblasts
    in cancer progression, 383–387
    carcinoma-associated, 383–387
    mammary, compared to mammary
        epithelial cells, 318–320
    in tumor induction and progression,
        344
Firestorm pattern of genomic change,
    57–59, 62
Fish. *See* Tks5 protein
Fluorescence in situ hybridization (FISH),
    51–62
Fluorescence molecular tomography, for
    lung cancer biomarker
    identification, 246
FSP1, and epithelial-to-mesenchymal
    transition, 384

G

Gastrointestinal stromal tumors, 419,
    479–480
Gefitinib (Iressa)
    clinical response in NSCLC
        predictive markers for, 483–486
        resistance to, 242–243, 419–425,
            526
    oncogene addiction and, 3–4, 26,
        43–44, 422–423
    relapse with, and differential
        sensitivity to, 75–77
Gene expression studies. *See* Epigenetics
Gene inactivation/expression, in cancer
    and preneoplasia, 329–332
Gene sequencing, of protein kinase gene
    family, in somatic
    mutations in human cancer,
    43–48, 527
Gene silencing
    aberrant, in tumor progression,
        427–431
    in cancer and preneoplasia, 329–332
    by promoter region methylation,
        329–330, 335
Genetic modifier screens, for kinase
    identification, 455–457
Genetic suppression, RNAi and cDNA
    screening of, 457
Genome-wide scans, polygenic inherited
    predisposition to breast
    cancer, 38–40
Genomic binding, by *Drosophila* Myc and
    Mnt transcription factors,
    299–305

Genomic instability
    metalloproteinases and, 350–351
    telomere dysfunction and, 197–203
Genomic profiles of human lung cancer
    subtypes, 11–22
Genomics
    in cancer research, 527–528
    and drug development, 499–510
    and lineage addiction in human
        cancer, 25–32
    lung cancer analysis and, 245–246
Genotype–phenotype relationships, in a
        mouse model for human
        small-cell lung cancer,
        225–231
Genotypes of cancer, 5–6
Genotypic progression, in liver tumor
        genesis, 217–223
Genotyping, DNA microarrays for, 26–27
GFAP gene, and T$_{121}$ expression, 284–285
Gleevec (imatinib). See Imatinib
Glial fibrillary acidic protein gene. See
        GFAP gene
Glioma, malignant
    EGFR mutations and amplification in,
        421
    kinase inhibitor therapy for, 480
Glucose-dependent metabolism, in
        growing cells, 361
Growth factors, in regulation of cell
        survival, 358–360

H

H1299 colorectal adenocarcinoma cell
        line, p53 and p73
        regulation in, 121–127
Haplo-insufficiency, 490
HCT116 colorectal adenocarcinoma cell
        line, p53 and p73
        regulation in, 121–127
Hemangioblastoma, pVHL tumor
        suppressor protein and,
        159, 161
Hematopoietic malignancies. See also
        Leukemia; Lymphoma
    leukemia/lymphoma genes, and solid
        tumor genesis, 83–90
    mouse model for, 277–279
    promoter region methylation in,
        329–330
Hematopoietic stem cells, and
        tumorigenesis, 187, 193,
        205–207
Hepatitis B and C viruses, and
        hepatocellular carcinoma,
        217, 251
Hepatocellular carcinoma
    genetically defined, generation and
        analysis of, 251–260
    mouse models of, 218–222
her2/neu oncogene overexpression in
        breast cancers, 375–380
Hereditary nonpolyposis colon cancer, 66
Hexokinase II, expression and binding of,
        in cancer cells, 363–364
HIC1 (hypermethylated-in-cancer 1) gene,
        429–430
HIF. See Hypoxia-inducible factor
Histone code, promoter region
        methylation and, 330
History of cancer genetics research, 83–90
HKI 272 experimental compound,
        424–425

Homology-directed repair pathway, in
        telomere-related genome
        instability, 199–200
Hormone-refractory prostate cancer,
        192–193
Hsp90 molecular chaperone inhibitors,
        378–380, 505–510
hTERT gene and hTERT protein
    in autosomal dominant dyskeratosis
        congenita, 205–207
    in telomerase regulation by human
        papillomaviruses, 209–214
hTR gene and hTR protein, in autosomal
        dominant dyskeratosis
        congenita, 205–207
Human cancer. See also specific cancer
        types, e.g., Breast cancer
    lineage-restricted DNA alterations in,
        27–32
    somatic mutations in, protein kinase
        gene family resequencing,
        43–48
Human papillomaviruses, telomerase
        regulation by, 209–214
Hypereosinophilic syndrome, 479–480
Hyper-/hypomethylation of DNA. See
        DNA methylation, altered
Hypermethylated-in-cancer 1 (HIC1)
        gene, 429–430
Hypoxia, in small Id-deficient breast
        tumors, 378
Hypoxia-inducible factor (HIF)
    in mouse model of mammary tumors,
        378
    von Hippel-Lindau tumor suppressor
        protein and, 159–162

I

Id proteins, loss of, and central necrosis of
        murine breast tumors,
        375–380
IGF2 gene, loss of imprinting and,
        335–340
Imaging technology
    for lung cancer biomarker
        identification, 246
    for murine lung cancer modeling,
        243–245
Imatinib (Gleevec)
    for chronic myelogenous leukemia,
        194
    as model for EGFR inhibitors, 419
    oncogene addiction and, 26, 43–44
    resistance to, 3, 242, 479–481, 526
Immortalization of cells, viral
        oncoproteins and, 209–214
Imprinting, loss of. See Loss of imprinting
Inactive X chromosome (Xi)
    abnormalities in BRCA1
        mutant and sporadic basal-
        like breast cancer, 93–96
Individualized therapy. See Personalized
        molecular cancer
        therapeutics/diagnostics
Inflammation, chronic, and stromal
        promotion of cancer, 383
INK4 genes and INK4 proteins, 129–135
Ink4 genes and Ink4 proteins, 129–135,
        234. See also p16^{Ink4a}
        protein
Ink4a gene, in stem cell self-renewal and
        cancer cell proliferation,
        179–181

Insulin-like growth factor II, 335. See also
        IGF2 gene
Intrabodies. See Intracellular antibodies
Intracellular antibodies (intrabodies),
        mouse models for testing
        of, 275–276
Intrahepatic seeding of genetically
        modified liver progenitor
        cells, 254–255
Invadopodia, Tks5 and, 167–170
Invasion-metastasis cascade, 149–150,
        291–292
Invertor chromosomal translocation
        model, 275, 279–281
Iressa (gefitinib). See Gefitinib
Irradiation
    -induced cell death, AKT1 gene and
        AKT1 protein in, 114–118
    p53 response to, 491
    and stromal promotion of cancer, 383

J

c-Jun, apoptosis regulation by, 159,
        161–162

K

Kidney tumors. See Renal cell carcinoma;
        Wilms' tumor
Kinases. See Protein kinase family
Knockin gene fusion, for development of
        translocation mimics, 275,
        277, 280–281
Knudson hypothesis, epigenetic
        modification of, 337
K-ras murine models of lung cancer, 2–3,
        241–242, 245–246
K-ras protein. See also Ras effector
        pathways
    activation of, in tumor progression,
        283, 285–286
    p53 cooperative effects, 243
KRAS mutations
    in NSCLC, and response to EGFR
        inhibitors, 485–486
    in pancreatic ductal cancer, 65–70

L

Lentivirus vectors
    Cre-expressing, for T$_{121}$ induction,
        286–287, 289
    in RNAi and cDNA screening,
        451–454
Leukemia
    acute myeloid, 193
    acute promyelocytic, 85
    chronic myelogenous, 3, 193–194,
        419, 479–481, 526
    chronic myelomonocytic, 479–480
Leukemia cell lines, promoter region
        methylation in, 329–330
Leukemia/lymphoma genes, and genesis
        of solid tumors, 83–90
Lineage addiction in human cancer, 25–32
Lineage-restricted DNA alterations, in
        human tumors, 27–32
Lipid synthesis in growing cells, 361
LIT1 antisense transcript gene, loss of
        imprinting of, 335–337
Liver tumors
    hepatocellular carcinoma, 218–222,
        251–260

intrahepatic seeding of genetically
modified progenitor cells,
254–255
mouse models of, 217–223
in situ cancer generation, 255–256
L-myc amplification, in mouse model of
SCLC, 225–231
Loss of imprinting
and cancer risk, 337–339
IGF2 gene and, 335–339
mouse model of, 338–339
Lucentis (ranibizumab), 411
Lung cancer. See also Adenocarcinoma,
of lung; Non-small-cell
lung cancer
acquired treatment resistance in, 3,
73–79, 410–425, 479–481,
525–526
biomarkers of, 246
cancer stem cells in, 247–248
EGFR inhibitor response of, 3–4,
419–425
genomic profiles of subtypes of, 11–22
lineage-restricted DNA alterations in,
28–30
murine models of
non-small-cell lung cancer, 2–3, 5,
241–248
small-cell lung cancer, 225–231
Lung metastasis of breast cancer, site-
specific metastasis genes
and, 153–155
Lymphocytes
EBV-transformed human B-
lymphocyte cell line,
111–118
normal, promoter region methylation
in, 329–330
Lymphoma
Burkitt's, 84
leukemia/lymphoma genes, and
genesis of solid tumors,
83–90
primary CNS, epigenetic silencing in,
331

M

Macromolecular drugs, mouse models for
testing of, 275–276
Macrophages, in tumor induction and
progression, 344
Macular degeneration, age-related, 411,
414–415
Magnetic resonance imaging (MRI), in
murine lung cancer
modeling, 245
Malignant glioma. See Glioma, malignant
Malignant melanoma. See Melanoma,
malignant
Malignant peripheral nerve sheath tumors,
173, 175
Mammalian tissue-culture cells. See
Tissue-culture cells,
mammalian
Mammary cancer. See Breast cancer
Mammary epithelial cells
assays of, in 3-dimensional gels,
345–349
genetic and epigenetic changes in a
carcinogenic
subpopulation,
317–326
malignant transformation in, 343,
350–352

pRb pathway inactivation in, 283, 289
Mammary fibroblasts, compared to
mammary epithelial cells,
318–320
Mammary gland, extracellular matrix of,
in tumor induction and
progression, 345, 349–352
Markers of cancer. See Biomarkers of
cancer
Mathematical modeling of information
from protein microarray
studies, 517, 520–521
Matrix metalloproteinase-3 (MMP-3;
stromelysin-1), 343,
350–351
Matrix metalloproteinase-13 (MMP-13),
385
Mcl-1 in Bak regulation, 471–472,
474–475
Mdm2, blockage of p53 interaction with,
493
Melanocytes, transformed, metastatic
phenotype of, 295
Melanoma, malignant
induction by mutant Cdk4R24C
kinase, 235
lineage-dependent oncogene in, 25,
30–32
metastatic mechanisms in, 295
sorafenib for, 465–466
MET proto-oncogene, in liver tumor
development, 217–223
Metalloproteinase. See Matrix
metalloproteinase
Metastasis
mechanisms of, 149–150, 291–295, 527
site-specific genes for, in breast
cancer, 149–158
Tks5 protein in, 167–170
Methyl-guanine methyl transferase,
expression of, and promoter
region methylation, 330
MGMT gene, epigenetic inactivation of, 330
Micro-computed tomography (CT), in
murine lung cancer
modeling, 245
Microenvironment, in tumor induction and
progression, 343–352,
383–387, 526–527
MITF gene and MITF protein, 25, 30–32
Mitochondria
bioenergetics of, 365
defects of associated with cancer,
363–365
mtDNA variations in disease and
climatic adaptation, 365–367
in pathophysiology of aging and
cancer, 367–372
MLH1 gene, epigenetic inactivation of, 330
Mll and MLL genes, 277–278, 280–281
MMP. See Matrix metalloproteinase
Mnt transcription factor, in Drosophila,
299–305
Molecular chaperone Hsp90, inhibitors of,
378–380, 505–510
Molecular profiling, in oncology drug
discovery, 445–448
Mouse models
of astrocytoma, 283–287
of autosomal dominant dyskeratosis
congenita, 206
of breast tumors, and regression with
antiangiogenic stress,
375–380

in cancer research, overview, 526
in cyclin-dependent kinase studies,
235–239
Eμ-myc mutations, 84
of hepatocellular carcinoma, 251–259
of human cancer epigenetics,
338–340
human chromosome translocation
mimics, 275–281
imaging technology and, 243–245
of liver tumors, genomic progression
in, 217–223
of neurofibromatosis type 1 tumors,
173–175
of non-small-cell lung cancer, 2–3, 5,
241–248
Npm mutations, 87–89
in p53 research, 490–491
of pancreatic ductal and intraepithelial
neoplasms, 67–70
with pRb pathway inactivation,
283–289
of prostatic adenocarcinoma, 283,
287–289
of small-cell lung cancer, 225–231
of telomere dysfunction, 202–203
transgenic, with inducible oncogenes,
1–3
VHL mutations, 160–161
MRI. See Magnetic resonance imaging
mtDNA variations in disease and climatic
adaptation, 365–367
MTOR inhibitors, 480–481
Multiple mole and melanoma syndrome,
familial atypical, 66
Myc protein
dMyc transcriptional regulation,
299–305
in intrinsic tumor suppression and
tumor maintenance,
264–269
L-myc, in mouse model of SCLC,
225–231
c-Myc transcription, 210–211
c-myc proto-oncogene
inactivation of, and increased
thrombospondin-1
expression, 393–394
role in tumorigenesis, 83–84
MYC-oncogene family, in small-cell lung
cancer, 226
Myelogenous leukemia, chronic (CML).
See Chronic myelogenous
leukemia
Myeloid leukemia, acute (AML), 193
Myelomonocytic leukemia, chronic
(CMML), 479–480

N

NBS1 protein, in recruitment of ATM,
106–108
NC160 cancer cell line, 25–32
Neoplastic transformation. See
Tumorigenesis
Neovascularization. See also
Angiogenesis
mechanisms and control of, 399–400
Network-targeted combination therapy,
521–522
Neural crest cell factor, in melanocytes,
295
Neuroendocrine differentiation, in small-
cell lung cancer, 225–231

Neurofibromatosis type 1, mouse models for, 173–175
Neurofibromin, 173–175
Nexavar (sorafenib), 465–467, 500
NFX1-91 protein, as repressor of hTERT transcription, 211–214
NFX1-123 protein, in hTERT transcription, 213–214
Nonhomologous end-joining repair pathway, in telomere-related genome instability, 198–199
Non-small-cell lung cancer (NSCLC)
    chemotherapeutic resistance in, 3, 73–79, 480–483, 526
    and kinase screening in tissue culture, 455–456
    EGFR gene and EGFR protein in, 3–5, 242–243, 419–425
    EGFR inhibitor response in, 3–4, 419–425
    EGFR inhibitor therapy, and markers of predicted benefit, 483–486
    essential kinase screening in tissue culture, 454–455
    genomic profiles of, 11–22
    mouse models of, 2–3, 5, 241–248
    resequencing of protein kinase gene family in, 43–48
    subtypes of, and pulmonary cell niches, 247–248
Npm gene and Npm protein, 87–90
NPM (nucleophosmin; B23), 86–89, 132–133
NPM1 gene, 86
NPM-RARα fusion protein, 86–89
NSCLC. *See* Non-small-cell lung cancer
Nuclear export inhibitor activation of p53 protein, 494
Nucleophosmin. *See* NPM
Nutrient uptake in metazoan cells, 357–361

O

Ocular disease, VEGF Trap antiangiogenic therapy for, 411, 414–415
Oncogene addiction
    angiogenesis and, 389–396
    gefitinib response and, 422–423
    in human lung adenocarcinoma, 3–5
    overview, 1–5
    protein kinase inhibitors and, 43–44
    and tumor dependency, 25–26
Oncogene cooperation, 263–264
Oncogene-dependent tumor suppression, 177–182, 263–272
Organ-specific metastatic colonization, 149–158
Organ-specific tumorigenesis, 344
Ovarian epithelial cells, pRb pathway inactivation in, 283
Oxidative phosphorylation, alterations of, in cancer, 363–367, 370–372

P

p15ink4b/CDKN2B silencing in leukemia, 329–330
P16ink4a gene, epigenetic inactivation of, 330

p16^Ink4a^ protein
    and carcinogenesis in mammary epithelial cells, 317–326
    in stem cell self-renewal and cancer cell proliferation, 179–181
p19^Arf^ protein. See also *Arf* gene
    biochemistry of, 132–133
    p53 induction by, 129–130
    p53-independent functions of, 133–134
    in regulation of *Arf/p53* tumor surveillance network, 310–313
    in stem cell self-renewal and cancer cell proliferation, 179–181
    sumoylation induced by, 134–135
p21WAF1 gene, p53 activation of, 121–127
p53 gene
    deletion of, in mouse model of SCLC, 225–231
    sequencing of, 492
p53 Mdm2 interaction, blockage of, 493
p53 protein
    antibodies against, staining of, 491–492
    in apoptosis, 470
    in astrocytoma, 284
    -dependent transcription profile, 492–493
    -dependent tumor suppression, and telomere attrition, 201–203
    K-ras cooperative effects, 243
    as mediator of aging, 181
    mutant, reactivation of, 493
    nuclear export inhibitor activation of, 494
    p19^Arf^ induction of, 129–130
    in prostatic adenocarcinoma, 283, 288–289
    in response to radiation and chemotherapy, 491
    RNAi suppression of, 256–257
    structure, homologs, and activity of, 489–490
    transcriptional elongation inhibitor activation of, 494
    transcriptional regulation by, compared to p73, 121–127
    wild-type, activation of, 493
p53 tumor surveillance network
    and Arf tumor suppressor function, 129–135
    in diagnostics and therapy, 489–495
    E2F transcription factor in regulation of, 309–315
    gene single-nucleotide polymorphisms in, 111–118
    in tumor maintenance, 269–272
p53AIP1 gene, p53 activation of, 121–127
p73 gene, epigenetic inactivation of, 330
p73 protein, transcriptional regulation by, 121–127
p107 expression in cancer, 234
p130 expression in cancer, 234
Pancreatic β cells, Myc activation in, 265–267
Pancreatic ductal adenocarcinoma
    compared to non-small-cell lung cancer, 17–21
    epidemiology, genetics, and clinical considerations, 65–67
    mouse models of, 67–70
Pancreatic intraepithelial neoplasms
    genetics of, 65–66
    mouse models of, 67–70

Parent-of-origin-specific transmission, in Beckwith-Wiedemann syndrome, 336–337
Patient biopsies, proteomic profiling of, 517–523
Patient-tailored therapy. *See* Personalized molecular cancer therapeutics/diagnostics
Perp gene, single-nucleotide polymorphism in, 114–118
Personalized molecular cancer therapeutics/diagnostics
    for EGFR inhibitor therapy, in lung adenosarcoma, 73–79
    p53-selective, 517–523
    progress and challenges in development of, 499–510
    proteomic profiling of patient biopsies, 517–523
Peutz-Jeghers syndrome, 66
Phenotypic expression
    of Cdk family alterations, 234
    epigenetic silencing of regulatory genes and, 331
    of mutations in a mouse model for small-cell lung cancer, 225–231
    screens for, in mammalian tissue culture, 449–458
Pheochromocytoma, hereditary, pVHL tumor suppressor protein and, 159, 161–162
Phosphoinositide 3-kinase inhibitors, 504–505
PML-RARα fusion protein, 85–86
Podosomes, Tks5 and, 167–170
Poly (ADP-ribose) polymerase-1
    inhibition, in treatment of *BRCA1/2* cancer, 142–146
Polygenic inheritance, and breast cancer, 35–40
Poor prognosis signatures
    in breast cancer, 150, 152, 156–157
    and metastasis mechanism theories, 292–294
pRB
    in cell cycle regulation, 233
    E2F transcription factor regulation by, 309–315
    expression of, in cancer, 234
pRb pathway inactivation, in mouse models of astrocytoma and prostatic adenocarcinoma, 283–289
Preneoplasia, epigenetic changes in, 329–332, 335, 339–340
Primary CNS lymphoma, epigenetic silencing in, 331
Prognostic tools. *See also* Biomarkers of cancer; Poor prognosis signatures
    breast cancer
        gene signatures in primary tumors, 150, 152, 154–157
        ROMA CGH and FISH analysis of, 59–61
    EGFR inhibitor response in NSCLC, 483–486
Promoter region methylation, 329–332
Promyelocytic leukemia, acute (APL), 85
Prostaglandin-endoperoxide synthase 2 (COX-2), association with p16Ink4a hypermethylation, 322–324

Prostate cancer
  adenocarcinoma, mouse models of, 283, 287–289
  hormone-refractory, 192–193
  kinase inhibitor therapy for, 480
  prostate stem cells and, 187–194
Prostatic stem cells
  identification of, 188–190
  niche of, 190–192
  and prostate cancer, 192–194
Pro-survival proteins of Bcl-2 family, and apoptosis, 469–475
Protein kinase family. *See also names of specific kinases*
  identification by genetic modifier screens, 455–457
  RNAi and cDNA screening for, 449–458
  sequencing of somatic mutations in human cancer, 43–48, 527
Protein kinase inhibitor therapy. *See also specific drugs and drug classes*
  acquired resistance to, 3, 73–79, 419–425, 480–481, 525–526
  review of application of, 479–481
Protein microarrays, in protein signaling network analysis, 517–519
Proteins, microenvironmental, in tumor induction and progression, 346, 352–353
Protein-signaling network models, clinical proteomic analysis of, 517–523
Proteomics, clinical
  and lung cancer biomarker identification, 246
  protein signaling network analysis in, 517–523
Proto-oncogene activation, in stem cell self-renewal and cancer cell proliferation, 177–182
Pten tumor suppressor
  inactivation, in tumor progression, 283, 286–287
  in prostate cancer suppression, 287
PTEN tumor suppressor
  genetic mutations of gene for, 502
  and kinase inhibitor response, 480–481
  in neoplastic proliferation and aging, 181–182
PTEN/AKT signaling pathway dysregulation, in human prostate cancer, 187, 194
pVHL, in cancer and oxygen sensing, 159–162

R

Radiation. *See* Irradiation
Raf kinase inhibitors, 465–467, 500–501
Raf proteins, 461–467
Ranibizumab (Lucentis), 411
Rapamycin, 480
RARα gene fusions, 84
Ras effector pathways. *See also* K-ras murine models of lung cancer; K-ras protein
  activation, in tumor progression, 283, 285–286
  cancer targets in, 461–467
  deregulation of in neurofibromatosis

type 1, 174–175
  in tumorigenesis, 245
RASSF1a gene, epigenetic inactivation of, 330
Rb1 gene
  deletion of, in mouse model of SCLC, 225–231
  epigenetic inactivation of, 330
Reactive oxygen species (ROS)
  mitochondrial alterations and, 363, 365, 368, 370–372
  phenotypic alterations and genomic instability due to, 350–351
Renal cell carcinoma
  clear-cell, pVHL tumor suppressor protein and, 159, 161
  sorafenib for, 465
Representational oligonucleotide microarray analysis (ROMA), 51–62
Retinoblastoma proteins. *See* pRB
Retroviral vectors
  Cre-expressing, for T_{121} induction, 286–287, 289
  in RNAi and cDNA screening, 451–454
Reverse phase microarray, 518–519
RNA interference (RNAi)
  in cancer-signaling network studies, 435–441
  in gene suppression studies, 256–257
  as research tool, 527–528
  screens using, in mammalian tissue culture, 449–458
  synthetic lethal screens, 447–448
ROMA (representational oligonucleotide microarray analysis), 51–62
ROS. *See* Reactive oxygen species
R-Roscovitine (seliciclib; CYC202), 502–504
Rous sarcoma virus, 1, 344–345

S

Sca-1 antigen, as prostatic stem cell marker, 187–194
SCC. *See* Squamous cell carcinoma
SCLC (small-cell lung cancer), mouse models for, 225–231
Screens. *See also* Biomarkers of cancer
  cell-based, for novel p53 activators, 494
  genetic modifier, for kinase identification, 455–457
  synthetic lethal, 438–441, 445–448
  using RNAi and cDNA expression, 449–458
SDF-1α (stromal-cell derived factor 1 α; CXCL-12), 384
Secreted frizzled related proteins (SFRPs), 428–429
Seed and soil hypothesis of metastasis, 149
Seliciclib (CYC202; *R*-roscovitine), 502–504
Serum protein biomarkers, 481
SFRPs (secreted frizzled related proteins), 428–429
Shelterin, 198, 202
Short hairpin RNAs (shRNAs)
  in cancer-signaling network studies, 435–441
  screens using, in mammalian tissue culture, 449–458

in synthetic lethal screens, 447–448
Signaling pathways. *See* Cancer-signaling networks
Single-nucleotide polymorphism (SNP) arrays, 25–32
Single-nucleotide polymorphisms (SNPs)
  in genes encoding microenvironmental proteins, 346, 352–353
  in p53 pathway, 111–118
siRNAs. *See* Small interfering RNAs
Site-specific metastatic colonization, genes mediating, 149–158
Site-specific tumorigenesis, 344
Slug neural crest cell factor, in melanocytes, 295
Small interfering RNAs (siRNAs)
  in synthetic lethal screens, 447–448
  use in mammalian cells, 435–436
Small molecule drugs. *See* Erlotinib; Gefitinib; Imatinib
Small-cell lung cancer (SCLC), mouse models for, 225–231
SMC1 protein
  in cellular response to DNA damage, 102–105
  and mechanisms of DNA repair, 106–108
Smoking history in NSCLC, and response to EGFR inhibitors, 485–486
SNPs. *See* Single-nucleotide polymorphisms
Somatic mutations in human cancer, 43–48
Sorafenib (Nexavar), 465–467, 500
Sporadic cancers
  "BRCA-ness" of, 144–145
  inactive X chromosome abnormalities in basal-like breast cancer, 93–96
Squamous cell carcinoma (SCC)
  of esophagus, promoter region methylation and progression of, 332
  of lung, genomic profile of, 11, 16–17, 20
v-src gene, 1, 344
Src protein tyrosine kinase, 167–170
Stem cells
  adult
    assays for enrichment of, 188
    hematopoietic, 187, 193
    prostatic, 187–194
    self-renewal of, proto-oncogene and tumor suppressor activation and, 177–182
    in tissue regeneration, 188
    tumorigenesis potential of, 187, 192–193, 527
  cancer
    in lung cancer, 247–248
    telomerase activity in, 205–207
    in tumorigenesis, 193, 225
  embryonic murine, homologous recombination techniques in, 275–281
Stem cell theory of cancer, telomerase activity and, 205–207
Stroma, in tumor induction and progression, 343–352, 383–387
Stromal-cell derived factor 1 α (SDF-1α; CXCL-12), 384
Stromelysin-1 (MMP-3), 343, 350–351

Sumoylation, Arf induction of, 129, 134–135

Synthetic lethal screens, 438–441, 445–448

T

T_{121}
  induction of, new systems for, 284–286
  induction of using *Cre*-expressing lentivirus vectors, 286–287
  pRb inactivation by, 283–289
T790M mutation of *EGFR*, 423
TAp73 expression, in colorectal adenocarcinoma cell lines, 121–127
Tarceva (erlotinib). *See* Erlotinib
Telomerase
  cancer stem cells and, 205–207
  human papillomavirus regulation of, 209–214
  up-regulation of, and telomere dysfunction, 202–203
Telomere dysfunction induced foci, 200–201
Telomere hypothesis of cancer, 205–207
Telomeres
  dysfunction of, and genomic instability in human cancer, 197–203, 320–321
  human, molecular structure of, 197–198
  length of, in neoplastic proliferation and aging, 181
TERT gene and TERT protein, human. See *hTERT* gene and hTERT protein
Testicular germ-cell tumors, resequencing of protein kinase gene family in, 43–48
Tetraploidy, telomere-related, 200–201
TGF-β (transforming growth factor β)
  and cancer progression, 384–385
  in wound healing and tumorigenesis, 345
Therapeutic strategies for cancer. *See also* Chemotherapeutic drugs; Chemotherapeutic resistance
  Bcl-2 life/death switch in, 469, 473, 475
  BH3 mimetics in, 469, 473–475
  in *BRCA1/2* carriers, 139–146, 526
  combination therapy, network-targeted, 521–522
  kinase inhibitors, 3, 479–481
  p53-selective therapies, 489–495
  personalized. *See* Personalized molecular cancer therapeutics/diagnostics
  progress and challenges in development of, 499–510
Thrombospondin-1/2
  overexpression of, and suppression of tumor growth, 392–393
  structure and mechanism of action of, 400, 404–406
Tissue polarity, in regulation of chemotherapeutic resistance, 349

Tissue structure and function regulators, in tumor induction and progression, 343–352, 526–527
Tissue-culture cells, mammalian
  aneuploidy of p53 knockout mouse cells, 490–491
  chemotherapeutic resistance in breast cancer, and kinase screening, 455–456
  proteomic profiling of, 519–520
  RNAi and cDNA screening in, 449–458
  siRNA use in, 435–436
Tks4 protein, 167–168
Tks5 protein, and cancer cell invasiveness, 167–170
TP53. See *p53* gene; p53 protein
TR gene and TR protein, human. See *hTR* gene and hTR protein
Transcription profile, p53-dependent, 492–493
Transcriptional elongation inhibitor activation of p53 protein, 494
Transcriptional regulation
  by *Drosophila* Myc and Mnt transcription factors, 299–305
  by human papillomavirus, 446
  by p53 and p73 proteins, 121–127
Transforming growth factor β (TGF-β)
  and cancer progression, 384–385
  in wound healing and tumorigenesis, 345
Translocator mouse model, 275, 277–279, 281
Trp53 gene deletion, in mouse model of SCLC, 225–231
Tumor progression. *See also* Angiogenesis; Metastasis
  aberrant gene silencing in, 427–431
  Darwinian model of, 291–293
  extracellular matrix in, 343–352, 526–527
  fibroblasts and, 383–387
  microenvironmental proteins in, 346, 352–353
  need for studies on, 6–7
  promoter region methylation and, 329, 331–332
  Pten inactivation in, 283, 286–287
  Ras effector pathways in, 285–286
Tumor suppression, oncogene-dependent, 263–272
Tumor suppressors. *See also names of specific tumor suppressors*
  activation of, in stem cell self-renewal and cancer cell proliferation, 177–182
  and kinase inhibitor response, 480
  pleiotropic, 85–86
Tumor-associated macrophages, 344
Tumorigenesis
  Bcl-2 life/death switch in, 469, 472–473
  extracellular matrix in, 343–352, 526–527
  leukemia/lymphoma genes and, 83–90
  c-*myc* proto-oncogene and, 83–84

organ-specific metastasis genes in breast cancer and, 155–156
  promoter region methylation and, 329–332
  stem cell potential in, 187, 192–193, 527
  telomerase activity in cancer stem cells and, 205–207
  telomere-related genome instability in, 197–203
  viral oncoproteins in, 209–214, 217
Tumstatin, structure and mechanism of action, 400, 402–404
Type 1 collagen, and cancer progression, 385
Tyrosine kinase inhibitors. *See also specific drugs and drug classes*
  differential sensitivity to, in lung adenocarcinoma, 3–5, 73–79
  oncogene addiction and, 25–26, 43–44

V

Vascular basement membrane, in angiogenesis, 400
VEGF and VEGF family, 411–412
VEGF receptors, 412
VEGF Trap, as antiangiogenic treatment, 411–415
VEGF-R2 inhibitors, 465–467
VelociGene-based discovery of angiogenesis targets, 415
VHL gene, 159–162, 330
Viral oncogenes, 1, 344
Viral oncoproteins
  in liver tumor development, 217
  and telomerase regulation disruption, 209–214
Viral vectors
  Cre-expressing, for T_{121} induction, 286–287, 289
  in RNAi and cDNA screening, 451–454
von Hippel-Lindau tumor suppressor protein (pVHL), in cancer and oxygen sensing, 159–162
Von Recklinghausen's neurofibromatosis, 173–175

W

Wilms' tumors, 335–337
Wound healing, and tumorigenesis, 345

X

X chromosome, inactive (Xi), abnormalities in BRCA1 mutant and sporadic basal-like breast cancer, 93–96

Y

Yeast, synthetic lethal screens in, 446

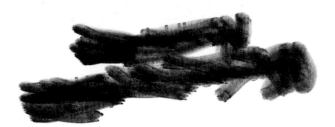

WITHDRAWN